THE MOLECULAR BASIS
OF HUMAN CANCER

THE MOLECULAR BASIS
OF HUMAN CANCER

Edited by

WILLIAM B. COLEMAN

Department of Pathology and Laboratory Medicine
University of North Carolina School of Medicine
Chapel Hill, NC

and

GREGORY J. TSONGALIS

Department of Pathology and Laboratory Medicine
Hartford Hospital
Hartford, CT

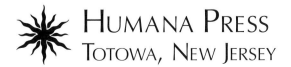

HUMANA PRESS
TOTOWA, NEW JERSEY

Cover Illustration: Liver tumor cells in culture (phase contrast, top left); A squamous cell lung carcinoma (hematoxylin and eosin stain, bottom middle); A CK18 immunostain of an invasive ductal carcinoma of the breast (top right); Agarose gels of primary and metastatic lung tumors showing the allelotype for D3S1744 and D15S822 (bottom left and top middle, respectively); Fluorescence in situ hybridization of the Rb1 locus on human chromosome 13 (bottom right).

Cover figure courtesy of William B. Coleman and Gregory J. Tsongalis.
(Thanks to Suzanne Tepper, Julie Howell, Chris Civalier, and Dr. William K. Funkhouser
for their contributions to the studies that produced these images.)

Cover design by Patricia F. Cleary.

Production Editor: Mark J. Breaugh.

This publication is printed on acid-free paper. ∞
ANSI Z39.48-1984 (American National Standards Institute) Permanence of Paper for Printed Library Materials.

Printed in the United States of America. 10 9 8 7 6 5 4 3 2 1

Library of Congress Cataloging-in-Publication Data

The molecular basis of human cancer / edited by William B. Coleman and Gregory J. Tsongalis.
  p. cm.
  Includes bibliographical references and index.
  ISBN 0-89603-634-0 (alk. paper)
  1. Carcinogenesis--Molecular aspects. 2. Cancer--Genetic aspects. 3. Mutation (Biology)
  I. Coleman, William B. II. Tsongalis, Gregory J.

RC268.5 .M6335 2001
616.99'4042--dc21   2001016560

PREFACE

The practice of medical oncology is in a period of significant positive change that owes primarily to advances in the basic science of oncology. In recent years, developments in molecular biology techniques have substantially increased our ability to detect and characterize genetic defects in human cells, resulting in significant increases in our understanding of the normal molecular mechanisms controlling cellular proliferation and differentiation. The advancement of our comprehension of these basic molecular mechanisms has been paralleled by comparable increases in our understanding of the molecular basis of the processes involved in neoplastic transformation and tumorigenesis. Information gleaned from studies conducted in basic molecular research laboratories is being applied with unprecedented speed to the development of new molecular tests for cancer diagnosis and prediction of clinical outcome, as well as to the development of new strategies for cancer prevention and treatment. Basic scientists, clinical scientists, and physicians have a need for a source of information on the current state of the art of the molecular biology of human neoplastic diseases. In this volume on *The Molecular Basis of Human Cancer* we attempt to provide such a source of current information, as well as provide a look to the future of the discipline and the potential impact of scientific advances on the practice of medical oncology. This book is directed primarily to advanced graduate students and medical students, postdoctoral trainees, and established investigators having basic research interests in the molecular basis of human neoplastic disease. However, it is also well suited for the non-expert with similar interests because it provides a broad overview of general themes in the molecular biology of cancer. To be sure, our understanding of the many processes of neoplasia and their molecular basis is far from complete, but few areas of thematic or conceptual consensus have developed. We have made an effort to integrate accepted principles with broader theoretic concepts in an attempt to present a current and comprehensive view of the molecular basis of human cancer. We hope that *The Molecular Basis of Human Cancer* will accomplish its purpose of providing students and researchers who already possess strong but diverse basic science backgrounds with unifying concepts, so as to stimulate new research aimed at furthering our understanding of neoplastic disease.

William B. Coleman
Gregory J. Tsongalis

DEDICATION

The information contained in this book represents the culmination of countless small success stories resulting from the ingenuity and hard work of cancer researchers from laboratories around the country and worldwide. This book is a tribute to the dedication, diligence, and perseverance of individuals who have contributed to advancements in our understanding of cancer pathogenesis and biology, especially the graduate students, laboratory technicians, and postdoctoral fellows, whose efforts are so frequently taken for granted and so often unrecognized.

The Molecular Basis of Human Cancer is dedicated to the memory of people we have known, who taught us through example about optimism, strength, and tenacity in the fight against cancer, including Samuel Apostola, Bobby G. Bell, Bobbie Coleman Clark, Jewell T. Coleman, George G. Gerding, Evelyn B. Hadden, Effie H. Helms, Joel C. Herren, Jean G. Herren, Kathleen M. Jackson, Gloria Morin, John Panu, Alexandria Rucho, Peter Rucho, and Ruth E. Trull. In particular, we dedicate this book to Dr. Eugene F. Hamer, a compassionate physician who worked tirelessly helping others all of his life, for demonstrating how much good one person can accomplish through selfless commitment to his profession. This book is also dedicated to the cancer survivors and those who continue to live with cancer, for their bravery and obstinacy, for the inspiration that they provide, and for reminding us that there is too much work left to be done for us to rest on our accomplishments.

We would also like to thank the many people that have played critical roles in our successes. We thank our teachers and our students; both have taught us much. We thank our scientific colleagues, past and present, for their camaraderie and support, and our scientific mentors for their example of research excellence. We thank our parents for believing in higher education, for encouragement through the years, and for helping make dreams into reality. We thank our brothers and sisters, and extended families, for the many years of love, friendship, and tolerance. We especially thank our wives, Monty and Nancy, for their unqualified love, unselfish support of our endeavors, understanding of our work ethic, and appreciation for what we do. Lastly, we thank our children for providing an unwavering bright spot in our lives, for their unbridled enthusiasm and boundless energy, for giving us a million reasons to take an occasional day off from work just to have fun.

William B. Coleman
Gregory J. Tsongalis

CONTENTS

CONTRIBUTORS

C. MARCELO ALDAZ • *Department of Carcinogenesis, The University of Texas M.D. Anderson Cancer Center, Smithville, TX*

GUADALUPE BILBAO • *Division of Human Gene Therapy, The University of Alabama at Birmingham, Birmingham, AL*

BRUCE M. BOMAN • *Division of Medical Genetics and Medicine, Jefferson Medical College, Thomas Jefferson University, Philadelphia, PA*

JOHN BUOLAMWINI • *Department of Pharmaceutical Sciences, College of Pharmacy, University of Tennessee Health Sciences Center, Memphis, TN*

KARIN BUTZ • *Angewandte Tumorvirologie, Deutsches Krebsforschungszentrum, Heidelberg, Germany*

APRIL CHARPENTIER • *Department of Carcinogenesis, The University of Texas M.D. Anderson Cancer Center, Smithville, TX*

ANU CHITTENDEN • *Department of Population Sciences, Dana-Farber Cancer Institute, Boston, MA*

SUSAN A. CHRYSOGELOS • *Department of Biochemistry and Molecular Biology, Lombardi Cancer Center, Georgetown University, Washington, DC*

WILLIAM B. COLEMAN • *Department of Pathology and Laboratory Medicine, University of North Carolina School of Medicine, Chapel Hill, NC*

DAVID T. CURIEL • *Division of Human Gene Therapy, The University of Alabama at Birmingham, Birmingham, AL*

MARIAROSARIA D'ERRICO • *Laboratory of Comparative Toxicology and Ecotoxicology, Istituto Superiore di Sanita', Rome, Italy*

EUGENIA DOGLIOTTI • *Laboratory of Comparative Toxicology and Ecotoxicology, Istituto Superiore di Sanita', Rome, Italy*

GIAN PAOLO DOTTO • *Cutaneous Biology Research Center, Massachusetts General Hospital, Harvard Medical School, Boston, MA*

JEREMY Z. FIELDS • *Center for Healthy Aging, St. Joseph Hospital, Chicago, IL*

KWUN M. FONG • *Department of Thoracic Medicine, The Prince Charles Hospital, Brisbane, Australia*

GARY GALLICK • *Department of Tumor Biology, University of Texas M.D. Anderson Cancer Center, Houston, TX*

ALLEN C. GAO • *Department of Pathology, University of Pittsburgh Cancer Institute and Medical Center, Pittsburgh, PA*

ARNOLD B. GELB • *Department of Pathology, Deltagen Inc., Menlo Park, CA*

JESÚS GÓMEZ-NAVARRO • *Division of Human Gene Therapy , The University of Alabama at Birmingham, Birmingham, AL*

JOE W. GRISHAM • *Department of Pathology and Laboratory Medicine, University of North Carolina School of Medicine, Chapel Hill, NC*

BRYAN HENRY • *Department of Biology, Boston University, Boston, MA*

ELAINE HILLER • *Department of Population Sciences, Dana-Farber Cancer Institute, Boston, MA*

FELIX HOPPE-SEYLER • *Angewandte Tumorvirologie, Deutsches Krebsforschungszentrum, Heidelberg, Germany*

JAMES HUFF • *Chemical Carcinogenesis, National Institute of Environmental Health Sciences, National Institutes of Health, Research Triangle Park, NC*

JOHN T. ISAACS • *Department of Urology, James Buchanan Brady Urologic Institute, The Johns Hopkins Oncology Center, The Johns Hopkins University School of Medicine, Baltimore, MD*

YVONNE JANSSEN-HEININGER • *Department of Pathology, University of Vermont College of Medicine, Burlington, VT*

J. MILBURN JESSUP • *Section of Surgical Oncology, University of Texas Health Science Center, San Antonio, TX*

STEPHANIE KIEFFER • *Department of Medical Genetics, University of Alberta Hospital, Edmonton, Canada*

BO LIU • *Department of Biochemistry and Molecular Biology, University of Pittsburgh Cancer Institute and Medical Center, Pittsburgh, PA*

EDWARD L. LOECHLER • *Department of Biology, Boston University, Boston, MA*

L. JEFFREY MEDEIROS • *Hemopathology Department, Division of Pathology and Laboratory Medicine, The University of Texas M.D. Anderson Cancer Center, Houston, TX*

LAEL MELCHERT • *Departments of Medical Genetics, Medicine, and Microbiology & Immunology, Jefferson Medical College, Thomas Jefferson University, Philadelphia, PA*

STEPHEN J. MELTZER • *Department of Medicine, Division of Gastroenterology, Baltimore Veteran's Affairs Hospital, The Marlene and Stewart Greenebaum Cancer Center, University of Maryland School of Medicine, Baltimore, MD*

JOHN D. MINNA • *Hamon Center for Therapeutic Oncology Research, University of Texas Southwestern Medical Center, Dallas, TX*

CATERINA MISSERO • *TIGEM– Telethon Institute of Genetics and Medicine, Napoli, Italy*

BROOKE T. MOSSMAN • *Department of Pathology, University of Vermont College of Medicine, Burlington, VT*

KAZUMA OHYASHIKI • *First Department of Internal Medicine, Tokyo Medical University, Tokyo, Japan*

ELIZABETH M. PETTY • *Division of Molecular Medicine and Genetics, Departments of Internal Medicine and Human Genetics, University of Michigan School of Medicine, Ann Arbor, MI*

SHARON COLLINS PRESNELL • *Department of Pathology and Laboratory Medicine, University of North Carolina School of Medicine, Chapel Hill, NC*

JOHN J. REINARTZ • *Department of Pathology, United Hospital, St. Paul, MN*

WILLIAM N. REZUKE • *Department of Pathology and Laboratory Medicine, Hartford Hospital, Hartford, CT*

KATHERINE SCHNEIDER • *Department of Population Sciences, Dana-Farber Cancer Institute, Boston, MA*

YOSHITAKA SEKIDO • *Department of Clinical Preventive Medicine, Nagoya University School of Medicine, Nagoya, Japan*

KWANG-YOUNG SEO • *Department of Biology, Boston University, Boston, MA*

KRISTEN SHANNON • *Hematology-Oncology Unit, Massachusetts General Hospital, Boston, MA*

TAKASHI SHIMAMOTO • *First Department of Internal Medicine, Tokyo Medical University, Tokyo, Japan*

KARA N. SMOLINSKI • *Department of Medicine, Division of Gastroenterology, Baltimore Veteran's Affairs Hospital, The Marlene and Stewart Greenebaum Cancer Center, University of Maryland School of Medicine, Baltimore, MD*

CYNTHIA R. TIMBLIN • *Department of Pathology, University of Vermont College of Medicine, Burlington, VT*

LORENZO TOMATIS • *National Institute of Environmental Health Sciences, Research Triangle Park, NC; International Society of Doctors for the Environment (ISDE), Arezzo, Italy.*

GREGORY J. TSONGALIS • *Department of Pathology and Laboratory Medicine, Hartford Hospital, Hartford, CT*

JAMES N. WELCH • *Tumor Biology, Department of Oncology, Lombardi Cancer Center, Georgetown University, Washington, DC*

BEVERLY M. YASHAR • *Division of Molecular Medicine and Genetics, Departments of Internal Medicine and Human Genetics, University of Michigan School of Medicine, Ann Arbor, MI*

INTRODUCTION 1

1 Cancer Epidemiology
Incidence and Etiology of Human Neoplasms

WILLIAM B. COLEMAN, PHD AND GREGORY J. TSONGALIS, PHD

INTRODUCTION

Cancer does not represent a single disease. Rather, cancer is a myriad collection of diseases with as many different manifestations as there are tissues and cell types in the human body, involving innumerable endogenous or exogenous carcinogenic agents, and various etiological mechanisms. What all of these disease states share in common are certain biological properties of the cells that compose the tumors, including unregulated (clonal) cell growth, impaired cellular differentiation, invasiveness, and metastatic potential. It is now recognized that cancer, in its simplest form, is a genetic disease, or more precisely, a disease of abnormal gene expression. Recent research efforts have revealed that different forms of cancer share common molecular mechanisms governing uncontrolled cellular proliferation, involving loss, mutation, or dysregulation of genes that positively and negatively regulate cell proliferation, migration, and differentiation (generally classified as proto-oncogenes and tumor suppressor genes). Essential to any discussion of the molecular mechanisms that govern disease pathogenesis for specific cancers is an appreciation for the distribution of these diseases among world populations, with consideration of specific risk factors and etiologic agents involved in disease causation. This introduction will describe cancer incidence and mortality for the major forms of human cancer, and will briefly review some of the known risk factors and/or causes of these cancers for specific at-risk populations.

CANCER INCIDENCE AND MORTALITY

Cancer is an important public health concern in the United States and world-wide. Owing to the lack of nationwide cancer registries for all countries, the exact numbers of the various forms of cancer occurring in the world populations are unknown. Nevertheless, estimations of cancer incidence and mortality are generated on an annual basis by several domestic

and world organizations. Estimations of cancer incidence and mortality for the United States are provided annually by the American Cancer Society (ACS) and the National Cancer Institute's Surveillance, Epidemiology, and End Results (SEER) program. Global cancer statistics are provided by the International Agency for Research on Cancer (IARC) and the World Health Organization (WHO). Monitoring of long-range trends in cancer incidence and mortality among different populations is important for investigations of cancer etiology. Given the long latency for formation of a clinically detectable neoplasm (up to 20–30 yr) following initiation of the carcinogenic process (exposure to carcinogenic agent), current trends in cancer incidence probably reflect exposures that occurred many years (and possibly decades) before. Thus, correlative analysis of current trends in cancer incidence with recent trends in occupational, habitual, and environmental exposures to known or suspect carcinogens can provide clues to cancer etiology. Other factors that influence cancer incidence include the size and average age of the affected population. The average age at the time of cancer diagnosis for all tumor sites is approx 67 yr (1). As a higher percentage of the population reaches age 60, the general incidence of cancer will increase proportionally. Thus, as the life expectancy of the human population increases due to reductions in other causes of premature death (due to infectious and cardiovascular diseases), the average risk of developing cancer will increase.

CANCER INCIDENCE AND MORTALITY IN THE UNITED STATES

GENERAL TRENDS IN CANCER INCIDENCE The ACS estimates that 1,221,800 new cases of invasive cancer were diagnosed in the United States in 1999 (2). This number of new cancer cases reflects 623,800 male cancer cases (51%) and 598,000 female cancer cases (49%). The estimate of total new cases of invasive cancer does not include carcinoma *in situ* occurring at any site other than in the urinary bladder, and does not include basal and squamous-cell carcinomas (SCCs) of the skin. In fact, basal and SCCs of the skin represent the most

From: *The Molecular Basis of Human Cancer* (W. B. Coleman and G. J. Tsongalis, eds.), © Humana Press Inc., Totowa, NJ.

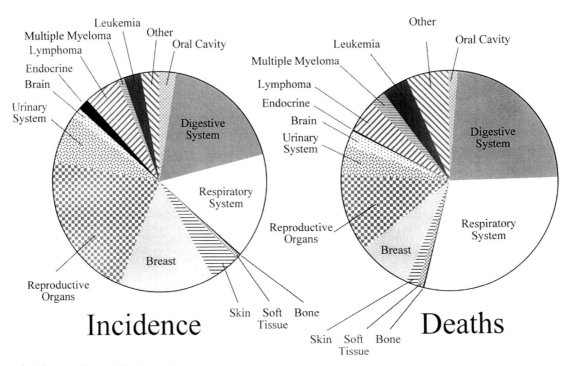

Fig. 1. Cancer incidence and mortality by site for both sexes (United States, 1999). The relative contributions of the major forms of cancer to overall cancer incidence and cancer-related mortality (both sexes combined) were calculated from data provided by Landis et al. *(2)*. Cancers of the reproductive organs include those affecting the prostate, uterine corpus, ovary, uterine cervix, vulva, vagina, testis, penis, and other organs of the male and female genital systems. Cancers of the digestive system include those affecting esophagus, stomach, small intestine, colon, rectum, anus, liver, gallbladder, pancreas, and other digestive organs. Cancers of the respiratory system include those affecting lung, bronchus, larynx, and other respiratory organs.

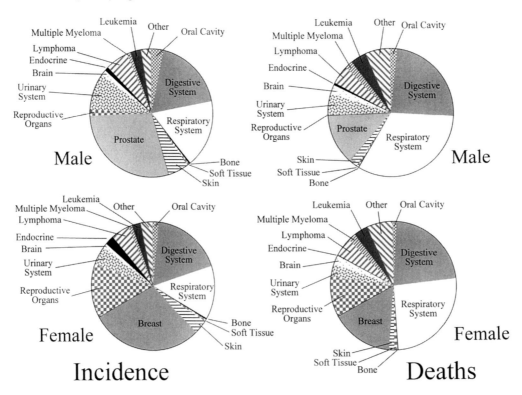

Fig. 2. Cancer incidence and mortality by site (United States, 1999). The relative contributions of the major forms of cancer to overall cancer incidence and cancer-related mortality for males and females were calculated from data provided by Landis et al. *(2)*. Cancers of the male reproductive organs include testis, penis, and other organs of the male genital system. Cancers of the female reproductive organs include those affecting the uterine corpus, ovary, uterine cervix, vulva, vagina, and other organs of the female genital systems. Cancers of the digestive system include those affecting esophagus, stomach, small intestine, colon, rectum, anus, liver, gallbladder, pancreas, and other digestive organs. Cancers of the respiratory system include those affecting lung, bronchus, larynx, and other respiratory organs.

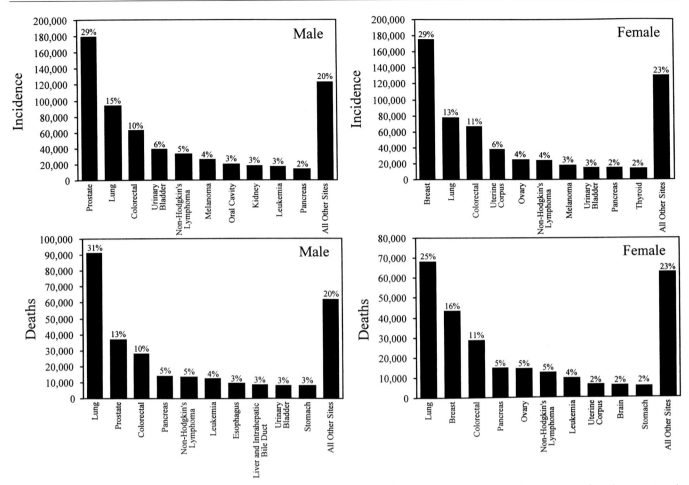

Fig. 3. Cancer incidence and mortality by leading site (United States, 1999). The numbers of cancers (and percentage of total cancers) and numbers of cancer-related deaths (and percentages of cancer-related deaths) for the leading sites for males and females were calculated from data provided by Landis et al. *(2)*. The numbers provided for lung include tumors of the lung and bronchus, and numbers for colorectal cancer include tumors of the colon and rectum.

frequently occurring neoplasms in the United States, with an estimated occurrence of approx 1 million total cases in 1999 *(2)*. Likewise, carcinoma *in situ* represents a significant number of new cancer cases with 39,900 newly diagnosed breast carcinomas *in situ* and 23,200 new cases of melanoma carcinoma *in situ* (2).

Estimated site-specific cancer incidence for both sexes combined are shown in Fig. 1. Cancers of the reproductive organs represent the largest group of newly diagnosed cancers in 1999 with 269,100 new cases. This group of cancers includes prostate (179,300 new cases), uterine corpus (37,400 new cases), ovary (25,200 new cases), and uterine cervix (12,800 new cases), in addition to other organs of the genital system (vulva, vagina, and other female genital organs; testis, penis, and other male genital organs). The next most frequently occurring tumors originated in the digestive tract (226,300 new cases), respiratory system (187,600 new cases), and breast (176,300 new cases). The majority of digestive system tumors involved colon (94,700 new cases), rectum (34,700 new cases), pancreas (28,600 new cases), stomach (21,900 new cases), liver and intrahepatic bile duct (14,500 new cases), and esophagus (12,500 new cases), in addition to the other digestive system organs (small intestine, gallbladder, and others). Most new cases of cancer involving the respiratory system affected the

lung and bronchus (171,600 new cases), with the remaining cases affecting the larynx or other components of the respiratory system. Other sites with significant cancer burden include the urinary system (86,500 new cases), lymphomas (64,000 new cases), skin (54,000 new cases), leukemias (30,200 new cases), and the oral cavity and pharynx (29,800 new cases).

Estimated cancer incidence by tumor site for males and females are shown in Fig. 2. Among men, cancers of the prostate, respiratory system (lung and bronchus), and digestive system (colon and rectum) occur most frequently. Together, these cancers account for 54% of all cancers diagnosed in men. Prostate is the leading site, accounting for 179,300 new cases and 29% of cancers diagnosed in men (Fig. 3). Among women, cancers of the breast, respiratory system (lung and bronchus), and digestive system (colon and rectum) occur most frequently. Cancers at these sites combine to account for 53% of all cancers diagnosed in women. Breast is the leading site for tumors affecting women, accounting for 175,000 new cases and 29% of all cancers diagnosed in women (Fig. 3).

GENERAL TRENDS IN CANCER MORTALITY IN THE UNITED STATES Mortality attributable to invasive cancers produced 563,100 cancer deaths in 1999. This reflects 291,100 male cancer deaths (52% of total) and 272,000 female cancer deaths (48% of total). Estimated numbers of cancer deaths by

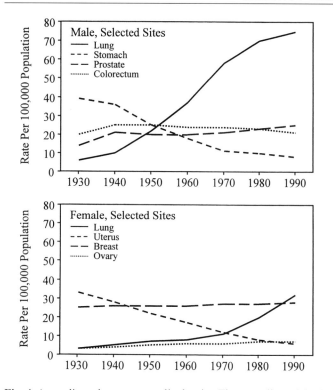

Fig. 4. Age-adjusted cancer mortality by site. The age-adjusted death rates for males and females for selected sites were adapted from the data provided by Landis et al. *(2)*. Death rates are per 100,000 population and are age-adjusted to the 1970 standard population of the United States.

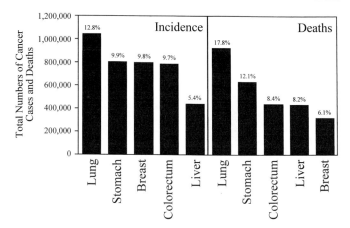

Fig. 5. World-wide cancer incidence and mortality by leading site. The numbers of cancers (and percentage of total cancers) and numbers of cancer-related deaths (and percentages of cancer-related deaths) for the leading sites world-wide were calculated from data provided by Parkin et al. *(3)*. The numbers provided for lung include tumors of the lung and bronchus and the numbers for colorectal cancer include tumors of the colon and rectum.

site for both sexes are shown in Fig. 1. The leading cause of cancer death involves tumors of the respiratory system (164,200 deaths), the majority of which are neoplasms of the lung and bronchus (158,900 deaths). The second leading cause of cancer deaths involve tumors of the digestive system (131,000 deaths), most of which are tumors of the colorectum (56,600 deaths), pancreas (28,600 deaths), stomach (13,500 deaths), liver and intrahepatic bile duct (13,500 deaths), and esophagus (12,200 deaths). Together, tumors of the respiratory and digestive systems account for 52% of cancer deaths.

Trends in cancer mortality among men and women mirror in large part cancer incidence (Fig. 2). Cancers of the prostate, lung and bronchus, and colorectum represent the three leading sites for cancer incidence and cancer mortality among men (Fig. 3). In a similar fashion, cancers of the breast, lung and bronchus, and colorectum represent the leading sites for cancer incidence and mortality among women (Fig. 3). Although cancers of the prostate and breast represent the leading sites for new cancer diagnoses among men and women (respectively), the majority of cancer deaths in both sexes are related to cancers of the lung and bronchus (Fig. 3). Tumors of the lung and bronchus are responsible for 31% of all cancer deaths among men and 25% of all cancer deaths among women (Fig. 3). The age-adjusted death rate for lung cancer among men has increased dramatically over the last 60–70 yr, whereas the death rates for other cancers (like prostate and colorectal) have remained relatively stable (Fig. 4). The lung cancer death rate for women has increased in an equally dramatic fashion since about 1960, becoming the leading cause of female cancer death in the

mid-1980s after surpassing the death rate for breast cancer (Fig. 4).

GLOBAL CANCER INCIDENCE AND MORTALITY

CURRENT TRENDS IN CANCER INCIDENCE AND MORTALITY WORLDWIDE The IARC estimates that 8,083,000 new cancer cases were diagnosed world-wide in 1990 *(3)*. This number of new cases represents 4,293,000 male cancer cases (53%) and 3,790,000 female cancer cases (47%). Mortality attributed to cancer for the same year produced 5,182,000 deaths world-wide. This reflects 2,957,000 male cancer deaths (57%) and 2,225,000 female cancer deaths (43%). The leading sites for cancer incidence and mortality world-wide in 1990 included tumors of the lung, stomach, breast, colorectum, and liver (Fig. 5). Lung cancer accounted for the most new cancer cases and the most cancer deaths during this period of time (Fig. 5). The leading sites for cancer incidence among males included lung (772,000 new cases), stomach (511,000 new cases), colorectum (402,000 new cases), prostate (396,000 new cases), and liver (316,000 new cases). Combined, cancers at these five sites account for nearly 56% of all cancer cases among men. The leading causes of cancer death among men included tumors of the lung (693,000 deaths), stomach (397,000 deaths), liver (306,000 deaths), colorectum (222,000 deaths), and esophagus (193,000 deaths). Deaths from these cancers account for 61% of all male cancer deaths. The leading sites for cancer incidence among females included breast (796,000 new cases), colorectum (381,000 new cases), cervix uteri (371,000 new cases), stomach (287,000 new cases), and lung (265,000 new cases). The leading causes of cancer death among females directly mirrors the leading causes of cancer incidence: breast (314,000 deaths), stomach (230,000 deaths), colorectum (215,000 deaths), lung (228,000 deaths), and uteri (190,000 deaths). Combined, these five cancer sites accounted for approx 56% of all female cancer cases and 53% of females cancer deaths.

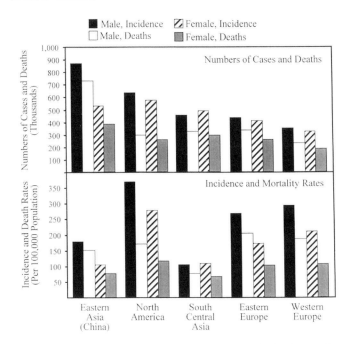

Fig. 6. World-wide cancer incidence and mortality for both sexes by world region. The total numbers of cancers and cancer-related deaths, and the total incidence of cancer and cancer-related mortality rates for selected world regions were calculated from data provided by Parkin et al. *(3).*

GEOGRAPHIC DIFFERENCES IN CANCER INCIDENCE AND MORTALITY Cancer incidence and mortality differs very little between developed and developing countries *(3)*. In 1990, developed countries account for 50.6% of new cancers and 55% of cancer deaths, whereas developing countries account for 49.4% of new cancers and 45% of cancer deaths. However, new cancer incidence and cancer-related mortality can differ tremendously from world area to world area, country to country, and even from region to region within a single country. The leading world areas for new cancer cases includes Eastern Asia/China (17.3% of new cases), North America (14.9% of new cases), South Central Asia (11.6% of new cases), Eastern Europe (10.4% of new cases), and Western Europe (8.3% of new cases). Collectively, Asia accounted for approx 40% of all new cancer cases world-wide in 1990. Recognizing the significant contribution of the population density of China and other regions of Asia to these numbers of cancers, it is appropriate to consider the cancer burden of these countries after correction for population. The numbers of cases/deaths and the incidence/mortality rates for these world regions are given in Fig. 6. It is evident from the data contained in Fig. 6 that there is a marked disparity between total numbers of cancer cases/deaths and the incidence/mortality rate for specific world regions. The North American male population exhibit the highest cancer incidence rate world-wide (370 cases per 100,000 population). While demonstrating the highest cancer incidence rate world-wide, this population ranks eighth for cancer mortality rate, possibly reflecting the relative quality and availability of healthcare and treatment options among the various world regions. The highest cancer mortality rate for males is found in Eastern Europe (205 deaths per 100,000 population), followed

by Western Europe (188 deaths per 100,000 population), Southern Africa (182 deaths per 100,000 population), Northern Europe (177 deaths per 100,000 population), Southern Europe (176 deaths per 100,000 population), and North America (171 deaths per 100,000 population). The North American female population shows the highest cancer incidence rate world-wide (278 cases per 100,000 population). The highest mortality rate for females world-wide is found in Northern Europe (125 deaths per 100,000 population), followed by North America (118 deaths per 100,000 population), Southern Africa (115 deaths per 100,000 population), tropical South America (111 deaths per 100,000 population), and Australia/New Zealand (109 deaths per 100,000 population).

POPULATION FACTORS CONTRIBUTING TO CANCER INCIDENCE AND MORTALITY

AGE-DEPENDENCE OF CANCER INCIDENCE AND MORTALITY Cancer is predominantly a disease of old age. Most malignant neoplasms are diagnosed in patients over the age of 65, making age the most important risk factor for development of many types of cancer *(4,5)*. The age-specific incidence and death rates for cancers of the prostate, breast (female), lung (both sexes combined), and colorectum (both sexes combined) for the period of 1992–1996 *(6)* are shown in Fig. 7. The trends depicted in this figure clearly show that the majority of each of these cancer types occur in individuals of advanced age. In the case of prostate cancer, 86% of all cases occur in men over the age of 65, and 99.5% occur in men over the age of 50. Likewise, 97% of prostate cancer deaths occur in men over the age of 65 (Fig. 7). In contrast, female breast cancer occurs much more frequently in younger individuals. Nonetheless, 63% of cases occur in women over the age of 65, and 88% occur in women over the age of 50 (Fig. 7). A notable exception to this relationship between advanced age and cancer incidence involves some forms of leukemia and other cancers of childhood. Acute lymphocytic leukemia (ALL) occurs with a bimodal distribution, with highest incidence among individuals less than 20 yr of age, and a second peak of increased incidence among individuals of advanced age (Fig. 8). The majority of ALL cases are diagnosed in children, with 40% of cases diagnosed in children under the age of 15, and 45% of cases occurring in individuals under the age of 20. Despite the prevalence of this disease in childhood, a significant number of adults are affected. In fact, 32% of ALL cases are diagnosed in individuals over the age of 65 yr of age. In contrast to ALL, the other major forms of leukemia demonstrate the usual pattern of age-dependence observed with solid tumors, with large numbers of cases in older segments of the population (Fig. 8).

CANCER INCIDENCE AND MORTALITY BY RACE AND ETHNICITY Cancer incidence and mortality can vary tremendously with race and ethnicity *(6)*. In the United States, African Americans and Caucasians are more likely to develop cancer than individuals of other races or ethnicity's (Fig. 9). African Americans demonstrated a cancer incidence for all sites combined of approx 443 cases per 100,000 population, and Caucasians exhibited a cancer incidence rate of 403 cases per 100,000 population. In contrast, American Indians showed the lowest cancer incidence among populations of the United States

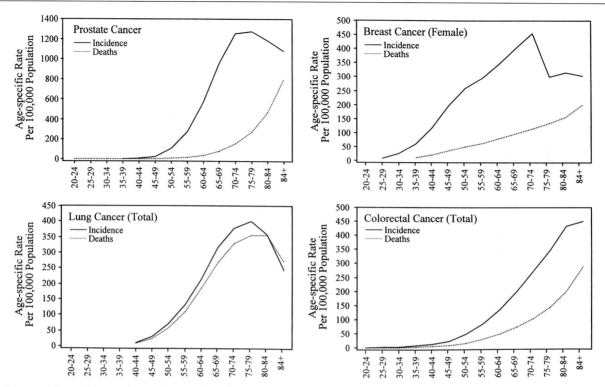

Fig. 7. Age-specific incidence and mortality rates for selected sites, 1992–1996. The age-specific rates for breast-cancer incidence and mortality are for females only. The age-specific rates for lung cancer and colorectal cancer are combined for both sexes. These data were adapted from Reis et al. *(6)*. Rates are per 100,000 population and are age-adjusted to the 1970 standard population of the United States.

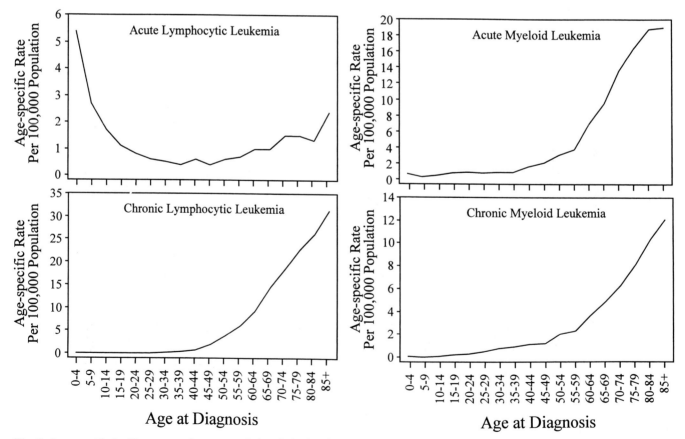

Fig. 8. Age-specific incidence rates for acute and chronic leukemias, 1992–1996. The age-specific rates for incidence and mortality for the major forms of leukemia are combined for both sexes. These data were adapted from Reis et al. *(6)*. Rates are per 100,000 population and are age-adjusted to the 1970 standard population of the United States.

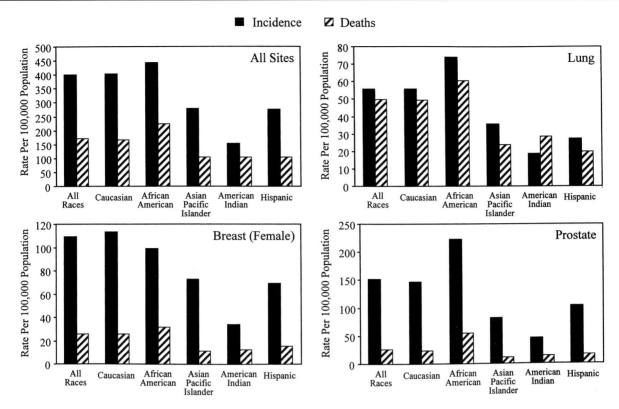

Fig. 9. Cancer Incidence and Mortality by Race and Ethnicity (United States, 1990–1996). The age-specific rates for cancer incidence and mortality for all races and select ethnicities residing in the United States are given for all cancer sites and select organ-specific cancer sites. The rates for all sites and lung cancer are for both sexes combined. These data were adapted from Reis et al. *(6).* Rates are per 100,000 population and are age-adjusted to the 1970 standard population of the United States.

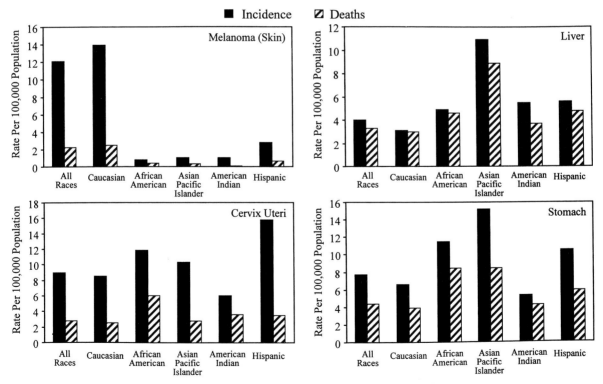

Fig. 10. Cancer incidence and mortality by race and ethnicity (United States, 1990–1996). The age-specific rates for cancer incidence and mortality for all races and select ethnicities residing in the United States are given for all cancer sites and select organ-specific cancer sites. The rates for melanoma, and cancers of the liver and stomach are for both sexes combined. These data were adapted from Reis et al. *(6).* Rates are per 100,000 population and are age-adjusted to the 1970 standard population of the United States.

with 153 cases per 100,000 population for all sites combined. Mortality due to cancer also differs among patients depending upon their race or ethnicity. Similar to the cancer incidence rates, mortality due to cancer is higher among African Americans (223 per 100,000 population) and Caucasians (167 deaths per 100,000 population) than other populations, including Asian/Pacific Islanders, American Indians, and Hispanics (Fig. 9). For both cancer incidence and mortality, racial and ethnic variations for all sites combined differ from those for individual cancer sites. African Americans and Caucasians demonstrate an excess of cancer incidence compared to the general population for a number of primary sites. African Americans exhibit high incidence rates for cancers of the prostate (223 cases per 100,000 population), lung (74 cases per 100,000 population for both sexes combined), colorectum (50 cases per 100,000 population), pancreas (13 cases per 100,000 population), oral cavity and pharynx (13 cases per 100,000), stomach (12 cases per 100,000 population), cervix uteri (12 cases per 100,000 population), and esophagus (8 cases per 100,000 population). The cancer incidence rates for lung, prostate, pancreas, and esophagus among African Americans are 33, 47, 50, and 115%, respectively, higher than those rates for the general population. Caucasians exhibit high incidence rates for cancers of the breast (113 cases per 100,000 population), corpus uterus (23 cases per 100,000 population), urinary bladder (18 cases per 100,000), ovary (16 per 100,000 population), and skin melanoma (14 cases per 100,000 population). The excess of melanoma in the Caucasian population compared with populations possessing darker skin pigmentation is clearly shown in Fig. 10. The Asian/Pacific Islander population exhibit high rates of liver cancer (11 cases per 100,000 population) and stomach cancer (15 cases per 100,000 population), which are 173 and 97%, respectively, higher than the rates for the general population (Fig. 10). The Hispanic population demonstrates high rates of incidence for cancers of the cervix uteri (16 cases per 100,000 population) and stomach (11 cases per 100,000 population). These rates are 78 and 36%, respectively, higher than rates for these cancers in the general population (Fig. 10).

TRENDS IN CANCER INCIDENCE AND MORTALITY FOR SPECIFIC SITES

LUNG CANCER Approximately 171,600 new cases of lung cancer were diagnosed in the United States in 1999, with 94,000 new cases among men and 77,600 new cases among women (2). The relative lung cancer incidence for men was estimated to be 75 cancers per 100,000 population in 1990 (WHO Mortality Database, http://www-dep.iarc.fr), down from the all-time high of 87 cases per 100,000 population in 1984 (1). The relative lung-cancer incidence rate among women continues to increase, reaching approx 40 cases per 100,000 in 1990 (WHO Mortality Database, http://www-dep.iarc.fr). Cancer of the lung and bronchus accounted for an estimated 158,900 deaths in 1999, which represents 28% of all cancer deaths (2). Furthermore, lung cancer is the leading cause of cancer deaths among men (31% of all cancer deaths) and women (25% of all cancer deaths) (Fig. 3).

Cancers of the lung and bronchus represent 91% of all respiratory system cancers (2). The remainder of respiratory sys-

tem cancers include tumors of the larnyx and nasal cavities. SCCs account for approx 35% of lung cancers (7). This histologic subtype of lung cancer is closely correlated with cigarette smoking and represents the most common type of lung cancer among men. SCCs display varying levels of differentiation, from tumors consisting of well-differentiated keratinized squamous epithelium to tumors consisting of undifferentiated anaplastic cells. Adenocarcinomas have increased in frequency in recent yr and now account for nearly 35% of lung cancers (7). These tumors grow faster than SCCs and frequently metastasize to the brain. Pulmonary adenocarcinomas can present as well-differentiated tumors consisting of well-differentiated glandular epithelium, or as undifferentiated tumors composed of highly mitotic anaplastic cells. Large-cell undifferentiated carcinomas account for approx 15% of all lung cancers (7). These tumors lack squamous- or glandular-cell characteristics and are typically composed of large anaplastic cells with frequent mitotic figures. Clinically, these tumors metastasize early and have a poor prognosis. Small-cell lung carcinomas (SCLC) make up the majority of the remaining cancers (10%) (7). These tumors are also associated with smoking history. SCLCs tend to produce a variety of neuroendocrine substances that can cause symptoms related to the biological activity of the hormonal substance. About 10% of SCLCs display a paraneoplastic phenotype related to production of these neuroendocrine effectors (8). These tumors grow rapidly, metastasize early, and have a very poor prognosis.

The majority of lung cancers are attributable to exposure to known carcinogenic agents, particularly cigarette smoke. Several lines of evidence strongly link cigarette smoking to lung cancer. Smokers have a significantly increased risk (11-fold to 22-fold) for development of lung cancer compared to nonsmokers (9), and cessation of smoking decreases the risk for lung cancer compared to continued smoking (9,10). Furthermore, heavy smokers exhibit a greater risk than light smokers, suggesting a dose-response relationship between cigarette consumption and lung-cancer risk (9,10). Numerous mutagenic and carcinogenic substances have been identified as constituents of the particulate and vapor phases of cigarette smoke, including benzo[a]pyrene, dibenza[a]anthracene, nickel, cadmium, polonium, urethane, formaldehyde, nitrogen oxides, and nitrosodiethylamine (11). There is also evidence that smoking combined with certain environmental (or occupational) exposures results in potentiation of lung-cancer risk. Urban smokers exhibit a significantly higher incidence of lung cancer than smokers from rural areas, suggesting a possible role for air pollution in development of lung cancer (12). Occupational exposure to asbestos, bis(chloromethyl) ether, and chromium have been associated with increased risk for development of lung cancer (13,14). Exposure to the radioactive gas radon has been suggested to increase the risk of lung cancer development. This gas is ubiquitous in the earth's atmosphere, creating the opportunity for exposure of vast numbers of people. However, passive exposure to the background levels of radon found in domestic dwellings and other enclosures are not sufficiently high to increase lung-cancer risk appreciably (15,16). High-level radon exposure has been documented among miners working in uranium, iron, zinc, tin, and fluorspar mines (17,18).

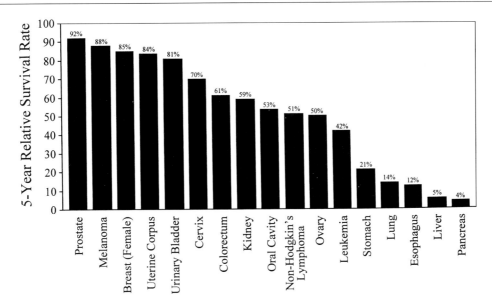

Fig. 11. Five-yr relative survival rates for invasive cancers (All Stages, 1989–1995). The average five-yr survival rates for select invasive cancers (including tumors diagnosed at all stages) among affected individuals residing in the United States for 1989–1995 are shown. These data were adapted from Reis et al. *(6).*

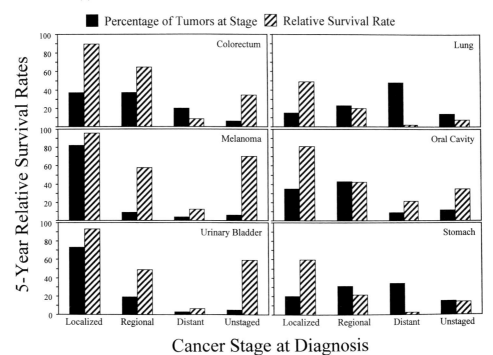

Fig. 12. Five-yr relative survival rates for selected sites by stage at diagnosis. The percentage of tumors for select invasive cancers according to tumor stage at diagnosis and the corresponding five-yr survival rates among affected individuals residing in the United States for 1989–1995 are shown. These data were adapted from Reis et al. *(6).*

These workers show an excess of lung cancer (compared to nonminers) that varies depending on the radon concentration encountered in the ambient air of the specific mine *(17,18).*

Therapy for lung cancer varies depending on the tumor type and other clinical variables (tumor stage, grade, location, and size). Surgery is the preferred treatment choice for SCC and adenocarcinoma, whereas SCLC is generally treated with chemotherapy. In some cases special treatment modalities are employed, such as chemotherapy followed by surgery or sur-

gery followed by radiation treatment. Despite the variety of treatment modalities that can be applied to lung-cancer management, the overall survival rates for affected individuals are not good (Fig. 11). The average five-yr survival rates for all patients and all stages of disease is only 13–14% *(6,19).* The survival rate increases to 49% if the disease is detected early (localized), but only 15% of tumors are discovered this early (Fig. 12). The majority of lung-cancer cases (48%) are not detected until after the development of distant metastases. The five-yr survival rate for these patients is only 2%. The overall poor probability of surviving lung cancer probably reflects the difficulty with early detection of this tumor (or the failure to detect tumors while localized) and the ineffectiveness of currently available therapies (radiation and chemotherapy).

COLORECTAL CANCER Approximately 129,400 new cases of colorectal cancer were diagnosed in the United States in 1999 (approx 11% of all cancers), with 62,400 new cases among men and 67,000 new cases among women (2). Colorectal cancer represent 57% of all digestive system tumors. The relative colorectal cancer incidence was estimated to be 20 cancers per 100,000 population for men and 19 cancers per 100,000 for women (WHO Mortality Database, http://www-dep.iarc.fr). Colorectal cancer accounted for an estimated 56,600 deaths in 1999, which represents 10% of all cancer deaths (2). Colorectal cancer is the third leading cause of death among men and women, accounting for 10% and 11% of all cancer deaths, respectively (Fig. 3).

Colorectal tumors are often first recognized as a polyp protruding from the wall of the bowel, which may be either hyperplastic (nondysplastic) or dysplastic (adenomatous). Hyperplastic polyps consist of large numbers of cells with normal morphology that do not have a tendency to become malignant (20). Adenomatous polyps contain dysplastic cells that fail to show normal intracellular and intercellular organization. Expanding adenomas become progressively more dysplastic and likely to become malignant. The majority of malignant tumors of the colon are thought to be derived from benign polyps. The malignant nature of colorectal tumors are defined by their invasiveness. The major histologic type of colorectal cancer is adenocarcinoma, which account for 90–95% of all colorectal tumors (21,22), although other rare epithelial tumor types do occur, including SCCs, adenosquamous carcinomas, and undifferentiated carcinomas, which contain no glandular structures or features such as mucinous secretions (21,23).

There are several recognized risk factors for development of colorectal cancer, some of which are genetic or related to benign pathological lesions of the colorectum, and others that are related to lifestyle or environment. Approximately 5–10% of colorectal cancers are thought to be related to an inherited predisposition. Familial colorectal cancer can arise in presence or absence of polyposis, which is characterized by the occurrence of multiple benign polyps lining the walls of the colon. Several polyposis syndromes have been described, the major form of which is familial adenomatous polyposis (FAP) (24). The hereditary nonpolyposis colorectal cancer (HNPCC) syndrome predisposes affected individuals to the development of colorectal cancer, as well as tumors at other tissue sites (25,26). These two hereditary syndromes account for a large percentage of familial colorectal cancers. Individuals affected by these syndromes carry mutations in one or more genes that function as tumor suppressor genes or that encode critical components of the DNA repair mechanisms that protect the genome from mutation (24). Patients with inflammatory bowel disease (ulcerative colitis) or Crohn's disease (granulomatous colitis) exhibit an increased risk for development of colorectal cancer (24,27). Epidemiologic studies indicate that individuals con-

suming diets that are high in animal fat and red meat (28–30), or low in fiber (31,32) are associated with increased risk for development of colorectal cancer. In addition, there is some evidence that alcohol intake and cigarette smoking can increase the risk for colorectal cancer (33,34).

Treatment for colorectal cancer may include surgery, radiation therapy, chemotherapy, or a combination of these treatment modalities. Chemotherapy alone is not very effective, but some drug combinations that are now employed show promise. In general, survival of colorectal cancer is closely correlated with early detection of localized disease, and the mortality due to this disease has been declining in recent years (2,35). The average five-yr relative survival rate for colorectal cancer is 61% (Fig. 11). The relative survival rate increases to nearly 90% if the tumor is detected early (localized), and remains relatively high (65% survival) when detected with regional metastasis (Fig. 12). In contrast, the five-yr survival is only 8% when the cancer is detected after development of distant metastases (6). Most colorectal cancers are now detected while localized (37% of tumors) or with limited regional spread (37% of tumors), which contributes to the generally favorable probability of survival for this form of cancer. Several screening methods are available for surveillance of patients that are at high risk for development of colorectal cancer, and some screening strategies are now routinely applied to the general population. These screening methods include digital rectal examination, fecal occult blood testing, and various forms of colonoscopy (36).

LIVER CANCER Hepatocellular carcinoma (HCC) is a relatively rare neoplasm in the United States, with 14,500 new cases diagnosed in 1999 (2). However, liver cancer occurs at high incidence when the world population is considered. In 1990, there were 437,000 new cases of liver cancer worldwide (3), which represents 5.4% of all cancers and the fifth leading site for cancer incidence (Fig. 5). Deaths attributed to liver cancer for the same year totaled 427,000, which represents 8.2% of all cancer deaths and the fourth leading site for cancer mortality (Fig. 5). The prevalence of primary liver cancer varies greatly from world region to world region (Fig. 13). The highest incidence of liver cancer world-wide is found in China, where men exhibit an incidence rate of approx 36 cases per 100,000 population (Fig. 13). High rates of liver cancer incidence are found throughout large portions of Asia and Africa, with much lower incidence rates for this tumor found in Europe and the Americas (Fig. 13). Early studies called attention to the extremely high incidence of hepatocellular carcinoma among black males in Mozambique (37,38), which demonstrate the highest incidence worldwide at 113 cases per 100,000 population (39). In fact, the incidence of this tumor among black Mozambican males aged 25–34 yr is over 500-fold higher than the incidence for comparably aged while males in the United States and United Kingdom (38,40). These statistics strongly suggest that factors related to genetic background and/or environmental exposure contribute significantly to the incidence of this tumor among world populations. Whereas the incidence rate for primary HCC in the united States has remained fairly low and stable over the last several decades, the occurrence of this neoplasm has been increasing in some countries. There has

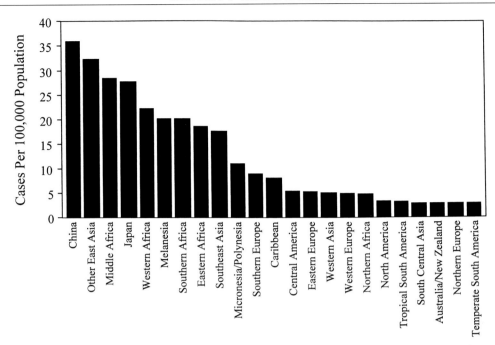

Fig. 13. Incidence of liver cancer among males by world region. The primary liver cancer incidence for 1990 for males residing in select world regions are shown. These data were adapted from Parkin et al. *(3),* and are expressed per 100,000 population.

been a dramatic rise in HCC incidence among Japanese men during the last 30 yr *(41),* possibly reflecting some significant change in risk factors or environmental exposures.

Liver cancer affects men more often than women. The ratio of male to female incidence in the United States is approx 2:1 *(2),* and world-wide is approx 2.6:1 *(3).* However, in high incidence countries or world regions, the male to female incidence ratio can be as high as 8:1 *(42,43).* This consistent observation suggests that sex hormones and/or their receptors may play a significant role in the development of primary liver tumors. Some investigators have suggested that hepatocellular carcinomas overexpress androgen receptors *(44),* and that androgens are important in the promotion of abnormal liver cell proliferation *(45,46).* Others have suggested that the male predominance of liver cancer is related to the tendency for men to drink and smoke more heavily than women, and are more likely to develop cirrhosis *(47).*

The etiology of HCC is clearly multifactorial *(48).* HCC is usually associated with chronic hepatitis *(49–52),* and 60–80% of HCC occurring world-wide develop in cirrhotic livers *(49,52–55),* most commonly nonalcoholic, posthepatitic cirrhosis *(56).* Numerous causative factors have been identified that are suggested to contribute to the development of HCC in humans, including exposure to naturally occurring carcinogens, industrial chemicals, pharmacologic agents, and various pollutants *(57,58).* In addition, viral infection, genetic disease, and life-style factors (like alcohol consumption) contribute to the risk for development of HCC *(57,58).* The most well-studied hepatocarcinogen is a natural chemical carcinogen known as aflatoxin B_1 that is produced by the *Aspergillus flavus* mold *(59,60).* This mold grows on rice or other grains (including corn) that are stored without refrigeration in hot and humid parts of the world. Ingestion of food that is contaminated with *Aspergillus flavus* mold results in exposure to potentially high

levels of aflatoxin B_1 *(61).* Aflatoxin B_1 is a potent, direct-acting liver carcinogen in humans, and chronic exposure leads inevitably to development of HCC *(60).* Numerous studies have shown a strong correlation between hepatitis B virus (HBV) infection and increased incidence of HCC *(39,62–64).* More recently, an association between chronic hepatitis C virus (HCV) infection and HCC has been recognized *(64–67).* In certain geographic areas (such as China), large portions of the population are concurrently exposed to aflatoxin B_1 and HBV, which increases their relative risk for development of liver cancer *(62).* Pharmacologic exposure to anabolic steroids and estrogens can lead to development of liver cancer *(68).* Several genetic diseases that result in liver pathology can increase the risk of development of a liver cancer, including hemochromatosis, hereditary tyrosinemia, glycogen storage disease types 1 and 3, galactosemia, Wilson's disease, and others *(69).* Chronic alcohol consumption is associated with an elevated risk for HCC *(70–73).* Alcohol is not directly carcinogenic to the liver; rather, it is thought that the chronic liver damage produced by sustained alcohol consumption (hepatitis and cirrhosis) may contribute secondarily to liver tumor formation *(74).* Other lifestyle factors may also contribute to risk for development of HCC, including tobacco smoking *(75,76).* Several chemicals, complex chemical mixtures, industrial processes, and/or therapeutic agents have been associated with development of HCC in exposed human populations *(58).* These include therapeutic exposure to the radioactive compound thorium dioxide (Thoratrast) for the radiological imaging of blood vessels *(77,78),* and exposures to certain industrial chemicals, such as vinyl chloride monomer *(79).*

Treatment of hepatocellular carcinoma may include surgery, chemotherapy, radiotherapy, or some combination of these treatments. The overall five-yr survival rate for HCC is only 5% (Fig. 11). The poor survival rate for HCC primarily reflects both the lack of effective treatment options and the advanced stage of disease at diagnosis. HCC is diagnosed as localized disease in approx 21% of cases, with region spread in 23% of cases, and with distant metastases in 22% of cases *(6)*. The five-yr survival for patients diagnosed with distant metastases is only 1.2%, and survival improves to only 14.7% when the patient presents with localized disease *(6)*. Most patients with HCC also have underlying cirrhosis, which makes surgical resection of the tumor very difficult. Furthermore, cirrhosis itself is a preneoplastic condition, which opens the possibility for development of additional secondary neoplasms in the unresected tissue after surgery. In fact, the recurrence rate after surgery for HCC was found to be 74% within five yr *(80)*. However, orthotopic liver transplantation can afford a complete cure for HCC if surgery is carried out prior to tumor spread from the liver *(81)*. Although the application of liver transplant in the treatment of HCC is not favored by transplant surgeons, the results emerging from such treatment are very encouraging in some cases. In one study of 17 patients *(82)*, liver transplant was performed to correct metabolic disorders of the liver (such as tyrosinemia) and small HCCs (without invasion or local spread) were incidentally discovered in the resected specimens. Of these patients, 90% survived >five yr without recurrence of the HCC *(82)*. Other studies have not produced such favorable results *(83)*, but it appears that certain types of HCC (such as fibrolamellar carcinoma) do very well after transplant, with >50% survival five yr after transplant *(84)*. A number of chemotherapeutic agents and combinations of these agents have been used to treat HCC. However, chemotherapy for HCC is generally not very effective and the response rates are very low, particularly when a single agent is used *(85)*. Nonetheless, there are occasional reports of dramatic responses using systemic chemotherapy, and some reports of complete remission *(86)*, suggesting that responsiveness of HCC to chemotherapy is totally unpredictable *(87)*. Radiation therapy for HCC can be effective at reduction of tumor size, but produces a number of serious side effects, including progressive atrophy of the liver parenchyma, which leads to fulminant liver failure in some patients *(87)*. More recent developments in radiation therapy have resulted in treatment modalities that limit collateral damage to the liver and surrounding tissues but are effective at reducing tumor burden *(88)*.

SKIN CANCER There are several major forms of skin cancer, including basal cell carcinoma (BCC), SCC, and malignant melanoma *(89)*. Nonmelanoma skin cancer represents the most frequently occurring tumor-type in the United States, with over 1 million total cases in 1999 *(2)*. These types of skin cancer tend to be slow growing, minimally invasive, not readily metastatic, and usually curable (given appropriate treatment). Thus, these forms of skin cancer are not typically included in cancer statistics for incidence, mortality, and survival rates. Nonetheless, the common occurrence of these tumors among the human population suggests that it is an important group of diseases to consider. BCC accounts for most cases of nonmelanoma skin cancer and is the most frequently occurring form of skin cancer. SCC is the second-most common form of skin cancer. BCC accounts for at least 75% of nonmelanoma skin cancers diagnosed each year in the United States, whereas SCCs account for approx 20% *(90)*. In contrast to the other forms of skin cancer,

malignant melanoma of the skin is an aggressive and invasive cancer that can metastasize to many tissue locations. The incidence of melanoma has been rising about 4%/yr in the United States. In 1999, there were 44,200 new cases of malignant melanoma, representing 4% of all male cancers (25,800 new cases) and 3% of all female cancers (18,400 new cases) (Fig. 3). Mortality due to malignant melanoma accounted for 7,300 deaths in 1999 *(2)*.

BCC is a malignant neoplasm of the basal cells of the epidermis and this tumor occurs predominately on sun-damaged skin. The carcinogenic agent that accounts for the neoplastic transformation of the basal cells is ultraviolet (UV) radiation. Thus, sun bathing and sun tanning using artificial UV light sources represent significant lifestyle risk factors for development of these tumors. BCC is now diagnosed in some people at very young ages (second or third decade of life), reflecting increased exposures to UV irradiation early in life. The incidence of this tumor increases with increasing age and increasing exposure to sunlight. Some researchers have suggested that the increasing frequencies of skin cancer can be partially attributed to depletion of the ozone layer of the earth's atmosphere *(91)*, which filters out (thereby reducing) some of the UV light produced by the sun. SCC is a malignant neoplasm of the keratinizing cells of the epidermis. It tends to occur later in life and is diagnosed more frequently in men than in women. Like BCC, extensive exposure to UV irradiation is the most important risk factor for development of this tumor. When left untreated, SCC can metastasize to regional lymph nodes and/or distant sites. Development of malignant melanoma occurs most frequently in fair-skinned individuals and is associated to some extent with exposure to UV irradiation. This accounts for the observation that Caucasians develop malignant melanoma at a much higher rate than individuals of other races and ethnicities (Fig. 10).

The preferred treatment of skin cancer is surgery. In fact, many, if not most, cases of BCC and SCC are treated with minor surgery in the setting of the physician's office. In the case of malignant melanoma, surgery is employed for localized disease, with radiotherapy used in the palliative treatment of metastasis to the central nervous system (CNS) and bone. Chemotherapy is employed for metastatic disease, but clinical responsiveness is limited to 15–20% of patients *(92)*. The five-yr survival rate for malignant melanoma is 88% (Fig. 11), reflecting the high rate of diagnosis (82%) of localized disease *(6)*. The five-yr survival of this disease drops precipitously with increasing spread of the tumor. Patients diagnosed with distant metastases exhibit a five-yr survival of only 13% *(6)*.

PROSTATE CANCER An estimated 179,300 new cases of prostate cancer were diagnosed in the United States in 1999 *(2)*, representing approx 150 cases per 100,000 population (Fig. 9), and 29% of all cancers in men (Fig. 3). The incidence rate for prostate cancer has been increasing in the last several decades at a rate of approx 4% per year, and this increase is paralleled by an increase in the mortality rate (Fig. 4). These increases are probably related to the increasing average age of the male population, increased reporting, and increased screening of older men *(93)*. Detection of prostate cancer can be achieved through the application of the digital rectal examination, screening based on detection of the prostate specific antigen (PSA) in

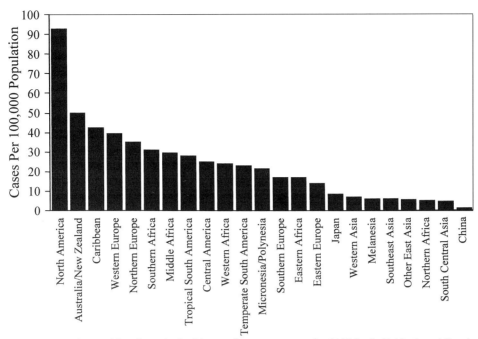

Fig. 14. Incidence of prostate cancer by world region. The incidence of prostate cancer for 1990 for individuals residing in select world regions are shown. These data were adapted from Parkin et al. *(3),* and are expressed per 100,000 population.

serum, and using ultrasonography. Elevations of PSA can be detected in both benign prostatic hypertrophy and in prostate cancer, but levels of this protein in the serum are markedly elevated in cancer. Although the serum PSA assay is extremely sensitive, it lacks specificity, which limits its usefulness as an definitive diagnostic for prostate cancer. However, when used in combination with the digital rectal exam and ultrasonography, PSA increases the ability to detect occult prostate cancer *(94).*

Cancer of the prostate provides a dramatic example of the age-dependent cancer development (Fig. 7). Tumors at this site occur with negligible frequency in men that are less than 55 yr of age, and the vast majority of cases (86%) occur in men over the age of 65 (Fig. 7). In addition, prostate cancer occurs with greatly varied frequency among men of different races and ethnicity (Fig. 9). In the United States, African-American men exhibit a significantly higher incidence of this tumor than Caucasian men, whereas American Indians demonstrate the lowest incidence of all groups (Fig. 9). The reason for these dramatic differences in prostate-cancer incidence are not readily apparent. However, differences in the levels of circulating testosterone among men from these different groups has been suggested as one factor contributing to the observed variations in prostate-cancer occurrence. The incidence of prostate cancer also varies widely from world region to world region, with the highest incidence among men living in North America (Fig. 14). It is notable that the incidence of prostate cancer among men from the various regions of Africa are significantly lower than the rates for African-American men living in the United States.

Treatment for prostate cancer includes surgical removal of the prostate, radiation therapy for locally invasive tumors, and hormone therapy. Strategies for hormone therapy in the treatment of prostate cancer include both administration of estrogenic hormones (such as diethylstilbesterol) or ablation of

androgenic hormones through surgical or chemical castration methods. The five-yr survival rate for prostate cancer has increased from 50% in the yr 1963–1965 to 93% in the yr 1989–1995 among Caucasian men *(6)*. This dramatic improvement in survival can be attributed to advances in early detection of this tumor. Currently, approx 79% of prostate cancers are detected while they are still localized with minimal regional spread, and the five-yr survival among this group >99% *(6)*. Although the overall survival of prostate cancer is excellent (Fig. 11), early diagnosis and treatment are essential. This point is highlighted by the observation that the five-yr survival among prostate cancer patients that have distant metastasis at the time of diagnosis drops to 9% *(6)*.

BREAST CANCER An estimated 175,000 new cases of breast cancer among women were diagnosed in the United States in 1999 *(2)*, accounting for 29% of all female cancers diagnosed (Fig. 3). During the 1980s, the number of new cases of breast cancer among women each year rose at a rate of about 4%/yr. However, the incidence of new cases has now apparently stabilized at approx 110 cases per 100,000 women *(6)*. The increases in breast-cancer incidence that were observed in the 1980s have been suggested to reflect increased early diagnosis as mammography screening became an established standard for surveillance of the general female population. Evidence supporting this suggestion includes the fact that the average primary breast tumor at diagnosis is of smaller size and earlier stage than those diagnosed more than a decade ago. The five-yr survival for breast cancer patients diagnosed in 1975 was approx 75%, compared to approx 85% for patients diagnosed in 1990 *(6)*. Nonetheless, the overall mortality rate for breast cancer has not changed substantially during this same period (Fig. 4), suggesting that earlier diagnosis has not significantly impacted patient outcome for this cancer. These observations suggest that the earlier diagnosis of smaller (and lower stage)

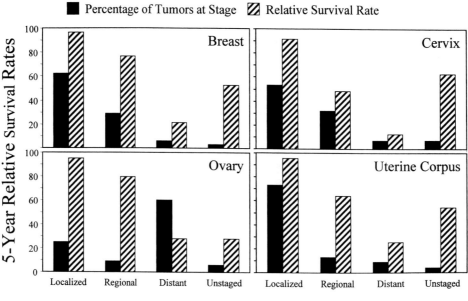

Cancer Stage at Diagnosis

Fig. 15. Five-yr relative survival rates for female cancers by stage at diagnosis. The percentage of tumors for select invasive female cancers according to tumor stage at diagnosis and the corresponding five-yr survival rates among affected individuals residing in the United States for 1989–1995 are shown. These data were adapted from Reis et al. *(6).*

tumors has impacted on the five-yr survival (Fig. 15), without affecting the overall survival for breast-cancer patients. In fact, it has been documented that breast cancer can recur after long periods of time, well after five-yr from the initial diagnosis. An estimated 43,300 women will die as a result of breast cancer during 1999 *(2),* making breast cancer the second leading cause of cancer death among women, accounting for 16% of all cancer deaths (Fig. 3).

Risk factors for development of breast cancer include, advancing age (over 50 yr of age), early age at menarche, late age at menopause, first childbirth after age of 35, nulliparity, family history of breast cancer, obesity, dietary factors (such as high-fat diet), and exposure to high-dose radiation to the chest before age 35 *(95–99).* In addition, fibrocystic breast disease is recognized as an established risk factor for breast cancer, especially when accompanied by cellular proliferation and atypia *(100).* Epidemiologic evidence has consistently pointed to family history as a strong and independent predictor of breast-cancer risk. A substantial amount of research has led to the discovery of several breast-cancer susceptibility genes, including *BRCA1, BRCA2,* and *p53 (101),* which may account for the majority of inherited breast cancers. It has been estimated that 5–10% of breast cancers occurring in the United States each year are related to genetic predisposition *(102).* Despite the recognition of multiple genetic and environmental risk factors for development of breast cancer, approx 50% of affected women have no identifiable risk factors other than being female and aging *(103).*

Treatment of breast cancer includes surgery, radiation therapy, chemotherapy, and hormone-modification therapy. Localized disease can very often be cured by partial mastectomy (lumpectomy) alone or in combination with localized radiation treatment. Total mastectomy remains a treatment of choice for more extensive localized disease, but breast-conserving surgery has been used with increasing frequency in recent years *(104).* Outcome data indicate that patients that undergo more conservative surgery with radiation therapy demonstrate survival rates that are similar to patients that are treated with total mastectomy for localized disease *(105).* Patients presenting with metastatic spread to regional lymph nodes are typically treated with chemotherapy. The anti-estrogenic drug tamoxifen is effective when used as a single agent or when used in combination with other chemotherapeutic agents in patients that are postmenopausal, have positive regional lymph-node involvement, and whose tumors express estrogen or progesterone receptors *(106).* Patients that receive adjuvant chemotherapy respond better to regimes that employ multiple drugs in combination. Commonly employed combinations include cyclophosphomide, methotrexate, and 5-fluorouracil (CMF), adriamycin plus cyclophosphomide, adriamycin followed by CMF, or one of these combinations with the addition of tamoxifen *(104).* The decision to use adjuvant chemotherapy depends on several variables (patient's age and general health), including the patient's estimated risk for recurrence. Typically, patients with a risk for recurrence of less than 10–15% are spared adjuvant chemotherapy, while all others are expected to benefit from the adjuvant treatment *(104).*

OVARIAN CANCER An estimated 25,200 new cases of ovarian carcinoma will be diagnosed in the United States in 1999 *(2),* accounting for 4% of all female cancers (Fig. 3). The majority of these cancers are diagnosed in postmenopausal women. Recognized risk factors for development of ovarian cancer include advancing age (>60 yr old), infertility, use of fertility drugs (such as clomiphene), history of breast cancer and other genetic predispositions, as well as some lifestyle and dietary factors *(107–114).* Pregnancy decreases the risk for ovarian cancer and multiple pregnancies increase the protective effect *(115)*. In addition, the use of oral contraceptives in nulliparous women reduces the risk for ovarian cancer to that for parous women *(116)*.

Treatment for ovarian cancer typically involves surgical removal of the ovaries, the uterus, and fallopian tubes. This is usually accomplished as part of a comprehensive staging laparotomy, after which the clinical findings and histologic evaluation of the tumor are used to select appropriate postoperative therapy. A subset of patients (stage IA or IB, with well-differentiated or moderately well-differentiated tumors) exhibit excellent long-term, disease-free survival in the absence of adjuvant therapy *(117)*. Several options exist for treatment of early-stage ovarian cancer with unfavorable prognosis, including radiation (external beam radiotherapy or intraperitoneal radioisotope) and chemotherapy. However, it is a matter of controversy whether treatment should be immediate or delayed until the disease begins to progress. The generally accepted therapy for advanced ovarian cancer is surgery followed by chemotherapy. The standard chemotherapy combination consist of paclitaxel and one of several platinum compounds (such as cisplatin or carboplatin).

Ovarian cancer accounted for 14,500 deaths in 1999 *(2)*, making this the leading cause of death among the cancers of the female reproductive tract (Fig. 3). Contributing to the significant mortality associated with this cancer is the fact that there are no obvious symptoms in affected patients until late in the disease. This is reflected in the poor five-yr survival rate (28%) for patients with distant metastases at the time of diagnosis is only (Fig. 15). In contrast, the five-yr survival rates for patients diagnosed with localized disease or regional disease are 95 and 80%, respectively (Fig. 15). However, most patients are diagnosed after development of distant metastases; 34% of cases are diagnosed as localized/regional disease, whereas 60% of cases present with distant metastases *(6)*. The overall five-yr survival rate for ovarian cancer is 50% (Fig. 11). Successful screening for ovarian cancer would be expected to decrease mortality by increasing the percentage of affected individuals that are diagnosed early in the progression of the disease. However, the currently available screening techniques (ovarian palpation, transvaginal ultrasonography, and serum CA125 measurements) lack sufficient specificity and sensitivity to allow for routine screening *(118)*.

LEUKEMIA Approximately 30,200 new cases of leukemia were diagnosed in the United States in 1999 *(2)*. These new cases were divided fairly evenly between myeloid (48%) and lymphocytic (52%) forms of the disease, with chronic forms of the disease representing slightly more than half of all leukemias (56 vs 44% for the acute leukemias). The major types of leukemia include acute lymphocytic leukemia (ALL), chronic lymphocytic leukemia (CLL), acute myeloid leukemia (AML), and chronic myeloid leukemia (CML). AML represents the most common form of leukemia (10,100 new cases), followed by CLL (7,800 new cases), CML (4,500 new cases), and ALL (3,100 new cases). Rarer forms of leukemia include monocytic, basophilic, eosinophilic, and erythroid leukemia. Although it is commonly regarded as a childhood cancer, leukemia affects more adults than children on an annual basis *(6)*. Development

of leukemia has been linked to certain environmental and genetic risk factors, including exposure to radiation (such as atomic bomb radiation), toxic chemicals (such as benzene), previous exposures to chemotherapeutic agents (mutagenic drugs), Down's syndrome, genetic disorders associated with chromosomal instability (Fanconi's anemia, Bloom syndrome, ataxia telangiectasia [AT]), and some viral infections *(119–124)*. Cigarette smoking has also been linked causally to development of leukemia, particularly in patients of advancing age *(125,126)*. Exposure to electromagnetic radiation or fields has been suggested as a risk factor for development of leukemia *(127)*, but a causal relationship has not been firmly established *(124)*.

Acute leukemia is relatively rare, representing approx 1% of all cancers *(2)*. However, the acute leukemias are the leading cause of cancer-related mortality in the United States for persons less than 35 yr of age *(128,129)*. In 1993, leukemias accounted for 3.9% of total cancer-related deaths among men in the United States *(130)*. However, leukemias were responsible for approx 37% of cancer-related deaths among men less than 15 yr of age, and approx 22% of cancer-related deaths among men less than 35 yr of age *(130)*. Likewise, in 1997, leukemia was responsible for approx 33% of all cancer-related deaths (both sexes combined) among individuals <20 yr of age *(131)*. Figure 8 shows the age-specific incidence rates for the major forms of leukemia. ALL occurs with an incidence of >5 cases per 100,000 population for children that are less than four yr old, declining with increasing age to approx 1 case per 100,000 population in individuals over 15 yr of age *(6)*. In fact, ALL accounts for the majority (approx 80%) of childhood leukemias. In contrast, AML is rare in individuals less than 40 yr of age, but increases with advancing age from approx 1.6 cases per 100,000 population at age 40 to >13 cases per 100,000 at age 70 *(6)*. Likewise, CML occurs very rarely in individuals less than 40 ($\leq$1 case per 100,000 population), but increase to >6 cases per 100,000 population in individuals over age 70 *(6)*. The incidence of CLL is strictly age-dependent, occurring only rarely in individuals less than 45 yr of age, increasing with advancing age to 6 cases per 100,000 population by age 65 yr, and to >31 cases per 100,000 population in individuals over 85 yr old *(6)*.

Conventional treatment of leukemia involves aggressive chemotherapy. Postremission therapy can involve bone marrow ablation (through high dose chemotherapy or whole-body radiation) with allogeneic bone marrow transplant. A variety of drugs and drug combinations have been evaluated for treatment efficacy in various forms of leukemia *(132,133)*. Appropriate drug regimens are chosen based on various diagnostic and prognostic factors, including the nature of chromosomal rearrangements in the leukemic clone *(134)*. Improvements in chemotherapeutic drugs and drug regimens for leukemia have dramatically improved treatment success rates for several forms of leukemia. Whereas childhood ALL was nearly uniformly fatal in the 1950s, today the majority (90–95%) of affected children achieve complete remission, and long-term survival (five-yr survival) for patients diagnosed at <45 yr of age is approx 69% *(6)*. The overall five-yr survival rate for patients with CLL is approx 71%, but is somewhat lower (58%) among older patients (diagnosed at ≥75 yr of age). In contrast, the overall five-yr survival rates for AML (approx 15%) and CML (approx 32%) remain dismally low despite improvements in treatments during the last 25 yr *(6).* With the exception of CLL, the long-term survival of older leukemia patients is dramatically lower than that of younger patients. In fact, most adult patients with acute leukemia ultimately succumb to their disease *(135).* The five-yr survival of patients older than 65 yr of age is approx 6% for ALL, compared to 63% for patients younger than 65 yr of age *(6).* Likewise, the five-yr survival of patients older than 65 yr of age is approx 3% for AML, compared to 25% for patients younger than 65 yr of age, and 35% for patients younger than 45 yr of age (6).

LYMPHOMA Approximately 64,000 new cases of lymphoma were diagnosed in the United States in 1999 *(2).* The majority of lymphomas are classified as non-Hodgkin's lymphoma (56,800 new cases), representing 89% of all lymphomas diagnosed *(2),* and the remaining cases are classified as Hodgkin's disease. Non-Hodgkin's lymphoma is a broad category consisting of several distinct lymphoid neoplasms *(136),* 85% of which are B-cell lymphomas (including follicular lymphoma, diffuse large B-cell lymphoma, mantle cell lymphoma, and several others), and 15% of which are T-cell lymphomas (including peripheral T-cell lymphoma, anaplastic large-cell lymphoma, and several others). Risk factors associated with non-Hodgkin's lymphoma include immunodeficiency associated with congenital diseases (such as AT, severe combined immunodeficiency [SCID], and X-linked lymphoproliferative disorder), acquired immunodeficiency (related to HIV infection, bone marrow transplant, or organ transplant with iatrogenic immunosuppression), various autoimmune disorders, infectious agents (Epstein-Barr virus [EBV], human T-cell leukemia virus [HTLV-1], and others), and chemical and physical agents (diphenylhydantoin, certain herbicides, radiation) *(136).* Hodgkin's disease is a unique form of neoplasm consisting of small numbers of putative neoplastic cells (known as Reed-Sternberg cells) in an inflammatory background *(137).* Most immunophenotypic and genetic data suggest that Reed-Sternberg cells represent some form of altered B-cell *(137),* whereas other evidence supports the suggestion that these cells represent a novel lymphoid cell type *(138).* Risk factors for development of Hodgkin's disease have not been definitively characterized. However, increased incidence of this disease is associated with HIV infection, other immunodeficiency syndromes (such as AT), autoimmune disorders (such as rheumatoid arthritis [RA]), certain genetic factors, and viral infections (such as EBV) *(139–142).*

Therapeutic approaches for the treatment of non-Hodgkin's lymphoma are based on a number of factors, including the specific lymphoid neoplasm, tumor stage, prognostic factors, and the physiologic status of the patient. Treatment options include radiotherapy alone, single-agent chemotherapy, or combination chemotherapy (mild or aggressive). The majority of patients with aggressive forms of non-Hodgkin's lymphoma require aggressive combination chemotherapy, often with additional radiotherapy. Treatment of Hodgkin's disease involves radiation therapy, radiation and chemotherapy, or chemotherapy alone. The results from a large number of randomized

trials suggest some advantages of combine modality radiation/chemotherapy in the treatment of Hodgkin's disease over radiation alone *(143).* However, there was no significant difference in the overall survival of patients between these approaches to treatment *(143,144).* Chemotherapy is effective against Hodgkin's disease. However, the use of drugs in combination is essential to effect complete and lasting remission of the disease *(145–147).*

Approximately 27,000 deaths were attributed to lymphoma in 1999, including 1300 deaths related to Hodgkin's disease and 25,700 deaths related to non-Hodgkin's lymphoma *(2).* Lymphoma affects more men than women on an annual basis, and non-Hodgkin's lymphoma represents a leading site for cancer-related mortality among men. Non-Hodgkin's lymphoma is the leading site for cancer-related mortality among men 20–39 yr of age, accounting for 13% of cancer deaths *(131).* Furthermore, non-Hodgkin's lymphoma accounts for significant numbers of cancer-related deaths among men <20 yr old (7% of cancer deaths), and 40–79 yr old (5% of cancer deaths). The overall five-yr survival rate for non-Hodgkin's lymphoma is 51% (Fig. 11). In general terms, long-term survival among non-Hodgkin's lymphoma patients does not differ with age. In contrast, there is a clear age-related difference in long-term survival among patients with Hodgkin's disease. Hodgkin's disease patients under the age of 65 display a five-yr survival rate of nearly 87%, whereas patients older than 65 have a five-yr survival rate of only 45%, and patients older than 75 exhibit a five-yr survival of only 31% *(6).*

REFERENCES

1. Hankey, B. F., Gloeckler-Ries, L. A., Miller, B. A., and Kosary, C. L. (1992) Overview. *In: Cancer Statistics Review 1973–1989.* NIH Publication No. 92-2789, I.1–17.
2. Landis, S. H., Murray, T., Bolden, S., and Wingo, P. A. (1999) Cancer statistics, 1999. *Ca Cancer J. Clin.* **49:**8–31.
3. Parkin, D. M., Pisani, P., and Ferlay, J. (1999) Global cancer statistics. *Ca Cancer J. Clin.* **49:**33–64.
4. Newell, G. R., Spitz, M. R., and Sider, J. G. (1989) Cancer and age. *Semin. Oncol.* **16:**3–9.
5. Miller, R. A. (1991) Gerontology as oncology. Research on aging as the key to the understanding of cancer. *Cancer* **68:**2496–2501.
6. Reis, L. A. G., Kosary, C. L., Hankey, B. F., Miller, B. A., Clegg, L., and Edwards, B. K. (eds.) (1999) *SEER Cancer Statistics Review, 1973-1996.* National Cancer Institute, Bethesda, MD.
7. Faber, L. P. (1991) Lung cancer. *In: Clinical Oncology* (Holleb, A. I., Fink, D. J., and Murphy, G. P., eds.), American Cancer Society Inc., Atlanta, pp. 194–212.
8. Bunn, P. A., Jr. and Minna, J. D. (1985) Paraneoplastic syndromes. *In: Principles and Practice of Oncology* (DeVita, V. T., Hellman, S., and Rosenberg, S. A., eds.), J.B. Lippincott, Philadelphia, pp. 1797–1842.
9. Shopland, D. R., Eyre, H. J., and Pechacek, T. F. (1991) Smoking-attributable cancer mortality in 1991: Is lung cancer now the leading cause of death among smokers in the United States? *J. Natl. Cancer Inst.* **83:**1142–1148.
10. Garfinkel, L. and Silverberg, E. (1991) Lung cancer and smoking trends in the United States over the past 25 yr. *Ca Cancer J. Clin.* **41:**137–145.
11. Public Health Service (1982) *The Health Consequences of Smoking-Cancer: A Report of the Surgeon General.* U.S. Department of Health and Human Services, Office on Smoking and Health, Rockville, MD.

12. Haenszel, W., Loveland, D. B., and Sirken, M. G. (1962) Lung cancer mortality as related to residence and smoking histories: I. White males. *J. Natl. Cancer Inst.* **28**:947–1001.

13. Hammond, E. C., Selikoff, I. J., and Seidman, H. (1979) Asbestos exposure, cigarette smoking, and death rates. *Ann. NY Acad. Sci.* **330**:473–490.

14. International Agency for Research on Cancer (1980) Report of an IARC working group : An evaluation of chemicals and industrial processes associated with cancer in humans based on human and animal data: IARC Monographs Vols. 1 to 20. *Cancer Res.* **40**:1–12.

15. Schoenberg, J. and Klotz, J. (1989) *A Case-Control Study of Radon and Lung Cancer among New Jersey Women.* New Jersey State Department of Health Technical Report, Phase I, Trenton, NJ.

16. Blot, W. J., Xu, Z.-Y., Boice, J. D., Jr., Zhao, D.-Z., Stone, B. J., Sun, J., et al. (1990) Indoor radon and lung cancer in China. *J. Natl. Cancer Inst.* **82**:1025–1030.

17. Archer, V. E., Gillam, J. D., and Wagoner, J. K. (1976) Respiratory disease mortality among uranium workers. *Ann. NY Acad. Sci.* **271**:280–293.

18. Harley, N. H. and Harley, J. H. (1990) Potential lung cancer risk from indoor radon exposure. *Ca Cancer J. Clin.* **40**:265–275.

19. Kessler, L. A. (1992) Lung and bronchus. *In: Cancer Statistics Review 1973–1989.* NIH Publication No. 92-2789, pp. XV.1–13.

20. Kent, T. H., Mitros, F. A. (1991) Polyps of the colon and small bowel, polyp syndromes, and the polyp-carcinoma sequence. *In: Pathology of the Colon, Small Intestine, and Anus,* 2nd ed. (Norris, H. T., ed.), Churchill Livingstone, New York, pp. 189–224.

21. Cooper, H. S. (1983) Carcinoma of the colon and rectum. *In: Pathology of the Colon, Small Intestine, and Anus,* 2nd ed. (Norris, H. T., ed.), Churchill Livingstone, New York, pp. 225–262.

22. Spjut, H. J. (1984) Pathology of neoplasms. *In: Neoplasms of the Colon, Rectum, and Anus: Mucosal and Epithelial* (Spratt, J. S., ed.), W.B. Saunders, Philadelphia, pp. 159–204.

23. DiSario, J. A., Burt, R., Kendrick, M. L., and McWhorter, W. P. (1994) Colorectal cancers of rare histologic types compared with adenocarcinoma. *Dis. Colon Rectum* **37**:1277–1280.

24. Kinzler, K. W. and Vogelstein, B. (1998) Colorectal tumors. *In: The Genetic Basis of Human Cancer* (Vogelstein, B. and Kinzler, K. W., eds.), McGraw-Hill, New York, pp. 565–587.

25. Lynch, H. T., Smyrk, T., and Jass, J. R. (1995) Hereditary nonpolyposis colorectal cancer and colonic adenomas: aggressive adenomas? *Semin. Surg. Oncol.* **11**:406–410.

26. Lynch, H. T., Smyrk, T., and Lynch, J. F. (1996) Overview of natural history, pathology, molecular genetics and management of HNPCC (Lynch Syndrome). *Int. J. Cancer* **69**:38–43.

27. Hamilton, S. R. (1985) Colorectal carcinoma in patients with Crohn's disease. *Gastroenterology* **89**:398–407.

28. Armstrong, B. and Doll, R. (1975) Environmental factors and cancer incidence and mortality in different countries, with special reference to dietary practices. *Int. J. Cancer* **15**:617–631.

29. Pickle, L. W., Greene, M. H., Zeigler, R. G., Toledo, A., Hoover, R., Lynch, H. T., et al. (1984) Colorectal cancer in rural Nebraska. *Cancer Res.* **44**:363–369.

30. Willett, W. C., Stampfer, M. J., Colditz, G. A., Rosner, B. A., and Speizer, F. E. (1990) Relation of meat, fat, and fiber intake to the risk of colon cancer in a prospective study among women. *N. Engl. J. Med.* **323**:1664–1672.

31. Burkitt, D. P. (1971) Epidemiology of cancer of the colon and rectum. *Cancer* **28**:3–13.

32. Bingham, S., Williams, D. R., Cole, T. J., and James, W. P. (1979) Dietary fibre and regional large-bowel cancer mortality in Britain. *Br. J. Cancer* **40**:456–463.

33. Martinez, M. E., McPherson, R. S., Annegers, J. F., and Levin, B. (1995) Cigarette smoking and alcohol consumption as risk factors for colorectal adenomatous polyps. *J. Natl. Cancer Inst.* **87**: 274–279.

34. Giovannucci, E., Rimm, E. B., Ascherio, A., Stampfer, M. J., Colditz, G. A., and Willett, W. C. (1995) Alcohol, low methionine low folate diets, and the risk of colon cancer in men. *J. Natl. Cancer Inst.* **87**:265–273.

35. Gloeckler Ries, L. A. (1992) Colon and rectum. *In: Cancer Statistics Review 1973–1989.* NIH Publication No. 92-2789, pp. VI.1–2.

36. Cohen, A. M., Minsky, B. D., and Schilsky, R. L. (1997) Cancer of the colon. *In: Cancer: Principles and Practice of Oncology,* 5th ed, (DeVita, V. T., Jr., Hellman, S., and Rosenberg, S. A., eds.), Lippincott-Raven, Philadelphia, pp. 1144–1197.

37. Berman, C. (1951) *Primary Carcinoma of the Liver.* London, Lewis.

38. Higginson, J. (1963) The geographical pathology of primary liver cancer. *Cancer Res.* **23**:1624–1633.

39. Munoz, N. and Bosch, X. (1987) Epidemiology of hepatocellular carcinoma. *In: Neoplasms of the Liver* (Okuda, K. and Ishak, K. G., eds.), Springer-Verlag, Tokyo, pp. 3–19.

40. Munoz, N. and Linsell, A. (1982) Epidemiology of primary liver cancer. *In: Epidemiology of Cancer of the Digestive Tract* (Correa, P. and Haenszel, W., eds.), Martinus Nijhoff, The Hague, pp. 161–195.

41. Okuda, K., Fujimoto, I., Hanai, A., and Urano, Y. (1987) Changing incidence of hepatocellular carcinoma in Japan. *Cancer Res.* **47**:4967–4972.

42. Stevens, R. G., Merkle, E. J., and Lustbader, E. D. (1984) Age and cohort effects in primary liver cancer. *Int. J. Cancer* **33**:453–458.

43. Simonetti, R. G., Camma, C., Fiorello, F., Politi, F., d'Amico, G., and Pagliari, L. (1991) Hepatocellular carcinoma: a worldwide problem and major risk factors. *Dig. Dis. Sci.* **36**:962–972.

44. Eagon, P. K., Francavilla, A., Di Leo, A., Elm, M. S., Gennari, L., Mazzaferro, V., et al. (1991) Quantitation of estrogen and androgen receptors in hepatocellular carcinoma and adjacent normal human liver. *Dig. Dis. Sci.* **36**:1303–1308.

45. Ohnishi, S., Murakami, T., Moriyama, T., Mitamura, K., and Imawari, M. (1986) Androgen and estrogen receptors in hepatocellular carcinoma and in surrounding non-cancerous liver tissue. *Hepatology* **3**:440–443.

46. Carr, B. I. and Van Theil, D. H. (1990) Hormonal manipulation of human hepatocellular carcinoma. *J. Hepatology* **11**:287–289.

47. Lai, C.-L., Gregory, P. B., Wu, P.-C., Lok, A. S. F., Wong, K.-P., and Ng, M. M. T. (1987) Hepatocellular carcinoma in Chinese males and females: possible causes of the male predominance. *Cancer* **60**:1107–1110.

48. Harris, C. C. and Sun, T.-T. (1984) Multifactorial etiology of human liver cancer. *Carcinogenesis* **5**:697–701.

49. Edmondson, H. A. and Steiner, P. E. (1954) Primary carcinoma of the liver. a Study of 100 cases among 48,900 necropsies. *Cancer* **7**:462–503.

50. Popper, H., Thug, S. N., McMahon, B. J., Lanier, A. P., Hawkins, I., and Alberts, S. B. (1988) Evolution of hepatocellular carcinoma associated with chronic hepatitis B virus infection in Alaskan Eskimos. *Arch. Pathol. Lab. Med.* **112**:498–504.

51. Unoura, M., Kaneko, S., Matsushita, E., Shimoda, A., Takeuchi, M., Adachi, H., et al. (1993) High-risk groups and screening strategies for early detection of hepatocellular carcinoma in patients with chronic liver disease. *Hepato-Gastroenterology* **40**:305–310.

52. Altmann, H. W. (1994) Hepatic neoformations. *Pathol. Res. Pract.* **190**:513–577.

53. Johnson, P. J. and Williams, R. (1987) Cirrhosis and the etiology of hepatocellular carcinoma. *J. Hepatol.* **4**:140–147.

54. Craig, J. R., Peters, R. L., and Edmondson, H. A. (1988) *Tumors of the Liver and Intrahepatic Bile Ducts.* Armed Forces Institute of Pathology, Washington, DC.

55. Tiribelli, C., Melato, M., Croce, L. S., Giarelli, L., Okuda, K., and Ohnishi, K. (1989) Prevalence of hepatocellular carcinoma and relation to cirrhosis: comparison of two different cities in the world: Trieste, Italy and Chiba, Japan. *Hepatology* **10**:998–1002.

56. Okuda, K. and Okuda, H. (1999) Primary liver cell carcinoma. *In: Oxford Textbook of Clinical Hepatology,* 2nd ed. (Bircher, J., Benhamou, J. P., McIntyre, N., Rizzetto, M., and Rodes, J., eds.), Oxford University Press, New York, pp. 1491–1530.

57. Grisham, J. W. (1995) Liver. *In: Pathology of Environmental and Occupational Disease* (Craighead, J. E., ed.), Mosby, St. Louis, pp. 491–509.

58. Grisham, J. W. (1997) Interspecies comparison of liver carcinogenesis: Implications for cancer risk assessment. *Carcinogenesis* **18**:59–81.

59. International Agency for Research on Cancer (1994) *IARC Monographs on the Evaluation of Carcinogenic Risks to Humans, Volume 56, Some Naturally Occurring Substances: Food Items and Constituents, Heterocylic Aromatic Amines and Mycotoxins.* IARC Scientific Publications, Lyon, France

60. International Agency for Research on Cancer (1994) *IARC Monographs on the Evaluation of Carcinogenic Risks to Humans, Volume 58, Aflatoxins.* IARC Scientific Publications, Lyon, France.

61. Linsell, C. A. (1979) Environmental and chemical carcinogens and liver cancer. *In: Liver Carcinogenesis* (Lapis, K. and Johannessen, J. V., eds.), Hemisphere Publishing Co., Washington, DC.

62. Lutwick, L. I. (1979) Relation between aflatoxins and hepatitis B virus and hepatocellular carcinoma. *Lancet* **1**:755–757.

63. Beasley, R. P., Hwang, L.-Y., Lin, C. C., and Chien, C.-S. (1981) Hepatocellular carcinoma and hepatitis B virus. A prospective study of 22707 men in Taiwan. *Lancet* **2**:1129–1133.

64. International Agency for Research on Cancer (1994) *IARC Monographs on the Evaluation of Carcinogenic Risks to Humans, Volume 59, Hepatitis Viruses.* IARC Scientific Publications, Lyon, France.

65. Stroffolini, T., Chiaramonte, M., Tiribelli, C., Villa, E., Simonetti, R. G., Rapicetta, M., et al. (1992) Hepatitis C virus infection, HbsAg carrier state and hepatocellular carcinoma, relative risk and population attributable risk from a case-control study in Italy. *J. Hepatol.* **16**:360–363.

66. Benvegnu. L., Fattivich, G., Noventa, F., Tremolada, F., Chemello, L., Cecchetto, A., et al. (1994) Concurrent hepatitis B and C virus infection and risk of hepatocellular carcinoma in cirrhosis. *Cancer* **74**:2442–2448.

67. Okuda, K. (1995) Hepatocellular carcinomas associated with hepatitis B and C virus infections: Are they different? *Hepatology* **22**:1883–1885.

68. Henderson, B. E., Preston-Martin, S., Edmondson, H. A., Peters, R. L., and Pike, M. C. (1983) Hepatocellular carcinoma and oral contraceptives. *Br. J. Cancer* **48**:437–440.

69. Cox, D. W. (1995) a_1-Antitrypsin deficiency. *In: The Metabolic and Molecular Bases of Inherited Disease,* 7th ed. (Scriver, C. R., Beaudet, A. L., Sly, W. S., and Valle, D., eds.), McGraw-Hill Inc., New York, pp. 4125–4158.

70. International Agency for Research on Cancer (1988) *IARC Monographs on the Evaluation of Carcinogenic Risks to Humans, Volume 44, Alcohol Drinking.* IARC Scientific Publications, Lyon, France.

71. Ikeda, K. Saitoh, S., Koida, I., Arase, Y., Tsubota, A., Chayaman, K., et al. (1993) A multivariant analysis of risk factors for hepatocellular carcinogenesis: a prospective observation of 795 patients with viral and alcoholic cirrhosis. *Hepatology* **18**:47–53.

72. Nalpas, B., Feitelson, M., Brechot, C., and Rubin, E. (1995) Alcohol, hepatotropic viruses and hepatocellular carcinoma. *Alcohol. Clin. Exp. Res.* **19**:1089–1095.

73. Noda, K., Yoshihara, H., Suzuki, K., Yamada, Y., Kasahara, A., Haynashi, N., et al. (1996) Progression of type C chronic hepatitis to liver cirrhosis and hepatocellular carcinoma: its relationship to alcohol drinking and age of transfusion. *Alcohol. Clin. Exp. Res.* **20**:95A–100A.

74. Lieber, C. S. (1990) Interactions of alcohol and other drugs and nutrients: implication for the therapy of alcoholic liver disease. *Drugs* **40**:23–44.

75. Trichopoulos, D., MacMahon, B., Sparros, L., and Merikas, G. (1980) Smoking and hepatitis B-negative hepatocellular carcinoma. *J. Natl. Cancer Inst.* **65**:111–114.

76. Chen, C.-J., Liang, K.-Y., Chang, A.-S., Chang, Y.-C., Lu, S.-N., Liaw, Y.-F., et al. (1991) Effects of hepatitis B virus, alcohol drinking, cigarette smoking, and familial tendency on hepatocellular carcinoma. *Hepatology* **13**:398–406.

77. Andersson, M. and Storm, H. H. (1992) Cancer incidence among Danish Thoratrast-exposed patients. *J. Natl. Cancer Inst.* **84**:1318–1325.

78. Andersson, M., Vyberg, M., Visfeldt, J., Carstensen, B., and Storm, H. H. (1994) Primary liver tumors among Danish patients exposed to Thoratrast. *Radiation Res.* **137**:262–273.

79. Vainio, H. and Wilbourn, J. (1993) Cancer etiology: Agents associated with human cancer. *Pharmacol. Toxicol.* **72**:S4–S11.

80. Takayasu, K., Wakao, F., Moriyama, N., Muramatsu, Y., Yamazaki, S., Kosuge, T., et al. (1992) Postresection recurrence of hepatocellular carcinoma treated by arterial embolization: analysis of prognostic factors. *Hepatology* **16**:906–911.

81. Mazzaferro, V., Regalia, E., Doci, R., Andreola, S., Pulvirenti, A., Bozzetti, F., et al. (1996) Liver transplantation for the treatment of small hepatocellular carcinomas in patients with cirrhosis. *N. Engl. J. Med.* **334**:693–699.

82. Iwatsuki, S., Starzl, T. E., Gordon, R. D., Esquivel, C. O., Tzakis, A. G., Makowka, T. L., et al. (1988) Experience in 1,000 liver transplants under cyclosporine-steroid therapy: a survival report. *Transplant Proc.* **20**(Suppl. 1):498–504.

83. Scharschmidt, B. F. (1984) Human liver transplantation: Analysis of data on 540 patients from four centers. *Hepatology* **4**:95S–106S.

84. O'Grady, J. G., Polson, R. J., Rolles, K., Calne, R. Y., and Williams, R. (1988) Liver transplantation for malignant disease: Results from 93 consecutive patients. *Ann. Surg.* **207**:373–379.

85. Simonetti, R. G., Liberati, A., Angiolini, C., and Pagliaro, L. (1997) Treatment of hepatocellular carcinoma: a systemic review of randomized controlled trials. *Ann. Oncol.* **8**:117–1136.

86. Harada, T., Makisaka, Y., Nishimura, H., and Okuda, K. (1978) Complete necrotization of hepatocellular carcinoma by chemotherapy and subsequent intravascular coagulation. *Cancer* **42**:67–73.

87. Okuda, K. and Okuda, H. (1999) Primary liver cell carcinoma. *In: Oxford Textbook of Clinical Hepatology,* 2nd ed. (Bircher, J., Benhamou, J.-P., McIntyre, N., Rizzetto, M., and Rodes, J., eds.), Oxford University Press, New York, pp. 1491–1530.

88. Matsuzaki, Y., Osuga, T., Saito, Y., Chuganii, Y., Tanaka, N., Shoda, J., et al. (1994) A new, effective, and safe therapeutic option using proton irradiation for hepatocellular carcinoma. *Gastroenterol.* **106**:1032–1041.

89. Marks, R. (1995) An overview of skin cancers: Incidence and causation. *Cancer* **75**:607–612.

90. Boring, C. C, Squires, T. S., and Tong, T. (1992) Cancer Statistics 1992. *Ca Cancer J. Clin.* **42**:19–38.

91. Friedman, R. J., Rigel, D. S., Berson, D. S., and Rivers, J. (1991) Skin cancer: Basal cell an d squamous cell carcinoma. *In: Clinical Oncology* (Holleb, A. I., Fink, D. J., and Murphy, G. P., eds.), American Cancer Society, Atlanta, GA, pp. 290–305.

92. Singletary, S. E. and Balch, C. M. (1991) Malignant melanoma. *In: Clinical Oncology* (Holleb, A. I., Fink, D. J., and Murphy, G. P., eds.), American Cancer Society, Atlanta, GA, pp. 263–270.

93. Miller, B. A. and Potosky, A. L. (1992) Prostate. *In: Cancer Statistic Review, 1973–1989.* NIH Publication Number 92-2789, XXII. 1–8.

94. Littrup, P. J., Lee, F., and Mettlin, C. (1992) Prostate cancer screening: Current trends and future implications. *Ca Cancer J. Clin.* **42**:198–211.

95. Kelsey, J. L. and Berkowitz, G. S. (1988) Breast cancer epidemiology. *Cancer Res.* **48**:5617–5623.

96. Hsieh, C.-C., Trichopoulos, D., Katsouyanni, K., and Yuasa, S. (1990) Age at menarche, age at menopause, height and obesity as risk factors for breast cancer: Associations and interactions in an international case-control study. *Int. J. Cancer* **46**:796–800.

97. Scanlon, E. F. (1991) Breast cancer. *In: Clinical Oncology* (Holleb, A. I., Fink, D. J., and. Murphy, G. P, eds.), American Cancer Society, Atlanta, GA, pp. 177–193.

98. Kelsey, J. L., Gammon, M. D., and John, E. M. (1993) Reproductive factors and breast cancer. *Epidemiol. Rev.* **15**:36–47.

99. Lipworth, L. (1995) Epidemiology of breast cancer. *Eur. J. Cancer Prev.* **4**:7–30.

21

100. Dupont, W. D., Page, D. L. (1985) Risk factors for breast cancer in women with proliferative breast disease. *N. Engl. J. Med.* **312**:146–151.
101. Gayther, S. A., Pharoah, P. D., and Ponder, B. A. (1998) The genetics of inherited breast cancer. *J. Mammary Gland Biol. Neoplasia* **3**:365–376.
102. Sutcliffe, S., Pharoah, P. D., Easton, D. F., and Ponder, B. A. (2000) Ovarian and breast cancer risks to women in families with two or more cases of ovarian cancer. *Int. J. Cancer* **87**:110–117.
103. Madigan, M. P., Zeigler, R. G., Benichou, J., Byrne, C., and Hoover, R. N. (1995) Proportion of breast cancers cases in the United States explained by well established risk factors. *J. Natl. Cancer Inst.* **87**:1681–1685.
104. Morris, J., Morrow, M., and Norton, L. (1997) Malignant tumors of the breast. *In: Cancer: Principles and Practice of Oncology,* 5th ed. (DeVita, V. T., Jr., Hellman, S., and Rosenberg, S. A., eds.), Lippincott-Raven, Philadelphia, pp. 1557–1616.
105. Pierce, S. M. and Harris, J. R. (1991) The role of radiation therapy in the management of primary breast cancer. *Ca Cancer J. Clin.* **41**:85–91.
106. National Cancer Institute Clinical Announcement. (1995) Adjuvant therapy of breast cancer: tamoxifen update. National Institutes of Health, U.S. Department of Health and Human Services, Washington, DC.
107. Lynch, H. T., Bewtra, C., Lynch, J. F. (1986) Familial ovarian cancer. Clinical nuances. *Am. J. Med.* **81**:1073–1076.
108. Schildkraut, J. M. and Thompson, W. D. (1988) Familial ovarian cancer: population-based case-control study. *Am. J. Epidemiol.* **128**:456–466.
109. Whittemore, A. S., Wu, M. L., Paffenbarger, R. S., Sarles, D. L., Kampert, J. B., Grosser, S., et al. (1989) Epithelial ovarian cancer and the ability to conceive. *Cancer Res.* **49**:4047–4052.
110. Piver, M. S., Baker, T. R., Piedmonte, M., and Sandecki, A. M. (1991) Epidemiology and etiliology of ovarian cancer. *Semin. Oncol.* **18**:177–185.
111. Gusberg, S. B. and Runowicz, C. D. (1991) Gynecologic cancer. *In: Clinical Oncology* (Holleb, A. I., Fink, D. J., and Murphey, G. P., eds.), American Cancer Society, Atlanta, GA, pp. 481–497.
112. Yancik, R. (1993) Ovarian cancer: age contrasts in incidence, histology, disease stage at diagnosis, and mortality. *Cancer* **71**:517–523.
113. Rossing, M. A., Daling, J. R., Weiss, N. S., Moore, D. E., and Self, S. G. (1994) Ovarian tumors in a cohort of infertile women. *N. Engl. J. Med.* **331**:771–776.
114. Whittemore, A. S. (1994) The risk of ovarian cancer after treatment for infertility. *N. Engl. J. Med.* **331**:805–806.
115. Greene, M. H., Clark, J. W., and Blayney, D. W. (1984) The epidemiology of ovarian cancer. *Semin. Oncol.* **11**:209–226.
116. Gross, T. P. and Schlesselman, J. J. (1994) The estimated effect of oral contraceptive use on the cumulative risk of epithelial ovarian cancer. *Obstet. Gynecol.* **83**:419–424.
117. Young, R. C., Walton, L. A., Ellenberg, S. S., Homesley, H. D., Wilbanks, G. D., Decker, D. G., et al. (1990) Adjuvant chemotherapy in stage I and stage II epithelial ovarian cancer: Results from two prospective randomized trials. *N. Engl. J. Med.* **322**:1021–1027.
118. Ozols, R. F., Schwartz, P. E., and Eifel, P. J. (1997) Ovarian cancer, fallopian tube carcinoma, and peritoneal carcinoma. *In: Cancer: Principles and Practice of Oncology,* 5th ed. (DeVita, V. T., Jr., Hellman, S., and Rosenberg, S. A., eds.), Lippincott-Raven, Philadelphia, pp. 1502–1539.
119. Austin, A., Delzell, E., and Cole, P. (1988) Benzene and leukemia: a review of the literature and risk assessment. *Am. J. Epidemiol.* **127**:419–439.
120. Kojima, S., Matsuyama, T., Sato, T., Horibe, K., Konishi, S., Tsuchida, M., et al. (1990) Down's syndrome and acute leukemia in children: an analysis of phenotype by use of monoclonal antibodies and electron microscopic platelet peroxidase reaction. *Blood* **76**:2348–2353.
121. Feuer, G. and Chen, I. S. Y. (1992) Mechanisms of human T-cell leukemia virus-induced leukemogenesis. *Biochim. Biophys. Acta* **1114**:223–233.
122. Pui, C.-H., Raimondi, S. C., Borowitz, M. J., Land, V. J., Behm, F. G., Pullen, D. J., et al. (1993) Immunophenotypes and karyotypes of leukemic cells in children with Down syndrome and acute lymphoblastic leukemia. *J. Clin. Oncol.* **11**:1361–1362.
123. Preston, D. L., Kusumi, S., Tomonaga, M., Izumi, S., Ron, E., Kuramoto, A., et al. (1994) Cancer incidence in atomic bomb survivors. III. Leukemia, lymphoma and multiple myeloma. *Radiat. Res.* **137**:S68–S97.
124. Sandler, D. P. (1995) Recent studies in leukemia epidemiology. *Curr. Opin. Oncol.* **7**:12–18.
125. Kabat, G. C., Augustine, A., and Herbert, J. R. (1988) Smoking and adult leukemia: a case-control study. *J. Clin. Epidemiol.* **41**:907–914.
126. Siegel, M. (1993) Smoking and leukemia: evaluation of a causal hypothesis. *Am. J. Epidemiol.* **138**:1–9.
127. Feychting, M. and Ahlbom, A. (1993) Magnetic fields and cancer in children residing near Swedish high-voltage power lines. *Am. J. Epidemiol.* **138**:467–481.
128. Hernandez, J. A., Land, K. J., and McKenna, R. W. (1995) Leukemias, myeloma, and other lymphoreticular neoplasms. *Cancer* **75**:381–394.
129. Wingo, P. A., Tong, T., and Bolden, S. (1995) Cancer statistics, 1995. *Ca Cancer J. Clin.* **45**:8–30.
130. Parker, S. L., Tong, T., Bolden, S., and Wingo, P. A. (1997) Cancer statistics, 1997. *Ca Cancer J. Clin.* **47**:5–27.
131. Greenlee, R. T., Murray, T., Bolden, S., and Wingo, P. A. (2000) Cancer statistics, 2000. *Ca Cancer J. Clin.* **50**:7–33.
132. Scheinberg, D. A., Maslak, P., and Weiss, M (1997) Acute leukemias. *In: Cancer: Principles and Practice of Oncology,* 5th ed. (DeVita, V. T., Jr., Hellman, S., and Rosenberg, S. A., eds.), Lippincott-Raven, Philadelphia, pp. 2293–2321.
133. Deisseroth, A. B., Kantarjian, H., Andreeff, M., Talpaz, M., Keating, M. J., Khouri, I., et al. (1997) Chronic leukemias. *In: Cancer: Principles and Practice of Oncology,* 5th ed. (DeVita, V. T., Jr., Hellman, S., and Rosenberg, S. A., eds.), Lippincott-Raven, Philadelphia, pp. 2321–2343.
134. Khouri, I., Sanchez, F. G., and Deisseroth, A. (1997) Molecular biology of the leukemias. *In: Cancer: Principles and Practice of Oncology,* 5th ed. (DeVita, V. T., Jr., Hellman, S., and Rosenberg, S. A., eds.), Lippincott-Raven, Philadelphia, pp. 2285–2293.
135. Brincker, H. (1985) Estimates of overall treatment results in acute non-lymphocytic leukemia based on age-specific rates of incidence and of complete remission. *Cancer Treat. Rep.* **69**:5–11.
136. Shipp, M. A., Mauch, P. M., and Harris, N. L. (1997) Non-Hodgkin's lymphomas. *In: Cancer: Principles and Practice of Oncology,* 5th ed. (DeVita, V. T., Jr., Hellman, S., and Rosenberg, S. A., eds.), Lippincott-Raven, Philadelphia, pp. 2165–2220.
137. DeVita, V. T., Mauch, P. M., and Harris, N. L. (1997) Hodgkin's disease. *In: Cancer: Principles and Practice of Oncology,* 5th ed. (DeVita, V. T., Jr., Hellman, S., and Rosenberg, S. A., eds.), Lippincott-Raven, Philadelphia, pp. 2242-2283.
138. Delsol, G. Meggetto, F., Brousett, P., Cohen-Knafo, E., al Saati, T., Rochaix, P., et al. (1993) Relation of follicular dendritic reticular cells to Reed-Sternberg cells of Hodgkin's disease with emphasis on the expression of CD21q antigen. *Am. J. Pathol.* **142**:1729–1738.
139. Connelly, R. R. and Chistene, B. W. (1974) A cohort study of cancer following infectious mononucleosis. *Cancer Res.* **34**:1172–1178.
140. Graff, K. S., Simon, R. M., Yankee, R. A., DeVita, V. T., and Rogentine, G. N. (1974) HL-A antigens in Hodgkin's disease: histopathologic and clinical correlations. *J. Natl. Cancer Inst.* **52**:1087–1090.
141. Biggar, R. J., Horm, J., Goedert, J. J., and Melbye, M. (1987) Cancer in a group at risk of acquired immunodeficiency syndrome (AIDS) through 1984. *Am. J. Epidemiol.* **126**:578–586.

142. Robertson, S. J., Lowman, J. T., Grufferman, S., Kostyu, D., van der Horst, C. M., Matthews, T. J., et al. (1987) Familial Hodgkin's disease: a clinical and laboratory investigation. *Cancer* **59**: 1314–1319.

143. Specht, L., Carde, P., Mauch, P., Magrini, S. M., and Santarelli, M. T. (1992) Radiotherapy versus combined modality in early stages. *Ann. Oncol.* **3**:77–81.

144. Nissen, N. I. and Nordentoft, A. M. (1982) Radiotherapy versus combined modality treatment of stage I and II Hodgkin's disease. *Cancer Treat. Rep.* **66**:799–803.

145. DeVita, V. T., Serpick, A. A., and Carbone, P. P. (1970) Combination chemotherapy in the treatment of advanced Hodgkin's disease. *Ann. Intern. Med.* **73**:881–895.

146. Klimo, P. and Conners, J. M. (1985) MOPP/ABV hybrid program: combination chemotherapy based on early introduction of seven effective drugs for advanced Hodgkin's disease. *J. Clin. Oncol.* **3**:1174–1182.

147. Prosnitz, L. R., Farber, L. R., Scott, J., Bertino, J. R., Fischer, J. J., and Cadman, E. C. (1988) Combine modality therapy for advanced Hodgkin's disease: a 15-year follow-up data. *J. Clin. Oncol.* **6**:603–612.

ESSENTIAL CONCEPTS IN MOLECULAR BIOLOGY

II

2 Essential Concepts and Techniques in Molecular Biology

SHARON COLLINS PRESNELL, PHD

THE BIOLOGY OF NUCLEIC ACIDS

COMPOSITION AND STRUCTURE OF DNA

Deoxyribonucleic acid (DNA) is formed by the linear polymerization of nucleotides, which are composed of a nitrogen-containing base and a phosphorylated sugar. The four nitrogenous bases found in DNA are either purines (adenine or guanine) or pyrimidines (cytosine or thymine), and the backbone of the DNA polymer is formed by linkage of these bases via phosphate groups (Fig. 1). The informational content of DNA is governed by the sequential arrangement and primary structure of the nucleotide polymer. The DNA strand is polar, with no nucleotide attached to the 5′ position of the deoxyribose at the 5′ end, and no nucleotide attached to the 3′ hydroxyl group at the 3′ end.

The DNA within the nucleus is arranged in a double-stranded helix composed of two strands of opposing polarity. The helix is stabilized by the formation of hydrogen bonds between complementary bases (A-T and G-C), by pi bonding that occurs when the bases are stacked together, and by the association of proteins (1,2). In eukaryotic cells, most of the DNA is in the B-form, a right-handed helix with bases on the inside where they are protected from damage by oxidating or alkylating agents. The Z-form of DNA occurs when a left-handed helix is formed, and is usually associated with portions of the DNA that are highly methylated and are not transcribed actively. Enzymatic reactions within the nucleus are responsible for conversion of DNA from the B-form to the Z-form and vice versa (3).

The DNA in each eukaryotic cell must be compressed to fit within the nucleus, which is only about 10μm in diameter. The DNA is segmented into 46 discreet structural units, termed chromosomes. Chromosomal DNA is condensed by the formation of nucleosomes; a group of small basic proteins (histones) around which 160–180 base pairs of DNA are wrapped (4). Formation of nucleosomes is not sequence-dependent and it

From: *The Molecular Basis of Human Cancer* (W. B. Coleman and G. J. Tsongalis, eds.), © Humana Press Inc., Totowa, NJ.

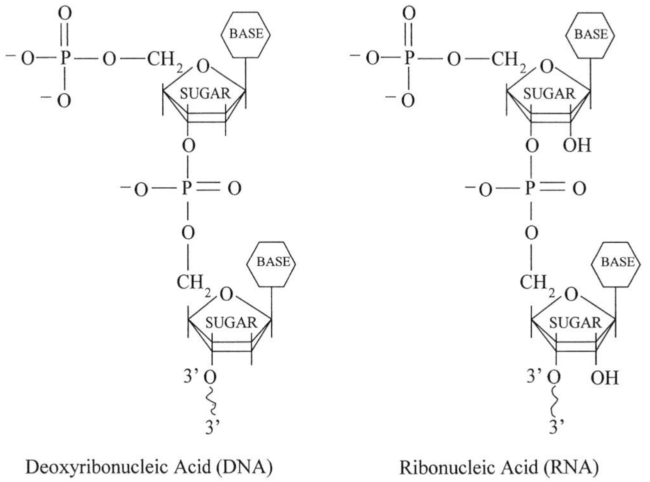

Fig. 1. DNA and RNA structure. Strands of nucleic acids are formed by the linkage of nitrogenous bases (purines and pyrimidines) via their phosphate groups. Note the presence of the extra hydroxyl group on the ribose component of RNA.

occurs in mammalian, bacterial, and viral DNA (5). Nucleosomes are wound into a left-handed helix for further condensation of the DNA, and higher orders of structure include supercoils and/or rosettes (2). Ultra-condensed DNA (heterochromatin) is inactive metabolically, and is found primarily in the periphery of the nucleus, whereas less condensed DNA (euchromatin) is readily accessible by transcription machinery and is located in the center of the nucleus (6).

GENE ORGANIZATION

The majority of genes that are transcribed into mRNA and translated into cellular proteins exist as two copies in the nucleus of each cell, one maternal and one paternal copy. Some genes are present at a high copy number (100–250 copies) within the genome, including the genes that encode for transfer RNA (tRNA), ribosomal RNA (rRNA), and the histone proteins (7). These tandemly repeated genes are present on several chromosomes and associate in the nucleus to form the nucleolus (8). Highly repetitive sequences with thousands of copies, called satellite DNAs, are found at the telomeric ends of chromosomes and around the centromeres (9). It is likely that the centromeric sequences play a role in the establishment and maintenance of chromosome structure. Telomeric repeats are involved in completing replication of chromosome ends (10), and it has been demonstrated that the length of the telomeric repeat sequences decreases with life-span of cultured human cells (11). The evidence of telomeric shortening in normal cells along with observations that immortalized or transformed cells display limited telomere degeneration has led to the hypothesis that telomeric shortening is involved in the cellular aging process (11). Other repetitive sequences, such as the *Alu* sequences, are found throughout chromosomes; their function is largely unknown, but a role in regulation of gene function has been proposed (12).

Simple polymorphic repetitive elements composed of dinucleotide or trinucleotide repeats are present in the human genome and have been associated with cancer and other diseases such as muscular dystrophy, Fragile X syndrome, Huntington's disease (HD), and spinocerebellar ataxia (13,14). Symptomatic problems arise when the affected DNA is inappropriately methylated and inactivated (as in Fragile X syndrome) (15), or when the repeats cause detrimental changes in the encoded protein (as in HD) (16).

DNA REPLICATION AND CELL DIVISION

In order for the DNA in a cell to be replicated prior to cell division, it must be single-stranded. This is accomplished by an enzyme (helicase), which denatures the DNA and allows DNA-binding proteins to associate with the DNA and prevent reformation of the DNA helix (17). A small strand of RNA 10–20 nucleotides in length acts as a primer, initiating synthesis of new complementary strands of DNA from multiple replication starting points. Deoxynucleotide triphosphates (dNTPs) are added to the primer by DNA polymerase, the RNA primers are removed, the gaps are filled in with dNTPs by DNA polymerase, and the nucleotide strands are joined by DNA ligase. The enzymatic action of topoisomerase removes twists generated during denaturation of the helix and allows the helix to re-form (18). DNA replication is complete when the telomerase enzyme has added the nucleotide repeats to the telomeres at the 5′ end of the DNA strands.

As a new strand of DNA is synthesized, dNTPs are selected based on hydrogen bonding to complementary dNTPs in the template strand, which results in an error rate of 1 in 10^4–10^5 (2). Eukaryotic cells employ a proofreading mechanism that removes mispaired dNTPs in the strand before the next dNTP is added, which decreases the error rate to 1 in 10^6–10^7 (2,19). Prior to cell division, another error correction system recognizes and repairs mismatched nucleotides and decreases the error rate further to 1 in 10^8–10^9 (2,19). Several inherited disorders are due to dysfunctional DNA damage-repair, including ataxia telangectasia (A-T), Fanconi's anemia, and xeroderma pigmentosum (XP) (20).

The DNA within the nucleus of a eukaryotic cell can be replicated completely in about eight h, during S phase of the cell cycle. Resting cells (G_0) receive a mitotic stimulus, which causes transition into G_1 phase, where the cell prepares for DNA synthesis (S phase). The G_2 phase occurs after replication but before division, and mitosis (M) involves actual nuclear and cellular division. The cell cycle is pivotal in cellular and organismal homeostasis, so it is tightly controlled by phosphorylation and dephosphorylation of kinases and cyclins, and by two major checkpoints (21,22). The first checkpoint occurs between G_1 and S, and can prevent cells with damaged or unrepaired DNA from entering S phase. The second checkpoint occurs between G_2 and M, and can prevent the initiation of mitosis (21).

STRUCTURE AND COMPOSITION OF RNA

RNA, or ribonucleic acid, is a linear polymer of ribonucleotides linked by 5′-3′ phosphodiester bonds (Fig. 1). RNA differs from DNA in that the sugar group of RNA is ribose, rather than deoxyribose, thymine is replaced by uracil (U) as one of the four bases, and RNA molecules are usually single-stranded. Because of the extra hydroxyl group present on the ribose, RNA is more susceptible than DNA to nucleases. Single-stranded RNA molecules form complex secondary structures, such as hairpin stems and loops, via Watson-Crick base pairing between adenine and uracil, and between guanine and cytosine.

RNA molecules are classified by function and cellular location, and there are three major forms of RNA in eukaryotic cells. Ribosomal RNA (rRNA) is the most stable and most abundant RNA. rRNA is highly methylated, and complexes with proteins to form ribosomes upon which proteins are synthesized (23). In eukaryotic cells, two major species of rRNA are present, 28S and 18S, as well as two minor species of 5.8S and 5S. Transfer RNA (tRNA) is responsible for carrying the amino acid residues that are added to a growing protein chain during protein synthesis. All tRNAs form secondary structures consisting of four stems and three loops, and many bases found in tRNA are modified by methylation, ethylation, thiolation, and acetylation (24,25). Messenger RNA (mRNA) mediates gene expression by carrying coding information from the DNA to the ribosomes, where proteins are synthesized. mRNA is the most heterogeneous type of RNA, and also has the shortest half-life. Other RNA species in eukaryotic cells include heterogeneous nuclear RNAs (hnRNA), which are the precursors to mature mRNA (26), and small nuclear RNAs, which are involved in the synthesis/processing of mRNA (27).

TRANSCRIPTION OF RNA

Even simple eukaryotic organisms, such as yeast, contain a large number of genes (~2,000), and higher eukaryotes, such as mammals, have ~100,000 genes (28). Clearly, the proteins encoded by all genes are not expressed simultaneously at any given time. Transfer of genetic information from DNA to protein begins with synthesis of RNA molecules from a DNA template by RNA polymerase, a process termed transcription. The RNA polymerase holoenzyme works processively, building an RNA chain with ribonucleoside triphosphates (ATP, GTP, CTP, UTP) (29). Initiation of transcription involves association of the transcription machinery (RNA polymerase and transcription factors) with the DNA template and the synthesis of a small ribonucleotide primer from which the RNA strand will be polymerized *(30)*. Initiation of transcription is not random, but occurs at specific sequences called promoters that are located at the 5′-end of genes. Every gene initiates transcription independently at its own promoter, therefore the efficiency of the process varies greatly depending on the strength of the promoter. Once RNA polymerase binds to a promoter, the DNA helix is opened and an RNA primer is synthesized. Elongation occurs as the RNA polymerase moves along the DNA strand, opening the DNA helix and conducting DNA-directed RNA synthesis until the gene is transcribed *(29)*. Termination of transcription is poorly understood in eukaryotes, but takes place at sites that include a stretch of T's on the nontemplate strand of the gene *(31)*.

RNA PROCESSING

The majority of eukaryotic RNAs require extensive modifications before they attain their mature structure and function. RNA strands may be modified by: 1) the removal of RNA sequences, 2) the addition of RNA sequences, or 3) the covalent modification of specific bases. The long, relatively unstable mRNA precursor strand (hnRNA) is synthesized and remains in the nucleus where it is subjected to several stability-enhancing processes. With the exception of mitochondrial mRNAs, the 5′-ends of eukaryotic mRNA precursor molecules are capped, which involves removal of the terminal phosphate group of the 5′-nucleoside triphosphate and subsequent linkage of the 5′-diphosphate group to a GTP molecule *(32)*. The cap structure is covalently modified by methylation of the newly added guanine. The hnRNA is also modified at the 3′ end by the addition of a poly-A tail, a string of 50–250 adenine residues. The poly-A tail serves to extend the life of the mRNA by protecting the 3′-end of the molecule from 3′-exonucleases, and may also act as a translational enhancer *(33)*. The mRNA molecule is stabilized further by the association of a ~70 kDa protein with the poly-A tail *(34)*.

The majority of protein-encoding eukaryotic genes contain intervening sequences, termed introns, which do not encode any portion of the protein. These introns are maintained during transcription of the hnRNA molecule, which results in production of a long hnRNA that must be modified in order to become a continuous template for synthesis of the encoded protein. Maturation of the hnRNA requires removal of the introns in conjunction with the joining of the coding sequences, termed exons. Introns may be between 65–10,000 base pairs, and short consensus sequences are found at either end and within the intron near the 3′-end *(35)*. The consensus sequences mark splice sites and act as targets for the spliceosome, a large multisubunit protein complex comprised of 45 proteins and thousands of snRNAs *(35)*. The spliceosome catalyzes removal of introns and rejoining of exons, ultimately resulting in the formation of a protein-encoding mRNA. Some genes encode for more than one protein, which is accomplished by alternative splicing of the primary hnRNA transcript. One mechanism of alternative splicing involves removal of one or more exons during splicing when the spliceosome ignores one or more intron-exon boundaries *(36)*. Alternative transcripts may also be generated by the use of a secondary polyadenylation site *(37)*.

RNA processing is not limited to mRNA. Eukaryotic tRNAs are modified post-transcriptionally, as are eukaryotic rRNAs *(38)*. Introns present within rRNAs are classified as Group I or Group II introns. Group I introns are removed as linear molecules by a self-splicing mechanism that requires magnesium and guanosine as cofactors *(39)*. Group II introns are also self-splicing, are removed as a lariat structure, and require spermidine as a cofactor *(40)*.

CONTROL OF GENE EXPRESSION

Gene expression in eukaryotes may be controlled at the level of mRNA stability, translational frequency, splicing, or protein stability. However, the predominant mechanism for expression control is at the level of transcription. Some genes, called housekeeping genes, are needed by cells at all times regardless of the metabolic needs of the cell. These genes are transcribed at about the same rate at all times, and are therefore expressed constitutively. Other genes are controlled stringently at the level of transcription, and their expression may be induced or repressed depending on the metabolic state of the cell. Some experimental models have taken advantage of this phenomenon by constructing expression vectors in which a promoter that can be modulated metabolically drives expression of a specific gene. For example, vectors have been constructed in which specific genes are placed under control of the metallothionein promoter, which is zinc-inducible *(41)*. When cells containing the metallothionein-promoted expression vector are exposed to Zn^{++}, the level of transcription of the gene of interest is induced, so that the effects of expression of that gene on the host cells can be evaluated in a controlled environment.

BASIC MOLECULAR ANALYSIS AND INTERPRETATION

Investigations into the molecular mechanisms of disease depend on the analysis of cellular DNA and RNA to identify and characterize the genes involved. Target genes can be identified, localized to specific chromosomes, amplified by cloning, and subjected to sequence analysis. DNA analyses are used practically in the identification of individuals and in the search for gene mutations, amplifications, and deletions, and RNA analyses are employed frequently in the characterization of gene expression.

DENATURATION AND HYBRIDIZATION The majority of techniques used in molecular analyses require single-stranded nucleic acids as starting material. Prior to hybridization with a complementary nucleotide sequence such as an oligonucleotide primer or a nucleic acid probe, double-stranded DNAs and single-stranded RNAs must be denatured to generate single strands and eliminate secondary structure. Denaturation of nucleic acids is rapid, and can be induced by various conditions, including extremes of pH (pH <4.0 or pH >10.0), hydrogen-bond disrupting agents (such as urea or formamide), or heat *(42)*. The melting point (T_m) of a specific double-stranded DNA sequence is reached when 50% of the hydrogen bonds are disrupted, and is related linearly to the percent G + C content of the DNA. The denaturation process is easily monitored by spectrophotometry, because the absorbance of the DNA at 260 nm increases as denaturation progresses (42).

Hybridization of nucleic acid strands is a slow process and the rate is governed by the relative concentration of strands with complementary sequences and by the temperature. When two complementary strands are aligned properly, hydrogen bonds form between the opposing complementary bases and the strands are joined. Target nucleic acid sequences can hybridize to a complementary DNA (cDNA) or RNA strand, or to other complementary sequences such as oligonucleotide primers or nucleic acid probes. Hybridization between two complementary RNA molecules is strongest, followed by RNA:DNA hybrids, and DNA:DNA hybrids (43).

CONCEPTS AND APPLICATIONS OF SOUTHERN BLOTTING The technique of Southern blotting is widely used in a clinical or forensic setting to identify individuals, determine relatedness, and to detect genes associated with genetic abnormalities or viral infections. Southern blot analysis is also used in basic scientific research to confirm the presence of an exogenous gene, evaluate gene copy number, or to identify genetic aberrations in models of disease.

The first step in successful Southern blotting is to obtain DNA that is reasonably intact. DNA that has been degraded by excessive exposure to the elements or mishandling will not produce a good quality Southern blot because it cannot be fragmented uniformly prior to the blotting procedure. The test DNA must be fragmented with restriction enzymes, which cut the double strands of DNA at multiple sequence-specific sites, creating a set of fragments of specific sizes that represent the regions of DNA between restriction sites. The fragmented DNAs are size-fractionated via agarose gel electrophoresis and are subsequently denatured, which enables them to later be hybridized to complementary nucleic acid probes. The DNAs are transferred to a solid support such as a nylon or nitrocellulose membrane via capillary action or electrophoretic transfer and are bound permanently to the membrane by brief ultraviolet (UV) crosslinking or by prolonged exposure to temperatures at 80°C. Blots at this stage may be stored for later use or may be probed immediately. For detailed protocols, the reader is referred to other sources (43,44).

The analysis of Southern blots requires the grasp of a few simple concepts. Interpretation is easy when the question is whether or not a gene is present in a particular sample, as long as appropriate positive and negative controls were included (a sample of DNA known to be positive and a sample of DNA known to be negative). The presence of multiple copies of a gene indicates gene amplification, which may occur in oncogenes during cancer development (45,46), or in genes such as the multidrug resistance gene (MDR1) during treatment with pharmacological agents (47). Amplifications are obvious on a Southern blot as a band or bands that are more intense than the normal single-copy control; numerical values that reflect intensity may be assigned to bands using a densitometer or phosphorimager. Structural aberrations in a gene of interest can be detected by Southern blotting, including the insertion or deletion of nucleotides or gene rearrangements. When nucleotides are mutated, inserted, or deleted, the ladder of fragments produced may be abnormal due to the obliteration of restriction sites, the generation of novel restriction sites, or alterations in fragment size due to an increase or decrease in the number of nucleotides between restriction sites. The majority of these aberrations are obvious on Southern blots as an abnormal banding pattern on the autoradiogram (Fig. 2). The Southern blot remains a useful and reliable way to obtain definitive data on gene structure.

THE POLYMERASE CHAIN REACTION (PCR) The development of PCR has increased the speed and accuracy of DNA analysis, and has resulted in the rapid development of new and creative techniques for detecting, replicating, and modifying DNA. Since it was described originally (48,49), PCR has evolved to encompass an enormous array of specific applications. This section will cover the basic concepts of PCR and several applications that are useful in molecular analyses of cancer. For a complete technical description of PCR techniques, the reader is referred to a more detailed source (50).

Principles of PCR Any PCR reaction must start with a DNA template. The DNA may be genomic DNA isolated directly from experimental or patient material, or it may be cDNA that has been synthesized from a DNA or RNA template by polymerase or reverse transcriptase. The target for any PCR reaction is dictated by specific oligonucleotide primers that anneal to two sites at either end of the region of interest, on opposite template strands. The primers are extended in the $5' \rightarrow 3'$ direction by DNA polymerase to yield overlapping copies of the original template. PCR is a cyclic process, consisting of three steps: denaturation of template (94∞C), annealing of primers (temperature is sequence-dependent), and extension of primers (72∞C). The three steps are repeated, with each cycle resulting in amplification of the target sequence. By the end of the third cycle, a new double-stranded molecule is formed in which the $5'$- and $3'$-ends coincide exactly with the primers (48,49). These double-stranded molecules accumulate exponentially during subsequent cycles of PCR, so that the majority of products are of a defined size and are seen clearly as a sharp band upon electrophoretic separation. Accumulation of target molecules reaches a plateau eventually; the initial number of target sequences and the efficiency of primer extension determine the upper limits of amplification. Due to the incredible sensitivity of PCR, even a miniscule amount of contaminating DNA can result in misinterpretation.

Design of Primers for PCR When constructing primers for PCR, it is important to keep in mind a few basic concepts. Primer length can influence target specificity and efficiency of hybridization. A long primer may be more specific for the target sequence, but is less efficient at hybridization, whereas a short primer is efficient at hybridization but less specific for the target sequence. As a general guideline, primers should be 20–30 nucleotides in length. Whenever possible, both primers should be the same length because primer length is considered when calculating an appropriate annealing temperature. The base composition of the primers is also important, because annealing temperature is governed in part by the percent G + C content of the primers. Ideally, G + C content is between 40–60%, and the percent G +C should be the same in any primer pair. A simple formula can be used to calculate an appropriate annealing temperature for any given primer: $T_m = 69.3 +$

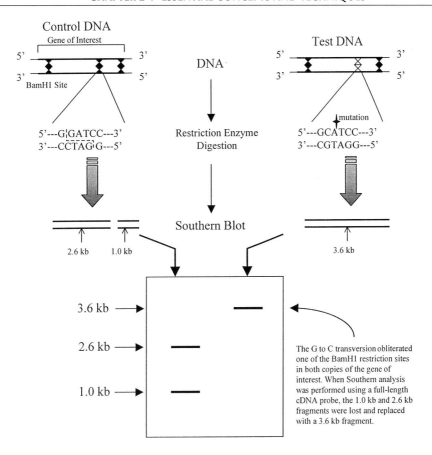

Fig. 2. Southern blot analysis. Double-stranded DNA of interest is fragmented with restriction enzymes and size-fractionated by agarose gel electrophoresis. The resulting ladder of fragments is transferred to a nylon or nitrocellulose membrane, which is then probed with a complementary RNA or DNA probe specific for the gene(s) of interest. In this example, the G‡C mutation present in the test DNA resulted in the loss of one of the *Bam*H1 restriction sites in the gene of interest, resulting in the loss of the 2.6 and 1.0 kb bands and appearance of a 3.6 kb band.

$0.41 (\%G + C) - (650/L)$, where L = primer length in bases *(51)*. Repetitive or palindromic sequences should be avoided in a primer, and primer pairs should not contain sequences complementary to each other.

The Role of Polymerase in PCR A DNA polymerase enzyme is essential for the primer extension step of PCR. Early PCR experiments employed the Klenow fragment of *E. coli* DNA polymerase I, but this enzyme is heat-labile and must be replenished with each amplification cycle. The developments of thermostable DNA polymerase and commercially available thermal cyclers have greatly improved the efficacy of PCR methodology. *Taq* DNA polymerase was isolated from *Thermus aquaticus*, and is characterized by its $5' \rightarrow 3'$ exonuclease activity, thermostability, and optimum performance at 70–80∞C *(52,53)*. Temperature, pH, and concentration of Mg^{++} may influence the activity of *Taq* polymerase, and extremely high denaturation temperatures (>97∞C) will significantly reduce its active lifetime. Lower divalent cation (Mg^{++}) concentrations decrease the rate of dissociation of enzyme from template by stabilizing the enzyme-nucleic acid interaction *(54)*. The optimum pH for a given PCR reaction will be between 8.0 and 10.0 (usually ~8.3), but must be determined empirically. While *Taq* DNA polymerase is ideal for routine PCR, there are many other DNA polymerases with unique qualities

that make them useful for special PCR applications such as amplification of long pieces of DNA or high-fidelity amplification *(54)*.

Visualization of PCR Products Once the PCR is complete, the products must be visualized for analysis and interpretation. Amplification products of routine PCR reactions can be separated by standard agarose gel electrophoresis and visualized by staining with ethidium bromide or other DNA dye. When finer resolution is needed, such as in the analysis of very small (<100 bp) products, polyacrylamide gel electrophoresis (PAGE) is standard. Recent technological advances have resulted in the development of gel-free quantification methods that are useful in high-throughput applications *(55)*.

Modifications and Improvements of PCR Hot-start PCR was developed to reduce background from nonspecific amplification by preventing polymerization of new DNA during the initial phase of the reaction when nonspecific binding may occur between primers and other DNAs in the mixture *(56,57)*. Hot start may be achieved by limiting the initial Mg^{++}, dNTP, or enzyme concentration, or by separating the components with a barrier, such as wax beads that melt as the mixture is heated. Alternatively, antibodies to the polymerase enzyme can be added to the reaction mixture; they prevent premature polymerization and are destroyed once the denaturation temperature is reached. The key concept in hot-start PCR is to achieve a temperature greater than the annealing temperature before the reaction components are allowed to initiate polymerization.

Touch-down PCR was developed to enhance amplification of the desired target sequences while reducing amplification of artifacts (58,59). The initial cycle begins with an annealing temperature that is greater than the expected T_m of the primer and the annealing temperature is lowered progressively with each cycle. As a result, the desired amplicon will accumulate preferentially while the amplification of undesired products is minimal.

Performing nested PCR can increase both the sensitivity and specificity of amplification (49). The amplification product(s) generated in the first PCR reaction are used as the template for a second PCR reaction, in which primers are used that are internal, or nested, within the first primer pair. Nonspecific products that are produced within the first round of PCR are not likely to contain sequences complementary to the nested primers, so that spurious products are eliminated during the second round of PCR. Extremely rare target sequences can be detected using nested PCR, because the first round of PCR effectively amplifies the specific template for the second round of PCR. Due to the sensitive nature of nested PCR, special care must be taken in order to avoid contamination.

It is possible to amplify sequences as large as 50 kb using long-distance PCR (LD-PCR) (60). One step toward successful LD-PCR is the use of thermostable, long-life polymerases that are capable of generating long strands of cDNA. The first LD-PCR was accomplished by using a 5′-endonuclease deficient, N-terminal deleted variant of *Taq* DNA polymerase in combination with *Pfu* DNA polymerase in a 180:1 ratio (61). Many special DNA polymerases capable of performing well in LD-PCR are now available commercially. Other prerequisites for successful LD-PCR are high-quality DNA for use as template, and carefully constructed primers with matching melting temperatures (T_m).

Quantitative PCR provides a quick and simple alternative to Southern- or Northern-blot analysis for the evaluation of gene copy number or gene expression levels (62). The underlying premise for quantitative PCR is that the accumulation of amplified products occurs exponentially and follows a predictable curve. The overall profile of product accumulation throughout the course of a reaction may be reproducible enough to extrapolate the amount of starting material. Accurate quantification requires that the analysis be done during the exponential (sloped) part of the curve, and not during the plateau. Accurate quantitative PCR experiments must include control template fragments, which may be synthesized or may be isolated from other sources. The control fragments should have priming sites and secondary structure that is identical to the test DNA, but should be sufficiently different in size that they can be discriminated upon electrophoretic separation. In a typical quantitative PCR reaction, replica tubes are prepared with a fixed concentration of test DNA; then known quantities of control DNA are added in a range of concentrations, PCR is conducted, and the samples are subjected to gel electrophoresis. When one template is in excess, it will yield a greater abundance of PCR product; but when the concentration of both the control and test

templates are equal, amplification will occur at equal rates, ultimately producing two bands of equal intensity on the gel. Quantitative approaches to PCR are useful when careful attention is paid to experimental reproducibility. For other aspects of quantitative PCR, see the following references (62,63).

Cloning PCR Products Some PCR reactions are intended to provide information that is gleaned from gel electrophoresis and visualization alone. However, PCR products can be cloned and used for sequence analysis, construction of molecular probes, mutation analysis, in vitro mutagenesis, studies of gene expression, and many other applications. PCR fragments can be introduced into suitable vectors via several methods (54), where they can be expanded and/or manipulated. A cloning strategy should be planned prior to the PCR reaction because modifications of the product, such as the insertion of restriction sites, are sometimes necessary to allow insertion of the product into the intended vector. Care should also be taken to verify the size and purity of the PCR product prior to cloning. With careful planning and the inclusion of appropriate controls, the conventional techniques of recombinant DNA technology can be replaced almost entirely with PCR-based methods.

DNA LIBRARIES In order to identify mutations or genetic alterations that are associated with disease, but are not detectable by Southern blot or PCR-based mutational analyses, the DNA of interest must be amplified so that a sufficient quantity is available for sequence analysis. One method for amplifying DNA is to clone the DNA of interest from a genomic DNA library or a cDNA library. Conceptually, genomic libraries represent the complete DNA from a specific source that has been divided into relatively small pieces ("books") that can be examined individually. cDNA libraries are constructed by synthesizing cDNA from the mRNAs that are expressed by a specific tissue or cell line, so that only the DNA that encodes expressed genes is represented. When screening a DNA library, the first task is to explore the library and identify the "book" that contains the DNA sequence of interest. Then, that particular piece of DNA must be isolated and amplified so that it may be examined in detail.

Construction of DNA Libraries DNA libraries may be constructed in bacteriophage vectors or cosmid vectors using genomic DNA that has been fragmented into large pieces by partial digestion with a restriction enzyme and ligated into the vector DNA and ultimately packaged into bacteriophage particles (43). Cosmid vectors are constructed by modification of a plasmid by addition of *cos* DNA sequences that enable the vector to be packaged in bacteriophage λ particles (64). The bacteriophage act simply as vehicles for delivery of the DNA into the host, where it replicates as a plasmid. Cosmid libraries are more difficult to construct using genomic DNA because the vector DNA often becomes concatenated and fails to incorporate the foreign eukaryotic DNA, and the foreign DNA sequences frequently undergo recombination, which results in rearrangement or loss of cloned segments of eukaryotic DNA. Although problems with cosmid vectors may be alleviated somewhat by additional steps such as the use of multiple restriction enzymes and treatment with phosphatases to prevent vector concatemerization, the additional steps required make cosmid vectors undesirable for routine cloning (43). Nonetheless, cosmid vectors are useful for cloning and propagation of single, complete eukaryotic genes that contain a large number of introns and are therefore too large (33–45 kb) to be propagated in bacterophage λ vectors *(64)*. Cosmid vectors may also be used to analyze a region of eukaryotic DNA that contains a gene family *(65)*. Gene families are typically spread over 70–300 kb, and can be cloned by using a segment of nonrepetitive DNA isolated from one end of a recombinant as a probe to identify recombinants containing the adjacent sequence. This process, called chromosome walking, is repeated until all recombinants comprising the region of interest are identified. Because the maximum size of foreign DNA that can be carried in cosmid vectors (~45 kb) is twice the maximum size for bacteriophage λ vectors, chromosome walking is expedited greatly by cosmid cloning.

Bacteriophage λ vectors are employed commonly in the construction of genomic and cDNA libraries because they are easy to manipulate and screen *(66)*. Bacteriophage λ infect *Escherichia coli* by adsorbing to receptors that transport maltose into the cells. In the majority of hosts the 50 kb double-stranded λ genome is transcribed extrachromosomally, generating the structural units of mature bacteriophage particles, which are ultimately responsible for lysis of the host bacterium and release of progeny *(43)*. However, a small percentage of bacterial hosts incorporate the λ DNA into their genome and do not undergo lysis. When constructing a library, there are many bacteriophage vectors to choose from (Charon, λgt, EMBL, and λZap, to name a few). The choice is made based on which restriction enzymes will be used, the size of foreign DNA fragments, and whether or not the foreign DNA is to be expressed by the bacterial host.

It is possible for DNA libraries to provide a means for both propagation and expression of inserted foreign DNA sequences *(67)*. Some plasmid-based and bacteriophage-based vectors, such as pUR, pEX, λgt11, or λORF8, allow expression of foreign cDNA sequences by carrying a portion of the *E. coli* β-galactosidase gene including the elements necessary for its expression. Foreign DNA is inserted into the carboxy-terminal coding region of the β-galactosidase gene, resulting in a chimeric gene that encodes for a fusion protein between β-galactosidase and the protein encoded by the foreign DNA. This approach ultimately provides a means of producing antisera to the foreign DNA-encoded protein and allows the expression library to be screened by immunological rather than nucleic acid probes.

Screening of DNA Libraries Once a DNA library has been generated, the sequence or gene of interest must be identified among all of the recombinants. The methods of screening recombinants vary depending on the type of vector that is used, but in theory they are similar. When cosmids are used, host bacteria are plated on agar plates containing an antibiotic that corresponds with the antibiotic resistance gene included on the plasmid vector. Ideally, the bacterial colonies should be far enough apart that it is simple technically to distinguish one from another. Grunstein and Hogness have described a methodology that allows *in situ* lysis of bacterial colonies onto nitrocellulose or nylon membranes, which can then be probed for sequence(s) of interest using labeled nucleic acid probes *(68)*.

When positive signals are obtained, the signal is traced back to a specific colony on the bacterial plates, which is then expanded and used for amplification of the foreign DNA sequences of interest.

Screening of bacteriophage λ DNA libraries involves infection of host bacteria with recombinant phage and plating them onto the surface of an agar plate. The bacteria grow to form a lawn on the surface of the plate and those that are infected with bacteriophage will undergo lysis, releasing progeny that in turn infect and lyse surrounding bacteria. The end result is the formation of cleared plaques on the lawn of bacteria, with each plaque representing the genetic material from a single recombinant *(43)*. Again, it is important that the number of infective bacteriophage used is adjusted so that the plaques are sufficiently separate from each other to be distinguished individually. Phage DNA within the plaques can be transferred easily by absorption onto a nitrocellulose or nylon membrane, and can be probed using labeled nucleic acid probes. Positive signals are traced back to a specific plaque, which is picked from the plate and used to infect more host bacteria, thus amplifying the recombinant phage DNA containing the foreign DNA sequence(s) of interest.

Screening of expression libraries is accomplished by using antibodies to identify specific proteins expressed by recombinant clones in either plasmid or bacteriophage vectors *(69)*. When bacteriophage λ is used, the debris in the plaques (which contains the expressed protein) is transferred directly to nitrocellulose filters and screened for immunoreactive material using antibodies to the protein of interest. Because plasmid libraries are maintained as bacterial colonies, they must be lysed prior to fixation on nitrocellulose membranes. Therefore, plasmid vectors may be advantageous because the conditions for lysis can be altered so that the structure and conformation of the expressed protein is preserved.

CLONING STRATEGIES FOR LARGE DNAS: YACS, BACS, AND PACS

The Yeast Artificial Chromosome System While cosmid and bacteriophage λ vectors are powerful tools for isolation of cDNAs and some eukaryotic genes, limitations on insert size (<45 kb) have precluded cloning and analysis of larger eukaryotic genes or chromosomal regions. Several advances were imperative in the development of the yeast artificial chromosome (YAC) system: 1) *cis*-acting elements required for chromosomal stability in yeast were identified and characterized by Szostak and Blackburn *(70)*; 2) a system was developed that enabled yeast to be transformed at high efficiency *(71)*; and 3) pulsed-field gel electrophoresis was developed, which provided a method for resolving DNA fragments up to 10,000 kb. The YAC library is constructed by ligating large fragments of DNA to the two arms of a YAC vector, which is then introduced into yeast via transformation *(72,73)*. The YAC vector carries antibiotic resistance as well as DNA sequences that function as telomeres, a centromere, and an origin of replication. Transformants that take up and stably maintain an artificial chromosome can be identified as colonies on agar plates that possess characteristics (i.e., antibiotic resistance, etc.) encoded on the YAC vector. Some problems associated with the use of YAC vectors include insert instability, the presence of chimeric clones within the YAC libraries, and difficulties in DNA manipulation.

The Bacterial Artificial Chromosome System The bacterial artificial chromosome (BAC) cloning system is based on the *E. coli* fertility plasmid (F-factor), into which foreign DNA sequences up to 300 kb are inserted *(74)*. The F-plasmids are introduced into host *E. coli* via electroporation where they are maintained at a low copy number, which limits detrimental recombination events. Although the BAC system offers some advantages over YAC vectors, there are significant limitations, such as the lack of positive selection for recombinants and low yields of recombinant DNA due to limited copy number of the F plasmid *(74)*.

The P1 Artificial Chromosome System Successful cloning of very large (up to 300 kb) pieces of DNA can be accomplished by employing a bacteriophage P1-based cloning system, or PAC *(75)*. The vector was created by combining a modified pAd10SacBII vector and a modified pUC19 plasmid, resulting in a vector that 1) allows insertion of large DNA fragments, 2) provides control of insert copy number, 3) allows discrimination of recombinant vs nonrecombinant vectors, and 4) provides stable recombinants with little to no occurrence of chimerism *(75)*. High molecular weight foreign DNA is modified by the ligation of specific restriction endonuclease sites to both the 5′- and 3′-ends, enabling the foreign DNA to be inserted into cloning sites within the PAC. The primary limiting step in PAC cloning is integrity of the foreign DNA inserted into the vector.

DNA SEQUENCE ANALYSIS DNA that has been isolated by screening of a genomic DNA or cDNA library or by PCR can be subjected to sequence analysis by either of two methods. Maxam-Gilbert analysis involves chemical cleavage at a specific base, followed by electrophoresis of the DNA, which produces a series of bands of various sizes, each ending in the targeted base *(76)*. The fragmentation procedure is done four times (once for each base) and the separate reactions are subjected to PAGE simultaneously, generating a ladder of bands from which the DNA sequence is read top to bottom.

In the Sanger sequencing method, a labeled primer is annealed to the DNA to be sequenced and the DNA is replicated in a reaction that contains a limiting concentration of one of the four nucleotides *(77)*. The reaction contains a dideoxynucleotide corresponding to the specific nucleotide that is in low concentration, resulting in termination of replication upon incorporation of the dideoxynucleotide, which has no 3′-hydroxyl group upon which another nucleotide may be added. The result is a set of DNA fragments, each of which ends in a specific base. The reaction is done four times, one reaction with a limiting concentration of each nucleotide, followed by denaturation and PAGE analysis. A ladder of bands is apparent as in the Maxam-Gilbert method, and the sequence is read bottom to top. Note that the sequence obtained by the Sanger method is the cDNA sequence, whereas the Maxam-Gilbert method yields the direct DNA sequence. When adequate normal controls are included, sequence analysis can reveal point mutations as well as other anomalies such as insertions and deletions. It is also possible to discern whether an individual is heterozygous or homozygous for a specific mutation by evaluating whether both a normal and

mutated allele are present in the sequence, which would indicate heterozygosity.

Recent advancements have significantly improved sequence analysis by eliminating the tedious task of reading sequencing autoradiographs. Fluorescent dyes have replaced radiolabeled isotopes used in the Sanger sequencing method *(78)*, and instruments have been devised that can image fluorescent dye-labeled DNA fragments during electrophoresis *(79,80)*. Automated DNA sequencing instruments shuttle sequence data into a computer, where it is assimilated and output. The development of improved DNA-labeling techniques and the introduction of more efficient DNA polymerases continue to streamline DNA sequencing procedures *(78,81)*, improving the quality and efficacy of high-throughput sequence analysis.

ELECTROPHORETIC SEPARATION OF NUCLEIC ACIDS

Standard Electrophoresis of Nucleic Acids Gel electrophoresis of DNA is widely used in procedures such as Southern blotting and PCR, where separation of a population of DNA fragments is an essential step in the analytical process. In some cases, a significant amount of information can be gleaned from relatively simple electrophoretic procedures that take advantage of the various properties of DNA molecules (i.e., charge, size, and conformation). Gels employed in electrophoretic techniques are generally composed of agarose or polyacrylamide. Agarose gels are useful for routine Southern blotting and analysis of PCR products >100 base pairs. However, when very small DNA fragments are to be analyzed, special agarose formulations (MetaPhor®, NuSieve®) are available with enhanced sieving properties that aide in the resolution of small fragments and/or fragments that differ in size by as little as 1%. Some mutational analyses require special gels, such as MDE™ (mutation detection enhancement) gels, that can resolve DNA fragments based on differences in conformation. MDE gels can be nondenaturing, which maintains single-stranded nucleic acids in their native conformation, or denaturing agents, such as formamide, hydroxide ions, or urea, can be added to the gel or sample buffer, resulting in elimination of secondary structure in the nucleic acid strand. The following sections discuss several widely used electrophoretic techniques that are capable of extracting valuable information from genomic DNA samples or from cDNA samples that were generated by PCR.

Separation of RNA for Northern-blot analysis is typically accomplished by electrophoresis through a 1–2% agarose gel containing formaldehyde, which maintains the denatured state of the RNA strands. When secondary structure of an RNA molecule is to be investigated, samples are subjected to nondenaturing PAGE.

Pulsed-Field Gel Electrophoresis Conventional gel electrophoresis techniques are not useful for separation of extremely long pieces of DNA, because the constant current eventually unravels the DNA strands completely so that they travel, end first, through the gel at a rate that is independent of their length. Pulsed-field gel electrophoresis (PFGE) overcomes this challenge by periodically switching the orientation of the electric fields with respect to the gel, thus preventing the DNA strands from losing secondary structure and allowing long strands to be size-differentiated *(82)*. PFGE is often used in the identification of pathogens *(83)*, i.e., differentiating between strains of bacteria. Other applications include chromosomal length polymorphism analysis, and large-scale restriction and deletion mapping in DNA that is hundreds or thousands of kb in length. The effectiveness of PFGE is dependent on high-integrity starting material, and DNA that is degraded or sheared will not yield informative results. High-quality DNA is often generated by embedding the cells of interest in agarose plugs, lysing cell membranes with detergent, and removing proteins enzymatically, leaving intact DNA that can be digested by restriction enzymes *in situ* and easily loaded into a gel apparatus *(82,84)*. In a typical analysis, PFGE will produce a pattern of DNA fragments that range in size from 10–800 kb.

Field-inversion gel electrophoresis (FIGE) is a type of PFGE that allows clear, reliable separation of large DNA fragments from 100 kb to several megabases *(85)*. FIGE devices are constructed so that periodic reversals of the electric field cause the DNA to alternate between forward and reverse migration through the gel *(86)*. Net forward movement of the DNA through the gel is achieved by making the duration of the forward pulse longer than the duration of the reverse pulse, or by using a greater voltage for the forward current than for the reverse current. Resolution of fragments less than 200 kb is achieved best by using greater voltage for the forward current rather than longer forward pulse duration *(86)*.

MUTATION ANALYSIS DNA sequencing is the most reliable way to detect a mutation, but it is an expensive and complex screening method. Mutations that involve single base changes are detectable by Southern-blot analysis or restriction fragment length polymorphism (RFLP) analysis when the change destroys or creates a restriction site *(87)*, and mutations may be identified directly by PCR when primers are designed to detect a specific mutation *(88)*. However, the success of these methods relies on some knowledge of the mutation, i.e., the restriction site that is altered or the location of the mutation in the gene sequence. Broader mutational analyses may be conducted using PCR and electrophoretic separation; the most commonly used techniques include heteroduplex analysis (HA), single-strand conformation polymorphism (SSCP), denaturing gradient gel electrophoresis (DGGE), and thermal gradient gel electrophoresis (TGGE).

SSCP Analysis SSCP analysis can detect mutations when the nucleotide sequence influences the secondary structure, or conformation, of a single strand of DNA *(89)*. Conformation polymorphisms may be detected as a change in the relative mobility of the DNA in a gel. Initially, the DNA of interest is purified and amplified via PCR using end-labeled primers. After denaturation, which generates single DNA strands, the DNA is subjected to nondenaturing PAGE. Mutations in sequences that govern the secondary structure of the single-strand result in conformation polymorphisms. Polymorphisms are evident on the gel as bands that migrate slower or faster than the control normal DNA, which must be included in the assay for interpretation (Fig. 3).

Heteroduplex Analysis HA is accomplished by mixing denatured DNA fragments from a wild-type (control) sample and a test DNA sample. The fragments reanneal, producing

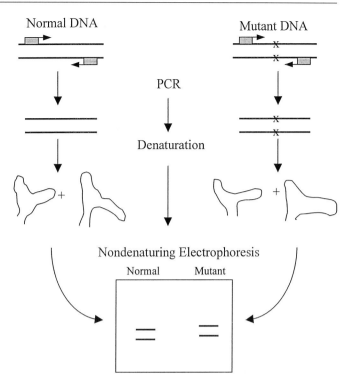

Fig. 3. SSCP analysis. Control and test DNA samples are subjected to PCR to amplify the region of interest. Single strands are generated by denaturation, and electrophoretic mobility of the strands are analyzed by nondenaturing PAGE. In this example, mutant DNA strands have altered conformations that are evident on the gel as a slight decrease in electrophoretic mobility when compared to normal control DNA.

either 1) wild-type:wild-type homoduplexes, 2) test:test homoduplexes, or 3) wild-type:test heteroduplexes. If a mutation is present in the test DNA, the heteroduplex will contain a bulge (in the case of an insertion or deletion) or a bubble (in the case of a point mutation) *(90)*. Bulge heteroduplexes are easily observed by agarose gel electrophoresis or PAGE, where they migrate slower than homoduplexes and result in the formation of a doublet on the gel (Fig. 4). However, bubble heteroduplexes are more difficult to visualize, and usually require the use of specialty gel matrices *(91,92)*.

DGGE and TGGE Analyses Some mutations in DNA can be detected by DGGE *(93)*. Denaturation of double-stranded DNA into single-stranded DNA occurs in steps as temperature rises or concentration of denaturant increases. Regions of DNA with the highest A + T content denature first, and denaturation continues until the region with the highest G + C content denatures, leaving completely single-stranded DNA. Mutations that change the denaturation profile of a region of DNA may be detected by DGGE. As test DNA migrates through a polyacrylamide gel containing a transverse gradient of denaturant, domains that denature yield partially single-stranded DNA fragments that have a decreased rate of migration *(94)*. The sensitivity of DGGE analysis may be increased by generating heteroduplexes between the test DNA sample and control DNA fragments of known sequence (Fig. 5). A mismatch between the test DNA and control DNA causes the heteroduplex to melt early compared to control DNA (Fig. 5). Once the area contain-

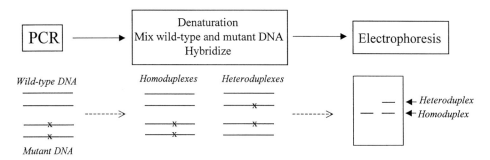

Fig. 4. Heteroduplex analysis. When wild-type DNA and test DNA are denatured, mixed, and hybridized, three types of double-stranded molecules are formed: 1) homoduplexes consisting of two strands of wild-type DNA, 2) homoduplexes consisting of two strands of test DNA, and 3) heteroduplexes consisting of one wild-type and one test strand. When mutations, insertions, or deletions are present in the test DNA, heteroduplexes that form do not align perfectly with the wild-type DNA strand, resulting in the formation of double-stranded DNA molecules with bulges or bubbles in the region of unpaired bases. Partially denatured heteroduplexes migrate more slowly than fully hybridized homoduplexes, resulting in the appearance of a doublet upon PAGE analysis. When the sequence of wild-type and test DNA is identical, heteroduplexes migrate at the same rate as homoduplexes and a single band is produced.

ing the mutation is defined and the melting profile generated by the mutation is characterized, DGGE analysis may be simplified by electrophoresing samples through MDE or polyacrylamide gels with a denaturant gradient in the same direction as electrophoresis; heteroduplexes with a mismatch exhibit slower mobility, producing a doublet in the gel similar to that seen in heteroduplex analysis (Fig. 4). TGGE is conducted essentially as DGGE, except the denaturing gradient is established by increasing temperatures rather than increasing concentrations of a chemical denaturant *(95)*.

BASIC RNA ANALYSIS AND INTERPRETATION

Isolating High-Quality RNA The success of any RNA-based molecular analysis rests largely on the quality of the RNA to be tested. Careful handling is essential to ensure that the RNA molecules remain intact during the isolation process. Total cellular RNA may be isolated reliably by centrifugation through cesium chloride gradients, or by acidic phenol extraction of cellular lysates *(96)*. For detailed protocols, *see* Sambrook et al. *(43)*. Contamination with RNAses (ubiquitous enzymes that readily degrade RNA) is frequently the cause of poor sample integrity. The quality of total RNA can be monitored by agarose gel electrophoresis of RNA samples, followed by ethidium bromide staining and UV visualization. The upper (or 28S) and lower (or 18S) ribosomal bands should be present at 5.0 kb and 1.87 kb, respectively, and there should be little to no degraded RNA evident. Samples lacking a clear upper or lower ribosomal RNA band or containing significant amounts of low molecular-weight (degraded) RNA should be considered suspect.

The poly-A tail present on mRNA strands provides an effective means of purifying mRNA from total cellular RNA, the bulk of which is rRNA. Isolation of mRNA is advantageous because it increases the proportion of mRNAs in the sample while lessening the concentration of other RNAs that may lead to background and interference in RNA analysis. Messenger RNA isolation techniques employ short stretches of thymidine or uracil residues (oligodT or oligodU) that are linked covalently to magnetic beads or resin. The total cellular RNA is exposed to the oligodT, and the poly-A tail of the mRNA hybridizes to the complementary thymidine or uracil residues. Unhybridized tRNA and rRNA are washed away, and the poly-A mRNA is eluted from the oligodT in a low-salt buffer. In typical eukaryotic cells, only 1–5% of the total cellular RNA is mRNA.

Northern Blotting Northern blotting involves the analysis of RNA without first converting the RNA to cDNA. Through Northern analysis, one can evaluate whether a gene is expressed, the relative level of expression, the size of the mRNA, and the presence of alternatively spliced transcripts. Total cellular RNA or mRNA is denatured, electrophoretically separated, and transferred to a solid support, such as nitrocellulose or positively charged nylon. The membrane-bound RNA is then probed with a labeled, complementary DNA or RNA probe. Visualization of positive signals is accomplished by generating autoradiograms, which can be analyzed quantitatively using a scanning densitometer, or, if ^{32}P-labeled probes were used, a phosphoimager. Simultaneous or subsequent probing of the RNA blot with a probe for a constitutively expressed housekeeping gene, such as *β-actin* or *cyclophilin*, will allow true quantitative assessment of expression of the gene of interest. For a more detailed description of Northern blot analysis and related protocols, see the following references *(43,44)*. Northern blots may be advantageous over other methods of gene-expression analysis, such as reverse transcription polymerase chain reaction (RT-PCR), when true quantitative results are desired, because there are fewer experimental artifacts associated with Northern blot analysis.

RNA ANALYSIS INVOLVING CDNA SYNTHESIS RNA is inherently unstable in comparison to DNA, therefore techniques have been developed that provide a means of analyzing RNA by first converting it to complementary DNA (cDNA). RNA-derived cDNA is used routinely in many analyses, including construction of gene-expression libraries, PCR amplification, sequence analysis, and vector construction. By taking a population of mRNAs from a cell line and converting them to cDNAs, a gene-expression fingerprint is created, which can

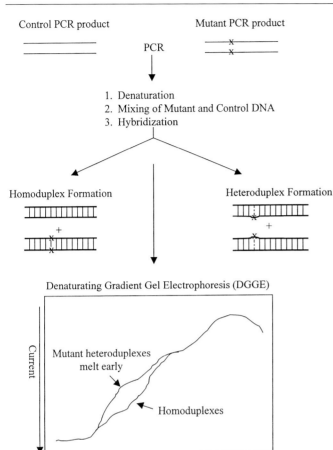

Fig. 5. DGGE analysis. Mutations may be identified in a test DNA sample by comparing the melting profile of test DNA to control wild-type DNA. In this example, heteroduplexes are generated between test DNA and wild-type DNA. The hybridized mixture is then loaded into a single trough-like well that extends the width of the gel, which contains a transverse concentration of a chemical denaturant. As the sample is electrophoresed, the double-stranded DNA molecules denature, or melt, in domains. The higher the concentration of denaturant, the more rapidly the DNA strands melt. Double-stranded molecules that are hybridized fully migrate rapidly, but electrophoretic mobility of partially denatured strands is slowed. When mutations are present in the test DNA, the melting profile of the heteroduplexes is altered so that the DNA melts at a lower concentration of denaturant when compared to the control homoduplexes, resulting in the formation of a bubble on the gel. Once the DNA strands are denatured fully, they migrate very rapidly through the gel at a rate that is independent of their sequence.

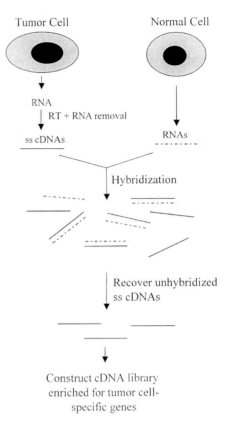

Fig. 6. Constructing a subtraction library. Subtraction libraries are often constructed to enrich for a population of cDNAs that may be involved in a specific biological process, such as malignant transformation. In this example, mRNA was isolated from a normal cell line and from a derived tumor cell line. The tumor cell mRNA was subjected to reverse transcription and the remaining RNAs were eliminated by enzymatic treatment with DNAse-free RNAse, leaving single-stranded cDNA molecules. A hybridization step is performed between the single-stranded cDNAs and mRNA isolated from the normal cells. Unhybridized mRNAs represent expressed genes that are probably unique to the normal cells, whereas unhybridized cDNAs represent genes that are expressed only by the tumor cells. Unhybridized single-stranded cDNAs are recovered and used to construct a cDNA library that is enriched for genes that may be involved in the malignant transformation of this cell line.

then be compared to other fingerprints. The following sections will discuss the process of cDNA generation and several technical applications.

Generating cDNA from RNA The process of RNA-directed cDNA synthesis relies on an enzyme called reverse transcriptase, which is a retroviral enzyme capable of synthesizing DNA using RNA as a template *(97)*. RNA that is isolated from cells or tissue is incubated in the presence of reverse transcriptase and all four deoxynucleotides, along with an oligonucleotide primer upon which the cDNA will be built. When mRNA is the intended template, the primer can be a short sequence of deoxythymidine residues that targets the poly-A tail.

Alternatively, primers specific for internal sequences may be used, or, when sequence information is unknown, random oligonucleotide primers are used. The primer provides a 3′-OH group to which the reverse transcriptase enzyme adds deoxynucleotides to the growing cDNA strand. As the reverse transcriptase transcribes RNA into DNA, it degrades the template RNA, leaving a single-stranded DNA that is complementary and in the opposite orientation (5′ to 3′).

Using cDNA to Construct Libraries A population of RNAs isolated from a specific cell type or tissue may be reverse transcribed, yielding a population of cDNAs that is representative of the RNAs expressed. The cDNAs can then be used to construct DNA libraries. These libraries can be screened repeatedly to identify and isolate cDNAs corresponding to genes that are expressed by the cell type or tissue. To enrich for RNAs expressed specifically during a particular biological process, a subtraction library can be prepared *(43,98)*. For example, suppose the goal is to detect genes that are expressed in a particular cell during malignant transformation. In this scenario, mRNA would be isolated from a control normal cell or tissue, and then mixed with cDNA prepared from the transformed cells or tumor tissue. Hybridization occurs between cDNAs and complementary RNAs, leaving unhybridized cDNAs that are expressed uniquely by the transformed cells or tumor tissue (Fig. 6). The unhybridized cDNAs are purified and used to produce a cDNA library that is enriched for genes that may be involved in the transformation process *(43)*. As an alternative approach, subtraction libraries may be constructed from the unhybridized mRNA that remains after hybridization between the cDNA and mRNA *(98)*.

RT-PCR   PCR methodology can be exploited in the analysis of gene expression *(99)*. Typically, mRNA is reverse transcribed using an oligo-dT primer, generating a cDNA strand complementary to the RNA sequence beginning at the 3′-end of the mRNA *(100)*. Subsequently, a second strand is synthesized using the cDNA as a template, resulting in a double-stranded DNA molecule. If the mRNA is long, reverse transcription with an oligo-dT primer may not generate a cDNA that extends through the 5′-end of the mRNA. When specific sequence information is known, internal sequence-specific primers may be used for the reverse transcription reaction. Alternatively, when no 5′-sequence information is available, random oligonucleotides may be used to prime the cDNA synthesis *(99)*. Once the desired cDNA is obtained, specific oligonucleotide primers are used to amplify target sequences using the reverse transcribed cDNA as a template. The amplified product(s) can be visualized by agarose gel electrophoresis or PAGE, and information on gene expression can be extracted.

Successful reverse transcription of sample mRNA with oligo-dT primers requires that the poly-A tail be relatively intact. Therefore, it is imperative that high quality mRNA is used as starting material for RT reaction or sufficient cDNA template will not be generated for the subsequent PCR reaction. Inclusion of appropriate controls when setting up a RT-PCR experiment will allow a semi-quantitative assessment of gene expression. Fixed concentrations of control template can be amplified along with the test template to provide standards against which the amount of test amplification product is gauged. Alternatively, amplification of housekeeping genes, such as actin or cyclophilin, may provide a mechanism for quantification similar to the approach used in Northern blot analysis. See Larrick and Siebert for more information on quantitative approaches to RT-PCR *(99)*.

MOLECULAR PROBES FOR NUCLEIC ACID ANALYSIS
There are several methods for generating molecular probes to be used in analysis of DNA or RNA. The central concept behind the use of nucleic-acid probes is hybridization. Probes may be made of RNA or DNA, and can be labeled with colorimetric, fluorescent, enzymatic, or radioactive molecules for visualization purposes. Labeled nucleic acid probes are frequently used in Southern blotting, Northern blotting, and screening of DNA libraries.

Generation of DNA Probes   DNA probes are useful for most routine procedures, because they are easy to generate and are very stable. Nick translation is one method for generating

labeled DNA probes *(101)*. The first step in nick translation is to generate nicks in the phosphodiester backbone of a double-stranded DNA template by treatment with pancreatic DNAase I, which produces free 3′-hydroxyl termini along the strand. DNA polymerase I extends the 3′-OH termini in the 3′-direction, using its 5′→3′ exonuclease activity to hydrolyze the nontemplate strand. There are many disadvantages associated with nick translation, including the requirement for a large amount (0.5 µg) of DNA template, and the need for strict time and temperature limits in the protocol. Consequently, most DNA probes are generated using alternative methodologies.

An easy and effective method for generating DNA probes is random primer extension. Oligonucleotide primers of random sequence are annealed to denatured DNA template strands, followed by primer extension by the Klenow fragment of DNA polymerase or by T7 DNA polymerase in the presence of labeled nucleotides *(101)*. Random primer extension is advantageous because of the small amount of template required (~25 ng), the high specific activity of probes generated, the ability to generate probes from very large or very small templates, and the ease in preparation.

Probes generated from double-stranded DNA templates are effective when target sequences are present in sufficient quantity and the probe hybridizes strongly to the target sequences. When hybridization between the probe and target is weak, unwanted hybridization may occur between the complementary sequences in the probe. Single-stranded probes provide a means to detect specific target sequences without the danger of reannealing probe, and are particularly useful when target sequences are rare or are only weakly homologous to the probe *(101)*. Recombinant bacteriophage M13 are composed of single-stranded DNA molecules that can serve as templates for synthesis of single-stranded DNA probes. Oligonucleotide primers are designed and annealed to viral DNA sequences upstream from the inserted template sequences, followed by primer extension with the Klenow fragment of DNA Polymerase I in the presence of labeled dNTPs. Labeled probe is often separated from unlabeled DNA by gel electrophoresis or alkaline chromatography, but the resulting probe has an extremely high specific activity.

Generation of RNA Probes   The RNA:RNA hybrid is much more stable than RNA:DNA hybrids or DNA:DNA hybrids. Therefore, single-stranded RNA probes (termed riboprobes) are advantageous when probing Northern blots or when detecting signals that are weak by other probing methods. The template DNA is inserted into a plasmid vector that contains one or more strong bacteriophage promoters (SP6, T7, or T3) that are recognized by bacteriophage-specific, DNA-dependent RNA polymerases *(102,103)*. In the presence of labeled NTPs, these polymerases synthesize a single-stranded riboprobe that is complementary to the target sequence and has a high specific activity. DNA is eliminated from the reaction by treatment with RNAse-free DNAase I. Riboprobes are a more sensitive and efficient alternative to double-stranded or single-stranded DNA probes.

Molecules for the Labeling of Probes   The majority of conventional probe-labeling practices involve incorporation of nucleotides that are labeled with a radioactive molecule, such as [32]P. Radioactive nucleotides may be incorporated into the probe during synthesis; three unlabeled (or cold) deoxynucleotides are added to the labeling mixture (dATP, dGTP, and dTTP), along with radiolabeled (or hot) ^{32}P-CTP. The radioactive molecule is incorporated into the nucleic acid probe, and positive signals are detected by autoradiography. As an alternative, radiolabeled dNTPs may be attached to the 3′-termini of a DNA probe using bacteriophage T4 DNA polymerase or to the 5′-termini using bacteriophage T4 polynucleotide kinase *(43)*. In general, a higher specific activity is achieved when the label is incorporated rather than attached to the ends of the probe.

Many nonradioactive labeling alternatives have been developed, reflecting concerns about the environment, safety, and cost. The most widely used methodologies involve incorporation or end-labeling of probes with molecules such as digoxigenin, biotin, or fluorescein, that can be detected using immunological methods or visualized by chemiluminescence *(104,105)*. This methodology generates an autoradiograph identical to those produced by traditional radioactive probes *(106)*.

PRACTICAL MOLECULAR BIOLOGY IN CANCER RESEARCH AND CLINICAL LABORATORY SCIENCE

In some cases, the tools of molecular biology are used to provide simple answers that aid in the diagnostic and/or prognostic evaluation of patient material or experimental specimens. Examples of such analysis include the analysis of genes that are associated with an increased risk of development of breast cancer such as *BRCA1* and *BRCA2 (107,108)*, or analysis of genes, that are associated with the development of a subset of colon cancers, such as *MSH2* and *MLH1 (109)*. For these types of analysis, PCR, Southern-blot analysis, or Northern-blot analysis may suffice. However, in many cases, especially in experimental models of cancer where there are many unknowns, the quest for information is not straightforward. For example, if one wishes to know the molecular differences between normal and cancerous tissue, or between a normal cell line and one that has been transformed by a carcinogenic treatment. Answers to such questions are dependent on the development of efficient techniques for screening large numbers of genes from two or more sources simultaneously (Fig. 7). While Southern blots, Northern blots, PCR, and RT-PCR may be used for such large-scale comparisons, it is time-consuming, and it requires that some information about potential target genes be known. The development of micro array technology has provided a new way to evaluate expression of a large number of genes in a small amount of time. In addition, techniques such as differential display RT-PCR (RT-PCR/DD) and comparative genomic hybridization (CGH) have created methods for comparing the genetic composition and gene expression patterns of two or more populations simultaneously.

MICROARRAY TECHNOLOGY Microarrays provide a means for screening samples for presence or expression of very large numbers of genes simultaneously *(110)*. Several approaches have been developed for construction of arrays. In one approach, hundreds of cDNA targets are immobilized

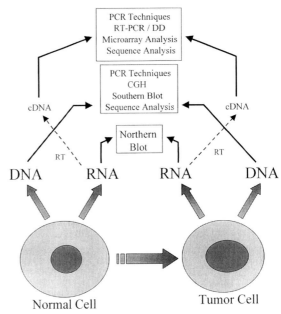

Fig. 7. Comparative analyses in molecular biology. In vivo and in vitro models of cancer, and the analysis of patient samples, often involve a comparative analysis between normal cells and tumor cells. Cellular RNA and DNA may be compared through a large variety of methods, including several (RT-PCR/DD, microarray analysis, CGH) that allow a broad comparative survey of genetic differences.

robotically on glass slides and hybridized to fluorescent ssDNA probes produced by reverse transcription from total mRNA of interest *(111)*. Positive hybridization signals are identified and compared to an internal standard with a laser scanner and displayed as a colored map, where the colors are indicative of relative expression level. A larger-scale analysis may be accomplished by immobilization of up to 30,000 cDNA or genomic DNA targets on large nylon membranes using automation *(112)*. Test DNA or cDNA is used to generate short ^{32}P-labeled oligonucleotide probes that are hybridized to the nylon membranes and imaged with a phosphoimager. In a similar approach, GeneChips have been constructed that contain nearly 100,000 probes per chip (10^6 probes per cm^2). Test DNA samples are labeled fluorescently, hybridized to the GeneChip, and analyzed by confocal epifluorescence microscopy and computer digitization *(113)*.

DNA microarrays have been employed successfully in studies of gene expression in yeast, plants, and mammalian cells. De Risi et al. investigated the molecular basis of tumorigenicity in a human melanoma cell line (UACC-903) by comparing tumorigenic and nontumorigenic derivatives of the cells by microarray technology. This approach resulted in the identification of several genes that are associated with suppression of tumorigenicity in UACC-903 cells *(114)*. In addition, a GeneChip containing 96,000 oligonucleotide probes was used successfully to detect heterozygous mutations in exon 11 of the *BRCA1* gene in patient samples *(113)*. Microarray technology is advancing rapidly, and has proven to be effective in diagnostics, gene-expression studies, gene mapping, and gene discovery.

DIFFERENTIAL DISPLAY RT-PCR RT-PCR/DD was introduced in 1992 as a technique for the comparison, identification, and isolation of genes that are expressed uniquely among

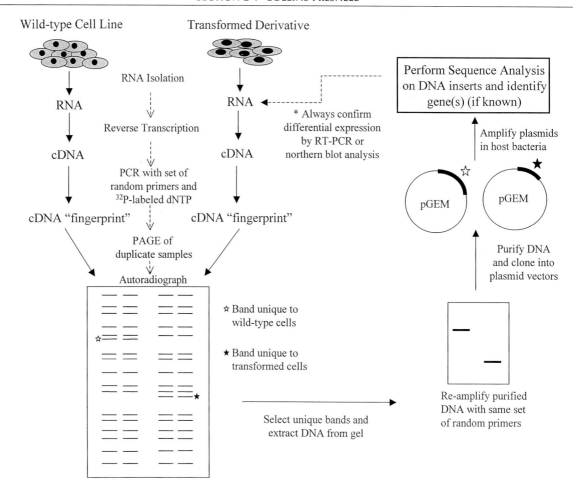

Fig. 8. Differential display RT-PCR analysis. RT-PCR/DD is a useful technique for evaluating differences in gene expression between two or more related cell lines. mRNA is isolated from the cells to be compared and subjected to reverse transcription with oligo-dT anchored primers. PCR is then conducted with a set of random oligonucleotide primers in the presence of ^{32}P-dNTP, generating a cDNA fingerprint composed of a ladder of labeled fragments that represents a subset of the genes expressed by the cell. The cDNA fingerprints from each sample to be compared are loaded onto a polyacrylamide gel and subjected to electrophoretic separation and autoradiography. Unique bands are extracted from the gel, purified, reamplified, and cloned into plasmid vectors where they can be amplified further, manipulated, stored, and sequenced. Sequence analysis often identifies the differentially expressed genes, and differential expression should always be confirmed by quantitative RT-PCR or Northern-blot analysis.

two or more cell populations (115). RT-PCR/DD has been used successfully in the identification of differentially expressed genes in cancers and other diseases, in cells after treatment with specific growth factors, and in many other situations (116). The basic scheme of RT-PCR/DD is shown in Fig. 8. Briefly, high-quality cellular RNA is reverse-transcribed into complementary single-stranded DNA using an anchored oligo-dT primer. Subsequently, PCR is conducted on the DNA in the presence of a labeled nucleotide (^{35}S-dNTP or ^{32}P-dNTP) using an anchored oligo-dT primer in combination with an arbitrary decamer, thus amplifying the 3′-ends of mRNAs. The labeled cDNAs produced by PCR are displayed on a gel such as a DNA sequencing gel, with each set of primers producing between 100–200 bands that are usually between 100–500 base pairs in length. Bands of interest are eluted from the gel and reamplified, after which they can be cloned and sequenced or used as probes in Northern blot analyses or cDNA library screening.

Since the original description of RT-PCR/DD, several improvements have been made that have increased the efficacy of the technique. The anchored oligo-dT RT primer may be modi-

fied regarding the base composition of the anchor or the number of anchored bases, allowing subdivision of the pool of mRNAs into several groups, thereby simplifying the screening of an entire mRNA pool (117). Also, restriction sites may be incorporated into the 5′-ends of the PCR primers, thus facilitating manipulation of the amplified cDNAs during cloning (117). Lastly, the use of fluorescein as an alternative label for RT-PCR/DD yields fluorescent products that can be read on an automated DNA sequencer (118).

Although RT-PCR/DD is used widely for comparative analyses of gene expression, there are several caveats associated with the technique that should be considered before choosing the method. The major drawback to RT-PCR/DD is the large number of false-positives that may appear; on average, ~25–30% of bands are not differentially expressed when evaluated by Northern blot analysis or quantitative RT-PCR, which emphasizes the importance of confirming differential expression before proceeding with further analysis (119). False-positives are frequently due to the inherent randomness of the technique paired with the extreme sensitivity that accompanies the 35–40 cycles of PCR. The number of false-positives can be reduced by including 3–4 independent replicates of each sample and by employing a stringent band-selection strategy.

Another potential problem is that the 3´-untranslated region is preferentially amplified using RT-PCR/DD *(119)*. Thus, the sequence of a selected band may not match any known sequence in the database because the 3´-untranslated sequence of previously identified genes may not be included in the database. When a differentially expressed band does not match a sequence in the database, it may be identified by screening an appropriate cDNA library. However, library screening is a relatively inefficient means of identifying large numbers of differentially expressed genes.

Lastly, the selection of appropriate samples for RT-PCR/DD comparison is an important step in ensuring meaningful results. Two unrelated samples, such as a prostate cancer cell line and a patient prostate tumor sample, would be poor candidates for RT-PCR/DD due to the large number of genetic differences between individuals. Companion RT-PCR/DD samples should be related, for example, patient tumor tissue and surrounding normal tissue from the same patient, or a cell line +/- a growth factor. Comparisons between multiple individuals or between multiple cell lines derived from different species will likely produce too many differentially expressed bands to analyze.

A related method, RNA arbitrary primed PCR (RAP-PCR), has been established as an alternative strategy for differential analysis of gene expression among multiple samples (120). In RAP-PCR, an alternative primer is used for cDNA synthesis that does not rely on recognition of the poly-A tail of mRNA. The arbitrary primer used for reverse transcription, usually ~20 base pairs in length, amplifies palindromic sequences typically found in large mRNAs *(120)*. A set of arbitrary primers are then used to amplify regions of the cDNA, as in RT-PCR/DD. With RAP-PCR, there are fewer mRNA bands generated, and the sequences that are amplified are more likely to correspond to mRNA coding regions than those amplified by traditional RT-PCR *(116)*. In addition, a typical RAP-PCR consists of a few initial cycles of low stringency annealing followed by cycles of high-stringency annealing, which increases reproducibility of the bands amplified. The main drawback of RAP-PCR is that mRNAs are not preferentially selected in the RT step, so that rRNAs and tRNAs may be amplified when total RNA is used as starting material *(116)*.

COMPARATIVE GENOMIC HYBRIDIZATION The technique of CGH was developed by Kallioniemi et al. in 1992, and has gained popularity as a tool for the detection of losses and gains in DNA copy number in the entire genome *(121)*. Tumor DNA is labeled with a green fluorochrome, normal reference DNA is labeled with a red fluorochrome, and the two samples are hybridized simultaneously to normal metaphase cells affixed to a slide *(121)*. Using a sensitive camera equipped with fluorescence detection and a computerized analysis system, the green:red ratios can be established along the length of each chromosome. Amplifications in tumor DNA result in an increase in the green:red ratio, while losses of DNA will decrease the green:red ratio of a specific region. For an amplification to be detected by CGH, the amplified DNA must total at least 2 Mb in size (i.e. amplicon size × degree of amplification ≥ 2 Mb) *(122)*. CGH has been used successfully to document chromosomal gains and losses in astrocytic tumors, to show amplification of the androgen receptor gene in recurrent prostate cancer, and to identify a large number of amplified cellular oncogenes in human neoplasms *(123)*.

REFERENCES

1. Watson, J. D. and Crick, F. H. C. (1953) Molecular structure of nucleic acids. A structure for deoxyribose nucleic acid. *Nature* **171**:737, 738.
2. Schumm, D. E. (1997) *Core Concepts in Clinical Molecular Biology.* Lippincott-Raven, Philadelphia.
3. Schumm, D. E. (1995) *Essentials of Biochemistry,* 2nd ed. Little & Brown, Boston.
4. Thoma, F. and Koller, T. (1977) Influence of histone H1 on chromatin structure. *Cell* **12**:101–107.
5. Varshavsky, A. J., Bakayev, V. V., Nedospasov, S. A., and Georgiev, G. P. (1978) On the structure of eukaryotic, prokaryotic, and viral chromatin. *Cold Spring Harbor Symp. Quant. Biol.* **42**:457–473.
6. Lamond, A. I. and Earnshaw, W. C. (1998) Structure and function in the nucleus. *Science* **280**:547–553.
7. Long, E. O. and Dawid, I. B. (1980) Repeated genes in eucaryotes. *Annu. Rev. Biochem.*, **49**, 727–764.
8. Jordan, E. G. (1978) *The Nucleolus,* 2nd ed. Oxford University Press, Oxford.
9. Tyler-Smith, C. (1993) Mammalian chromosome structure. *Curr. Opin. Genet. Dev.* **3**:390–397.
10. Biessmann, H. and Mason, J. M. (1994) Telomeric repeat sequences. *Chromosoma* **103**:154–161.
11. Counter, C. M. (1996) The roles of telomeres and telomerase in cell life span. *Mutation Res.* **366**.
12. Hanke, J. H., Hambor, J. E., and Kavathas, P. (1995) Repetitive Alu elements form a cruciform structure that regulates the function of the human CD8 alpha cell-specific enhancer. *J. Mol. Biol.* **246**:63–73.
13. Arzimanoglou, I. I., Gilbert, F., and Barber, H. R. (1998) Microsatellite instability in human solid tumors. *Cancer* **82**:1808–1820.
14. Sutherland, G. R. (1995) Simple tandem DNA repeats and human genetic disease. *Proc. Natl. Acad. Sci. USA* **92**:3636–3641.
15. Craig, I. (1991) Methylation and the fragile X. *Nature* **349**:742–743.
16. (HDCRG) Huntington's Disease Collaborative Research Group (1993) A novel gene containing a trinucleotide repeat that is unstable on Huntington's disease chromosomes. *Cell* **72**:971–983.
17. Hoffmann-Berling, H. (1982) DNA unwinding enzymes. *Prog. Clin. Biol. Res.* **102**:89–98.
18. Kato, S. and Kikuchi, A. (1998) DNA topoisomerase: the key enzyme that regulated DNA super structure. *Nagoya J. Med. Sci.* **61**:11–26.
19. Heywood, L. A. and Burke, J. F. (1990) Mismatch repair in mammalian cells. *Bioessays* **12**:473–477.
20. Auerbach, A. D. and Verlander, P. C. (1997) Disorders of DNA replication and repair *Curr. Opin. Pediat.* **9**:600–616.
21. Nojima, H. (1997) Cell cycle checkpoints, chromosome stability and the progression of cancer. *Human Cell* **10**:221–230.
22. Fotedar, R. and Fotedar, A. (1995) Cell cycle control of DNA replication. *Prog. Cell Cycle Res.* **1**:73–89.
23. Green, R. and Noller, H. F. (1997) Ribosomes and translation. *Ann. Rev. Biochem.* **66**:679–716.
24. Persson, B.C. (1993) Modification of tRNA as a regulatory device. *Mol. Microbiol.* **8**:1011-1016.
25. Sharp, S. J., Schaack, J., Cooley, L., Burke, D. J., and Soll, D. (1985) Structure and transcription of eukaryotic tRNA genes. *Crit. Rev. Biochem.* **19**:107–144.
26. Goldberg, S., Schwartz, H., and Darnell, J. E. (1977) Evidence from UV transcription mapping in HeLa cells that heterogeneous nuclear

RNA is the messenger RNA precursor. *Proc. Natl. Acad. Sci. USA* **74**:4520–4523.

27. Sharp, P. A. (1988) RNA splicing and genes. *JAMA* **260**:3035–3041.
28. Lewin, B. (1994) Genome size and genetic content. *In: Genes V* (Lewin, B., ed.), Oxford University Press, New York, pp. 657–674.
29. Chou, K. C. and Kezdy, F. J. (1994) Kinetics of processive nucleic acid polymerases and nucleases. *Anal. Biochem.* **221**:217–230.
30. Kollmar, R. and Farnham, P. J. (1993) Site-specific initiation of transcription by RNA polymerase II. (Review). *Proc. Soc. Exp. Biol. Med.* **203**:127–139.
31. Tantravahi, J. and Alvira, M. (1993) Characterization of the mouse beta globin transcription termination region: a spacing sequence is required between the poly(A) signal sequence and multiple downstream termination elements. *Mol. Cell. Biol.* **13**:578–587.
32. Varani, G. (1997) A cap for all occasions. *Structure* **5**:855–858.
33. Munroe, D. and Jacobson, A. (1990) Tales of poly(A): A review. *Gene* **91**:151–158.
34. Gorlach, M., Burd, C. G., and Dreyfuss, G. (1994) The mRNA poly(A)-binding protein: localization, abundance, and RNA-binding specificity. *Exp. Cell Res.* **211**:400–407.
35. Balvay, L., Libri, D., and Fiszman, M. Y. (1993) Pre-mRNA secondary structure and the regulation of splicing. *Bioessays* **15**:165–169.
36. Staley, J. P. and Guthrie, C. (1998) Mechanical devices of the spliceosome: Motors, clocks, springs, and things. *Cell* **92**:315–326.
37. Edwalds-Gilbert, G., Veraldi, K. L., and Milcarek, C. (1997) Alternative poly(A) site selection in complex transcription units: means to an end? (Review). *Nucleic Acids Res.* **25**:2547–2561.
38. Morrissey, J. P. and Tollervey, D. (1995) Birth of the snRNPs: the evolution of RNase MRP and the eukaryotic pre-rRNA-processing system. *Trends Biochem. Sci.* **20**:78–82.
39. Cech, T. R. (1990) Self-splicing of group I introns. *Ann. Rev. Biochem.* **59**:543–568.
40. Jacquier, A. (1990) Self-splicing group II and nuclear pre-mRNA introns: how similar are they? *Trends Biochem. Sci.* **15**:351–354.
41. Suzuki, K. and Watanabe, M. (1994) Modulation of cell growth and mutation induction by introduction of the expression vector of human hsp70 gene. *Exp. Cell Res.* **215**:75–81.
42. Thomas, R. (1993) The denaturation of DNA. *Gene* **135**:77–79.
43. Sambrook, J., Fritsch, E. F., and Maniatis, T. (1989) *Molecular Cloning: A Laboratory Manual,* 2nd ed. Cold Spring Harbor Laboratory Press, Cold Spring Harbor, NY.
44. Presnell, S. C. (1997) Nucleic acid blotting techniques. *In: Molecular Diagnostics for the Clinical Laboratorian.* (Coleman, W. B. and Tsongalis, G. J., eds.), Humana Press, Totowa, NJ, pp. 63–88.
45. Boltz, E. M., Kefford, R. F., Leary, J. A., Houghton, C. E., and Friedlander, M. L. (1989) Amplification of c-ras-Ki oncogene in human ovarian tumours. *Int. J. Cancer* **43**:428–430.
46. Hynes, N. E. (1993) Amplification and overexpression of the erbB-2 gene in human tumors: its involvement in tumor development, significance as a prognostic factor, and potential as a target for cancer therapy. *Semin. Cancer Biol.* **4**:19–26.
47. Wang, S. J., Scavetta, R., Lenz, H. J., Danenberg, K., Danenberg, P. V., and Schonthal A. H. (1995) Gene amplification and multidrug resistance induced by the phosphatase-inhibitory tumor promoter, okadaic acid. *Carcinogenesis* **16**:637–641.
48. Saiki, R. K., Scharf, S., Faloona, F., Mullis, K., Horn, G., Erlich H., et al. (1985) Enzymatic amplification of beta-globin genomic sequences and restriction site analysis of sickle cell anemia. *Science* **230**:1350–1354.
49. Mullis, K. B. and Faloona, F. A. (1987) Specific synthesis of DNA in vitro via a polymerase-catalyzed chain reaction. *Methods Enzymol.* **155**:335–350.
50. Sorscher, D. H. (1997) DNA Amplification Techniques. *In: Molecular Diagnostics for the Clinical Laboratorian* (Coleman, W. B. and Tsongalis, G. J., eds), Humana Press, Totowa, NJ, pp. 89–101.
51. Wallace, R. B., Shaffer, J., Murphy, R. F., Bonner, J., Hirose, T., and Itakura, K. (1979) Hybridization of synthetic oligodeoxy-ribonucleotides to phi chi 174 DNA: the effect of single base pair mismatch. *Nucleic Acids Res.* **6**:3543–3557.
52. Lawyer, F. C., Stoffel, S., Saiki, R. K., Chang, S. Y., Landre, P. A., Abramson, R. D., et al. (1993) High-level expression, purification, and enzymatic characterization of full-length Thermus aquaticus DNA polymerase and a truncated form deficient in 5′ to 3′ exonuclease activity. *PCR Methods Appl.* **2**:275–287.
53. Lawyer, F. C., Stoffel, S., Saiki, R. K., Myambo, K., Drummond, R., and Gelfand, D. H. (1989) Isolation, characterization, and expression in Escherichia coli of the DNA polymerase gene from Thermus aquaticus. *J. Biol. Chem.* **264**:6427–6437.
54. Fanning, S. and Gibbs, R. A. (1997) PCR in Genome Analysis. *In: Genome Analysis. Volume 1: Analyzing DNA.* (Birren, B., Green, E. D., Klapholz, S., Myers, R. M., and Roskams, J., eds.) Cold Spring Harbor Laboratory Press, Plainview, NY, pp. 249–299.
55. Heid, C. A., Stevens, J., Livak, K. J., and Williams, P.M. (1996) Real time quantitative PCR. *Genome Res.* **6**:986–994.
56. Kaijalainen, S., Karhunen, P. J., Lalu, K., and Lindstrom, K. (1993) An alternative hot start technique for PCR in small volumes using beads of wax-embedded reaction components dried in trehalose. *Nucleic Acids Res.* **21**:2959–2960.
57. Bassam, B. J. and Caetano-Anolles, G. (1993) PCR using mineral oil and paraffin wax. *BioTechniques* **14**:30–34.
58. Roux, K. H. (1994) Using mismatched primer-template pairs in touchdown PCR. *BioTechniques* **16**:812–814.
59. Don, R. H., Cox, P. T., Wainwright, B. J., Baker, K., and Mattick, J. S. (1991) "Touchdown" PCR to circumvent spurious priming during gene amplification. *Nucleic Acids Res.* **19**:4008.
60. Foord, O. S. and Rose, E. A. (1994) Long-distance PCR. *Genome Res.* **3**:S149–61.
61. Barnes, W. M. (1994) PCR amplification of up to 35-kb DNA with high fidelity and high yield from lambda bacteriophage templates. *Proc. Natl. Acad. Sci. USA* **91**:2216–2220.
62. Ferre, F. (1992) Quantitative or semi-quantitative PCR: reality versus myth. *Genome Res.* **2**:1–9.
63. Raeymakers, L. (1996) A commentary on the practical applications of competitive PCR. *Genome Res.* **5**:91–94.
64. Lau, Y. F. and Kan, Y. W. (1983) Versatile cosmid vectors for the isolation, expression, and rescue of gene sequences: studies with the human alpha-globin gene cluster. *Proc. Natl. Acad. Sci. USA* **80**:5225–5229.
65. Lepourcelet, M., Andrieux, N., Giffon, T., Pichon, L., Hampe, A., Galibert, F., et al. (1996) Systematic sequencing of the human HLA-A/HLA-F region: establishment of a cosmid contig and identification of a new gene cluster within 37 kb of sequence. *Genomics* **37**:316–326.
66. Rowen, L., Kobori, J. A., and Scherer S. (1982) Cloning of bacterial DNA replication genes in bacteriophage lambda. *Mol. Gen. Genet.* **187**:501–509.
67. Young, R. A., Bloom, B. R., Grosskinsky, C. M., Ivanyi, J., Thomas, D., and Davis, R. W. (1985) Dissection of Mycobacterium tuberculosis antigens using recombinant DNA. *Proc. Natl. Acad. Sci.USA* **82**:2583–2589.
68. Grunstein, M. and Hogness, D. S. (1975) Colony hybridization: a method for the isolation of cloned DNAs that contain a specific gene. *Proc. Natl. Acad. Sci. USA* **72**:3961–3965.
69. Wang, S. Z. and Esen, A. (1985) Screening expression libraries with nonradioactive immunological probes. *Gene* **37**:267–269.
70. Szostak, J. W. and Blackburn, E. H. (1982) Cloning yeast telomeres on linear plasmid vectors. *Cell* **29**:245–255.
71. Burgers, P. M. and Percival, K. J. (1987) Transformation of yeast spheroplasts without cell fusion. *Anal. Biochem.* **163**:391–397.
72. Larin, Z., Monaco, A. P., and Lehrach, H. (1991) Yeast artificial chromosome libraries containing large inserts from mouse and human DNA. *Proc. Natl. Acad. Sci. USA* **88**:4123–4127.
73. Burke, D. T., Carle, G. F., and Olson, M. V. (1987) Cloning of large segments of exogenous DNA into yeast by means of artificial chromosome vectors. *Science* **236**:806–812.
74. Shizuya, H., Birren, B., Kim, U. J., Mancino, V., Slepak, T., Tachiiri, Y., et al. (1992) Cloning and stable maintenance of 300-

kilobase-pair fragments of human DNA in Escherichia coli using an F-factor-based vector. *Proc. Natl. Acad. Sci. USA* **89**:8794–9797.

75. Ioannou, P. A., Amemiya, C. T., Garnes, J., Kroisel, P. M., Shizuya, H., Chen, C., et al. (1994) A new bacteriophage P1-derived vector for the propagation of large human DNA fragments. *Nature Genet.* **6**:84–89.

76. Maxam, A. M. and Gilbert, W. (1977) A new method for sequencing DNA. *Proc. Natl. Acad. Sci. USA.* **74**:560–564.

77. Sanger, F., Nicklen, S., and Coulson, A. R. (1977) DNA sequencing with chain-terminating inhibitors. *Proc. Natl. Acad. Sci. USA* **74**:5463–5467.

78. Ju, J., Ruan, C., Fuller, C. W., Glazer, A. N., and Mathies, R. A. (1995) Fluorescence energy transfer dye-labeled primers for DNA sequencing and analysis. *Proc. Natl. Acad. Sci. USA* **92**:4347–4351.

79. Zimmerman, J. H., Voss, H., Schwager, C., Stegemann, J., and Ansorge, W. (1988) Automated Sanger dideoxy sequencing reaction protocol. *FEBS Lett.* **233**:432–436.

80. Mardis, E. R. and Roe, B. A. (1989) Automated methods for single-stranded DNA isolation and dideoxynucleotide DNA sequencing reactions on a robotic workstation. *BioTechniques* **7**:840–850.

81. Tabor, S. and Richardson, C. C. (1995) A single residue in DNA polymerases of the Escherichia coli DNA polymerase 1 family is critical for distinguishing between deoxy- and dideoxy-ribonucleotides. *Proc. Natl. Acad. Sci. USA* **92**:6339–6343.

82. Schwartz, D. C. and Cantor, C. R. (1984) Separation of yeast chromosome-sized DNAs by pulsed field gradient gel electrophoresis. *Cell* **37**:67–74.

83. Sader, H. S., Hollis, R. J., and Pfaller, M. A. (1995) The use of molecular techniques in the epidemiology and control of infectious diseases. *Clin. Lab. Med.* **15**:407–431.

84. Anand, R. (1986) Pulsed field gel electrophoresis: A technique for fractionating large DNA molecules. *Trends Genet.* **2**:278–286.

85. Turmel, C., Brassard, E., Slater, G.W., and Noolandi, J. (1990) Molecular detrapping and band narrowing with high frequency modulation of pulsed field electrophoresis. *Nucleic Acids Res.* **18**:569–575.

86. Carle, G. F., Frank, M., and Olson, M. V. (1986) Electrophoretic separation of large DNA molecules by periodic inversion of the electric field. *Science* **234**:1582–1585.

87. Pourzand, C. and Cerutti, P. (1993) Genotypic mutation analysis by RFLP/PCR. *Mutation Res.* **288**:113–121.

88. Newton, C. R., Graham, A., Heptinstall, L. E., Powell, S. J., Summers, C., Kalsheker, N., et al. (1989) Analysis of any point mutation in DNA. The amplification refractory mutation system (ARMS). *Nucleic Acids Res.* **17**:2503–2516.

89. Hayashi, K. (1992) PCR-SSCP: a method for detection of mutations. *Genet. Anal. Tech. Appl.* **9**:73–79.

90. Bhattacharyya, A. and Lilley, D. M. J. (1989) The contrasting structures of mismatched DNA sequences containing looped-out bases (bulges) and multiple mismatches (bubbles). *Nucleic Acids Res.* **17**:6821–6840.

91. Keen, J., Lester, D., Inglehearn, C., Curtis, A., and Bhattacharyya, S. (1991) Improved detection of heteroduplexes on Hydrolink gels. *Trends Genet.* **7**:5.

92. Molinari, R. J., Conners, M., and Shorr, R. G. (1993) Hydrolink gels for electrophoresis. *In: Advances in Electrophoresis,* Vol. 6 (Chrambach, A., Dunn, M. J. and Radola, B. J., eds.), VCH, New York, pp. 44–60.

93. Fodde, R. and Losekoot, M. (1994) Mutation detection by denaturing gradient gel electrophoresis (DGGE). *Human Mutation* **18**:83–94.

94. Myers, R. M., Maniatis, T., and Lerman, L. S. (1987) Detection and localization of single base changes by denaturing gradient gel electrophoresis. *Methods Enzymol.* **155**:501–510.

95. Riesner, D., Steger, G., Zimmat, R., Owens, R.A., Wagenhofer, M., Hillen, W., et al. (1989) Temperature-gradient gel electrophoresis of nucleic acids: Analysis of conformational transitions, sequence variations, and protein-nucleic acid interactions. *Electrophoresis* **10**:377–389.

96. Chomczynski, P. and Sacchi, N. (1987) Single-step method of RNA isolation by acid guanidinium thiocyanate-phenol-chloroform extraction. *Anal. Biochem.*, **162**, 156–159.

97. Kotewicz, M. L., D'Alessio, J. M., Driftmier, K. M., Blodgett, K. P., and Gerard, G. F. (1985) Cloning and overexpression of Maloney murine leukemia virus reverse transcriptase in Escherichia coli. *Gene* **35**:249–258.

98. Schraml, P., Shipman, R., Stulz, P., and Ludwig, C. U. (1993) cDNA subtraction library construction using a magnet-assisted subtraction technique (MAST). *Trends Genet.* **9**:70–71.

99. Larrick, J. W. and Siebert, P. D. (1995) Reverse Transcriptase PCR. *In: Ellis Horwood Series in Pharmaceutical Technology* (Rubinstein, M. H., ed.), Ellis Horwood Ltd., Hertfordshire, U.K.

100. Lai, C. J., Markoff, L. J., Zimmerman, S., Cohen, B., Berndt, J. A., and Chanock, R.M., R.M.C. (1980) Cloning DNA sequences from influenza viral RNA segments. *Proc. Natl. Acad. Sci. USA* **77**:210–214.

101. Kaguni, J. and Kaguni, L. S. (1992) Enzyme-labeled probes for nucleic acid hybridization. *Bioanal. Appl. Enzymes* **36**:115–127.

102. Studier, F. W., Rosenberg, A. H., Dunn, J. J., and Dubendorff, J. W. (1990) Use of T7 RNA polymerase to direct expression of cloned genes. *Methods Enzymol.* **185**:60–89.

103. Krieg, P. A. and Melton, D. A. (1987) In vitro RNA synthesis with SP6 RNA polymerase. *Methods Enzymol.* **155**:397–415.

104. Nakagami, S., Matsunaga, H., Oka, N., and Yamane, A. (1991) Preparation of enzyme-conjugated DNA probe and application to the universal probe system. *Anal. Biochem.* **198**:75–79.

105. Yamaguchi, K., Zhang, D., and Byrn R. (1994) A modified nonradioactive method for northern blot analysis. *Anal. Biochem.* **218**:343–346.

106. Isaac, P. G., Stacey, J., and Clee, C. M., C.M.C. (1995) Nonradioactive probes. *Mol. Biotechnol.* **3**:259-265.

107. Wooster, R., Neuhausen, S. L., Mangion, J., Quirk, Y., Ford, D., Collins, N., et al. (1994) Localization of a breast cancer susceptibility gene, BRCA2, to chromosome 13q12-13. *Science* **265**:2088–2090.

108. Bowcock, A. M. (1993) Molecular cloning of BRCA1: A gene for early onset familial breast and ovarian cancer. *Breast Cancer Res. Treat.* **28**:121–135.

109. Lynch, H. T. and Smyrk, T. (1996) Hereditary nonpolyposis colorectal cancer (Lynch syndrome): an updated review. *Cancer* **78**:1149–1167.

110. Ramsay, G. (1997) DNA chips: State-of-the art. *Nature Biotechnol.* **16**:40-44.

111. Shalon, D., Smith, J. S., and Brown, P. O. (1996) A DNA microarray system for analyzing complex DNA samples using two-color fluorescent probe hybridization. *Genome Res.* **6**:639–645.

112. Drmanac, S., Stavropoulos, N. A., Labat, I., Vonau, J., Hauser, B., Soares, M. B., et al. (1996) Gene-representing cDNA clusters defined by hybridization of 57,419 clones from infant brain libraries with short oligonucleotide probes. *Genomics* **37**, 29–40.

113. Hacia, G. H., Brody, L. C., Chee, M. S., Fodor, S. P. A., and Collins, F. S. (1996) Detection of heterozygous mutations in BRCA1 using high-density oligonucleotide arrays and two color fluorescence analysis. *Nature Genet.* **14**:441–447.

114. DeRisi, J. L., Iyer, V. R., and Brown, P. O. (1997) Exploring the metabolic and genetic control of gene expression on a genomic scale. *Science* **270**:680–686.

115. Liang, P. and Pardee, A. B. (1992) Differential display of eukaryotic messenger RNA by means of the polymerase chain reaction. *Science* **257**:967–971.

116. Liang, P. and Pardee, A. B. (1995) Recent advances in differential display. *Current Opin. Immunol.* **7**:274–280.

117. Liang, P., Zhu, W., Zhang, X., Guo, Z., O'Connell, R. P., and Averboukh, L. (1994) Differential display using one-base anchored oligo-dT primers. *Nucleic Acids Res.* **22**:5763–5764.

118. Ito, T., Kito, K., Adati, N., Mitsui, Y., Hagiwara, H., and Sakaki, Y. (1994) Fluorescent differential display: arbitrarily primed RT-PCR fingerprinting on an automated DNA sequencer. *FEBS Lett.* **351**:231–236.

119. Sunday, M. E. (1995) Differential Display RT-PCR for identifying gene expression in the lung. *Am. J. Phsiol.* **269**:L273–L284.

120. Welsh, J., Chada, K., Dalal, S. S., Chang, R., Ralph, D., and McClelland, M. M. (1992) Arbitrary primed PCR fingerprinting of RNA. *Nucleic Acids Res.* **20**:4965–4970.

121. Kallioniemi, A., Kallioniemi, O.-P., Sudar, D., Rutovitz, D., Gray, J.W., Waldman, F., et al. (1992) Comparative genomic hybridization for molecular cytogenetic analysis of solid tumors. *Science* **258**:818–821.

122. Kallioniemi, O.-P., Kallioniemi, A., Piper, J., Isola, J., Waldman, F. M., Gray, J. W., et al. (1994) Optimizing comparative genomic hybridization for analysis of DNA sequence copy number changes in solid tumors. *Genes Chromosomes Cancer* **10**:231–243.

123. Knuutila, S., Bjorkqvist, A.-M., Autio, K., Tarkkanen, M., Wolf, M., Monni, O., et al. (1998) DNA copy number amplifications in human neoplasms: review of comparative genomic hybridization studies. *Am. J. Pathol.* **152**:1107–1123.

MOLECULAR THEMES   III
IN ONCOGENESIS

3 Cancer Genes

JOHN J. REINARTZ, MD

INTRODUCTION

Although environmental factors certainly play a role, the dominant view regarding the molecular basis of human cancer currently rests on the concept that the accumulation of multiple mutations within genes of a single cell drive neoplastic transformation, ultimately leading to tumorigenesis. Mutations confer some form of selective advantage for cell growth to the affected cells, thereby contributing to the initiation of carcinogenesis and progression of human malignancies. Transforming mutations typically affect three major classes of genes: proto-oncogenes, tumor-suppressor genes, and DNA repair genes. The purpose of this chapter is to serve as an introduction to proto-oncogenes and tumor-suppressor genes, with the intent of providing both background information and a conceptual framework for the reader to gain a better general understanding of the types of genes involved in tumorigenesis, their mechanisms of activation or inactivation, and their normal cellular function(s).

The discovery of proto-oncogenes is one of the most fundamentally important discoveries of this century. Oncogenes are activated (frequently mutated) alleles of normally functioning wild-type genes (proto-oncogenes) that function in cell-cycle progression or cellular proliferation. Activated or mutated proto-oncogenes promote unregulated cell-cycle progression and cell proliferation, leading to cancer development. Proteins encoded by normal cellular proto-oncogenes function in all sub-cellular compartments including the nucleus, cytoplasm, and cell surface, and exert their function in most intracellular processes by acting as protein kinases, growth factors, growth-factor receptors, or membrane-associated signal transducers. Mutations in proto-oncogenes alter the normal structure and/or expression pattern, and the resulting oncogene acts in a dominant manner. That is, a mutation in only a single allele is re-

From: *The Molecular Basis of Human Cancer* (W. B. Coleman and G. J. Tsongalis, eds.), © Humana Press Inc., Totowa, NJ.

quired for activation of the proto-oncogene and loss of regulation of the proto-oncogene product. In genetic terms, this is typically referred to as a gain of function mutation.

While proto-oncogenes are normal cellular genes that act in a positive fashion to promote physiologic cell growth and differentiation, tumor-suppressor genes act as the cellular braking mechanism, regulating cell growth in a negative fashion. Normal tumor-suppressor proteins exhibit diverse functions and are found in all sub-cellular compartments. As alterations of tumor-suppressor protein function contribute to the development of cancer, their principle normal function is likely the control of cellular proliferation and differentiation. The specific types of mutations in these genes invariably lead to the inability of the encoded protein to perform its normal function. In general, neoplastic transformation requires loss of tumor-suppressor protein function, and this requires mutational inactivation or loss (deletion) of both alleles of the tumor-suppressor gene. Thus, tumor-suppressor genes are termed recessive and alterations of these genes are typically considered loss of function mutations.

VIRAL ONCOGENES AND CELLULAR PROTO-ONCOGENES

The discovery of proto-oncogenes is rooted in the study of mammalian viruses, and in particular, retroviruses. In the earlier years of the twentieth century, radiation, chemicals, and viruses were shown to induce cancer in experimental animals, and later, transform cells in culture. The study of so-called tumor viruses advanced quickly compared to studies of radiation-induced and chemical-induced carcinogenesis, for several reasons. Although both chemical carcinogens and radiation are potent inducers of neoplasia, it was found that tumor viruses could more efficiently and reproducibly transform cells in culture and induce tumors in experimental animals. Tumor viruses caused tumors to develop in a matter of days to weeks allowing rapid analysis following infection. Moreover, both radiation and chemical carcinogens act randomly on the cellular genome. Examining the cellular genome to determine the carcinogenic effect of these agents at a level of individual genes or DNA segments was a daunting task. In contrast to the mammalian cellular genome, the small genome of the tumor viruses offered a less complex model for identification of specific sequences responsible for induction and progression of tumors, and a more efficient system for elucidation of molecular mechanisms governing neoplastic transformation.

Six classes of DNA viruses and one class of RNA viruses (the retroviruses) have been shown to have oncogenic potential. The Shope papilloma virus was one of the first DNA tumor viruses to be described *(1)*. It causes benign papillomas that can progress to malignant carcinomas in cottontail rabbits. Papillomaviruses, along with other classes of DNA viruses such as the hepatitis B viruses (HBVs), have the ability to transform cells in their natural host. Most other DNA viruses, including adenoviruses, simian virus 40 (SV40), and polyomaviruses, lack transforming ability. In natural hosts, cells infected with these DNA viruses undergo cell death rather than transformation as a consequence of viral replication. However, these later viruses demonstrate their oncogenic potential in heterologous, nonpermissive species in which viruses cannot replicate. Each class of DNA virus has led to remarkable discoveries in proto-oncogenesis *(2)*.

The RNA retroviruses represent the class of tumor viruses that has contributed the most to our understanding of mammalian carcinogenesis. Retroviruses are the only currently known RNA viruses to have oncogenic potential. A feature common to these viruses is the ability to replicate in infected cells via a provirus intermediate. The proviral intermediate is generated through the action of a retroviral enzyme termed reverse transcriptase, which synthesizes a DNA copy of the retroviral RNA genome. RNA to DNA reverse transcription is obligatory for RNA retroviral replication in infected mammalian cells. The DNA transcript of the retroviral genome incorporates into the cellular genome where it replicates along with cellular DNA. The RNA polymerase enzyme of the host cells transcribes the provirus DNA, generating new RNA virions and retroviral mRNAs needed for synthesis of viral proteins. Importantly, unlike most of the DNA viruses, retroviruses are not cytotoxic or cytocidal to the host cells. This reflects the nature of the retroviral lifecycle, where new retroviral particles are released from the cell by budding rather than by cell lysis. Thus, RNA viruses can transform the same cells in which they replicate. The recombination event that occurs between the retroviral DNA (provirus) and host DNA as part of the replication cycle has significant implications for neoplastic transformation and tumor development *(3)*.

The first oncogenic retrovirus discovered was the Rous sarcoma virus (RSV). Peyton Rous inoculated chickens with a chicken sarcoma cellular extract and was able to demonstrate efficient transmission of an agent that propagated tumor growth *(4)*. Subsequent studies demonstrated that RSV had transforming properties in cultured cells. This was found to be in contrast to another well-studied retrovirus, the avian leukosis virus (ALV). ALV maintained the ability to induce tumors following innoculation in chickens (albeit after months, and not days to weeks compared to RSV), but did not demonstrate the ability to transform cells in culture *(4)*. The differences in induction efficiency in animals (in vivo activity) and ability to transform cells in culture (in vitro activity) form the basis for dividing retroviruses into two groups: 1) the acutely transforming oncogenic retroviruses, and 2) the weakly oncogenic or nontransforming retroviruses.

The differences between the acutely and weakly or nontransforming retroviruses are extremely important and provided clues towards recognition of the first proto-oncogene. In comparing RSV and ALV genomes, RSV was shown to be 1.5 kb greater in size than ALV. This additional segment was correctly postulated to be responsible for the rapid transforming properties of RSV. In 1971, Peter Vogt isolated RSV mutants that had the weakly oncogenic properties of ALV *(5)*. These weakly oncogenic RSV mutants were approximately the same size as ALV, did not have the ability to transform cultured cells, and did not efficiently induce sarcomas in animals, but maintained retroviral replication capabilities. The missing 1.5 kb sequence in these mutant RSV genomes was subsequently demonstrated to be required not only for initiation but also for maintenance of neoplastic transformation. Because different RSV mutants were not complimentary and did not lead to neoplastic transformation in cell culture, it was concluded that a single gene could be responsible for both in vitro transformation and *in vivo* oncogenesis. The first retroviral oncogene was named v-*src* for its sarcoma inducing action. Since then over 30 viral oncogenes have been discovered in over 40 transforming viruses *(2,5,6)*.

Similar to the discovery of the first oncogene, the discovery of the origin of retroviral oncogenes had monumental implications. The extra 1.5 kb of nucleic acid in RSV was not necessary for viral replication/growth. It was not clear where the apparently extraneous nucleic acid segment originated. The answer was obtained through the study of retroviruses from tumors of the very rare animal that developed tumors after being infected by a nontransforming retroviruses. These previously nontransforming retroviruses were found to have incorporated new genetic material in their RNA genome corresponding to a new oncogene that conferred capability for neoplastic transformation. The portion of the proviral genome corresponding to the newly recognized oncogene was used to probe for similar sequences in host cells. This analysis demonstrated that genes possessing the capability for neoplastic transformation were conserved among several different species. This observation suggested that host-cell DNA could be incorporated into the genome of a retrovirus during recombination in the infected cell. Further study of the cellular homologs of retroviral oncogenes showed that they are normal cellular genes that encode proteins involved in various aspects of cellular homeostasis, including cell proliferation and differentiation. The normal cellular counterpart of the retroviral oncogenes are referred to as cellular proto-oncogenes. The current paradigm holds that viral oncogenes originate from cellular proto-oncogenes, and that these genes have been altered in a manner that confers the ability to induce cellular neoplastic transformation in infected cells *(2,6)*. In like manner, cellular proto-oncogenes can be activated in various ways (point mutation, deletion, amplification, or rearrangement) that result in the synthesis of an oncogenic protein product *(2,6)*.

Table 1
Chromosomal Translocation Breakpoints and Genes[a]

Type	Affected gene	Disease	Rearranging gene
Nonfusions/hematopoietic tumors			
Basic-helix-loop-helix			
t(8;14)(q24;q32)	c-*myc* (8q24)	BL, BL-ALL	IgH, IgL
t(2;8)(p12;q24)			
t(8;22)(q24;q11)			
t(8;14)(q24;q11)	c-*myc* (8q24)	T-ALL	TCR-α
t(8;12)(q24;q22)	c-*myc* (8q24)	B-CLL/ALL	
	BTG (12q22)		
t(7;19)(q35;p13)	*lyl1* (19p13)	T-ALL	TCR-β
t(1;14)(p32;q11)	*tal1*/SCL	T-ALL	TCR-α
t(7;9)(q35;q34)	*tal2* (9q34)		
LIM proteins			
t(11;14)(p15;q11)	RBTN1/Ttg1 (11p15)	T-ALL	TCR-δ
t(11;14)(p13;q11)	RBTN2/Ttg2 (11p13)	T-ALL	TCR-δ/α/β
t(7;11)(q35;p13)			
Homeobox protein			
t(10;14)(q24;q11)	*hox11* (10q24)	T-ALL	TCR-a/β
t(7;10)(q35;q24)			
Zinc-finger protein			
t(3;14)(q27;q32)	*Laz3*/*bcl6* (3q27)	NHL/DLCL	IgH
t(3;4)(q27;p11)	*Laz3*/*bcl6* (3q27)	NHL	
Others			
t(11;14)(q13;q32)	*bcl1* (*PRAD-1*) (11q13)	B-CLL and others	IgH, IgL
t(14;18)(q32;21)	*bcl2* (18q21)	FL	TCR-Cα
inv14 & t(14;14)(q11;32)	*TCL-1* (14q32.1)	T-CLL	IgH
t(10;14)(q24;q32)	*lyt-10* (10q24)	B lymphoma	IgH
t(14;19)(q32;q13.1)	*bcl3* (19q13.1)	B-CLL	IgH
t(5;14)(q31;q32)	IL3 (5q31)	Pre-B-ALL	TCRβ
t(7;9)(q34;q34.3)	*tan1* (9q34.3)	T-ALL	TCRα
t(1;7)(p34;q34)	*lck* (1p34)	T-ALL	TCRα
t(X;14)(q28;11)	*C6.1B* (Xq28)	T-PLL	

Type	Affected gene	Protein domain	Fusion protein	Disease
Gene Fusions/Hematopoietic Tumors				
inv 14(q11;q32)	*TCR*-α (14q11)	TCR-Cα	VH-TCR-Cα	T/B-cell lymphoma
	VH (14q32)	Ig VH		
t(9;22)(q34;q11)	*CABL* (9q34)	tyrosine kinase	Serine + tyrosine kinase	CML/ALL
	bcr (22q11)	serine kinase		
t(1;19)(q23;p13.3)	*PBX1* (1q23)	HD	AD + HD	Pre-B-ALL
	E2A (19p13.3)	AD-bHLH		
t(17;19)(q22;p13)	*HLF* (17q22)	bZIP	AD + bZIP	Pro-B-ALL
	E2A (19p13)	AD-b-HLH		
t(15;17)(q21-q11-22)	*PML* (15q21)	Zinc finger	Zn-finger + RAR DNA	APL
	*RAR*α (17q21)	Retinoic acid receptor-α	and ligand binding	
t(11;17)(q23;q21.1)	*PLZF* (11q23)	Zinc-finger	Zn-finger + RAR DNA	APL
	*RAR*α (17q21)	Retinoic acid receptor-α	and ligand binding	
t(4;11)(q21;q23)	*mll* (11q23)	A-T hook/Zn-finger	A-T hook + Ser-pro	ALL/PreB-ALL/ ANLL
	AF4 (4q21)	Ser-Pro rich		
t(9;11)(q21;q23)	*AF9*/*MLLT3* (9p22)	(Ser-Pro rich)	A-T hook + (Ser-pro)	ALL/PreB-ALL/ ANLL
	mll (11q23)	A-T hook/Zn-finger		
t(11;19)(q23;p13)	*mll* (11q23)	A-T hook/Zn-finger	A-T hook + Ser-pro	Pre-B-ALL/ T-ALL/ANLL
	ENL (19p13)	Ser-Pro rich		
t(X;11)(q13;q23)	*AFX1* (Xq13)	(Ser-Pro rich)	A-T hook + (Ser-pro)	T-ALL
	mll (11q23)	A-T hook/Zn-finger		
t(1;11)(p32;q23)	*AF1P* (1p32)	Eps-15 homolog	A-T hook + ?	ALL
	mll (11q23)	A-T hook/Zn-finger		

Table 1 (Cont)

Type	Affected gene	Protein domain	Fusion protein	Disease
t(6;11)(q27;q23)	AF6 (6q27)	myosin homolog	A-T hook + ?	ALL
	mll (11q23)	A-T hook/Zn-finger		
t(11;17)(q23;q21)	mll (11q23)	A-T hook/Zn-finger	A-T hook + leucine zipper	AML
	AF17 (17q21)	Cys-rich/leucine zipper		
t(8;21)(q22;q22)	eto/MTG8 (8q22)	Zn-finger	DNA binding +	AML
	aml1/CBFα (21q22)	DNA binding Zn-fingers runt homology		
t(3;21)(q26;q22)	evi-1 (3q26)	Zn-finger	DNA binding +	CML
	aml1 (21q22)	DNA binding	Zn-fingers	
t(3;21)(q26;q22)	EAP (3q26)	Sn Protein	DNA binding +	Myelodysplasia
	aml1 (21q22)	DNA binding	out-of-frame EAP	
t(16;21)(p11;q22)	FUS (16p11)	Gln-Ser-Tyr/Gly-rich/ RNA binding	Gln-Ser-Tyr + DNA binding	Myeloid
	erg (21q22)	Ets-like DNA binding		
t(6;9)(p23;q34)	dek (6p23)	?	? + ZIP	AML
	can (9q34)	ZIP		
9;9?	set (9q34)	?	? + ZIP	AUL
	can (9q34)	ZIP		
t(4;16)(q26;p13)	IL2 (4q26)	IL2	IL2/TM	T-lymphoma
	BMC (16p13.1)	?/TM domain		
inv(2;2)(p13;p11.2-p14)	rel (2p13)	DNA binding-activator	DNA binding + ?	NHL
	NRG (2p11.2-p12)	?		
inv(16)(p13;q22)	myosin MYH11 (16p13)		DNA binding?	AML
	CBFβ (16q22)			
t(5;12)(q33;p13)	PDGFb (5q33)	Receptor kinase	Kinase + DNA binding	CMML
	TEL (12p13)	ets-like DNA binding		
t(2;5)(p23;q35)	NPM (5q35)	Nucleolar phosphoprotein	N-terminus NPM + kinase	NHL
	ALK (2p23)	Tyrosine kinase		
Gene fusions/solid tumors				
inv10(q11.2;q21)	ret (10q11.2)	tyrosine kinase	Unk + tyrosine kinase	Papillary thyroid carcinoma
	D10S170 (q21)	uncharacterized		
t(11;22)(q24;q12)	fli1 (11q24)	Ets-like DNA binding	Gin-Ser-Tyr + DNA binding	Ewing's sarcoma
	ews (22q12)	Gin-Ser-Tyr/Gly-rich/RNA		
t(21;22)(?;q12)	erg (21q22)	Ets-like DNA binding	Gin-Ser-Tyr + DNA binding	Ewing's sarcoma
	ews (22q12)	Gin-Ser-Tyr/Gly-rich/RNA binding		
t(12;22)(q13;q12)	AFT1 (12q13)	bZIP	Gin-Ser-Try-bZIP	Melanoma
	ews (22q12)	Gin-Ser-Tyr/Gly-rich/RNA binding		
t(12;16)(q13;p11)	CHOP (12q13)	(DNA binding?)/ZIP	Gin-Ser-Tyr	Liposarcoma
	FUS (16p11)	Gin-Ser-Tyr/Gly-rich/RNA binding		
t(2;13)(q35;q14)	PAX3 (2q35)	Paired box/homeodomain	+ (DNA binding?)/ZIP -sarcoma	Rhabdomyo
FKHR (13q14)	Forkhead domain			
t(X;18)(p11.2;q11.2)	SYT (18q11.2)	None identified	PB/HD + DNA binding	Synovial sarcoma
	SSX (Xp11.2)	None identified		

[a]Adapted from T. H. Rabbitts (94).

The discovery of the ability of genes to induce tumors in animals and humans linked the study of transforming retroviruses with the field of molecular biology of human cancers. However, it is clear that most human cancers are not caused by infection with transforming viruses. Shortly after it was established that specific virus-associated genes could cause cellular transformation, alterations in cellular proto-oncogenes were found to be responsible for human tumors. The first instance linking the possibility of a human proto-oncogene with cancer, when retroviral involvement could be eliminated, was reported in 1981 by two groups, who showed that DNA extracted from a human bladder-carcinoma cell line (EJ) could induce transformation in an immortalized but nontransformed mouse cell line NIH 3T3 (7,8). In 1982 the first human activated proto-oncogenes were isolated and identified from the EJ bladder carcinoma cell line and a human lung carcinoma. These genes were cellular homologs of the Harvey-ras and Kirsten-ras retroviral oncogenes, both of which had previously been shown to induce rat sarcomas (9). The discovery of proto-oncogenes solidified the link between genes and cancer, and

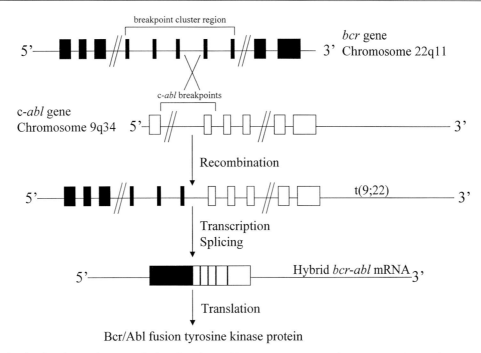

Fig. 1. bcr-abl translocation in chronic myelogenous leukemia. The c-*abl* proto-oncogene on chromosome 9 is translocated to the breakpoint cluster region (*bcr*) of chromosome 22. The result is a novel tyrosine kinase which functions independently of normal regulatory elements.

ushered in an era of genetic discovery focused on identification of genetic abnormalities that contribute to the development of human neoplasms.

MECHANISMS OF ACTIVATION OF CELLULAR PROTO-ONCOGENES

Cellular proto-oncogenes must become activated in order to express oncogenic potential leading to neoplastic transformation. Activation of cellular proto-oncogenes typically involves chromosomal translocation, amplification, or point mutation. The changes that result can be broadly categorized into: 1) changes to the structure of a proto-oncogene, which result in an abnormal gene product with aberrant function (examples include the *bcr-abl* translocation and c-*ras* point mutations, described below); and 2) changes to the regulation of gene expression, which result in aberrant expression or inappropriate production of the structurally normal growth-promoting protein (examples include translocations involving c-*myc*, amplification involving N-*myc* in neuroblastomas, and some point mutations in c-*ras*).

PROTO-ONCOGENE ACTIVATION THROUGH CHROMOSOMAL TRANSLOCATION

Translocation Leading to Structural Alteration of bcr-abl Evolving techniques in cytogenetics over the last century have led to increased resolution of individual chromosomes. Abnormalities in chromosomes were known to occur in neoplastic cells from at least 1914, when Boveri noted somatic alterations in the genetic material of sea-urchin eggs fertilized by two sperm. The abnormal cells looked similar to tumors, and he hypothesized that cancer might result from cellular aberrations that produced abnormal mitotic figures *(10)*. However, it was not clear whether chromosomal abnormalities represented primary oncogenic events, or accumulated errors secondary to

neoplastic transformation. Initially, the plethora of chromosomal abnormalities favored the latter scenario, as no consistent chromosomal abnormality was identified upon examination of many tumors and similar tumors from different individuals. That changed in 1960 when Nowell and Hungerford described the first reproducible tumor-specific chromosomal aberration in chronic myelogenous leukemia *(11)*. They observed the presence of a shortened chromosome 22, subsequently named the Philadelphia chromosome after the city in which it was discovered. It was found in cancer cells from over 90% of patients with chronic myelogenous leukemia (CML). This observation suggested that: 1) the abnormality may have imparted some form of growth advantage over other cells and may be causally related to the development of tumors, and 2) other neoplasms may also harbor their own specific chromosomal or genetic aberrations. Since the first recognition of common chromosomal abnormalities in specific human tumors, numerous translocations involving important genes have been characterized (Table 1).

Consequent to rapid advances in cytogenetic resolution techniques, Rowley in 1973 *(12)* found that the Philadelphia chromosome actually resulted from a reciprocal translocation involving the long arms of chromosomes 9 (9q34) and 22 (22q11). Analysis of the affected region on chromosome 9 revealed a proto-oncogene, c-*abl (13)*, which when translocated to chromosome 22 generates a fusion gene. The c-*abl* proto-oncogene has 11 exons that encode for a 145 kDa protein with tyrosine kinase activity. The chromosomal breakpoint within the c-*abl* gene consistently involves one of two alternatively spliced exons. Breakpoints along the functional gene on chromosome 22 are clustered near the center in a 6 kb region termed the breakpoint cluster region (*bcr*). Upon translocation, nearly the entire c-*abl* proto-oncogene is placed under *bcr* promoter

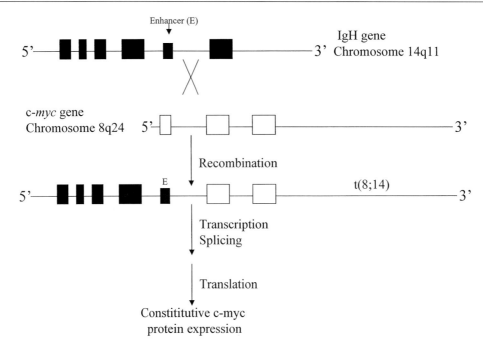

Fig. 2. The t(8;14) translocation. The c-*myc* gene of chromosome 8 is normally not expressed in differentiated B cells. After translocation, it comes under the control of either a cryptic promoter in intron 1 or an enhancer from the immunoglobulin locus of chromosome 14, leading to constitutive expression of the normal c-myc protein (exon 1 is noncoding).

activity. Transcription and splicing yield a long mRNA transcript that encodes a chimeric 210 kDa protein that expresses increased tyrosine kinase activity, likely because it is less responsive to normal regulatory elements (Fig. 1). A similar translocation exists in some acute lymphoblastic leukemias, although the breakpoint occurs further upstream in the *bcr* gene, which results in a smaller chimeric protein (190 kDa), which has also been shown to have increased tyrosine kinase activity *(14–18)*.

Translocation Leading to Dysregulation of c-myc Investigation into the role of the c-*myc* proto-oncogene in neoplastic transformation led to development of a model of proto-oncogene activation based on insertional mutagenesis. This mechanism of proto-oncogene activation emerged from studies of acutely transforming retroviruses and weakly oncogenic or nontransforming retroviruses. The primary differences between these two classes of retrovirus reflect the amount of time necessary for induction of tumors after infection of cells and the genomic content of their proviral DNA. Acutely transforming retroviruses have oncogenes incorporated into their genome whereas nontransforming retroviruses do not. Thus, the transformation potential of weakly oncogenic and nontransforming retroviruses depend on insertion adjacent to a cellular proto-oncogene. Although retroviruses insert randomly, in independently derived tumors retroviral sequences were found incorporated into similar chromosomal locations in the host genomic DNA. The site of insertion then became the focus of attention, and cellular homologs of known retroviral oncogenes and their surrounding sequences were studied intensely. Finally, Hayward and Astrin demonstrated that nonacutely transforming retroviruses insert adjacent to and cause activation of the cellular proto-oncogene c-*myc (2,19).*

Insertional mutagenesis is based on the ability of proviral DNA to insert into host genomic DNA and cause either activation or inactivation of host genes, independent of expression of retroviral genes (as in the case of acutely transforming viruses). In the case of insertional activation of cellular genes, the proviral DNA may provide a promoter or enhancer for the cellular gene, resulting in an alteration in the normal regulation and expression pattern of the affected gene.

In the early 1980s data on c-*myc* activation by nonacutely transforming retroviruses in chicken lymphomas merged with data accumulating on translocations in Burkitt's lymphoma (BL), a high-grade B-lymphocyte neoplasm. It was reasoned that if proviral sequences were capable of altering host cellular gene expression to cause tumors, chromosomal alterations that juxtapose promoter or enhancing sequences and cellular proto-oncogenes (through chromosomal translocation) were likely to promote neoplastic transformation. The best studied translocations at the time involved those of BL, in which a portion of the long arm of chromosome 8 is consistently translocated to either chromosome 14, 2, or 22, adjacent to the loci for immunoglobulin heavy chain, κ light chain, and λ light chain, respectively. The immunoglobulin loci on chromosomes 14, 2, and 22 were postulated to be good partner candidates to be coupled with and cause activation of a proto-oncogene that was suspected to reside on chromosome 8. Tumor DNA was directly probed for c-*myc* sequences. The gene was detected on chromosome 8, and found to be translocated to chromosomes 14, 2, and 22 in Burkitt's lymphoma and in some plasmacytomas. In plasmacytomas, a form of the c-*myc* proto-oncogene lacking the untranslated exon 1 is involved in the chromosomal translocation (Fig. 2). The breakpoints within the c-*myc* gene are more varied in BL. Nonetheless, the translocation results in abnor-

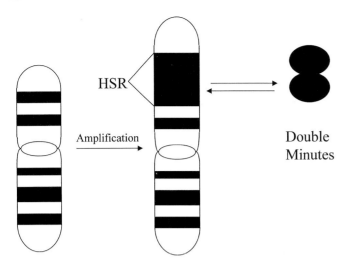

Fig. 3. DNA amplification. When DNA is amplified by repeated DNA replication events, the results can sometimes be seen cytogenetically as homogeneously staining regions (HSRs) or double minutes (DMs). DMs represent the extrachromosomal manifestation of HSRs. DMs can insert into a chromosome other than that from which they are derived.

Table 2
Oncogene Amplification in Human Tumors

Oncogene	Neoplasm
c-*myc* Family	
c-*myc*	Leukemias, breast, stomach, lung, and colon carcinomas, neuroblastomas and glioblastomas
N-*myc*	Neuroblastomas, rhabomyosarcomas, retinoblastomas, lung carcinomas
L-*myc*	Lung carcinomas
c-*erb*B Family	
c-*erb*B1	Glioblastomas, medulloblastomas, renal cell, squamous cell, breast, gastric, and esophageal carcinomas
c-*erb*B2	Breast, salivary gland, gastric esophageal, lung, colon, and ovarian carcinomas
c-*ras* Family	
c-H-*ras*	Bladder carcinoma
c-K-*ras*	Breast, lung, and head and neck carcinomas
Other Proto-oncogenes	
*int*2	Breast and squamous-cell carcinomas
hst	Breast and squamous-cell carcinomas
PRAD-1	Breast and squamous-cell carcinomas
c-*abl*	K562 chronic myelogenous leukemia cell line
c-*myb*	Colon and breast carcinomas, leukemias
*ets*1	Lymphoma, breast cancers
gli	Glioblastomas
K-*sam*	Stomach carcinomas
*mdm*2	Sarcomas
11q13 locus	Breast, gastric, esophageal, squamous, ovarian, bladder carcinomas, and melanoma

mal (constitutive) expression of a c-*myc* coding sequence identical to its normal allele in both types of tumor. This observation strongly suggested the chromosome translocation-mediated activation of the c-*myc* proto-oncogene as a causal event in human tumorigenesis *(2,20–23)*.

Proto-oncogene Activation Through Gene Amplification Activation of cellular proto-oncogenes can occur as a consequence of DNA amplification, resulting in overexpression of the amplified proto-oncogene, which confers a proliferative advantage to affected cells. Amplified gene segments can be discerned cytogenetically as double-minute chromosomes (DMs) and homogeneously staining regions (HSRs). Proto-oncogenes (and other genetic loci) are amplified by repeated DNA replication events that can result in an abnormal homogeneous staining pattern in a karyotypic analysis of affected cells; for example, rather than the familiar chromosomal staining pattern in R-banded or G-banded chromosome spreads. Instead, HSRs appear as abnormally extended R-bands or G-bands (Fig. 3). The tandem arrays of amplified DNA forming HSRs may be excised from the chromosome to form double minutes, which are small chromosomal structures lacking centromeres that do not replicate during cell division. DMs may integrate into other chromosomes to create additional stable HSRs able to propagate upon cell division *(24,25)*.

In the same way that investigation of the c-*myc* proto-oncogene formed the underpinnings of our current understanding of proto-oncogene activation by means of chromosomal translocation, studies of the c-*myc* proto-oncogene led to the unraveling of proto-oncogene activation through gene amplification in human neoplasms *(26)*. DNA amplification represents one mechanism leading to drug resistance in mammalian cells *(27)*. Through direct probing for c-*myc* it was discovered that DMs and HSRs contained amplified copies of the oncogene in human colon carcinoma cells *(28)*. The c-*myc* gene has been shown to be amplified and overexpressed in a number of human

neoplasms supporting the role of DNA amplification as a major mechanism for cellular proto-oncogene activation in neoplastic transformation.

Although the precise mechanism for gene amplification has not been entirely determined, the role amplification plays in cellular transformation in human malignancies is clear, particularly from studies of neuroblastomas and studies involving neoplastic transformation of cells in vitro *(29)*. Neuroblastoma is one of the most common childhood extracranial solid tumors accounting for approx 15% of all childhood cancer deaths *(30)*. Neuroblastomas exhibit DMs and HSRs that hybridize with probes to the c-*myc* gene. The hybridizing sequences were determined to be related to but distinct from c-*myc* and was designated N-*myc* *(31)*. The N-*myc* gene is transcribed at higher levels in neuroblastomas that demonstrate gene amplification. N-*myc* amplification is now a major prognostic determinant in neuroblastomas, with high levels of transcription from either a single copy or more commonly from increased gene copy number in the form of DMs or HSRs correlating with poor patient survival *(32)*. The demonstration of the link between high N-*myc* expression and poor clinical prognosis, and its demonstrated ability to cause neoplastic transformation in cell culture, provides strong evidence for the importance of gene amplification in the activation of cellular proto-oncogenes. Table 2 lists other cellular proto-oncogenes that have been shown to be amplified in human neoplasms.

Proto-oncogene Activation Through Point Mutation Several cellular proto-oncogenes have been shown to be activated through point mutation. However, the c-*ras* family of proto-oncogenes represent the most important subset of proto-oncogenes that are activated through this mechanism. The c-*ras* genes were the first human proto-oncogenes identified using gene-transfer assays *(7,8)*. This family includes the cellular homologs of the Harvey-*ras* (H-*ras*) and Kirsten-*ras* (K-*ras*) retroviral oncogenes, both of which had previously been shown to induce sarcomas in rats *(9)*. DNA extracted from various human tumor cell lines have been shown to induce transformation of mouse fibroblast cell lines in vitro, and the most commonly isolated sequences responsible for neoplastic transformation are members of the c-*ras* family of proto-oncogenes *(33,34)*. The activated form of c-*ras* (oncogenic) exhibits markedly different transforming properties from that of the normal c-*ras* proto-oncogene. The activated form consistently and efficiently induces neoplastic transformation in cultured cells, whereas the normal proto-oncogene does not. The critical molecular difference between the two forms of c-*ras* was found in the nucleic acid sequence: the activated form of c-*ras* harbors a point mutation in codon 12 of exon 1, which results in a glycine to valine amino acid substitution *(35–37)*. Up to 30% of all human neoplasms are now known to harbor c-*ras* mutations, and mutations in c-H-*ras*, c-K-*ras*, and N-*ras* reflect specific alterations affecting only codon 12 (most mutations), codon 13, or codon 61. An additional mutation in an intron of c-H-*ras* has been shown to upregulate production of the structurally normal gene product, resulting in increased transforming activity *(38)*. A common theme of c-*ras* mutations is that a single point mutation is capable of drastically altering the biological activity of a normal protein product into one with efficient transforming properties. Mutations of c-*ras* are found in a large number of human tumor types, including thyroid *(39–41)*, gastrointestinal tract *(42–46)*, uterus *(47–51)*, lung *(52–56)*, myelodysplastic syndromes *(57)*, and leukemias *(58–61)*. The incidence of c-K-*ras* gene mutations is highest for exocrine pancreas and bile-duct carcinomas, which has lead to the development of ancillary diagnostic techniques for the detection of pancreatic and bile-duct carcinomas *(62–64)*.

ONCOGENE MECHANISM OF ACTION: PROTEIN PRODUCTS OF ONCOGENES

Proto-oncogene protein products regulate cell proliferation and differentiation. Oncogene protein products often closely resemble their proto-oncogene protein products, but differ in that they act independently of normal regulatory elements. Events that occur as a part of normal cell growth and differentiation can be simplified into a series of four steps, all of which involve proto-oncogenes normally, and each of which is subject to disruption during neoplastic transformation: 1) an extracellular growth factor binds to a specific receptor on the plasma membrane; 2) the growth factor receptor is transiently activated, leading to a cascade of signaling cellular events, many of which involve signal-transducing proteins on the plasma

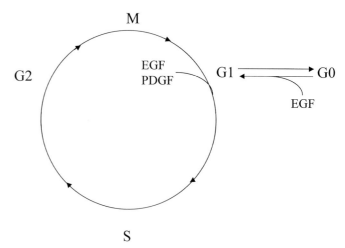

Fig. 4. Epidermal growth factor (EGF) and platelet-derived growth factor (PDGF) interactions with the cell cycle.

membrane; 3) the signal/message is transmitted from the plasma membrane to the nucleus via secondary messenger molecules; and 4) the nuclear regulatory machinery is induced/activated to initiate cell replication and transcription. Within these pathways, there are three major biochemical mechanisms through which these oncoproteins function *(65,66)*. The first of these mechanisms involves the phosphorylation of target proteins at serine, tyrosine, and threonine amino acid residues. The second mechanism involves intracellular signal transmission through proteins with GTPase activity. The last of these involves the transcriptional regulation of structural genes in the nucleus.

THE FIBROBLAST GROWTH-FACTOR FAMILY The discovery of growth factors in the early 1960s led to the isolation of a diverse group of factors affecting all cells. Growth factors are grouped into families that share significant sequence homology and cell-surface receptors. One example is the epidermal growth factor (EGF) family, which includes, among others, EGF and the transforming growth factor alpha TGF-α *(67,68)*. EGF, one of the earlier growth factors discovered, was shown to be a polypeptide of 53 amino acids that stimulated proliferation of a variety of different cell types. Growth factors were not only capable of promoting growth, but some also concurrently promoted differentiation *(69)*. In normal cells, growth factors induce cells to exit the resting or G_0 phase and enter the cell cycle, or they may stimulate cells already cycling (Fig. 4). It follows that the biochemical and physiologic effect of aberrant expression of growth factors leads to constitutive stimulation of cell growth, potentiating the process of cell transformation.

Platelet-derived growth factor (PDGF) is another growth factor shown to have transforming potential, and has an important history in that it provided the first link between two originally disparate tracks of research: biochemical studies of the regulation of cell proliferation (growth factors), and molecular analysis of neoplastic transformation (oncogenes) *(70)*. In the early 1980s, two groups working independently reported PDGF was the protein product of an oncogene *(2,71,72)*. Each group determined a partial amino acid-sequence of PDGF, and with a computer search of a protein sequence data base, amino acid

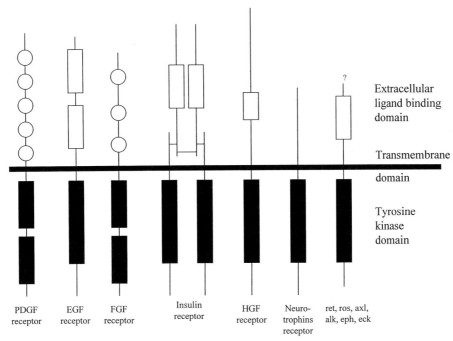

Fig. 5. Transmembrane tyrosine kinases. Growth-factor receptors with tyrosine kinase activity share similar overall structure with extracellular binding domains, transmembrane domains, and cytoplasmic tyrosine kinase domains. Each receptor is designated according to its prototype ligand. Open circles illustrate immunoglobulin-like repeats. Open boxes denote cytosine-rich domains. Black boxes represent conserved tyrosine kinase domains. Adapted from Aaronson *(67)*.

sequence homology was demonstrated with the predicted sequence of v-*sis*, the simian sarcoma virus. From this initial work, oncogenes activated by mechanisms described previously frequently have been shown to encode growth factors that participate in mitogenic signaling and cell transformation *(67)*.

Further understanding the mechanism of action of transforming growth factors came from a hypothesis forwarded in 1977 by George Todaro *(73)*. He suggested that because transformed cells are capable of producing growth factors, autocrine stimulation of cell growth could be, at least in part, responsible for transformation *(73)*. An individual cell abnormally overexpressing a growth factor to which it responds would result in continuous cell proliferation. This hypothesis gained credence with the discovery of the homology between PDGF and the protein product of v-*sis* as well as from work on the EGF family of growth factors (EGF and TGF-α, among others). Several human tumors are known to overexpress TGF-a as well as its receptor, the epidermal growth-factor receptor (EGFR), which substantiated the autocrine mechanism *(74,75)*. The transfection of TGF-α genes into cultured cells could induce transformation *(76,77)*. Finally, the link between mitogenic signaling and cell-transformation properties of growth factors and oncogenes was strengthened by data showing TGF-a overexpression in transgenic mice results in the development of tumors *(2,78,79)*. Additional growth factors with oncogenic potential are listed in Table 3.

THE EGFR FAMILY OF GROWTH-FACTOR RECEPTORS   The EGFR family is one of many growth-factor families capable of promoting neoplastic transformation. The EGFR family includes c-*erb*B1, c-*erb*B2 (also known as *neu*), and c-*erb*B3, and are structurally related to other transmembrane

Table 3
Growth Factors with Oncogenic Potential[a]

PDGF family
 A chain
 B chain (c-*sis*)
FGF family
 acidic FGF (aFGF)
 basic FGF (bFGF)
 Int-2
 hst (KS3)
 Fgf-5
EGF family
 EGF
 TGF-α
Wnt family
 Wnt-1
 Wnt-3
Neurotrophins
 NGF
 BDNF
 NT-3
Hematopoietic growth factors
 Interleukin-2
 Interleukin-3
 M-CSF
 GM-CSF

[a]Adapted from G. M. Cooper *(2)*.

tyrosine kinase proteins with an external ligand-binding domain, a transmembrane domain, and an internal tyrosine kinase domain (Fig. 5). These receptors are activated by binding of a ligand, which is followed by transduction of a signal into the cell through the kinase activity of the intracellular domain of

Table 4
Receptor Protein-Tyrosine Kinases[a]

EGF receptor family
     erbB1 (c-*erb*B)
     erbB2 (*neu*)
     erbB3
     erbB4
FGF receptor family
     FGF receptor-1 (*fig*)
     FGF receptor-2 (K-*sam*)
     FGF receptor-3
     FGF receptor-4
PDGF receptor family
     PDGF α-receptor
     PDGF β-receptor
     CSF-1 receptor (c-*fms*)
     SLF receptor (c-*kit*)
Insulin receptor family
     Insulin receptor (α, β)
     IGF-1 receptor (c-*ros*)
Hepatocyte growth ractor receptor family
     HGF receptor (*met*) (α, β)
     c-*sea* (ligand unknown) (α, β)
Neurotrophin receptor family
     NGF receptor (*trk*)
     BDNF and NT4 receptor (*trk*-B)
     NT3 receptor (*trk*-C)
Ligands unknown
     eph/elk
     VEGF receptor
     eck
     c-*ret*
     ax

[a]Adapted from S. A. Aaronson (67).

Table 5
Proto-oncogenes that Encode for Cytoplasmic Serine/ threonine Kinases and Nonreceptor Tyrosine Kinases with Oncogenic Potential[a].

Serine/threonine kinases
     c-*raf* family
          raf-1
          A-*raf*
          B-*raf*
     Protein Kinase C family
          PKC-β1
          PKC-γ
          PKC-ε
          PKC-ζ
     Other serine-threonine kinases
          mos
          pim-1
          akt
          cot
          tpl-2

Nonreceptor tyrosine kinases
     yes
      fgr
      fyn
      lck
      abl
      fps/fes

[a]Adapted from G. M. Cooper (2) and T. Yamamoto (163).

the receptor protein. Kinase enzymes regulate protein function by phosphorylation of tyrosine, serine, or threonine amino acid residues. Examples of these receptor tyrosine kinase proteins are listed in Table 4. The EGFR was implicated as playing a central role as a regulator of normal cellular growth and differentiation, primarily because the kinase activity of the EGFR is stimulated by EGF or TGF-a binding (80,81). Also, the human *EGFR* gene was linked via significant sequence homology to a known avian erythroblastosis virus oncogene, v-*erb*B. Eventually it was determined that the v-*erb*B gene product was a truncated protein derived from the *EGFR* gene. The v-*erb*B gene product lacks the extracellular ligand-binding domain (the amino-terminal half of the normal protein) that is present in the normal EGFR protein. This structural aberration results in a constitutively activated protein with tyrosine kinase activity. The constitutive cell signaling activity of the truncated receptor drives signal transduction and cell proliferation in the absence of growth-factor stimulation. Thus, an oncogene was shown to correspond to a known growth factor receptor, which established a direct link between the two (2,82–86).

Although structural aberrations play and important role in EGFR-mediated neoplastic transformation, a more common mechanism is overexpression of the normal proto-oncogene product, as is seen in breast cancers. Overexpression occurs not only as a result of gene amplification, but also in the absence of gene amplification, suggesting another as yet undetermined mechanism. Overexpression of EGFR has been found to have prognostic significance in several human tumors (75,87).

PROTEINS INVOLVED IN SIGNAL TRANSDUCTION: C-ABL AND C-RAS Once a cell receives a signal via plasma membrane-bound receptors, it is transmitted to the cell nucleus by a cascade of messenger molecules. Because abnormal growth factor receptors can function as oncoproteins by stimulating cell proliferation, it follows that protein messengers coupled to receptors, or even proteins involved in signal transduction that are not associated with receptors, can act as equally potent oncoproteins. In fact, many such oncoproteins have been identified, and they have been shown to mimic the normal function of signal-transducing proteins. The signal-transducing proteins can be widely grouped into two categories (Table 5): protein kinases (nonreceptor- associated tyrosine kinases, such as the c-*abl* protein product, and cytoplasmic serine/threonine kinases) and receptor-associated GTP-binding proteins (which include the c-ras proteins). The c-*abl* protein product is present on the inner surface of the plasma membrane. However, its tyrosine kinase activity is not dependent on coupling with a plasma membrane-bound receptor. Rather, negative regulatory domains are lost when c-*abl* of chromosome 9 is translocated to the breakpoint cluster region of chromosome 22. The hybrid protein product has increased enzymatic activity responsible for phosphorylating downstream substrates. This constitutive activity drives cells to proliferate, contributing to neoplastic growth. This form of molecular aberration characterizes CML and some forms of acute lymphoblastic leukemia (ALL).

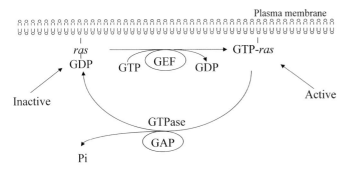

Fig. 6. c-ras mechanism of action. The c-ras protein is active when complexed with GTP, and this interaction is facilitated by GEFs in response to growth-factor stimulation. Although c-ras has it own GTPase activity, its inactivation by GTP hydrolysis is stimulated by GAPs, such as neurofibromin. Mutated c-ras protein has a decreased ability to hydrolyze GTP, or an increased rate of exchange of bound GDP for free GTP. By either mechanism, the result is increased activated c-ras.

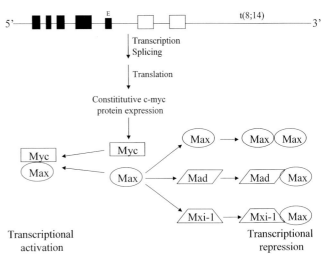

Fig. 7. The myc/max/mad/mxi-1 transcription network in Burkitt's lymphoma. The c-myc protein is expressed constitutively as a result of the chromosomal translocations t(8;14), t(8;22), and t(2;8). The t(8;14) translocation is depicted above. The c-myc protein dimerizes with max, which activates transcription. The max protein can homodimerize, or form complexes with mad or mxi-1. Each of these complexes inhibit transcription. Constitutive expression of c-myc leads to a shift in the equilibrium in favor of transcriptional activation.

The larger category of signal-transducing proteins is associated with membrane bound receptors, such as the GTP-binding proteins (G proteins), which include the c-ras family of proteins. There are many similarities between these latter two sets of proteins. G proteins are located on the inner face of the cell membrane, where they couple signals received from activated plasma-membrane receptors to other, mainly cytoplasmic, second messengers in a cascade ultimately culminating in the cell nucleus. Cell signaling through G proteins requires GTP binding. Hydrolysis of the bound GTP terminates signaling through a specific G protein molecule.

The c-*ras* proto-oncogenes are activated by point mutations. As would be predicted, the point mutations alter the function of the GTPase activity of its protein product. The mutated protein has a decreased ability to hydrolyze GTP, or has an increased rate of exchange of bound GDP for free GTP (Fig. 6). The decreased ability to hydrolyze GTP results from interactions between c-ras and GTPase activating proteins (GAPs), an example of which is neurofibromin, the gene product of the tumor-suppressor gene neurofibromatosis 1 (NF1). GAPs inactivate normal c-ras protein by augmenting the conversion of GTP-ras (active form) to GDP-ras (inactive form). The activated c-ras oncoproteins bind GAP, but their GTPase activity is stunted, leading to upregulation of active GTP-ras. Given the central role of GAPs in c-ras regulation, it is not surprising that the loss of activity of the GAP neurofibromin also results in upregulation of ras-GTP in affected cells. In response to growth-factor stimulation, c-ras is activated by guanine nucleotide-releasing or exchange factors (GEFs). They are responsible for the exchange of GDP for GTP (converting inactive ras-GDP to active ras-GTP). The increased exchange of GDP for GTP produces the same result: constitutively active c-ras protein bound to GTP. Interestingly, a GEF domain is present in the *bcr* protein product as well as in the *bcr-abl* fusion protein product created in the t(9;22) translocation, suggesting a possible role in c-ras regulation *(2,33,88–92)*.

The c-myc Family of Nuclear Regulatory Proteins The final steps in the mitogenic signaling pathways involve signal

entry into and the subsequent events that occur in the nucleus. The protein products of many proto-oncogenes (and tumor-suppressor genes) are localized to the nucleus, and function to control the transcription of growth-related genes through interaction with specific regulatory DNA sequences. Regulation of transcription is a key mechanism through which proto-oncogenes and tumor-suppressor genes exert control over cell proliferation. Nuclear proteins involved in these processes generally bind upstream to a specific gene and function as a transcription factor. Once bound to a specific DNA sequence, they act to increase expression of the target gene by interacting with other proteins involved in transcription. In order to be able to straddle the interaction between DNA and other proteins, most transcription factors have two functional domains: 1) a DNA binding domain, and 2) a protein binding domain. The DNA binding domain is often either a cysteine-rich region, the secondary structure of which binds zinc and forms looped structures (called zinc fingers), or a stretch of basic amino acids proximal to leucine zipper motifs (ZIP) or basic helix-loop-helix (bHLH) domains. The leucine zipper is composed of a stretch of hydrophobic leucine residues and functions in protein dimerization. The bHLH motif is composed of two amphipathic a-helical regions separated by a loop and also functions in protein dimerization *(3)*.

Because the c-*myc* oncogene is commonly involved in human tumors, there has been tremendous research activity into its mechanism of action. The c-*myc* proto-oncogene is expressed in nearly all eukaryotic cells and its mRNA synthesis is rapidly induced when quiescent cells receive a signal to divide. The C-terminal region of c-myc proteins has one basic DNA binding domain followed by bHLH and ZIP domains. The c-myc protein was suggested to function as a transcription

Table 6
Putative and Cloned Tumor-Suppressor Genes

Gene	Chromosomal location	Inherited cancer	Sporadic cancer
Rb1	13q14	retinoblastoma	Retinoblastoma, sarcomas, bladder, breast, esophageal, and lung carcinomas
p53	17p13	Li-Fraumeni cancer family syndrome	Bladder, breast, colorectal, esophageal, liver, lung, and ovarian carcinomas, brain tumors, sarcomas, lymphomas, and leukemias
DCC	18q21	———	Colorecetal carcinomas
MCC	5q21	———	Colorecetal carcinomas
APC	5q21	Familial adenomatous polyposis	Colorectal, stomach, and pancreatic carcinomas
WT1	11p13	Wilms tumor	Wilms tumor
WT2	11p15	Weidemann-Beckwith syndrome	Renal rhabdoid tumors, embryonal rhabdomyosarcoma
WT3	16q	Wilms tumor	———
NF1	17q11	Neurofibromatosis type 1	Colon carcinoma and astrocytoma
NF2	22q12	Neurofibromatosis type 2	Schwannoma and meningioma
VHL	3p25	von Hippel-Lindau syndrome	Renal cell carcinomas
MEN1	11q23	Multiple endocrine neoplasia type 1 (MEN1)	Endocrine tumors such as pancreatic adenomas
nm23	17q21	———	Melanoma, breast, colorectal, prostate, meningioma, others
MTS1	9p21	Melanoma	Melanoma, brain tumors, Leukemias, sarcomas, bladder, breast, kidney, lung, and ovarian carcinomas

factor based on the pattern of transient expression following cell stimulation by growth factors and sequence similarities with other DNA-binding transcription factors. However, it was found that the c-myc protein by itself does not bind DNA well. Rather, c-myc protein binds to DNA with greater affinity when dimerized with another protein possessing c-myc-like bHLH and ZIP domains, called max (Fig. 7). Max is a small protein that forms homodimers, interacts with all members of the c-myc family, and forms heterodimers with other proteins called mad and mxi1. Although c-myc, max, and mad share sequence domains, they differ in that c-myc has a transcriptional activation domain at its amino terminus. Thus, the myc-max heterodimer represents the functional form of c-myc, and upon binding to specific CACGTG DNA sequences, stimulates expression of genes involved in cell proliferation.

Max-max homodimers and heterodimers composed of max-mad and max-mxi1 also bind DNA efficiently. These other max-containing complexes compete with myc-max heterodimers for DNA binding. However, the proteins that compose these complexes lack a transcriptional activation domain. Therefore, DNA binding by any of these other complexes results in repression of transcription. The control over cell proliferation is influenced by the balance between transcriptional activation by myc-max heterodimers and transcriptional repression by max-max, max-mad, and max-mxi1. A

common theme of c-*myc* activation by chromosome translocation, insertional mutagenesis, or amplification, is overexpression of the c-myc protein. Overexpression of the c-myc protein leads to a shift in equilibrium toward myc-max dimers, activating transcription, promoting cell proliferation, and thereby contributing to neoplastic transformation *(2,93–101)*.

TUMOR-SUPPRESSOR GENES

Normal cellular proliferation is regulated by proto-oncogenes that encode for proteins that stimulate cell proliferation, and tumor-suppressor genes, which encode for proteins that inhibit, constrain, or suppress cell proliferation. Genetic alterations in proto-oncogenes leading to their activation, produce abnormal proteins or overexpression of normal proteins, which drive cells to enter the cell cycle and proliferate. In contrast, inactivating alterations or the physical or functional loss of both alleles of tumor-suppressor genes frees the cell from constraints imposed by their protein products. Tumor-suppressor genes act recessively, and alterations in these genes are commonly referred to in genetic terms as loss of function mutations. A list of known or putative tumor-suppressor genes is given in Table 6.

In the mid and late 1960s theories about the genesis of malignant tumors were enormously influenced by studies of virus- and gene-transfer experiments. Introduction of a virus into

Table 7
Characteristics of Oncogenes and Tumor-Suppressor Genes

Characteristic	Oncogenes	Tumor-suppressor gene
Number of mutational events required to contribute to cancer development	One	Two
Function of the mutant allele	Dominant (gain of function)	Recessive (loss of function)
Activity demonstrated in gene-transfer assays	Yes	Yes
Associated with hereditary syndromes (inheritance of germ-line mutations)	Seldom (c-*ret* proto-oncogene)	Often
Somatic mutations contribute to cancer development	Yes	Yes
Tissue specificity of mutational event	Some	In inherited cases, there is often a tissue preference

cultured cells added new genetic information that led to transformation. Most investigators believed at the time that neoplastic transformation resulted from a simple gain of genetic information, rather than from a loss of some cellular gene. In Mendelian terms, malignancy was thought to be a dominant characteristic. Henry Harris of the University of Oxford in collaboration with George Klein of Stockholm forwarded another approach *(102)*. Cells from mouse tumor cell lines were fused with nonmalignant cells, and the resulting hybrids were evaluated for their tumorigenic potential in appropriate hybrid animals. The hybrid cells produced very few tumors compared with the malignant parent cells. These results were interpreted to mean that normal cells contain one or more genes that act as negative regulators of the neoplastic phenotype. They postulated that malignancy was determined by a loss and not a gain of genetic information. At the time, these results were vigorously challenged *(103)*.

Additional cell-hybrid studies strengthened the concept that normal cellular genes can function to suppress the tumorigenic potential of neoplastically transformed cells. A cytogenetic analysis of cell hybrids that re-expressed tumorigenic potential established the chromosomal location of one of the normal genes in mouse that suppressed the malignant phenotype *(104,105)*. Similar studies in human hybrid cells derived from the fusion of normal fibroblasts and HeLa cells (cervical carcinoma cell line) showed that reversion to the tumorigenic phenotype followed the loss of chromosome 11. Introduction of the wild-type allele by fusion with a normal cell once again suppressed malignancy, suggesting the presence of a tumor-suppressor gene on this chromosome *(2,106,107)*.

Some generalizations about tumor-suppressor genes can be made (Table 7), and are further illustrated with specific examples below. Tumor-suppressor gene mutations or deletions are often found as germline mutations associated with hereditary syndromes that predispose to the development of specific tumors. Mutations or deletions in the same genes involved in cancers arising in the setting of these hereditary syndromes are also found in sporadic tumors (tumors that arise in individuals known not to have germline mutations). Commonly, these somatic mutations can be found in tumors not related to those associated with hereditary syndromes. These latter findings in sporadic tumors suggest a broader role for these genes in tum-

origenesis. In many but not all cases, tumor-suppressor activity can be demonstrated in gene-transfer assays. Tumor-suppressor gene products are integral components of cell-signaling pathways, in addition to having roles in cell-cell and cell-matrix interactions. Their role in the development of cancers has been demonstrated to be as significant as the role played by proto-oncogenes.

MECHANISM OF TUMOR-SUPPRESSOR GENE INACTIVATION IN RETINOBLASTOMA

Although by the mid 1970s, cell-hybrid studies clearly established that malignancy is at least in part due to loss of function of critical regulatory genes in malignant cells, the identification of tumor-suppressor genes at the molecular level did not occur until more than a decade later. As the prototypic tumor-suppressor gene, the mechanism of inactivation and loss of function associated with the retinoblastoma gene (*Rb1*) are illustrative of the whole class of tumor-suppressor genes. The inactivation of both alleles of the retinoblastoma gene is required for development of retinoblastoma, an eye malignancy occurring in the very young. Until the end of the nineteenth century, this tumor was uniformly fatal. During the twentieth century, more of these tumors were recognized and diagnosed at an earlier stage, permitting surgical cure. It was noted that the offspring of retinoblastoma patients cured by surgery developed retinoblastoma at a very high frequency. Pedigree analysis of these families suggested a dominant pattern of Mendelian inheritance *(108,109)*.

The suggestion that a specific gene was responsible for the disease stemmed not from molecular or cell-hybrid analyses, but rather from epidemiological data first reported by Alfred Knudson *(110)*. He noted that 40% of the cases of retinoblastoma were bilateral and occurred in young infants (mean age 14 mo), who if cured went on to develop secondary tumors (often osteosarcomas). In these patients, there was often a relevant family history of retinoblastoma. In contrast, the remaining 60% of cases were unilateral and occurred in older children (mean age 30 mo), who if cured did not develop secondary malignancies. These patients generally lacked a relevant family history. Knudson proposed that the first group inherited a mutant allele (germline mutation), which conferred a dominant predisposition to cancer to this group of patients. In these patients, a second somatic mutation in retinal cells resulted in retinoblastoma. The second nonfamilial, later-onset form was very rare (occurring in 1 in 30,000 people). Knudson suggested that these patients did not inherit a mutant gene, but rather two independent somatic mutations in retinal cells occurred to give rise to retinoblastoma.

The two-hit model proposed by Knudson did not address the mechanism of action of the gene(s) involved. There were at least two possible explanations. The first is that a dominant mutation of a single proto-oncogene allele is insufficient for the development of neoplasia, or that a second mutation, perhaps in a second proto-oncogene, is required. The second possibility, which proved to be correct, is that two mutations are required for development of retinoblastoma and that these mutations are inactivating mutations. Thus, the loss of both functional copies of the *Rb1* gene is necessary for neoplastic transformation and tumor formation. This conclusion is based on numerous studies involving cytogenetic, linkage, and restriction fragment-length polymorphism (RFLP) analyses of constitutional and tumor DNAs from affected individuals.

Cytogenetic studies demonstrated a loss of the long arm (13q14 region) of chromosome 13 in retinoblastoma tumors, and in the germline of patients with a hereditary predisposition to retinoblastoma development *(111)*. Esterase D, a gene present on chromosome 13q14, was used in linkage-analysis studies. Assuming that a mutant *Rb1* is closely linked to one of the two esterase D alleles that can be traced back to an affected parent, one can detect offspring who have inherited the mutant *Rb1* allele. Tumors arising in these individuals were shown to be homozygous for one form of esterase D, and by extension, homozygous for the mutant *Rb1* gene *(112)*. Similar conclusions were drawn from RFLP analysis of retinoblastomas arising in patients with familial predisposition, by comparing tumor DNA with germline DNA. Paralleling the findings using Esterase D, homozygosity was found in these tumors as well *(108,113)*. Shortly thereafter, probes from the 13q14 region were used to screen retinoblastomas, and several demonstrated homozygous deletions for at least 25 kb of DNA.

Molecular cloning of the gene was accomplished using probes to human 13q14 to isolate genomic DNA clones corresponding to flanking DNA. The genomic DNA clones from the tumor-suppressor gene region were then used as probes against RNA to compare the pattern of mRNA expression between retinoblastoma and normal retinal cells. The retinoblastoma gene was found to have 27 exons extending over approx 200 kb of DNA and to encode a 928 amino acid protein *(114–116)*. Once the *Rb1* gene was isolated, mechanisms of inactivation were found and included deletions and inactivating point mutations *(117,118)*. Importantly, tumor cell lines into which a cloned normal *Rb1* gene was introduced lost their malignant phenotype, confirming the tumor-suppressing action of *Rb1* *(119)*. These studies definitively established the role of deletion and/or loss of function as a major genetic mechanism involved with neoplastic transformation, and solidified the existence of a new class of genes, the tumor-suppressor genes.

The *Rb1* gene has since been found to be associated with many human neoplasms, usually through a genetic mechanism involving mutations or deletions. Most other tumor-suppressor genes have similar mechanisms of inactivation as described for *Rb1*. Specifically, any alterations in DNA or functional inacti-

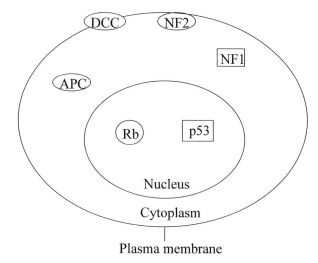

Fig. 8. Intracellular localization of select tumor-suppressor gene protein products.

vation of the gene-protein product that results in a loss of function of both copies or alleles of the gene is required for the development of tumors. These alterations include inactivating point mutations, deletions, or insertions. In general, all of these mechanisms have been described for many of the tumor-suppressor genes, and it is possible to find in one inactivated gene of a clonal-cell population a combination of two mechanisms of inactivation, a different one for each allele.

MECHANISM OF TUMOR-SUPPRESSOR GENE ACTION

The mechanism of action for the products of tumor-suppressor genes is diverse and not fully understood. Conceptually, the products of tumor-suppressor genes can be thought of as functioning to receive and process growth inhibitory signals from their surroundings. When a cell loses components of this signaling network, or loses responsiveness to extracellular growth-inhibitory signals, the cellular consequences are the same as for unchecked stimulation of cell growth, neoplasia. The tumor-suppressor gene products function in parallel with the protein products of proto-oncogenes, but work instead to suppress cell proliferation through the regulation of signal transduction and nuclear transcription. Not all tumor-suppressor gene products conform to the growth inhibitory concept. Cell-surface and cell-matrix molecules are responsible for normal cell morphology, cell-cell interactions, and cell-extracellular matrix (ECM) interactions. Tumor-suppressor genes encode for such proteins (Fig. 8), and mutations in these genes lead to altered cellular morphology, loss of normal intracellular-signaling pathways, and loss of normal intercellular interactions, all of which are features of neoplastic cells.

TUMOR-SUPPRESSOR GENE PRODUCTS THAT REGULATE SIGNAL TRANSDUCTION An example of a tumor-suppressor gene whose product regulates signal transduction is the gene product of neurofibromatosis 1 (NF1), which is responsible for the clinical syndrome Neurofibromatosis or von Recklinghausens's disease. Neurofibromatosis is one of the more common autosomal dominant disorders in humans and is clinically associated with café-au-lait spots (brown skin macules), benign neurofibromas, and other abnormalities. Patients with Neurofibromatosis have a higher incidence of malignant tumors, including neurofibrosarcomas, pheochromocytomas, optic nerve gliomas, and malignant myeloid diseases *(120)*.

The product of the *NF1* gene (neurofibromin) encodes for a GTPase activating protein (GAP). GAP proteins interact with c-ras proteins, which in normal cells are transiently activated upon exchange of bound GDP for bound GTP (Fig. 6). The c-ras proteins have intrinsic GTPase activity which is significantly increased upon binding with GAP proteins. Mutations in c-*ras* alter the GTPase activity, of its protein product. The ras-GTP oncoprotein is significantly less responsive to GAP-augmented hydrolysis *(2,33,88–92)*. It follows that mutations in genes that encode for GAP proteins, such as *NF1*, should be similarly deleterious to affected cells. In fact, *NF1* mutations are associated with and may contribute to the development of not only those tumors found in *NF1*, but also adenocarcinomas of the colon, anaplastic astrocytomas, and myeloid malignancies, among others *(120,121)*.

TUMOR-SUPPRESSOR GENE PRODUCTS THAT REGULATE TRANSCRIPTION Examples of tumor-suppressor genes whose products regulate transcription include *Rb1* and *p53*, the latter representing the gene most frequently involved in human cancers *(122)*. The discovery of the *Rb1* gene resulted in an intense research effort to understand the mechanism of action of its gene product. In studies of cell cycle regulation, the *Rb1* tumor-suppressor gene product was found to be active in an hypophosphorylated state, and inactive in a hyperphosphorylated state. Further, the active hypophosphorylated gene product was present in abundance in the G_0/G_1 stage of the cell cycle as compared to the finding of abundant inactive hyperphosphorylated pRb protein in late G_1, S, G_2, and M, suggesting a role for pRb as a suppressor of cell proliferation between the G_0/G_1 and S phase of the cell cycle. This was found to be true. The pRb protein binds transcription factors, and in particular, the E2F family of transcription factors as well as the product of the c-*myc* oncogene *(123,124)*. Cyclin-dependent kinases are responsible for phosphorylating pRb (resulting in inactivation) when cells are stimulated to divide by exogenous growth factors or other mitogenic signals. The pRb protein dissociates from sequestered/bound transcription factors, allowing the cell to progress from G_0/G_1 to the S phase. After mitosis, a phosphatase returns pRb to its active, hypophosphorylated form. Unlike other regulators of transcription, pRb does not directly interact with DNA *(108,125,126)*.

The inability of pRb to bind and negatively regulate the function of certain transcription factors leads to unregulated cell proliferation, and this can result from deletion or mutation of the *Rb1* gene, or functional inactivation of the pRb protein. In general, mutation of the *Rb1* gene results in truncated and unstable proteins *(120)*. As might be expected, the significant mutations or deletions in the *Rb1* gene occur in the transcription factor binding domain, also known as the pRb pocket. Functional inactivation of pRb was first recognized in studies of viral oncogenes. DNA viral oncogene products from animals (SV40 large T antigen) and humans (human papilloma virus [HPV] E7, adenovirus E1A) inhibit pRb function by binding

and occupying the pRb pocket. Gene mutations or occupation of the pRb pocket/transcription binding domain have, as a common result, the liberation of activating transcription factors with subsequent uncontrolled cell proliferation. The interplay between the products of these viral oncoproteins and pRb is an illustration of their mutual cooperation, which serves as a paradigm of the multistep nature of oncogenesis. Inhibition of tumor-suppressor genes represents an important way in which oncogenes exert their neoplastic potential *(127–129)*.

The *p53* gene is briefly mentioned because of its important and frequent involvement in human neoplasia *(122,130)*. Like the *Rb1* gene product, p53 is a nuclear phosphoprotein and functions primarily as a regulator of transcription. Specifically, when the genome sustains mutagenic damage (from radiation or a chemical insult) wild-type p53 protein accumulates in the nucleus where it binds DNA and causes cells to halt in the G_1 phase of the cell cycle, where the genetic damage is repaired. If the damage is not repaired, p53 induces apoptosis *(131)*. When first discovered, *p53* was thought to be a proto-oncogene because overexpression of cloned *p53* genes was shown to be related to transformation in gene-transfer assays. It was later shown that the clones used were actually mutant forms of the *p53* gene. When the wild-type gene was cloned and used in similar transfection studies, it did not demonstrate the ability to participate in the neoplastic transformation of normal cells. Rather, overexpression led to inhibition of neoplastic transformation, suggesting it to be a tumor-suppressor gene.

The tumor-suppressor function of p53 can be inactivated by either mutational events or through negative protein-protein interactions. The *p53* gene is composed of 11 exons spanning 20 kb of genomic DNA, encoding a protein of 393 amino acids. Mutations have been described for each exon, but appear to be most common in exons 5–9. A similar distribution of mutations is found in the Li-Fraumeni syndrome, in which patients inherit a germline mutation in the *p53* gene. This syndrome is characterized by a familial predisposition to many tumor types, including breast (among other epithelial) carcinomas, soft tissue sarcomas, brain neoplasms, and leukemias *(132)*. Mutant p53 protein products lose their ability to suppress transformation, and gain the ability to inactivate wild-type p53. A cell with one mutant and one wild-type copy of p53 behaves as if it has no wild-type p53 at all. This type of mutation is referred to as dominant-negative because the mutant allele acts in a dominant fashion to alter the functioning of the normal allele *(133,134)*. The half-life of mutant species of the p53 protein tend to be increased compared to the very short half-life of the wild-type protein. This increase in protein half-life enhances the dominant-negative effects of the mutant protein. Furthermore, when complexed with oncoprotein products such as from DNA tumor viruses (SV40 large T antigen, adenovirus E1B protein, and the E6 protein of HPV), the p53 protein is functionally inactivated in a manner analogous to the oncoprotein inactivation of the pRb *(135)*.

TUMOR-SUPPRESSOR GENE PRODUCTS THAT FUNCTION AS CELL SURFACE/CELL MATRIX MOLECULES Properties of malignant cells include not only uncontrolled proliferation capabilities, but also changes in cell morphology, loss of contact inhibition or cell-cell interactions, and loss of cell-ECM interactions. This results in an altered phenotype, including morphologic changes, which allow recognition by microscopy as malignant, inability to process inhibitory or other signals from adjacent cells, and loss of adhesion properties resulting in metastatic potential. Cell-surface and cell-matrix molecules thought to play a role in these processes include products from the neurofibromatosis 2 (*NF2*) gene, the adenomatous polyposis coli (*APC*) gene, and the deleted in colon cancer (*DCC*) gene, among others.

The *APC* gene was isolated in 1991 and is responsible for the familial adenomatous polyposis (FAP) syndrome, an uncommon autosomal dominant disease affecting approx 1 in 8000 individuals *(136,137)*. Patients with FAP typically develop 500–2500 adenomas of the colonic mucosa. The frequency of progression to colon adenocarcinoma approaches 100%, necessitating prophylactic colectomy by the second or third decade of life, and early surveillance of siblings and first degree relatives *(138)*. The *APC* gene was found to be located on the long arm of chromosome 5 (5q21), a locus known to be deleted frequently in colonic adenocarcinomas. Patients with FAP carry germline *APC* mutations leading to the production of truncated APC proteins, the detection of which has provided a diagnostic assay *(139)*. In addition to its role in the development of hereditary FAP, *APC* mutations have been found in sporadic adenomas, the majority of sporadic colorectal cancers *(140,141)*, and other human malignancies of the pancreas, esophagus, stomach, and lung *(142–145)*. Sporadic mutations also lead to the production of truncated proteins. Tumor-suppressor activity has not been demonstrated in gene-transfer assays using the *APC* gene.

The *APC* gene is large, extending over 8500 nucleotides, and encodes a protein of approx 2840 amino acids. The protein interacts with catenins, which are cytoplasmic proteins thought to play a role in signal transduction because of their interactions with cadherins, a family of cell-surface molecules. Cadherins have been shown to regulate cell-cell interactions and morphogenesis. Based on these observations, it has been postulated that the APC-catenin complex plays a role in cell adherence, and possibly signal transduction such as contact inhibition of cell growth *(146)*. In FAP, mutations in the 5′-portion of the gene have been shown to correlate with an attenuated form of the disease *(147)*, whereas mutations at codon 1309 are associated with an early onset of colon cancer in FAP families *(120,148)*.

The *DCC* gene was discovered using polymorphic DNA markers that showed a loss of heterozygosity (LOH) of the long arm of chromosome 18 in colorectal tumors *(44)*. The gene was subsequently isolated and shown to be composed of more than 29 exons spanning more than 1×10^6 nucleotides *(149)*. The *DCC* gene encodes for a transmembrane molecule with unknown function which has homology to cell-adhesion molecules (CAMs) involved in cell-cell or cell ECM interactions. It may play a role in transmitting negative signals, and inactivation of *DCC* function through deletion or mutation (a rare event) may lead to loss of contact inhibition and subsequent uncontrolled cellular proliferation *(150,151)*. LOH at the 18q locus was initially described in colorectal carcinomas as one of several steps involved in the sequence of events from premalig-

nant adenomas to invasive carcinomas. Although no hereditary conditions involving germline alterations of the gene have been described (in contrast to most other tumor-suppressor genes), *DCC* abnormalities are associated with several tumor types other than colon cancer, including stomach cancer, pancreatic cancer, and leukemias (152–155). The *DCC* gene has not been formally classified as a tumor-suppressor gene because the predicted tumor-suppressor activity has not been demonstrated in gene-transfer assays *(2,156,157)*.

NF2 is genetically and clinically distinct from NF1 discussed earlier. It is a rare autosomal dominant disorder in which patients develop bilateral schwannomas affecting the vestibular branch of the eighth nerve (acoustic neuromas), and other tumors of the central nervous system (CNS) such as meningiomas and ependymomas (hence its designation as central neurofibromatosis). The gene is located on the long arm of chromosome 22 (22q22) and was isolated in 1993 *(158,159)*. Mutations of the *NF2* gene have been found in tumors (breast carcinomas and melanomas) other than those associated with the NF2 syndrome *(160)*, as well as in sporadic meningiomas and ependymomas *(161,162)*, suggesting a role in tumorigenesis extending beyond that played in NF2. Its protein product (schwannomin or merlin) shows sequence homologies to proteins that act as linkers between cytoskeletal scaffolding components and proteins in the cell membrane. On this basis schwannomin is thought to play a role in cell shape, cell-cell interactions, and cell-matrix interactions *(158,159)*. Inactivation of the *NF2* gene may lead to changes in cell shape and loss of contact inhibition *(120)*.

ACKNOWLEDGMENT

The author thanks John Mendiola, PhD and Stanley McCormick, MD for critical review of this chapter.

REFERENCES

1. Shope, R. E. (1933) Infectious papillomatosis of rabbits. *J. Exp. Med.* **58**:607–624.
2. Cooper, G. M. (1995) *Oncogenes,* 2nd ed. Jones and Bartlett Publishers, Sudbury, MA.
3. Watson, J. D., Gilman, M., Witkowski, J., and Zoller, M. (1992) *Recombinant DNA,* 2nd ed. W.H. Freeman and Co., New York.
4. Rous, P. (1911) A sarcoma of the fowl transmissible by an agent separable from the tumor cells. *J. Exp. Med.* **13**:397–411.
5. Vogt, P. K. (1971) Spontaneous segregation of nontransforming viruses from cloned sarcoma viruses. *Virology* **46**:939–946.
6. Weis, R., Teich, N., Varmus, H., and Coffin, J. (eds.) (1985) *Molecular Biology of Tumor Viruses: RNA Tumor Viruses,* 2nd ed. Cold Spring Harbor Laboratory Press, Cold Spring Harbor, New York.
7. Cooper, G. M., Okenquist, S., and Silverman, L. (1980) Transforming activity of DNA of chemically transformed and normal cells. *Nature* **284**:418–421.
8. Shih, C., Shilo, B. Z., Goldfarb, M. P., Dannenberg, A., and Wienberg, R. A. (1979) Passage of phenotypes of chemically transformed cells via transfection of DNA and chromatin. *Proc. Natl. Acad. Sci. USA* **76**:5714–5718.
9. Der, C. J., Krontiris, T. G., and Cooper, G. M. (1982) Transforming genes of human bladder and lung carcinoma cell lines are homologous to the *ras* genes of Harvey and Kirsten sarcoma viruses. *Proc. Natl. Acad. Sci. USA* **79**:3637–3640.
10. Boveri, T. (1929) *The Origin of Malignant Tumors.* Williams and Wilkins, Baltimore, MD.

11. Nowell, P. C. and Hungerford, D. A. (1960) A minute chromosome in chronic granulocytic leukemia. *Science* **132**:1497–1498.

12. Rowley, J. D. (1973) A new consistent chromosomal abnormality in chronic myelogenous leukemia identified by quinacrine fluorescence and Giemsa staining. *Nature* **243**:290–293.

13. DeKlein, A., van Kessel, A. G., Grosveld, G., Bartram, C. R., Hagemeijer, A., Bootsma, D., et al. (1982) A cellular oncogene is translocated to the Philadelphia chromosome in chronic myelocytic leukemia. *Nature* **300**:765–767

14. Copelan, E. A. and McGuire, E. A. (1995) The biology and treatment of acute lymphoblastic leukemia in adults. *Blood* **85**:1151–1168.

15. Kurzrock, R., Gutterman, J. U., and Talpaz, M. (1988) The molecular genetics of Philadelphia chromosome-positive leukemias. *N. Engl. J. Med.* **319**:990–998.

16. Vardiman, J. W. (1992) Chronic myelogenous leukemia and the myeloproliferative disorders. *In: Neoplastic Hematopathology* (Knowles, D. M., ed.), Williams and Wilkins, Baltimore, MD, pp. 1405–1438.

17. Rezuke, W. N. and Abernathy, E. C. (1997) Molecular genetics in the laboratory diagnosis of hematologic malignancies. *In: Molecular Diagnostics for the Clinical Laboratorian* (Coleman, W. B. and Tsongalis, G .J., eds.), Humana Press, Totowa, NJ, pp. 317–339.

18. Shtivelman, E., Lifshitz, B., Gale, R. P., and Canaani, E. (1985) Fused transcript of abl and bcr genes in chronic myelogenous leukaemia. *Nature* **315**:550–554.

19. Hayward, W. S., Neel, B. G., and Astin, S. M. (1981) Activation of a cellular *onc* gene by promoter insertion in ALV-induced lymphoid leukemias. *Nature* **290**:475–480.

20. Marcu, K. B., Bossone, S. A., and Patel, A. J. (1992) *myc* function and regulation. *Ann. Rev. Biochem.* **61**:809–860,

21. Solomon, E., Borrow, J., and Goddard, A. D. (1991) Chromosome aberrations and cancer. *Science* **254**:1153–1160.

22. Dalla-Favera, R., Bregni, M., Erickson, J., Patterson, D., Gallo, R. C., and Croce, C. M. (1982) Human c-*myc onc* gene is located on the region of chromosome 8 that is translocated in Burkitt lymphoma cells. *Proc. Natl. Acad. Sci. USA* **79**:7824–7827.

23. Taub, R., Kirsch, I., Morton, C., Lenoir, G., Swan, D., Tronick, S., et al. (1982) Translocation of the c-*myc* gene into the immunoglobulin heavy chain locus in human Burkitt lymphoma and murine plasmacytoma cells. *Proc. Natl. Acad. Sci. USA* **79**:7837–7841.

24. Cowell, J. K. (1982) Double minutes and homogeneously staining regions: gene amplification in mammalian cells. *Ann. Rev. Genet.* **16**:21–59.

25. Barker, P. E. (1982) Double minutes in human tumor cells. *Cancer Genet. Cytogenet.* **5**:81–94.

26. Collins, S. and Groudine, M. (1982) Amplification of endogenous myc-related DNA sequences in a human myeloid leukaemia cell line. *Nature* **298**:679–681.

27. Biedler, J. L. and Spengler, B. A. (1976) Metaphase chromosome anomaly: association with drug resistance and cell specific products. *Science* **191**:185–187.

28. Alitalo, K., Schwab, M., Lin, C. C., Varmus, H. E., and Bishop, J. M. (1983) Homogeneously staining chromosomal regions contain amplified copies of an abundantly expressed cellular oncogene (c-*myc*) in malignant neuroendocrine cells from a human colon carcinoma. *Proc. Natl. Acad. Sci. USA* **80**:1707–1711.

29. Schwab, M., Varmus, H. E., and Bishop, J. M. (1985) Human N-*myc* gene contributes to neoplastic transformation of mammalian cells in culture. *Nature* **316**:160–162.

30. Woods, W. G., Tuchman, M., Bernstein, M. L., Leclerc, J. M., Brisson, L., Look, T., et al. (1992) Screening for neuroblastoma in North America. 2-year results from the Quebec Project. *Am. J. Ped. Hematol. Oncol.* **14**:312–319.

31. Schwab, M., Alitalo, K., Klempnauer, K. H., Varmus, H. E., Bishop, J. M., Gilbert, F., et al. Amplified DNA with limited homology to *myc* cellular oncogene is shared by human neuroblastoma cell lines and a neuroblastoma tumour. *Nature* **305**:245–248.

32. Shimada, H. (1992) Neuroblastoma: pathology and biology. *Acta Pathol. Jpn.* **42**:229–241.

33. Feig, L. A. (1993) The many roads that lead to Ras. *Science* **260**:767–768.

34. Bos, J. L. (1989) Ras oncogenes in human cancer: a review. *Cancer Res.* **49**:4682–4689.

35. Reddy, E. P., Reynolds, R. K., Santo, E., and Barbacid, M. (1982) A point mutation is responsible for the acquisition of transforming properties by the T24 human bladder carcinoma oncogene. *Nature* **300**:149–152.

36. Tabin, C. J., Bradley, S. M., Bargmann, C. K., Weinberg, R. A., Papageorge, A. G., Scolnick, E. M., et al. (1982) Mechanism of activation of a human oncogene. *Nature* **300**:143–149.

37. Taparowsky, E., Suard, Y., Fasano, O., Shimizu, K., Goldfarb, M., and Wigler, M. (1982) Activation of the T24 bladder carcinoma-transforming gene is linked to a single amino acid change. *Nature* **300**:762–765.

38. Cohen, J. B. and Levinson, A. D. (1988) A point mutation in the last intron responsible for increased expression and transforming activity of the c-Ha-*ras* oncogene. *Nature* **334**:119–124.

39. Capella, G., Matias-Guiu, X., Ampudia, X., de Leiva, A., Perucho, M., and Prat, J. (1996) *ras* oncogene mutations in thyroid tumors: polymerase chain reaction-restriction-fragment-length polymorphism analysis from paraffin-embedded tissues. *Diagnostic Mol. Pathol.* **5**:5–52.

40. Sciacchitano, S., Paliotta, D. S., Nardi, F., Sacchi, A., Andreoli, M., and Pontecorvi, A. (1994) PCR amplification and analysis of *ras* oncogenes from thyroid cytologic smears. *Diagnostic Mol. Pathol.* **3**:114–121.

41. Moley, J. F., Brother, M. B., Wells, S. A., Spengler, B. A., and Beider, J. L. (1991) Low frequency of *ras* gene mutations in neuroblastomas, pheochromocytomas, and medullary thyroid cancers. *Cancer Res.* **51**:1559–1569.

42. Wright, P. A., Lemoirre, N. R., Mayall, E. S., Hughes, D., and Williams, E. D. (1989) Papillary and follicular thyroid carcinomas show a different pattern of *ras* oncogene mutations. *Br. J. Cancer* **60**:576–577.

43. Bos, J. L., Fearon, E. R., Hamilton, S. R., Verlaan-de Vries, M., van Boom, J. H., van der Eb, A. J., et al. (1987) Prevalence of *ras* gene mutations in human colorectal cancers. *Nature* **327**:293–297.

44. Vogelstein, B., Fearon, E. R., Hamilton, S. R., Kern, S. E., Preisinger, A. C., and Leppert, M. (1988) Genetic alterations during colorectal development. *N. Engl. J. Med.* **319**:525–532.

45. Neuman, W. L. (1991) Evidence for a common molecular pathogenesis in colorectal, gastric, and pancreatic cancer. *Genes Chromosomes Cancer* **3**:468–473.

46. Shen, C, Chang, J. G., Lee, L. S., Yang, M. J., Chen, T. C., Link, Y., et al. (1991) Analysis of *ras* mutations in gastrointestinal cancers. *J. Formosan Med. Assoc.* **90**:1149–1154.

47. Grendys, E. C., Jr., Barnes, W. A., Weitzel, J., Sparkowski, J., and Schlegel, R. (1997) Identification of H, K, and N-*ras* point mutations in stage IB cervical carcinoma. *Gynecol. Oncol.* **65**:343–347.

48. Tenti, P., Romagnoli, S., Silini, E., Pellegata, N. S., Zappatore, R., Spinillo, A., et al. (1995) Analysis and clinical implications of K-*ras* gene mutations and infection with human papillomavirus types 16 and 18 in primary adenocarcinoma of the uterine cervix. *Int. J. Cancer* **64**:9–13,

49. Semczuk, A., Berbec, H., Kostuch, M., Kotarski, J., Wojcierowski, J. (1997) Detection of K-*ras* mutations in cancerous lesions of human endometrium. *Eur. J. Gynaecol. Oncol.* **18**:80–83.

50. Varras, M. N., Koffa, M., Koumantakis, E., Ergazaki, M., Protopapa, E., Michalas, S., et al. (1996) *ras* gene mutations in human endometrial carcinoma. *Oncology* **53**:505–510.

51. Sasaki, H., Nishii, H., Takahashi, H., Tada, A., Furusato, M., Terashima, Y., et al. (1993) Mutation of the Ki-*ras* protooncogene in human endometrial hyperplasia and carcinoma. *Cancer Res.* **53**:1906–1910.

52. Gao, H. G., Chen, J. K., Stewart, J., Song, B., Rayappa, C., Whong, W. Z., et al. (1997) Distribution of p53 and K-*ras* mutations in human lung cancer tissues. *Carcinogenesis* **18**:473–478.

53. Rodenhuis, S., Slebos, R. J. C., Boot, A. J. M., Evers, S. G., Mooi, M. J., and Wagenaar, S. C. C. (1988) Incidence and possible clinical

significance of K-*ras* oncogene activation in adenocarcinoma of the human lung. *Cancer Res.* **48**:5738–5741.

53. Rodenhuis, S., van de Wetering, M. L., Mooi, W. J., Evers, S. G., van Zandwjk, W., and Bos, J. L. (1987) Mutational activation of the K-*ras* oncogenes: a possible pathogenetic factor in adenocarcinoma of the lung. *N. Engl. J. Med.* **317**:929–935.

54. Visscher, D. W., Yadrandji, S., Tabaczka, P., Kraut, M., and Sarkar, F. H. (1997) Clinicopathologic analysis of k-*ras*, p53, and erbB-2 gene alterations in pulmonary adenocarcinoma. *Diagnostic Mol. Pathol.* **6**:64–69.

55. Urban, T., Ricci, S., Lacave, R., Antoine, M., Kambouchner, M., Capron, F., et al. (1996) Codon 12 Ki-*ras* mutation in non-small-cell lung cancer: comparative evaluation in tumoural and non-tumoural lung. *Br. J. Cancer* **74**:1051–1055.

56. Neubauer, A., Greenberg, P., Negrin, R., Ginzton, N., and Liu, E. (1984) Mutations in the *ras* proto-oncogenes in patients with myelodysplastic syndromes. *Leukemia* **8**:638–641

57. Gougopoulou, D. M., Kiaris, H., Ergazaki, M., Anagnostopoulos, N. I., Grigoraki, V. Spandidos, D. A. (1996) Mutations and expression of the *ras* family genes in leukemias. *Stem Cells* **14**:725–729.

58. Farr, C. J., Saiki, R. K., Erlich, H. A., McCormick, F., and Marshall, C. J. (1988) Analysis of *ras* gene mutations in acute myeloid leukemia by PCR and oligonucleotide probes. *Proc. Natl. Acad. Sci. USA* **85**:1629–1633.

59. Aurer, I., Labar, B., Nemet, D., Ajdukovic, R., Bogdanic, V., Gale, R. P. (1994) High incidence of conservative *ras* mutations in acute myeloid leukemia. *Acta Haematologica* **92**:123–125.

60. Kawamura, M., Kikuchi, A., Kobayashi, S., Hanada, R., Yamamoto, K., Horibe K., et al. (1995) Mutations of the p53 and *ras* genes in childhood t(1;19)-acute lymphoblastic leukemia. *Blood* **85**:2546–2552.

61. Reinartz, J. J., Yakshe, P., Nelson, D., Trenckner, S., Meier, P., Niehans, G., et al. (1998) Detection of K-*ras* mutations in pancreatic and biliary samples to aid in the diagnosis of malignancy: a prospective study. Submitted.

62. Levi, S., Urbano-Ispizua, A., Gill, R., Thomas, D. M., Gilbertson, J., Foster, C., et al. (1991) Multiple K-*ras* codon 12 mutations in cholangiocarcinomas demonstrated with a sensitive polymerase chain reaction technique. *Cancer Res.* **51**:3497–3502.

63. Van Laethem, J. L., Vertongen, P., Deviere, J., Van Rampelbergh, J., Rickaert, F., Cremer, M., et al. (1995) Detection of c-Ki-*ras* gene codon 12 mutations from pancreatic duct brushings in the diagnosis of pancreatic tumours. *Gut* **36**:781–787.

64. Weinberg, R. A. (1994) Oncogenes and tumor-suppressor genes. *Recent Results Cancer Res.* **136**:35–47.

65. Bishop, J. M. (1991) Molecular themes in oncogenesis. *Cell* **64**:235–248.

66. Aaronson, S. A. (1991) Growth factors and cancer. *Science* **254**:1146–1153.

67. Cohen, S. (1986) Nobel lecture. Epidermal growth factor. *Biosci. Rep.* **6**:1017–1028.

68. Metcalf, D. (1989) The molecular control of cell division, differentiation commitment and maturation in haemopoietic cells. *Nature* **339**:27–30.

69. Westermark, B. and Heldin, C. H. (1991) Platelet derived growth factor in autocrine transformation. *Cancer Res.* **51**:5087–5092.

70. Doolittle, R. F., Hunkapiller, M. W., Hood, L. E., Devare, S. G., Bobbins, K. C., Aaronson, S. A., et al. (1983) Simian sarcoma virus *onc* gene, v-*sis*, is derived from the gene (or genes) encoding a platelet-derived growth factor. *Science* **221**:275–277.

71. Waterfield, M. D., Scrace, G. T., Whittle, N., Stroobant, P., Johnsson, A., Wasteson, A., et al. (1983) Platelet derived growth factor is structurally related to the putative transforming protein p28sis of simian sarcoma virus. *Nature* **304**:35–39.

72. Todaro, G. J., De Larco, J. E., Nissley, S. P., and Rechler, M. M. (1977) MSA and EGF receptors on sarcoma virus transformed cells and human fibrosarcoma cells in culture. *Nature* **267**:526–528.

73. Derynck, F., Goeddel, D. V., Ullrich, A., Gutterman, J. U., Williams, R. D., Bringman, T. S., et al. (1987) Synthesis of messenger

RNAs for transforming growth factors a and b and the epidermal growth factor receptor by human tumors. *Cancer Res.* **47**:707–712.

74. Reinartz, J. J., George, E., Lindgren, B. R., and Niehans, G. A. (1994) Expression of p53, transforming growth factor alpha, epidermal growth factor receptor, and c-erbB-2 in endometrial carcinoma and correlation with survival and known predictors of survival. *Human Pathol.* **25**:1075–1083.

75. Rosenthal, A., Lindquist, P. B., Bringman, T. S., Goeddel, D. V., and Derynck, R. (1986) Expression in rat fibroblasts of a human transforming growth factor a cDNA results in transformation. *Cell* **46**:301–309.

76. Watanabe, S., Lazar, E., and Sporn, M. B. (1987) Transformation of normal rat kidney (NRK) cells by an infectious retrovirus carrying a synthetic rat type a transforming growth factor gene. *Proc. Natl. Acad. Sci. USA* **84**:1258–1262.

77. Jhappan, C., Stahle, C., Harkins, R. N., Fausto, N., Smith, G. H., and Merlino, G. T. (1990) TGF-a overexpression in transgenic mice induces liver neoplasia and abnormal development of the mammary gland and pancreas. *Cell* **61**:1137–1146.

78. Matsui, Y., Halter, S. A., Holt, J. T., Hogan, B. L. M., and Coffey, R. J. (1990) Development of mammary hyperplasia and neoplasia in MMTV-TGF-a transgenic mice. *Cell* **61**:1147–1155.

79. Carpenter, G., King, L., and Cohen, S. (1978) Epidermal growth factor stimulates phosphorylation in membrane preparations *in vitro*. *Nature* **276**:409–410.

80. Ushiro, H., and Cohen, S. (1980) Identification of phophotyrosine as a product of epidermal growth factor-activated protein kinase in A431 cell membranes. *J. Biol. Chem.* **255**:8363–8365.

81. Downward, J., Yarden, Y., Mayes, E., Scrace, G., Totty, N., Stockwell, P., et al. (1984) Close similarity of epidermal growth factor receptor and v-*erb*B oncogene protein sequences. *Nature* **307**:521–527.

82. Segatto, O., King, C. R., Pierce, J. H., Di Fiore, P. P., and Aaronson, S. A. (1988) Different structural alterations upregulate in vitro tyrosine kinase activity and transforming potency of the erB-2 gene. *Mol. Cell Biol.* **8**:5570–5574.

83. Wells, A. and Bishop, J. M. (1988) Genetic determinants of neoplastic transformation by the retroviral oncogene v-erbB. *Proc. Natl. Acad. Sci. USA* **85**:7597–7601.

84. Di Fiore, P. P., Pierce, J. H., Flemming, T. P., Hazan, R., Ullich, A., King, C. R., et al. (1987) Overexpression of the human EGF receptor confers an EGF-dependent transformed phenotype to NIH 3T3 cells. *Cell* **51**:1063–1070.

85. Di Fiore, P. P., Pierce, J. H., Kraus, M. H., Segatto, O., King, C. R., and Aaronson, S. A. (1987) ErbB-2 is a potent oncogene when overexpressed in NIH 3T3 cells. *Science* **237**:178–182.

86. Slamon, D. J., Clark, G. M., Wong, S. G., Levin, W. J., Ullrich, A., and McGuire, W. L. (1987) Human breast cancer: correlation of relapse and survival with amplification of the HER-2/neu oncogene. *Science* **235**:177–182.

87. McCormick, F. (1993) How receptors turn Ras on. *Nature* **363**:15–42.

88. Polakis, P. and McCormick, F. (1992) Interaction between p21ras proteins and their GTPase activating proteins. *Cancer Surv.* **12**:25.

89. Ballester, R., Marchuk, D., Bofuski, M., Saulino, A., Letcher, R., Wigler, M., et al. (1990) The NF1 locus encodes a protein functionally related to mammalian GAP and yeast IRA proteins. *Cell* **63**:851–859.

90. Martin, G. A., Wiskochil, D., Bollag, G., McCabe, P. C., Crosier, W. J., Hanubruck, H., et al. (1990) The GAP-related domain of the neurofibromatosis type 1 gene product interacts with ras p21. *Cell* **63**:843–849.

91. Shoug, C., Farnsworth, C. L., Neel, B. G., and Feig, L. A. (1992) Molecular cloning of cDNAs encoding a guanine-nucleotide-releasing factor for Rasp21. *Nature* **358**:351–354.

92. Rabbitts, T. H. (1994) Chromosomal translocations in human cancer. *Nature* **373**:143149.

93. Amanti, B., Brooks, M. W., Bevy, N., Littlewood, T. D., Evan, G. I., and Land, H. (1993) Oncogenic activity of the c-*myc* protein requires diermization with Max. *Cell* **72**:233–245.

94. Ayer, D. E., Kretzner, L., and Eisenman, R. N. (1993) Mad: a heterodimeric protein partner for Max that antagonizes Myc transcriptional activity. *Cell* **72**:211–222.

95. Zervos, A. S., Gyuris, J., and Brent, R. (1993) Mxi1, a protein that specifically interacts with Max to bind Myc-Max recognition sites. *Cell* **72**:223–232.

96. Blackwell, T. K., Kretzner, L., Blackwood, E. M., Eisenman, R. N., and Weintraub, H. (1990) Sequence specific DNA binding by the c-Myc protein. *Science* **250**:1149–1151.

97. Blackwood, E. M. and Eisenman, R. N. (1991) Max: a helix-loop-helix zipper protein that forms a sequence-specific DNA-binding complex with Myc. *Science* **251**:1211–1217.

98. Kato, G. J., Barrett, J., Villa, G. M., and Dang, C. V. (1990) An amino-terminal c-*myc* domain required for neoplastic transformation activates transcription. *Mol. Cell Biol.* **10**:5914–5920.

99. Kretzner, L., Blackwood, E. M., and Eisenman, R. N. (1992) Myc and Max possess distinct transcriptional activities. Nature **359**:426–429.

100. Marcu, K. B., Bossone, S. A., and Petel, A. J. (1992) Myc function and regulation. *Ann. Rev. Biochem.* **61**:809–860.

101. Harris, H., Miller, O. J., Klein, G., Worst, P., and Tachibana, T. (1969) Suppression of malignancy by cell fusion. *Nature* **223**:363–368.

102. Ephrussi, B., Davidson, R. L., Weiss, M. C., Harris, H., and Klein, G. (1969) Malignancy of somatic cell hybrids. *Nature* **224**:1314–1316.

103. Jonasson, J., Povey, S., and Harris, H. (1977) The analysis of malignancy by cell fusion. VII. Cytogenetic analysis of hybrids between malignant and diploid cells and of tumours derived from them. *J. Cell Sci.* **24**:217–254.

104. Evans, E. P., Burtenshaw, M. D., Brown, B. B., Hennion, R., and Harris, H. (1982) The analysis of malignancy by cell fusion. IX. Reexamination and clarification of the cytogenetic problem. *J. Cell Sci.* **56**:113–130.

105. Stanbridge, E. J., Flandermeyer, R. R., Daniels, D. W., and Nelson Rees, W. A. (1981) Specific chromosome loss associated with the expression of tumorigenicity in human cell hybrids. *Somatic Cell Mol. Genet.* **7**:699–712.

106. Stanbridge, E. J. (1976) Suppression of malignancy in human cells. *Nature* **260**:17–20.

107. Weinberg, W. A. (1995) The molecular basis of oncogenes and tumor-suppressor genes. *Ann. NY Acad. Sci.* **758**:331–338.

108. Sparkes, R. S. (1985) The genetics of retinoblastoma. *Biochim. Biophys. Acta* **780**:95–118.

109. Knudson, A. G., Jr. (1971) Mutation and cancer: statistical study of retinoblastoma. *Proc. Natl. Acad. Sci. USA* **68**:820–828.

110. Yunnis, J. J. and Ramsay, N. (1978) Retinoblastoma and subband deletion of chromosome 13. *Am. J. Dis. Children* **132**:161–163.

111. Sparkes, R. S., Murphree, A. L., Lingua, R. W., Sparkes, M. C., Field, L. L., Funderburk, S. J., et al. (1983) Gene for hereditary retinoblastoma assigned to human chromosome 13 by linkage to esterase D. *Science* **219**:971–973.

112. Dryja, T. P., Cavenee, W., White, R., Rapaport, J. M., Petersen, R., Albert, D. M., et al. (1984) Homozygosity of chromosome 13 in retinoblastoma. *N. Engl. J. Med.* **310**:550–553.

113. Lee, W. H., Bookstein, R., Hong, F., Young, L. J., Shew, J. Y., Lee, E. Y. H. P. (1987) Human retinoblastoma susceptibility gene: cloning, identification, and sequence. *Science* **235**:1394–1399.

114. Friend, S. H., Bernards, R., Rogelj, S., Weinberg, R. A., Rapaport, J. M., Albert, D. M., et al. (1986) A human DNA segment with properties of the gene that predisposes to retinoblastoma and osteosarcoma. *Nature* **323**:643–646.

115. Hong, Y. K. T., Huang, H. J. S., To, H., Young, L. J. S., Oro, A., Bookstein, R., et al. (1989) Structure of the human retinoblastoma gene. *Proc. Natl. Acad. Sci. USA* **85**:5502–5506.

116. Dunn, J. M., Phillips, R. A., Becker, A. J., and Gallie, B. L. (1988) Identification of germline and somatic mutations affecting the retinoblastoma gene. *Science* **241**:1797–1800.

117. Horowitz, J. M., Yandell, D. W., Park, S. H., Canning, S., Whyte, P., Buchkovich, K., et al. (1989) Point mutational inactivation of the retinoblastoma antioncogene. *Science* **243**:937–940.

118. Huang, H. J. S., Yee, J. K., Shew, J. Y., Chen, P. L., Bookstein, R., Friedmann, T., et al. (1988) Suppression of the neoplastic phenotype by replacement of the RB gene in human cancer cells. *Science* **242**:1562–1566.

119. Hoppe-Seyler, F. and Butz, K. (1994) Tumor-suppressor genes in molecular medicine. *Clin. Invest.* **72**:619–630.

120. Seizinger, B. R. (1993) NF1: A prevalent cause of tumorigenesis in human cancers? *Nature Genet.* **3**:97–99.

121. Nigro, J. M., Baker, S. J., Preisinger, A. C., Jessup, J. M., Hostetter, R., Cleary, K., et al. (1989) Mutations in the p53 gene occur in diverse human tumor types. *Nature* **342**:705–708.

122. Goodrich, D. W. and Lee, W. (1992) Abrogation by c-*myc* of G1 phase arrest inducted by Rb protein by not by p53. *Nature* **360**:177–180.

123. Wiman, K. (1993) The retinoblastoma gene: role in cell cycle control and cell differentiation. *FASEB J.* **7**:841-845.

124. Chen, P. L., Scully, P., Shew, J. Y., Wang, J. Y. J., and Lee, W. H. (1989) Phosphorylation of the retinoblastoma gene product is modulated during the cell cycle and cellular differentiation. *Cell* **58**:1193–1198.

125. Ludlow, J. W., Shon, J., Pipas, J. M., Livingston, S. M., and DeCaprio, J. A. (1990) The retinoblastoma susceptibility gene product undergoes cell cycle dependent dephosphorylation and binding to and release from SV40 large T. *Cell* **60**:387–396.

125. Whyte, P. K., Buckovich, K. J., Horowitz, J. M., Friend, S. H., Raybuck, M., Weinberg, R. A., et al. (1988) Association between an oncogene and an anti-oncogene: retinoblastoma gene product. *Nature* **334**:124–129.

127. Chellapan, S., Kraus, V., Kroger, B., Munger, K., Howley, P. M., Phelps, W. C., et al. (1992) Adenovirus E1A, simian virus 40 tumor antigen, and human papillomavirus E7 protein share the capacity to disrupt the interaction between transcription factor E2F and the retinoblastoma gene product. *Proc. Natl. Acad. Sci. USA* **89**:4549–4553.

128. Goodrich, D. W. and Lee, W. (1993) Molecular characterization of the retinoblastoma susceptibility gene. *Biochim. Biophys. Acta* **1155**:43–61.

129. Levine, A. J. (1997) P53, the cellular gatekeeper for growth and division. *Cell* **88**:323–331.

130. Zambetti, G. P. and Levine, A. J. (1993) A comparison of the biologic activities of wild type and mutant p53. *FASEB J.* **7**:855–864.

131. Malkin, D., Li, F. P., Strong, L. C., Fraumeni, J. F., Jr., Nelson, C. E., Kim, D. H., et al. (1990) Germ line p53 mutations in a familial syndrome of breast cancer, sarcomas, and other neoplasms. *Science* **250**:1233–1238.

132. Weinberg, R. A. (1991) Tumor-suppressor gene. *Science* **254**:1138–1146.

133. Levine, A. J. (1993) The tumor-suppressor genes. *Ann. Rev. Biochem.* **62**:623–651.

134. Hollstein, M., Sidransky, D., Vogelstein, B., and Harris, C. C. (1991) p53 mutations in human cancers. *Science* **253**:49–53.

135. Burt, R. and Samowitz, W. (1988) The adenomatous polyp and the hereditary polyposis syndromes. *Gatroenterol. Clin. North Am.* **17**:657–678.

136. Groden, J., Thiveris, A., Samowotz, W., Carlson, M., Gelbert, L., Albertsen, H., et al. (1991) Identification and characterization of the familial adenomatous polyposis coli gene. *Cell* **66**:589–600.

137. Lynch, H. T., Watson, P., Smyrk, T. C., Lanspa, S. J., Boman, B. M., Boland, C. R., et al. (1992) Colon cancer genetics. *Cancer* **70**:1300–1312.

138. Poell, S. M., Petersen, G. M., Krush, A. J., Booker, S., Jen, J., Giardiello, F. M., et al. (1993) Molecular diagnosis of familial adenomatous polyposis. *N. Engl. J. Med.* **329**:1982–1987.

139. Miyoshi, Y., Nagase, H., Ando, H., Horii, A., Ichii, S., Nakatsuru, S., et al. (1992) Somatic mutations of the APC gene in colorectal tumors: mutation cluster region in the APC gene. *Human Mol. Genet.* **1**:229–233.

140. Powell, S. M., Nilz, N., Beazer-Barclay, Y., Bryan, T. M., Hamilton, S. R., Thibodeau, S. M., et al. (1992) APC mutations occur early during colorectal tumorigenesis. *Nature* **359**:235–237.

141. Horii, A., Nakatsuru, S., Miyoshi, Y., Ichii, S., Nagase, H., Ando, H., et al. (1992) Frequent somatic mutations of the APC gene in human pancreatic cancer. *Cancer Res.* **52**:3231–3233.

142. Boynton, R. F., Bount, P. L., Yin, J., Brown, V. L., Huang, Y., Tong, Y., et al. (1992) Loss of heterozygosity involving the APC and MCC genetic loci occurs in the majority of human esophageal cancers. *Proc. Natl. Acad. Sci. USA* **89**:3385–3388.

143. Horii, A., Nakatsuru, S., Miyoshi, Y., Ichii, S., Nagase, H., Kato, Y., et al. (1992) The APC gene, responsible for familial adenomatous polyposis, is mutated in human gastric cancer. *Cancer Res.* **52**:3231–3233.

144. D'Amico, D., Carbone, D. P., Johnson, B. E., Meltzer, S. J., and Minna, J. D. (1992) Polymorphic sites within the MCC and APC loci reveal very frequent loss of heterozygosity in human small cell cancer. *Cancer Res.* **52**:1996–1999.

145. Pfeifer, M. (1993) Cancer, catenins, and cuticle pattern: a complex connection. *Science* **262**:1667–1668.

146. Spirio, L., Olschwang, S., Groden, G., Robertson, M., Samowitz, W., Joslyn, G., et al. Alleles of the APC gene: an attenuated form of familial polyposis. *Cell* **75**:951–957.

147. Caspari, R., Friedl, W., Mandl, M., Moslein, G., Kadmon, M., Knapp, M., et al. (1994) Familial adenomatous polyposis: mutation at codon 1309 and early onset of colon cancer. *Lancet* **343**:629–632.

148. Fearon, E. R., Cho, K. R., Nigro, J. M., Kern, S. E., Simons, J. W., Ruppert, J. M., et al. (1990) Identification of a chromosome 18q gene that is altered in colorectal cancers. *Science* **247**:49–56.

149. Cho, K. R., Oliner, J. D., Simons, J. W., Hedrick, L., Fearon, E. R., Preisinger, A. C., et al. (1994) The DCC gene: structural analysis and mutations in colorectal carcinomas. *Genomics* **19**:525–531.

150. Cho, K. R. and Fearon, E. R. (1995) DCC: Linking tumor-suppressor genes and altered cell surface interactions in cancer? *Curr. Opin. Genet. Dev.* **5**:72–78.

151. Uchino, S., Tsuda, H., Noguchi, M., Yokota, J., Terada, M., Saito, T., et al. (1992) Frequent loss of heterozygosity at the DCC locus in gastric cancer. *Cancer Res.* **52**:3099–3102.

152. Hohne, M. W., Halatsch, M. E., Kahl, G. F., and Weinel, R. J. (1992) Frequent loss of expression of the potential tumor-suppressor gene DCC in ductal pancreatic adenocarcinoma. *Cancer Res.* **52**:2616–2619.

153. Porfiri, E., Secker-Walker, L. M., Hoffbrand, A. V., and Hancock, J. F. (1993) DCC tumor-suppressor gene is inactivated in hematologic malignancies showing monosomy 18. *Blood* **81**:2696–2701.

154. Fearon, E. R. (1995) Oncogenes and tumor-suppressor genes. *In: Clinical Oncology* (Abeloff, M. D., ed.), Churchill Livingston, New York, pp. 11–40.

155. Fearon, E. R. (1992) Genetic alterations underlying colorectal tumorigenesis. *Cancer Surv.* **12**:119–136.

156. Fearon, E. R. and Vogelstein, B. (1990) A genetic model for colorectal tumorigenesis. *Cell* **61**:759–767.

157. Rouleau, G. A., Merel, P., Lutchman, M., Sanson, M., Zucman, J., Marineau, C., et al. (1993) Alteration in a new gene encoding a putative membrane-organizing protein cause neurofibromatosis 2. *Nature* **363**:515–521.

158. Trofatter, J. A., MacCollin, M. M., Rutter, J. L., Murell, J. R., Duyao, M. P., Parry, D. M., et al. (1993) A novel Moesin-, ezrin-, radixin-like gene is a candidate for the neurofibromatosis 2 tumor suppressor. *Cell* **72**:791–800.

159. Bianchi, A. B., Hara, T., Ramesh, V., Gao, J., Klein-Szanto, A. J. P., Morin, F., et al. Mutations in transcript isoforms of the neurofibromatosis 2 gene in multiple human tumor types. *Nature Genet.* **6**:185–192.

160. Rubio, M. P., Correa, K. M., Ramesh, V., MacCollin, M. M., Jacoby, L. B., von Deimling, A., et al. (1994) Analysis of the neurofibromatosis 2 gene in human ependymomas and astrocytomas. *Cancer Res.* **54**:45–47.

161. Ruttledge, M. H., Sarrazin, J., Fangaratnam, S., Phelan, C. M., Twist, E., Merel, P., et al. (1994) Evidence for the complete inactivation of the NF2 gene in the majority of sporadic meningioms. *Nature Genet.* **6**:180–184.

162. Yamamoto, T. (1993) Molecular basis of cancer: Oncogenes and tumor-suppressor genes. *Microbiol. Immunol.* **37**:11–22.

4 Positive Mediators of Cell Proliferation in Neoplastic Transformation

JAMES N. WELCH, PhD AND SUSAN A. CHRYSOGELOS, PhD

INTRODUCTION

Cancer is not a single disease, but a collection of diseases all of which are related by a common root cause: the loss of controlled cell growth. Cancer begins as a clonal disease, that is, it stems from the genetic corruption of a single cell. This conversion of a normal cell into the neoplastic state is a multi-step phenomenon called neoplastic transformation and requires the accumulation of several genetic mutations. Some of these mutations enhance the activity of growth-promoting cellular processes, whereas other mutations undermine regulatory mechanisms designed to keep replication in check. Transformed cells differ from normal cells with respect to many observable characteristics, including alterations in growth parameters and cellular behavior. Damage to growth-regulation and DNA repair mechanisms permit acquired somatic mutations to remain uncorrected and to accumulate. As the tumor population grows, the specific genetic mutations acquired vary from one cell to the next, causing tumor progression from a clonal entity to a genetically and phenotypically heterogeneous population of cells.

Metastasis is the spread of the tumor from the primary site to one or more secondary sites at distant locations throughout the body. Between the primary transformation event and the establishment of secondary metastases lies a series of complicated steps, including: 1) growth at the primary site, 2) invasion of the surrounding tissue and blood supply, 3) dissemination through the circulatory system, and 4) establishment of growth at a secondary site. Cells making this journey must acquire specialized functions (largely due to accumulated mutations) that allow them to evade destruction and exploit their surroundings at each stage. Positive mediators of carcinogenesis can therefore be defined as those molecular players which enhance the progression of a cell through one or more stages of neoplastic transformation or metastatic growth.

PROTO-ONCOGENES AND CARCINOGENESIS

An oncogene is a gene that encodes a protein product (an oncoprotein) that stimulates uncontrolled cellular proliferation. Oncogenes are derivatives of normal cellular genes, which encode critical (and tightly regulated) molecular participants in cell growth. The unaltered progenitor genes are referred to as proto-oncogenes, denoting their potential to be mutated into dysfunctional forms. A proto-oncogene to oncogene conversion can occur by a variety of mechanisms ranging from dramatic genetic alterations (such as chromosomal translocations) to subtle point mutations. However, the overall effect in each case is the same: a gain-of-function. In some cases, the gain-of-function occurs through increased expression of the gene product. In other instances, mutations that alter the gene coding region can yield a gain-of-function by changing the physical structure of the protein product. Some proto-oncogene to oncogene conversions involve both mechanisms. Establishment of a gene as a proto-oncogene requires demonstration that a mutated form can transform cells such as immortalized fibroblasts in culture. However, oncogenes can also exert their effects after transformation has occurred, enhancing neoplastic progression.

Mutations in proto-oncogenes act in concert with each other and with other accumulated genetic defects affecting tumor-suppressor genes and DNA repair genes. Tumor-suppressor proteins and DNA repair enzymes play important roles in preventing carcinogenesis. Mutations derailing these molecular players result in a loss of normal function, removing their restrictive influence over cell proliferation. Tumor suppressors and DNA-repair enzymes are classified as negative mediators of carcinogenesis. What is important to bear in mind is that alterations in the normal functions of both positive and negative mediators are required for a noncancerous cell to be transformed to the neoplastic state.

RETROVIRUSES AND THE DISCOVERY OF PROTO-ONCOGENES

Proto-oncogenes are evolutionarily conserved, reflecting their importance in normal cellular function. This conservation proved critical to the discovery of proto-

From: *The Molecular Basis of Human Cancer* (W. B. Coleman and G. J. Tsongalis, eds.), © Humana Press Inc., Totowa, NJ.

oncogenes through the study of oncogenic retroviruses in animals *(1,2)*. A retrovirus contains an RNA genome (instead of DNA) composed of three genes: *GAG* (encodes the core protein for the retrovirus), *POL* (encodes the enzyme reverse transcriptase), and *ENV* (encodes the envelope protein). The retroviral genome also contains long terminal repeats at each end that function as promoter and enhancer sequences. Retroviruses can cause proto-oncogene to oncogene conversion in host cells by one of two mechanisms: transduction or insertional mutagenesis.

Transduction is the acquisition of a small portion of genomic DNA from the host cell chromosome by the infecting retrovirus. During normal retroviral replication, a reverse transcriptase enzyme copies the RNA genome into a duplex DNA form (called a provirus) *(3)*. Through integration of the provirus into the host genome and recombination between the host and viral DNA, a segment of host cell DNA can be taken into the viral genome. The expression of this transduced gene sequence is then placed under the control of the highly active retroviral promoter. Transduction is a consequence of the normal retroviral life cycle and is associated with carcinogenesis when the acquired DNA segment contains part or all of a proto-oncogene. Transduction is not limited to proto-oncogenes. Any segment of the host genome is probably susceptible to this process, but most other cases do not result in an observable phenotype. In the case of proto-oncogene transduction, the subsequent infection of a new host cell by the now-oncogenic retrovirus results in transformation of the host cell. The acquired proto-oncogene segment can lead to an oncogenic gain-of-function if either: 1) the gene is expressed to an abnormally high degree because of its association with the retroviral promoter, or 2) the acquired gene is structurally altered during transduction to yield a protein product with activity that differs from its normal cellular counterpart. These structural alterations range from point mutations and/or small deletions to the fusion of a portion of the proto-oncogene to one of the retroviral genes, resulting in a hybrid protein product *(4)*.

Insertional mutagenesis does not involve the acquisition of host-gene sequences. Instead, the retrovirus corrupts a cellular proto-oncogene without removing it from the host genome. As stated earlier, insertion of the provirus within the host genome is a part of the viral replication cycle. The location of the provirus insertion is random, but can be oncogenic if the insertion occurs proximal to a proto-oncogene locus. Again, conversion of the proto-oncogene to an oncogene can result by either placing the expression of the oncogene under the influence of the retroviral promoter elements or by disrupting the coding region of the gene resulting in a structurally abnormal protein product with altered function *(5)*.

Retroviruses have been the tools of discovery for many oncogenes in animals, but only rarely have they been established as carcinogenic agents in humans. However, protein and gene homology studies of animal oncogenes discovered via retroviruses has led to the discovery of a long list of human counterparts. A full treatment of this topic is beyond the scope of this chapter. However, several important examples of retroviral oncogenes and their mammalian counterparts are described.

MECHANISMS OF PROTO-ONCOGENE TO ONCOGENE CONVERSION IN HUMANS

Because retroviruses are believed not to be the primary cause of proto-oncogene to oncogene conversion in humans, other mechanisms must be involved. These mechanisms include chromosomal translocations, point mutations, gene amplification, and gene overexpression.

CHROMOSOMAL TRANSLOCATION Chromosomal translocations involve the joining of two previously distinct chromosomal segments. The segments can originate from different chromosomes or from within a single chromosome (specifically referred to as chromosomal inversion). Oncogenic chromosomal translocations are similar to retroviral insertional mutagenesis in that they can cause oncogenic gain-of-function if either: 1) a proto-oncogene is relocated near a strong promoter, or 2) a section of a proto-oncogene is fused to another gene to create a hybrid gene product.

Chromosomal translocations are common mutagenic events underlying B- and T-cell leukemias and lymphomas, but are found much less frequently in solid tumors. Leukemias and lymphomas are derived from B and T cells, which employ gene rearrangement processes as a method of generating immune-cell diversity. The immunoglobin and T-cell receptor recombination events, which take place in B and T cells, respectively, can result in the accidental rearrangement of chromosomal segments containing proto-oncogenes. Specifically, these oncogenic recombination events involve the movement of a proto-oncogene away from its own regulatory structures to within the proximity of a highly active promoter for a constitutively expressed gene *(6)*. In the case of B-cell tumors, the translocation usually involves an immunoglobin gene, whereas in T-cell tumors, genes encoding the cell-surface antigen receptors are generally involved *(7,8)*. Many novel proto-oncogenes have been identified in association with chromosomal translocations within B- and T-cell malignancies *(9)*.

Genetic characterization of Burkitt's lymphoma (BL) provided one of the first examples of an oncogenic gain-of-function caused by increased gene expression due to a chromosomal translocation *(10)*. The c-*myc* proto-oncogene is invariably disrupted in BL. This gene encodes a transcription factor that promotes the expression of a variety of growth stimulatory genes *(11)*. The aberrant translocation leads to the positioning of c-*myc* proximal to an immunoglobin gene promoter. Immunoglobin genes are highly expressed in B-cells, and the translocation of the c-*myc* gene near an immunoglobin promoter region results in overexpression (and therefore increased activity) of c-*myc* *(12)*.

The Philadelphia chromosome, which is characteristic of two specific forms of leukemia, was one of the first characterized examples of a chromosomal translocation resulting in the fusion of two genes to produce a gain-of-function hybrid protein product. The hybrid protein contains the beginning of the *bcr* (for breakpoint cluster region) gene product and the catalytic portion of the c-*abl*, which encodes a protein tyrosine kinase involved in cellular growth. This combination yields a very specialized oncoprotein product containing functional domains from both the *bcr* and c-*abl* segments, which contribute to oncogenesis *(13)*. The bcr domain, which replaces the regulatory domain of the c-abl protein, provides an oligomerization motif, a domain that acts specifically on the c-abl segment to activate its kinase activity, and binding sites for other intracellular proteins involved in cell growth, thus integrating this overactive mutant tyrosine kinase with several growth-related signaling pathways *(14)*. Chromosomal translocations that generate the Philadelphia chromosome employ alternative breakpoints in the *bcr* gene to render a pair of differently sized chimeric proteins: the larger p210 bcr-abl is characteristic of chronic myelogenous leukemia (CML) and the smaller p185 bcr-abl is characteristic of acute lymphocytic leukemia (ALL). The smaller protein product lacks a domain believed necessary for actin stress fiber stabilization and this disparity is implicated in the association of each form with a different type of leukemia *(15)*.

In some cases of acute myeloid leukemia (AML), a specific chromosomal translocation may actually be of some benefit. Inversion of chromosome 16 is common in AML patients. Some AML patients display a loss of the multi-drug resistance gene as a consequence of the use of an alternative breakpoint in the inversion process *(16)*. The multi-drug resistance gene (*mdr*) encodes a transmembrane pump called p-glycoprotein that is involved in the export of many cytotoxic drugs administered in chemotherapy *(17)*. The p-glycoprotein pump greatly enhances the ability of cancer cells to survive exposure to chemotherapeutic agents, and its deletion in a subset of AML patients provides a potential therapeutic advantage.

POINT MUTATION Subtle alterations of a gene's nucleotide sequence can have dramatic effects on the structure and function of the encoded protein. DNA point mutations, changes in single base pairs, are caused mainly by exposure to carcinogens and by infrequent but inevitable errors occurring during DNA replication and repair *(18)*. A single residue change in the amino acid sequence can have drastic effects on the three dimensional structure of the protein product, altering affinity for regulatory partners and/or substrates. Conversely, mutations of catalytic residues can alter enzymatic activity without having an observable effect on the overall protein structure. DNA point mutations are a very common mechanism of proto-oncogene to oncogene conversion. Well-studied examples of point mutations causing oncogenic conversions occur in the c-*ras* and the c-*ret* proto-oncogenes. The c-*ras* genes encode signaling proteins that mediate growth and other cellular functions, and are mutated in a wide range of human cancers. Likewise, the c-ret gene encodes a receptor tyrosine kinase that is involved in cell signaling and proliferation.

GENE AMPLIFICATION AND GENE OVEREXPRESSION Gene amplification is the result of abnormal reduplication of a select chromosomal region. The reduplicated chromosomal section can be present in as much as 100-fold to 1000-fold excess. Amplified genes are commonly found in tumors but the mechanisms leading to this abnormality are not fully understood *(19)*. Amplification of a proto-oncogene can result in oncogenic conversion without otherwise altering the gene should the amplified gene product be expressed at such a high level that it simply overwhelms the normal cellular regu-

latory machinery. However, in many cases the gene is mutated before being amplified, which can increase the potency of the overexpressed gene product. Gene amplification is generally thought to be a post-transformation event, most likely occurring as a result of the genomic instability that is characteristic of neoplastic cells. Amplification is probably not selective for specific genes, but the amplification of certain genes can provide a growth advantage for tumor cells. Amplification of the c-*myc* gene results in enhanced transactivation of growth-related genes, and is frequently found in small cell lung carcinomas, and to a lesser extent in breast and colorectal cancers *(20)*. Selection for amplification of the androgen receptor gene has been observed in some prostate-cancer patients receiving androgen-deprivation therapy. This appears to be an acquired means of resistance by allowing the cancer cells to exploit the remaining low levels of androgens to sustain cell growth *(21)*. A more common example is the aforementioned multidrug resistance gene. Overexpression of *mdr* as a result of gene amplification provides an obvious survival advantage for tumor cells and so it is logical that this specific gene-amplification event is a common feature of many human tumors as well as tumor-derived cell lines selected for resistance to chemotherapeutic compounds in vitro *(17)*.

A gain-of-function can also be achieved through dysregulated expression of an otherwise normal proto-oncogene. Although this can result from a variety of mechanisms, most often it involves the disruption of the regulatory machinery that governs transcription of the gene. Some cases involve genetic damage, which alters or removes the gene-promoter region, as is found with chromosomal translocations. Discrete changes within the promoter region, such as point mutations and small deletions, can disrupt the binding patterns of regulatory protein factors and lead to increased or even constitutive transcription. Some proteins are found to be overexpressed in many tumors types (with respect to their normal tissue counterparts) without a common attributable mechanism. Overexpression of the epidermal growth-factor receptor (EGFR) is a prime example. Increased EGFR levels are associated with more aggressive forms of many tumors, but the mechanisms underlying this phenomenon are varied, including gene amplification, gene rearrangement, and altered transcriptional regulation *(22)*.

EXTRACELLULAR SIGNALS AND CELL-SURFACE RECEPTORS

Cells interpret and respond to changes in their microenvironment through the use of a complex intracellular-communication network process collectively referred to as signal transduction. Extracellular signals such as hormones, cytokines, and other molecules interact with specific receptors that translate and funnel messages into intracellular-signaling cascades. These cascades require the formation of multi-protein complexes and the generation of second messengers to convey the signal from the receptor to the target point within the cell. The target in most cases is the transcription machinery in the nucleus. Put simply, most signal transduction events evoke particular changes in gene expression, which allow the cell to respond to biological commands and changes in its surrounding microenvironment.

Many proto-oncogenes encode proteins involved in signal-transduction pathways that stimulate cell growth. Because these proteins are normally tightly regulated, conversion of the proto-oncogene to an oncogene involves an altered or overexpressed signal-transduction component that defies regulation and leads to uncontrolled signal-cascade activity, and as the end result, a continuously proliferating cell. Proto-oncogenes are found at every level of signal transduction, from the extracellular signals and receptors, through the cytoplasmic signaling cascade components, to the transcriptional effector targets.

EXTRACELLULAR SIGNALING Extracellular signals that are received and interpreted by their target cells come in a variety of forms including proteins and small peptides, steroid compounds, and ions. One class of secreted extracellular signaling molecules that are particularly prevalent in cancer development and progression are hormones. The term hormone describes a diverse spectrum of secreted macromolecules that bind with high affinity to their cognate receptors on the surface or within a target cell. Only those cells that express the cognate receptor for a specific hormone are able to recognize and respond to that extracellular signal. Receptors are proteins that bind to extracellular signaling molecules with high affinity and initiate a cellular response. In most cases involving receptors, the extracellular signal is conveyed into the cell by an intracellular signaling cascade. As with other proto-oncogenes, receptors can function in an oncogenic capacity if: 1) the receptor is overexpressed, leading to signal amplification; or 2) the structure of the receptor is altered such that it is constitutively activated, circumventing the requirement for hormone binding, and generating a perpetual signal.

A hormone is usually synthesized at some point distant from its target cell (endocrine stimulation) or by a neighboring cell (paracrine stimulation). In some cases, a hormone can be synthesized and secreted by a cell that also expresses the cognate receptor for that hormone (autocrine stimulation), resulting in a cell with a self-sustained stimulation loop (Fig. 1). Endocrine, paracrine, and autocrine signaling can contribute to transformation if the extracellular signal is abnormally expressed and stimulates a growth response.

A prominent example of autocrine stimulation associated with transformation involves the *v-sis* oncogene. *v-sis* is the transforming component of the simian sarcoma virus, the human homolog of which is the gene encoding the B-chain of platelet-derived growth factor, PDGF-B *(9)*. Infection by the simian sarcoma virus in animal hosts or cultured cells results in the unscheduled production and secretion of PDGF-BB dimers. When this virus infects a cell that naturally expresses the PDGF-receptor, the consequence is autocrine growth stimulation and transformation of the cell. Aberrant PDGF/PDGF-receptor expression is a common characteristic of many human cancers. Close to 170 human cell lines (derived from over 25 different tumor types) have thus far been reported to express PDGF-A or PDGF-B chains and greater than 50 of these cell lines also express the cognate receptor. Although a clear relationship between PDGF stimulation and transformation remains to be determined in most of these cell lines, the commonality of

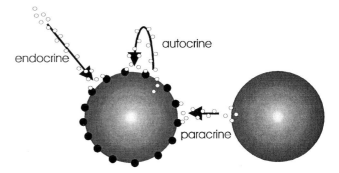

Fig. 1. Mechanisms of hormonal signaling. In endocrine signaling the hormone (white circles) is synthesized at a point distant from the target cell expressing the cognate receptor (black circles). In paracrine signaling, the hormone is synthesized by a neighboring cell. In autocrine signaling, the same cell produces the hormone and expresses the cognate receptor.

PDGF/PDGF-receptor expression in so many tumor-derived cell lines indicates that PDGF stimulation may be a prevalent autocrine/paracrine mechanism underlying tumorigenesis in a spectrum of cancers *(24–26)*. PDGF expressing tumor cells have also been shown to induce expression of the PDGF receptor by stromal components within certain tumors, such as basal-cell carcinomas *(27)* and neuroendocrine (NE) tumors of the digestive system *(28)*, establishing a paracrine communication link between stromal and neoplastic tumor components. Communication between tumor cells and stromal tissues allows tumors to manipulate their microenvironment in order to enhance their ability to grow, spread, and survive. Paracrine communication between tumor and normal tissues is vital to metastatic processes.

Receptor Tyrosine Kinases Growth factors are a specific subset of peptide hormones, which influence cell growth by binding a specific class of membrane receptors: receptor tyrosine kinases (RTKs) *(29)*. RTKs are a family of structurally related transmembrane receptors expressed on the plasma membrane. All the RTK family members share common features that are critical to their function and regulation, including: 1) a ligand- (hormone) binding domain that is specific for one or a small set of related hormones; 2) a dimerization motif; 3) a short transmembrane domain that anchors the receptor to the plasma membrane; and 4) tyrosine kinase catalytic domains and substrate domains, which are found within the cytoplasmic portion of the receptor (Fig. 2). Activation of an RTK occurs through the following ordered steps: (Step 1) hormone (growth factor) binding and subsequent dimerization with an identical or closely related RTK; (Step 2) tyrosine autophosphorylation, which is actually *trans*-phosphorylation by each dimerized partner upon the other at specific tyrosine residues; (Step 3) release of inhibition of further tyrosine autophosphorylation activity, creating phosphotyrosine motifs within the RTK cytoplasmic domain; (Step 4) the cytoplasmic phosphotyrosine motifs bind to cytoplasmic proteins with specific affinity for the phosphotyrosine motifs in the activated receptor. This binding of an intracellular effector initiates the signal-transduction cascade that transmits the extracellular signal to the appropriate target(s) within the cell (Fig. 3) *(30,31)*.

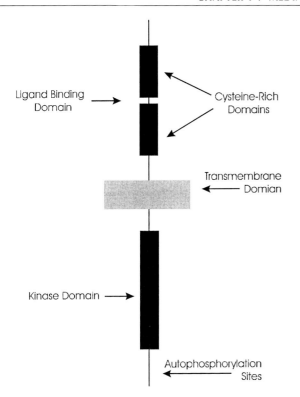

Fig. 2. Common structural features of receptor tyrosine kinases (RTK).

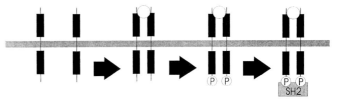

Fig. 3. The ordered steps in RTK activation. Step 1, Ligand binding followed by receptor dimerization. Step 2, Autophosphorylation. Step 3, Intracellular signaling through interaction with other cellular signaling proteins (like binding to an SH2 domain protein).

Overexpression or structural mutation are the two mechanisms by which oncogenic alteration of an RTK can occur. EGFR, the prototype member of the type one tyrosine kinase family, exhibits both of these mechanisms in different forms of cancer. The deletion-mutant form, designated EGFRvIII, lacks 267 amino acids from the extracellular domain resulting in the removal of the ligand-binding domain. EGFRvIII exhibits different behaviors from the wild-type EGFR, including ligand-independent activation, and an inability to be internalized and downregulated. These differences, perhaps in combination, are thought to have oncogenic effects in several forms of cancer, including breast, lung, and ovarian carcinomas, and various forms of gliomas *(32)*.

Overexpression of EGFR is a far more common event than is mutation of the receptor. Increased EGFR levels can result from either gene amplification or upregulated gene expression. Overexpression by either means results in increased EGFR signaling which is thought to drive the cell to a higher rate of proliferation. Accordingly, increased levels of EGFR are associated with more aggressive forms of a variety of cancers including those of the breast, bladder, and pancreas, as well as melanomas and nonsmall-cell lung carcinoma *(22,33–36)*.

Oncogenic activation of RTKs can also be achieved by chromosomal rearrangements yielding gain-of-function fusion proteins. For example, the tpr-met chimera protein, originally isolated from a human osteogenic sarcoma cell line, combines the amino terminal region of the so-called translocated promoter region *(tpr)* with the carboxy-terminal region of c-*met* (which encodes the hepatocyte growth factor/scatter factor). The tpr amino-terminal domain replaces the ligand binding site and dimerization domain of the met receptor with a leucine-

zipper structure that can dimerize without the need for hormone binding. Unregulated dimerization then permits autophosphorylation within the met-derived portion, leading to continuous activation and signaling from the tpr-met oncoprotein *(37)*. Tpr sequences have also been discovered fused to other kinase domains in different tumor types including c-*trk* (a nerve growth factor kinase proto-oncogene isolated from human thyroid papillary carcinomas) and c-*raf* (a serine/threonine kinase proto-oncogene). It seems likely that tpr-fusion events represents common oncogenic mechanisms affecting many proto-oncogenes, but that has yet to be demonstrated *(37)*.

A similar and well-characterized example of an oncogenic RTK is the Npm-ALK fusion protein that is prevalent in cases of non-Hodgkin's lymphoma *(38)*. In this case, the amino-terminal portion of nucleophosmin (Npm) provides a dimerzation motif and is fused to the carboxy-terminal region of the RTK ALK, which contributes the tyrosine kinase catalytic/signaling regions. Like tpr-met, dimerzation and activation of the ALK tyrosine kinase domain leads to unregulated signaling. The Npm-ALK and tpr-fusion examples illustrate a common mechanism for RTK oncogenic activation: gene rearrangement resulting in the combination of a novel amino-terminal gene sequence (providing nonregulated dimerization capacity) with the kinase/substrate signaling domain from an RTK gene.

A unique example of an RTK involved in transformation is the protein product of the c-*ret* proto-oncogene. This gene is expressed in neural crest cell lineages and binds a glial cell line-derived neurotrophic factor *(39)*. The ret protein is believed to function normally in embryogenesis, but the details have yet to be elucidated *(40)*. The oncogenic conversion of ret is unique because distinct mutations of the c-*ret* proto-oncogene are linked to three different thyroid-associated cancer syndromes *(41–43)*. More surprising, mutations in the c-*ret* gene associated with all three syndromes can be inherited or acquired somatically. This is highly unusual because the inheritance of any constitutively active proto-oncogene would presumably interfere with normal cellular processes essential to viable embryonic development. Hereditary cancers are almost always associated with the inheritance of genetic defects attenuating tumor-suppressor or DNA-repair enzyme functions. The mutations affecting the c-*ret* proto-oncogene reflect a variety of mechanisms: deletions, nonsense mutations, and point mutations resulting in loss of function. Of particular note is a point mutation that removes a cysteine residue that is thought to be necessary for the formation of an intramolecular disulfide bond. The loss of one cysteine residue leaves an orphaned cysteine that is hypothesized to cross-link with its orphaned cysteine counterpart on another mutant receptor molecule, thereby permitting receptor dimerization and activation without hormone binding. This particular point mutation is of special interest because it might reflect a common mechanism of oncogenic activation for many RTKs.

CYTOPLASMIC SIGNAL TRANSDUCTION

Receptor Tyrosine Kinase Signaling Through c-ras The discovery of the ras signaling cascade was of fundamental importance to the study of cancer. Mutations affecting c-*ras* and genes encoding related proteins are common to a diverse array of tumors, whereas mutations in c-*ras* itself are found in about 30% of all cancers *(44)*. The ras protein is an important signal-transduction effector because it serves as a convergence point, responding to a diverse array of signals, and can interact with several targets, acting as a signaling branch point to extend its influence over many cellular responses and functions *(45)*. Ras-associated pathways, depending on the cell context, control events related to cytoskeletal rearrangement, stress responses, intracellular vesicle transport, and most notably mitogenic responses. Not every ras-mediated pathway has an established oncogenic role. However, oncogenic pathways that are ras-mediated typically involve proto-oncogene derived protein components in addition to c-ras *(46)*. Most of these proteins were first identified through their involvement in neoplastic transformation before their normal cellular function and connection to ras signaling pathways were elucidated.

Ras is a small G-protein that is anchored to the cytoplasmic side of the plasma membrane. Intracellular signals are carried from the cytoplasmic domain of an activated RTK to ras by a pair of proteins. These proteins form a physical and catalytic connection between the RTK and ras. The first is a noncatalytic adapter protein that binds the RTK, and the second is a catalytic factor that acts on c-ras after binding the adapter protein. The adaptor, Grb2, is an SH2 (for src homology 2) domain protein, a class of intracellular proteins that bind to activated RTKs by recognizing the phosphotyrosine residues in the cytoplasmic domain *(47)*. The protein product of c-*src* is the prototype for this family *(48)*. The SH2 domain is a relatively well conserved structure, usually about 100 amino acids in length. Proteins in this family function to link activated RTKs to a wide range of intracellular signaling cascades that catalyze an array of cellular responses. All SH2 domains are similar in their ability to bind to phosphotyrosine motifs, but the pairing of a particular SH2 domain protein and an activated RTK depends on the amino acid sequence surrounding the phosphotyrosine residues. The specificity of this interaction between activated RTKs and SH2 domain proteins determines the ultimate cellular response brought about by the activation of a specific receptor.

Some SH2 domain proteins possess catalytic activity whereas others serve as adapter proteins, binding both the activated receptor and a separate catalytic protein. Adapter SH2 domain proteins usually have a second protein binding motif, called an SH3 domain, that binds to specific proline-containing motifs. Grb2 functions as an adapter, possessing one SH3 domain flanked by two SH2 domains. Grb2 binds to hSOS1 (the human homolog of the *Drosophila* son of sevenless protein), a guanine nucleotide exchange factor that serves to activate the

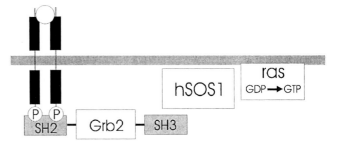

Fig. 4. Protein intermediates required for RTK signaling through the c-ras pathway. The interaction between an activated RTK and c-ras protein is mediated by an SH2 domain protein (like Grb2), and a guanine nucleotide exchange protein (like hSOS1). In this example, the hSOS1 protein is recruited by RTK-bound Grb2, which activates c-ras by accelerating the GDP/GTP exchange reaction.

ras protein *(49)*. It is believed that the binding of hSOS1 to Grb2 activates hSOS1 primarily by bringing it into close proximity to membrane-anchored ras protein (Fig. 4).

The c-*ras* gene product is a GTP-binding protein that shares some limited similarity with the larger heterotrimeric G-protein components of G-protein coupled receptors *(50)*. Ras exists in either an inactive GDP-bound form or an active GTP-bound form *(51)*. It cycles between these states by exchanging bound GDP for GTP (which exists in excess in the cytoplasm), followed by GTP hydrolysis. The three-dimensional conformation of the inactive and active forms of c-ras differ. In the active (GTP-bound) form an effector loop between amino acid residues 32 and 40 is exposed and accessible; whereas this portion of the peptide structure is not exposed and accessible in the inactive GDP-bound state. The c-ras protein is capable of cycling between these forms without the participation of other protein factors, but only very slowly. To cycle at an appreciable rate, separate catalytic proteins interact with ras to accelerate each reaction (Fig. 5). This allows tight regulation of both the activation and inactivation of ras. hSOS1 serves to activate ras by catalyzing GDP/GTP exchange, while ras-GAPs (GTPase activating proteins) inactivate ras by catalyzing the hydrolysis of ras-bound GTP to GDP. In its activated form, ras presumably interacts directly with its downstream effectors to activate them. However, the exact nature of how ras interacts with and activates its substrates is not known.

Three distinct c-*ras* genes have been identified thus far: c-H-*ras*, c-K-*ras*, and c-N-*ras*. All three are very similar in form and function and all three are oncogenically activated by similar mechanisms *(52)*. The oncogenic activation of c-*ras* occurs through permanent trapping of the ras protein in its active GTP-bound state. This can be accomplished in one of three ways: 1) mutations within c-*ras* itself that lock the conformation of the protein in the active GTP-bound form, 2) hyperactivity of a ras-guanine nucleotide exchange factor (like hSOS1), or 3) inactivation of the ras-GAPs responsible for accelerating the downregulation of ras activity. Each of these mechanisms has been observed in different forms of cancer, but all three have the same net effect: the over-stimulation of ras-mediated signaling.

Mutations within c-*ras* itself represent the most common mechanism leading to deregulation of ras protein function.

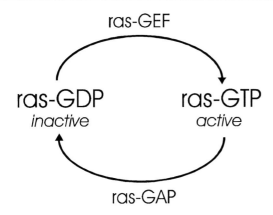

Fig. 5. Regulatory proteins modulate c-ras activity. The c-ras signaling protein cycles between an inactive GDP-bound form and an active GTP-bound form. This cycle is accelerated by the guanine nucleotide exchange factors that target c-ras protein (ras-GEF), and GTPase activating proteins that target c-ras protein (ras-GAP). The ras-GEF catalyzes the GDP/GTP exchange, and the ras-GAP speeds the GTP hydrolysis reaction.

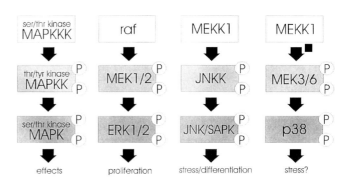

Fig. 6. MAPK modules function through the action of multiple protein kinases. A MAPK module consists of three protein kinases, which act in series. Step 1, A serine/threonine kinase (MAPKKK) phosphorylates and activates a threonine/tyrosine kinase (MAPKK). Step 2, The activated threonine/tyrosine kinase phosphorylates and activates another serine/threonine kinase (MAPK). Step 3, The final activated serine/threonine kinase phosphorylates the final protein substrates, which produce effects. The ERK1/ERK2, JNK/SAPK, and p38 kinase cascades are activated through a similar set of reactions as the MAPK modules. The cellular effects of these cascades are indicated.

Specific ras-activating-point mutations within c-*ras* have been identified (most commonly at codons 12, 13, and 61), all of which result in single amino acid substitutions that leave the ras protein intact and active, but completely unable to hydrolyze bound GTP. Ras GTPase activity requires a nucleophilic water molecule to hydrolyze the γ phosphate group of GTP. The amino acids at positions 12 and 13 are glycine residues and are a part of a small loop that contacts the α and β phosphate groups of the bound guanine nucleotide. The amino acid at position 61 is a glutamine, and is located in the putative GTPase catalytic region. Amino acid substitutions at this position are believed to subtly alter the architecture of the catalytic domain so as to exclude the water molecule, thus disrupting the GTP-hydrolysis reaction *(53)*.

Activating mutations of hSOS1 have not yet been established in any form of cancer. However, aberrant levels of hSOS1 activity are observed in conjunction with constitutively active RTK signaling, confirming the functional role of these proteins in RTK-mediated ras activation. Conversely, loss of ras-GAP function has been shown to disable downregulation of ras activity. Most prominent among the ras-GAP family members in this regard is neurofibromin, the product of the *NF1* tumor-suppressor gene, the activity of which has been observed to be reduced or abolished is several human cancers.

Ras-Mediated Oncogene Pathway Components Ras serves as a vital signaling branch point. One very important ras substrate is c-*raf-1*, the prototype member of a small family of serine/threonine kinases (which also includes genes encoding A-raf and B-raf). The Raf-1 protein, which is activated by ras, also serves as a signaling branch point, mediating pathways governing cell growth, differentiation, cytoskeletal architecture, and apoptosis. Ras-raf-1 signaling is stimulated by an array of extracellular signals that are mediated through RTK activation in a cell-specific manner. Raf-1 is an important component of the ERK1/ERK2 MAP kinase (for mitogen-activated protein kinase) module. There are three known MAP kinase modules, which share functional similarities among their components (Fig. 6), but evoke different cellular responses *(54)*.

The ERK1/ERK2 module which elicits responses involving gene transcription, growth, phospholipid metabolism, and protein synthesis *(55)*. The MAP kinase signaling pathway, which transmits signals from membrane to nucleus via ras and ERK1/ERK2, is well-characterized and has been strongly implicated in oncogenesis (owing to its role in promoting growth and its interactions with other known oncoproteins).

The JNK/SAPK and p38 protein kinase cascades are parallel MAP kinase modules that are involved in differentiation and stress response. The JNK/SAPK pathway is also ras-mediated and both modules activate some of the same transcription factors as the ERK module. However, neither the JNK/SAPK or p38 signaling pathways have been shown to have an oncogenic role in any form of cancer *(46)*.

Ras-mediated signaling also influences changes in cytoskeletal architecture. This involves the Rho family of small G-proteins, which influence various aspects of actin-structure assembly and plasma membrane topology *(57)*. Three prominent members of the Rho gene family are *rho* (which stimulates actin stress-fiber assembly), *rac* (which stimulates membrane ruffling and lammellipoda formation), and *cdc42* (which stimulates filopodia formation). As a part of their function, Rho family proteins activate the JNK/SAPK and p38 signaling pathways *(46)*. Although none of the Rho family members have yet been classified as proto-oncogenes, they appear to negotiate important transformation-associated changes in the cytoskeletal architecture. Such differences between transformed and nontransformed cells include changes in expression patterns of cytoskeletal proteins, decreased organization of the actin cytoskeleton, and the acquisition of anchorage-independent growth. Strengthening the association between Rho activity and transformation is the recent emergence of a growing family of mutant GDP/GTP exchange factors that interact with and constitutively activate Rho family members and have fibroblast-transforming capabilities. These exchange factors activate Rho family members in a similar manner to that of hSOS1

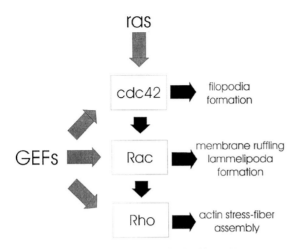

Fig. 7. Functions of the Rho G-protein family and interactions with oncoproteins. The Rho family members cdc42, rho, and rac influence different aspects of cytoskeletal changes in response to neoplastic transformation. These small G-proteins have not been designated proto-oncogene products, but are influenced by various oncoproteins (gray arrows). C-ras activates cdc42, which can stimulate rac and rho (as shown). In addition, all three Rho family members have been shown to respond to stimulation by oncogenic GEF proteins.

and ras, but provide an oncogenic mode of Rho activation that is ras-independent *(58)* (Fig. 7).

Ras-Independent RTK Signaling Proto-oncogenes RTK signaling through ras is only one of numerous intracellular signaling cascades triggered by receptor activation *(59)*. Many SH2 proteins that bind activated receptors function in ras-independent pathways *(60)*. In addition, not all membrane -receptor mediated cascades involve SH2 protein binding. For example, phosphotidyl-insitol-3-kinase (PI3K) signaling is a prominent pathway that is mediated by RTK activity in a ras-independent manner. PI3K can be stimulated by many extracellular signals (not exclusively by RTK signaling) and acts specifically to generate phosphoinositide second messengers. Avian sarcoma virus (ASV16) carries an oncogene encoding a transforming fusion protein called GAG-P3K, which combines portions of the viral GAG protein and PI3K, while retaining PI3K activity *(46)*. PI3K signaling governs a range of cellular responses, including stimulation of protein synthesis, chemotaxis, and membrane ruffling cell survival. In addition, PI3K is also known to activate the serine-threonine protein-kinase AKT, which is related to members of the protein kinase C family and contains an SH2-like domain. AKT (also known as protein kinase B) is thought to be activated by specific interaction with one PI3K phosphoinsitide second messenger, which promotes its membrane association and activation. Paralleling the interaction/activation of AKT is the oncogenic product of the AKT8 murine retrovirus oncogene v-*Akt*, which is myristolated, constitutively membrane associated, and activated *(61)*. AKT acts upstream of the S6 kinase to enhance protein synthesis and plays a role in cellular protection against apoptosis *(62)*.

Other Membrane Receptors as Oncoproteins RTKs are the most clearly understood form of receptors involved in carcinogenesis, but other receptor types are known to play oncogenic roles in human cancer as well. Several types of receptors have been implicated as proto-oncogenes, including steroid hormone receptors (which function within the nucleus), membrane-bound G-protein coupled receptors, and cytokine receptors.

Cytokine receptors (CRs) and their ligands are essential to the development of hematopoietic cells *(63)*. CRs have broad similarities to RTKs in that they are activated by ligand binding followed by assembly into multi-subunit complexes, which is usually a homodimer where the partners share binding to a single ligand molecule. In addition, both CR and RTK activation result in cytoplasmic tyrosine kinase activity. CRs, however, do not have intrinsic tyrosine kinase activity and must interact with separate catalytic subunits upon activation. This lack of intrinsic tyrosine kinase activity may account for the observation that very few activating mutations have been identified in CRs as compared to RTKs. CR signaling overlaps RTK signaling, sharing features such as ras activation and induction of common transcription factors in the nucleus *(64,65)*. Thus far, only four types of activating mutations in CRs have been found *(66)*, affecting: 1) the erythropoietin receptor, 2) the thrombopoietin receptor, 3) the common β-subunit structure shared by granulocyte-macrophage colony-stimulating factor (GM-CSF), interleukin 3 (IL-3), and IL-5 receptors, and 4) the prolactin receptor. Mutations affecting these receptors enable ligand-independent dimerization, and include deletions of ligand-binding domains and point mutations that replace amino acid residues within the normal structure with cysteine residues that can form intermolecular disulfide bonds with similarly mutated receptor proteins. In all cases, the ligand-independent activation of the mutant CRs allows for factor-independent proliferation of hematopoietic cells and are associated with cancers derived from these cell types, such as leukemias and lymphomas.

G-protein coupled receptors are large plasma-membrane proteins that span the lipid bilayer seven times and are thus commonly referred to as serpentine receptors. These receptors contain multiple extracellular and cytoplasmic loops, which connect the seven transmembrane segments. The extracellular loops interact with signaling molecules such as hormones and ions. The intracellular loops interact with heterotrimeric G-proteins, which consist of three subunits (α,ß,γ) and relay the signal from the activated receptor to intracellular effectors. G-proteins are divided into four categories based on broad structural and functional similarities of the α subunits: $G\alpha_s$, $G\alpha_i$, $G\alpha_q$, and $G\alpha_{12}$/$G\alpha_{13}$ *(67)*. The α subunit cycles between an inactive GDP bound state and an active GTP bound state. A ligand-bound/activated serpentine receptor facilitates the conversion of the inactive GDP-bound a subunit to the activated GTP-bound version. The GTP-bound a subunit dissociates from the ß/γ components (which remain dimerized) and both the α and ß/γ components are capable of interacting with downstream effectors. Mitogenic G-protein signaling employs an array of intracellular cascades, including ras-mediated pathways *(68)*.

The α subunit has intrinsic GTPase activity, and thus governs its own inactivation. Oncogenic mutations in the α subunit have been found that abolish the intrinsic GTP hydrolysis activity, resulting in constitutive activation of associated G-protein signaling pathways. Oncogenic mutations have also been found within the serpentine receptor structure, and such mutations drive ligand-independent stimulation of downstream signaling pathways *(69)*.

One example that illustrates the effects of mutations in both the Gα subunit and the serpentine receptor involves the thyroid stimulating hormone (TSH) receptor and its associated G-protein. TSH normally stimulates the growth/differentiation and function of thyrocytes via $Gα_s$ and cAMP-dependent regulatory pathways *(70,71)*. Point mutations in the $Gα_s$ protein (the oncogenic form, which is designated gsp) have been associated with about 30% of hyperfunctioning thyroid adenomas and another 30% have activating mutations in the TSH serpentine receptor *(72,73)*. The *gsp* proto-oncogene is involved in some pituitary growth hormone-secreting tumors, which are growth stimulated by intracellular cAMP-directed pathways *(74)*.

Autocrine stimulation of G-protein receptor-mediated signaling promotes carcinogenesis in small-cell lung carcinoma (SCLC). A characteristic of SCLC is the heterogeneous expression and secretion of many hormones and neuropeptides *(75,76)*. The neuropeptides, most commonly bombesin-like peptides, are thought to be mitogenic for SCLC by completing an autocrine loop, which signals through naturally expressed G-protein receptors to enhance cell growth. This autocrine stimulation funnels through $Gα_q$-stimulated phospholipase C activation and possibly through c-ras signaling involving $Gα_{12}$/$Gα_{13}$ and activation of the MAPK pathway *(77)*.

NUCLEAR ONCOPROTEINS

The ultimate goal of most signal-transduction pathways is to induce alterations in gene-expression patterns. Oncogenic corruption of signal-transduction cascades at any level has functional consequences within the nucleus that involve changes in the level or activity of key transcriptional regulators *(78)*. Many nuclear proteins have been found to be oncogenic in a variety of cancers *(79)*. Nuclear proto-oncogenes have common characteristics that reflect the vital nature of their tight regulation. The induction of their expression in response to growth stimuli is rapidly activated but transient in duration, leading to short bursts of transcription. Nuclear proto-oncogene mRNA and protein products have very short half-lives, preventing prolonged growth-promoting activity in the absence of stimuli. In addition, the activity of the protein products is often modulated by phosphorylation or by association with other nuclear proteins, providing an additional level of post-translational control.

The nuclear targets of mitogenic pathways triggered by membrane-bound receptors are transcription factors that promote the expression of proteins required for cell-cycle progression. Three such transcription factors that play central roles in growth-related and oncogenic transcriptional events are c-*myc*, c-*fos*, and c-*jun*. Characterization of these transcription factors has provided insights into how the regulation of transcriptional events governing growth relies on a careful balance between activation and repression.

The c-*myc* gene product is a nuclear protein that has been shown to be oncogenically activated via many mechanisms leading to overexpression, including gene amplification, increased transcription, and increased mRNA stability. The oncogenic capacity of c-*myc* is reinforced by its involvement in the chromosomal translocation underlying Burkitt's Lymphoma. Functioning as a transcription factor, c-myc is believed to induce genes associated with cell-cycle progression, although the identities of c-myc-target genes remain largely unknown *(10,80)*. Bursts of c-*myc* gene expression are correlated with passage of cells from G_0 into the cell cycle, and loss of one c-*myc* allele has been found to result in slower cell-cycle progression and delayed entry into S-phase.

The c-myc protein functions as a transcription factor by heterodimerizing with a related protein, called max. Protein complexes consisting of myc-max heterodimers bind to specific DNA sequences (termed E boxes) to promote transcription of c-myc-regulated genes *(81)*. The c-myc protein cannot activate transcription without complexing with max, and c-myc protein competes with other factors, (such as mad, mxi, and max itself) for binding to max *(82)*. Unlike myc-max, other max-containing heterodimers cannot activate transcription; some complexes, such as mad-max heterodimers have transcriptional repressor activity. Overexpression of c-myc, as illustrated in the case of Burkitt's lymphoma, results in an imbalance of the ratio of c-myc and max protein. This leads to increased myc-max pairing, increasing transcription of growth-promoting genes that are regulated by c-myc.

The c-*fos* and c-*jun* proto-oncogenes encode nuclear oncoproteins, which heterodimerize to form the transcription factor AP-1 *(83)*. Although the c-jun protein can homodimerize to generate an alternative form of AP-1, the fos-jun heterodimer exhibits higher affinity for the AP-1 binding site. Both the c-fos and c-jun protiens contribute to the transcriptional activation capacity of AP-1, and both are the products of immediate early genes *(84)*. These genes are upregulated at the transcriptional level in response to a range of stimuli including mitogens, pharmacological agents (including phorbol compounds), stress, and heat shock. AP-1 is also post-translationally regulated, being functionally enhanced by phosphorylation on both jun (through the JNK/SAPK pathway) and fos (through the MAPK pathway).

Like c-*myc*, c-*fos*, and c-*jun* were designated as proto-oncogenes through identification of their retroviral oncogene counterparts *(85)*. Both are members of protein families, and heterodimers composed of different members of each family appear to have specific transcriptional regulation capabilities. Although the details are still forthcoming, these interactions between fos and jun family members and their competition for promoter elements indicate the importance of precisely controlled levels of c-*fos* and c-*jun* expression in maintaining the normal cellular state. It has been demonstrated that ras-mediated cellular transformation and malignancy require c-*jun* expression *(86)*. Clinically, dysregulated (elevated) activity of AP-1 is associated with reduced survival for lung-cancer patients, and increased activity of the p-glycoprotein multidrug resistance pump *(87)*. Interestingly, asbestos treatment of trachial epithelial cells has been shown to result in persistant induction of c-*fos* and c-*jun*, providing a potential mechanistic basis for the action of this carcinogen *(88)*.

Steroid hormone/receptor complexes function directly as transcription factors, without the use of an intracellular signaling cascade as in intermediary *(89)*. Steroid hormones are lipid-soluble cholesterol derivatives that pass easily through the plasma membrane and bind to their cognate receptors within the cell. Upon entry into the nucleus, the steroid hormone/receptor complex binds hormone-response elements contained within the promoter sequences of certain genes. Steroid hormone/receptor complexes promote the transcription of a variety of genes, the products of which are involved in many cellular processes depending on the type of cell. Tumors that are derived from hormone-responsive tissues are frequently growth-stimulated and sometimes highly dependent on hormones for growth *(90)*. For example, estrogen is a well-established growth promoter for breast tumors and androgens are established growth promoters for prostate tumors *(91,92)*.

Not all nuclear oncoproteins that regulate transcription are activators. Some transcriptional repressors have been designated as oncogene products. A common feature of these oncogenic repressors is their ability to block expression of genes related to differentiation, thus directing the cell away from differentiation and towards proliferation. The prototype nuclear oncoprotein repressor is the v-*erbA* oncogene component of the avian erythroblastosis virus. This retrovirus, which induces erythroleukemia and sarcomas in chickens, is unusual in that it also contains a second viral oncogene, v-*erbB*, whose cellular counterpart, c-*erbB*, encodes the EGFR. These two viral oncogenes act synergistically to transform infected cells. Although v-*erbB* has transforming activity on its own, v-*erbA* does not. However, v-*erbA* has provided insights into a mechanism by which transcriptional repression of differentiation contributes to oncogenesis *(93,94)*. The c-*erbA* gene encodes the thyroid hormone receptor (TR). The protein product of the v-*erbA* gene is unable to bind thyroid hormone due to point mutations in the hormone-binding site, but is still able to bind the promoter regions within thyroid hormone-responsive genes, which include erythroid differentiation genes. Thyroid hormone-bound c-erbA/TR activates the transcription of genes that regulate erythroid differentiation, whereas the v-*erbA* gene product represses expression of these genes. The c-erbA/TR protein can heterodimerize with other receptors, particularly those of the retinoid family (which are also involved in promoting differentiation). This provides v-*erbA* an additional mechanism for blocking differentiation by acting in a dominant negative fashion to suppress transcription factor activity. Thus, v-*erbA* promotes proliferation indirectly by preventing differentiation *(95)*. Additionally, c-erbA/TR can repress the activity of AP-1, which promotes the transcription of growth-related genes. In contrast, v-*erbA* lacks this repressive ability, further shifting the cell away from differentiation and towards proliferation *(96)*.

Some nuclear oncoproteins do not bind directly to DNA. Proteins that influence chromatin assembly can have broad effects on gene- expression patterns. One example is Bmi1, one of many chromatin structural proteins, which is overexpressed in MuLV-induced thyomas. Bmi1 (and other nuclear proteins with similar functions) is involved in large-scale chromatin architectural changes, which are believed to repress gene expression within large chromatin sections. Bmi1 overexpression is specifically implicated in downregulation of expression of genes required for lymphoid differentiation *(97)*.

REGULATION OF APOPTOSIS AND ONCOGENESIS

Apoptosis, the process of programmed cell death, is mediated by a group of proteins known as the bcl2 family. The bcl2 family consists of both promoters and inhibitors of apoptosis that work together in a carefully balanced design as mediators between survival and suicide *(98)*. In addition, the bcl2 proteins interact with several other intracellular effectors, allowing the apoptotic machinery to communicate with and react to different intracellular signals. Apoptosis plays an extremely important role in preventing carcinogenesis by functioning to remove cells with irreparable DNA damage from the population. Apoptotic malfunction has emerged as an important process underlying carcinogenesis, and dysfunction of bcl2 proteins is central to this process *(99)*.

The exact functions of the bcl2 proteins are being uncovered. The anti-apoptotic family members such as *bcl2* and *bcl-X_L* act in part to shut down mitochondrial permeability. This process involves the opening of membrane pores in the mitochondria to permit the release of oxygen free radicals, calcium ions, and protease activators (the true effectors of cellular destruction) *(100)*. The pro-apoptotic members such as *bad* and *bax*, are proposed to interfere with *bcl2* and *bcl-X_L* by binding them directly, resulting in the formation of nonfunctional heterodimers *(101)*.

Oncogenic changes can deter cells from undergoing apoptosis through direct and indirect means. An imbalance favoring apoptosis inhibitors is the ultimate requirement. This can be established through overexpression or hyperactivity of the anti-apoptotic proteins, or by loss of pro-apoptotic proteins. Altered expression patterns of bcl2 proteins have been observed in some instances. For example, bcl2, the prototype anti-apoptotic protein, is overexpressed in follicular B-cell lymphoma, due to transcriptional deregulation resulting from a chromosomal translocation. Proteins of the bcl2 family are also targets for oncogenic signaling pathways. As shown in Fig. 8, the raf-1 kinase is capable of phosphorylating bad protein, which dissociates from bcl2, allowing bcl2 inhibition of apoptosis to proceed *(102)*. So oncogenic forms of raf-1 can promote neoplastic growth both by promoting growth (through MAPK signaling) and by blocking cell suicide. PI3K-stimulated AKT has also been shown to phosphorylate bad, promoting cell survival in the same manner as raf-1 *(103)*. As the study of apoptosis continues, more connections between oncogenic signaling pathways and the bcl2 protein family are sure to emerge.

POSITIVE MEDIATORS OF METASTASIS

Thus far, the discussion has been limited to the initiation and preliminary growth of the tumor at the primary site. However, the traits that permit neoplastic transformation and early growth of a tumor are insufficient to support progression to a fully metastatic disease. The acquisition of new attributes determines the ultimate ability of a tumor to metastasize. As a tumor grows at the primary site, genetic instability and the continuous accumulation of mutations creates a genetically and phenotypically heterogeneous tumor population. Thus, subsets of cells within

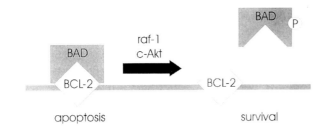

Fig. 8. Regulation of apoptosis by bcl2 family proteins and other oncoproteins. Prevention of apoptosis by bcl2 is promoted by the dissociation of the pro-apoptotic protein bad. The bcl2 protein is attached to the mitochondrial membrane and is suppressed through binding to bad protein. The bcl2 protein is activated following release from bad, which results from phosphorylation of the bad protein by signaling molecules such as raf-1 and c-akt.

the population acquire new traits, resulting in a tumor composed of sub-populations of cells with varying abilities to cope with and manipulate their tissue microenvironment.

Not all tumor types metastasize, but most do. Upon diagnosis, about 30% of patients exhibit detectable metastasis and an equal number are estimated to have already developed undetectable occult metastases. The process of metastasis involves multiple stages, which are collectively referred to as the metastatic cascade *(104)*. The ordered stages of the metastatic cascade are: 1) growth at the primary site, 2) vascularization of the primary tumor, 3) invasion of the surrounding tissue, 4) entry into the circulation, 5) aggregation with circulatory elements and dissemination, 6) arrest within the capillary bed at a secondary site, (7) invasion of the secondary-site tissue, and 8) growth at the secondary site. Each stage of the metastatic cascade is a separate test of survival, and very few cells that begin the process survive to generate a secondary growth. Those tumor cells that possess qualities that enhance their ability to survive at each stage will have the greatest chance of producing a secondary metastasis.

Angiogenesis A primary tumor cannot exceed a certain minimal size (about 2 cm in diameter) without gaining access to the circulatory system. This provides the tumor with both nutrients and waste-disposal capacity. The process of tumor vascularization involves the generation of new blood vessels (angiogenesis) that connect the tumor to the existing circulatory system. Normally, angiogenesis occurs only in specific instances, such as during embryogenesis, wound healing, and the proliferative phase of the female reproductive cycle. Tumor cells can initiate angiogenesis by secreting angiogenic factors, which act in a paracrine manner to stimulate the extension of new blood vessels into the tumor from local branches of the circulatory system *(105,106)*. The number of identified angiogenic factors continues to rise, although the mechanisms of secretion and activity for every factor are not fully understood. Tumor cells release both inducers and inhibitors of angiogenesis and it is thought that the balance between these opposing factors allows a tumor to carefully control neovascularization *(107)*. Some angiogenic factors have wide-spread mitogenic activity, whereas others have more specific roles. For example, vascular endothelial growth factor (VEGF) has specific mito-

genic activity for vascular endothelial cells, whereas basic and acidic fibroblast growth factors (bFGF and aFGF) are pleotropic, stimulating endothelial and epithelial cells, smooth-muscle cells, and fibroblasts. How the expression of angiogenic factors is induced in the neoplastic states remains to be determined, but one intriguing possibility involves regulation by oncogenic signaling pathways that are already known to be associated with growth. For example, VEGF has been shown to be induced by oncogenic mutant forms of c-*ras*, as well as by v-*src* and v-*raf (108)*. Once the primary tumor gains access to the circulatory system, growth at the primary site is no longer limited.

Extracellular Proteases Metastasis requires that tumor cells break away from the primary tumor. For this to occur, loss of cell-to-cell adhesion and gain of cell motility must occur *(109)*. Increased cell motility is also associated with the alteration of cytoskeletal elements (as influenced by Rho family member signaling, for example) *(110)*. Invasion also requires degradation of the basement membranes and interstitial connective tissue that comprise the surrounding tissue. Basement membranes are primarily composed of type IV collagen, but include other important components such as laminin, enactin, osteonectin, and proteoglycans *(111)*. Invasive cells usually traverse basement membranes at least three times during the metastatic process: 1) when escaping the primary growth site, 2) when entering the bloodstream, and 3) when exiting the bloodstream. Interstitial connective tissue consists of cells distributed in a meshwork of collagen fibers, glycoproteins, proteoglycans, and hyaluronic acid. Extracellular proteases are secreted enzymes that mediate the breakdown of basement membranes and interstitial tissue. Those tumor cells with a greater capacity for synthesizing and secreting extracellular proteases will more easily invade surrounding tissues. As one might expect, the highest concentrations of proteases are usually found at the tumor-invasion front, reflecting their role in clearing pathways for dissemination.

A myriad of extracellular proteases are employed by tumor cells. Well-characterized examples include the urokinase-type plasminogen activator (uPA), cathepsins B and D, and various metalloproteases. uPA is a serine protease that converts inactive plasminogen into active plasmin. Plasmin, in turn, is a broad-spectrum protease that catalyzes the degradation of extracellular- tissue components such as fibrin, laminin, fibronectin, and others. The plasminogen to plasmin reaction requires binding of uPA by a membrane-bound receptor that is often expressed at high levels on tumor cells. The presence of the uPA receptor not only accelerates the plasminogen-to-plasmin conversion but also focuses the concentration of active plasmin around the advancing tumor cells *(112)*.

Matrix metalloproteinases (MMPs) are a family of extracellular matrix-degrading zinc-dependent and calcium-dependent proteolytic enzymes *(113)* that have roles in angiogenesis, tissue invasion, and intravasation and extravasation of the circulatory and lymphatic systems. MMPs are secreted by tumors cells and by host stroma tissue in response to tumor cell invasion in a process that is similar to wound healing, demonstrating that metastasis involves communication between tumor and stromal cells. Growth factors, such as EGF, bFGF, PDGF, and

TGF-γ have all been demonstrated to stimulate MMP production by tumors in vivo, providing a potential link between oncogenic signaling through these growth factor-stimulated pathways and the increased expression of MMPs by tumor cells (114).

Routes of Metastatic Dissemination The breakdown of surrounding tissue provides tumor cells with access to one of three routes for dissemination: 1) the lymphatic system, 2) the circulatory system, and 3) direct invasion into surrounding body cavities. There is mounting evidence that the routes taken by different forms of cancer are selective and nonrandom. For example, dissemination through the lymphatic system is characteristic of carcinomas. The walls of lymphatic channels are easily penetrable, and invading cells can be arrested and form tumors within lymph nodes. Lymph-node metastases can then break off and enter the blood stream. Tumor cells can directly invade the circulatory system by a process that is dependent on the vascularization of the primary tumor. Blood vessels recruited by growing tumors are weaker and more easily penetrated than normal blood vessels. Direct invasion into the body cavities by expanding tumor masses usually involves the pleural and peritoneal spaces (115).

Procoagulants and Circulatory Survival The circulatory system is a hazardous place for disseminating tumor cells. Factors that reduce tumor cell survival in the circulatory system include both host immune responses such as macrophage and natural killer (NK) cell activity, and microenvironmental challenges such as blood turbulence and shearing forces within capillaries. Nitric oxide (NO) produced by cytokine-activated endothelial cells is thought to play a range of anti-tumor roles, controlling factors like vasodilation and apoptosis, as well as being directly cytotoxic to tumor cells. Positive mediators at this stage help a tumor cell ward off these challenges. Expression of specific cell-surface and secreted molecules enables disseminating tumor cells to generate a safety cushion that surrounds and protects the cells. This process, called thrombus formation, involves the aggregation of platelets and fibrin deposits around the cell. Tumor cells secrete procoagulents to enhance blood-coagulation mechanisms. They also express receptors (called thrombin receptors) that are thought to be connected to as yet undefined intracellular signaling pathways that activate the tumors cells and increase their adhesive properties. Thrombin stimulation has also been shown to activate platelets and increase their adhesiveness as well, presenting the interesting possibility that tumor-cell/platelet activation is a synergistic process (116).

Aggregation with platelets not only helps protect tumor cells in the circulatory system, but also promotes their arrest within capillary beds at secondary sites (117). Damage to microvessels induced by normal wear and tear and by endothelial-cell shedding creates gaps that are bound by circulating platelets. The binding of tumor cell-associated platelets to these gaps provides a mechanism of tumor-cell arrest. In addition, large tumor-cell aggregates can be trapped within very narrow microvessels. Disseminating tumor cells frequently express adhesion receptors/molecules that enhance their binding and interactions with the endothelial cells and extracellular matrix proteins at secondary sites. A wide range of these cell surface molecules are involved, including integrins, selectins, immunoglobulins, cadherins, and proteoglycans (118).

Secondary-site Growth of Tumors Finally, invasion and growth at the secondary site must be achieved to complete the metastatic cascade. The same mechanisms that promote invasion at the primary site, such as degradation of the surrounding tissue and increased cell motility, are again needed to promote invasion into the secondary site. Furthermore, the ability to colonize a secondary tissue site might require a specific cellular phenotype that is compatible with the tissue microenvironment at that site. This requirement will be dictated by differences in the tissue microenvironments between the primary and secondary sites. Certain secondary sites will provide more suitable microenvironment for specific tumor-cell types (119). This has been reflected in experiments employing animal models that have demonstrated that there are indeed consistent patterns of secondary-site selection for a variety of primary tumor-cell types (120). Despite having microenvironment-specific requirements, the general mechanisms employed by positive mediators to promote growth at the secondary site are very similar to those necessary for growth at the primary site. These include response to specific growth factors, autocrine and paracrine stimulation, and expression of adhesion molecules specific for the secondary site microenvironment (121).

REFERENCES

1. Huebner, R. J. and Todaro, G. J. (1969) Oncogenes of RNA tumor viruses as determinants of cancer. *Proc. Natl. Acad. Sci. USA* **64**:1087–1094.
2. Bishop, J. M. (1983) Cellular oncogenes and retroviruses. *Ann. Rev. Biochem.* **52**:301–354.
3. Varmus, H. E. (1982) Form and function of retroviral proviruses. *Science* **216**:812–820.
4. Robinson, H. L. (1992) Oncogene transduction and activation. *Dev. Biol. Stand.* **76**:165–169.
5. Jonkers, J. and Berns, A. (1996) Retroviral insertional mutagenesis as a strategy to identify cancer genes. *Biochim. Biophys. Acta.* **1287**:29–57.
6. Cory, S. (1986) Activation of cellular oncogenes in hemopoietic cells by chromosome translocation. *Adv. Cancer Res.* **47**:189–234.
7. Cotter, F. E. (1993) Molecular pathology of lymphomas. *Cancer Surv.* **16**:157–174.
8. Kluin, P. M. and van Krieken, J. H. (1991) The molecular biology of B-cell lymphoma: clinicopathologic implications. *Ann. Hematol.* **62**:95–102.
9. Korsmeyer, S. J. (1992) Chromosomal translocations in lymphoid malignancies reveal novel proto-oncogenes. *Ann. Rev. Immunol.* **10**:785–807.
10. Taub, R., Kirsch, I., Morton, C., Lenoir, G., Swan, D., Tronick, S., et al. (1982) Translocation of the c-myc gene into the immunoglobulin heavy chain locus in human Burkitt lymphoma and murine plasmacytoma cells. *Proc. Natl. Acad. Sci. USA* **79**:7837–7841.
11. Kato, G. J. and Dang, C. V. (1992) Function of the c-Myc oncoprotein. *FASEB J.* **6**:3065–3072.
12. de The, G. (1993). The etiology of Burkitt's lymphoma and the history of the shaken dogmas. *Blood Cells* **19**:667–673.
13. Gishizky, M. L. (1996) Molecular mechanisms of Bcr-Abl-induced oncogenesis. *Cytokines Mol. Ther.* **2**:251–261.
14. Pendergast, A. M., Quilliam, L. A., Cripe, L. D., Basssing, C. H., Dai, Z., Der, C. J., et al. (1993) BCR-ABL-induced oncogenesis is mediated by direct interaction with the SH2 domain of the Grb-2 adaptor protein. *Cell* **75**:175–185.

15. McWhirter, J. R. and Wang J. Y. (1997) Effect of Bcr sequences on the cellular function of the Bcr-Abloncoprotein. *Oncogene.* **15**:1625–1634.

16. Kuss, B. J., Deeley, R. G., Cole, S. P., Willman, C. L., Kopecky, K. J., Wolman, S. R., et al. (1996) The biological significance of the multidrug resistance gene MRP in inversion 16 leukemias. *Leukemia Lymphoma* **20**:357–364.

17. Fardel, O., Lecureur, V., and Guillouzo, A. (1996) The P-glycoprotein multidrug transporter. *Gen. Pharmacol.* **27**:1283–1291.

18. Strauss, B. S. (1992) The origin of point mutations in human tumor cells. *Cancer Res.* **52**:249–253.

19. Alitalo, K. and Schwab, M. (1986) Oncogene amplification in tumor cells. *Adv. Cancer Res.* **47**:235–281.

20. Takahashi, T., Obata, Y., Sekido, Y., Hida, T., Ueda, R., Watanabe, H., et al. (1989) Expression and amplification of myc gene family in small-cell lung cancer and its relation to biological characteristic. *Cancer Res.* **49**:2683–2688.

21. Koivisto, P., Visakorpi, T., and Kallioniemi, O. P. (1996) Androgen receptor gene amplification: a novel molecular mechanism forendocrine therapy resistance in human prostate cancer. *Scand. J. Clin. Lab. Invest. Suppl.* **226**:57–63.

22. Gullick, W. J. (1991) Prevalence of aberrant expression of the epidermal growth factor receptor in human cancers. *Br. Med. Bull.* **47**:87–98.

23. Leal, F., Williams, L. T., Robbins, K. C., and Aaronson, S .A. (1985) Evidence that the v-sis gene product transforms by interaction with the receptor for platelet-derived growth factor. *Science* **230**:327–330.

24. Potapvoa, O., Fakhrai, H., and Mercola, D., (1996) Growth factor PDGF-B/v-sis confers a tumorigenic phenotype to human tumor cells bearing PDGF receptors but not to cells devoid of receptors: evidence for an autocrine, but not a paracrine, mechanism. *Int. J. Cancer.* **66**:669–677.

25. Westermark, B. and Heldin, C. H. (1986) Platelet-derived growth factor as a mediator of normal and neoplastic cell proliferation. *Med. Oncol. Tumor Pharmacother.* **3**:177–183.

26. Heldin, C. H., Betsholtz, C., Johnsson, A., Nister, M., Ek, B., Ronnstrand, L., et al. (1985) Platelet-derived growth factor: mechanism of action and relation to oncogenes. *J. Cell. Sci. Suppl.* **3**:65–76.

27. Ponten, F., Ren, Z., Nister, M., Westermark, B., and Ponten, J. (1991) Epithelial-stromal interactions in basal cell cancer. *J. Invest. Dermatol.* **102**:304–309.

28. Chaudhry, A., Funa, K., and Oberg, K. (1993) Expression of growth factor peptide and their receptors in neuroendocrine tumors of the digestive system. *Acta Oncol.* **32**:107–144.

29. Boyle, W. J. (1992) Growth factors and tyrosine kinase receptors during development and cancer. *Curr. Opin. Oncol.* **4**:156–162.

30. Kazlauskas, A. (1994) Receptor tyrosine kinases and their targets. *Curr. Opin. Genet. Dev.* **4**:5–14.

31. Lemmon, M. A. and Schlessinger, J. (1994) Regulation of signal transduction and signal diversity by receptor oligomerization. *Trends Biochem. Sci.* **19**:459–463.

32. Voldborg, B. R., Damstrup, L., Spang-Thomsen, M., and Poulsen, H. S. (1997) Epidermal growth factor receptor (EGFR) and EGFR mutations, function and possible role in clinical trials. *Ann. Oncol.* **8**:1197–1206.

33. Eccles, S. A., Modjtahedi, H., Box, G., Court, W., Sandle, J., and Dean, C. J. (1994) Significance of the c-erbB family of receptor tyrosine kinases in metastatic cancer and their potential as targets for immunotherapy. *Invasion Metastasis* **14**:337–348.

34. Yamanaka, Y., Friess, H., Kobrin, M. S., Buchler, M., Beger, H. G., and Korc, M. (1993) Coexpression of epidermal growth factor and its ligands in human pancreatic cancer is associated with enhanced tumor aggressiveness. *Anticancer Res.* **13**:565–570.

35. Harris, A. L., Nicholson, J. R. C., Sainsbury, D., Neal, D., Smith, K., Horne, C. H. W., et al. (1991) Epidermal growth factor: a marker of early relapse in breast cancer and tumor stage progression in bladder cancer: interaction with neu. *Cancer Cells* **7**:353–357.

36. Harris, A. L., Nicholson, S., Sainsbury, R., Wright, C., and Farndon, J. (1992) Epidermal growth factor and other oncogenes as prognostic markers. *J. Natl. Cancer Inst.* **11**:181–198.

37. Rodrigues, G. A. and Morag, P. (1993) Dimerization mediated through a leucine zipper activates the oncogenic potential of *met* receptor tyrosine kinase. *Mol. Cell. Biol.* **13**:6711–6722.

38. Morris, S. W. Kirsten, M. N., Valentine, M. B., Dittmer, K. G., Shapiro, D. N., Saltman, D. L., et al. (1994) Fusion of a kinase gene, *ALK*, to a nucleolar protein gene, *NPM*, in non-Hodgkins lymphoma. *Science* **263**:1281–1284.

39. Edery, P., Eng, C., Munnich, A., and Lyonnet, S. (1997) RET in human development and oncogenesis. *BioEssays* **19**:389–395.

40. van Heyningen, V. (1994) One gene : four syndromes. *Nature* **367**:319–320.

41. Komminoth, P. (1997) The RET proto-oncogene in medullary and papillary thyroid carcinoma. Molecular features, pathophysiology and clinical implications. *Virchows Arch.* **431**:1–9.

42. Schuchardt, A., D'Agati, V., Larsson-Blomberg, L., Costantini, F., and Pachnis, V. (1994) Defects in the kidney and enteric nervous system of mice lacking the tyrosine kinase receptor Ret. *Nature* **367**:380–383

43. Hofstra, R. M., Landsvater, R. M., Ceccherini, I., Stulp, R. P., Stelwagen, T., Luo, Y., et al. (1994) A mutation in the *RET* proto-oncogene associated with multiple endocrine neoplasia type 2B and sporadic medullary thyroid carcinoma. *Nature* **367**:375–383.

44. Hockenbery, D. M. (1992) The bcl-2 oncogene and apoptosis. *Semin. Immunol.* **4**:413–420.

45. Joneson, T. and Bar-Sagi, D. (1997) Ras effectors and their role in mitogenesis and oncogenesis. *J. Mol. Med.* **75**:587–593.

46. Hunter, T. (1997) Oncoprotein networks. *Cell* **88**:333–346.

47. Lowenstein, E. J., Daly, R. J., Batzer, A. G., Li, W., Margolis, B., Lammers, R., et al. (1992) The SH2 and SH3 domain-containing protein GRB2 links receptor tyrosine kinases to ras signaling. *Cell* **70**:431–442.

48. Thomas, S. M. and Brugge, J. S. (1997) Cellular functions regulated by src family kinases. *Ann. Rev. Cell. Dev. Biol.* **13**:513–609.

49. Rozakis-Adcock, M., Fernley, R., Wade, J., Pawson, T., and Bowtell, D. (1993) The SH2 and SH3 domains of mammalian Grb2 couple the EGF receptor to the Ras activator mSos1. *Nature* **363**:83–85.

50. Khosravi-Far, R., Campbell, S., Rossman, K. L., and Der, C. J. (1998) Increasing complexity of Ras signal transduction: involvement of Rho family proteins. *Adv. Cancer Res.* **72**:57–107.

51. Downward, J. (1996) Control of ras activation. *Cancer Surv.* **27**:87–100.

52. Bos, J. L. (1989) ras oncogenes in human cancer: a review. *Cancer Res.* **49**:4682–4689.

53. Pai, E. F., Krengel, U., Petsko, G. A., Goody, R. S., Kabsch, W., and Wittinghofer, A. (1990) Refined crystal structure of the triphosphate conformation of H-ras p21 at 1.35 A resolution: implications for the mechanism of GTP hydrolysis. *EMBO J.* **9**:2351–2359.

54. Pelech, S. L. and Sanghera, J. S. (1992) Mitogen-activated protein kinases: versatile transducers for cell signaling. *Trends. Biochem. Sci.* **17**:233–238.

55. Williams, N. G., Paradis, H., Agarwal, S., Charest, D. L., Pelech, S. L., and Roberts, T. M. (1993) Raf-1 and p21v-ras cooperate in the activation of mitogen-activated protein kinase. *Proc. Natl. Acad. Sci. USA* **90**:5772–5776.

56. Williams, N. G. and Roberts T. M. (1994) Signal transduction pathways involving the Raf proto-oncogene. *Cancer Metastasis Rev.* **13**:105–116.

57. Khosravi-Far, R., Campbell, S., Rossman, K. L., and Der, C. J. (1998) Increasing complexity of Ras signal transduction: involvement of Rho family proteins. *Adv. Cancer Res.* **72**:57–107.

58. Olson, M. F. (1996) Guanine nucleotide exchange factors for the Rho GTPases: a role inhuman disease? *J. Mol. Med.* **74**:563–57.

59. Weiss, F. U., Daub, H., and Ullrich, A. (1997) Novel mechanisms of RTK signal generation. *Curr. Opin. Genet. Dev.* **7**:80–86.

60. Birge, R. B., Knudsen, B. S., Besser, D., and Hanafusa, H. (1996) SH2 and SH3-containing adaptor proteins: redundant or indepen-

dent mediators of intracellular signal transduction? *Genes Cells* **1**:595–613.

61. Ahmed, N. N., Franke, T. F., Bellacosa, A., Datta, K., Gonzalez-Portal, M. E., Taguchi, T., et al. (1993) The proteins encoded by c-akt and v-akt differ in post-translational modification, subcellular localization and oncogenic potential. *Oncogene.* **8**:1957–1963.

62. Burgering, B. M. and Coffer, P. J. (1995) Protein kinase B (c-Akt) in phosphatidylinositol-3-OH kinase signal transduction. *Nature* **376**:599–602.

63. Drachman, J. G. and Kaushansky, K. (1995) Structure and function of the cytokine receptor superfamily. *Curr. Opin. Hematol.* **2**:22–28.

64. Itoh, T., Muto, A., Watanabe, S., Miyajima, A., Yokota, T., and Arai, K. (1996) Granulocyte-macrophage colony-stimulating factor provokes RAS activation and transcription of c-fos through different modes of signaling. *J. Biol. Chem.* **271**:7587–7592.

65. Cohen, P. (1996) Dissection of protein kinase cascades that mediate cellular response to cytokines and cellular stress. *Adv. Pharmacol.* **36**:15–27.

66. Gonda, T. J. and D'Andrea, R. J. (1997) Activating mutations in cytokine receptors: implications for receptor function and role in disease. *Blood* **89**:355–369.

67. Wess, J. (1997) G-protein-coupled receptors: molecular mechanisms involved in receptor activation and selectivity of G-protein recognition. *FASEB J.* **11**:346–354.

68. Bokoch, G.M. (1996) Interplay between Ras-related and heterotrimeric GTP binding proteins: lifestyles of the BIG and little. *FASEB J.* **10**:1290–1295.

69. Dhanasekaran, N., Heasley, L. E., and Johnson, G. L. (1995) G protein-coupled receptor systems involved in cell growth and oncogenesis. *Endocrinol. Rev.* **16**:259-270.

70. Uyttersprot, N., Allgeier, A., Baptist, M., Christophe, D., Coppee, F., Coulonval, K., et al. (1997) The cAMP in thyroid: from the TSH receptor to mitogenesis and tumorigenesis. *Adv. Second Messenger Phosphoprotein Res.* **31**:125–140.

71. Duh, Q. Y. and Grossman, R. F. (1995) Thyroid growth factors, signal transduction pathways, and oncogenes. *Surg. Clin. North Am.* **75**:421–43.

72. Vallar, L. (1990) GTPase-inhibiting mutations activate the alpha-chain of Gs in human tumours. *Biochem. Soc. Symp.* **56**:165–170.

73. Parma, J., Duprey, L., Van Sande, J., Cochaux, P., Gervy, C., Mochel, J., et al. (1993) Somatic mutations in the thyrotropin receptor gene cause hyperfuntioning thyroid adenomas. *Nature* **365**:649–651.

74. Vallar, L. (1996) Oncogenic role of heterotrimeric G-proteins. *Cancer Surv.* **27**:325–338.

75. Sorenson, G. D., Bloom, S. R., Ghatei, M. A., Del Prete, S. A., Cate, C. C., and Pettengill, O. S. (1982) Bombesin production by human small cell carcinoma of the lung. *Regul. Pept.* **4**:59–66.

76. Sorenson, G. D., Pettengill, O. S., Brinck-Johnsen, T., Cate, C. C., and Maurer, L. H. (1981) Hormone production by cultures of small-cell carcinoma of the lung. *Cancer* **47**:1289–1296.

77. Woll, P. J. and Rozengurt, E. (1989) Multiple neuropeptides mobilise calcium in small cell lung cancer: effects of vasopressin, bradykinin, cholecystokinin, galanin and neurotensin. *Biochem. Biophys. Res. Commun.* **164**:66–73.

78. Lewin, B. (1991) Oncogenic conversion by regulatory changes in transcription factors. *Cell* **64**:303–12.

79. Lucibello, F. C. and Muller R. (1992) Transcription factor encoding oncogenes. *Rev. Physiol. Biochem. Pharmacol.* **119**:226–257.

80. Schmidt, E. V. (1996) MYC family ties. *Nature Genet.* **14**:8–10.

81. Kato, G. J., Wechsler, D. S., and Dang, C. V. (1992) DNA binding by the Myc oncoproteins. *Cancer Treat. Res.* **63**:313–325.

82. Henriksson, M. and Luscher, B. (1996) Proteins of the Myc network: essential regulators of cell growth and differentiation. *Adv. Cancer. Res.* **68**:109–182.

83. Ransone, L. J., Verma, I. M. (1990) Nuclear proto-Oncogenes Fos and Jun. *Ann. Rev. Cell Biol.* **6**:539–57.

84. Weisz, A. and Bresciani, F. (1993) Estrogen regulation of proto-oncogenes coding for nuclear proteins. *Crit. Rev. Oncogen.* **4**:361–388.

85. Rahmsdorf, H. J. (1996) Jun: transcription factor and oncoprotein. *J. Mol. Med.* **74**:725–774.

86. Johnson, R., Spiegelman, B., Hanahan, D., and Wisdom, R. (1996) Cellular transformation and malignancy induced by ras require c-jun. *Mol. Cell. Biol.* **16**:4504–4511.

87. Volm, M. (1993) P-glycoprotein associated expression of c-fos and c-jun products in human lung carcinoma. *Anticancer Res.* **13**:375–378.

88. Heintz, N. H., Janssen, Y. M., and Mossman, B. T. (1993) Persistent induction of c-Fos and c-Jun expression by asbestos. *Proc. Natl. Acad. Sci. USA* **90**:3299–3303.

89. Vedeckis, W. V. (1992) Nuclear receptors, transcriptional regulation, and oncogenesis. *Proc. Soc. Exp. Biol. Med.* **199**:1–12.

90. Schuchard, M., Landers, J. P., Sandhu, N. P., and Spelsberg, T. C. (1993) Steroid hormone regulation of proto-oncogenes. *Endocrine Rev.* **14**:659–669.

91. Griffiths, K., Morton, S., and Nicholson, R. I. (1997) Androgens, androgen receptors, antiandrogens and the treatment of prostate cancer. *Eur. Urol.* **32**:24–40.

92. Greene, G. L., Sharma, V., and Cheng, L. (1996) Estrogen receptor structure and function in breast cancer cells. *Accompl. Cancer Res.* pp. 147–165.

93. Damm, K. (1993) ErbA: Tumor suppressor turned oncogene? *FASEB J.* **7**:904–909.

94. Renkaitz, R. (1993) Repression mechanism of v-*erbA* and other members of the steroid receptor superfamily. *Ann. NY Acad. Sci.* **684**:1–10.

95. Schroeder, C., Gibson, L., Zenke, M., and Beug, H. (1992) Modulation of normal erythroid differentiation by the endogenous thyroid hormone and retinoic acid receptors: A possible target for v-erbA oncogene action. *Oncogene* **7**:217–227.

96. Desbois, C., Aubert, D., Legrand, C., Pain, B., and Samarut, J. (1991) A novel mechanism of action for v-ErbA: abrogation of the inactivation of transcription factor AP-1 by retinoic acid and thyroid hormone receptors. *Cell* **67**:731–40.

97. Gunster, M.. J, Satijn, D. P., Hamer, K. M., den Blaauwen, J. L., de Bruijn, D., Alkema, M. J., et al. (1997) Identification and characterization of interactions between the vertebrate polycomb-group protein BMI1 and human homologs of polyhomeotic. *Mol. Cell. Biol.* **17**:2326–2335.

98. Brown, R. (1997) The bcl-2 family of proteins. *Br. Med. Bull.* **53**:466–477.

99. Williams, G. T. (1991) Programmed cell death: apoptosis and oncogenesis. *Cell* **65**:1097–1098.

100. Mignotte, B. and Vayssiere, J. L. (1998) Mitochondria and apoptosis. *Eur. J. Biochem.* **252**:1–15.

101. Jacobson, M. D. (1997) Apoptosis: Bcl-2-related proteins get connected. *Curr. Biol.* **7**:R277–R281.

102. Pritchard, C. and McMahon, M. (1997) Raf revealed in life-or-death decisions. *Nature Genet.* **16**:214–215.

103. Franke, T. F. and Cantley, L. C. (1997) A Bad kinase makes good. *Nature* **390**:116–117.

104. Ahmad, A. and Hart, I. R. (1997) Mechanisms of metastasis. *Crit. Rev. Oncol. Hematol.* **26**:163–173.

105. Pluda, J. M. (1997) Tumor-associated angiogenesis: mechanisms, clinical implications, and therapeutic strategies. *Semin. Oncol.* **24**:203–218.

106. Folkman, J. and Shing, Y. (1992). Angiogenesis (minireview). *J. Biol. Chem.* **267**:10931–10934.

107. Kumar, R., Yoneda, J., Bucana, C. D., and Fidler, I. J. (1998) Regulation of distinct steps of angiogenesis by different angiogenic molecules. *Int. J. Oncol.* **12**:749–757.

108. Rak, J., Filmus, J., Finkenzeller, G., Grugel, S., Marme, D., and Kerbel, R. S. (1995) Oncogenes as inducers of tumor angiogenesis. *Cancer Metastasis Rev.* **14**:263–277.

109. Tang, D. G. and Honn, K. V. (1994) Adhesion molecules and tumor metastasis: an update. *Invasion Metastasis.* **14**:109–122.

110. Button, E., Shapland, C., and Lawson, D. (1995) Actin, its associated proteins and metastasis. *Cell Motility Cytoskeleton* **30**:247–251.

111. Tryggvason, K., Hoyhtya, M., and Salo, T. (1987) Proteolytic degradation of extracellular matrix in tumor cell invasion. *Biochim. Biophys. Acta.* **907**:191–207.

112. Andreasen, P. A., Kjoller, L., Christensen, L., and Duffy, M. J. (1997) The urokinase-type plasminogen activator system in cancer metastasis: a review. *Int. J. Cancer.* **72**:1–22.

113. Matrisan, L. M. (1992) The matrix-degrading metalloproteases. *Bioessays* **14**:455–463.

114. Birkedal-Hansen, H., Moore, W. G., Bodden, M. K., Windsor, L. J., Birkedal-Hansen, B., DeCarlo, A., et al. (1993) Matrix metalloproteinases: a review. *Crit. Rev. Oral. Biol. Med.* **4**:197–250.

115. Morgan-Parkes, J. H. (1995) Metastases: mechanisms, pathways, and cascades. *Am. J. Roentgenol.* **164**:1075–1082.

116. Ordinas, A., Diaz-Ricart, M., Almirall, L., and Bastida, E. (1990) The role of platelets in cancer metastasis. *Blood Coagulation Fibrinolysis* **1**:707–711.

117. Pauli, B. U., Augustin-Voss, H.G., el-Sabban, M. E., Johnson, R. C., and Hammer, D. A. (1990) Organ-preference of metastasis. The role of endothelial cell adhesion molecules. *Cancer Metastasis Rev.* **9**:175–189.

118. Albelda, S. M. and Buck, C. A. (1990) Integrins and other cell adhesion molecules. *FASEB. J.* **4**:2868–2880.

119. Auerbach, R. (1998) Patterns of tumor metastasis: organ selectivity in the spread of cancer cells. *Lab. Invest.* **58**:361–364.

120. Togo, S., Wang, X., Shimada, H., Moossa, A. R., and Hoffman, R. M. (1995) Cancer seed and soil can be highly selective: human-patient colon tumor lung metastasis grows in nude mouse lung but not colon or subcutis. *Anticancer Res.* **15**:795–798.

121. Nicolson, G. L. (1998) Organ specificity of tumor metastasis: role of preferential adhesion, invasion and growth of malignant cells at specific secondary sites. *Cancer Metastasis Rev.* **7**:143–188.

5 Inactivation of Negative Growth Regulators During Neoplastic Transformation

Kara N. Smolinski, MD, PhD and Stephen J. Meltzer, MD

INTRODUCTION

THE ROLE OF ABNORMAL CELL PROLIFERATION IN TUMORIGENESIS One of the hallmarks of cancer cells is their capacity for unchecked growth and clonal expansion, which leads to the progressive accumulation of tumor cells. The etiology of tumor cell development has been the subject of intensive scientific investigation and speculation for centuries and has spawned a fascinating litany of theories *(1)*. The first modern physician to advance a comprehensive clinical definition of cancer was Dr. R.A. Willis, who stated in the introduction to his 1950 text, *Pathology of Tumours*, that "a tumour is an abnormal mass of tissue, the growth of which exceeds and is uncoordinated with that of the normal tissues, and persists in the same excessive manner after cessation of the stimuli which evoked the change" *(2)*. We now know that this increased proliferative potential is the result of the dysregulation of several cellular processes, including disruption of cellular differentiation, abnormal communication between tumor cells and their microenvironment, failure of induction of programmed cell death, and loss of response to the normal regulators of cell proliferation.

Increased cell proliferation is considered to be not only a result of cell transformation, but is also an active contributor to its development. According to the current multistage model, tumor progression is driven by the accumulation of multiple somatic genetic changes. Tumor initiation occurs as a result of an irreversible, mutagenic event, whereas tumor promotion involves the proliferation of initiated cells in response to mitogenic stimuli. An increase in cell proliferation confers a small but appreciable risk for the generation of mutations in cancer-related genes through a combination of errors in DNA replication and repair and abnormal chromosome segregation. The resultant genetic instability and cell heterogeneity, and the expansion of one or more clonal populations under selective pressure from the host, then leads to the development of a fully malignant phenotype.

Many clinically recognized risk factors for cancer are factors that stimulate cell proliferation, including the hormones estrogen and testosterone, infectious agents such as hepatitis B virus (HBV) and human papilloma virus (HPV), and sites of chronic irritation and/or inflammation as seen in ulcerative colitis, reflux esophagitis, or asbestosis. Many regulatory proteins involved in the transduction of growth-stimulatory signals are also implicated in the development of cancer; in their tumorigenic or activated form they are called oncogenes. These include growth factors such as epidermal growth factor (EGF), growth-factor receptors like the EGF receptor (EGFR), cytoplasmic signal transducers such as the c-*ras* family of GTP-binding proteins, and nuclear transcription factors like c-*fos* and c-*myc*.

NEGATIVE REGULATORS OF CELL PROLIFERATION In light of the role of increased cell proliferation in tumor development, it is not surprising that many factors negatively regulating cell proliferation are targets of inactivation or loss in tumor cells. These factors display a wide range of cellular activities, including regulation of cell-cycle progression, DNA repair, stimulation of apoptosis, transcriptional regulation, and intercellular communication. Many individual cell-growth regulators have multiple functions and interact with each other in a complex and dynamic fashion. It is apparent that the coordinated and integrated response of the cell to the highly variable composite of growth signals is quite sophisticated.

During the last 10 years, numerous genes have been shown to be deleted and/or mutated in human cancer. Although many are considered putative tumor-suppressor genes, not all have met the rigorous definition of this gene class. Characteristics of tumor-suppressor genes include: 1) homozygous loss or inactivation in a significant proportion of human tumors or tumor types; 2) demonstrated function related to negative regulation of cell growth, survival, or differentiation; and 3) ability to suppress tumorigenicity in cells that do not have normal alleles of the gene in question. A comparison of the properties of tu-

From: *The Molecular Basis of Human Cancer* (W. B. Coleman and G. J. Tsongalis, eds.), © Humana Press Inc., Totowa, NJ.

Table 1
Characteristic Properties of Proto-oncogenes and Tumor-Suppressor Genes

Property	Proto-oncogenes	Tumor-suppressor genes
Number of mutational events required	One	Two
Function of mutation	Dominant (gain of function)	Recessive (loss of function)
Germline inheritance	No	Yes
Effect on cell growth	Stimulates cell growth	Suppresses cell growth
Types of mutation	Activating point mutations Gene rearrangements Gene amplification	Frameshift mutations, Point mutations Homozygous deletion
Types of epigenetic alteration	?	Promoter methylation

mor-suppressor genes and proto-oncogenes is provided in Table 1.

Mutations in several tumor-suppressor genes segregate with disease in hereditary cancer syndromes, and it was through the careful study of affected families that many important tumor-suppressor genes were identified. One of the hallmarks of tumor-suppressor gene inactivation is mutation of one allele accompanied by deletion of the other allele. These deletions often span many megabases of genomic DNA and may be detectable by routine cytologic or molecular techniques, allowing researchers to identify common regions of loss from a large panel of tumors. Such regions are suspected to harbor one or more important suppressor genes, and are screened for open reading frames that are lost or mutated in a high proportion of tumors. The ultimate test for a tumor-suppressor gene is its ability to suppress tumorigenicity when re-introduced into cells that have lost the normal gene function.

Regulation of cell proliferation involves a complex system designed to integrate internal and external growth signals. In general, cell proliferation is predominantly regulated at the level of the cell cycle and involves the regulation of the retinoblastoma protein (pRb) by the cyclin-dependent kinases (cdk) and their inhibitors. This pathway functions in all normal, dividing cells to coordinate cell growth with DNA replication and cell division. The growth of many cells is inhibited by exposure to transforming growth factor-β (TGF-β) ligand, and the TGF-β signaling pathway can interact with the Rb pathway to alter cell-cycle kinetics. Under conditions in which the cell is stressed or damaged, cell division ceases and the damaged cell is repaired or eliminated. The most well-characterized damage-response pathway involves the p53 tumor-suppressor protein, which is involved in many cellular functions, including the cell cycle, apoptosis, and DNA repair. The p53 damage-response pathway interacts with several distinct cellular pathways, including the Rb pathway. Disturbances of one or more of these three signaling pathways—the Rb cell-cycle pathway, the TGF-β growth inhibition pathway, and the p53 damage-response pathway—are implicated in the majority of human cancers, underscoring their importance in restraining cell proliferation and in suppressing cell transformation.

THE RB PATHWAY

THE RETINOBLASTOMA-SUSCEPTIBILITY GENE The
Rb pathway is central to cell-cycle control and its components are common targets of modulation by regulators of cell proliferation. The retinoblastoma-susceptibility protein (pRb) is the prototype tumor suppressor. It is worthwhile to elaborate on the discovery of the *Rb1* gene, as it serves as an excellent model for the role of this class of genes in human cancer.

In 1971, Alfred Knudson, a pediatrician, developed a theory to explain the genesis of retinoblastoma, a pediatric tumor that involves the retinal epithelium, based on his observations of the clinical presentation of the disease *(3)*. Knudson noted that retinoblastoma occurred either as a single, unilateral tumor, which usually presented in toddlers, or as a multi-tumor, bilateral disease seen in infants. Familial cases of retinoblastoma were also reported that were bilateral and multifocal. He proposed his now-famous "two-hit hypothesis," wherein the development of retinoblastoma required two mutations to occur in the same cell. Knudson predicted that one of these mutations was inherited in the germline of patients with hereditary or multifocal disease, increasing the relative risk for the disease in these patients. In 1973, Knudson's hypothesis was expanded by David Comings, who proposed that inactivation of only a single gene was responsible for tumor formation *(4)*. The development of a sporadic tumor required inactivating mutations to occur in both somatic alleles of the same cell; familial and multifocal cases would be transmitted through the inheritance of one mutated allele, with only a single somatic mutation required for neoplastic transformation. Multifocal disease occurs as a result of a new mutation that develops in one of the germ cells of the patient's parents prior to fertilization; thus, the parents are not affected.

The substantiation of Knudson's hypothesis culminated 16 yr later after a substantial amount of ceaseless investigation, and is a triumph of molecular medicine. Restriction-fragment length polymorphism (RFLP) analysis of genomic DNA from a series of retinoblastoma tumors had revealed a small conserved region of genomic DNA loss at chromosome 13q14. Several laboratories painstakingly analyzed this region for the

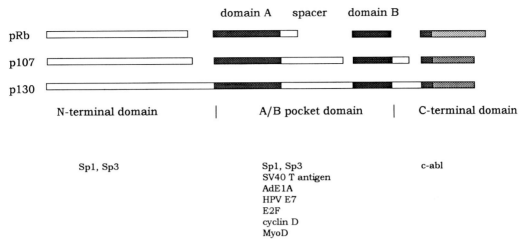

Fig. 1. The pRB family of cell-cycle regulators. pRb and the related proteins p107 and p130 possess three defined domains: an N-terminal domain, an A/B pocket domain, and a C-terminal domain. p107 and p130 also contain a spacer domain within the A/B pocket domain. Several proteins known to interact with specific pRb domains are indicated.

presence of candidate *Rb* genes, which were then analyzed for changes in expression patterns in retinoblastoma and other tumor cell lines. The *Rb1* gene was identified in 1986–1987 by three independent investigators *(5–7)*, and was subsequently shown to be biallelically lost or mutated in all cases of sporadic and hereditary retinoblastoma and to suppress tumorigenicity when reintroduced into nullizygous cell lines *(8)*, thus fulfilling two important criteria for the identification of the predisposing suppressor gene. Expression of a normal pRb has not been detected in any case of primary retinoblastoma or in any retinoblastoma tumor cell line. The importance of *Rb1* in the regulation of cell proliferation has been demonstrated by the involvement of dysregulation of the Rb pathway in the majority of human cancers. Knudson's original two-hit hypothesis has now been expanded into a multi-hit model in which cancer is believed to result from the accumulation of mutations in many genes. The most well-characterized multi-hit model for the development of a human cancer is that proposed by Fearon and Vogelstein for colorectal carcinoma, which predicts that colorectal carcinoma develops as a results of an ordered progression of mutations in specific oncogenes and tumor-suppressor genes, including *APC*, c-K-*ras*, and *p53* *(9)*.

STRUCTURE AND FUNCTION OF THE RB TUMOR-SUPPRESSOR PROTEIN The *Rb1* gene encodes a 4.7 kb mRNA that is translated into a 928 amino acid protein. pRb is ubiquitously expressed in all tissues *(7)*. pRb contains three major domains: the N-terminal domain, the A/B pocket domain, and the C-terminal domain *(8,10,11)*, as shown in Fig. 1. The half-life of pRb is relatively long *(12)*, implying that functional regulation is accomplished primarily by post-transcriptional mechanisms, the most important of which is phosphorylation.

Several characteristics of pRb function that were demonstrated soon after its discovery suggested that this protein is an important modulator of the cell cycle *(8,10,11)*. The retinoblastoma protein was localized to the nucleus, where it appeared to be tethered through binding to nuclear lamins A and C. pRb was shown to interact with several cell-cycle regulatory proteins, including the cellular proteins c-myc, E2F, cdc2, cdk2, and ATF-2, as well as with the DNA virus transforming oncoproteins SV40 large T antigen, HPV E7, and adenovirus E1A. Phosphorylation of pRb was shown to oscillate with the phases of the cell cycle and was recognized as an important modulator of Rb function. The viral oncoproteins and other pRb-binding proteins were demonstrated to complex preferentially with the hypophosphorylated form of pRb.

Hyperphosphorylated forms of pRb predominate during the S, G_2, and M phases of the cell cycle, whereas hypophosphorylated pRb is present in cells during G_0/G_1. Serum stimulation increases pRb phosphorylation in many different cell types, whereas antiproliferative agents such as TGF-β, cAMP, and interferon-α (IFN-α) decrease pRb phosphorylation, illustrating an association between pRb phosphorylation and the cell cycle *(10)*. Injection of pRb into normal monkey kidney CV-1 cells and human Saos-2 osteosarcoma cells during early G_1, but not during late G_1 or early S phase, prevents induction of DNA synthesis *(13)*. Thus, the active form of pRb is the hypophosphorylated form that is present during G_1 and the hyperphosphorylated form of pRb is inactive, allowing cell-cycle progression.

Multiple different phosphorylated forms of pRb are detected in vivo, suggesting that the function of pRb can be modified by the phosphorylation of specific sites, some of which may be targets of kinases other than cdks. Phosphorylation occurs on at least seven serine and threonine residues in the amino-terminal and carboxy-terminal domains of the protein, inactivating the ability of pRb to suppress entry into S phase *(10,14,15)*. pRb is phosphorylated by cyclin-cdk complexes during different phases of the cell cycle *(15)*; the existence and identity of other physiologic pRb kinases remain speculative. The rapid dephosphorylation of pRb that occurs in M phase is believed to be mediated by one or more type 1 protein phosphatases (PP-1) *(10)*. Two candidate pRb phosphatases have been identified in mitotic cell extracts: a novel type 1 protein phosphatase *(16)* and the PP-1δ isoform *(17)*.

THE RB PATHWAY IN CELL-CYCLE CONTROL Progression through the cell cycle is tightly controlled by cell-cycle checkpoints in phases G_1 and G_2 *(18,19)*. The

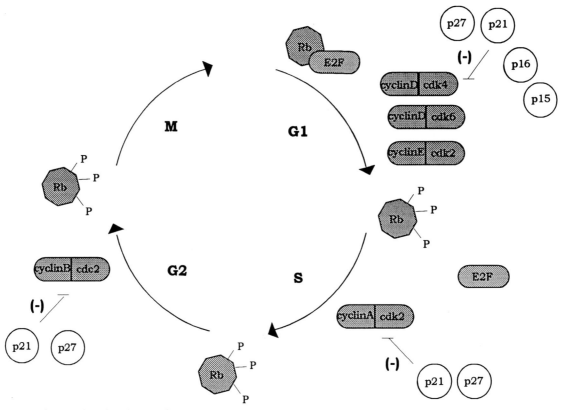

Fig. 2. The pRb pathway. Phosphorylation of pRb during G_1 by cyclin D-cdk complexes relieves repression of E2F-mediated transcription and allows DNA replication to proceed during S phase. Phosphorylation of pRb is maintained throughout S and G_2, then pRb is rapidly dephosphgorylated during mitosis. E2F is again sequestered by hypophosphorylated pRb during G_1. The cyclin-cdk targets of the cdk inhibitors p15, p16, p21, and p27 are indicated.

commitment to the cell-cycle occurs during G_1, when cells pass the restriction point and prepare for DNA replication during S phase. G_1 progression is dependent on positive regulatory signals and is responsive to growth-inhibitory signals such as contact inhibition and antiproliferative cytokines. From its inception as the major cell-cycle checkpoint, the restriction point was proposed to be involved in the prevention of cell transformation *(20,21)*. Inappropriate initiation of DNA synthesis or mitosis can have detrimental effects on cell fate. An inability to repair damaged DNA before initiation of S phase can allow mutations to become incorporated into the genome or can result in cell death if DNA damage is severe. Premature entry into the cell cycle may also prevent cells from responding to external signals that regulate quiescence, differentiation, apoptosis, or intercellular communication, interfering with normal cellular function and fate. pRb controls progression past the restriction point and regulates coordinated expression of genes required for DNA synthesis *(22)*. The importance of the restriction point in cell-cycle control is confirmed by the demonstration that the key regulators of this checkpoint (the D-type cyclins, cdk4, pRb, and p16^{INK4A}) are targets of mutation in many human tumors.

Based on numerous experimental observations, a simplified model for the critical role of pRb in cell-cycle regulation has been devised *(14,15)*. The phosphorylation of pRb during G_1 by cyclin D-cdk4 and cyclin D-cdk6 complexes serves as the primary target of cell-cycle control (Fig. 2). Expression of D-type cyclins increases during G_1 in response to mitogenic

stimuli, and cyclin D complexes with cdk4 or cdk6, whose levels remain relatively stable during the cell cycle. Cyclin D-cdk complexes phosphorylate pRb during G_1, and just prior to S-phase initiation, cyclin E-cdk2 complexes appear and target pRb for additional phosphorylation. Forced overexpression of cyclin D, but not cyclin E, is able to trigger entry into S phase *(23)*, indicating that cyclin D activity is required for cell-cycle progression. Phosphorylatiopn of pRb reaches a critical threshhold late in G_1, resulting in inactivation of pRb and initiation of S phase. In the absence of functional pRb, cyclin D is not required for cell-cycle progression *(24)*, whereas loss of cyclin D in normal cells prevents S-phase entry *(25)*. Cyclin A-cdk and cyclin B-cdk complexes maintain the hyperphosphorylation of pRb during S, G_2, and M phases, after which pRb is rapidly dephosphorylated and inactivated as cells re-enter the G_0/G_1 phase of the cell cycle *(14,15)*.

MODULATION OF E2F ACTIVITY BY pRb   The primary targets of cell-cycle regulation by pRb appear to be the E2F family of transcription factors *(10,14,15)*. The *E2F-1* gene was first cloned based on its ability to bind to pRb *(26–28)*, although the E2F protein had been previously identified as a cellular protein that was required for transcription of adenovirus *E2* genes. Four additional members of the *E2F* gene family have been identified and have been designated *E2F-2* through *E2F-5*. *E2F-4* and *E2F-5* are more closely related to each other than to *E2F-1*, *E2F-2*, and *E2F-3*, as the protein products of the former lack part of the N-terminal domain and have an extended spacer region between the A and B domains that mediates binding to cyclins A and E. E2F factors activate transcription of numerous genes involved in DNA replication, including c-*myc*, b-*myb*, cyclin A, dihydrofolate reductase, thymidine kinase, and DNA polymerase-α *(15)*.

E2F proteins form functional heterodimers with the related proteins dimerization protein-1 (DP-1) and DP-2, and binding of these complexes is restricted to specific pRb family members: E2F-1, E2F-2, and E2F-3 bind to pRb, E2F-4 binds p107, and E2F-5 binds p107 and p130 *(15,29)*. These complexes are also associated with specific cell-cycle phases. E2F-1, E2F-2, and E2F-3 are bound to pRb during G_1 and released during S phase. p107-E2F-4 complexes are present throughout the cell cycle, but are bound to cyclin E-cdk2 during G_1 phase and to cyclin A-cdk2 during S phase. p130-E2F-4 and p130-E2F-5 complexes predominate during G_0 in quiescent cells, and disappear when cells enter the cell cycle. These observations suggest that individual E2F proteins have distinct functions during the cell cycle, which are controlled by interaction with specific Rb proteins.

E2F proteins bind to the A/B pocket domain of hypophosphorylated pRb and to the pRb-related proteins p107 and p130 *(10,14,15)*. The A/B pocket domain, along with part of the C-terminal region, is required for binding of viral oncoproteins and cellular proteins and for growth suppression. Inactivation of pRb by cyclin-cdk-dependent phosphorylation, viral inactivation, or mutation releases E2F and allows cell-cycle progression. Sequestration of E2F may be the predominant target of pRb activity during cell-cycle arrest, as overexpression of *E2F-1* in Saos-2 osteosarcoma cells arrested in G_1 by pRb can overcome these effects *(30)*. It appears that pRb suppresses cell cycling by direct repression of E2F-mediated transcription during G_1: pRb may be recruited to some promoters by E2F, where it proceeds to bind to and inactivate other bound transcription factors *(31)*. Recently, pRb has been shown to recruit the histone deacetylase HDAC1 to the pRb-E2F complex, which results in repression of the E2F-regulated cyclin E promoter. HDAC1 binds to the LXCXE motif of pRb that is recognized by the viral-transforming proteins *(32,33)*. This suggests that the HDAC1-pRb complex may modify the chromatin structure by deacetylation, resulting in transcriptional repression. pRb-mediated transrepression may be important in preventing transcription of S-phase genes during the other phases of the cell cycle or in regulating differentiation.

INTERACTION OF pRb WITH OTHER CELLULAR PROTEINS

In addition to its ability to regulate the activity of the E2F family of transcription factors, pRb can interact with a wide range of other nuclear factors. An Rb control element (RCE) has been identified in the promoters of several genes, including c-*myc*, c-*fos*, *IGF-2*, and *TGF*-β *(14)*. pRb can activate or repress transcription via the RCE by a mechanism that appears to involve superactivation of the transcription factors Sp1/Sp3 *(34,35)*. Other transcription factors shown to interact with pRb include the lymphoid-specific transcription factor Elf-1, the transcription factor Id-2, the muscle-specific factor MyoD, the macrophage/B cell specific factor PU.1, c-myc, and the general enhancer ATF-2 *(10,14,15)*. Some of these interactions involve the A domain of pRb, which shares considerable homology with a domain in the TATA-binding protein of the basal transcription factor TFIID, suggesting that pRb may compete for binding to these proteins *(36,37)*. Interactions between pRb and BRG1 and hBRM1, two proteins believed to be involved in inducing changes in chromatin structure *(15)*, is believed to be involved in the stimulation of transcription. During G_1 phase, pRb binds to and inhibits the nuclear tyrosine kinase c-*abl*, and overexpression of c-*abl* in Saos-2 cells can overcome pRb-mediated growth suppression, indicating that pRb and c-abl have reciprocal functions during early cell-cycle progression *(38,39)*. Interestingly, pRb has also been shown to interact with mdm2, a negative regulator of p53-mediated transactivation, suggesting that mdm2 plays an important role in coordinating the activities of pRb and p53 *(40)*.

pRb also possesses the ability to directly modulate RNA polymerase II transcription, tRNA synthesis, and rRNA synthesis (14). In vitro, pRb forms a complex with the trancription factor UBF, preventing UBF from stimulating RNA polymerase I and impairing rRNA transcription *(41,42)*. pRb has also been shown to interact with the TAFII250 subunit of TFIID *(43,44)* and with DNA polymerase-α *(45)*, suggesting a potential mechanism by which pRb may modulate RNA polymerase activity. Finally, pRb can restrict RNA polymerase III activity, presumably by binding to the general polymerase III factors TFIIIB and TFIIIC2 *(46–48)*. The ability of pRb to interact with such a wide variety of proteins, including nuclear matrix proteins, transcription factors, cyclins, and cdks suggests that it may function predominantly as a molecular matchmaker, bringing together proteins in a context-dependent fashion *(10)*.

pRb AS A TUMOR SUPPRESSOR

In order to confirm the role of Rb as a tumor suppressor, wild-type *Rb1* has been expressed in several *Rb1*-mutant cell lines, including those derived from osteosarcoma (Saos-2), bladder carcinoma (HTB9 and J82), breast carcinoma (MD468), cervical carcinoma (C33A), and prostate carcinoma (DU145) *(10,11)*. Results indicate that although most *Rb1*-transfected cell lines show little or no in vitro evidence of reduced growth rate, tumorigenicity in nude mice is diminished in some, but not all, of the cell lines. This suggests that pRb function is highly context-dependent and that loss may occur early in tumorigenesis, with progression of tumorigenesis involving loss of additional growth regulators and an inability to restore responsiveness to pRb.

Rb-deficient mouse models have been created that also raise questions about the importance of pRb in regulating cell proliferation. Heterozygous null mice show an increased incidence of pituitary tumors but not of retinoblastoma, and homozygous null mice develop normally until 13–15 d of gestation, when they die *in utero* of massive neuronal and hematopoietic destruction *(49–51)*. Unregulated E2F-1 activity appears to be a major contributor to the development of pituiatry tumors in cells that have lost wild-type pRb function, as $Rb^{+/-}/E2F\text{-}1^{-/-}$ mice develop fewer pituitary tumors and display an extended lifespan when compared to $Rb^{+/-}$ mice *(52)*. It appears that pRb may have diverse functions related to cell growth, differentiation, and development, many of which are context-dependent. Most studies of pRb function have concentrated on the role of the A/B pocket domain in growth suppression, as this region interacts with viral oncoproteins and many cellular proteins and is conserved between the three known pRb family mem-

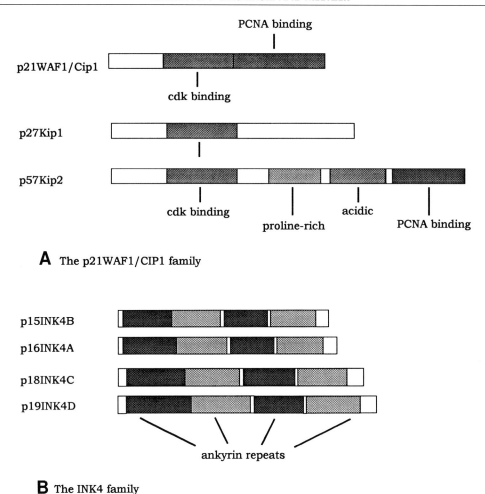

A The p21WAF1/CIP1 family

B The INK4 family

Fig. 3. The p21[WAF1/CIP1] and INK4A families of cyclin-dependent kinase inhibitors. **(A)** p21, p27, and p57 inhibit the activity of all cyclin-cdk complexes. **(B)** p15, p16, p18, and p19 specifically inhibit the association of cdk4 and cdk 6 with the G_1 cyclins.

bers. Recently, however, transgenic mouse models of N-terminal pRb deletions have been constructed that support a role for this region in proper embryonic development and in tumor suppression *(53)*. Thus, interactions between pRb and other growth-regulatory proteins may involve multiple protein domains, and the principal function of pRb may be to provide a link between higher level regulatory networks and the basic cell-cycle clock *(8)*.

Inactivating mutations in *Rb1* have been described in a wide variety of tumors, including osteosarcomas, soft-tissue sarcomas, leukemias, small-cell lung carcinomas (SCLCs), breast carcinomas, esophageal carcinomas, and prostate and renal cancers *(8,15,54)*. Many of these occur within the A/B pocket domain and are predicted to prevent interaction with E2F. The transforming proteins of the DNA tumor viruses also interact with the A/B pocket domain. In human tumors, missense mutations, deletions, and splice-site mutations are common, but no hotspots of mutation are evident *(55,56)*. Mutations have also been detected in the N-terminal domain that may account for at least some families displaying low-penetrance inheritance of retinoblastoma *(57,58)*. Other small deletions or missense mutations that result in partial inactivation of pRb have also been reported in families with low-penetrance retinoblastoma *(59–62)*. The spectrum of mutations seen in human tu-

mors further supports the idea that pRb has multiple functions involved in growth suppression.

THE pRb-RELATED PROTEINS p107 AND p130 Two proteins that share structural similarities with pRb have been identified: p107 *(63)*, and pRb2/p130 *(64–66)*. All three proteins possess the A/B pocket region that is responsible for mediating many of the protein-protein interactions in which these proteins are involved (Fig. 1). Like pRb, p107 and p130 form complexes with specific E2F family members, and appear to regulate the transcription of different sets of E2F-responsive genes *(67)*. p107 binds preferentially to E2F-4 and E2F-5, whereas p130 binds only to E2F-5 *(10,14,15)*. Both p107 and p130 are able to induce G_1 arrest in some cell types when overexpressed, and are inactivated by the DNA tumor virus oncoproteins. Similar to pRb, p107 and p130 are phosphorylated by cyclin D-cdk complexes in mid-G_1; however, hypophosphorylated p107 and p130 accumulate coincident with S-phase entry. Unlike pRb, p107 and p130 contain a region within the spacer that binds to cyclin E-cdk2 and cyclin A-cdk2 complexes, and it appears as though p107 and p130 inactivate these cyclin-cdk complexes, in contrast to the cyclin-cdk complex-mediated inactivation of pRb *(15)*.

It has been suggested that in some cell types p107 and p130 can compensate for loss of pRb function, but the different interactions of p107 and p130 with target proteins argues that this redundancy cannot be complete. Mice that are nullizygous for *p107* are viable and show no obvious abnormalities. However, *Rb⁺/⁻/p107⁻/⁻* mice exhibit growth retardation and increased neonatal mortality, and *Rb⁻/⁻/p107⁻/⁻* homozygous mice die *in utero* two d earlier than *Rb⁻/⁻* embryos *(68)*. Mice that are null for *p130* show no major abnormal phenotype, whereas *p107⁻/⁻/p130⁻/⁻* mice display abnormalities in limb development and increased neonatal lethality *(69)*. The expression of *Rb*, *p107*, and *p130* during murine embryogenesis reveals that *Rb* expression is abundant in neural tissue, hematopoietic cells, myocytes, and the ocular lens and retina, whereas *p107* expression is highest in heart, lung, kidney, and intestine *(70)*. *Rb* and *p107* were both expressed in the liver and central nervous system (CNS), whereas *p130* was low in all tissues. Inactivation of *Rb* is common in human tumors, loss of *p107* has never been reported, and loss of *p130* has only been reported in a single cell line *(71)*.

Cdk INHIBITIORS: THE INK4 FAMILY AND THE p21^WAF1/CIP1 FAMILY

During the cell cycle and in response to growth signals, modulation of pRb activity occurs primarily through phosphorylation by cyclin-cdk complexes. The activity of these cyclin-cdk complexes is also subject to regulation, which is achieved partly through the activity of two families of cdk inhibitors: 1) the INK4 family, and 2) the p21^WAF1/CIP1/p27^KIP1/p57^KIP2 family (Fig. 3). p21^WAF1/CIP1, p27^KIP1, and p57^KIP2 are universal cdk inhibitors that bind to all known cyclin-cdk complexes and inhibit their activation and kinase activity, whereas the INK4 inhibitors bind only to the cyclin D kinases (cdk4 and cdk6) and inhibit their association with cognate cyclins *(14,55)*. These two families of cdk inhibitors play distinctly different roles in the regulation of the cell cycle. However, all cdk inhibitors are capable of arresting the cell cycle under the proper circumstances.

p21^WAF1/CIP1 was the first cdk inhibitor identified, and it was independently discovered by several investigators. p21^WAF1/CIP1 was isolated as part of a quaternary complex with cyclin D1-cdk4 and proliferating cell nuclear antigen (PCNA) *(72)*, by its interaction with cyclin-cdk2 complexes *(73)*, and as a p53-inducible transcript *(74,75)*. Analysis of purified p21^WAF1/CIP1 protein revealed its ability to inhibit cdk activity and to induce cell-cycle arrest in vitro *(55)*. The cdk-inhibitory domain resides in the amino-terminus of p21^WAF1/CIP1, while PCNA binds to part of the C-terminal domain. These multiprotein complexes exhibit cdk activity when p21^WAF1/CIP1 is present in equimolar amounts; inactivation of cdk activity requires an excess of p21^WAF1/CIP1 as a result of either an increase in p21^WAF1/CIP1 levels or a decrease in cyclin-cdk complex formation *(76,77)*. p21^WAF1/CIP1 expression is low in G₁ and increases as the cell-cycle progresses such that the proper growth stimulus must be present during G₁ in order to induce a parallel increase in cyclin D-cdk complexes that can overcome the inhibitory effects of p21^WAF1/CIP1. p21^WAF1/CIP1 is also elevated in cells undergoing differentiation and during cell senescence *(55)*. Furthermore, this cdk inhibitor is believed to be responsible for mediating cell-cycle arrest in response to stressors such as DNA damage and during permanent states of cell-cycle arrest such as occur during quiescence and senescence.

The interaction of p21^WAF1/CIP1 with PCNA, a processivity factor associated with the polymerase-δ DNA-replication apparatus, is believed to contribute to cell-cycle arrest in response to DNA damage. In vitro, p21^WAF1/CIP1 directly inhibits PCNA-dependent DNA replication but not PCNA-dependent DNA repair *(78)*. Recent evidence suggests that inactivation of PCNA-dependent DNA replication is required for p21^WAF1/CIP1-mediated cell-cycle arrest *(79)*. p21^WAF1/CIP1 expression is induced by p53 in response to DNA damage, but p21^WAF1/CIP1 expression is not fully dependent on functional p53, and can be expressed at high levels in the absence of p53. Induction of p21^WAF1/CIP1 has been reported to occur by p53-independent, BRCA1-dependent transactivation in association with cell-cycle arrest *(80)*. Germline mutations in BRCA1 are associated with familial breast and ovarian cancer, and the structure of the BRCA1 protein suggests that it is a transcription factor of the RING finger family that may also be involved in DNA recombination and repair *(81)*. Recently, p21^WAF1/CIP1 has been shown to inhibit the mitogen-activated kinase SAPK *(82)* and to complex with gadd45, a nuclear protein also induced by p53 in response to DNA damage *(83)*, indicating that p21^WAF1/CIP1 may have many functions involved in cellular homeostasis.

Despite the seemingly critical role of p21^WAF1/CIP1 in cell-cycle control, mutations in p21^WAF1/CIP1 are extremely rare in primary human tumors (84–87). It may be more likely that during tumorigenesis, p21^WAF1/CIP1 function is lost indirectly due to epigenetic changes that may occur as a result of the loss of p53 or some other regulatory protein. In vivo studies indicate that p21^WAF1/CIP1 is not critical for normal growth and development. p21^WAF1/CIP1 deficient mice develop normally and do not exhibit and increased incidence of tumors. However, *p21^WAF1/CIP1-/-* embryonic fibroblasts are partially deficient in G₁ arrest in response to DNA damage and grow to high cell density *(88)*.

p27^KIP1 was isolated from TGF-β-treated Mv1Lu mink-lung epithelial cells on the basis of its ability to interact with and inhibit cyclin E-cdk2 complexes *(89,90)*, and by virtue of its ability to bind to cyclin D-cdk4 *(91)*. p27^KIP1 shares with p21^WAF1/CIP1 an amino-terminal cdk-inhibitory domain and can inhibit the activity of cyclin D-, E-, A-, and B-dependent kinases in vitro. In contrast to p21^WAF1/CIP1, p27^KIP1 levels are high in quiescent cells and decline as cells progress from G₁ to S phase *(14,55)*. The increase in cyclin D-cdk complexes during late G₁ effectively overwhelms p27^KIP1 levels, permitting cell-cycle progression. p27^KIP1 levels are variably affected by treatment with antiproliferative agents such as TGF-β, which inhibits cdk4 synthesis in mink lung epithelial cells, increasing the level of free p27^KIP1 *(92)*, and cAMP, which increases p27^KIP1 synthesis and inhibits its degradation in cultured macrophages *(93)*. It is believed that p27^KIP1 responds to physiologic signals such as growth-factor stimulation, and in vitro inactivation of p27^KIP1 in a fibroblast cell line allowed cells to continue cycling even in the absence of serum mitogens *(94)*. Cell-cycle arrest by p27^KIP1 does not appear to be dependent on the presence of functional pRb or p53. Mice that are null for p27^KIP1 display a complex phenotype of macrosomia, multiorgan hyperplasia, retinal dysplasia, female sterility, and pituitary tumors *(95,96)*, indicating that p27^KIP1 plays an important role in the growth regulation of many tissues. Mutations in p27^{KIP1} have not been described in human tumors, but heterozygous deletion involving the p27^{KIP1} locus on chromosome 12p12-p13 is detected with high frequency in human leukemias, leading to speculation that p27^{KIP1} haplo-insufficiency may prevent accumulation of the critical threshold level required to restrain cell proliferation in these cells (97).

The third general cdk inhibitor known to date, p57^{KIP2}, contains four structurally distinct domains: 1) an amino-terminal cdk-inhibitory domain, 2) a proline-rich domain, 3) an acidic domain, and 4) a carboxy-terminal domain that shares sequence similarity to p27^{KIP1} (98,99). Like p21$^{WAF1/CIP1}$, p57^{KIP2} has been shown to interact with PCNA, and this function is important in the ability of p57^{KIP2} to suppress cellular transformation (100). In contrast to p21$^{WAF1/CIP1}$ and p27^{KIP1}, p57^{KIP2} expression is restricted to selective tissues and appears highest in well-differentiated cells, suggesting that p57^{KIP2} may have a specialized role in coordinating cell-cycle arrest with differentiation. Transfection of p57^{KIP2} into Saos-2 osteosarcoma cells induces a G$_1$ arrest that does not appear to require pRb or p53 (98).

The role of p57^{KIP2} in cell growth, differentiation, and development appears complex. p57^{KIP2} is located on chromosome 11p15, a region involved in several types of cancer including Wilms' tumor and rhabdomyosarcoma. Although mutations in p57^{KIP2} have not been observed in Wilms' tumor, several mutations have been described in Beckwith-Wiedemann syndrome (BWS), a fetal organ overgrowth syndrome also linked to chromosome 11p15 and associated with an increased predisposition to childhood tumors, including Wilms' tumor (101–104). p57$^{KIP2-/-}$ mice display multiple severe developmental defects, including abnormal endochondral ossification, cleft palate, abdominal muscle defects, and gastrointestinal abnormalities (105,106), several features of which are also common in BWS. p57^{KIP2} has been demonstrated to be paternally imprinted, and loss of the maternally expressed allele has been reported to occur in human lung cancer (107).

The INK4 family members (p16^{INK4A}, p15^{INK4B}, p18^{INK4C}, and p19^{INK4D}) are distinguished by the presence of an ankyrin-like repeat domain, which binds to cdk4 and cdk6 at the expense of cyclin D. The INK4 prototype, p16^{INK4A}, was originally identified as a cdk4-binding protein in cells lacking functional pRb (108), whereas p15^{INK4B} was discovered on the basis of its marked induction by TGF-β in human keratinocytes (109). p18^{INK4C} and p19^{INK4D} were discovered later and have also been shown to inhibit cdk4 and cdk6 activity (110,111). Because the INK4 proteins selectively target cyclin D-cdk activity, they are dependent on functional pRb in order to control G$_1$ cell-cycle progression. p16^{INK4A} is able to induce growth arrest when introduced into deficient cell lines, but only in cells that have wild-type pRb (112,113). It has been proposed that the primary function of p16^{INK4A} may be to downregulate cdk4 and cdk6 activity after progression to S phase (109), or to prevent accidental activation of cyclin D-cdk complexes and maintain states of quiescense and differentiation (93). The importance of p16^{INK4A} in regulating cell proliferation is verified by the high frequency of tumors that develop in mice that are null for p16^{INK4A} (114). Although p16^{INK4A} can be consid-

ered an intrinsic cell-cycle regulator, p15^{INK4B} appears to function as an inducible cdk inhibitor that responds to extracellular signals. p15^{INK4B} expression is induced in keratinocytes in response to TGF-β, where it acts to sequester cdk4 and cdk6 (109). The functions of p18^{INK4C} and p19^{INK4D} are less well-understood. p18^{INK4C} and p19^{INK4D} are highly expressed during embryogenesis, and p15^{INK4B}, p18^{INK4C}, and p19^{INK4D} expression is detectable in many adult tissues. In contrast, p16^{INK4A} expression appears to be more restricted (115). Expression of p19^{INK4D} is induced as cells enter S phase, suggesting that it may also function to downregulate cyclin D-cdk activity after pRb phosphorylation (110). The exact role of each of the INK4 proteins and whether they exhibit any functional overlap at all remains unknown.

Inactivation of p16^{INK4A} is frequent in many primary human tumors, including gliomas, leukemias, and pancreatic and esophageal carcinomas (55,113). The frequency of p16^{INK4A} mutation in human tumors is second only to mutation of p53, underscoring the importance of p16^{INK4A} as a tumor-suppressor protein. Soon after its discovery as a modulator of cdk4 activity, p16^{INK4A} was independently identified as the multiple tumor suppressor (MTS) gene that was mutated in many different tumor types (116). p16^{INK4A} inactivation was later shown to be associated with familial melanoma (117,118). However, while a high rate of loss of heterozygosity for the p16^{INK4A} locus is also seen in sporadic melanomas, mutation of the remaining allele has been difficult to document, raising the possibility that either a second tumor-suppressor gene may be linked to p16^{INK4A} or that other mechanisms account for p16^{INK4A} inactivation in sporadic melanoma. The primary mechanism of p16^{INK4A} inactivation in gliomas, adult T-cell leukemias, and T-cell acute lymphocytic leukemia (ALL) is through homozygous deletion, which may also involve the p15^{INK4B} locus, which is located within 30 kb of p16^{INK4A} on chromosome 9q21 (113). In other tumor types p16^{INK4A} point mutations predominate, but frameshift mutations and splice-site mutations also occur (119). Promoter methylation has emerged as an important silencer of p16^{INK4A} expression in some tumors (120–124). In an effort to define the role of p16^{INK4A} in human cancer, a database of information on 146 human somatic and germline p16^{INK4A} mutations has been created (125). In vitro support for the role of p16^{INK4A} as a tumor-suppressor protein is evidenced by the ability of adenovirus-mediated p16^{INK4A} expression to induce cell-cycle arrest in tumor cells lines with mutant p16^{INK4A} and wild-type pRb (126,127). Concomitant loss of p15^{INK4B} with p16^{INK4A} occurs frequently in deletion mutants, and methylation of p15^{INK4B} has also been reported in gliomas and leukemias (128–130). As expected, loss of p15^{INK4B} and p16^{INK4A} is restricted to tumors that retain normal pRb. Mutations of p18^{INK4C} or p19^{INK4D} have not been described in human tumors, although p18^{INK4C} is located at chromosome 1p32, a region frequently altered in some human tumors.

The p16^{INK4A} gene has recently been shown to encode a second protein, p19^{ARF}, via splicing of alternate first exons (131). p19^{ARF} is also a growth suppressor and its germline inactivation predisposes to the development of cancer in mice (132). New evidence suggests that cell-cycle arrest mediated by p19^{ARF} requires functional p53, and that p19^{ARF} interacts with mdm2, a key regulator of p53 activity, to prevent degradation of p53 and enhance p53-dependent transactivation (132–134). The INK4A locus may represent an important mechanistic link between two key pathways involved in cell-growth regulation: the p16^{INK4A}/cyclin D/cdk4/pRb pathway, which controls cell-cycle progression, and the p19^{ARF}/mdm2/p53 pathway, which regulates growth arrest and induction of apoptosis in response to cell damage.

THE ROLE OF PRB IN APOPTOSIS AND CELLULAR DIFFERENTIATION Although pRb is known to play a key role in the ability of cells to pass the restriction point and commit to the cell cycle, it also appears to function in several other prominent physiological pathways including differentiation and apoptosis. The main function of pRb may be as a coordinator of the cellular events that lead to differentiation at the expense of proliferation. It has been proposed that a pRb-mediated arrest of the cell cycle is required before induction of differentiation or senescence (22). pRb expression increases during induction of differentiation and in response to cytokines such as TGF-β and IFN-γ (14,15), suggesting that quantitative levels of pRb may modulate cell fate. In addition, dephosphorylation of pRb, an increase in p21$^{WAF1/CIP1}$, and G$_0$/G$_1$ arrest occur prior to induction of differentiation in many cell types (11,14), implying that pRb-mediated cell-cycle arrest may be a prerequisite for differentiation. Loss of pRb function can induce even terminally differentiated cells to reenter the cell cycle, suggesting that pRb is required to maintain the differentiated phenotype (14). The ability to induce differentiation appears to be dissociated from growth suppression (135).

Rb is believed to exert a protective effect against apoptosis (14), and re-expression of Rb in Rb$^{-/-}$/p53$^{-/-}$ tumor cells results in cellular senescence, a permanant cell-cycle arrest (136). Homozygous Rb null mice die at 13–15 d of gestation secondary to massive neuronal and hematopoietic cell death (49–51). The developing mouse lens has been used as a model for studying the role of pRb in apoptosis. In cells lacking functional pRb, induction of apoptosis occurs by a p53-dependent response (137). This may explain why a significant proportion of human tumors have lost both of these suppressor genes, as only when both pRb and p53 are inactivated can the apoptotic cascade be averted. Additional studies have confirmed these findings in other cell systems and further suggest that unrestrained E2F-1 activity is an important modulator of apoptosis in this context (14).

THE P53 DAMAGE RESPONSE PATHWAY

p53 AS A MASTER REGULATOR p53 is a multifunctional protein that plays a key role in protecting the integrity of the cellular genome. p53 coordinates the cellular response to DNA damage and other forms of genotoxic stress by regulating cell-cycle progression, modulating DNA damage-repair responses, inducing differentiation, and triggering apoptosis in cases of severe genetic compromise. In this manner, p53 prevents the accumulation of deleterious mutations and protects against cellular transformation. The importance of p53 in growth control and genomic stability is evidenced by the prevalence of p53 mutations in the majority of human cancers (138,139). Mutations in p53 have been found in 50% of all human cancers, and

cells lacking normal p53 exhibit genetic instability and defects in cell-cycle control. p53 is also involved in the induction of differentiation and in cellular senescence, two alternative states for cells that have left the cycling compartment (140,141). Thus, p53 is a master regulator of cell fate that determines whether a cell will divide, senesce, differentiate, or die.

The p53 protein was originally identified in 1979 by virtue of its ability to bind to the SV40 T-antigen oncoprotein (142–144). Early studies of p53 function were based on mutant forms of p53, which led to the proposition that p53 was a proto-oncogene. Later studies using the wild-type protein demonstrated that transfection of p53 prevented virally-induced transformation and inhibited the growth of tumor cell lines (145–150). This growth arrest was then shown to involve a reversible inhibition of cell-cycle progression (151–153). Mutations in p53 were found in many primary human tumors and tumor cell lines (138), and functional studies indicated that cell lines lacking functional p53 protein exhibited defects in cell-cycle control and chromosomal stability (148,154,155). Levels of p53 protein were shown to increase in vitro following treatment with DNA-damaging agents, and a link between DNA damage, p53, and cell-cycle arrest was postulated (156–160).

STRUCTURE AND ACTIVATION OF p53 p53 is a 393 amino acid protein that functions as a classic transcription factor and as a modulator of DNA repair (140,161–163). Structurally, p53 is divided into four functional domains: 1) an acidic N-terminal transcriptional activation domain that interacts with the basal transcriptional apparatus; 2) a sequence-specific DNA-binding domain; 3) an oligomerization domain; and 4) a C-terminal domain rich in basic amino acids that binds to DNA with limited specificity, including damaged DNA or RNA intermediates, and transmits structural changes that activate the sequence-specific DNA-binding domain. The p53 gene contains five evolutionarily conserved regions, four of which are located in the sequence-specific DNA-binding domain (Fig. 4). The native form of p53 is a tetramer, which is stabilized via interactions involving the C-terminal oligomerization domain. The normal half-life of p53 in the cell is short, on the average of 20–30 min, and the level of p53 in a cell under normal conditions is low. Maintenance of low levels of p53 are acheived through a combination of ubiquitin-mediated proteolysis and a negative feedback mechanism in which p53 downregulates translation of its own mRNA (164,165).

In response to DNA damage from ultraviolet (UV) irradiation, γ-irradiation, or chemical damage, p53 levels increase through a combination of increased stability and increased translational activity. The interaction of p53 with other proteins accounts for at least some of the increased stability of p53 in response to cellular damage. The amino terminus of p53 contains a proline-rich region that is recognized by src-homology 3 (SH3)-domain binding proteins, which is required for cell-cycle arrest and apoptosis (166). Binding of p53 to DNA may also prevent its degradation (167). Thus, it is not surprising that several proteins that associate with damaged DNA, such as the product of the ATM (mutated in ataxia telangiectasia; AT) gene, are known to interact with p53. Hypoxia (168), nitric oxide (NO) (169), heat shock (170), and diminished ribonucleotide triphosphate pools (171) have also been shown to

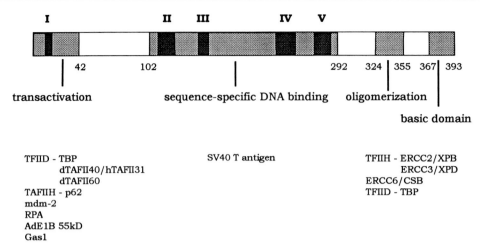

Fig. 4. The structure of human p53. The p53 protein contains an amino-terminal transactivation domain, a sequence-specific DNA-binding domain, an oligomerization domain, and a carboxy-terminal domain rich in basic amino acids that binds RNA and DNA with limited sequence specificity. Regions I–V indicate evolutionarily conserved regions; II–V are hotspots for inactivating mutations. Several proteins that are known to interact with specific regions of p53 are indicated.

activate p53, indicating that p53 responds to several distinct types of cellular stress. p53 levels also increase in response to cell adhesion and decrease upon loss of cell anchorage, suggesting a role for p53 in mediating contact inhibition of cell growth (172,173).

Negative regulation of p53 activity is mediated in large part through interaction with the mdm2 protein, which binds to the N-terminal transactivation domain of p53 and inhibits transcriptional activation (174–176). Mdm2 also promotes the rapid degradation of p53 (175,177) and is transcriptionally upregulated by p53 activation itself, forming an autoregulatory feedback loop (178,179). The mdm2 gene has been shown to be amplified in some tumors, notably sarcomas (180), and mdm2 overexpression inhibits p53-dependent G_1 arrest (181). Recently, p19^{ARF} was shown to bind to mdm2 and prevent degradation of p53 (133,134). Several oncogenic DNA tumor viruses also encode proteins that bind to and inactivate p53, including SV40 T antigen, adenovirus E1B 55 kDa protein, and HPV E6 protein (162,182).

TRANSCRIPTIONAL ACTIVATION BY p53 The most well-characterized role of p53 is as a transcriptional activator. The p53-response element consists of two copies of the decameric consensus sequence RRRC(A/T)(T/A)GYYY, where R = A or G and Y = C or T (140). This sequence is recognized by the sequence-specific DNA-binding domain, which is the primary site for inactivating p53 mutations in human tumors. The oligomerization domain also appears to be required for sequence-specific DNA binding to some target sites. The basic C-terminal domain appears to allosterically regulate the ability of p53 to bind to DNA by mediating conversion from an inactive form of p53, which is prevented from sequence-specific DNA binding, to an active form (163).

Activation of the sequence-specific DNA-binding activity of p53 may be triggered by interaction with other proteins, phosphorylation, or other events. p53 is known to be phosphorylated in vivo on several serine and threonine residues in both the amino and carboxy terminus (183,184). Kinase enzymes capable of phosphorylating p53 in vitro include MAP kinase,

jun-N-terminal kinase (JNK), protein kinase C (PKC), cyclin A-cdk2, and cyclin B-cdc2. C-terminal phosphorylation of p53 is believed to relieve the allosteric inhibition of sequence-specific DNA binding (162). N-terminal phosphorylation has been shown to correlate with nuclear translocation and transactivation (185) and with release of inhibition by mdm2 (186). Recent evidence suggests that differential phosphorylation on both the amino and carboxy terminus is involved in the regulation of DNA-binding and transactivation (187).

Although many genes have been suggested to be regulated by p53, to date only a handful have demonstrated p53-dependent, cis-acting DNA elements, including p21$^{WAF1/CIP1}$ (73,74), mdm2 (178), gadd45 (160), cyclin G (188), bax (189), and IGF-BP3 (190). With the exception of mdm2 and bax, these effectors are involved in cell-cycle regulation. Other genes that are candidates for transcriptional regulation by p53 include those that encode thrombospondin-1, TGF-a, PCNA, Fas/Apo1, cyclin D, pRb, and the EGFR (163).

p53 can also repress transcription of some genes that lack p53 response elements, including bcl2, c-fos, Rb, IL-6, nitric oxide synthase, thrombospondin-1, and several serum-inducible genes (163). The mechanism of p53-dependent transcriptional repression appears to depend on sequestering, or squelching, of TATA-binding protein (TBP) or a TBP-associated factor (TAF) and therefore is a feature of TATA-dependent promoters (191,192). Thus, p53 may function as a general repressor of many genes during the cellular response to genotoxic stress. The amino and the carboxy terminus, which can each interact with TBP, are required for transcriptional repression by p53 (193–195).

Interaction of the N-terminal transactivation domain of p53 with other components of the basal transcription complex may be important in the coordination of transcriptional regulation and nucleotide excision repair. Two RNA polymerase II-associated transcription factor complexes that interact with p53 are TFIID and TFIIH. p53 binds to the TBP (193), which is part of the general transcription factor TFIID. Several TAFs that are part of TFIID have also been shown to bind to p53, including human TAFII31 *(196),* and the *Drosophila* TAFII40 and TAFII60 proteins *(197).* In vitro, TFIIH can phosphorylate p53 and activate its sequence-specific DNA-binding capacity *(198).* p53 binds to the p62, ERCC2, and ERCC3 subunits of the TFIIH transcription factor, and ERCC2 and ERCC3 are inhibited by wild-type p53 *(199–202).* The ERCC2 and ERCC3 DNA helicases are involved in DNA excision repair and are mutated in some patients with xeroderma pigmentosum (XP), an hereditary condition that predisposes to UV-induced skin tumors. It has been shown that mutant p53 proteins such as those found in human tumors are less potent inhibitors of ERCC2 and ERCC3 than wild-type p53 *(202).* In addition, p53 binds to another helicase implicated in XP, the strand-specific repair factor CSB/ERCC6 *(201).* p53 recognizes RP-A *(203–205),* a single-stranded DNA-binding protein that is part of the eukaryotic DNA polymerase complex. Recently, p53 has been shown to form a DNA-binding complex with the related transcription factors p300 and CBP, which possess histone acetyltransferase activity. Disruption of this complex by viral oncoproteins such as E1A and SV40 T antigen may contribute to cell transformation *(206–209).* Further, p53 is acetylated by p300, which activates its sequence-specific DNA-binding activity *(210).*

p53 AND CELL-CYCLE REGULATION Cell-cycle regulation by p53 has been the subject of intense investigation since the discovery of an association between p53 induction and G_1 phase arrest. However, the ability of p53 to suppress cell growth via regulation of the cell cycle does not appear to fully account for its tumor-suppressive activities *(211).* Tumor suppression involves other functions of p53 such as induction of apoptosis. The exact role of p53-dependent pathways in tumor suppression depends on the cell type and the expression of other cellular effectors. The predominant hypothesis regarding the significance of p53-mediated cell-cycle arrest in response to DNA damage assumes that the cell-cycle arrest allows time for DNA repair. However, recent evidence suggests that p53-dependent G_1 arrest is involved in eliminating cells with damaged chromosomes from the proliferating cell compartment, rather than repairing them *(212).*

Early studies demonstrated that reintroduction of *p53* into p53-null cell lines was sufficient to induce a reversible growth arrest, which occurred prior to the G_1 restriction point in cultured human tumor cells *(163).* Growth suppression by p53 requires both the N-terminal transactivation domain and the C-terminal domain involved in oligomerization/nonspecific DNA-binding *(213).* Loss of either the transactivation domain *(214,215)* or the carboxy terminus *(216)* results in reduced growth suppression. Thus, cell-cycle regulation and growth suppression are dependent on transcriptional activity.

The current model for cell-cycle arrest by p53 in response to irreparable DNA damage involves transactivation of key cell-cycle regulatory genes, most notably the cyclin-dependent kinase inhibitor p21[WAF1/CIP1] *(74,75).* p21[WAF1/CIP1] inhibits several cyclin-cdk complexes required for cell-cycle progression, including cyclin D-cdk4, cyclin E-cdk2, and cyclin A-cdc2 *(55).* p21[WAF1/CIP1] also binds to PCNA, a DNA polymerase processivity factor, and inhibits DNA replication but not DNA repair activities *(72,78).* Loss of cyclin-cdk activity in G_1 phase prevents phosphorylation of pRb, and the hypophosphorylated

pRb retains its ability to sequester E2F and prevents initiation of DNA synthesis. In vitro studies confirm that after DNA damage in cells with wild-type p53, pRb is found predominantly in the hypophosphorylated form, and abrogation of pRb activity by HPV E7 prevents G_1 arrest *(217–220).* The central importance of the pRb pathway in the regulation of cell proliferation, and the importance of p53 in monitoring cell-cycle parameters, is demonstrated by the prevalence of mutations of both p53 and pRb in human cancers.

In support of a key role for p53-mediated induction of p21[WAF1/CIP1] in cell-cycle arrest, deletion of p21[WAF1/CIP1] from some colorectal-carcinoma cell lines containing wild-type p53 results in a total loss of cell-cycle arrest in response to DNA damage and in induction of apoptosis *(221).* In vitro, overexpression of p21[WAF1/CIP1] arrests cell growth *(73),* indicating that an increase in p21[WAF1/CIP1] in response to p53 induction may be sufficient to inhibit growth. However, p21[WAF1/CIP1] does not appear to be absolutely required for p53-mediated growth arrest, as *p21[WAF1/CIP1]* null mice develop normally and exhibit only a partial defect in cell-cycle arrest in response to DNA damage *(88,222).* Although *p21[WAF1/CIP1]* expression in response to DNA damage appears to depend on p53, *p21[WAF1/CIP1]* expression can also be induced in the absence of p53 *(223,224).*

Several other proteins appear to be involved in the p53-mediated growth arrest. The gadd45 protein is induced by p53 in response to DNA damage, binds to PCNA, and inhibits cell growth *(225).* The c-abl nonreceptor protein kinase has also been shown to be involved in p53-mediated cell-cycle arrest and to enhance transactivation by p53 *(226–229).* Although the exact function of c-abl is not known, c-abl activity increases during S phase in response to genotoxic stress *(230).* c-abl was recently identified as a downstream effector of the ATM DNA damage-response pathway *(231,232)* and may represent part of a common pathway for both p53-dependent and ATM-dependent growth inhibition. Another growth-arrest pathway that involves p53 is the Gas1 pathway. Gas1 is a cell membrane protein that is expressed during G_1 and is associated with cell-cycle arrest. p53 is required for Gas1-mediated growth arrest, but not through transactivation of *Gas1.* Rather, Gas1 appears to bind to a proline-rich motif in the amino terminus of p53 *(233,234).* A novel type 2C protein phosphatase, Wip1, is induced by p53 and suppresses cell growth in vitro *(235).* A role for phosphatases in regulation of cell proliferation has long been suspected based on the prominant role of proliferative signaling via protein kinases *(236).* Recently, the tumor suppressor BRCA1 was shown to co-immunoprecipitate with p53 and to enhance p53-mediated transactivation *(237).* BRCA1-mediated cell-cycle arrest requires p21[WAF1/CIP1] activity, which can be induced by both p53-dependent and p53-independent mechanisms *(80).* The *WT1* gene product, a transcription factor and a tumor-suppressor gene implicated in the development of Wilms' tumor, also interacts with p53, stimulates p53 transcriptional activity, and inhibits apoptosis when both are overexpressed *(238).* Finally, the recently identified growth suppressor p33ING1 has been shown to complex with p53 and to be required for p53-dependent p21[WAF1/CIP1] induction and growth arrest *(239).* It is apparent that the role of p53 in cell-

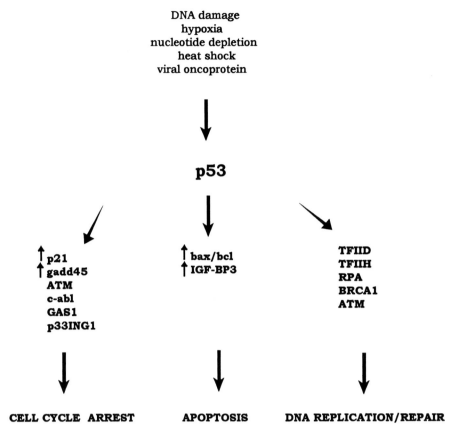

Fig. 5. The p53 damage-response pathway. Induction and stabilization of p53 occurs in response to many cellular stressors. Activated p53 induces expression of genes such as *p21*, *gadd45*, *bax*, and *IGF-BP3*. Activated p53 also interacts with other cellular proteins (like TFIIH, p33ING1, and BRCA1) to coordinate cell cycle arrest, DNA repair, and apoptosis.

cycle arrest is complex and can involve interactions with many other effector proteins (Fig. 5).

p53 has also been implicated in cellular senescence, a permanent growth arrest that occurs in normal cells after a predetermined number of cell divisions *(240)*, and in the G_2/M checkpoint that prevents premature entry into mitosis when DNA synthesis has not been completed or when the DNA damage is detected *(241)*. p53 can induce senescence in response to oncogenic c-*ras* activation *(243)*, and overexpression of p53 has been shown to induce senescence in the p53-deficient EJ bladder carcinoma cell line *(243)*. p53-mediated transactivation appears to be required for senescence to occur *(244)*. The role of p53 in G_2 arrest *(245–247)* and in centrosome function and mitotic spindle stability *(248,249)* has been suggested to account for the increased propensity of p53-deficient cells to develop an aneuploid chromosomal content and to undergo gene amplification. Upregulation of cyclin G and p21[WAF1/CIP1] *(250–252)* have been suggested to play a role in p53-mediated G_2 arrest. Chromosomal instability is observed in cells from *p53*-null mice *(248,253,254)* and in *p53*-deficient human tumor cells *(154,155)*. p53 downregulates expression of topoisomerase IIα *(255,256)*, a key enzyme involved in chromosome segregation, and inhibits RAD51 *(257)*, the mammalian homolog of RecA, a key mediator of homologous recombination. These studies suggest that p53 functions to coordinate multiple cell-cycle events involved in the preservation of genomic stability.

p53 AND APOPTOSIS Elimination of damaged cells is an important defense against cellular transformation and cancer. It is believed that p53 induces apoptosis in response to irreparable or overwhelming nuclear damage or loss of required growth-stimulatory signals, but that apoptosis during normal growth and development is controlled by other factors *(258)*. The ability of p53 to influence cell-cycle arrest, differentiation, senescence, and apoptosis indicates that the damage response pathway is complex and variable. The decision to induce apoptosis instead of cell-cycle arrest is influenced by the severity of the perturbation that activates p53 and by the specific cell type. The activity of other growth regulators such as those involved in the pRb pathway are important in determining whether cell-cycle arrest or apoptosis occurs. p16[INK4A] has been shown to cooperate with p53 in inducing apoptosis in several cell lines *(259)*. Overexpression of p53 protein prevents p21[WAF1/CIP1]-mediated cell-cycle arrest and induces apoptosis in H1299 non-SCLC cells *(260)*. However, excess pRb can prevent p53-induced apoptosis in HeLa cells, indicating that other factors can contribute to cell-type specific control over apoptosis *(261)*.

p53 is able to induce apoptosis in response to many signals, including DNA damage, hypoxia, growth-factor withdrawal, and uncontrolled proliferation as a result of unregulated activity of oncoproteins like c-myc, adenovirus E1A, or E2F-1 *(140,162,163)*. Overexpression of p53 can induce apoptosis in many cell types *(263)*. The importance of p53-dependent apoptosis is illustrated by the clinical correlation between p53 status and tumor regression after γ-irradiation secondary to apoptosis (265). Recently, an analysis of gene transcripts that increased after p53 induction but before the onset of apoptosis identified several proteins involved in the cellular generation of, or response to, oxidative stress (264). This lends support to the proposal that p53-mediated apoptosis may involve the generation of reactive oxygen species (ROS) with subsequent oxidative damage to mitochondrial components. ROS have been demonstrated to be produced during p53-dependent apoptosis (265).

p53-dependent apoptosis appears to have both transcription-dependent and transcription-independent components. The function that predominates depends on 1) the cell type, 2) p53 level, and 3) the environmental context. p53 can induce apoptosis without transcriptional activation in GHFT1 pituitary cells and in HeLa cells (266,267), although transactivation of target genes probably does occur in other forms of p53-dependent apoptosis. p53-mediated apoptosis does not require prior cell-growth arrest (268,269), and a p53 mutant that is deficient in apoptosis but not cell-cycle arrest has been described (270), indicating that these two functions are distinct. Mutations in the N-terminus of p53 that abrogate apoptosis in some cell types have also been described (193,271), and both the N-terminus and C-terminus of p53 appear to be required for p53-dependent apoptosis (272). Recently, a poly-proline region, located between the transactivation domain and the DNA-binding domain, has been shown to be required for apoptosis but not for growth arrest (273). These studies suggests that p53-mediated cell growth arrest and apoptosis are distinct, and that interaction with other proteins is required for apoptosis.

In general, apoptosis is believed to be dependent on the activation of latent effector proteins already present within the cell and therefore to function independently of transcription and translation. The interaction of p53 with other proteins also appears to play an important role in some forms of apoptosis. However, not all forms of apoptosis are dependent on p53. Transcriptional repression by p53 may be involved in p53-dependent apoptosis, as both the adenovirus E1B 19 kD protein and bcl2 (which inhibit p53-dependent apoptosis) prevent the downregulation of transcription by p53 (192,274). The transforming proteins of DNA tumor viruses, including adenovirus E1B 55 kD protein, SV40 T antigen, and HPV E6, also bind to p53 and prevent apoptosis (162).

p53 is known to regulate directly two genes that are important in the control of apoptosis: bax (189,275,276) and insulin-like growth factor binding protein-3 (IGFBP-3) (190) (Fig. 5). p53 has also been reported to induce expression of a third pro-apoptotic factor, Fas/Apo1 (277). Bax is a member of the bcl2 family of apoptosis proteins. However, whereas bcl2 is a pro-apoptotic factor, bax exerts anti-apoptotic effects (258,278). Active bcl2 exists as a homodimer or a heterodimer with a second bcl2 anti-apoptotic family member. Heterodimerization with bax or another pro-apoptotic family member results in apoptosis. Recent evidence for a tumor-suppressive role of bax has been demonstrated in a transgenic mouse brain tumor model in which tumor growth is accelerated and p53-dependent apoptosis is reduced in bax-deficient mice (279).

Although overexpression of bcl2 can override induction of apoptosis by p53 (280), overexpression of bax is not sufficient to induce apoptosis (281), suggesting that other effectors are required for p53-dependent apoptosis. Direct repression of bcl2 from a p53-dependent silencer has been reported (282,283) and may be important in p53-mediated apoptosis. Bax is not always expressed during p53-mediated apoptosis (284), and it is therefore apparent that the cell type determines which activities of p53 are required for apoptosis. Transcription-dependent functions of p53 may be required only in cell types that have low endogenous levels of bax that must be increased in order to titrate out bcl2 activity; in cells where bax levels are high, other functions of p53 may predominate during apoptosis. Mutations in bax have been detected in two leukemia cell lines (285) and in several colon cancer cell lines. Furthermore, mutations of the bax gene have been reported in a significant proportion of primary colorectal carcinomas exhibiting microsatellite instability (286), where it has been suggested to account for the low frequency of somatic p53 mutations in these cancers.

IGFBP-3 has several growth-suppressive effects (288). IGFBP-3 binds to the insulin-like growth factor-1 (IGF-1) and prevents activation of the IGF-1 receptor. IGFBP-3 is also believed to have growth-suppressive effects that are independent of its ability to sequester IGF-1 and appear to involve induction of apoptosis (287–289). The type V TGF-β receptor has been suggested to be a receptor for IGFBP-3 (290), and a link between TGF-β-mediated growth inhibition and IGFBP-3 has been suggested (291).

COORDINATION OF CELL-CYCLE ARREST AND DNA REPAIR BY p53 AND ATM Decreased ability to repair damaged DNA has been reported in cells with mutant p53 (292–294), and p53 binds directly to damaged DNA, including single-stranded DNA ends and DNA mismatches (162,163). Loss of p53 can result in increased DNA damage in vitro, but p53-deficient mouse fibroblasts and human p53⁻/⁻ fibroblasts from Li-Fraumeni syndrome patients display normal transcription-coupled DNA repair (200,292,295–298). However, nucleotide excision repair is defective in p53-deficient cells (292,299), although the interaction of p53 with TFIIH has not been shown to affect DNA repair in vitro (201). With respect to its role as a DNA damage detector, it is expected that p53 may interact with or recruit other proteins involved in the repair of damaged DNA (Fig. 5). For instance, the tumor suppressor BRCA1 co-immunoprecipitates with p53 and is suggested to enhance p53-mediated transactivation (237).

Recent studies also suggest that the ATM gene is part of the p53 DNA repair pathway. AT is an autosomal recessive disorder characterized by cerebellar ataxia, immune dysfunction, premature aging, growth retardation, and a predisposition to certain malignancies, including leukemia, lymphoblastic lymphoma, and breast cancer. Cells from affected patients exhibit defects in complete cell-cycle arrest, increased frequency of chromosomal aberrations, and extreme sensitivity to DNA damage by ionizing radiation (300). Based on these observations, it was suspected that the primary defect responsible for AT involved DNA repair mechanisms. The ATM gene encodes a 13 kb mRNA expressed in many tissues and producing a protein of 350 kDa (301,302). The ATM protein belongs to a family of proteins that share a region of homology to the catalytic subunit of phosphotidylinositol-3 kinase (PI-3 kinase). This family of proteins, which includes DNA-protein kinase and several yeast proteins, is involved in cell-cycle control, DNA repair, and DNA recombination *(300)*.

Cells from AT patients have been shown to display impaired induction of p53 and its downstream targets p21$^{WAF1/CIP1}$, mdm2, and gadd45 in response to ionizing radiation *(160,284,303)*. This implies that the *ATM* gene product and p53 are effectors in the same DNA repair pathway, and that ATM is involved in activating p53 in response to ionizing radiation. However, AT cells are also deficient in other cell-cycle checkpoints, suggesting that the *ATM* gene may regulate multiple cell-cycle activities. Thymocytes from *ATM*$^{-/-}$ mice do not demonstrate induction of p53 and display defects in cell-cycle arrest in response to ionizing radiation, although apoptosis and induction of *bax* occur normally *(304–306)*. This suggests that ATM activates only a subset of p53-dependent functions. ATM and p53 appear to regulate different target cdk-cyclin activities during the G$_1$/S checkpoint *(307)*. Like *p53*$^{-/-}$ mice, *ATM*$^{-/-}$ mice develop lymphomas with high frequency (305), but p53$^{-/-}$/ATM$^{-/-}$ mice exhibit a marked acceleration of tumor formation *(308)*, indicating that ATM has independent tumor-suppressor functions. In contrast to p53, ATM levels remain constant after exposure to γ-irradiation *(309)*, suggesting that it may have a constitutive role in maintaining genomic integrity. Recently, wild-type ATM has been shown to interact with and activate the tyrosine kinase c-abl during the response to ionizing radiation *(231,232)*, indicating that c-abl is a common downstream effector of both the ATM and p53 DNA damage response pathways that preserve genomic integrity.

p53 AND HUMAN CANCER Greater than half of all human tumors have mutations in the *p53* gene, and the majority of mutations occur as missense mutations, which are found in four highly conserved regions of the sequence-specific DNA binding domain *(138,139)*. These mutational hotspots occur in codons corresponding to amino acids in the p53 structure that are in direct contact with DNA, as determined from the crystal structure of p53 *(310)*. As with loss of many tumor-suppressor genes, one allele is usually deleted and the second allele is mutated. Some tumors, however, such as testicular teratocarcinomas, never develop mutations in p53 *(311)*. An extensive database of over 570 p53 mutations from greater than 8,000 human tumors and cell lines is available through the International Agency for Research on Cancer *(312)*, and a database of germline p53 from 122 pedigrees has also been generated *(313)*.

Although mutations in p53 are common in human tumors, some tumors appear to inactivate the p53 response pathway by other mechanisms. Overexpression of mdm2 is seen in a proportion of human sarcomas *(180)*. Several DNA tumor viruses encode proteins that inactivate p53 and are associated with human cancer, including adenovirus in nasopharyngeal carcinoma, HPV in anogenital cancer, herpes simplex virus (HSV)-8 in Kaposi's sarcoma KS, and Epstein-Barr virus (EBV) in lymphoid malignancies *(314)*. Exclusion of p53 from the nucleus has been reported to account for loss of p53 activity in neuroblastomas and breast carcinomas *(315,316)*, although there is conflicting data regarding the effects of cytoplasmic sequestration on p53 function *(317,318)*.

Germline mutations in p53 are responsible for the Li-Fraumeni syndrome, a hereditary cancer syndrome characterized by an increased incidence of breast cancer, sarcomas, and adrenal carcinomas, which occur at a relatively young age *(319)*. A Li-Fraumeni family must contain a member with a childhood sarcoma who has two first-degree relatives who develop cancer before the age of 45. This definition is a strict one, and some families that do not meet these criteria have been found to contain germline p53 mutations, indicating that p53 germline mutations can produce a spectrum of clinical phenotypes.

Mutations in p53 may result in a loss of part or all normal p53 function, a dominant-negative effect via oligomerization with wild-type p53, or a gain of oncogenic properties. Loss of function mutations and dominant negative effects of tumor-derived mutant p53 proteins have been extensively documented in vitro. p53 mutants, which have an increased oncogenic capacity in vitro or in vivo, have also been described *(320,321)*. Several *p53*-knockout mouse models have been generated that demonstrate the complexity of p53 functions. *p53*-null mice primarily display an increased frequency of lymphoma, whereas mice that are heterozygous for *p53* are prone to the development of osteosarcomas and soft tissue sarcomas *(254,322–324)*. The genetic background of the transgenic animal can also influence the phenotype of loss-of-function mutants. An in vivo model of a *p53* mutant with a dominant-negative mutation has been generated in heterozygous transgenic mice, which show increased tumor incidence and decreased survival compared to nontransgenic mice *(325)*. In addition to lymphomas, p53$^{-/-}$/pRb$^{+/-}$ mice also develop endocrine tumors, indicating that p53 and Rb have distinct but cooperative functions *(326,327)*. These different phenotypes support the idea that the functions of p53 are highly context-dependent. The prevalence of missense mutations in human tumors, as opposed to nonsense mutations or frameshift mutations, suggests that many mutant p53 proteins may have acquired novel or modified functions that are important in cell transformation.

p73, A NEW p53 FAMILY MEMBER The importance of p53 in maintaining genomic integrity has argued for the existence of related proteins with similar functions. Only recently was the first p53-related protein, p73, identified *(328)*. p73 exhibits 63% identity with the DNA-binding domain of p53 and exact homology of the residues in direct contact with DNA, which are the most frequently mutated regions of p53. Lower sequence similarity is present in the transactivation domain and the oligomerization domain, and the carboxy terminal domain of p73 is distinct. Preliminary studies indicate that p73 can form oligomers, although this interaction has not been shown to involve the oligomerization domain. Overexpression of p73 inhibited the growth of a neuroblastoma cell line and of the Saos-2 osteosarcoma cell line. Overexpression of p73 has also been shown to activate transcription of p21$^{WAF1/CIP1}$ and to induce apoptosis *(329)*, indicating that at least some of the functions of p53 may also be achieved by p73.

The *p73* gene has been localized to chromosome 1p36, a region frequently deleted in neuroblastomas, suggesting that loss of p73 may play a role in the development of these tumors *(328)*. Low levels of *p73* expression are detected in all normal tissues but not present in neuroblastomas that show deletion of 1p36. Mutations have not been detected in the remaining allele, however, but there is some indication that p73 may be paternally imprinted. Thus mutation of the remaining allele would not be expected, nor would it be required for complete loss of p73 function. p73 remains a putative tumor-suppressor gene and the subject of intense scrutiny with regard to its normal function, role in tumorigenesis, and potential redundancy with p53.

THE TGF-β SIGNALING PATHWAY

TGF-β AND HUMAN CANCER TGF-β is the prototype member of a large superfamily of cytokines that exhibit diverse effects on cell proliferation, differentiation, embryonal development, immune-system modulation, cell-matrix production, and apoptosis *(330)*. TGFβ1 is the most extensively studied member of this family and its antiproliferative effects on many types of cells (epithelial, endothelial, and lymphohematopoietic) have been well-documented *(331–333)*. However, TGFβ1 is able to stimulate the growth of some cells, suggesting that its effects on cell proliferation are highly dependent on cell type, state of differentiation, and growth conditions. Two additional TGF-β species, TGFβ2 and TGFβ3, have been identified and are encoded by distinct genes. They exhibit similar structure to TGFβ1 but different patterns of expression and activity and are much less well-characterized.

Many primary tumors and tumor cell lines have lost responsiveness to the growth inhibitory effects of TGFβ1 *(333–336)*, indicating that TGFβ1 may play a significant role in regulating the proliferative capacity of many cell types. Loss of responsiveness to the effects of TGFβ1 on growth regulation appears to occur relatively late in tumorigenesis and to correlate with increasing clinical aggressiveness and invasiveness *(336)*. Our understanding of the intracellular events that mediate TGFβ1 activity has been augmented by the observation that several key molecules in the TGFβ1 signaling pathway, including the type II TGFβ1 receptor (TGFβRII) and the cytoplasmic effector Smad4/DPC4, are mutated in some types of human cancer.

PRODUCTION AND ACTIVATION OF TGF-β TGFβ1 is synthesized as an inactive latent complex, and its activation represents a critical step in the regulation of its physiologic activity. The active form of TGFβ1 is a 25 kDa disulfide-linked homodimer. Proteolytic processing of latent TGFβ1 occurs intracellularly, where the propeptide, also known as the latency-associated peptide (LAP), is removed *(337)*. The LAP remains noncovalently associated with the TGFβ1 homodimer and renders it biologically inactive. Outside of the cell, TGFβ1 exists as the large latent TGFβ1 complex, consisting of TGFβ1, the LAP, and the latent TGFβ1 binding protein (LTBP). TGFβ1 must be liberated from this complex in order to exert its biologic activity.

The in vitro activation of TGFβ1 has been characterized in cocultures of bovine endothelial cells and smooth muscle cells, and requires several factors, including the cation-dependent mannose-6-phosphate/insulin-like growth factor-2 receptor (M6P/IGF-2R), type II tissue transglutaminase, plasminogen,

urokinase plasminogen activator (uPA), and the uPA receptor *(337)*. These factors serve to localize key components in the proteolytic process to the cell surface or matrix compartment. Latent TGFβ1 binds to the M6P/IGF-2R via two mannose phosphate moieties on the LAP, wherease the uPA receptor concentrates the serine protease uPA at the cell surface. The localization process enables plasminogen to be activated to plasmin, which cleaves the LAP/LTBP fragment from the large latent complex, freeing active TGFβ1.

THE M6P/IGF-2 RECEPTOR IN HUMAN CANCER The recent identification of mutations in the M6P/IGF-2R in several types of tumors suggests that this multi-functional receptor may be involved in the tumorigenic process in some tumors. Mutations of the M6P/IGF-2R have been documented in colorectal, gastric, and endometrial carcinomas exhibiting microsatellite instability (338–340), as well as in breast and hepatocellular carcinomas without microsatellite instability (340–342).

In addition to its proposed role in the activation of TGF-β, the M6P/IGF-2R also mediates the binding, internalization, and degradation of IGF-2 ligand *(343)*, which is itself a mitogen for many tumor cell types *(344)*. IGF-2 is a potent growth stimulatory factor through its interaction with its cognate receptor, the insulin-like growth factor-1 receptor (IGF-1R). The IGF-1R also mediates positive growth signals via IGF-1 and plays an important role in the growth stimulation of many tumors *(345)*. Thus, the IGF-2R is proposed to act as a tumor-suppressor gene in the genesis or progression of human malignancies by removing the normal growth-controlling effects of activation of TGFβ1 and degradation of IGF-2 ligand. In support of this contention, immunohistochemical analysis of several tumors with mutation of the M6P/IGF-2R revealed increased levels of latent TGFβ1 and IGF-2, and decreased levels of active TGFβ1 *(346)*.

EFFECTS OF TGF-β ON CELL-CYCLE PROGRESSION The most well-characterized growth inhibitory effects of TGFβ1 involve regulation of cell-cycle progression. When administered in the G_1 phase of the cell cycle, TGFβ1 reversibly arrests cells in late G_1, by preventing phosphorylation of pRb by cyclin-cdk complexes *(347)*. After progression from G_1 to S phase, cells become unresponsive to the growth-inhibitory effects of TGFβ1. Cell-cycle arrest is primarily accomplished by a either inhibition of cdk4 expression or induction of p15^{INK4B}. The inhibition of *cdk4* expression in response to TGFβ1 appears to occur primarily in cells emerging from quiescence, whereas induction of *p15^{INK4B}* predominates in actively proliferating cells *(89,92,109,348–351)*. Overexpression of *cdk4* can render cells resistant to the inhibitory effects of TGFβ1 *(92)*. Interestingly, in the human melanoma cell line WM35, which lacks *p15^{INK4B}*, TGFβ1 treatment, resulted in reduced expression of *cyclin D1, cyclin A,* and *cdk4*, and increased levels of *p21$^{WAF1/CIP1}$* and *p27^{KIP1}* in cells emerging from quiescence, rather than in asynchronously replicating cells, suggesting that compensatory mechanisms may exist when *p15^{INK4B}* is not functional *(352)*. Inhibition of *cyclin D* expression has been reported in several cell lines *(351,353)*, whereas induction of the cdk inhibitor *p21$^{WAF1/CIP1}$*, an effector of the apoptotic response with p53-dependent and p53-inde-

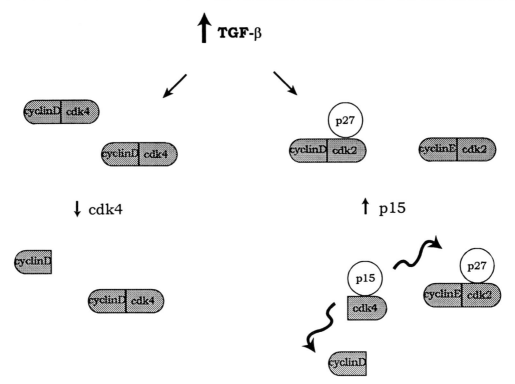

Fig. 6. Effects of TGFß1 on G1 phase progression. TGFß1 can decrease *cdk4* expression and prevent the formation of cyclin D-cdk4 complexes in quiescent cells. In proliferating cells, TGFß1 increases *p15* expression, p15 inhibits cyclin D-cdk activity and displaces p27, which is able to inhibit any active cyclin E-cdk complexes. The overall effect of TGFß1 is to decrease cyclin-cdk activity during the G_1 phase of the cell cycle and prevent S-phase entry.

pendent activity, has been observed in several different cell types *(349,354–357)*. TGFβ1 also causes a rapid decline in c-*myc* expression *(358)*, and overexpression of c-*myc* can prevent TGFβ1-mediated growth suppression *(359)*. Decreased c-myc protein expression may also stabilize p27[KIP1] activity, leading to decreased cyclin E-Cdk2 activity *(360)*. TGFβ1 inhibits expression of the cdk tyrosine phosphatase *cdc25A*, which maintains cdk4 and cdk6 in an inactive phosphorylated state *(361)*. This inhibition is also believed to result from a direct repression of c-*myc* expression *(362)*. TGFβ1 may also have indirect effects on other cell-cycle components that are cell-type specific. In HaCaT keratinocytes, TGFβ1 inhibits the induction of *cyclin E, cyclin A,* and *cdk2* expression *(350)*. The pRb-related protein p130 also appears to be a target of TGFβ1 activity in keratinocytes, where TGFβ1 treatment results in the formation of complexes between p130 and E2F, inhibition of cdk2, and inhibition of cell-cycle progression *(363)*.

The general model for TGFβ1-induced cell-cycle arrest depends on the proliferation status of the cell, although certain cell-type specific modifiers may be important *(364)* (Fig. 6). In quiescent cells where cyclin and cdk levels are low, TGFβ1 treatment prevents cdk4 expression and functional cyclin D-cdk4 complexes are not formed. However, in actively proliferating cells, cyclin-cdk complexes are present and their activity is modulated by p27[Kip1]. TGFβ1 exposure increases levels of p15[INK4B], which bind to and inhibit cyclin D-cdk4 and cyclin D-cdk6, preventing phosphorylation of pRb and displacing p27[Kip1] from cyclin D-cdk4 complexes. In this manner, p27[Kip1] is able to bind to and inhibit cyclin E-cdk2 complexes, which keeps pRb hypophosphorylated and able to sequester the tran-

scriptional activator E2F *(349,365)*, whose activity is required for S phase. Thus, once E2F has been activated, TGFβ1 is without effect. Overexpression of E2F-1 *(366)* or loss of functional pRb *(367)* can prevent TGFβ1-mediated growth arrest in some cell lines.

INDUCTION OF IGFBP-3 BY TGF-β The complex relationship between TGFβ1 and IGF signaling is further complicated by recent studies that show that expression of insulin-like growth-factor binding protein-3 (IGFBP-3) is induced by TGFβ1. At least 10 IGFBPs have been identified to date, and they were originally discovered as binding factors for IGF-1 and IGF-2 that prevent activation of IGF-1R-mediated cell proliferation *(344)*. Several studies have demonstrated that IGFBP-3 possesses antiproliferative functions that are independent of its ability to sequester IGFs *(368,369)*, and IGFBP-3 inhibits the growth of fibroblasts with a targeted disruption of the IGF-1R *(370)*. The identification of the cell-surface receptor for IGFBP-3 that mediates its growth suppressive effects remains elusive. TGFβ1 has been shown to induce expression of IGFBP-3 in Hs578T and MDA-MB-231 breast-cancer cells *(371,372)*, and IGFBP-3 induces apoptosis in PC-3 prostate-carcinoma cells *(289)* and MCF7 breast-cancer cells *(373)*. IGFBP-3 is also induced by p53 *(192)*, but not by a mutant p53 that is unable to induce apoptosis *(374)*, suggesting a mechanistic link between IGFBP-3 and apoptosis.

TGFβ1 SIGNALING VIA THE TGF-β RECEPTOR TGFβ1 signal transduction occurs through interaction with a heteromeric complex of high affinity TGFβ1 cell surface receptors *(375)*. The type I and type II TGFβ1 receptors are required for signaling activity and are structurally related

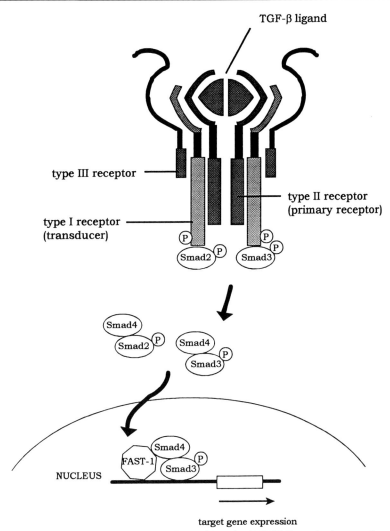

Fig. 7. Signaling through the TGFß receptor complex. Binding of TGFß1 to the TGFßRII results in transphosphorylation and activation of the TGFßRI, which then phosphorylates the cytoplasmic signal transducers Smad2 and Smad 3. Smad4/DPC4 binds to activated Smad2 and Smad3 proteins and these complexes translocate to the nucleus, where they interact with other transcription factors, such as FAST-1.

single-pass transmembrane proteins with serine-threonine kinase activity. The type III receptor, also known as betaglycan, appears to play a role in presenting ligand to the signaling complex when localized to the cell surface; a secreted form appears to sequester TGFβ1 from the receptor complex. The type I, II, and III receptors all form homodimers in a ligand-independent manner, but only the type II receptors are constitutively autophosphorylated. The TGFβRII is the major determinant of ligand-binding specificity, whereas the TGFβRI is unable to bind ligand alone and requires association with the TGFβRII. However, it is the TGFβRI that is the effector of the TGFβ1 response.

The current model for the activation of the TGF-β receptor complex, based on analysis of ^{125}I-labelled TGFb1 crosslinked to its receptor *(376)*, predicts that ligand binding to the type II receptor recruits the type I receptor to form a heterotetrameric complex of two type I and two type II receptors *(377)*. In this complex, the cytoplasmic domain of the TGFβRI is phosphorylated by the TGFβRII in a glycine- and serine-rich region, termed the GS domain *(378,379)*. The activated TGFβRI then phosphorylates its target proteins, including members of the

recently discovered Smad family of signal transducers *(380)*. Activated Smads dimerize and translocate to the nucleus, where they are believed to function as transcriptional regulators (Fig. 7).

Several observations have led to the proposal that TGFβ1 receptor signaling is more complex than is evident at first glance. The growth-inhibitory and gene-induction pathways appear to diverge somewhere downstream of receptor activation, such that they can become uncoupled when signaling effectors are perturbed. Many tumors have been reported to express increased levels of TGFβ1 *(334,335)*, and it has been suggested that TGFβ1 can facilitate tumor growth and metastasis by increasing expression of angiogenic factors and ECM molecules. Overexpression of truncated TGFβRII suppresses the inhibitory but not the gene-induction response, suggesting that TGFβRI plays an important role in gene induction *(381)*. Several cell lines that lack functional TGFβRII and are not growth-inhibited respond to TGFβ1 by synthesis of ECM components *(382)*. A threshold model has therefore been proposed in which quantitative levels of both type I and type II receptors are required to mediate both the antiproliferative and gene-induction responses. A decrease in TGFβRII will first affect the growth-inhibitory response without affecting gene induction, whereas loss of TGFβRI activity abolishes both responses *(383)*.

INACTIVATION OF THE TGFβRII IN HUMAN CAN-CER Mutations in *TGFβRII* gene were first described in colorectal carcinomas displaying microsatellite instability (MSI) *(384,385)*. In these tumors, one or two adenosine residues are inserted or deleted within a 10-basepair deoxy(A) tract spanning nucleotides 709–718. Tumors that demonstrate MSI, mutations within short repetitive tracts of DNA, are associated with defects in DNA base mismatch repair *(386)*. Most MSI occurs within noncoding regions of genomic DNA, and presumably has little or no significance with regard to cell viability. The *TGFβRII* gene was the first gene shown to contain MSI within the protein-coding region of the genomic DNA sequence, and was said to be a target of MSI as the mutation has functional significance. Mutations in target genes containing coding-region microsatellites appear to be actively selected for, as other genes containing microsatellite sequences do not display the high incidence of these mutations *(387)*.

Many MSI-positive colorectal tumors display this type of mutation in both alleles of the *TGFβRII* gene, but in some tumors the second mutation occurs at a different location *(387)*. The resultant frameshift mutation is predicted to produce truncated receptors, and indeed no surface receptors were detected by chemical crosslinking using radiolabeled TGFβ1 *(385)*. These mutations within the *TGFβRII* gene have also been detected with strikingly high frequency in gastric adenocarcinomas with MSI but only sporadically in MSI-positive endometrial tumors *(388)*, and not at all in MSI-positive lung cancers *(389)* or MSI-positive pancreatic adenocarcinomas *(340)*. This finding emphasizes the nonrandom occurrence of these mutations in MSI-positive gastric and colorectal tumors and suggests that other effectors of the TGFβ1 response may be targets for inactivation in other tumors. Mutation or loss of expression of the *TGFβRII* occurs infrequently in sporadic colorectal tumors lacking MSI *(385,387,390)*. Other *TGFβRII* mutations have been identified in MSI-negative gastric tumors *(388,391)*, and inactivating mutations in the kinase domain of the *TGFβRII* gene have been reported in head and neck squamous carcinomas *(392,393)*. Loss of expression of both type I and type II receptors has been reported in prostate cancer *(394)*, and reduced expression of the type II receptor is seen in thyroid carcinomas *(395)* and esophageal cancers *(396)*. A dominant-negative mutation that inhibits the assembly and activation of the TGF-β receptor complex has been described in a cutaneous T-cell lymphoma cell line *(397)*. Proof that inactivation of the TGFβRII contributes to the malignant phenotype has been demonstrated by transfection of the wild-type receptor into cell lines containing mutant receptor; these cell lines express surface receptor, which binds TGFβ1, is growth-inhibited by TGFβ1, and shows decreased tumorigenicity in nude mice *(385,398–400)*.

INACTIVATION OF TGFβRI AND TGFβRIII IN HUMAN CANCER Mutations in the *TGFβRI* have been reported to occur in the prostate carcinoma cell line LNCaP, and restoration of the wild-type receptor results in growth inhibi-

tion by TGFβ1 *(401)*. Loss of TGFβRI expression has also been reported in KS *(402)*. The LMC19 rat bladder carcinoma cell line expresses undetectable levels of the TGFβRI and is insensitive to growth inhibition by TGFβ1. Transfection of the wild-type *TGFβRI* into these cells restores TGFβ1 binding and markedly reduces tumorigenicity *(403)*, suggesting that the TGFβRI may also function as a tumor suppressor. Mutations in the *TGFβRIII* have not been reported to occur in cancer, but transfection of the *TGFβRIII* into two breast-cancer cell lines with reduced endogenous expression levels restores TGFβ1 responsiveness in vitro and reduces tumorigenicity in vivo *(404,405)*, suggesting that in at least some tissues the TGFβRIII may play an important role in controlling the ability of the TGF-β signaling receptor complex to interact with TGF-β ligand.

THE SMAD FAMILY OF TGF-β SIGNAL TRANS-DUCERS The Smads are evolutionarily conserved signaling molecules that are phosphorylated and activated by members of the TGF-β superfamily. The designation Smad is derived from a fusion of the names for the homologous TGF-β signaling genes in *Caenorhabditis Elegans* (the *sma* genes) and *Drosophila* (the *mad* genes). To date, nine human Smads have been identified, five of which appear to function in a pathway-restricted manner; the remaining three are involved in signaling by all members of the TGF-β superfamily, two as inhibitory molecules. Signaling by the Smads involves heterodimerization of a pathway-restricted Smad with the common partner Smad4/DPC4 *(380)*.

The Smads range from 42–60 kDa in size and share two regions of amino acid homology located at the amino and carboxy terminals. These conserved domains are the Mad-homology domains MH1 and MH2, respectively (Fig. 8). These domains are important in regulating the interactions of Smad molecules with each other. Smad2 and Smad3 are the pathway-restricted Smads that are involved in signaling through the TGFβRI *(406–408)*. Pathway-restricted Smads bind directly to TGFβRI and are phosphorylated at a C-terminal SSXS motif *(409)*. Phosphorylated Smad2 and Smad3 form hetero-oligomers with the common mediator Smad4, and the complex translocates to the nucleus *(377,410)*. Smad4/DPC4 lacks a C-terminal SSXS phosphorylation motif and does not interact directly with the TGFβRI *(377,407)*. Targeted deletion of Smad4/DPC4 in colorectal cancer cells abolishes TGF-β signaling, confirming the role of Smad4/DPC4 as a common mediator of signaling by the TGF-β superfamily *(411)*.

The MH1 domain of Smad4, and probably other Smads, functions as a autorepressor of hetero-oligomer formation by interacting with the MH2 domain *(412)*. The MH2 domain of Smad2 and Smad3 mediates hetero-oligomer interactions with Smad4 *(412,413)*. Mutations in MH1 domains at R-133 in Smad2 and R-100 in Smad4, which increase the affinity of the MH1 domain for the cognate MH2 domain and therefore prevent hetero-oligomer formation have been identified in certain cancers *(406,414)*. Structural and functional data suggest that the active Smad complex may consist of hexamers or other configurations. The three-dimensional structure of Smad4 is a trimer *(415)*, and Smad2 and Smad3 can interact with each

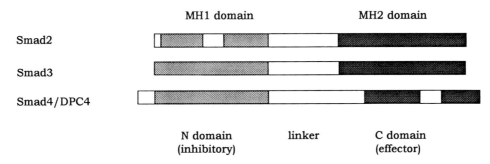

Fig. 8. Structure of the Smad proteins. Smad2, Smad3, and Smad4/DPC4 are involved in TGF-ß signalling. The Smad proteins contain a C-terminal effector domain (MH2) and an N-terminal autoinhibitory domain (MH1).

other, as well as with Smad4, in a TGF-β-dependent manner *(408)*.

While the Smads are proposed to function as DNA-binding transcription factors, the genomic targets of Smad transcriptional regulation are not yet known. The induction of p21$^{WAF1/CIP1}$ in response to TGFβ1 is dependent on functional Smad4/DPC4 *(416)*, and the Smad3/Smad4 complex appears to recognize a bipartite binding site within TGFβ1-responsive promoters and to potentiate the activity of the AP-1 transcription factor *(417)*. In *Xenopus*, Smad2/Smad4 appears to form a transcriptionally active complex with the winged helix protein FAST-1 *(418)*, suggesting that the Smads may interact with multiple other DNA binding proteins to coordinate signaling responses. Smad4/DPC4 mediates binding of an Smad2/Smad4/FAST-1 complex to DNA and promotes transactivation *(418)*.

SMADS IN HUMAN CANCER Smads appear to play a role in the development of certain human cancers, reflecting the importance of a functional TGF-β signaling pathway in controlling cell proliferation. Smad4/DPC4 was first identified as a tumor-suppressor gene that was mutated in 20% and homozygously deleted in another 30% of pancreatic tumors *(419)*. Mutations frequently occur in the MH2 domain, leading to truncation of the protein product or prevention of interactions with heteromeric partner Smads. Inactivation of Smad4/DPC4 also occurs in 30% of colorectal carcinomas *(420)*, but appears very infrequently in other tumors, including those of lung, esophagus, and breast cancers *(414,421–424)*. Loss of Smad4/DPC4 expression has been noted in several TGF-β-resistant cell lines, and transfection of Smad4/DPC4 into these cells restores TGF-β sensitivity *(408,414,425)*, confirming the role of Smad4/DPC4 as a tumor suppressor. Mutations in Smad2 have been detected in a few colorectal and lung cancers *(406,426)*. To date, mutations have not been identified in Smad3, the other partner in the TGF-β signaling pathway *(424)*, or in other Smads. The predominance of mutations in Smad4/DPC in pancreatic cancer underscores its role as a key modulator of responsiveness to TGF-β in this cell type. However, the targets of inactivation that are responsible for TGF-β-insensitivity in other systems remain to be identified.

OTHER TGFβ-MEDIATED CELLULAR RESPONSES TGFβ1 stimulation results in the transcriptional activation of several genes through other transcription factors whose relationships to the Smads are not known. For example, TGFβ1 induces transcription of the cyclin-dependent kinase inhibitors

p21$^{WAF1/CIP1}$ and p15^{INK4B} via the nuclear factors AP-1 *(427)* and Sp1 *(428)*, respectively. Growth inhibition by TGF-β is linked to stimulation of c-*ras* *(429)*. Several MAP kinases, including ERK-1, ERK-2, and SAPK/JNK *(430–432)* have been reported to be activated by TGF-β, and expression of dominant-interfering mutants of various components of the SAPK/JNK signaling cascade blocks TGF-β-mediated and DPC4-mediated gene induction *(433)*. TAK-1, a MAPKK kinase has also been shown to be activated by TGF-β *(434)*.

Recently, TGF-β has been shown to downregulate expression of the candidate tumor suppressor *PTEN* (for phosphatase and tensin homolog deleted on chromosome 10, also known as *MMAC1* for mutated in multiple advanced cancers 1) *(435)*. PTEN is a protein tyrosine phosphatase and mutations in the *PTEN* gene are observed in many primary human cancers and cell lines, including gliomas, and tumors of the breast, prostate, endometrium, and kidney *(436–439)*. In addition, germline mutations of *PTEN* are associated with Cowden disease and Bannayan-Zonana syndrome, disorders that confer an elevated risk for breast, thyroid, and skin cancers, and hamartomatous intestinal polyps and lipomas, respectively *(440,441)*. Growth suppression is observed in glioma cell lines transfected with wild-type *PTEN (442)*. Based on these observations, it has been suggested that PTEN phosphatase activity is important in regulating tyrosine signaling by one or more critical tyrosine kinases involved in cell proliferation and cell adhesion. It is probable that the multitude of effects of TGF-β on cell functions is mediated through cross-talk between several signaling pathways.

CONCLUSIONS

Regulation of cell proliferation is a crucial mechanism by which cells maintain homeostasis, regulate growth and differentiation, and monitor genomic integrity. Loss of control over the cell cycle is a hallmark of cellular transformation and predisposes to the development of cancer. Proper regulation depends on a complex interaction between multiple factors, most of which participate in one or more of three key regulatory pathways: 1) the pRb cell-cycle pathway, 2) the p53 damage-response pathway, or 3) the TGF-β growth-inhibition pathway (Fig. 9).

pRb is a central cell-cycle regulator that controls the G_1/S phase transition and responds to both external and internal growth signals. p53 is a key component of the DNA damage-

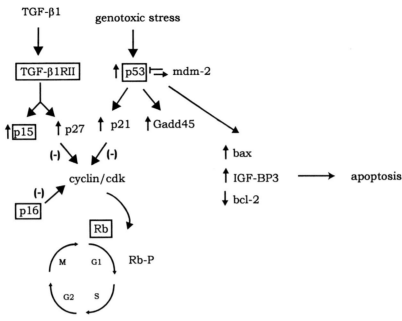

Fig. 9. TGFß1, p53, and pRb cooperate to insure regulated cell proliferation in normal cells. Loss or mutation of key regulators of cell proliferation can lead to dysregulated cell growth, which can contribute to tumorigenesis. Common targets of inactivation in human tumors are boxed in this schematic.

response pathway, which induces cell-cycle arrest in G_1, monitors mitotic spindle assembly, coordinates DNA repair, and induces apoptosis. TGF-β is a potent inhibitor of cell proliferation in many cell types that influences cell-cycle progression during G_1. Together, these three regulators cooperate to prevent aberrant cell proliferation via a complex network of intracellular signaling molecules. Dysregulation of at least one of these three key regulatory pathways is present in virtually all human cancers, emphasizing the importance of regulation of both cell-cycle dynamics and apoptosis in preventing neoplasia.

ACKNOWLEDGMENTS

We would like to thank John Abraham for his critical review of this manuscript. This work was supported by NIH grants DK47717, CA85069, CA77057, DK53620, CA78843, and the Medical Research Service of the Department of Veterans' Affairs. We apologize to all authors whose work could not be cited due to space constraints, or whose work was inadvertently overlooked.

REFERENCES

1. Wolff, J. (1989) *The Science of Cancerous Disease from Earliest Times to the Present.* Science History Publications/USA,Canton, MA.
2. Willis, R. A. (1948) Definition of tumour. *In: Pathology of Tumours.* The C.V. Mosby Co., St. Louis, MO, pp.1–8.
3. Knudson, A. G. (1971) Mutation and cancer: statistical study of retinoblastoma. *Proc. Natl. Acad. Sci. USA* **68**:820–823.
4. Comings, D. E. (1973) A general theory of carcinogenesis. *Proc. Natl. Acad. Sci. USA* **70**:3324–3328.
5. Friend, S. H., Bernards, R., Rogelj, S., Weinberg, R. A., Rapaport, J. M., Albert, D. M., et al. (1986) A human DNA segment with properties of the gene that predisposes to retinoblastoma and osteosarcoma. *Nature* **323**:643–646.
6. Fung, Y. K., Murphee, A. L., T'Ang, A., Qian, J., Hinrichs, S. H., and Benedict, W. F. (1987) Structural evidence for the authenticity of the human retinoblastoma gene. *Science* **236**:1657–1661.
7. Lee, W. H., Bookstein, R., Hong, F., Young, L. J., Shew, J. Y., and Lee, E. Y. (1987) Human retinoblastoma susceptibility gene: cloning, identification, and sequence. *Science* **235**:1394–1399.
8. Goodrich, D. W. and Lee, W. H. (1993) Molecular characterization of the retinoblastoma susceptibility gene. *Biochim. Biophys. Acta* **1155**:43–61.
9. Fearon, E. R. and Vogelstein, B. (1990) A genetic model for colorectal tumorigenesis. *Cell* **61**:759–761.
10. Wang, J. Y. J., Knudsen, E. S., and Welch, P .J. (1994) The retinoblastoma tumor suppressor protein. *Adv. Cancer Res.* **64**:25–85.
11. Riley, D. J., Lee, E. Y., and Lee, W. H. (1994) The retinoblastoma protein: more than a tumor suppressor. *Ann. Rev. Cell Biol.* **10**:1–29.
12. Chen, P. L., Scully, P., Shew, J. Y., Wang, J. Y .J., and Lee, W. H. (1989) Phosphorylation of the retinoblastoma gene product is modulated during the cell cycle and cellular differentiation. *Cell* **58**:1193–1198.
13. Goodrich, D. W., Wang, N. P., Qian, Y. W., Lee, E. Y. H. P., and Lee, W. H. (1991) The retinoblastoma gene product regulates progression through the G1 phase of the cell cycle. *Cell* **67**:293–302.
14. Herwig, S. and Strauss, M. (1997) The retinoblastoma protein: a master regulator of cell cycle, differentiation, and apoptosis. *Eur. J. Biochem.* **246**:581–601.
15. Beijersbergen, R. L. and Bernards, R. (1996) Cell cycle regulation by the retinoblastoma family of growth inhibitory proteins. *Biochim. Biophys. Acta* **1287**:103–120.
16. Nelson, D. A., Krucher, N. A., and Ludlow, J. W. (1997) High molecular weight protein phosphatase type 1 dephosphorylates the retinoblastoma protein. *J. Biol. Chem.* **272**:4528–4535.
17. Puntoni, F. and Villa-Moruzzi, E. (1997) Association of protein phosphatase-1delta with the retinoblastoma protein and reversible phosphatase activation in mitotic HeLa cells and in cells released from mitosis. *Biochem. Biophys. Res. Commun.* **235**:704–708.
18. Elledge, S. J. (1996) Cell cycle checkpoints: preventing an identity crisis. *Science* **274**:1664–1672.
19. Sherr, C. J. (1996) Cancer cell cycles. *Science* **274**:1672–1677.
20. Pardee, A. B. (1974) A restriction point for control of normal animal cell proliferation. *Proc. Natl. Acad. Sci. USA* **71**:1286–1290.
21. Pardee, A. B. (1989) G1 events and regulation of cell proliferation. *Science* **246**:603–608.

22. Weinberg, R. A. (1995) The retinoblastoma protein and cell cycle control. *Cell* **81**:323–330.
23. Zhu, L., van den Heuvel, S., Helin, K., Fattaey, A., Ewen, M. E., Livingston, D. M., et al. (1993) Inhibition of cell proliferation by p107, a relative of the retinoblastoma protein. *Genes Develop.* **7**:1111–1125.
24. Lukas, J., Muller, H., Bartkova, J., Spitkovsky, D., Kjerulff, A. A., Jansen, D. P., et al. (1994) DNA tumor virus oncoproteins and retinoblastoma gene mutations share the ability to relieve the cell's requirement for cyclin D1 function in G1. *J. Cell. Biol.* **125**:625–638.
25. Baldin, V., Lukas, J., Marcote, M. J., Pagano, M., and Draetta, G. (1993) Cyclin D1 is a nuclear protein required for cell cycle progression in G1. *Genes Dev.* **7**:812–821.
26. Helin, K., Lees, J. A., Vidal, M., Dyson, N., Harlow, E., and Fattaey, A. (1992) A cDNA encoding a pRb-binding protein with properties of the transcription factor E2F. *Cell* **70**:337–350.
27. Kaelin, W. G., Jr, Krek, W., Sellers, W. R., DeCaprio, J. A., Ajchenbaum, F., Fuchs, C. S., et al. (1992) Expression cloning of a cDNA encoding a retinoblastoma-binding protein with E2F-like properties. *Cell* **70**:351–364.
28. Shan, B., Zhu, X., Chen, P. L., Durfee, T., Yang, Y., Sharp, D., et al. (1992) Molecular cloning of cellular genes encoding retinoblastoma-associated proteins: identification of a gene with properties of the transcription factor E2F. *Mol. Cell. Biol.* **12**:5620–5631.
29. Sanchez, I. and Dynlacht, B. D. (1996) Transcriptional control of the cell cycle. *Curr. Opin. Cell Biol.* **8**:318–324.
30. Qin, X. Q., Livingston, D. M., Ewen, M., Sellers, W. R., Arany, Z., and Kaelin, W. G. (1995) The transcription factor E2F-1 is a downstream target of RB action. *Mol. Cell. Biol.* **15**:742–755.
31. Weintraub, S. J., Chow, K. N., Luo, R. X., Zhang, S. H., He, S., and Dean, D. C. (1995) Mechanism of active transcriptional repression by the retinoblastoma protein. *Nature* **375**:812–815.
32. Magnaghi-Jaulin, L., Groisman, R., Naguibneva, I., Robin, P., Lorain, S., Le Villain, J. P., et al. (1998) Retinoblastoma protein represses transcription by recruiting a histone deacetylase. *Nature* **391**:601–605.
33. Brehm, A., Miska, E. A., McCance, D. J., Reid, J. L., Bannister, A. J., and Kouzarides, T. (1998) Retinoblastoma protein recruits histone deacetylase to repress transcription. *Nature* **391**:597–601.
34. Udvadia, A. J., Templeton, D. J., and Horowitz, J. M. (1995) Functional interactions between the retinoblastoma (Rb) protein and Sp-family members: superactivation by Rb requires amino acids necessary for growth suppression. *Proc. Natl. Acad. Sci. USA* **92**:3953–3957.
35. Kennett, S. B., Udvadia, A. J., and Horowitz, J. M. (1997) Sp3 encodes multiple proteins that differ in their capacity to stimulate or repress transcription. *Nucleic Acids Res.* **25**:3110–3117.
36. Hateboer, G., Timmers, H. T., Rustgi, A. K., Billaud, M., van't Veer, L. J., and Bernards, R. (1993) TATA-binding protein and the retinoblastoma gene product bind to overlapping epitopes on c-myc and adenovirus E1A protein. *Proc. Natl. Acad. Sci. USA* **90**:8489–8493.
37. Hagemeier, C., Bannister, A. J., Cook, A., and Kouzarides, T. (1993) The activation domain of transcription factor PU.1 binds the retinoblastoma (RB) protein and the transcription factor TFIID in vitro: RB shows sequence similarity to TFIID and TFIIB. *Proc. Natl. Acad. Sci. USA* **90**:1580–1584.
38. Welch, P. J. and Wang, J. Y. (1993) A C-terminal protein-binding domain in the retinoblastoma protein regulates nuclear c-abl tyrosine kinase in the cell cycle. *Cell* **75**:779–790.
39. Welch, P. J. and Wang, J. Y. (1995) Abrogation of retinoblastoma protein function by c-abl tyrosine kinase-dependent and -independent mechanisms. *Mol. Cell. Biol.* **15**:5542–5551.
40. Xiao, Z. X., Chen, J., Levine, A. J., Modjtahedi, N., Xing, J., Sellers, W. R., et al. (1995) Interaction between the retinoblastoma protein and the oncoprotein MDM2. *Nature* **375**:694–698.
41. Voit, R., Schafer, K., and Grummt, I. (1997) Mechanism of repression of RNA polymerase I transcription by the retinoblastoma protein. *Mol. Cell. Biol.* **17**:4230–4237.
42. Cavanaugh, A. H., Hempel, W. M., Taylor, L. J., Rogalsky, V., Todorov, G., and Rothblum, L. I. (1995) Activity of RNA polymerase I transcription factor UBF blocked by Rb gene product. *Nature* **374**:177–180.
43. Shao, Z., Siegert, J. L., Ruppert, S., and Robbins, P. D. (1997) Rb interacts with TAF(II)250/TFIID through multiple domains. *Oncogene* **15**:385–392.
44. Shao, Z., Ruppert, S., and Robbins, P. D. (1995) The retinoblastoma-susceptibility gene product binds directly to the human TATA-binding protein-associated factor TAFII250. *Proc. Natl. Acad. Sci. USA* **92**:3115–3119.
45. Takemura, M., Kitagawa, T., Izutu, S., Wasa, J., Takai, A., Akiyama, T., et al. (1997) Phosphorylated retinoblastoma protein stimulates DNA polymerase alpha. *Oncogene* **15**:2483–2492.
46. White, R. J., Trouche, D., Martin, K., Jackson, S. P., and Kouzarides, T. (1996) Repression of RNA polymerase III transcription by the retinoblastoma protein. *Nature* **382**:88–90.
47. Larminie, C. G., Cairns, C. A., Mital, R., Martin, K., Kouzarides, T., Jackson, S. P., et al. (1997) Mechanistic analysis of RNA polymerase III regulation by the retinoblastoma protein. *EMBO J.* **16**:2061–2071.
48. Chu, W. M., Wang, Z., Roeder, R. G., and Schmid, C. W. (1997) RNA polymerase III transcription repressed by Rb through its interactions with TFIIIB and TFIIIC2. *J. Biol. Chem.* **272**:14755–14761.
49. Clarke, A. R., Mandaag, E. R., van Roon, M., van der Lugt, N. M. T., van der Valk, M., Hooper, M. L., et al. (1992) Requirement for a functional Rb-1 gene in murine development. *Nature* **359**:328–330.
50. Jacks, T., Fazeli, A., Schmitt, E. M., Bronson, R. T., Goodell, M. A., and Weinberg, R. A. (1992) Effects of an Rb mutation in the mouse. *Nature* **359**:295–300.
51. Lee, E. Y. H. P., Chang, C. Y., Hu, N., Wang, Y. C. J., Lai, C. C., Herrup, K., et al. (1992) Mice deficient for Rb are nonviable and show defects in neurogenesis and haematopoiesis. *Nature* **359**:288–294.
52. Yamaskai, L., Bronson, R., Williams, B. O., Dyson, N. J., Harlow, E., and Jacks, T. (1998) Loss of E2F-1 reduces tumorigenesis and extends the lifespan of Rb1 (+/-) mice. *Nature Genet.* **18**:360–363.
53. Riley, D. J., Liu, C. Y., and Lee, W. H. (1997) Mutations in the N-terminal regions render the retinoblastoma protein insufficient for functions in development and tumor suppression. *Mol. Cell. Biol.* **17**:7342–7352.
54. Hamel, P. A., Phillips, R. A., Muncaster, M., and Gallie, B. L. (1992) Speculations on the roles of RB1 in tissue specific differentiation, tumor initiation, and tumor progression. *FASEB J.* **7**:846–854.
55. Sherr, C. J. and Roberts, J. M. (1995) Inhibitors of mammalian cyclin-dependent kinases. *Genes Dev.* **9**:1149–1163.
56. Bookstein, R. and Lee, W. H. (1991) Molecular genetics of the retinoblastoma suppressor gene. *Crit. Rev. Oncogen.* **2**:211–227.
57. Dryja, T. P., Rapaport, J., McGee, T. L., Nork, T. M., and Schwartz, T. L. (1993) Molecular etiology of low-penetrance retinoblastoma in two pedigrees. *Am. J. Hum. Genet.* **52**:1122–1128.
58. Hogg, A., Bia, B., Onadim, Z., and Cowell, J. K. (1993) Molecular mechanisms of oncogenic mutations in tumors from patients with bilateral and unilateral retinoblastoma. *Proc. Natl. Acad. Sci. USA* **90**:7351–7355.
59. Kratzke, R. A., Otterson, G. A., Hogg, A., Coxon, A. B., Geradts, J., Cowell, J. K., et al. (1994) Partial inactivation of the RB product in a family with incomplete penetrance of familial retinoblastoma and benign retinal tumors. *Oncogene* **9**:1321–1326.
60. Lohman, D. R., Brandt, B., Hopping, W., Passarge, E., and Horsthemke, B. (1994) Distinct RB1 gene mutations with low penetrance in hereditary retinoblastoma. *Human Genet.* **94**:349–354.

61. Otterson, G. A., Chen, W. D., Coxon, A. B., Khleif, S. N., and Kaye, F. J. (1997) Incomplete penetrance of familial retinoblastoma linked to germ-line mutations that result in partial loss of RB function. *Proc. Natl. Acad. Sci. USA* **94**:12036–12040.

62. Bremner, R., Du, D. C., Connolly-Wilson, M. J., Bridge, P., Ahmad, K. F., Mostachfi, H., et al. (1997) Deletion of RB exons 24 and 25 causes low-penetrance retinoblastoma. *Am. J. Human Genet.* **61**:556–570.

63. Ewen, M. E., Xing, Y. G., Lawrence, J. B., and Livingston, D. M. (1991) Molecular cloning, chromosomal mapping, and expression of the cDNA for p107, a retinoblastoma gene product-related protein. *Cell* **66**:1155–1164.

64. Hannon, G. J., Demetrick, D., and Beach, D. (1993) Isolation of the Rb-related p130 through its interaction with CDK2 and cyclins. *Genes Dev.* **7**:2378–2391.

65. Li, Y., Graham, C., Lacy, S., Duncan, A. M., and Whyte, P. (1993) The adenovirus E1A-associated 130-kD protein is encoded by a member of the retinoblastoma gene family and physically interacts with cyclins A and E. *Genes Dev.* **7**:2366–2377.

66. Mayol, X., Grana, X., Baldi, A., Sang, N., Hu, Q., and Giordano, A. (1993) Cloning of a new member of the retinoblastoma gene family (pRb2) which binds to the E1A transforming domain. *Oncogene* **8**:2561–2566.

67. Hurford, R. K., Jr., Cobrink, D., Lee, M. H., and Dyson, N. (1997) pRB and p107/p130 are required for the regulated expression of different sets of E2F responsive genes. *Genes Dev.* **11**:1447–1463.

68. Lee, M. H., Williams, B. O., Mulligan, G., Mukai, S., Bronson, R. T., Dyson, N., et al. (1996) Targeted disruption of p107: functional overlap between p107 and Rb. *Genes Dev.* **10**:1621–632.

69. Cobrinik, D., Lee, M. H., Hannon, G., Mulligan, G., Bronson, R. T., Dyson, N., et al. (1996) Shared role of the pRB-related p130 and p107 proteins in limb development. *Genes Dev.* **10**:1633–644.

70. Jiang, Z., Zacksenhaus, E., Gallie, B. L., and Phillips, R. A. (1997) The retinoblastoma gene family is differentially expressed during embryogenesis. *Oncogene* **14**:1789–1797.

71. Helin, K., Holm, K., Niebuhr, A., Eiberg, H., Tommerup, N., Hougaard, S., et al. (1997) Loss of the retinoblastoma protein-related p130 protein in small cell lung carcinoma. *Proc. Natl. Acad. Sci. USA* **94**:6933–6938.

72. Xiong, Y., Zhang, H., and Beach, D. (1992) D-type cyclins associate with multiple protein kinases and the DNA replication and repair factor PCNA. *Cell* **71**:505–514.

73. Harper, J. W., Adami, G. R., Wei, N., Keyomarsi, K., and Elledge, S. J. (1993) The p21 cdk-interacting protein Cip1 is a potent inhibitor of G1 cyclin-dependent kinases. *Cell* **75**:805–816.

74. El-Deiry, W. S., Tokino, T., Velculescu, V. E., Levy, D. B., Parsons, R., Trent, J. M., et al. (1993) WAF1, a potent mediator of p53 tumor suppression. *Cell* **75**:817–825.

75. El-Deiry, W. S., Harper, J. W., O'Connor, P. M., Velculescu, V. E., Canman, C. E., Jackman, J., et al. (1994) WAF1/CIP1 is induced in p53-mediated G1 arrest and apoptosis. *Cancer Res.* **54**:1169–1174.

76. Harper, J. W., Elledge, S. J., Keyomarsi, K., Dynlacht, B., Tsai, L. H., Zhang, P., et al. (1995) Inhibition of cyclin-dependent kinases by p21. *Mol. Biol. Cell* **6**:387–400.

77. Zhang, H., Hannon, G. J., and Beach, D. (1994) p21-containing cyclin kinases exist in both active and inactive states. *Genes Dev.* **8**:1750–1758.

78. Li, R., Waga, S., Hannon, G. J., Beach, D., and Stillman, B. (1994) Differential effects by the p21 cdk inhibitor on PCNA-dependent DNA replication and repair. *Nature* **371**:534–537.

79. Cayrol, C., Knibiehler, M., and Ducommun, B. (1998) p21 binding to PCNA causes G1 and G2 cell cycle arrest in p53-deficient cells. *Oncogene* **16**:311–320.

80. Somasundaram, K., Zhang, H., Zeng, Y. X., Houvras, Y., Peng, Y., Zhang, H., et al. (1997) Arrest of the cell cycle by the tumour-suppressor BRCA1 requires the CDK-inhibitor p21WAF1/CIP1. *Nature* **389**:187–190.

81. Feunteun, J. and Lenoir, G. M. (1996) BRCA1, a gene involved in inherited predisposition to breast and ovarian cancer. *Biochim. Biophys. Acta* **1242**:177–180.

82. Shim, J., Lee, H., Park, J., Kim, H., and Choi, E. J. (1996) A non-enzymatic p21 protein inhibitor of stress-activated protein kinases. *Nature* **381**:804–806.

83. Kearsey, J. M., Coates, P. J., Prescott, A. R., Warbrick, E., and Hall, P. A. (1995) Gadd45 is a nuclear cell cycle regulated protein which interacts with p21Cip1. *Oncogene* **11**:1675–1683.

84. Gao, X., Chen, Y. Q., Wu, N., Grignon, D. J., Sakr, W., Porter, A. T., et al. (1995) Somatic mutations of the WAF1/CIP1 gene in primary prostate cancer. *Oncogene* **11**:1395–1398.

85. Watanabe, H., Fukuchi, K., Takagi, Y., Tomoyasu, S., Tsuruoka, N., and Gomi, K. (1995) Molecular analysis of the Cip1/Waf1 (p21) gene in diverse types of human tumors. *Biochim. Biophys. Acta* **1263**:275–280.

86. Balbin, M., Hannon, G. J., Pendas, A. M., Ferrando, A. A., Vizoso, F., Fueyo, A., et al. (1996) Functional analysis of a p21WAF1,CIP1,SDI1 mutant (Arg94ÆTrp) identified in a human breast carcinoma. Evidence that the mutation impairs the ability of p21 to inhibit cyclin-dependent kinases. *J. Biol. Chem.* **271**:15782–15786.

87. Lacombe, L., Orlow, I., Silver, D., Gerald, W. L., Fair, W. R., Reuter, V. E., et al. (1996) Analysis of p21WAF1/CIP1 in primary bladder tumors. *Oncol. Res.* **8**:409–414.

88. Deng, C., Zhang, P., Harper, J. W., Elledge, S. J., and Leder, P. (1995) Mice lacking p21CIP1/WAF1 undergo normal development, but are defective in G1 checkpoint control. *Cell* **82**:675–684.

89. Polyak, K., Kato, J. Y., Solomon, M. J., Sherr, C. J., Massague, J., Roberts, J. M., et al. (1994) 27Kip1, a cyclin-cdk inhibitor, links transforming growth factor-beta and contact inhibition to cell cycle arrest. *Genes Dev.* **8**:9–22.

90. Polyak, K., Lee, M., Erdjument-Bromage, H., Koff, A., Roberts, J. M., Tempst, P., et al. (1994) Cloning of p27[KIP1], a cyclin-dependent kinase inhibitor and a potential of extracellular antimitogenic signals. *Cell* **78**:59–66.

91. Toyoshima, H. and Hunter, T. (1994) p27, a novel inhibitor of G1 cyclin-cdk protein kinase activity, is related to p21. *Cell* **78**:67–74.

92. Ewen, M. E., Sluss, H. K., Whitehouse, L. L., and Livingston, D. M. (1993) TGF beta inhibition of Cdk4 synthesis is linked to cell cycle arrest. *Cell* **74**:1009–1020.

93. Kato, J. Y., Matsuoka, M., Polyak, K., Massague, J., and Sherr, C. J. (1994) Cyclic AMP-induced G1 phase arrest mediated by an inhibitor (p27Kip1) of cyclin-dependent kinase 4 activation. *Cell* **79**:487–496.

94. Coats, S., Flanagan, W. M., Nourse, J., and Roberts, J. M. (1996) Requirement of p27Kip1 for restriction point control of the fibroblast cell cycle. *Science* **272**:877–880.

95. Nakayama, K., Ishida, N., Shirane, M., Inomata, A., Inoue, T., Shishido, N., et al. (1996) Mice lacking p27(Kip1) display increased body size, multiple organ hyperplasia, retinal dysplasia, and pituitary tumors. *Cell* **85**:707–720.

96. Fero, M. L., Rivkin, M., Tasch, M., Porter, P., Carow, C. E., Firpo, E., et al. (1996) A syndrome of multiorgan hyperplasia with features of gigantism, tumorigenesis, and female sterility in p27(Kip1)-deficient mice. *Cell* **85**:733–744.

97. Pietenpol, J. A., Bohlander, S. K., Sato, Y., Papadopoulos, N., Liu, B., Friedman, C., et al. (1995) Assignment of the human p27Kip1 gene to 12p13 and its analysis in leukemias. *Cancer Res.* **55**:1206–1210.

98. Matsuoka, S., Edwards, M. C., Bai, C., Parker, S., Zhang, P., Baldini, A., et al. (1995) p57KIP2, a structurally distinct member of the p21CIP1 cdk inhibitor family, is a candidate tumor-suppressor gene. *Genes Dev.* **9**:650–662.

99. Lee, M. H., Reynisdottir, I., and Massague, J. (1995) Cloning of p57KIP2, a cyclin-dependent kinase inhibitor with unique domain structure and tissue distribution. *Genes Dev.* **9**:639–649.

100. Watanabe, H., Pan, Z. Q., Schreiber-Agus, N., DePinho, R. A., Hurwitz, J., and Xiong, Y. (1998) Suppression of cell transformation by the cyclin-dependent kinase inhibitor p57 (KIP2) requires binding to proliferating cell nuclear antigen. *Proc. Natl. Acad. Sci. USA* **95**:1392–1397.

101. Hatada, I., Ohashi, H., Fukushima, Y., Kaneko, Y., Inoue, M., Komoto, Y., et al. (1996) An imprinted gene p57KIP2 is mutated in Beckwith-Wiedemann syndrome. *Nature Genet.* **14**:171–173.
102. Lee, M. P., DeBaun, M., Randhawa, G., Reichard, B. A., Elledge, S. J., and Feinberg, A. P. (1997) Low frequency of p57KIP2 mutation in Beckwith-Wiedemann syndrome. *Am. J. Human Genet.* **61**:04–309.
103. Hatada, I., Nabetani, A., Morisaki, H., Xin, Z., Ohishi, S., Tonoki, H., et al. (1997) New p57KIP2 mutations in Beckwith-Wiedemann syndrome. *Human Genet.* **100**:681–683.
104. O'Keefe, D., Dao, D., Zhao, L., Sandrson, R., Warburton, D., Weiss, L., et al. (1997) Coding mutations in p57KIP2 are present in some cases of Beckwith-Wiedemann syndrome but are rare or absent in Wilms tumors. *Am. J. Human Genet.* **61**:295–303.
105. Yan, Y., Frisen, J., Lee, M. H., Massague, J., and Barbacid, M. (1997) Ablation of the cdk inhibitor p57Kip2 results in increased apoptosis and delayed differentiation during mouse development. *Genes Dev.* **11**:973–983.
106. Zhang, P., Liegeois, N. J., Wong, C., Finegold, M., Hou, H., Thompson, J. C., et al. (1997) Altered cell differentiation and proliferation in mice lacking p57KIP2 indicates a role in Beckwith-Wiedemann syndrome. *Nature* **387**:151–158.
107. Kondo, M., Matsuoka, S., Uchida, K., Osada, H., Nagatake, M., Takagi, K., et al. (1996) Selective maternal-allele loss in human lung cancers of the maternally expressed p57KIP2 gene at 11p15.5. *Oncogene* **12**:1365–1368.
108. Serrano, M., Hannon, G. J., and Beach, D. (1994) A new regulatory motif in cell-cycle control causing specific inhibition of cyclin D-cdk4. *Nature* **366**:704–707.
109. Hannon, G. J. and Beach, D. (1994) p15INK4B is a potential effector of TGF-beta-induced cell cycle arrest. *Nature* **371**:257–261.
110. Hirai, H., Roussel, M. F., Kato, J. Y., Ashmun, R. A., and Sherr, C. J. (1995) Novel INK4 proteins, p19 and p18, are specific inhibitors of the cyclin D-dependent kinases cdk4 and cdk6. *Mol. Cell. Biol.* **15**:2672–2681.
111. Chan, F. K., Zhang, J., Cheng, L., Shapiro, D. N., and Winoto, A. (1995) Identification of human and mouse p19, a novel cdk4 and cdk6 inhibitor with homology to p16ink4. *Mol. Cell. Biol.* **15**:2682–2688.
112. Lukas, J., Parry, D., Aagaard, L., Mann, D. J., Bartkova, J., Strauss, M., et al. (1995) Retinoblastoma-protein-dependent cell-cycle inhibition by the tumour suppressor p16. *Nature* **375**:503–506.
113. Shapiro, G. I. and Rollins, B. J. (1996) p16INK4A as a human tumor suppressor. *Biochim. Biophys. Acta* **1242**:165–169.
114. Serrano, M., Lee, H., Chin, L., Cordon-Cardo, C., Beach, D., and DePinho, R. A. (1996) Role of the INK4a locus in tumor suppression and cell mortality. *Cell* **85**:27–37.
115. Zindy, F., Quelle, D. E., Roussel, M. F., and Sherr, C. J. (1997) Expression of the p16INK4a tumor suppressor versus other INK4 family members during mouse development and aging. *Oncogene* **15**:203–211.
116. Kamb, A., Gruis, N. A., Weaver-Feldhaus, J., and Liu, Q. (1994) A cell cycle regulator potentially involved in the genesis of many tumor types. *Science* **264**:436–440.
117. Hussussian, C. J., Struewing, J. P., Goldstein, A. M., Higgins, P. A., Ally, D. S., Sheahan, M. D., et al. (1994) Germline p16 mutations in familial melanoma. *Nature Genet.* **8**:15–21.
118. Kamb, A., Shattuck-Eidens, D., Eeles, R., Liu, Q., Gruis, N. A., Ding, W., et al. (1994) Analysis of the p16 gene (CDKN2) as a candidate for the chromosome 9p melanoma susceptibility locus. *Nature Genet.* **8**:22–26.
119. Foulkes, W. D., Flanders, T. Y., Pollock, P. M., and Hayward, N. K. (1996) The CDKN2 (P16) gene and human cancer. *Mol. Med.* **3**:5–20.
120. Herman, J. G., Merlo, A., Mao, L., Lapidus, R. G., Issa, J. P., Davidson, N. E., et al. (1995) Inactivation of the CDKN2/p16/MTS1 gene is frequently associated with aberrant DNA methylation in all common human cancers. *Cancer Res.* **55**:4525–4530.
121. Gonzalez-Zulueta, M., Bender, C. M., Yang, A. S., Nguyen, T., Beart, R. W., Van Tornout, J. M., et al. (1995) Methylation of the 5′ CpG island of the p16/CDKN2 tumor-suppressor gene in normal and transformed human tissues correlates with gene silencing. *Cancer Res.* **55**:4531–4535.
122. Pollock, P. M., Pearson, J. V., and Hayward, N. K. (1996) Compilation of somatic mutations of the CDKN2 gene in human cancers: non-random distribution of base substitutions. *Genes Chromosomes Cancer* **15**:77–88.
123. Shapiro, G. I., Park, J. E., Edwards, C. D., Mao, L., Merlo, A., Sidransky, D., et al. (1995) Multiple mechanisms of p16INK4A inactivation in non-small cell lung cancer cell lines. *Cancer Res.* **55**:6200–6209.
124. Merlo, A., Herman, J.'G., Mao, L., Lee, D. J., Gabrielson, E., Burger, P. C., et al. (1995) 5′CpG island methylation is associated with transcriptional silencing of the tumour suppressor p16/CDKN2/MTS1 in human cancers. *Nature Med.* **1**:686–692.
125. Smith-Sorensen, B. and Hovig, E. (1996) CDKN2A (p16INK4A) somatic and germline mutations. *Human Mutat.* **7**:294–303.
126. Craig, C., Kim, M., Ohri, E., Wersto, R., Katayose, D., Li, Z., et al. (1998) Effects of adenovirus-mediated p16INK4A expression on cell cycle arrest are determined by endogenous p16 and Rb status in human cancer cells. *Oncogene* **16**:265–272.
127. Fueyo, J., Gomez-Manzano, C., Yung, W. K., Clayman, G. L., Liu, T. J., Bruner, J., et al. (1996) Adenovirus-mediated p16/CDKN2 gene transfer induces growth arrest and modifies the transformed phenotype of glioma cells. *Oncogene* **12**:103–110.
128. Herman, J. G., Jen, J., Merlo, A., and Baylin, S. B. (1996) Hypermethylation-associated inactivation indicates a tumor suppressor role for p15INK4B. *Cancer Res.* **56**:722–727.
129. Iravani M, Dhat R, and Price C. M. (1997) Methylation of the multi tumor-suppressor gene-2 (MTS2, CDKN1, p15INK4B) in childhood acute lymphoblastic leukemia. *Oncogene* **15**:2609–2614.
130. Herman, J. G., Civin, C. I., Issa, J. P., Collector, M. I., Sharkis, S., and Baylin, S. B. (1997) Distinct patterns of inactivation of p15INK4B and p16INK4A characterize the major types of hematological malignancies. *Cancer Res.* **57**:837–841.
131. Quelle, D. E., Zindy, F., Ashmun, R. A., and Sherr, C. J. (1995) Alternative reading frames of the INK4a tumor-suppressor gene encode two unrelated proteins capable of inducing cell cycle arrest. *Cell* **83**:993–1000.
132. Kamijo, T., Zindy, F., Roussel, M. F., Quelle, D. E., Downing, J. R., Ashmun, R. A., et al. (1997) Tumor suppression at the mouse INK4a locus mediated by the alternative reading frame product p19ARF. *Cell* **91**:649–659.
133. Pomerantz, J., Schreiber-Agus, N., Liegeois, N. J., Silverman, A., Alland, L., Chin, L., et al. (1998) The Ink4a tumor-suppressor gene product, p19Arf, interacts with MDM2 and neutralizes MDM2's inhibition of p53. *Cell* **92**:713–723
134. Zhang, Y., Xiong, Y., and Yarbrough, W. G. (1998) ARF promotes MDM2 degradation and stabilizes p53: ARF-INK4a locus deletion impairs both the Rb and p53 tumor suppression pathways. *Cell* **92**:725–734.
135. Sellers, W. R., Novitch, B. G., Miyake, S., Heith, A., Otterson, G. A., Kaye, F. J., et al. (1998) Stable binding to E2F is not required for the retinoblastoma protein to activate transcription, promote differentiation, and suppress tumor cell growth. *Genes Dev.* **12**:95–106.
136. Wu, X. J., Zhou, Y., Ji, W., Parng, G. S., Kruzelock, R., Kong, C. T., et al. (1997) Reexpression of the retinoblastoma protein in tumor cells induces senescence and telomerase inhibition. *Oncogene* **15**:2589–2596.
137. Morgenbesser, S. D., Williams, B. O., Jacks, T., and DePinho, R. A. (1994) p53-dependent apoptosis produced by Rb-deficiency in the developing mouse lens. *Nature* **371**:72–74.
138. Hollstein, M., Sidransky, D., Vogelstein, B., and Harris, C. (1991) p53 mutations in human cancers. *Science* **253**:49–53.
139. Greenblatt, M. S., Bennett, W. P., Hollstein, M., and Harris, C. C. (1994) Mutations in the p53 tumor-suppressor gene: clues to cancer etiology and molecular pathogenesis. *Cancer Res.* **54**:4855–4878.

140. Levine, A. J. (1997) p53, the cellular gatekeeper for growth and division. *Cell* **88**:323–331.

141. Almog, N. and Rotter, V. (1997) Involvement of p53 in cell differentiation and development. *Biochim. Biophys. Acta* **1333**:F1–F27.

142. Linzer, D. I. H. and Levine, A. J. (1979) Characterization of a 54 K dalton cellular SV40 tumor antigen present in SV40-transformed cells and uninfected embryonal carcinoma cells. *Cell* **17**:43–52.

143. Lane, D. and Crawford, L. (1979) T antigen is bound to a host protein in SV40-transformed cells. *Nature* **278**:261–263.

144. DeLeo, A. B., Jay, G., Appella, E., Dubois, G. C., Law, L. W., and Old, L .J. (1979) Detection of a transformation-related antigen in chemically induced sarcomas and other transformed cells of the mouse. *Proc. Natl. Acad. Sci. USA* **76**:2420–2424.

145. Eliyahu, D., Michalovitz, D., Eliyahu, S., Pinhasi-Kimhi, O., and Oren, M. (1989) Wild-type p53 can inhibit oncogene-mediated focus formation. *Proc. Natl. Acad. Sci. USA* **86**:8763–8767.

146. Finlay, C. A., Hinds, P. W., and Levine, A. J. (1989) The p53 proto-oncogene can act as a suppressor of transformation. *Cell* **57**:1083–1093.

147. Baker, S. J., Markowitz, S., Fearon, E. R., Willson, J. K., and Vogelstein, B. (1990) Suppression of human colorectal carcinoma cell growth by wild-type p53. *Science* **249**:912–915.

148. Diller, L., Kassel, J., Nelson, C. E., Gryka, M. A., Litwak, G., Gebhardt, M., et al. (1990) p53 functions as a cell cycle control protein in human osteosarcomas. *Mol. Cell. Biol.* **10**:5772–5781.

149. Mercer, W. E., Shields, M. T., Amin, M., Sauve, G. J., Appella, E., Romano, J. W., et al. (1990) Negative growth regulation in a glioblastoma tumor cell line that conditionally expresses human wild-type p53. *Proc. Natl. Acad. Sci. USA* **87**:6166–6170.

150. Chen, P. L., Chen, Y., Bookstein, R., and Lee, W. H. (1991) Genetic mechanisms of tumor suppression by the human p53 gene. *Science* **250**:1576–1580.

151. Mercer, W. F., Shields, M. T., Amin, M., Sauve, G. J., Appella, E., Romano, J. W., et al. (1990) Negative growth regulation in a glioblastoma tumor cell line that conditionally expresses human wild type p53. *Proc. Natl. Acad. Sci. USA* **87**:6166–6170.

152. Michalovitz, D., Halevy, O., and Oren, M. (1990) Conditional inhibition of transformation and of cell proliferation by a temperature-sensitive mutant of p53. *Cell* **62**:671–680.

153. Martinez, J., Georgoff, I., Martinex, J., and Levine, A. J. (1991) Cellular localization and cell cycle regulation by a temperature-sensitive p53 protein. *Genes Dev.* **5**:151–159.

154. Livingstone, L. R., White, A., Sprouse, J., Livanos, E., Jacks, T., and Tlsty, T. (1992) Altered cell cycle arrest and gene amplification potential accompany loss of wild-type p53. *Cell* **70**:923–935.

155. Yin, Y., Tainsky, M. A., Bischoff, F. Z., Strong, L. C., and Wahl, G. M. (1992) Wild-type p53 restores cell cycle control and inhibits gene amplification in cells with mutant p53 alleles. *Cell* **70**:937–948.

156. Maltzmann, W. and Czyzyk, L. (1984) UV irradiation stimulates levels of p53 cellular tumor antigen in nontransformed mouse cells. *Mol. Cell. Biol.* **4**:1689–1694.

157. Kastan, M. B., Onyekwere, O., Sidransky, D., Vogelstein, B., and Craig, R. W. (1991) Participation of p53 protein in the cellular response to DNA damage. *Cancer Res.* **51**:6304–6311.

158. Fritsche, M., Haessler, C., and Brandner, G. (1993) Induction of nuclear accumulation of the tumor-suppressor protein p53 by DNA-damaging agents. *Oncogene* **8**:307–318.

159. Kuerbitz, S. J., Plunkett, B. S., Walsh, W. V., and Kastan, M. (1992) Wild-type p53 is a cell cycle checkpoint determinant following irradiation. *Proc. Natl. Acad. Sci. USA* **89**:7491–7495.

160. Kastan, M. B., Zhan, Q., El-Deiry, W. S., Carrier, F., Jacks, T., Walsh, W. V., et al. (1992) A mammalian cell cycle checkpoint pathway utilizing p53 and GADD45 is defective in ataxia-telangiectasia. *Cell* **71**:587–597.

161. Wang, X. W. and Harris, C. C. (1997) p53 tumor-suppressor gene: clues to molecular carcinogenesis. *J. Cell. Physiol.* **173**:247–255.

162. Gottlieb, T. M. and Oren, M. (1996) p53 in growth control and neoplasia. *Biochim. Biophys. Acta* **1287**:77–102.

163. Ko, L. J. and Prives, C. (1996) p53: puzzle and paradigm. *Genes Dev.* **10**:1054–1072.

164. Mosner, J. T., Mummernbraur, T., Bauer, C., Sczakiel, G., Grosse, F., and Deppart, W. (1995) Negative feedback regulation of wild-type p53 biosynthesis. *EMBO J.* **14**:4442–4449.

165. Deffie, A., Wu, H., Reinke, V., and Lozano, G. (1993) The tumor suppressor p53 regulates its own transcription. *Mol. Cell. Biol.* **13**:3415–3423.

166. Walker, K. K. and Levine, A. J. (1996) Identification of a novel p53 functional domain which is necessary for efficient growth suppression. *Proc. Natl. Acad. Sci. USA* **93**:15335–15340.

167. Molinari, M. and Milner, J. (1995) p53 in complex with DNA is resistant to ubiquitin-dependent proteolysis in the presence of HPV-16 E6. *Oncogene* **10**:1849–1854.

168. Graeber, A. J., Osmanian, C., Jack, T., Housman, D. E., Koch, C. J., Lowe, S. W., et al. (1996) Hypoxia-mediated selection of cells with diminished apoptotic potential in solid tumors. *Nature* **379**:88–91.

169. Forrester, K., Ambs, S., Lupold, S. E., Kapust, R. B., Spillare, E. A., Weinberg, W. C., et al. (1996) Nitric oxide-induced p53 accumulation and regulation of inducible nitric oxide synthase (NOS2) expression by wild-type p53. *Proc. Natl. Acad. Sci. USA* **93**:2442–2447.

170. Nitta, M., Okamura, H., Aizawa, S., and Yamaizumi, M. (1997) Heat shock induces transient p53-dependent cell cycle arrest at G1/S. *Oncogene* **15**:561–568.

171. Linke, S. P., Clarkin, K. C., DiLeonardo, A., Tsou, A., and Wahl, G. M. (1996) A reversible, p53-dependent G0/G1 cell cycle arrest induced by ribonucleotide depletion in the absence of detectable DNA damage. *Genes Dev.* **10**:934–947.

172. Nigro, J. M., Aldape, K. D., Hess, S. M., and Tlsty, T. D. (1997) Cellular adhesion regulates p53 protein levels in primary human keratinocytes. *Cancer Res.* **57**:3635–3639.

173. Wu, R. C. and Schonthal, A. H. (1997) Activation of p53-p21waf1 pathway in response to disruption of cell-matrix interactions. *J. Biol. Chem.* **272**:29091–29098.

174. Momand, J., Zambetti, G. P., Olson, D.C., George, D., and Levine, A. J. (1992) The mdm-2 oncogene product forms a complex with the p53 protein and inhibits p53-mediated transactivation. *Cell* **69**:1237–1245.

175. Kubbutat, M. H., Jones, S. N., and Vousden, K. H. (1997) Regulation of p53 stability by mdm2. *Nature* **387**:299–303.

176. Piette, J., Neel, H., and Marechal, V. (1997) Mdm2: keeping p53 under control. *Oncogene* **15**:1001–1010.

177. Haupt, Y., Maya, R., Kazaz, A., and Oren, M. (1997) Mdm2 promotes the rapid degradation of p53. *Nature* **387**:296–299.

178. Barak, Y., Juven, T., Haffner, R., and Oren, M. (1993) Mdm2 expression is induced by wild type p53 activity. *EMBO J.* **12**:461–468.

179. Wu, X., Bayle, J. H., Olson, D., and Levine, A. J. (1993) The p53-mdm2-autoregulatory feedback loop. *Genes Dev.* **7**:1126–1132.

180. Oliner, J. D., Kinzler, K. W., Meltzer, P. S., George, D., and Vogelstein, B. (1992) Amplification of a gene encoding a p53-associated protein in human sarcomas. *Nature* **358**:80–83.

181. Chen, C. Y., Oliner, J. D., Zhan, Q., Fornace, A. J., Vogelstein, B., and Kastan, M. B. (1994) Interactions between p53 and mdm2 in a mammalian cell cycle checkpoint pathway. *Proc. Natl. Acad. Sci. USA* **91**:2684–2688.

182. Neil, J. C., Cameron, E. R., and Baxter, E. W. (1997) p53 and tumour viruses: catching the guardian off-guard. *Trends Microbiol.* **5**:115–120.

183. Meek, D. (1994) Post-translational modification of p53. *Semin. Cancer Biol.* **5**:203–210.

184. Steegenga, W. T., van der Eb, A. J., and Jochemsen, A. G. (1996) How phosphorylation regulates the activity of p53. *J. Mol. Biol.* **263**:103–113.

185. Martinez, J. D., Craven, M. T., Joseloff, E., Milczarek, G., and Bowden, G. T. (1997) Regulation of DNA binding and transactivation in p53 by nuclear localization and phosphorylation. *Oncogene* **14**:2511–2520.

186. Shieh, S. Y., Ikeda, M., Taya, Y., and Prives, C. (1997) DNA damage-induced phosphorylation of p53 alleviates inhibition by mdm2. *Cell* **91**:325–334.

187. Lohrum, M. and Scheidtmann, K. H. (1996) Differential effects of phosphorylation of rat p53 on transactivation of promoters derived from different p53 responsive genes. *Oncogene* **13**:2527–2539.

188. Okamoto, K. and Beach, D. (1994) Cyclin G is a transcriptional target of the p53 tumor suppressor protein. *EMBO J.* **13**:4816–4822.

189. Miyashita, T. and Reed, J. C. (1995) Tumor suppressor p53 is a direct transcriptional activator of the human bax gene. *Cell* **80**:293–299.

190. Buckbinder, L., Talbott, R., Velasco-Miguel, S., Takenaka, I., Faha, B., Seizinger, B. R., et al. (1995) Induction of the growth inhibitor IGF-binding protein-3 by p53. *Nature* **377**:646–649.

191. Mack, D. H., Vartikar, J, Pipas, J. M., and Laimins, L. (1993) Specific repression of TATA-mediated but not initiator-mediated transcription by wild-type p53. *Nature* **363**:281–283.

192. Sabbatini, P., Lin, J., Levine, A. J., and White, E. (1995) Essential role for p53-mediated transcription in E1A-induced apoptosis. *Genes Dev.* **9**:2184–2192.

193. Horikoshi, N., Usheva, A., Chen, J., Levine, A. J., Weinmann, R., and Shenk, T. (1995) Two domains of p53 interact with the TATA-binding protein, and the adenovirus 13S E1A protein disrupts the association, relieving p53-mediated transcriptional repression. *Mol. Cell. Biol.* **15**:227–234.

194. Shaulian, E., Haviv, I., Shaul, Y., and Oren, M. (1995) Transcriptional repression by the C-terminal domain of p53. *Oncogene* **10**:671–680.

195. Subler, M. A., Martin, D. W., and Deb, S. (1994) Overlapping domains on the p53 protein regulate its transcriptional activation and repression functions. *Oncogene* **9**:1351–1359.

196. Lu, H. and Levine, A. J. (1995) Human TAF31 protein is a transcriptional coactivator of the p53 protein. *Proc. Natl. Acad. Sci. USA* **92**:5154–5158.

197. Thut, C. J., Chen, J. L., Klemin, R., and Tijan, R. (1995) p53 transcriptional activation mediated by coactivators TAFII40 and TAFII60. *Science* **267**:100–104.

198. Lu, H., Fisher, R. P., Bailey, P., and Levine, A. J. (1997) The CDK7-cycH-p36 complex of transcription factor IIH phosphorylates p53, enhancing its sequence-specific DNA binding activity in vitro. *Mol. Cell. Biol.* **17**:5923–5934.

199. Xiao, H., Pearson, A., Coulombe, B., Truant, R., Zhang, S., Reiger, J. L., et al. (1994) Binding of basal transcription factor TFIIH to the acidic activation domains of VP16 and p53. *Mol. Cell. Biol.* **14**:7013–7024.

200. Wang, X. W., Forrester, K., Yeh, Y., Feitelson, M. A., Gu, J. R., and Harris, C. C. (1994) Hepatitis B virus X protein inhibits p53 sequence-specific DNA binding, transcriptional activity and association with transcription factor ERCC3. *Proc. Natl. Acad. Sci. USA* **91**:2230–2234.

201. Wang, X. W., Yeh, H., Schaeffer, L., Roy, R., Moncollin, V., Egly, J. M., et al. (1995) p53 modulation of TFIIH-associated nucleotide excision repair activity. *Nature Genet.* **10**:188–193.

202. Leveillard, T., Andera, L., Bissonette, N., Schaeffer, L., Bracco, L., Egly, J. M., et al. (1996) Functional interactions between p53 and the TFIIH complex are affected by tumour-associated mutations. *EMBO J.* **15**:1615–1624.

203. Dutta, A., Ruppert, S. M., Aster, J. C., and Winchester, E. (1993) Inhibition of DNA replication factor RPA by p53. *Nature* **365**:79–82.

204. He, Z., Brinton, B. T., Greenblatt, J., Hassell, J. A., and Ingels, C. J. (1993) The transactivator proteins VP16 and GAL4 bind replication factor A. *Cell* **73**:1223–1232.

205. Li, R. and Botchan, M. R. (1993) The acidic transcriptional activation domains of VP16 and p53 bind the cellular replication protein A and stimulate in vitro BPV-1 DNA replication. *Cell* **73**:1207–1221.

206. Lill, N. L., Grossman, S. R., Ginsberg, D., DeCaprio, J., and Livingston, D. M. (1997) Binding and modulation of p53 by p300/CBP coactivators. *Nature* **387**:823–827.

207. Gu, W., Shi, X. L., and Roeder, R. G. (1997) Synergistic activation of transcription by CBP and p53. *Nature* **387**:819–823.

208. Avantaggiati, M. L., Ogryzko, V., Gardner, K., Giordano, A., Levine, A. S., and Kelly, K. (1997) Recruitment of p300/CBP in p53-dependent signal pathways. *Cell* **89**:1175–1184.

209. Scolnick, D. M., Chehab, N. H., Stavridi, E. S., Lien, M. C., Caruso, L., Moran, E, et al. (1997) CREB-binding protein and p300/CBP-associated factor are transcriptional coactivators of the p53 tumor suppressor protein. *Cancer Res.* **57**:3693–3696.

210. Gu, W. and Roeder, R. G. (1997) Activation of p53 sequence-specific DNA binding by acetylation of the p53 C-terminal domain. *Cell* **90**:595–606.

211. Hansen, R. S. and Braithwaite, A. W. (1996) The growth-inhibitory function of p53 is separable from transactivation, apoptosis and suppression of transformation by E1A and ras. *Oncogene* **13**:995–1007.

212. Linke, S. P., Clarkin, K. C., and Wahl, G. M. (1997) p53 mediates permanent arrest over multiple cell cycles in response to gamma-irradiation. *Cancer Res.* **57**:1171–1179.

213. Pietenpol, J. A., Toniko, T., Thiagalingam, S., El-Deiry, W. S., Kinzler, K. W., and Vogelstein, B. S. (1994) Sequence-specific transcriptional activation is essential for growth suppression by p53. *Proc. Natl. Acad. Sci. USA* **91**:1998–2002.

214. Unger, T., Mietz, J. A., Scheffner, M., Yee, C. L., and Howley, P. M. (1993) Functional domains of wild-type and mutant p53 proteins involved in transcriptional regulation, transdominant inhibition, and transformation suppression. *Mol. Cell. Biol.* **13**:5186–5194.

215. Crook, T., Marston, N. J., Sara, E. A., and Vousden, K. H. (1994) Transcriptional activation by p53 correlates with suppression of growth but not transformation. *Cell* **79**:817–827.

216. Shaulian, E., Haviv, I., Shaul, Y., and Oren, M. (1995) Transcriptional repression by the C-terminal domain of p53. *Oncogene* **10**:671–680.

217. Demers, G. W., Foster, S. A., Halbert, C. L., and Galloway, D. A. (1994) Growth arrest by induction of p53 in damaged keratinocytes is bypassed by human papillomavirus 16 E7. *Proc. Natl. Acad. Sci. USA* **91**:4382–4386.

218. Hickman, E. S., Picksley, S. M., and Vousden, K. H. (1994) Cells expressing HPV16 E7 continue cell cycle progression following DNA damage induced p53 activation. *Oncogene* **9**:2177–2181.

219. Slebos, R. J., Lee, M. H., Plunkett, B. S., Kessis, T. D., Williams, B. O., Jacks, T., et al. (1994) p53-dependent G1 arrest involves pRB-related proteins and is disrupted by the human papillomavirus 16 E7 oncoprotein. *Proc. Natl. Acad. Sci. USA* **91**:5320–5324.

220. Dulic, V., Kaufmann, W. K., Wilson, S. J., Tlsty, T. D., Lees, E., Harper, J. W., et al. (1994) p53-dependent inhibition of cyclin-dependent kinase activities in human fibroblasts during radiation-induced G1 arrest. *Cell* **76**:1013–1023.

221. Polyak, K., Waldman, T., He, T. C., Kinzler, K. W., and Vogelstein, B. (1996) Genetic determinants of p53-induced apoptosis and growth arrest. *Genes Dev.* **10**:1945–1952.

222. Brugarolas, J., Chandrasekaran, C., Gordon, J. I., Beach, D., Jacks, T., and Hannon, G. J. (1995) Radiation-induced cell cycle arrest compromised by p21. *Nature* **377**:552–557.

223. MacLeod, K. F., Sherry, N., Hannon, G., Beach, D., Tokino, T., Kinzler, K. W., et al. (1995) p53-dependent and independent expression of p21 during cell growth, differentiation, and DNA damage. *Genes Dev.* **9**:935–944.

224. Michieli, P., Chedid, M., Lin, D., Pierce, J. H., Mercer, W. E., and Givol, D. (1994) Induction of WAF1/CIP1 by a p53-independent pathway. *Cancer Res.* **54**:3391–3395.

225. Zhan, Q., Lord, K. A., Alamo, I., Jr., Hollander, M. C., Carrier, F., Ron, D., et al. (1994) The gadd and myoD genes define a novel set of mammalian genes encoding acidic proteins that synergistically suppress cell growth. *Mol. Cell. Biol.* **14**:2361–2371.

226. Goga, A., Liu, X., Hambuch, T. M., Senechal, K., Major, E., Berk, A. J., et al. (1995) p53-dependent growth suppression by the c-abl nuclear tyrosine kinase. *Oncogene* **11**:791–799.

227. Yuan, Z. M., Huang, Y., Whang, Y., Sawyers, C., Weichselbaum, R., Kharbanda, S., et al. (1996) Role for c-abl tyrosine kinase in growth arrest response to DNA damage. *Nature* **382**:272–274.

228. Wen, S. T., Jackson, P. K., and Van Etten, R. A. (1996) The cytostatic function of c-abl is controlled by multiple nuclear localization signals and requires the p53 and Rb tumor-suppressor gene products. *EMBO J.* **15**:1583–1592.

229. Yuan, Z. M., Huang, Y., Fan, M. M., Sawyers, C., Kharbanda, S., and Kufe, D. (1996) Genotoxic drugs induce interaction of the c-abl tyrosine kinase and the tumor suppressor protein p53. *J. Biol. Chem.* **271**:26457–26460.

230. Liu, Z. G., Baskaran, R., Lea-Chou, E. T., Wood, L. D., Chen, Y., Karin, M., et al. (1996) Three distinct signaling responses by murine fibroblasts to genotoxic stress. *Nature* **384**:273–276.

231. Baskaran, R., Wood, L. D., Whitaker, L. L., Canman, C. E., Morgan, S. E., Xu, Y., et al. (1997) Ataxia telangiectasia mutant protein activates c-abl tyrosine kinase in response to ionizing radiation. *Nature* **387**:516–519.

232. Shafman, T., Khanna, K. K., Kedar, P., Spring, K., Kozlov, S., Yen, T., et al. (1997) Interaction between ATM protein and c-abl in response to DNA damage. *Nature* **387**:520–523.

233. Del Sal, G. D., Ruaro, E. M., Utrera, R., Cole, C. N., Levine, A. J., and Schneider, C. (1995) Gas1-induced growth suppression requires a transactivation-independent p53 function. *Mol. Cell. Biol.* **15**:7152–7160.

234. Ruaro, E. M., Collavin, L., Del Sal, G., Haffner, R., Oren, M., Levine, A. J., et al. (1997) A proline-rich motif in p53 is required for transactivation-independent growth arrest as induced by Gas1. *Proc. Natl. Acad. Sci. USA* **94**:4675–4680.

235. Fiscella, M., Zhanag, H., Fan, S., Sakaguchi, K., Shen, S., Mercer, W. E., et al. (1997) Wip1, a novel human protein phosphatase that is induced in response to ionizing radiation in a p53-dependent manner. *Proc. Natl. Acad. Sci. USA* **94**:6048–6053.

236. Parsons, R. (1998) Phosphatases and tumorigenesis. *Curr. Opin. Oncol.* **10**:88–91.

237. Ouchi, T., Monteiro, A. N. A., August, A., Aaronson, S. A., and Hanafusa, H. (1998) BRCA1 regulates p53-dependent gene expression. *Proc. Natl. Acad. Sci. USA* **95**:2302–2306.

238. Maheswaran, S., Englert, C., Bennett, P., Hedrich, G., and Haber, D. A. (1995) The WT1 gene product stabilizes p53 and inhibits p53-mediated apoptosis. *Genes Dev.* **9**:2143–2156.

239. Garkavtsev, I., Grigorian, I. A., Ossovskaya, V. S., Chernov, M. V., Chumakov, P. M., and Gudkov, A. V. (1998) The candidate tumor suppressor p33ING1 cooperates with p53 in cell growth control. *Nature* **391**:295–298.

240. Vojta, P. J. and Barrett, J. C. (1995) Genetic analysis of cellular senescence. *Biochim. Biophys. Acta* **1242**:29–41.

241. O'Connor, P. M. (1997) Mammalian G1 and G2 phase checkpoints. *Cancer Surv.* **29**:151–182.

242. Serrano, M., Lin, A. W., McCurrach, M. E., Beach, D., and Lowe, S. W. (1997) Oncogenic ras provokes premature cell senescence associated with accumulation of p53 and p16INK4a. *Cell* **88**:593–602.

243. Sugrue, M. M., Shin, D. Y., Lee, S. W., and Aaronson, S. A. (1997) Wild-type p53 triggers a rapid senescence program in human tumor cells lacking functional p53. *Proc. Natl. Acad. Sci. USA* **94**:9648–9453.

244. Bond, J., Haughton, M., Blaydes, J., Gire, V., Wynford-Thomas, D., and Wyllie, F. (1996) Evidence that transcriptional activation by p53 plays a direct role in the induction of cellular senescence. *Oncogene* **13**:2097–2104.

245. Agarwal, M. L., Agarwal, A., Taylor, W. R., and Stark, G. G. (1995) p53 controls both the G2/M and the G1 cell cycle checkpoints and mediates reversible growth arrest in human fibroblasts. *Proc. Natl. Acad. Sci. USA* **92**:8493–8497.

246. Stewart, N., Hicks, G. G., Paraskevas, F., and Mowat, M. (1995) Evidence for a second cell cycle block at G2/M by p53. *Oncogene* **10**:109–115.

247. Guillouf, C., Rosselli, F., Krishnaraju, K., Moustacchi, E., Hoffman, B., and Liebermann, D. A. (1995) p53 involvement in control of G2 exit of the cell cycle: role in DNA damage-induced apoptosis. *Oncogene* **10**:2263–2270.

248. Cross, S. M., Sanchez, C. A., Morgan, C. A., Schimke, M. K., Ramel, S., Idzerda, R. L., et al. (1995) A p53-dependent mouse spindle checkpoint. *Science* **267**:1353–1356.

249. Lanni, J. S. and Jacks, T. (1998) Characterization of the p53-dependent postmitotic checkpoint following spindle disruption. *Mol. Cell. Biol.* **18**:1055–1064.

250. Shimizu, A., Nishida, J., Ueoka, Y., Kato, K., Hachiya, T., Kuriaki, Y., et al. (1998) CyclinG contributes to G2/M arrest of cells in response to DNA damage. *Biochem. Biophys. Res. Commun.* **242**:529–533.

251. Dulic, V., Stein, G. H., Far, D. F., and Reed, S. I. (1998) Nuclear accumulation of p21Cip1 at the onset of mitosis: a role at the G2/M-phase transition. *Mol. Cell. Biol.* **18**:546–557.

252. Niculescu, A. B., 3rd, Chen, X., Smeets, M., Hengst, L., Prives, C., and Reed, S. I. (1998) Effects of p21 (Cip1/Waf1) at both the G1/S and the G2/M cell cycle transitions: pRb is a critical determinant in blocking DNA replication and in preventing endoreduplication. *Mol. Cell. Biol.* **18**:629–643.

253. Harvey, M., Sands, A. T., Weiss, R. S., Hegi, M. E., Wiseman, R. W., Pantazis, P., et al. (1993) In vitro growth characteristics of embryo fibroblasts isolated from p53-deficient mice. *Oncogene* **8**:2457–2467.

254. Purdie, C. A., Harrison, D. J., Peter, A., Dobbie, L., White, S., Howie, S. E. M., et al. (1994) Tumour incidence, spectrum and ploidy in mice with a large deletion in the p53 gene. *Oncogene* **9**:603–609.

255. Sandri, M. I., Isaacs, R. J., Ongkeko, W. M., Harris, A. L., Hickson, I. D., Broggini, M., et al. (1996) p53 regulates the minimal promoter of the human topoisomerase II alpha gene. *Nucleic Acids Res.* **24**:4464–4470.

256. Wang, Q., Zambetti, G. P., and Suttle, D. P. (1997) Inhibition of DNA topoisomerase II alpha gene expression by the p53 tumor suppressor. *Mol. Cell. Biol.* **17**:389–397.

257. Sturzbecher, H. W., Donzelmann, B., Henning, W., Knippschild, U., and Buchhop, S. (1996) p53 is linked directly to homologous recombination processes via RAD51/RecA protein interaction. *EMBO J.* **15**:1992–2002.

258. White, E. (1996) Life, death, and the pursuit of apoptosis. *Genes Develop.* **10**:1-15.

259. Sandig, V., Brand, K., Herwig, S., Lukas, J., Bartek, J., and Strauss, M. (1997) Adenovirally transferred p16INK4/CDKN2 and p53 genes cooperate to induce apoptotic tumor cell death. *Nature Med.* **3**:313–319.

260. Kagawa, S., Fujiwara, T., Hizuta, A., Yasuda, T., Zhang, W. W., Roth, J. A., et al. (1997) p53 expression overcomes p21WAF1/CIP1-mediated G1 arrest and induces apoptosis in human cancer cells. *Oncogene* **15**:1903–1909.

261. Haupt, Y., Rowan, S., and Oren, M. (1995) p53-mediated apoptosis in HeLa cells can be overcome by excess pRb. *Oncogene* **10**:1563–1571.

262. Oren, M. (1994) Relationship of p53 to the control of apoptotic death. *Semin. Cancer Biol.* **5**:221–227.

263. Lowe, S. W., Bodis, S., McClatchey, A., Remington, L., Ruley, H. E., Fisher, D. E., et al. (1994) p53 status and the efficacy of cancer therapy in vivo. *Science* **266**:807–810.

264. Polyak, K., Xia, Y., Zwier, J. L., Kinzler, K. W., and Vogelstein, B. (1997) A model for p53-induced apoptosis. *Nature* **389**:300–305.

265. Johnson, T. M., Yu, Z. X., Ferrans, V. J., Lowenstein, R. A., and Finkel, T. (1996) Reactive oxygen species are downstream mediators of p53-dependent apoptosis. *Proc. Natl. Acad. Sci. USA* **93**, 11848–11852.

266. Caelles, C., Helmberg, A., and Karin, M. (1994) p53-dependent apoptosis in the absence of transcriptional activation of p53-dependent target genes. *Nature* **370**:220–223.

267. Haupt, Y., Rowan, S., Shaulian, E., Vousden, K., and Oren, M. (1995) Induction of apoptosis in HeLa cells by transcription-deficient p53. *Genes Dev.* **10**:1563–1571.

268. Yonish-Rouach, E., Grunwald, D., Wilder, S., Kimchi, A., May, E., Lawrence, J. J., et al. (1993) p53-mediated cell death: relationship to cell cycle control. *Mol. Cell. Biol.* **13**:1415–1423.

269. Kelley, L. I., Green, W. F., Hicks, G. G., Bondurant, M. C., Koury, M. J., and Ruley, H. E. (1994) Apoptosis in erythroid progenitors deprived of erythropoietin occurs during the G1 and S phases of the cell cycle without growth arrest or stabilization of wild-type p53. *Mol. Cell. Biol.* **14**:4183–4192.

270. Rowan, S., Ludwig, R. L., Haupt, Y., Bates, S., Lu, X., Oren, M., et al. (1996) Specific loss of apoptotic but not cell cycle arrest function in a human tumor derived p53 mutant. *EMBO J.* **15**:827–838.

271. Yonish-Rouach, E., Deguin, V., Zaitchouk, T., Breugnot, C., Mishal, Z., Jenkins, J., et al. (1995) Transcriptional activation plays a role in the induction of apoptosis by transiently transfected wild-type p53. *Oncogene* **11**:2197–2205.

272. Chen, X., Ko, L. J., Jayaraman, L., and Prives, C. (1996) p53 levels, functional domains, and DNA damage determine the extent of the apoptotic response of tumor cells. *Genes Dev.* **10**:2438–2451.

273. Sakamuro, D., Sabbatini, P., White, E., and Prendergast, G. C. (1997) The polyproline region of p53 is required to activate apoptosis but not growth arrest. *Oncogene* **15**:887–898.

274. Shen, Y. and Shenk, T. (1994) Relief of p53-mediated transcriptional repression by the adenovirus E1B 19-kDa protein or the cellular bcl-2 protein. *Proc. Natl. Acad. Sci. USA* **91**:8940–8944.

275. Selvakumaran, M., Lin, H. K., Miyashita, T., Wang, H. G., Krajewsky, S., Reed, J. C., et al. (1994) Immediate early up-regulation of bax expression by p53 but not TGF-beta 1: a paradigm for distinct apoptotic pathways. *Oncogene* **9**:1791–1798.

276. Zhan, Q., Fan, S., Bae, I., Guillof, C., Liebermann, D. A., O'Connor, P. M., et al. (1994) Induction of bax by genotoxic stress in human cell correlates with normal p53 status and apoptosis. *Oncogene* **9**:3743–3751.

277. Owen-Schaub, L., Zhang, W., Cusack, J. C., Angelo, L. S., Santee, S. M., Fujiwara, T., et al. (1995) Wild-type human p53 and a temperature-sensitive mutant induce Fas/Apo-1 expression. *Mol. Cell. Biol.* **15**:3032–3040.

278. Kroemer, G. (1997) The proto-oncogene bcl-2 and its role in regulating apoptosis. *Nature Med.* **3**:614–620.

279. Yin, C., Knudson, C. M., Korsmeyer, S. J., and Van Dyke, T. (1997) Bax suppresses tumorigenesis and stimulates apoptosis in vivo. *Nature* **385**:637–640.

280. Chiou, S. K., Rao, S. L., and White, E. (1994) Bcl-2 blocks p53-dependent apoptosis. *Mol. Cell. Biol.* **14**:2556–2563.

281. Oltvai, Z. N., Milliman, C. L., and Korsmeyer, S. J. (1993) Bcl-2 heterodimerizes in vivo with a conserved homolog, bax, that accelerates programmed cell death. *Cell* **74**:609–619.

282. Miyashita, T., Krajewski, S., Krajewski, M., Wang, H. G., Lin, H. K., Liebermann, D. A., et al. (1994) Tumor suppressor p53 is a regulator of bcl-2 and bax gene expression in vitro and in vivo. *Oncogene* **9**:1799–1805.

283. Miyashita, T., Harigai, M., Hanada, M., and Reed, J. C. (1994) Identification of a p53-dependent negative response element in bcl-2 gene. *Cancer Res.* **54**:3131–3135.

284. Canman, C., Gilmer, T. M., Coutts, S. B., and Kastan, M. B. (1995) Growth factor modulation of p53-mediated growth arrest versus apoptosis. *Genes Dev.* **9**:600–611.

285. Meijerink, J. P. P., Smetsers, T. F. C. M., Sloetjes, A. W., Linders, E. H. P., and Mensink, E. J. B. M. (1995) Bax mutations in cell lines derived from hematological malignancies. *Leukemia* **9**:1828–1832.

286. Rampino, N., Yamamoto, H., Ionov, Y., Li, Y., Sawai, H., Reed, J. C., et al. (1997) Somatic frameshift mutations in the bax gene in colon cancers of the microsatellite mutator phenotype. *Science* **275**:967–969.

287. Rechler, M. M. (1997) Editorial: growth inhibition by insulin-life growth factor (IGF) binding protein-3 – what's IGF got to do with it? *Endocrinol.* **138**:2645–2647.

288. Rajah, R., Valentis, B., and Cohen, P. (1997) Insulin-like growth factor binding protein-3 induces apoptosis and mediates the effects of transforming growth factor-β1 on programmed cell death through a p53- and IGF-independent mechanism. *J. Biol. Chem.* **272**:12181-12188.

289. Gill, Z. P., Parks, C. M., Newcomb, P. V., and Holly, J. M. (1997) Insulin-like growth factor-binding protein (IGFBP-3) predisposes breast cancer cells to programmed cell death in a non-IGF-dependent manner. *J. Biol. Chem.* **272**:25602–25607.

290. Rajah, R., Valentinis, B., and Cohen, P. (1997) Insulin-like growth factor (IGF)-binding protein-3 induces apoptosis and mediates the effects of transforming growth factor-beta1 on programmed cell death through a p53- and IGF-independent mechanism. *J. Biol. Chem.* **272**:12181–12188.

291. Leal, S. M., Liu, Q., Huang, S. S., and Huang, J. S. (1997) The type V transforming growth factor beta receptor is the putative insulin-like growth factor-binding protein 3 receptor. *J. Biol. Chem.* **272**:20572–20576.

292. Oh, Y., Muller, H. L., Ng, L., and Rosenfeld, R. G. (1995) Transforming growth factor-beta-induced cell growth inhibition in human breast cancer cells is mediated through insulin-like growth factor binding protein-3 action. *J. Biol. Chem.* **270**:13589–13592.

293. Ford, J. M. and Hanawalt, P. C. (1995) Li-Fraumeni syndrome fibroblasts homozygous for p53 mutations are deficient in global DNA repair but exhibit normal transcription-coupled repair and enhanced UV-resistance. *Proc. Natl. Acad. Sci. USA* **92**:8876–8880.

294. Smith, M. L., Chen, I. T., Zhan, Q., O'Connor, P. M., and Fornace, A. J. (1995) Involvement of the p53 tumor suppressor in repair of UV-type DNA damage. *Oncogene* **10**:1053–1059.

295. Li, G., Mitchell, D. L., Ho, V. C., Reed, J. C., and Tron, V. A. (1996) Decreased DNA repair but normal apoptosis in UV-irradiated skin of p53 transgenic mice. *Am. J. Pathol.* **4**:1113–1123.

296. Havre, P. A., Yuan, J., Hedrick, L., Cho, K. R., and Glazer, P. M. (1995) p53 inactivation by HPV16 results in increased mutagenesis in human cells. *Cancer Res.* **55**:4420–4424.

297. Smith, M. L., Chen, I. T., Zhan, Q., O'Connor, P. M., and Fornace, A. J. (1995) Involvement of the p53 tumor suppressor in repair of u.v.-type DNA damage. *Oncogene* **10**:1053–1059.

298. Ishizaki, K., Ejima, Y., Matsunaga, T., Hara, R., Sakamoto, A., Ikenaga, M., et al. (1994) Increased UV-induced SCEs but normal repair of DNA damage in p53-deficient mouse cells. *Int. J. Cancer* **57**:254–257.

299. Ford, J. M. and Hanawalt, P. C. (1997) Expression of wild-type p53 is required for efficient global genomic nucleotide excision repair in UV-irradiated human fibroblasts. *J. Biol. Chem.* **272**:28073–28080.

300. Morgan, S. E. and Kastan, M. B. (1997) p53 and ATM: cell cycle, cell death, and cancer. *Adv. Cancer Res.* **71**:1–25.

301. Savitsky, K., Bar-Shira, A., Gilad, S., Rotman, G., Ziv, Y., Vanagaite, I., et al. (1995) A single ataxia-telangiectasia gene with a product similar to PI-3 kinase. *Science* **268**:1749–1753.

302. Savitsky, K., Sfez, S., Tagle, D. A., Sartiel, A., Collins, F. S., Shiloh, Y., et al. (1995) The complete sequence of the coding region of the ATM gene reveals similarity to cell-cycle regulators in different species. *Human Mol. Genet.* **4**:2025–2032.

303. Khanna, K. K. and Lavin, M. F. (1993) Ionizng radiation and UV induction of p53 protein by different pathways in ataxia-telangiectasia. *Oncogene* **8**:3307–3312.

304. Barlow, C., Brown, K. D., Deng, C. X., Tagle, D. A., and Wynshaw-Boris, A. (1997) Atm selectively regulates distinct p53-dependent cell-cycle checkpoint and apoptotic pathways. *Nature Genet.* **17**:453–456.

305. Barlow, C., Hirotsune, S., Paylor, R., Liyanage, M., Eckhaus, M., Collins, F., et al. (1996) Atm deficient mice: a paradigm of ataxia-telangiectasia. *Cell* **86**:159–171.

306. Xu, Y. and Baltimore, D. (1996) Dual roles of ATM in the cellular response to radiation and in cell growth control. *Genes Dev.* **10**:2401–2410.

307. Xie, G., Habbersett, R. C., Jia, Y., Peterson, S. R., Lehnert, B. E., Bradbury, E. M., et al. (1998) Requirements for p53 and the ATM gene product in the regulation of G1/S and S phase checkpoints. *Oncogene* **16**:721–736.

308. Westphal, C. H., Rowan, S., Schmaltz, C., Elson, A., Fisher, D. E., and Leder, P. (1997) Atm and p53 cooperate in apoptosis and suppression of tumorigenesis, but not in resistance to acute radiation toxicity. *Nature Genet.* **17**:397–401.

309. Brown, K. D., Ziv, Y., Sadanandan, S. N., Chessa, L., Collins, F. S., Shiloh, Y., et al. (1997) The ataxia-telangiectasia gene product, a constitutively expressed nuclear protein that is not upregulated following genome damage. *Proc. Natl. Acad. Sci. USA* **94**:1840–1845.

310. Cho, Y., Gorina, S., Jeffrey, P. D., and Pavletich, N. P. (1994) Crystal structure of a p53 tumor suppressor-DNA complex: understanding tumorigenic mutations. *Science* **265**:346–355.

311. Lutzker, S. and Levine, A .J. (1996) A functionally inactive p53 protein in embryonal carcinoma cells is activated by DNA damage or cellular differentiation. *Nature Med.* **2**:804–810.

312. Hainault, P., Hernandez, T., Robinson, A., Rodriguez-Tome, P., Flores, T., Hollstein, M., et al. (1994) IARC database of p53 gene mutations in human tumors and cell lines: updated compilation, revised formats and new visualization. *Nucleic Acids Res.* **26**:205–213.

313. Sedlacek, Z., Kodet, R., Poustka, A., and Goetz, P. (1998) A database of germline p53 mutations in cancer prone families. *Nucleic Acids Res.* **26**:214–215.

314. Hoppe-Seyler, F. and Butz, K. (1995) Molecular mechanisms of virus-induced carcinogenesis: the interaction of viral factors with cellular tumor suppressor proteins. *J. Mol. Med.* **73**:529–538.

315. Moll, U., LaQuaglia, M., Benard, J., and Riou, G. (1995) Wild-type p53 protein undergoes cytoplasmic sequestration in undifferentiated neuroblastomas but not in differentiated tumors. *Proc. Natl. Acad. Sci. USA* **92**:4407–4411.

316. Moll, U. M., Riou, G., and Levine, A. J. (1992) Two distinct mechanisms alter p53 in breast cancer: mutation and cytoplasmic sequestration. *Proc. Natl. Acad. Sci. USA* **89**:7262–7266.

317. Moll, U. M., Ostermeyer, A. G., Haladay, R., Winkfield, B., Frazier, M., and Zambetti, G. (1996) cytoplasmic sequestration of wild-type p53 impairs the G1 checkpoint after DNA damage. *Mol. Cell. Biol.* **16**:1126–1137.

318. Goldman, S. C., Chen, C. Y., Lansing, T. J., Gilmer, T. M., and Kastan, M. B. (1996) The p53 signal transduction pathway is intact in human neuroblastoma despite cytoplasmic localization. *Am. J. Pathol.* **148**:1381–1385.

319. Malkin, D. (1994) p53 and the Li-Fraumeni syndrome. *Biochim. Biophys. Acta* **1198**:197–213.

320. Hsiao, M., Low, J., Dorn, E., Ku, D., Pattengale, P., Yeargin, J., and Haas, M. (1994) Gain-of-function mutations of the p53 gene induce lymphohematopoietic metastatic potential and tissue invasiveness. *Am. J. Pathol.* **145**:702–714.

321. Dittmer, D., Pati, S., Zambetti, G., Chu, S., Teresky, A. K., Moore, M., et al. (1993) Gain of function mutations in p53. *Nature Genet.* **4**:42–45.

322. Donehower, L. A., Harvey, M., Slagle, B. L., McArthur, M. J., Montgomery, C. A., Jr., Butel, J.S., et al. (1992) Mice deficient for p53 are developmentally normal but susceptible to spontaneous tumors. *Nature* **356**:215–221.

323. Harvey, M., McArthur, M. J., Montgomery, C. A., Bradley, A., and Donehower, L. A. (1993) Genetic background alters the spectrum of tumors that develop in p53-deficient mice. *FASEB J.* **7**:938–943.

324. Jacks, T., Remington, L., Williams, B. O., Schmitt, E. M., Halachmi, S., Bronson, R. T., et al. (1994) Tumor spectrum analysis in p53-mutant mice. *Curr. Biol.* **4**:1–7.

325. Harvey, M., Vogel, H., Morris, D., Bradley, A., Bernstein, A., and Donehower, L. A. (1995) A mutant p53 transgene accelerates tumor development in heterozygous but not nullizygous p53-deficient mice. *Nature Genet.* **9**:305–311.

326. Harvey, M., Vogel, H., Lee, E. Y., Bradley, A., and Donehower, L. A. (1995) Mice deficient in both p53 and Rb develop tumors primarily of endocrine origin. *Cancer Res.* **55**:1146–1151.

327. Williams, B. O., Remington, L., Albert, D. M., Mukai, S., Bronson, R. T., and Jacks, T. (1994) Cooperative tumorigenic effects of germline mutations in Rb and p53. *Nature Genet.* **7**:480–484.

328. Kaghad, M., Bonnet, H., Yang, A., Creancier, L., Bascan, J. C., Valent, A., et al. (1997) Monoallelically expressed gene related to p53 at 1p36, a region frequently deleted in neuroblastoma and other human cancers. *Cell* **90**:809–819.

329. Jost, C. A., Marin, M. C., and Kaelin, W. G., Jr. (1997) p73 is a human p53-related protein that can induce apoptosis. *Nature* **389**:191–194.

330. Massague J. (1990) The transforming growth factor-beta family. *Ann. Rev. Cell Biol.* **6**:597–641.

331. Moses, H. L., Yang, Y., and Pietenpol, J. A. (1990) TGF-beta stimulation and inhibition of cell proliferation: new mechanistic insights. *Cell* **63**:245–247.

332. Roberts, A. B. and Sporn, M. B. (1993) Physiological actions and clinical applications of transforming growth factor-beta (TGF-beta). *Growth Factors* **8**:1–9.

333. Ravitz, M. J. and Wenner, C. E. (1997) Cyclin-dependent kinase regulation during G1 phase and cell cycle regulation by TGF-β. *Adv. Cancer Res.* **71**:165–207.

334. Arrick, B. A. and Derynck, R. (1996) The biological role of transforming growth factor-β in cancer development. In: *Molecular Endocrinology of Cancer* (Waxman, T., ed.), Cambridge University Press, Cambridge, UK, pp. 51–78.

335. Markowitz, S. D. and Roberts, A. B. (1996) Tumor suppressor activity of the TGF-β pathway in human cancers. *Cytokine Growth Factor Rev.* **7**:93–102.

336. Fynan, T. M. and Reiss, M. (1993) Resistance to inhibition of cell growth by transforming growth factor-beta and its role in oncogenesis. *Crit. Rev. Oncog.* **4**:493–540.

337. Nunes, I., Munger, J. S., Harpel, J. C., Nagano, Y., Shapiro, R. L., Gleizes, P. E., et al. (1996) Structure and activation of the large latent transforming growth factor-β complex. *Int. J. Obes.* **20**:S4–S8.

338. Souza, R. F., Appel, R., Yin, J., Wang, S., Smolinski, K. N., Abraham, J. M., et al. (1996) Microsatellite instability in the insulin-like growth factor II receptor gene in gastrointestinal tumours. *Nature Genet.* **14**:255–257.

339. Chung, Y. J., Park, S. W., Song, J. M., Lee, K. Y., Seo, E. J., Choi, S. W., et al. (1997) Evidence of genetic progression in human gastric carcinomas with microsatellite. *Oncogene* **15**:1719–1726.

340. Ouyang, H., Shiwaku, H. O., Hagiwara, H., Miura, K., Abe, T., Kato, Y., et al. (1997) The insulin-like growth factor II receptor gene is mutated in genetically unstable cancers of the endometrium, stomach, and colon. *Cancer Res.* **57**:1851–1854.

341. DeSouza, A. T., Hankins, G. R., Washington, M. K., Orton, T. C., and Jirtle, R. L. (1995) M6P/IGF2R gene is mutated in human hepatocellular carcinomas with loss of heterozygosity. *Nature Genet.* **11**:447–449.

342. Hankins, G. R., DeSouza, A. T., Bentley, R. C., Patel, M. R., Marks, J. R., Iglehart, J. D., et al. (1996) M6P/IGF2R receptor: a candidate breast tumor-suppressor gene. *Oncogene* **12**:2003–2009.

343. Oka, Y., Rozek, L. M., and Czech, M. P. (1985) Direct demonstration of the rapid insulin-like growth factor II receptor internalization and recycling in rat adipocytes. *J. Biol. Chem.* **260**:9435–9442.

344. Werner, H. and LeRoith, D. (1996) The role of the insulin-like growth factor system in human cancer. *Adv. Cancer Res.* **68**:183–223.

345. Baserga, R., Resnicoff, M., and Dews, M. (1996) The IGF-I receptor and cancer. *Endocrine* **7**:99–102.

346. Wang, S., Souza, R. F., Kong, D., Yin, J., Smolinski, K. N., Zou, T. T., et al. (1997) Deficient transforming-growth factor beta1 activation and excessive insulin-like growth factor II (IGFII) expression in IGFII receptor mutant tumors. *Cancer Res.* **57**:2543–2546.

347. Laiho, M., DeCaprio, J. A., Ludlow, J. W., Livingston, D. M., and Massague, J. (1990) Growth inhibition by TGF-β linked to suppression of retinoblastoma protein phosphorylation. *Cell* **62**:175–185.

348. Geng, Y. and Weinberg, R. A. (1993) Transforming growth factor-β effects on expression of G1 cyclins and cyclin-dependent kinases. *Proc. Natl. Acad. Sci. USA* **90**:10315–10319.

349. Reynisdottir, I., Polyak, K., Iavarone, A., and Massague, J. (1995) Kip/Cip and Ink4-cdk inhibitors cooperate to induce cell cycle arrest in response to TGF-β. *Genes Develop.* **9**:1831–1845.

350. Geng, Y. and Weinberg, R. A. (1993) Transforming growth factor beta effects on expression of G1 cyclins and cyclin-dependent protein kinases. *Proc. Natl. Acad. Sci. USA* **90**:10315–10319.

351. Ko, T. C., Sheng, H. M., Reisman, D., Thompson, E. A., and Beauchamp, R. D. (1995) Transforming growth factor–beta 1 inhibits cyclin D1 expression in intestinal epithelial cells. *Oncogene* **10**:177–184.

352. Florenes, V. A., Bhattacharya, N., Bani, M. R., Ben-David, Y., Kerbel, R. S., and Slingerland, J. M. (1996) TGF-beta mediated G1 arrest in a human melanoma cell line lacking p15INK4B: evidence for cooperation between p21Cip1/WAF1 and p27Kip1. *Oncogene* **13**:2447–2457.

353. Ko, T. C., Sheng, H. M., Reisman, D., Thompson, E. A., and Beauchamp, R. D. (1995) Transforming growth factor–beta 1 inhibits cyclin D1 expression in intestinal epithelial cells. *Oncogene* **10**:177–184.

354. Li, C. Y., Suardet, L., and Little, J. B. (1995) Potential role of WAF1/Cip1/p21 as a mediator of TGF-beta cytoinhibitory effect. *J. Biol. Chem.* **270**:4971–4974.

355. Datto, M. B., Li, Y., Panus, J. F., Howe, D. J., Xiong, Y., and Wang, X. F. (1995) Transforming growth factor beta induces the cyclin-dependent kinase inhibitor p21 through a p53-independent mechanism. *Proc. Natl. Acad. Sci. USA* **92**:5545–5549.

356. Elbendary, A., Berchuck, A., Davis, P., Havrilesky, L., Bast, R. C., Jr., Inglhart, J. D., et al. (1994) Transforming growth factor beta 1 can induce CIP1/WAF1 expression independent of the p53 pathway in ovarian cancer cells. *Cell Growth Diff.* **5**:1301–1307.

357. Malliri, A., Yeudall, W. A., Nikolic, M., Crouch, D. H., Parkinson, E. K., and Ozanne, B. (1996) Sensitivity to transforming growth factor beta1-induced growth arrest is common in human squamous cell carcinoma cell lines: c-myc down-regulation and p21waf1 induction are common events. *Cell Growth Diff.* **7**:1291–1304.

358. Alexandrow, M. G. and Moses, H. L. (1995) Transforming growth factor-β and cell cycle regulation. *Cancer Res.* **55**:1452–1457.

359. Alexandrow, M. G., Kawabata, M., Aakre, M. E., and Moses, H. L. (1995) Overexpression of the c-myc oncoprotein blocks the growth-inhibitory response but is required for the mitogenic effects of transforming growth factor β1. *Proc. Natl. Acad. Sci. USA* **92**:3239–3243.

360. Alexandrow, M. G. and Moses, H. L. (1997) Kips off to myc: implications for TGFβ signaling. *J. Cell Biochem.* **66**:427–432.

361. Iavarone, A. and Massague, J. (1997) Repression of the CDK activator Cdc25A and cell cycle arrest by cytokine TGF-β in cells lacking the CDK inhibitor p15. *Nature* **387**:417–422.

362. Galaktionov, K., Chen, X., and Beach, D. (1996) Cdc25A cell-cycle phosphatase as a target of c-myc. *Nature* **382**:511–517.

363. Herzinger, T., Wolf, D. A., Eick, D., and Kind, P. (1995) The pRb-related protein p130 is a possible effector of transforming growth factor beta 1 induced cell cycle arrest in keratinocytes. *Oncogene* **10**:2079–2084.

364. Polyak, K. (1996) Negative regulation of cell growth by TGF-β. *Biochim. Biophys. Acta* **1241**:185–199.

365. Sandhu, C., Garbe, J., Bhattacharya, N., Daksis, J., Pan, C. H., Yaswen, P., et al. (1997) Transforming growth factor beta stabilizes p15INK4B protein, increases p15INK4B-cdk4 complexes, and inhibits cyclin D1-cdk4 association in human mammary epithelial cells. *Mol. Cell. Biol.* **17**:2458–2467.

366. Schwarz, J. K., Bassing, C. H., Kovesdi, I., Datto, M. B., Blazing, M., George, S., et al. (1995) Expression of the E2F1 transcription factor overcomes type beta transforming growth factor-mediated growth suppression. *Proc. Natl. Acad. Sci. USA* **92**:483–487.

367. Herrera, R. E., Makela, T. P., and Weinberg, R. A. (1996) TGF beta-induced growth inhibition in primary fibroblasts requires the retinoblastoma protein. *Mol. Biol. Cell.* **7**:1335–1342.

368. Oh, Y., Muller, H. L., Pham, H., and Rosenfeld, R. G. (1993) Demonstration of receptors for insulin-like growth factor binding protein-3 on Hs587T human breast cancer cells. *J. Biol. Chem.* **268**:26045–26048.

369. Oh, Y., Muller, H. L., Lamsom, G., and Rosenfeld, R. G. (1993) Insulin-like growth factor (IGF)-independent action of IGF-binding protein-3 in Hs578T human breast cancer cells. Cell surface binding and growth inhibition. *J. Biol. Chem.* **268**:14964–14971.

370. Valentis, B., Bhala, A., DeAngelis, T., Baserga, R., and Cohen, P. (1995) The human insulin-like growth factor (IGF) binding protein-3 inhibits the growth of fibroblasts with a targeted disruption of the IGF-I receptor gene. *Mol. Endocrinol.* **9**:361–367.

371. Gucev, Z. S., Oh, Y., Kelley, K. M., and Resonfeld, R. G. (1996) Insulin-like growth factor binding protein-3 mediates retinoic acid- and transforming growth factor beta2-induced growth inhibition in human breast cancer cells. *Cancer Res.* **56**:1545–1550.

372. Oh, Y., Muller, H. L., Ng, L., and Rosenfeld, R. G. (1995) Transforming growth factor-beta-induced cell growth inhibition in human breast cancer cells is mediated through insulin-like growth factor-binding protein-3 action. *J. Biol. Chem.* **270**:13589–13592.

373. Nickerson, T., Huynh, H., and Pollack, M. (1997) Insulin-like growth factor binding protein-3 induces apoptosis in MCF-7 breast cancer cells. *Biochem. Biophys. Res. Commun.* **237**:690–693.

374. Friedlander, P., Haupt, Y., Prives, C., and Oren, M. (1996) A mutant p53 that discriminates between p53-responsive genes cannot induce apoptosis. *Mol. Cell. Biol.* **16**:4961–4971.

375. Derynck, R. and Feng, X. H. (1997) TGF-beta receptor signaling. *Biochim. Biophys. Acta* **1333**:F105–F150.

376. Yamashita, H., ten Dijke, P., Franzen, P., Miyazono, K., and Heldin, C. H. (1994) Formation of hetero-oligomeric complexes of type I and type II receptors for transforming growth factor-β. *J. Biol. Chem.* **269**:20172–20178.

377. Lagna, G., Hata, A., Hammati-Brivanlou, A., and Massague, J. (1996) Partnership between DPC4 and SMAD proteins in TGF-β signaling pathways. *Nature* **383**:832-836.

378. Wrana, J.L., Attisano, L., Wieser, R., Ventura, F., and Massague, J. (1994) Mechanism of activation of the TGF-β receptor. *Nature* **370**:341–347.

379. Souchelnytskyi, S., ten Dijke, P., Miyazono, K., and Heldin, C. H. (1996) Phosphorylation of Ser165 in TGF-β type I receptor modulates TGF-β1-induced cellular responses. *EMBO J.* **15**:6231–6240.

380. Heldin, C. H., Miyazono, K., and ten Dijke, P. (1997) TGF-β signaling from cell membrane to nucleus through SMAD proteins. *Nature* **390**:465–471.

381. Chen, R. H., Ebner, R., and Derynck, R. (1993) Inactivation of the type II receptor reveals two receptor pathways for the diverse TGF-beta activities. *Science* **260**:1335–1338.

382. Fafeur, V., O'Hara, B., and Bohlen, P. (1993) A glycosylation-deficient cell mutant with modified responses to transforming growth factor-β and other growth inhibitory cytokines: evidence for multiple growth inhibitory signal transduction pathways. *Mol. Biol. Cell.* **4**:135–144.

383. Feng, X. H., Filvaroff, E. H., and Derynck, R. (1995) Transforming growth factor-β (TGF-β)-induced downregulation of cyclin A expression requires a functional TGF-β receptor complex. Characterization of chimeric and truncated type I and type II receptors. *J. Biol. Chem.* **270**:24237–24245.

384. Wang, J., Sun, L., Myeroff, L., Wang, X., Gentry, L. E., Yang, J., et al. (1995) Demonstration that mutation of the type II TGF-β receptor inactivates its tumor suppressor activity in replication error-positive colon carcinoma cells. *J. Biol. Chem.* **270**:22044–22049.

385. Markowitz, S. A., Wang, J., Myeroff, I., Parsons, R., Sun, L., Lutterbaugh, J., et al. (1995) Inactivation of the type II TGF-β receptor in colon cancer cells with microsatellite instability. *Science* **268**:1336–1338.

386. Loeb, L. A. (1998) Cancer cells exhibit a mutator phenotype. *Adv. Cancer Res.* **72**:25–56.

387. Parsons, R., Myeroff, B., Liu, B., Wilson, J. K. V., Markowitz, S. A., Kinzler, K. W., et al. (1995) Microsatellite instability and mutations of the transforming growth factor-β type II receptor gene in colorectal cancer. *Cancer Res.* **55**:5548–5550.

388. Myeroff, L., Parsons, R., Kim, S. J., Hedrick, L., Cho, K., Ooth, K., et al. (1995) A TGF-β type II receptor mutation common in colon and gastric but rare in endometrial cancers with microsatellite instability. *Cancer Res.* **55**:5545–5547.

389. Takenoshita, S., Hagiwara, K., Gemma, A., Nagashima, M., Ryberg, D., Lindstedt, B. A., et al. (1997) Absence of mutations in the transforming growth factor beta type II receptor in sporadic lung cancers with microsatellite instability and rare H-ras1 alleles. *Carcinogenesis* **18**:1427–1429.

390. Takenoshita, S., Tani, M., Nagashima, M., Hagiwara, K., Bennett, W. P., Yokota, J., et al. (1997) Mutation analysis of coding sequences of the entire transforming growth factor beta type II receptor gene in sporadic human colon cancer using genomic DNA and intron primers. *Oncogene* **14**:1255–1258.

391. Park, J., Kim, S. J., Bang, Y. J., Park, J. G., Kim, N. K., Roberts, A. B., and Sporn, M. B. (1994) Genetic changes in the transforming growth factor-β (TGF-β) type II receptor gene in human gastric cancer cells: correlation with sensitivity to growth inhibition by TGF-β. *Proc. Natl. Acad. Sci. USA* **91**:8772–8776.

392. Garrigue-Antar, L., Munoz-Antonia, T., Antonia, S. J., Gesmonde, J., Velluci, V. F., and Reiss, M. (1995) Missense mutations of the transforming growth factor-β type II receptor in human head and neck squamous carcinoma cells. *Cancer Res.* **55**:3982–3987.

393. Wang, D., Song, H., Evans, J. A., Lang, J. C., Schuller, D. E., and Weghorst, C. M. (1997) Mutation and downregulation of the transforming growth factor beta type II receptor gene in primary squamous cell carcinomas of the head and neck. *Carcinogenesis* **18**:2285–2290.

394. Guo, Y., Jacobs, S. C., and Kyprianou, N. (1997) Down-regulation of protein and mRNA expression for transforming growth factor-beta (TGF-beta1) type I and type II receptors in human prostate cancer. *Int. J. Cancer* **71**:573–579.

395. Lazzereschi, D., Ranieri, A., Mincione, G., Taccogna, S., Nardi, F., and Colletta, G. (1997) Human malignant thyroid tumors display reduced levels of transforming growth factor beta receptor type II messenger RNA and protein. *Cancer Res.* **57**:2071–2076.

396. Garrigue-Antar, L., Souza, R. F., Vellucci, V. F., Meltzer, S. J., and Reiss, M. (1996) Loss of transforming growth factor-beta type II receptor gene expression in primary human esophageal cancers. *Lab. Invest.* **75**:263–272.

397. Knaus, P. I., Lindemann, D., DeCoteau, J. F., Perlman, H., Yankelev, M., Hille, M. E., et al. (1996) A dominant inhibitory mutant of the type II transforming growth factor-β receptor in the malignant progression of a cutaneous T-cell lymphoma. *Mol. Cell. Biol.* **16**:3480–3489.

398. Damstrup, L., Rygaard, K., Spang-Thomsen, M., and Poulson, H. S. (1993) Expression of transforming growth factor-β (TGF-β) receptors and expression of TGF-β1, TGF-β2, and TGF-β3 in human small cell cancer cell lines. *Br. J. Cancer* **67**:1015–1021.

399. Sun, L., Wu, G., Wilson, J. K. V., Zborowska, E., Yang, J., Rajkarunanayake, I., et al. (1994) Expression of transforming growth factor-β type II receptor leads to reduced malignancy in human breast cancer MCF-7 cells. *J. Biol. Chem.* **269**:26449–26455.

400. Chang, J., Park, K., Bang, Y. J., Kim, W. S., Kim, D., and Kim, S. J. (1997) Expression of transforming growth factor beta type II receptor reduces tumorigenicty in human gastric cancer cells. *Cancer Res.* **57**:2856–2859.

401. Kim, I. Y., Ahn, H. J., Zelner, D. J., Shaw, J. W., Sensibar, J. A., Kim, J. H., et al. (1996) Genetic change in transforming growth factor-β (TGF-β) receptor type I gene correlates with insensitivity to TGF-β in human prostate cancer cells. *Cancer Res.* **56**:44–48.

402. Ciernik, I. F., Ciernik, B., Cockerell, C., Minna, J., Gazdar, A., and Carbone, D. (1995) Expression of transforming growth factor-β and transforming growth factor-β receptors on AIDS-associated Kaposi sarcoma. *Clin. Cancer Res.* **1**:1119–1124.

403. Okamoto, M. and Oyasu, R. (1997) Overexpression of transforming growth factor beta type I receptor abolishes malignant phenotype of a rat bladder carcinoma cell line. *Cell Growth Diff.* **8**:921–926.

404. Sun, L. and Chen, C. (1997) Expression of transforming growth factor beta type III receptor suppresses tumorigenicty of human breast cancer MDA-MB-231 cells. *J. Biol. Chem.* **272**:25367–25372.

405. Chen, C., Wang, X. F., and Sun, L. (1997) Expression of transforming growth factor beta (TGFbeta) type III receptor restores autocrine TGFbeta1 activity in human breast cancer MCF-7 cells. *J. Biol. Chem.* **272**:12862–12867.

406. Eppert, K., Scherer, S. W., Ozcelik, H., Pirone, R., Hoodless, P., Kim, H., et al. (1996) MADR2 maps to 18q21and encodes a TGF-β-regulated MAD-related protein that is functionally mutated in colorectal carcinoma. *Cell* **86**:543–552.

407. Zhang, Y., Feng, X. H., Wu, R. Y., and Derynck, R. (1996) Receptor-associated Mad homologs synergize as effectors of the TGF-β response. *Nature* **383**:168–172.

408. Nakao, A., Imamura, T., Souchelnytskyi, S., Kawabata, M., Ishisaki A, Oeda E, et al. (1997) TGF-β receptor-mediated signaling through Smad2, Smad3, and Smad4. *EMBO J.* **16**:5353–5362.

409. Marcias-Silva, M., Abdollah, S., Hoodless, P. A., Pirone, R., Attisano, L., and Wrana, J. L. (1996) MADR2 is a substrate of the TGF-β receptor and its phosphorylation is required for nuclear accumulation and signaling. *Cell* **87**:1215–1224.

410. Wu, R. Y., Zhang, Y., Feng, X. Y., and Derynck, R. (1997) Heteromeric and homomeric interactions correlate with signaling activity and functional cooperativity of Smad3 and Smad4/DPC4. *Mol. Cell. Biol.* **17**:2521–2528.

411. Zhou, S., Buckhaults, P., Zawel, L., Bunz, F., Riggins, G., Le Dai, J., et al. (1998) Targeted deletion of Smad4 shows it is required for transforming growth factor beta and activin signaling in colorectal cancer cells. *Proc. Natl. Acad. Sci. USA* **95**:2412–2416.

412. Hata, A., Lo, R. S., Wotton, D., Lagna, G., and Massague, J. (1997) Mutations increasing autoinhibition inactivate tumor suppressors Smad2 and Smad4. *Nature* **388**:82–87.

413. Zhang, Y., Musci, T., and Derynck, R. (1997) The tumor suppressor Smad4/DPC4 as a central mediator of Smad function. *Curr. Biol.* **7**:270–276.

414. Schutte, M., Hruban, R. H., Hedrick, L., Cho, K. R., Nadasdy, G. M., Weinstein, C. L., et al. (1996) DPC4 gene in various tumor types. *Cancer Res.* **56**:2527–2530.

415. Shi, Y., Hata, A., Lo, R. S., Massague, J., and Pavletich, N. P. (1997) A structural basis for mutational inactivation of the tumor suppressor Smad4. *Nature* **388**:87–93.

416. Grau, A. M., Zhang, L., Wang, W., Ruan, S., Evans, D. B., Abbruzzese, J. L., et al. (1997) Induction of p21waf1 expression and growth inhibition by transforming growth factor beta involve the tumor-suppressor gene DPC4 in human pancreatic adenocarcinoma cells. *Cancer Res.* **57**:3929–3934.

417. Yingling, J. M., Datto, M. B., Wong, C., Frederick, J. P., Liberati, N. T., and Wang, X. F. (1997) Tumor suppressor Smad4 is a transforming growth factor beta-inducible DNA binding protein. *Mol. Cell. Biol.* **17**:7019–7028.

418. Liu, F., Pouponnot, C., and Massague, J. (1997) Dual role of the Smad4/DPC4 tumor suppressor in TGFbeta-inducible transcriptional complexes. *Genes Dev.* **11**:3157–3167.

419. Hahn, S. A., Schutte, M., Hoque, A. T., Moskaluk, C. A., da Costa, L. T., Rozenblum, E., et al. (1996) DPC4, a candidate tumor-suppressor gene at human chromosome 18q21.1. *Science* **271**:350–353.

420. Thiagalingam, S., Lengauer, C., Leach, F. S., Schutte, M., Hahn, S. A., Overhauser, J., et al. (1996) Evaluation of candidate tumor-suppressor genes on chromosome 18 in colorectal cancers. *Nature Genet.* **13**:343–346.

421. Nagatake, M., Takagi, Y., Osada, N., Uchida, K., Mitsudomi, T., Saji, S., et al. (1996) Somatic in vivo alterations of the DPC4 gene at 18q21 in human lung cancers. *Cancer Res.* **56**:2718–2720.

422. Kim, S. K., Fan, Y., Papadimitrakopoulou, V., Clayman, G., Hittleman, W. N., Hong, W. K., et al. (1996) DPC4, a candidate tumor-suppressor gene, is altered infrequently in head and neck squamous carcinoma. *Cancer Res.* **56**:2519–2521.

423. Barrett, M. T., Schutte, M., Kern, S. E., and Reid, B. J. (1996) Allelic loss and mutational analysis of the DPC4 gene in esophageal adenocarcinoma. *Cancer Res.* **57**:4351–4353.

424. Riggins, R. G., Kinzler, K. W., Vogelstein, B., and Thiagalingam, S. (1997) Frequency of Smad gene mutations in human cancers. *Cancer Res.* **57**:2578–2580.

425. de Caestecker, M. P., Hemmati, P., Larisch-Bloch, S., Ajmera, R., Roberts, A. B., and Lechleider, R. J. (1997) Characterization of the functional domains within Smad4/DPC4. *J. Biol. Chem.* **272**:13690–13696.

426. Riggins, J. G., Thiagalingam, S., Rozenblum, E., Weinstein, C. L., Kern, S. E., Hamilton, S. R., et al. (1996) Mad-related genes in the human. *Nature Genet.* **13**:347–349.

427. Datto, M. B., Yu, Y., and Wang, X. F. (1995) Functional analysis of the transforming growth factor-β responsive elements in the WAF1/Cip1/p21 promoter. *J. Biol. Chem.* **270**:28623–28628.

428. Li, J. M., Nichols, M. A., Chandrasekharan, S., Xiong, Y., and Wang, X. F. (1995) Transforming growth factor-β activates the promoter of cyclin-dependent kinase inhibitor p15/INK4B through an Sp1 consensus site. *J. Biol. Chem.* **270**:26750–26753.

429. Hartsough, M. T. and Mulder, K. M. (1997) Transforming growth factor-beta signaling in epithelial cells. *Pharmacol. Ther.* **75**:21–41.

430. Atfi, A., Djelloul, S., Chatstre, E., Davis, R. R., and Gesbach, C. (1997) Evidence for a role of Rho-like GTPases and stress-activated protein kinase/c-jun N-terminal kinase (SAPK/JNK) in transforming growth factor beta-mediated signaling. *J. Biol. Chem.* **272**:1429–1432.

431. Frey, R. S. and Mulder, K. M. (1997) Involvement of extracellular signal-regulated kinase-2 and stress-activated protein kinase/Jun N-terminal kinase activation by transforming growth factor-β in the negative growth control of breast cancer cells. *Cancer Res.* **57**:628–633.

432. Yan, Z., Winawer, S., and Friedman, E.. (1994) Two different signal transduction pathways activated by transforming growth factor beta 1 in epithelial cells. *J. Biol. Chem.* **269**:13231–13237.

433. Atfi, A., Buisine, M., Mazars, A., and Gesbach, C. (1997) Induction of apoptosis by DPC4, a transcriptional factor regulated by transforming growth factor-beta through stress-activated protein kinase/ c-Jun N-terminal kinase (SAPK/JNK) signaling pathway. *J. Biol. Chem.* **272**:24731–24734.

434. Yamaguchi, K., Shirakabe, K., Shibuya, H., Irie, K., Oishi, I., Ueno, N., et al. (1995) Identification of a member of the MAPKKK family as a potential mediator of TGF-β signal transduction. *Science* **270**:2008–2011.

435. Li, D. M. and Sun, H. (1997) TEP1, encoded by a candidate tumor suppressor locus, is a novel protein tyrosine phosphatase regulated by transforming growth factor beta. *Cancer Res.* **57**:2124–2129.

436. Li, J., Yen, C., Liaw, D., Podsypanina, K., Bose, S., Wang, S. I., et al. (1997) PTEN, a putative protein tyrosine phosphatase gene mutated in human brain, breast, and prostate cancer. *Science* **275**:1943–1947.

437. Steck, P. A., Pershouse, M. A., Jasser, S. A., Yung, W. K. A., Lin, H., Ligon, A. H., et al. (1997) Identification of a candidate tumor-suppressor gene, MMAC1, at chromosome 10q23.3 that is mutated in multiple advanced cancers. *Nature Genet.* **15**:356–362.

438. Kong, D., Suzuki, A., Zou, T. T., Sakurada, A., Kemp, L. W., Wakatsuki, S., et al. (1997) PTEN is frequently mutated in primary endometrial carcinomas. *Nature Genet.* **17**:143–144.

439. Tashiro, H., Blazes, M. S., Wu, R., Cho, K. R., Bose, S., Wang, S. I., et al. (1997) Mutations in PTEN are frequent in endometrial carcinoma but rare in other common gynecologic malignancies. *Cancer Res.* **57**:3935–3940.

440. Liaw, D., Marsh, D. J., Li, J., Dahia, P. L. M., Wang, S. I., Zheng, Z., et al. (1997) Germline mutations of the PTEN gene in Cowden disease, an inherited breast and thyroid cancer syndrome. *Nature Genet.* **16**: 64–67.

441. Marsh, D. J., Dahia, P. L. M., Zheng, Z., Liaw, D., Parsons, R., Gorlin, R. J., et al. (1997) Germline mutations in PTEN are present in Bannayan-Zonana syndrome. *Nature Genet.* **16**:333–334.

442. Furnari, F. B., Lin, H., Huang, H. J. S., and Cavanee, W. K. (1997) Growth suppression of glioma cells by PTEN requires a functional phosphatase catalytic domain. *Proc. Natl. Acad. Sci. USA* **94**:12479–12484.

MECHANISMS IV
OF MUTATION

6 The Role of Genomic Instability in the Development of Human Cancer

WILLIAM B. COLEMAN, PHD AND GREGORY J. TSONGALIS, PHD

INTRODUCTION

Cancer development is a multi-step process through which cells acquire increasingly abnormal proliferative and invasive behaviors. Furthermore, cancer represents a unique form of genetic disease, characterized by the accumulation of multiple somatic mutations in a population of cells undergoing neoplastic transformation *(1–5)*. Several forms of molecular alteration have been described in human cancers, including gene amplifications, deletions, insertions, rearrangements, and point mutations *(5,6)*. In many cases specific genetic lesions have been identified that are associated with the process of neoplastic transformation and/or tumor progression in a particular tissue or cell type *(4)*. Statistical analyses of age-specific mortality rates for different forms of human cancer predict that multiple (three to eight) mutations in specific target genes are required for the genesis and outgrowth of most clinically diagnosable tumors *(7)*. In accordance with this prediction, it has been suggested that tumors grow through a process of clonal expansion driven by mutation *(1,2,8–10)*. In this model, the first mutation leads to limited expansion of progeny of a single cell, and each subsequent mutation gives rise to a new clonal outgrowth with greater proliferative potential. The idea that carcinogenesis is a multi-step process is supported by morphologic observations of the transitions between premalignant (benign) cell growths and malignant tumors. In some tumor systems (such as colon), the transition from benign to malignant can be easily documented and occurs in discernible stages, including benign adenoma, carcinoma *in situ*, invasive carcinoma, and eventually local and distant metastasis *(11,12)*. Moreover, specific genetic alterations have been shown to correlate with each of these well-defined histopathologic stages of tumor development and progression *(13,14)*. However, it is important to recognize that it is the accumulation of multiple genetic alterations in affected cells, and not necessarily the order in which these

changes accumulate, that determines tumor formation and progression. These observations suggest strongly that the molecular alterations observed in human cancers represent integral (necessary) components of the process of neoplastic transformation and tumor progression.

In this chapter, we review the evidence that genomic instability plays an important role in the genesis of various human cancers. Furthermore, we attempt to define more clearly the possible molecular pathways to tumorigenesis in humans, and we examine how different forms of genomic instability impinge on these pathways.

MUTATIONS AND CANCER

MUTATIONS DRIVE NEOPLASTIC TRANSFORMATION AND TUMOR PROGRESSION
Mutation is the ultimate source of variability for individual cells (and organisms), and is an essential component of the process of natural selection *(9)*. Tumorigenesis can be viewed simply as a natural selection process in which cells develop a growth advantage that allows them to proliferate and invade under conditions where other (normal) cells cannot, and the acquisition of this ability is driven by mutation. In other words, tumor progression represents a form of somatic evolution, at the ultimate expense of the host organisms *(15,16)*.

The idea that somatic mutation could significantly contribute to cancer development was suggested by Boveri early in this century (reviewed in *17*). At about the same time, De Vries proposed that certain forms of radiation (Röntgen rays) may be mutagenic (reviewed in *16*), suggesting that mutation rates could be influenced by exogenous factors. Evidence in support of the idea that multiple somatic mutations occur in and contribute to the step-wise process of neoplastic transformation and tumorigenesis has been provided by several investigators *(18–21)*. In early studies, the nature of the mutations and the contribution of these mutations to tumorigenesis were not at all clear. Nonetheless, the presence of multiple mutations in cancer cells could be observed in the form of karyotypic alterations and abnormal chromosome numbers in tumor cells *(22–25)*.

From: *The Molecular Basis of Human Cancer* (W. B. Coleman and G. J. Tsongalis, eds.), © Humana Press Inc., Totowa, NJ.

More recent studies utilizing comparative genomic hybridization extended these observations by identifying both gross (cytogenetically detectable) and subtle chromosomal abnormalities in several types of human tumors, including breast *(26)*, colon *(27–29)*, ovarian *(30)*, and liver *(31)*. Subsequently, numerous positive and negative mediators (protooncogenes and tumor-suppressor genes) of cell growth and differentiation have been identified and characterized, defining the basic role for these critical genetic elements in neoplastic transformation and tumorigenesis *(3,4,32,33)*.

HOW MANY MUTATIONS ARE REQUIRED FOR NEOPLASTIC TRANSFORMATION AND TUMORIGENESIS? The exact number of critical mutations required for neoplastic transformation of normal cells is not known. Investigations involving the statistical analysis of human tumor incidence and natural history in sporadic and inherited human tumors formed the basis for the two-hit model of cancer induction *(34–36)*. In this model, a genetic predisposition for developing a specific tumor is conferred on an individual that either inherits or otherwise acquires a germline mutation in one allele of a critical target (such as a tumor-suppressor gene), constituting the first "hit." The second "hit" represents an acquired somatic mutation in the remaining normal allele of the critical gene. Accumulation of two hits alters (or eliminates) normal gene function in affected cells, which proliferate to form a tumor. Although the kinetics of tumorigenesis for some tumor types are consistent with this model, it is now recognized that neoplastic transformation involves the mutational alteration or aberrant expression of multiple genes that function in cell proliferation or differentiation. In recent years, a reexamination of the number of critical mutations needed for cancer development has led to the suggestion that as many as six to eight mutations may be necessary for progression to an invasive tumor *(7,13,37)*. These analyses provide estimates of the numbers of mutations involving genes that control proliferation and differentiation of specific cell types that may be necessary for neoplastic transformation of that cell type. However, numerous lines of evidence support the suggestion that tumors are mutation-prone and/or accumulate large numbers of mutations *(10,38,39,40)*, and some investigators have estimated that tumor cells may contain thousands or tens of thousands of mutations *(15,39,41)*.

THE NATURE OF MUTATIONS Mutations can be categorized into two major groups: 1) chromosomal abnormalities, and 2) nucleotide sequence abnormalities. There has been some debate in the literature as to which forms of mutation (chromosomal or nucleotide sequence) are more prevalent in cancer cells and/or constitute the foundation of the molecular mechanism of neoplastic transformation *(42)*. However, there is abundant evidence that representations of both of these major categories of genetic abnormalities exist in most tumor cells, and that both can contribute to the neoplastic transformation.

Chromosomal abnormalities include the gain or loss of one or more chromosomes (aneuploidy), chromosomal rearrangements resulting from DNA strand breakage (translocations, inversions, and other rearrangements), and gain or loss of portions of chromosomes (amplification, large-scale deletion). The direct result of chromosomal translocation is the movement of

some segment of DNA from its natural location into a new location within the genome, which can result in altered expression of the genes that are contained within the translocated region. If the chromosomal breakpoints utilized in a translocation are located within structural genes, then hybrid (chimeric) genes can be generated. The major consequence of chromosomal deletion (involving a whole chromosome or a large chromosomal region) is the loss of specific genes that are localized to the deleted chromosomal segment, resulting in changes in the copy number of the affected genes. Likewise, gain of chromosome number or amplification of chromosomal regions results in an increase in the copy numbers of genes found in these chromosomal locations.

Nucleotide sequence abnormalities include changes in individual genes involving single nucleotide changes (missense and nonsense), and small insertions or deletions (some of which result in frameshift mutations). Single nucleotide alterations that involve a change in the normal coding sequence of the gene (point mutations) can give rise to an alteration in the amino acid sequence of the encoded protein. Missense mutations alter the translation of the affected codon, whereas nonsense mutations alter codons that encode amino acids to produce stop codons. This results in premature termination of translation and the synthesis of a truncated protein product. Small deletions and insertions are typically classified as frameshift mutations, because deletion or insertion of a single nucleotide (for instance) will alter the reading frame of the gene on the 3'-side of the affected site. This alteration can result in the synthesis of a protein that bears very little resemblance to the normal gene product, or production of a abnormal/truncated protein due to the presence of a stop codon in the altered reading frame. In addition, deletion or insertion of one or more groups of three nucleotides will not alter the reading frame of the gene, but will alter the resulting polypeptide product, which will exhibit either loss of specific amino acids or the presence of additional amino acids within its primary structure.

DNA DAMAGE AND MUTATION Mutations in critical targets leading to neoplastic transformation can result from exogenous insults (carcinogens, radiation) or from endogenous mutagenic factors *(38,43)*. DNA damage can result from spontaneous alteration of the DNA molecule or from the interaction of numerous chemical and physical agents with the structural DNA molecule. Spontaneous lesions occur during normal cellular processes such as DNA replication, DNA repair, or gene rearrangement *(44)*, or through chemical alterations of the DNA molecule itself as a result of hydrolysis, oxidation, or methylation *(10,45,46)*. In most cases, DNA lesions create nucleotide mismatches that lead to point mutations. Nucleotide mismatches can result from the formation of apurinic or apyrimidinic sites after depurination or depyrimidation reactions *(45)*, from nucleotide conversions involving deamination reactions *(44)*, or in rare instances from the presence of a tautometric form of an individual nucleotide in replicating DNA. Deamination of nucleotide bases that contain exocyclic amino groups results in the conversion of cytosine to uracil, adenine to hypoxanthine, and guanine to xanthine *(44)*. However, the most common nucleotide deamination reaction involves methylated cytosines. The deamination of 5-methylcytosine, which results in the formation thymine, accounts for a large percentage of spontaneous mutations in human disease *(47–49)*.

Interaction of DNA with physical agents, such as ionizing radiation (X-rays), can lead to single-strand or double-strand breaks through sission of phosphodiester bonds on one or both polynucleotide strands of the DNA molecule *(44)*. Ultraviolet (UV) light can produce cyclobutane pyrimidine dimers between adjacent pyrimidine bases on the same DNA strand. Less frequently, UV light produces noncyclobutane-type pyrimidine dimers or 6-4 photoproducts between adjacent nucleotides in TC, CC, and TT pyrimidine dimers. Other minor forms of DNA damage caused by UV light include strand breaks and cross-links *(44)*. Nucleotide base modifications can result from exposure of the DNA to various chemical agents, such as *N*-nitroso compounds and polycyclic aromatic hydrocarbons *(44)*. Among the numerous sites in the chemical structure of the nucleotides subject to modification by alkylating chemicals, the N^7 position of guanine and the N^3 position of adenine are the most frequently altered. DNA damage can also be caused by chemicals that intercalate the DNA molecule and/or cross-link the DNA strands *(44)*. Bifunctional alkylating agents can cause both intrastrand and interstrand cross-links in the DNA molecule.

ARE NEOPLASTIC CELLS PRONE TO MUTATION? It is widely accepted that cancer cells accumulate numerous genetic abnormalities (consisting of chromosomal alterations and/or nucleotide sequence mutations) during the protracted interval between the initial carcinogenic insult and the outgrowth of a tumor. Although there is evidence that at least a portion of the genetic changes occurring in neoplasia are related to the underlying molecular mechanism of neoplastic transformation *(13,14,50,51)*, whether the myriad genetic lesions found in cancer cells are the causes or consequences of neoplastic transformation continues to be the subject of debate *(52,53)*. In addition, some investigators have suggested that the intrinsic mutation rate in mammalian cells is insufficient to account for the many genetic changes observed in cancer cells, leading to the suggestion that an early (and possibly essential) step in neoplastic transformation is the development of a condition of hypermutability or genetic instability *(38,39,54,55)*. In the past, increased rates of mutation in preneoplastic or neoplastic cells would have been attributed to exposure of these cells to exogenous mutagenic agents *(56)*. However, more recent analyses of the nature and frequency of mutations occurring in human tumors suggests that a significant proportion are the result of spontaneous mutational mechanisms *(57–59)*. This observation strengthens the suggestion that cancer cells may exhibit diminished capacities for surveillance and repair of DNA lesions, leading to increased rates of spontaneous mutation and/or increased susceptibility to mutation following exposure to some exogenous carcinogenic agent. However, some investigators suggest that increased rates of mutation are not necessary for accumulation of large numbers of genetic lesions in cancer cells, but that selection of advantageous mutations represents a more important feature of the process of tumorigenesis *(60)*.

Spontaneous Mutation Rates in Normal Cells The measured spontaneous mutation rate of mammalian cells depends on the exact experimental conditions employed and the nature of the cells and target sequence examined *(61)*. Somatic mutation rates have been determined for a variety of cultured cell types through examination of the spontaneous mutation frequency at one of several specific loci, such as the hypoxanthine-guanine phosphoribosyltransferase gene *(62–65)*, the Na^+-K^+-ATPase gene *(64)*, or the adenine phosphoribosyltransferase gene *(66)*. Using the results from several of these studies *(63–65)*, the spontaneous mutation frequency at the hypoxanthine-guanine phosphoribosyltransferase locus can be estimated to be approx 2.7×10^{-10} to 1×10^{-9} mutations/nucleotide/cell generation in untransformed human cells. This is consistent with calculations made by others for this same locus where the spontaneous mutation rate was estimated to be 1.4×10^{-10} mutations/nucleotide/cell generation *(39)*. The latter mutation rate is sufficient to yield approx three mutations per cell over the life span of an individual, but is suggested to be too low to account for the number of mutations thought to be required for carcinogenesis *(38,39)*. This observation led to the hypothesis that an early event in neoplastic transformation may involve an increase in the spontaneous mutation rate in cells that are progressing through this multi-step pathway *(39)*. Cells expressing the "mutator phenotype" accumulate mutations more rapidly than normal cells, and would therefore be more likely to sustain mutations in critical genes required for enhanced growth and tumorigenesis *(67,68)*.

Mutation Rates in Neoplastic Cells Some investigators have found the measured mutation rate in malignant cells to be significantly higher than that of corresponding normal cells. In some cases the elevated mutation rates were as much as 100-fold higher than in untransformed cells *(69–71)*. Some tumor cell lines that are deficient for DNA repair exhibit mutation rates that are 750-fold higher than that displayed by DNA repair-proficient tumors *(72)*. In addition, the rate of gene amplification in malignant cells is much higher than in normal cells *(73–75)*. However, other studies find no difference in the spontaneous mutation rate between normal and malignant cells *(63–65)*. Thus, some cancer cells may express a "mutator phenotype" and exhibit an enhanced mutation rate compared to normal cells *(39)*, whereas other cancers may exhibit multiple mutations in the absence of any appreciable increase in mutation frequency. These observations suggest the possibility that multiple molecular mechanisms are needed to reconcile the occurrence of multiple mutations in human cancers and the expression of a mutator phenotype with elevated mutational frequency in only a subset of these tumors.

DEFINING GENOMIC INSTABILITY IN HUMAN CANCER

An appropriate definition of genomic instability is needed before a complete understanding of the interconnecting causes and consequences of genomic instability can be developed, and the contribution of this phenomenon to neoplastic transformation can be appreciated. The observation that most cancer cells contain discernible genetic abnormalities (chromosomal aberrations and/or DNA sequence abnormalities) suggests that all

Spontaneous or Induced
DNA Damage

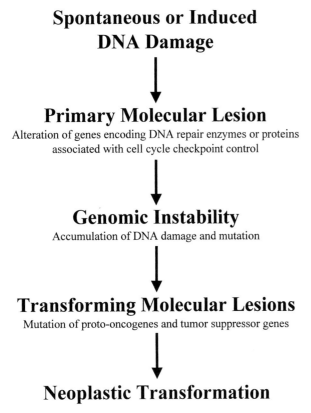

Primary Molecular Lesion

Alteration of genes encoding DNA repair enzymes or proteins
associated with cell cycle checkpoint control

Genomic Instability

Accumulation of DNA damage and mutation

Transforming Molecular Lesions

Mutation of proto-oncogenes and tumor suppressor genes

Neoplastic Transformation

Fig. 1. DNA damage, genomic instability, and neoplastic transformation. A simple model for neoplastic transformation involving primary molecular lesions that give rise to genomic instability
(accumulation of DNA damage and mutations), leading to neoplastic
transformation.

neoplastically transformed cells have sustained genetic damage and may have experienced some form of genomic instability during their development (Fig. 1). Normal human cells
demonstrate a remarkable degree of genomic integrity, which
reflects the combined contributions of high-fidelity DNA replication processes, and the expression of multiple mechanisms
that recognize and repair DNA damage. Nonetheless, it is recognized that rare spontaneous mutations can occur in cells that
are proficient for both DNA replication and repair. The observation that neoplastic cells contain variable numbers of mutations reflecting specific forms of DNA damage, and that tumors
develop over widely variable periods of time (from initiation of
the transformation process to the outgrowth of a clinically detectable tumor) suggests the possible involvement of different
pathogenic mechanisms that may reflect multiple distinct mutagenic pathways to neoplastic transformation. Tumors are
highly variable with respect to their growth characteristics;
some tumors become clinically evident early in the human life
span, whereas others present later in life. This discrepancy could
reflect individual differences among tumors and tumor types
with respect to the relative rapidity of their development and
progression. Consistent with the proposal that tumors form
through clonal expansion driven by mutation *(1,2,8)*, tumors
displaying early onset and rapid progression may accumulate a
critical level of genetic damage more quickly than tumors with
later onset and more indolent course.

Tumors tend to display genetic damage in one of two general
forms: 1) chromosomal alterations (karyotypic abnormalities
and/or numerical changes), and 2) DNA sequence alterations
(involving single nucleotide pairs or short segments of DNA).
Although these forms of genetic damage are not mutually exclusive, the evidence available suggests the involvement of
different mutagenic mechanisms *(76–80)*. Nonetheless, it is
likely that the same groups of target genes might be involved in
tumorigenesis driven by the accumulation of either form of
genetic damage. Inactivation of the p53 tumor-suppressor gene
(loss of function) can be accomplished through point mutation
at numerous nucleotide sites *(33,57)* or through deletion of the
locus on 17p *(81)*. Likewise, activation of proto-oncogene function can be accomplished by point mutation, as with the H-*ras*
gene *(82)*, or by chromosomal translocation, as with the c-*myc*
gene *(83,84)*.

Based on these observations, a unifying hypothesis is needed
to describe the possible mechanisms of genomic instability that
can account for the disparate numbers of mutations (specific
loci vs widespread mutation) and diverse nature of genetic
damage (types of mutations) that characterize various human
cancers. We propose that at least two broad categories of genomic instability may exist: 1) progressive (persistent) genomic
instability, and 2) episodic (transient) genomic instability (Fig.
2). Evidence supporting the existence of these forms of genetic
instability has emerged from studies in bacteria *(85)*, and good
examples of each of these forms of genomic instability have
been identified in subsets of human neoplasms. Progressive or
persistent instability defines an ongoing mutagenic process,
with new mutations occurring in each cell generation. This
form of genomic instability is associated with cells that are
compromised in their ability to safeguard the integrity of their
genome. This form of genomic instability would be transmitted
from cell generation to cell generation as a heritable trait *(85)*.
For instance, tumor cells from patients with hereditary
nonpolyposis colorectal cancer (HNPCC) exhibit progressive
genomic instability, which is manifest as alterations in
microsatellite sequences *(86–90)*. In contrast to progressive
instability, episodic or transient instability describes sporadic
genetic damage in cells that are otherwise proficient in the
various pathways that govern genomic homeostasis. This form
of instability is associated with tumors that contain specific
mutations and/or chromosomal alterations, in the absence of
wide-spread damage to the genome. The transient mutator state
may account for a large portion of adaptive mutations occurring in cells *(85)*. For instance, cells exposed to high levels of
oxidative or nutritional stress may incur and accumulate adaptive mutations that enable the altered cells to thrive under highly
selective conditions. These mutations may occur in cells in the
absence of cell proliferation *(67,68)*. Nonetheless, such adaptive mutations would facilitate clonal expansion of an altered
clone in response to subsequent selection pressures *(60)*. Cells
exposed to high levels of reactive oxygen species (ROS) may
accumulate mutations in this manner *(91–94)*. Numerous sporadic tumor types could exemplify this form of instability, including sporadic colorectal tumors of the tumor-suppressor
pathway *(37,95)*, or the microsatellite mutator pathway *(91)*. It
can be envisioned that both chromosomal abnormalities and

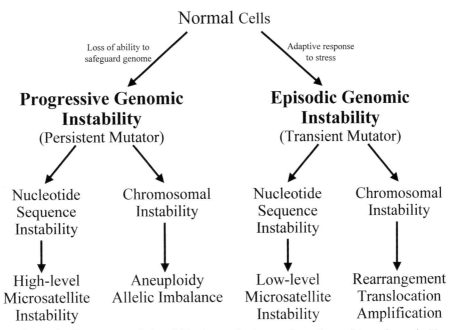

Fig. 2. Possible molecular pathways leading to genomic instability in neoplastic transformation and tumorigenesis. Normal cells accumulate numerous molecular alterations during neoplastic transformation and tumorigenesis. Cells that exhibit a deficiency for DNA repair or otherwise lose the ability to safeguard their genomic DNA may develop a progressive genomic instability characterized by wide-spread genomic mutation. These mutations may involve DNA sequence alterations (as in microsatellite instability; MSI) or large-scale alterations (chromosomal aberrations). Alternatively, cells with apparently normal DNA repair and replication mechanisms may accumulate sporadic transforming molecular alterations through an episodic or transient mutator process. This pathway may give rise to tumors that exhibit low-level (sporadic) MSI or that display characteristic chromosomal alterations (numerical or structural).

DNA sequence abnormalities could result from the expression of either of these forms of genomic instability during neoplastic transformation (Fig. 2).

ABNORMAL DNA REPAIR CONTRIBUTES TO GENOMIC INSTABILITY AND CANCER PREDISPOSITION

The ability to repair damaged DNA is fundamental to all biological processes because damaged sites in the genome can be converted to permanent mutations during DNA replication. The susceptibility of a particular cell type to carcinogenesis is related to its relative abilities to metabolize genotoxic carcinogens and to repair damaged DNA (96). Furthermore, it has been suggested that susceptibility to genotoxic damage partially depends on the temporal relationship between DNA damage, DNA repair, and DNA replication (45,97). It follows that there are aspects of several normal cellular processes that can contribute indirectly to genetic mutation in normal cells, including: 1) slow repair of damaged DNA in specific gene sequences, and 2) timing of replication of specific genes (reviewed in 98). DNA damage is repaired through one of several distinct pathways, including enzymatic reversal repair, nucleotide excision repair, and postreplication repair. An extensive review of each of these DNA-repair pathways is beyond the scope of this chapter. Several excellent reviews are available for interested readers (44,99–105).

FAULTY DNA-REPAIR SYNDROMES PREDISPOSE CANCER DEVELOPMENT Genetic alterations that affect normal DNA-repair mechanisms would necessarily lead to an accelerated accumulation of DNA damage and mutation in affected cells. Numerous genes have been identified that encode proteins involved with DNA repair and are required for the maintenance of the stability of the genome. Mutation of any of these genes might lead to genetic instability and a mutation-prone phenotype, contributing to the multiplicity of mutations observed in human tumors (39,106). Evidence for this suggestion comes from studies of several rare genetic disorders identified in humans that involve dysfunctional DNA-repair pathways. These disorders include xeroderma pigmentosum (XP), Cockayne's syndrome, trichothiodystrophy, ataxia telangiectasia (AT), Bloom's syndrome, and Fanconi's anemia. Of these disorders, XP, AT, Bloom's syndrome, and Fanconi's anemia predispose affected individuals to the development of various malignancies when exposed to specific DNA damaging agents. Patients with XP display hypersensitivity to UV light and increased incidence of several types of skin cancer, including basal-cell carcinoma, squamous-cell carcinoma (SCC), and malignant melanoma (107,108). Patients with AT exhibit hypersensitivity to ionizing radiation and chemical agents, and are predisposed to the development of B-cell lymphoma, chronic lymphocytic leukemias (CLL) (109,110), and affected women demonstrate an increased risk of developing breast cancer (110,111). Patients with Fanconi's anemia demonstrate sensitivity to DNA cross-linking agents and are predisposed to malignancies of the hematopoietic system, particularly acute myelogenous leukemia (AML) (112). Patients with Bloom's syndrome demonstrate an increased incidence of several forms of cancer, including leukemia, skin cancer, and breast cancer (113,114). These patients exhibit

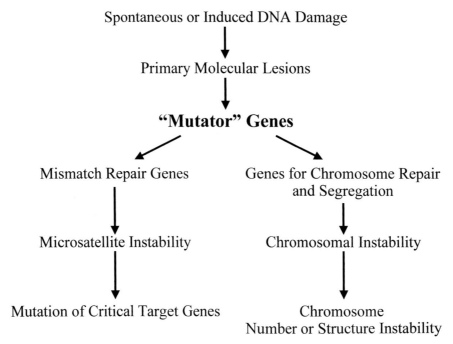

Fig. 3. Mutation of different sets of mutator genes lead to different forms of genomic instability. Primary molecular lesions affecting mismatch repair genes can lead to MSI, precipitating frameshift mutations in critical target genes that contain microsatellite repeats. Primary molecular lesions affecting genes that regulate chromosome segregation can lead to chromosomal instability and the generation of chromosome number and/or structure abnormalities.

chromosomal instability manifest as abnormally high levels of sister chromotid exchange *(114–116).*

The molecular basis of several of these genetic DNA-repair deficiencies has been partially determined through genetic complementation analyses. Each complementation group identified represents a different genetic defect that eliminates a specific functional aspect of a DNA-repair pathway. Seven complementation groups have been identified for XP *(107),* four complementation groups have been identified for ataxia telangiectasia *(117),* and four complementation groups have been identified for Fanconi's anemia *(118).* The molecular defect in Bloom's syndrome has been suggested to involve faulty regulation of DNA-repair processes rather than faulty DNA-repair enzymes *(113).* The candidate Bloom's syndrome gene product is an enzyme with helicase activity *(119).* Candidate genes for each of the XP complementation groups have now been cloned. Each of these genes encode proteins involved with various aspects of DNA nucleotide excision repair (NER), including proteins that function in the recognition of DNA damage, and factors that couple the processes of transcription and repair *(107).* Recently, a candidate AT susceptibility gene (termed *ATM*) has been identified, cloned, and characterized *(120).* The *ATM* gene product is similar to several mammalian phosphotidylinositol kinases that are involved in mitogenic signal transduction, meiotic recombination, and cell cycle control *(120).*

GENETIC INSTABILITY IN HEREDITARY COLORECTAL CANCER INVOLVES DEFECTIVE DNA REPAIR
Colorectal cancer is a fairly common disease worldwide, and particularly in populations from Western nations *(121).* A substantial fraction of colorectal cancers exhibit a genetic component and several familial colorectal cancer syndromes are

recognized, including familial adenomatous polyposis (FAP) and HNPCC. Genes associated with each of these conditions have been identified and characterized. Of these familial colorectal cancer syndromes, HNPCC has been determined to be related to defective DNA repair (reviewed in *122*). HNPCC is characterized by the occurrence of predominately right-sided colorectal carcinoma with an early age of onset and an increased risk for the development of certain extracolonic cancers, including cancers of the endometrium, stomach, urinary tract, and breast *(122–124).* Tumors associated with HNPCC exhibit a form of genomic instability, which represents a unique mechanism for a genome-wide tendency for instability in short repeat sequences (microsatellites), which was originally termed the "replication error phenotype" *(90,125,126).* This form of genetic instability and mutation is not limited to neoplasms occurring in HNPCC patients. Rather, phenotypically normal cells from these individuals also display characteristics of genomic instability manifest as microsatellite mutations *(127).* The molecular defect responsible for microsatellite instability (MSI) in HNPCC involves the genes that encode proteins required for normal mismatch repair *(128–132).*

Two addition familial cancer syndromes have been described that exhibit clinical features similar to that of HNPCC or FAP. The Muir-Torre syndrome is defined by the development of at least one sebaceous gland tumor and a minimum of one internal tumor *(134),* which is frequently colorectal carcinoma *(134).* This syndrome shares several features with HNPCC syndromes Lynch I and Lynch II (reviewed in *135*), including the occurrence of MSI in a subset of tumors *(135).* This observation suggests the possible involvement of abnormal mismatch-repair mechanisms (MMR) in the genesis of a subset of Muir-Torre syndrome tumors. Turcot's syndrome is defined by the occurrence of a primary brain tumor and multiple colorectal adenomas *(136)*. The molecular basis for this syndrome has been suggested to involve mutation of the *APC* gene or mutation of a MMR gene in tumors exhibiting microsatellite instability *(137)*.

CHROMOSOMAL ABNORMALITIES IN CANCER

The majority of human cancers (including solid tumors, leukemias, and lymphomas) contain chromosomal abnormalities, consisting of either numerical changes (aneuploidy) and/or structural aberrations (138–142). These two general types of chromosomal damage may reflect two distinct mechanisms of chromosomal instability *(5)*: 1) chromosome number instability, and 2) chromosome structure instability. In some forms of cancer, chromosomal instabilities predominate over nucleotide sequence instabilities, suggesting that these mechanisms of genetic instability may not significantly overlap (Fig. 3).

Detailed karyotypic studies have been carried out on a large number of tumor types, but most of these studies have examined chromosomal alterations in leukemia and lymphoma *(138– 140)*, partially reflecting the difficulty of performing traditional cytogenetic analysis on solid tumors. While technical advances have increased the number of solid tumors examined cytogenetically (by chromosome banding), additional methods have been applied to examination of chromosomal abnormalities in these tumors *(142)*. A large number of studies have investigated allelic LOH in various human solid tumors using Southern-blot analysis or polymerase chain reaction (PCR) *(81,143–145)*. Although these methods do not provide the same information as karyotypic analysis, the indication of large-scale deletions can be inferred from the loss of multiple markers on a specific chromosomal arm. In addition, flow cytometry is now widely employed for determination of tumor ploidy *(146)*, and fluorescence *in situ* hybridization (FISH) is used to examine specific chromosome numbers and alterations (reviewed in *147*). A detailed review of chromosomal alterations in human cancer is beyond the scope of this chapter. Several recent reviews are available *(24,140–142)*.

INSTABILITY OF CHROMOSOME NUMBER Numerical alterations of chromosomes can involve both loss of entire chromosomes or allelic losses, which may be accompanied by duplication of the opposite allele. This phenomenon results in the generation of a tumor with normal karyotype, but an abnormal allelotype *(148)*. Several studies have produced evidence that suggest that tumors arising in various tissues share a common chromosome number instability and may lose a significant number (25–50%) of alleles during neoplastic transformation and tumorigenesis *(148–153)*. These large-scale genomic changes may be due to some form of progressive chromosomal instability. In support of this suggestion are studies showing that gains and losses of multiple chromosomes occur in aneuploid colorectal-cancer cell lines 10-fold to 100-fold more frequently than in diploid-cancer cell lines of the same histological subtype *(77,154)*. In other studies, the rate of LOH at marker loci proximal to a selectable gene (adenine phosphoribosyl transferase) was increased 10-fold in colorectal cancer cell lines that exhibit proficiency of MMR compared with cell lines that lack MMR *(155,156)*. In addition to these results, numerous

studies have combined to show that aneuploid cancers exhibit highly variable karyotypes *(140,141)* suggesting that new chromosomal variations are produced in a progressive manner during tumor outgrowth and evolution.

The absence of chromosomal instability in diploid cancers and/or cancers that exhibit nucleotide sequence alterations, argues against a nonspecific mechanism for chromosomal instability related to abnormal properties of neoplastic cells *(5)*. Further, the high rates of numerical chromosomal alterations in aneuploid cells do not simply reflect the ability of these cells to survive changes in chromosome number *(77)*. Likewise, tetraploid cells resulting from the fusion of diploid cancer cells retain a stable tetraploid chromosome number *(77)*, suggesting that the presence of a nondiploid chromosome number does not in and of itself precipitate progressive chromosomal instability. Rather, the evidence from the literature supports the existence of a specific form of genetic instability in cancer cells that results from dysfunction of a normal chromosomal homeostasis pathway producing numerical chromosomal abnormalities. Several possibilities have been investigated, including the involvement of: 1) mutant p53 protein, 2) abnormal centrosomes, 3) abnormal mitotic-spindle checkpoint function, or 4) abnormal DNA-damage checkpoint function *(5)*.

Inactivation of p53 and Numerical Chromosome Abnormalities The p53 tumor-suppressor protein has long been suggested to play significant roles in cell-cycle progression and cell-cycle checkpoint function in response to DNA damage *(157)*. The *p53* gene is commonly mutated in human cancers *(57–59)*, and these same cancers frequently exhibit abnormalities of chromosome number *(24,138,141)*. Thus, numerous studies have been performed in order to define the role of *p53* in maintenance of chromosomal stability in normal cells and instability in neoplastic cells. Cells in culture often become aneuploid concurrent with mutation or inactivation of *p53 (158,159)*, suggesting that loss of p53 function leads to abnormal regulation of mitosis and segregation of chromosomes *(160)*. However, several other lines of evidence do not support a direct role for *p53* mutation in the genesis of this form of chromosomal instability. For example, development of aneuploidy occurs very early in the process of neoplastic transformation and tumorigenesis, and *p53* mutation typically occurs later in the process *(37,144,161,162)*. In addition, some diploid-tumor cell lines that exhibit a stable karyotype also contain mutant *p53 (79)*. These observations combine to suggest that loss of normal p53 function may contribute significantly to chromosomal instability in certain forms of cancer, but does not represent the primary cause of this form of genomic instability.

Centrosomes and Numerical Chromosome Abnormalities Aneuploid tumors demonstrate significant numbers of chromosomal imbalances, whereas such imbalances are rare in diploid or near-diploid tumors. The abnormalities of chromosome number observed in aneuploid tumors are consistent with a mechanism involving dysfunction of chromosome segregation during mitosis. Several lines of evidence support the idea that the integrity of the centrosome plays an integral role in the development of aneuploidy. Human tumors and tumor-derived cell lines have been characterized to contain abnormal numbers of centrosomes, abnormally sized and shaped centrosomes, and multipolar spindles in a number of human tumor types, including breast, lung, prostate, colon, and brain (163,164). In addition, the numbers of centrosomes was elevated in 6/7 (85%) aneuploid colorectal-carcinoma cell lines evaluated, compared to diploid-tumor cell lines, which displayed normal centrosome numbers (154). Further, centrosome function was impaired in 4/5 (80%) aneuploid colorectal-cancer cell lines examined, whereas centrosome function was found to be intact in all diploid-tumor cell lines (154). These observations suggest that abnormal centrosome number and/or function are common among neoplastic cells that display aneuploidy, and may represent an essential component of chromosome number instability in human cancers.

The mechanism leading to formation of increased numbers of centrosomes in cancer cells remains undefined. However, abnormal centrosome number and function has been linked to the STK15 kinase in some cancers (165,166), and to a related kinase (PLK1) in others (167). The STK15 gene was found to be amplified in approx 12% of primary breast cancers, and in cell lines derived from neuroblastoma and tumors of the breast, ovary, colon, prostate, and cervix (165). Overexpression of STK15 (evidenced by immunostaining) was detected in 94% of invasive ductal carcinomas of the breast irrespective of histopathological subtype, suggesting that overexpression of this centrosome-associated kinase may be a common feature of breast cancers (168). In addition, overexpression of STK15 was found in cell lines that lacked evidence of gene amplification, and ectopic expression of STK15 in near-diploid human-breast epithelial cells produced centrosome abnormality accompanied by induction of aneuploidy (165). An alternative mechanism suggests that mutational inactivation of p53 or functional inactivation of p53 through binding by mdm2 results in abnormal centrosome numbers and induction of chromosomal instability (169). Furthermore, there is evidence that loss of BRCA2 can lead to centrosome amplification and chromosome segregation dysfunction (170). These studies combine to suggest that a number of different genes may contribute to centrosome function and homeostasis in normal cells, and that inactivation or dysregulation of one or more of them can lead to abnormal centrosome number/function.

Aberrant Mitotic-Spindle Checkpoint Function and Aneuploidy The mitotic-spindle checkpoint governs proper chromosome segregation by ensuring that chromatid separation does not occur prior to completion of alignment of all chromosomes along the mitotic spindle. It follows that if the mitotic-spindle checkpoint is defective, chromosome segregation during mitosis will occur asynchronously, potentially producing an unequal distribution of chromatids between the daughter cells (171). Evidence supporting a role for aberrant mitotic-spindle checkpoint function in the development of aneuploidy includes the observation that aneuploid cells respond inappropriately to agents that disrupt the spindle apparatus, such as colcemid. Normal cells respond to colcemid treatment by arresting in metaphase, whereas cells that display instability of chromosome numbers prematurely exit mitosis and initiate another round of DNA synthesis (80). The hallmark of mitotic spindle checkpoint defect is the inability to inhibit

entry into S phase when mitosis cannot be completed due to damage to the mitotic spindle (172,173). Mutation or aberrant expression of genes that encode proteins involved in mitotic spindle checkpoint function can eliminate proper checkpoint function in tumor cells, contributing to development of aneuploidy. A number of these genes have now been identified (174). Alterations in mitotic-spindle checkpoint genes have been documented in several human cancers, including decreased expression of hMAD2 in breast cancers (175), and mutations in the hBUB1 gene in colorectal cancers (80,176). However, these mitotic-spindle checkpoint genes are not implicated in all aneuploid cancers. Some aneuploid breast cancers lack mutations in hBUB1 and exhibit normal mRNA expression levels (177). Likewise, cancers of the respiratory tract, including head and neck cancers, small-cell lung carcinoma (SCLC), and non-SCLC, have not been shown to have significant numbers of mutations in hBUB1 (176,178,179), and sporadic tumors of the digestive tract rarely contain mutations of hBUB1 or hsMAD2 (180). The absence of mutations or significant alterations in expression of mitotic-spindle checkpoint genes in aneuploid cells suggests that additional genes and/or mechanisms of checkpoint inactivation are operational in the majority of cancers that demonstrate chromosomal instability. Certain p53 mutations have been described that are associated with gain-of-function and relaxed spindle checkpoint function in response to mitotic inhibitors, suggesting that both mutational inactivation of p53 and dominant gain-of-function mutations in p53 can contribute to genomic instability and aberrant chromosome segregation (181). In addition, defective checkpoint function has been demonstrated in patients with AT who carry mutations of the ATM gene (182). These studies combine to suggest that a variety of genes may function in normal control of the mitotic-spindle checkpoint, and when mutated or aberrantly expressed could contribute to chromosomal instability through inactivation of the mitotic-spindle checkpoint.

Abnormal DNA-Damage Checkpoint and Aneuploidy The DNA-damage checkpoint represents the major cellular mechanism that guards against the replication of damaged DNA or entry of cells with DNA damage into mitosis. The types of DNA damage that elicit checkpoint activation include polymerase errors remaining after DNA replication and other forms of incompletely repaired DNA, damage resulting from exposure to exogenous genotoxins (ionizing radiation, chemical mutagens, and others), and damage related to endogenous genotoxic insult (such as ROS). A number of genes have been implicated in the control of this checkpoint, including p53 (157), ATM (183,184), BRCA1 and BRCA2 (185), and some others (5). Functional inactivation of one or more of these genes through genetic or epigenetic mechanisms could result in a genomic instability related to the loss of the DNA-damage checkpoint. Loss of this checkpoint might then lead to development of aneuploidy directly resulting from abnormal segregation of damaged chromosomes (5).

INSTABILITY OF CHROMOSOME STRUCTURE The majority of human cancers exhibit chromosomal abnormalities, including marker chromosomes with altered structure. It is generally accepted that many (if not the majority) of the alterations of chromosome structure occurring in cancer cells confer some selective advantage to the evolving tumor. Thus, accumulation of a critical number of chromosomal aberrations or development of specific chromosomal abnormalities may represent essential steps in the process of neoplastic transformation. Three general forms of chromosomal alteration are observed in cancer cells: 1) gene amplifications, 2) rearrangements and translocations, and 3) large-scale deletions.

Gene Amplification Gene amplifications have been documented in some cancers and in many cancer cell lines (73–75,186–188), some of which involve cellular proto-oncogenes resulting in abnormal expression levels of the proto-oncogene products (reviewed in 189). In general, gene amplification occurs late in tumorigenesis and is associated with tumor progression. It is the recognized mechanism through which many tumors acquire resistance to chemotherapeutic agents. Thus, gene amplifications can profoundly affect tumor behavior, and can have prognostic significance for some cancers. However, gene amplifications probably are not involved with early genetic alterations in preneoplastic lesions leading to neoplastic transformation.

The mechanisms governing gene amplification have not been determined with any certainty. However, several studies suggest that gene amplification occurs at much higher rates in neoplastic cells than in normal cells (73–75). A role for the p53 tumor suppressor in gene amplification has been suggested by some investigators. Evidence supporting this suggestion includes the observation that gene amplification occurs more readily in cells following inactivation of p53 function (190,191). However, gene amplification can also occur in cells with normal p53 (190). One possibility for the role of p53 in this process is that amplification of a chromosomal segment in a normal cell may trigger apoptosis in response to perceived DNA damage (192), whereas in the absence of normal p53 function cells would not undergo apoptosis, but would continue to accumulate amplicons in subsequent rounds of replication (5). Thus, this form of chromosomal instability may involve a mechanism (or a mechanistic component) that increases the ability of an affected to survive the genetic alteration.

Chromosomal Rearrangements and Translocations Chromosomal rearrangements can take on several different forms, the most common of which are chromosomal translocations. Patterns of chromosomal translocation in human cancer can be classified as complex or simple (5). In some human cancers no consistent pattern of chromosomal abnormality can be discerned (complex translocations). These tumors exhibit complex-type translocations, which may appear to be random. Among individual tumors of one type, or individual cells of a single tumor, different chromosomal aberrations may be found. Very often, these rearrangements are accompanied by large-scale loss of chromosomal segments. Although it is possible that some of these chromosomal alterations are not essential to tumorigenesis, it is unlikely that any chromosomal alteration that does not confer a proliferative or adaptive advantage would be preserved in an evolving tumor. In some human cancers, specific chromosomal anomalies are consistently found in a high percentage of tumors (simple translocations). These recurrent chromosomal abnormalities may reflect molecular alterations that are essential and necessary to

the molecular pathogenesis of the specific tumor type. The discovery of the Philadelphia chromosome [trans(9;22)(q34;q11)] in the cancer cells of patients with chronic myelogenous leukemia (CML) was the first report suggesting the involvement of nonrandom chromosomal changes in the molecular pathogenesis of the disease (193). Subsequent studies suggest that the neoplastic cells of 80–90% of leukemia and lymphoma patients contain some sort of demonstrable karyotypic abnormality (141), and many of these are uniquely associated with morphologically or clinically defined subsets of these cancers (140). Similar relationships between chromosomal alterations (and other genetic changes) and definable stages of tumor development and progression have been established for some human solid tumors, including colorectal carcinoma (13,14), and proposed for others, including ovarian carcinoma (194) and pancreatic carcinoma (162). The role of chromosomal translocation in cancer pathogenesis has been suggested to involve activation of proto-oncogenes by repositioning of the gene adjacent to a heterologous genetic control element. Evidence for this type of proto-oncogene activation includes studies of chromosome translocations in Burkitt's lymphoma (BL) (139). In this cancer, the c-*myc* proto-oncogene is translocated from chromosome 8 to chromosome 14, proximal to the immunoglobulin enhancer sequences, resulting in abnormal constitutive expression of c-*myc* (83,84).

Large-Scale Deletions Large-scale deletions of whole chromosomes or chromosomal arms have been documented in many cancers. These deletions can contribute to the abnormal allelotype of tumors, and may accompany chromosomal rearrangements and/or translocations. In most cases, such deletions are thought to be related to the presence of a tumor-suppressor locus on the affected chromosomal arm. Large-scale deletions affecting several chromosomes have been documented in sporadic colorectal carcinoma, including deletions of 5q, 17p, and 18q (14). Each of these chromosomal arms contains a known tumor-suppressor locus; the adenomatous polyposis coli (*APC*) gene at 5q (196–197), the *p53* gene at 17p (81,144), and the *DCC* (for "deleted in colorectal cancer") gene at 18q (198).

MSI IN HUMAN CANCER

FREQUENCY OF MSI IN HUMAN NEOPLASMS MSI is characterized by alterations to simple repeated sequences, including both expansions (insertions) and contractions (deletions), typically resulting in frameshift mutations. Microsatellites are repetitive sequences that consist of variable numbers of repeated units of 1 to 4 (or more) nucleotides. Such sequences are numerous and randomly distributed throughout the human genome (199,200). Mutational alterations of numerous adenine mononucleotide repeat motifs (polyA tracts) distributed throughout the genome was the first characteristic used to define MSI in human tumors (125,201). These early studies of sporadic colorectal cancers suggested that 12% of all tumors harbor these mutations, with as many as 1×10^5 mutated polyA tracts per tumor (125). Subsequent studies demonstrated frequent microsatellite alterations in hereditary colorectal cancers (90) and sporadic tumors (126) when higher order repeated units were examined.

Table 1
Microsatellite Instability in Human Solid Tumors

Tumor type[a]	Micro-satellite instability (% tumors)	Altered micro-satellites (n)	Number of loci examined (n)	Reference(s)
Bladder	87/103 (84%)	≥2	17	(357)
	6/200 (3%)	≥1	7	(358)
	9/32 (28%)	≥1	52	(323)
	25/61 (41%)	≥1	4	(359)
	12/72 (17%)	≥1	10	(360)
	14/14 (100%)	≥8	22	(361)
	0/33 (0%)	NA[b]	3–6	(362)
Breast	11/37 (30%)	≥2	11	(248)
	20/81 (25%)	≥2	8	(250)
	5/28 (18%)	≥2	8	(249)
	11/75 (15%)	≥2	20	(149)
	6/88 (7%)	≥2	10	(251)
	6/23 (26%)[c]	≥2	19	(252)
	5/40 (13%)	≥2	8	(253)
	2/24 (8%)[d]	≥1	1–10	(363)
	8/100 (8%)	≥1	9	(364)
	5/93 (5%)	≥1	13	(365)
	1/26 (4%)	≥1	4	(366)
	4/20 (20%)	≥1	8	(367)
	4/78 (5%)	≥1	11	(368)
	11/104 (11%)	≥1	12	(369)
	10/528 (2%)	≥1	14	(370)
	20/69 (29%)	=1	5	(371)
	0/267 (0%)	NA	104	(372)
	0/107 (0%)	NA	15–18	(218)
	0/84 (0%)	NA	7–8	(205,210)
	0/20 (0%)	NA	5–8	(211)
	0/22 (0%)	NA	12	(221)
	0/22 (0%)	NA	42	(373)
Colorectal (carcinoma)	10/13 (77%)[e]	≥2	7	(86)
	9/11 (82%)[e]	≥2	2–17	(87)
	19/20 (95%)[e]	≥3	5	(88)
	25/29 (86%)[e]	≥2	7–11	(89)
	10/13 (77%)[e]	≥2	7	(90)
	37/39 (95%)[e]	≥2	6	(202)
	20/21 (95%)[e]	≥2	28	(203)
	11/13 (85%)[e]	≥2	13	(204)
	18/31 (58%)[f]	≥2	4–5	(217)
	53/80 (66%)[f]	≥2	5	(244)
	17/24 (71%)[g]	≥2	5	(243)
	12/49 (24%)[h]	≥2	3	(374)
	13/22 (59%)[h]	=3	3	(297)
	42/160 (26%)	≥2	>10	(218)
	17/39 (44%)	≥2	5–11	(230)
	4/35 (11%)	≥7	12	(232)
	5/19 (26%)	≥4	12	(223)
	11/65 (17%)	≥2	6	(234)
	22/76 (29%)	≥3	7	(235)
	37/201 (18%)	≥2	3	(228)
	35/92 (38%)	≥2	9	(226)
	21/230 (9%)	≥2	12	(224)
	25/114 (22%)	≥3	6	(219)
	18/57 (31%)	≥2	6	(202)
	19/158 (12%)	≥2	4–5	(217)
	8/49 (16%)	≥2	7–11	(89)
	6/46 (13%)	≥2	7	(90)
	15/90 (17%)	≥2	4	(126)
	21/100 (21%)	≥2	5–28	(206)
	11/56 (20%)	≥2	5	(214)
	82/508 (16%)	≥2	5–11	(207)

Table 1 (Continued)

Tumor type[a]	Micro-satellite instability (% tumors)	Altered micro-satellites (n)	Number of loci examined (n)	Reference(s)
	19/184 (10%)	≥2	5	(208)
	7/108 (6%)	≥2	5–15	(209)
	22/226 (10%)	≥2	7–8	(205,210)
	18/114 (16%)	≥2	5–8	(211)
	24/200 (12%)	≥2	5	(212)
	35/134 (26%)	≥2	32–100	(213)
	37/183 (20%)	≥2	2	(216)
	15/56 (27%)	>2	7–15	(215)
	5/79 (6%)	≥2	7–12	(220)
	6/25 (24%)	≥2	12	(221)
	3/23 (13%)	≥2	6	(222)
	9/62 (15%)	≥2	8	(225)
	11/116 (9%)	≥2	10	(227)
	5/32 (16%)	≥2	13	(204)
	22/191 (12%)	≥2	9	(229)
	13/148 (9%)[i]	≥2	5	(231)
	76/508 (15%)	≥2	11	(239)
	31/415 (8%)	≥2	4–6	(236)
	7/27 (26%)	≥2	6	(237)
	9/62 (15%)	≥2	8	(238)
	27/303 (9%)	≥2	6	(239)
	12/65 (18%)	≥2	5	(240)
	70/342 (20%)	≥2	6–12	(241)
	5/22 (22%)	≥2	4	(242)
	21/387 (5%)[j]	≥1	5	(88)
	24/82 (29%)	≥1	3	(375)
	17/168 (10%)	≥1	5	(88)
	2/18 (11%)	≥1	4	(366)
	19/110 (17%)	≥1	7	(376)
	10/46 (22%)	≥1	4	(377)
	20/79 (25%)	≥1	5	(378)
Colorectal (adenoma)	10/14 (71%)[e]	≥2	7	(86)
	9/12 (75%)[e]	≥2	3–17	(87)
	8/14 (57%)[e]	≥2	7–11	(89)
	16/30 (53%)[e]	≥2	9	(379)
	1/33 (3%)	≥2	7–11	(89)
	19/93 (20%)	≥1	10	(380)
	0/46 (0%)	NA	5–15	(209)
Endometrial	12/65 (18%)	≥3	7	(254)
	14/57 (25%)	≥3	5	(258)
	12/51 (24%)	≥3	5	(259)
	21/62 (34%)[k]	≥2	7	(257)
	9/29 (31%)[f]	≥2	5	(244)
	53/250 (21%)	≥2	7	(260)
	4/18 (22%)	≥2	8	(210)
	26/100 (26%)	≥2	5–8	(211)
	6/36 (17%)	≥2	71	(254)
	4/12 (33%)	≥2	12	(221)
	3/4 (75%)[e]	≥2	71	(254)
	3/17 (18%)	≥2	9	(226)
	4/12 (33%)	≥2	>10	(218)
	27/109 (25%)	≥1	8	(381)
Esophageal	17/35 (49%)	≥2	7	(262)
	7/21 (30%)	≥2	6	(237)
	1/36 (3%)	≥2	>10	(218)
	2/18 (11%)	≥1	17	(382)
	11/106 (10%)	≥1	5	(383)
	17/41 (42%)	≥1	7	(384)
Gastric	10/34 (29%)	≥3	12	(385)
	6/20 (30%)	≥3	8	(337)

Table 1 (*Continued*)

Tumor type[a]	Microsatellite instability (% tumors)	Altered microsatellites (n)	Number of loci examined (n)	Reference(s)
	17/117 (15%)	≥3	10–32	(386)
	33/108 (31%)[k]	≥2	6	(245)
	4/6 (67%)[k]	≥2	8	(246)
	6/18 (33%)	≥2	8	(210)
	12/81 (15%)	≥2	5–8	(211)
	15/52 (29%)	≥2	5	(387)
	12/40 (30%)	≥2	7	(388)
	35/152 (23%)	≥2	6	(335)
	14/61 (23%)	≥2	6	(389)
	5/24 (21%)	≥2	9	(390)
	30/205 (15%)	≥2	5	(352)
	20/93 (22%)	≥2	7–13	(313)
	9/14 (64%)[g]	≥2	3–6	(247)
	13/22 (59%)[g]	≥2	5	(243)
	19/167 (11%)	≥2	5	(338)
	19/63 (30%)	≥2	49	(391)
	8/49 (16%)	≥2	9	(226)
	5/28 (18%)[j]	≥2	6	(339)
	8/42 (19%)	≥2	12	(314)
	8/61 (13%)	≥2	5	(392)
	14/100 (14%)	≥2	10	(316)
	3/19 (16%)	≥2	6	(237)
	10/59 (17%)	≥2	>10	(218)
	18/41 (44%)	≥1	2	(315)
	22/57 (39%)	≥1	4	(366)
	15/50 (30%)	≥1	11	(393)
	25/76 (33%)	≥1	2	(394)
	4/22 (18%)	≥1	10	(395)
	4/23 (17%)	≥1	5	(396)
	13/20 (65%)[g]	≥1	4	(397)
	10/42 (24%)	≥1	4	(397)
	10/102 (10%)	≥1	5	(398)
Glioma	7/40 (18%)	≥1	4	(399)
	1/54 (2%)	≥1	12	(369)
	6/16 (38%)	≥1	17	(400)
	4/22 (18%)	≥2	5	(343)
	2/80 (3%)	≥2	24	(401)
	0/78 (0%)	NA	>10	(218)
	0/15 (0%)[l]	NA	7	(402)
Head and neck (squamous)	6/20 (30%)	≥2	25	(403)
	10/35 (29%)	≥1	52	(323)
Hodgkin's disease	5/16 (31%)	≥1	7	(404)
Leukemia	15/16 (94%)[m]	≥2	7	(405)
	9/14 (64%)[n]	≥2	11	(406)
	10/19 (53%)[o]	≥2	5	(407)
	11/30 (37%)[p]	≥2	5	(342)
	4/44 (9%)[g]	≥2	5	(342)
	2/43 (5%)[n]	≥2	5	(342)
	0/132 (0%)[n]	NA	3	(408)
	0/20 (0%)[r]	NA	5	(407)
	0/23 (0%)[s]	NA	9	(409)
Liver	2/4 (50%)[g]	≥2	5	(243)
	4/38 (11%)	≥2	29	(219)
	19/46 (41%)	≥2	9	(263)
	16/46 (35%)	≥1	16	(410)
	1/29 (3%)	≥1	4	(366)
	0/55 (0%)	NA	3	(411)
Lung (non-small cell)	28/68 (41%)	≥3	8	(268)

Table 1 (*Continued*)

Tumor type[a]	Microsatellite instability (% tumors)	Altered microsatellites (n)	Number of loci examined (n)	Reference(s)
	22/64 (34%)	≥2	8	(264)
	8/38 (21%)	≥2	16	(265)
	12/35 (34%)	≥2	8	(266)
	1/31 (3%)	≥2	34	(267)
	7/36 (19%)	≥2	4	(269)
	18/52 (33%)	≥1	6	(412)
	3/21 (15%)	≥1	3	(413)
	25/51 (49%)	≥1	4	(414)
	2/23 (9%)	≥1	52	(323)
	7/108 (6%)	≥1	6	(415)
	22/87 (25%)	≥1	6	(416)
	0/85 (0%)	NA	8	(210)
	0/27 (0%)[t]	NA	12	(221)
	0/43 (0%)	NA	1[v]	(417)
Lung (small cell)	5/10 (50%)	≥1	52	(323)
	15/33 (45%)	≥1	18-25	(418)
	6/37 (16%)	≥1	49	(150)
	0/16 (0%)[u]	NA	1[v]	(417)
Lymphoma (non-Hodgkin's)	3/12 (25%)[w]	≥2	5–9	(419)
	5/41 (12%)	=1	5	(420)
	1/17 (6%)[x]	≥2	5	(420)
Neuroblastoma	3/46 (7%)	≥2	8	(421)
	1/46 (2%)	=1	5	(422)
Oral (squamous cell)	6/91 (7%)	≥5	19	(423)
Ovarian	13/78 (17%)	≥2	10	(261)
	2/12 (17%)	≥2	12	(221)
	1/33 (3%)	≥2	9	(226)
	3/19 (16%)	≥1	4	(366)
	2/20 (10%)	≥1	12	(369)
	7/49 (14%)	≥1	13	(424)
	0/39 (0%)	NA	5–8	(211)
Pancreatic	7/51 (14%)	≥2	5–8	(211)
	6/9 (67%)	≥1	4	(366)
	8/13 (62%)	≥1	12	(425)
	14/21 (67%)	≥1	10	(222)
Prostatic	8/66 (12%)	≥2	8	(273)
	7/24 (29%)	≥2	9	(270)
	25/57 (44%)	≥2	18	(271)
	14/40 (35%)	≥2	36	(272)
	25/60 (42%)	≥2	10	(274)
	6/40 (15%)	>1	20	(426)
	18/40 (45%)	≥1	44	(427)
	0/49 (0%)	NA	>10	(218)
Sebaceous gland carcinoma	9/13 (69%)[y]	≥4	5	(428)
	0/8 (0%)	NA	5	(428)
Soft-tissue sarcoma	2/18 (11%)	≥1	12	(369)
	14/26 (54%)[z]	≥1	57	(429)
	2/7 (29%)[w]	≥2	5–9	(419)
Testicular	0/86 (0%)	NA	7–8	(205,210)
	12/66 (18%)	≥1	3	(430)
Thyroid	0/31 (0%)	NA	>10	(218)
Uterine-cervix	5/89 (6%)	≥2	30	(431)
	6/44 (14%)	≥2	9	(432)
	2/10 (20%)	≥2	>10	(218)
	2/13 (15%)	≥1	4	(366)

Table notes on following page

A large number of studies have now accumulated document-ing the occurrence of MSI in human neoplasms (Table 1). Tumors from patients diagnosed with HNPCC frequently ex-hibit MSI (141/159 tumors, 89%) at two or more loci *(86–90,202–204)*. In contrast, only 15% (887/5724 tumors) sporadic colorectal cancers demonstrate MSI at two or more loci *(89,90,126,202,204,205–242)*. However, sporadic colorectal cancers occurring in young patients (<35 yr of age) and in pa-tients with multiple primary tumors exhibit MSI at higher fre-quency (64% and 71% respectively) than sporadic colorectal tumors in general *(217,243,244)*. Sporadic gastric cancers ex-hibit microsatellite instability at two or more loci in 19% (276/1485) of tumors (Table 1). As observed with colorectal tumors, gastric carcinomas from patients with multiple primary tumors or familial predisposition exhibit an elevated frequency of MSI (61 and 32%, respectively) compared to sporadic tumors *(243,245–247)*. Several other cancers exhibit MSI at multiple microsatellite loci in 15–35% of tumors examined (Table 2). Sporadic breast cancers demonstrate microsatellite instability at two or more loci in 17% (64/372 tumors) of cases *(149,248–253)*, but this percentage varies widely from study to study. The combined results of six studies failed to detect MSI at even one locus among 522 tumors examined (Table 1), suggesting that the actual frequency of occurrence of MSI among breast can-cers is very low (Table 2). MSI at two or more loci has been documented in 24% (168/713) tumors of the endometrium *(210,211,218,221,226,254–260)*. Likewise, 13% (16/123) ova-rian cancers *(221,226,261)*, 27% (25/92) of esophageal tumors *(218,237,262)*, 28% (25/88) of liver tumors *(219,243,263)*, 29% (78/272) non-SCLCs *(264–269)*, and 32% (79/247) pros-tate cancers *(270–274)*, demonstrate MSI at two or more loci (Table 1). Hodgkin's disease and some forms of leukemia ex-hibit MSI in a high percentage of cases (Table 1). However, additional studies will be needed to determine more precisely the prevalence of this genetic abnormality in these neoplasms, particularly among the various forms of leukemia. MSI is rare (<10% tumors) among gliomas, neuroblastomas, and cancers of the testicles, thyroid, and uterine-cervix (Table 1). Evidence for the involvement of MSI in some other tumors has been produced, although the numbers of tumors examined and the numbers of studies conducted are limited (Table 1). Some tu-mor types exhibit extreme variability in the frequency of occur-rence of MSI (among different studies or groups of tumors), or show no significant level of MSI (Tables 1 and 2).

MMR Defects Give Rise to MSI The molecular defects responsible for the MSI in human tumors involve the genes that encode proteins required for normal MMR *(76,102,103)*. These include *hMSH2 (128,129)*, *hMSH3 (275)*, and *hMSH6/GTBP (276,277)*, which are human homologs of the bacterial *MutS* gene; and *hMLH1 (130,131)*, *hPMS1 (132)*, *hPMS2 (132)*, and *hMLH3 (278)*, which are human homologs of the bacterial MutL gene. One or more of these genes are mutated in the germline of the majority of individuals with *HNPCC (128–131,230,279–281)*, and somatic mutations have been identified in sporadic colorectal tumors that display MSI *(207,282–284)*. MMR gene defects have also been identified in other forms of cancer that exhibit MSI *(76,104,284,285)*.

The proteins involved with MMR operate in concert to rec-ognize mispaired or unpaired nucleotides, and facilitate their removal and repair *(104,286)*. This mechanism differs from NER, which recognizes and repairs abnormal (adducts) nucle-otides *(44,104)*. The observation that microsatellite mutations consist of expansion or contraction of the repeated sequence through insertion or deletion of variable numbers of repeat units has led to the suggestion that such mutations could arise through a slippage mechanism during replication of these simple repeat sequences *(287)*. Strand slippage of the primer at a repetitive sequence during replication generates a misaligned intermedi-

Table 1 Notes

[a]All tumors were reported to be sporadic unless noted otherwise.
[b]Not applicable.
[c]Patients with bilateral (synchronous or metachronous) breast tumors.
[d]Medullary breast carcinomas.
[e]From patients with hereditary nonpolyposis colorectal cancer.
[f]Sporadic colorectal tumors from patients <35 yr of age *(217)*, or <50 yr of age *(244)*.
[g]From patients with multiple primary tumors.
[h]Colorectal carcinoma cell lines.
[i]Neoplastic lesions associated with inflammatory bowel disease (ulcerative colitis or Crohn's disease).
[j]Tumors in patients with FAP.
[k]Tumors associated with familial predisposition.
[l]Pediatric brain tumors including examples of astrocytoma, craniopharyngioma, medulloblastoma, and hemagioblastoma.
[m]Acute leukemia related to prior radiotherapy, chemotherapy, or combination therapy.
[n]Acute myeloid leukemia *(408)*, acute lymphocytic leukemia *(406)*, or combined from acute and chronic myeloid leukemia cell lines *(342)*.
[o]Chronic myelogenous leukemia progressing from chronic phase to accelerated or blast phase.
[p]T-cell acute lymphoblastic leukemia cell lines.
[q]B-cell acute lymphoblastic leukemia cell lines.
[r]Chronic myelogenous leukemia in chronic phase.
[s]The majority of cases represent chronic lymphocytic leukemia.
[t]Histologic subtype of lung cancer was not specified.
[u]Including 3 primary small cell lung tumors and 13 small cell lung cancer cell lines.
[v]Microsatellite instability was assessed using the *BAT26* marker only.
[w]HIV[+] patients showed microsatellite instability in 2/5 (40%) Kaposi's sarcomas and in 3/6 (50%) non-Hodgkin's lymphomas.
[x]B-cell non-Hodgkin's lymphoma related to AIDS.
[y]Tumors from patients with Muir-Torre syndrome.
[z]Rhabdomyosarcoma.

Table 2
Frequency of Microsatellite Instability
Among Human Neoplasms

Tumor type	Microsatellite instability at ≥ 2 loci[a] (% tumors)	Microsatellite instability for all tumors examined[b] (% tumors)
Bladder	101/117 86% n = 2	101/515 20% n = 7
Breast	64/372 17% n = 7	64/1936 3% n = 22
Colorectal	887/5724 15% n = 42	887/6614 13% n = 49
Endometrial	168/713 24% n = 13	168/822 20% n = 14
Esophageal	25/92 27% n = 3	25/257 10% n = 6
Gastric	276/1485 19% n = 21	276/1918 14% n = 30
Glioma	6/102 6% n = 2	6/305 2% n = 7
Liver	25/88 28% n = 3	25/218 11% n = 6
Lung (Non-small cell)	78/272 29% n = 6	78/769 10% n = 15
Ovarian	16/123 13% n = 3	16/250 6% n = 7
Prostatic	79/247 32% n = 5	79/376 21% n = 8

[a]Average among studies that detected microsatellite instability at ≥2 loci (from Table 1).

[b]Average for all tumors examined, where tumors exhibiting microsatellite instability at a single locus are considered to be microsatellite stable. In some cases, the numbers of tumors with microsatellite alterations at ≥2 loci could not be determined from the published study. Thus, this average represents a minimum (likely an underestimation) of the actual microsatellite instability index for some tumors.

ate that is stabilized by correct base-pairing between discrete repeat units on the misaligned strand (reviewed in *284*). Such a misaligned intermediate is normally repaired through the proofreading function of the polymerase complex, or by postreplication repair mechanisms *(288)*. If the intermediate is not repaired, subsequent rounds of replication will generate insertion or deletion mutations in the newly synthesized DNA strands. The relative location of the unpaired repeat sequence in the replication intermediate determines whether an insertion or deletion will result (contraction or expansion of the microsatellite). Evidence for the involvement of a misaligned

replication intermediate has come from studies of MMR in bacteria *(289)*.

Novel Methods for Determination of Microsatellite Frameshift-Mutation Frequencies Several laboratories have developed reporter constructs and transfection systems for estimation of mutation frequencies in exogenous microsatellite sequences *(290,291)*. Most of these reporter constructs contain an antibiotic-resistance gene that is interrupted by a $(CA)_n$ repeat sequence, resulting in a frameshift mutation to the resistance gene. Thus, a frameshift mutation (contraction or expansion) of the microsatellite sequence restores the reading frame of the reporter gene, and the host cells develop antibiotic resistance. Using such a reporter system, the spontaneous mutation rate of a dinucleotide microsatellite-repeat sequence in normal human fibroblasts (NHF1 cells) has been estimated to be 12.7×10^{-8} mutations/cell/generation *(292)*, suggesting that dinucleotide-repeat sequences are remarkably stable in normal human cells. This selectable reporter system has been employed to assess the mutation frequency of dinucleotide-repeat sequences in tumor cell lines that exhibit MMR defects. The MMR proficient HT1080 fibrosarcoma cell line exhibited a mutation rate of 9.8×10^{-6} mutations/cell/generation, whereas MMR-deficient colorectal tumor cell lines H6 and LoVo gave mutations rates of 1.6×10^{-4} and 3.3×10^{-3} mutations/cell/generation, respectively *(293)*. The estimated mutation rates at the dinucleotide repeat in MMR-deficient tumor cells were 16-fold (H6) and 337-fold (LoVo) higher than that of the MMR-proficient HT1080 tumor cell line, and 1260-fold and 25,984-fold higher than that of the normal NHF1 fibroblast cell line *(292)*. These results highlight the propensity for spontaneous mutation at microsatellite repeat sequences of tumor cells that are deficient for MMR, and support the notion of a mutator phenotype in cells that have sustained lesions in their MMR systems.

More recently, a method was described that facilitates detection of small numbers of cells containing microsatellite alterations in a given tumor *(294)*. These investigators inserted a partial restriction enzyme recognition site into the 3′-end of one of the PCR primers used for a specific gene sequence, such as the poly(A) tract of TGFβII. In this case, the 3′-end of the primer contains ~TTTTTGATT-3′ *(294)*. When this primer anneals to and amplifies from a mutant (contracted) $(A)_9$ microsatellite repeat, the resulting product contains a 5′-GAATC sequence, which is recognized and cleaved by Hinf1. In contrast, when this primer amplifies from a normal $(A)_{10}$ microsatellite repeat, the resulting product contains a 5′-GAAATC sequence, which is not subject to restriction digestion by Hinf1. This method is capable of detecting an altered microsatellite repeat that occurs with very low frequency, on the order of 1×10^{-3} *(294)*.

Specific MMR Genes Are Responsible for Specific Types of MSI Genetic complementation studies have produced direct evidence for the involvement of specific chromosomal loci or specific genes in MMR-deficient tumor cells that exhibit MSI. Transfer of human chromosome 2, which contains the *hMSH2* and *hMSH6* genes, restores genetic stability and MMR proficiency to *hMSH2*-mutant HEC59 endometrial tumor cells *(295)*. Furthermore, the chromosome 2 containing cells demonstrate microsatellite stability at a triplet repeat locus (D7S1794) and at a dinucleotide repeat (D14S73), whereas clones containing other transferred chromosomes (such as chromosome 17) continue to exhibit instability at these loci *(295)*. Furthermore, transfer of chromosome 2 restores genetic stability to HCT15 or DLD1 colon-tumor cells which carry mutations of both *hMSH6* and DNA polymerase δ *(277,296)*. This result suggests that the DNA polymerase δ defect is not the primary determinant of genetic instability in these cell lines *(295)*. However, other studies question whether *hMSH6* plays a major role in MSI *(297–299)*. Transfer of chromosome 3, which contains *hMLH1*, into HCT116 colon-carcinoma cells that are homozygous for *hMLH1* mutation, restores MMR and stability to the D5S107 dinucleotide microsatellite repeat *(300)*. In similar studies, transfer of human chromosome 5 (containing *hMSH3*) or human chromosome 2, into HHUA human endometrial tumor cells resulted in partial correction of the MMR defect *(301)*. More recent studies have utilized single gene transfer to correct *dMMR* deficiency. HEC-1-A endometrial carcinoma cells, which are defective for mismatch repair due to an *hPMS2* mutation *(302)*, show increased microsatellite stability, reduced mutation rate at the hypoxanthine phosphoribosyltransferase locus, and cell extracts can perform strand-specific MMR following transfection with a wild-type *hPMS2* gene *(303)*. Likewise, transfection of HCT15 colon tumor cells with hMSH6 resulted in restoration of mismatch bind and repair capacities, increased stability of the *BAT26* polyA tract, and reduction in the mutation rate at the hypoxanthine phosphoribosyltransferase locus *(304)*.

Epigenetic Silencing of MMR Genes Results in MSI Mutational inactivation of MMR genes have been documented in numerous human tumors that display MSI *(76,285)*. However, in many cases the underlying molecular defect in MMR cannot be identified in cells that display MSI, suggesting that additional MMR genes exist, or that alternative mechanisms for microsatellite mutation are operational in these tumors. Recent studies have produced strong evidence that epigenetic regulation of MMR gene expression may be responsible for loss of MMR function in many tumors that display MSI. Initially, a strong correlation between general methylation status and MMR proficiency in colorectal-carcinoma cell lines was noted *(305,306)*. Cell lines that were deficient for MMR and showed MSI demonstrated hypermethylation of endogenous and exogenous DNA sequences *(305,306)*. Subsequently, several laboratories have examined expression of *hMLH1,* methylation of the *hMLH1* promoter region, and MSI status among sporadic colorectal carcinomas *(307–309)*. Tumors exhibiting high-level MSI, no detectable expression of *hMLH1,* and no *hMLH1* point mutation, also showed hypermethylation of the *hMLH1* promoter region *(307–309)*. In cell lines that exhibit loss of *hMLH1* and hypermethylation of the *hMLH1* promoter, treatment with 5-aza-2′-deoxycytidine resulted in re-expression of *hMLH1* and restoration of MMR capacity *(309)*. These results suggest that inactivation of *hMLH1* through hypermethylation of its promoter region may represent a principle mechanism of gene inactivation in sporadic colorectal carcinoma characterized by widespread MSI. Consistent with this suggestion, recent studies have shown that the *hMLH1* promoter is hypermethylated in 122/167 (73%) colorectal carcinomas with MSI, but in only 20/138 (14%) of microsatellite-stable colorectal cancers *(231,232,308, 309,310–312)*. Likewise, *hMLH1* promoter hypermethylation is observed in 87/97 (90%) gastric tumors with MSI, but in only 14/265 (5%) of microsatellite-stable tumors *(313–318)*. Although fewer tumors have been analyzed, this same relationship has been documented in endometrial carcinomas where 12/14 (86%) tumors with MSI show promoter hypermethylation vs 0/10 (0%) microsatellite-stable tumors *(260)*. In contrast to the relationship observed in sporadic cancers with MSI, tumors from HNPCC patients that harbor mutations in MMR genes do not show *hMLH1* promoter hypermethylation *(311)*.

DETERMINATION OF MMR IN HUMAN TUMORS

PATTERNS OF MSI IN HUMAN NEOPLASMS Tumors that express the microsatellite-mutator phenotype contain numerous altered microsatellite sequences. However, not all microsatellite sequences are altered in all tumors expressing the mutator phenotype (Table 3). In fact some studies have shown dramatic differences in susceptibility to mutation of individual microsatellite loci *(203,207,212)*. In addition, two distinct patterns of microsatellite alteration have been described in various human cancers that express the mutator phenotype, and specific microsatellite markers tend to be altered in a characteristic pattern *(207,319,320)*. Pattern 1 appears as a ladder-like banding pattern on electrophoresis, reflecting either expansion or contraction of the microsatellite-repeat unit *(207,319)*. In contrast, pattern 2 shows a minor alteration of the microsatellite-repeat unit, usually demonstrating a one-repeat unit expansion or contraction *(207,319)*. The pattern of alteration observed at a specific microsatellite locus may reflect the nature of the genomic instability displayed by a tumor (Fig. 2), as suggested by others *(207,320)*. Several factors might influence the probability of mutation at a specific microsatellite locus: 1) the type of repeated sequence (mononucleotide, dinucleotide, etc.), 2) the length of the microsatellite sequence (number of repeated units), 3) the location of the microsatellite sequence within the genome, and 4) the underlying molecular lesion. The results of several studies support these suggestions. Numerous polyA mononucleotide repeats have been evaluated in human cancers, and several of these have been shown to be useful in the determination of MSI *(212,213,218)*. However, some tumors that can be defined as exhibiting MSI exhibit no polyA tract alterations, and may only exhibit alterations in higher-order repeats *(212)*. Thus, no single type of microsatellite will be diagnostic for MSI in all tumors. A direct relationship has been observed between the length of polyA tracts and their mutation frequency among these genetically unstable tumors *(321)*, consistent with the suggestion that the probability of sustaining a mutation in an individual microsatellite sequence is proportional to the length of its sequence *(322)*. Extensive comparison of the mutation of dinucleotide vs higher-order repeat units (trinucleotide or tetranucleotide) in human tumors supports the suggestion that larger alleles are more susceptible to mutation in genetically unstable tumors *(323)*. Studies with cancer cell lines that harbor mutations of known MMR genes tend to demonstrate instability of specific classes of microsatellites. A cell line possessing a defect in *hPMS2* has been shown to exhibit instability of trinucleotide repeats *(302)*, whereas other cell lines deficient for *hMSH3* or *hMSH6* demonstrate an inability to correct mismatches in dinucleotide (or higher order) repeats *(324)*. Furthermore, cells lacking *hMSH6* (DLD-1 cells) demonstrate minimal levels of dinucleotide instability, while cell lines lacking *hMSH2* (LoVo cells) or *hMLH1* (HCT116 and SW48 cells) demonstrate profound dinucleotide instability *(325)*. These observations suggest that the individual MMR complexes may exhibit specificity for certain types of mismatches.

Criteria for Determination of MSI in Human Tumors Despite the large number of published studies on microsatellite mutations in human cancer, there is no consensus on a definition of MSI. Numerous studies have described MSI that is limited to one locus in human tumors (Table 1). However, it is clear that a more stringent definition of MSI is needed *(212,326,327)*. Generation of a uniform definition of MSI requires consideration of several important factors. These include: 1) the number of microsatellites examined, 2) the identity of the microsatellite markers employed, and 3) the number of altered sequences per tumor. The reports of MSI in human cancers that are contained in the literature demonstrate a widely variable number of microsatellite markers examined (Table 1). There is no convincing evidence that large numbers of markers (>20) are required to determine MSI in human tumors. Furthermore, it has been suggested that the absolute number of mutated microsatellite loci may not be as important as the overall frequency of unstable (altered) microsatellite markers *(207,212,327)*. Several lines of evidence suggest strongly that certain microsatellites are prone to mutation in specific types of cancers, and therefore may be highly informative in these tumors. An example of this is the high frequency of mutation of the *BAT26* polyA tract in colorectal tumors *(213,218)*. Multiple studies have shown *BAT26* to be a highly informative marker of MSI in cancers of the colorectum and stomach, as well as some others (Table 4). However, *BAT26* is not useful for determination of MSI in some other tumors, most notably breast *(252,328)*. These observations combine to suggest that strategies for determination of MSI in specific tumor types can be devised that combine a definition of instability (cutoff value for number of required alterations) and an appropriate battery of microsatellite markers (minimum number of specific microsatellite loci with high positive-predictive value required for accurate prediction). Using this approach, recommendations for a uniform method for determination of MSI in colorectal cancers have been developed by several laboratories *(202,212)*, and through a consensus conference *(327)*. In one study, it was suggested that a combination of mononucleotide and higher-order repeats should be evaluated, and that at least 40% of the loci should demonstrate instability for the tumor to be classified as unstable *(212)*. Furthermore, a group of 10 specific primer sets has been recommended that reliably detects MSI in colorectal tumors, including *APC, BAT25, BAT26, BAT40, D2S123, D10S197, D18S58, D18S69, mfd15*, and *MYCL1 (212)*. An alternative proposal recommends utilizing a reference panel consisting of mononucleotide and dinucleotide microsatellite markers (including *BAT25, BAT26, D2S123,*

D5S346, and *D17S250*) for initial screening of colorectal tumors *(202,326,327)*. Using this panel of markers, the authors suggest that alteration of one marker indicates low-level MSI, a shift of two or more loci indicates high- level MSI, and genetically stable tumors will exhibit no microsatellite alterations *(202)*. An additional number of microsatellite markers are recommended as alternative loci in the analysis of MSI in colorectal cancer *(327)*. When more than 5 loci are evaluated, alterations in at least 30–40% of the markers is required for an indication of high level MSI *(327)*. Additional research is needed before similar programs can be developed for determination of MSI in other human tumors.

MOLECULAR TARGETS OF MSI

Numerous simple repeat sequences are found in the human genome. Some of these occur within the coding regions of structural genes. These genes may be targets for mutation in cells that express the microsatellite-mutator phenotype. The *TGFβRII* gene contains two simple repeat sequences: 1) a 10 bp adenine mononucleotide tract at nucleotides 709–718, and 2) a 6 bp GT repeat at nucleotides 1931–1936 *(329)*. This gene represents the first recognized target for inactivation due to microsatellite mutations in human tumors and cell lines, and both of the simple repeat sequences contained within the gene have been shown to be subject to mutation *(330)*. Mutation of the $(GT)_3$ repeat region in one tumor by insertion of an additional GT repeat unit resulted in a frameshift that was predicted to significantly alter the carboxy-terminus of the receptor protein *(330)*. Additional mutations were documented in the $(A)_{10}$ repeat region of the *TGFβRII* gene (deletion of one or two bases) resulting in frameshifts that were predicted to give rise to truncated receptor proteins (330). Inactivating *TGFβRII* mutations involving these simple repeat regions have now been identified in a significant number of human tumors that exhibit MSI (Table 5), including sporadic and hereditary cancers of the colorectum *(202,223,226,229,237,241,242,297,331–334)*, as well as cancers of the stomach (226,237,316,333,335–341), endometrium *(333,340)*, and acute lymphoblastic leukemia (ALL) (342). However, cancers of the esophagus *(237)* and gliomas *(343)* display no mutation in the microsatellite repeats of the *TGFβRII* gene.

TGF-β is a multifunctional protein that acts on a wide range of cell types through interaction with specific cell-surface receptors *(344,345)*. Among its many functions, TGF-β has been shown to act as a dominant-negative growth regulator *(344–346)*. Thus, loss of TGF-β responsiveness could significantly contribute to uncontrolled cell proliferation and tumorigenesis in affected cells. The HCT116 colon-carcinoma cell line expresses the microsatellite mutator phenotype and harbors a 1 bp deletion of the *TGFβRII* $(A)_{10}$ microsatellite repeat *(347)*. Reconstitution of a functional TGF-β type II receptor through transfection with a functional *TGFβRII* gene results in modulation of the neoplastic phenotype of these cells, including decreased clonogenicity in soft-agar culture, and reduced/delayed tumorigenicity in athymic mice *(347)*. These results suggest that mutational inactivation of the *TGFβRII* gene may significantly contribute to the neoplastic phenotype of human colon tumors of the microsatellite mutator phenotype. Evidence

Table 3
Comparison of Various Microsatellite Markers for Determination of Microsatellite Instability in Hereditary Nonpolyposis Colorectal Cancer[a]

Microsatellite marker	Repeat type	Chromosomal location	Microsatellite alterations
BAT26	Mononucleotide	2p	10/10 (100%)
D2S123	Dinucleotide	2p16	8/10 (80%)
D18S35	Dinucleotide	18q21	8/10 (80%)
TP53	Dinucleotide	17p13	8/10 (80%)
BAT25	Mononucleotide	4q11-q12	7/10 (70%)
D1S2883	Dinucleotide	1q24	7/10 (70%)
D5S346	Dinucleotide	5q21	7/10 (70%)
VWF	Tetranucleotide	12p13.2-p13.3	7/10 (70%)
D3S1611	Dinucleotide	3p22	5/10 (50%)
D13S175	Dinucleotide	13q11	5/10 (50%)
D7S501	Dinucleotide	7q31	4/10 (40%)
D12S755E	Trinucleotide	12	4/10 (40%)
D17S250	Dinucleotide	17q11.2-q12	4/10 (40%)
D8S254	Dinucleotide	8p22	3/10 (30%)
TP53	Pentanucleotide	17p13	3/10 (30%)
D2S119	Dinucleotide	2p16	1/10 (10%)
D2S147	Dinucleotide	2p13.3	1/10 (10%)
D11S904	Dinucleotide	11p13-p14	1/10 (10%)

[a]Adapted from Frazier et al. *(203)*.

Table 4
Predictive Value of BAT26 in Determination of Microsatellite Instability in Gastrointestinal Neoplasms and Other Select Tumors

Tumor type[a]	Frequency of microsatellite instability (≥2 loci)	Mutation frequency at BAT26 (% MSI tumors)	Reference
Gastrointestinal tumors			
Colorectal	22/76 (29%)	22/22 (100%)	*(235)*
	11/65 (17%)	11/11 (100%)	*(334)*
	11/116 (9%)	11/11 (100%)	*(227)*
	35/134 (26%)	34/35 (97%)	*(213)*
	16/45 (36%)[b]	14/16 (88%)	*(204)*
	17/39 (44%)	13/17 (76%)	*(230)*
	9/62 (15%)	6/9 (67%)	*(225)*
	31/415 (7%)	25/31 (81%)	*(236)*
	42/160 (26%)	41/42 (98%)	*(218)*
	13/22 (59%)[c]	13/13 (100%)	*(297)*
	5/22 (22%)	5/5 (100%)	*(242)*
Gastric	19/63 (30%)	19/19 (100%)	*(391)*
	30/205 (15%)	30/30 (100%)	*(352)*
	10/59 (17%)	10/10 (100%)	*(218)*
	17/117 (13%)	10/17 (59%)	*(386)*
	26/50 (52%)	11/26 (42%)	*(433)*
Tumors at other sites			
Breast	7/46 (15%)	2/7 (29%)	*(252)*
Endometrium	4/12 (33%)	3/4 (75%)	*(218)*
Leukemia	17/117 (15%)	15/17 (88%)	*(342)*

[a]All tumors are sporadic unless otherwise noted.
[b]Includes some cases of hereditary nonpolyposis colorectal cancer.
[c]Colorectal carcinoma cell lines.

Table 5
Frameshift Mutations in Target Genes Among Human Tumors Exhibiting Microsatellite Instability

| | Tumor type and microsatellite status | | | | | | | |
| | Sporadic colorectal | | HNPCC[b] | | Sporadic gastric | | Sporadic endometrial | |
Target gene[a]	Microsatellite instability	Microsatellite stable	Microsatellite instability	Microsatellite stable	Microsatellite instability	Microsatellite stable	Microsatellite instability	Microsatellite stable
TGFβRII[c]	388/492	1/471	89/113	0/26	151/243	1/282	9/63	1/9
	79%	<1%	79%	0%	62%	<1%	14%	11%
IGF2R	44/193	0/9	2/16	0/30	27/152	0/145	9/41	ND
	23%	0%	13%	0%	18%	0%	22%	
BAX	125/280	0/9	31/58	0/12	65/180	0/220	7/48	ND
	45%	0%	53%	0%	36%	0%	15%	
hMSH3	132/316	0/23	14/27	0/10	49/116	0/183	14/41	ND
	42%	0%	52%	0%	42%	0%	34%	
hMSH6	80/300	2/9	9/27	0/10	31/113	0/183	7/41	ND
	27%	22%	33%	0%	27%	0%	17%	
E2F-4	39/78	0/48	12/17	0/1	20/63	0/86	4/24	ND
	50%	0%	71%	0%	32%	0%	17%	
TCF-4	58/161	1/72	ND	ND	2/22	ND	0/23	ND
	36%	~1%			9%		0%	

[a]These mutations involve the $(A)_{10}$ tract of TGFβRII, the $(G)_8$ tract of IGF2R, the $(G)_8$ tract of BAX, the $(A)_8$ tract of hMSH3, the $(C)_8$ tract of hMSH6, the $(CAG)_{13}$ tract of E2F-4, and the (A) tract of TCF-4. These were compiled from data in the literature (see refs. in the text).

[b]Hereditary nonpolyposis colorectal cancer.

[c]Data were compiled from references provided in the text, with additional data for sporadic colorectal cancers (434,435), HNPCC (436), and sporadic gastric tumors (437).

suggesting a significant role for *TGFβRII* mutation in colorectal tumorigenesis was obtained through examination of the relationship between MSI, tumor grade, and *TGFβRII* mutation status in early and late colonic adenomas (348). Mutations of *TGFβRII* were observed in high-grade dysplastic adenoma, but were absent from surrounding simple adenoma. These results suggest strongly that *TGFβRII* mutation represents a late event in colonic adenomas that express MSI and that these mutations correlate with progression from adenoma to carcinoma in the colon (348).

In addition to *TGFβRII*, several other genes that function in various aspects of normal cellular homeostasis (growth control and DNA repair) exhibit frameshift mutations at microsatellite loci (Table 5). These genes include *APC (349)*, *BAX (202,226, 241,297,316,331–336,338,340,350–352)*, *E2F-4 (202,206, 316,333,338,353,354)*, *IGF2R (226,241,316,332,333,335, 336,338,340,350,351,355,356)*, *hMSH3 (206,226,241,297, 316,331,333,334,337–340,350,351,355)*, and *hMSH6 (226, 241,297,316,331,333,334,337-340,350,351,355)*, *TCF-4 (332,340)*, *BLM (241,355)*, and some others (327). Mutation in these genes have been identified in a significant percentage (as high as 50–55%) of gastrointestinal cancers (HNPCC, sporadic colorectal, stomach) that exhibit MSI (Table 5). However, some other cancers that display MSI do not contain mutations of these particular genes (351), suggesting that these genes may be preferential targets in tumors of the gastrointestinal tract. Mutation of the *IGF2R* has been documented in some (~25%) ALL cell lines and gliomas that exhibit MSI (342,343), but the total numbers of cases examined was extremely low. A signifi-

cant percentage of ALL cell lines harbored mutations in *BAX* (14/17, 82%), *hMSH3* (7/17, 41%), and *hMSH6* (5/13, 38%) (342).

CONCLUSIONS

Considerable evidence has now been accumulated suggesting a genetic basis for the development of neoplastic disease in humans. However, the genetic damage that has been documented in various human cancers includes both large-scale alterations (chromosomal aberrations and ploidy changes) and DNA sequence alterations (single nucleotide changes or alterations in short segments of DNA). In addition, the patterns of genetic damage within a single tumor can vary from a few molecular alterations at specific loci to genome-wide mutations involving a large number of loci. We suggest that there may be several distinct forms of genomic instability that provide the molecular basis for neoplastic transformation in humans. In our model, we propose that tumors will exhibit genetic damage related to expression of a progressive genomic instability, or due to accumulation of genetic damage related to episodic (or transient) genomic instability. Further, we propose that transforming mutations may arise through either of these mechanisms to involve primarily chromosomal alterations or sequence alterations (point mutations and/or MSI), although these alterations may not be mutually exclusive. It is likely that this proposal is overly simplistic to fully account for the molecular mechanisms that govern neoplastic transformation and tumorigenesis in humans. Future studies will enable the present hypothesis to be stringently evaluated and further refined.

REFERENCES

1. Foulds, L. (1958) The natural history of cancer. *J. Chronic Dis.* **8**:2–37.
2. Nowell, P. C. (1976) The clonal evolution of tumor cell populations. *Science* **194**:23–28.
3. Weinberg, R. A. (1989) Oncogenes, antioncogenes, and the molecular bases of multistep carcinogenesis. *Cancer Res.* **49**:3713–3721.
4. Bishop, J. M. (1991) Molecular themes in oncogenesis. *Cell* **64**:235–248.
5. Lengauer, C., Kinzler, K. W., and Vogelstein, B. (1999) Genetic instabilities in human cancers. *Nature* **396**:643–649.
6. Cooper, D. N., Krawczak, M., and Antonarakis, S. E. (1998) The nature and mechanisms of human gene mutation. *In: The Genetic Basis of Human Cancer* (Vogelstein, B. and Kinzler, K.W., eds.), McGraw-Hill, New York, pp. 65–94.
7. Renan, M. J. (1993) How many mutations are required for tumorigenesis? Implications from human cancer data. *Mol. Carcinogenesis* **7**:139–146.
8. Cairns, J. (1975) Mutation, selection and the natural history of cancer. *Nature* **255**:197–200.
9. Crow, J.F. (1997) The high spontaneous mutation rate: is it a health risk? *Proc. Natl. Acad. Sci. USA* **94**:8380–8386.
10. Loeb, K. R. and Loeb, L. A. (2000) Significance of multiple mutations in cancer. *Carcinogenesis* **21**:379–385.
11. Sugarbaker, J. P., Gunderson, L. L., and Wittes, R. E. (1985) Colorectal cancer. *In: Cancer: Principles and Practice of Oncology* (De Vita, V. T., Hellman, S., and Rosenberg, S. A., eds,), J.B. Lippincott, Philadelphia, pp. 800–815.
12. Cohen, A. M., Minsky, B. D., and Schilsky, R. L. (1997) Cancer of the colon. *In: Cancer: Principles and Practice of Oncology,* 5th ed. (De Vita, V. T., Hellman, S., and Rosenberg, S. A., eds.), J.B. Lippincott, Philadelphia, pp. 1144-1197.
13. Fearon, E. R. and Vogelstein, B. (1990) A genetic model for colorectal tumorigenesis. *Cell* **61**:757–767.
14. Kinzler, K. W. and Vogelstein, B. (1995) Colorectal Tumors. *In: The Metabolic and Molecular Bases of Inherited Disease,* 7th ed. (Scriver, C. R., Beaudet, A. L., Sly, W. S., and Valle, D., eds.), McGraw-Hill, New York, pp. 643–663.
15. Stoler, D. L., Chen, N., Basik, M., Kahlenberg, M. S., Rodriguez-Bigas, M. A., Petrelli, N. J., et al. (1999) The onset and extent of genomic instability in sporadic colorectal tumor progression. *Proc. Natl. Acad. Sci. USA* **96**:15121–15126.
16. Cairns, J. (1998) Mutation and cancer: The antecedents to our studies of adaptive mutation. *Genetics* **148**:1433–1440.
17. Ruddon, R. W. (1995) *Cancer Biology,* 3rd ed. Oxford University Press, New York.
18. Fisher, J. C. and Holloman, J. H. (1951) A hypothesis for the origin of cancer foci. *Cancer* **4**:916–918.
19. Fisher, J. C. (1958) Multiple mutation theory of carcinogenesis. *Nature* **181**:651–652.
20. Strong, L. C. (1949) The induction of mutations by a carcinogen. *Br. J. Cancer* **3**:97–108.
21. Berenblum, I. and Shubik, P. (1949) An experimental study of the initiating stage of carcinogenesis, and a re-examination of the somatic cell mutation theory of cancer. *Br. J. Cancer* **3**:109–118.
22. Nowell, P. C. and Hungerford, D. A. (1960) Chromosome studies on normal and leukemic human leukocytes. *J. Natl. Cancer Inst.* **25**:85–109.
23. Rowley, J. D. (1973) A new consistent chromosomal abnormality in chronic myelogenous leukemia identified by quinacrine fluorescence and Giemsa staining. *Nature* **243**:290–293.
24. Solomon, E., Borrow, J., and Goddard, A. D. (1990) Chromosome aberrations and cancer. *Science* **254**:1153–1160.
25. Sen, S. (2000) Aneuploidy and cancer. *Curr. Opin. Oncol.* **12**:82–88.
26. Kallioniemi, A., Kallioniemi, O.-P., Piper, J., Tanner, M., Stoke, T., et al. (1994) Detection and mapping of amplified DNA sequences in breast cancer by comparative genomic hybridization. *Proc. Natl. Acad. Sci.USA* **91**:2156–2160.
27. Korn, W. M., Yasutake, T., Kuo, W. L., Warren, R. S., Collins, C., Tomita, M., et al. (1999) Chromosome arm 20q gains and other genomic alterations in colorectal cancer metastatic to liver, as analyzed by comparative genomic hybridization and fluorescence in situ hybridization. *Genes Chromosomes Cancer* **25**:82–90.
28. De Angelis, P. M., Clausen, O. P., Schjolberg, A., and Stokke, T. (1999) Chromosomal gains and losses in primary colorectal carcinomas detected by CGH and their associations with tumour DNA ploidy, genotypes and phenotypes. *Br. J. Cancer* **80**:526–535.
29. Ried, T., Knutzen, R., Steinbeck, R., Blegen, H., Schrock, E., Heselmeyer, K., et al. (1996) Comparative genomic hybridization reveals a specific pattern of chromosomal gains and losses during the genesis of colorectal tumors. *Genes Chromosomes Cancer* **15**:234–245.
30. Iwabuchi, H., Sakamoto, M., Sakunaga, H., Ma, Y.-Y., Carcangiu, M. L., Pinkel, D., et al. (1995) Genetic analysis of benign, low-grade, and high grade ovarian tumors. *Cancer Res.* **55**:6172–6180.
31. Wong, N., Lai, P., Pang, E., Fung, L.-F., Sheng, Z., Wong, V., et al. (2000) Genomic aberrations in human hepatocellular carcinomas of differing etiologies. *Clin. Cancer Res.* **6**:4000–4009.
32. Park, M. (1995) Oncogenes: Genetic abnormalities of cell growth. *In: The Metabolic and Molecular Bases of Human Disease,* 7th ed. (Scriver, C. R., Beaudet, A. L., Sly, W. S., and Valle, D., eds.), McGraw-Hill, New York, pp. 589–611.
33. Hussain, S. P. and Harris, C. C. (1998) Molecular epidemiology of human cancer: Contribution of mutation spectra studies of tumor suppressor genes. *Cancer Res.* **58**:4023–4037.
34. Armitage, P. and Doll, R. (1957) A two-stage theory of carcinogenesis in relation to the age distribution of human cancer. *Br. J. Cancer* **11**:161–169.
35. Knudson, A. G. (1971) Mutation and cancer: a statistical study of retinoblastoma. *Proc. Natl. Acad. Sci. USA* **68**:820–823.
36. Knudson, A. G. (1986) Genetics of human cancer. *Ann. Rev. Genetics* **20**:231–251.
37. Kinzler, K. W. and Vogelstein, B. (1998) Colorectal tumors. *In: The Genetic Basis of Human Cancer* (Vogelstein, B. and Kinzler, K. W., eds.). McGraw-Hill, New York, pp. 565–587.
38. Cheng, K. C. and Loeb, L. A. (1993) Genomic instability and tumor progression: mechanistic considerations. *Adv. Cancer Res.* **60**:121–156.
39. Loeb, L. A. (1991) Mutator phenotype may be required for multistage carcinogenesis. *Cancer Res.* **51**:3075–3079.
40. Jackson, A. L. and Loeb, L. A. (1998) The mutation rate and cancer. *Genetics* **148**:1483–1490.
41. Perucho, M. (1996) Cancer of the microsatellite mutator phenotype. *Biol. Chem.* **377**:675–684.
42. Orr-Weaver, T. L. and Weinberg, R. A. (1998) A checkpoint on the road to cancer. *Nature* **392**:223–224.
43. Christians, F. C., Newcomb, T. G., and Loeb, L. A. (1995) Potential sources of multiple mutations in human cancers. *Preventative Med.* **24**:329–332.
44. Friedberg, E. C. (1985) *DNA Repair.* W.H. Freeman, New York.
45. Ames, B. N., Shigenagan, M. K., and Gold, L. S. (1993) DNA lesions, inducible DNA repair, and cell division: three key factors in mutagenesis and carcinogenesis. *Environ. Health Perspect. Suppl.* **101**:35–44.
46. Lindahl, T. (1993) Instability and decay of the primary structure of DNA. *Nature* **362**:709–715.
47. Cooper, D. N. and Youssoufian, H. (1988) The CpG dinucleotide and human genetic disease. *Human Genet.* **78**:151–155.
48. Rideout, W. M., Coetzee, G. A., Olumi, A. F., and Jones, P. A. (1990) 5-Methylcytosine as an endogenous mutagen in the human LDL receptor and p53 genes. *Science* **249**:1288–1290.
49. Jones, P. A., Buckley, J. D., Henderson, B. E., Ross, R. K., and Pike, M. C. (1991) From gene to carcinogen: a rapidly evolving field in molecular epidemiology. *Cancer Res.* **51**:3617–3620.
50. Vogelstein, B., Fearon, E. R., Hamilton, S. R., Kern, S. E., Preisinger, A. C., Leppert, M., et al. (1988) Genetic alterations

during colorectal tumor development. *N. Engl. J. Med.* **319**:525–532.

51. Goyette, M. C., Cho, K., Fasching, C. L., Levy, D. B., Kinzler, K. W., Paraskeva, C., et al. (1992) Progression of colorectal cancer is associated with multiple tumor suppressor gene defects but inhibition of tumorigenicity is accomplished by correction of any single defect via chromosome transfer. *Mol. Cell. Biol.* **12**:1387–1395.

52. Prehn, R. T. (1994) Cancers beget mutations versus mutations beget cancers. *Cancer Res.* **54**:5296–5300.

53. Duesberg, P., Rausch, C., Rasnick, D., and Hehlmann, R. (1998) Genetic instability of cancer cells is proportional to their degree of aneuploidy. *Proc. Natl. Acad. Sci. USA* **95**:13692–13697.

54. Loeb, L. A. (1994) Microsatellite instability: marker of a mutator phenotype in cancer. *Cancer Res.* **54**:5059–5063.

55. Strauss, B. S. (1998) Hypermutability in carcinogenesis. *Genetics* **48**:1619–1626.

56. Ames, B. N., Durston, W., Yamasaki, E., and Lee, F. (1973) Carcinogens are mutagens: a simple test system combining liver homogenates for activation and bacteria for detection. *Proc. Natl. Acad. Sci. USA* **70**:2281–2285.

57. Greenblatt, M. S., Bennett, W. P., Hollstein, M., and Harris, C. C. (1994) Mutations in the p53 tumor suppressor gene: clues to cancer etiology and molecular pathogenesis. *Cancer Res.* **54**:4855–4878.

58. Hollstein, M., Sidransky, D., Vogelstein, B., and Harris, C. C. (1991) p53 mutations in human cancers. *Science* **253**:49–53.

59. Hollstein, M., Shomer, B., Greenblatt, M., Soussi, T., Hovig, E., Montesano, R., et al. (1996) Somatic point mutations in the p53 gene of human tumors and cell lines: updated compilation. *Nucleic Acids Res.* **24**:141–146.

60. Tomlinson, I. P. M., Novelli, M. R., and Bodmer, W. F. (1996) The mutation rate and cancer. *Proc. Natl. Acad. Sci. USA* **93**:14800–14803.

61. Boesen, J. J. B., Niericker, M. J., Dieteren, N., and Simons, J. W. I. M. (1994) How variable is a spontaneous mutation rate in cultured mammalian cells? *Mutation Res.* **307**:121–129.

62. Monnat, R. J., Jr. (1989) Molecular analysis of spontaneous hypoxanthine phosphoribosyltransferase mutations in thioguanine-resistant HL-60 human leukemia cells. *Cancer Res.* **49**:81–87.

63. Eldridge, S. R. and Gould, M. N. (1992) Comparison of spontaneous mutagenesis in early-passage human mammary cells from normal and malignant tissues. *Int. J. Cancer* **50**:321–324.

64. Elmore, E., Kakunaga, T., and Barrett, J. C. (1983) Comparison of spontaneous mutation rates of normal and chemically transformed human skin fibroblasts. *Cancer Res.* **43**:1650–1655.

65. Wittenkeller, J. L., Storer, B., Bittner, G., and Schiller, J. H. (1997) Comparison of spontaneous and induced mutation rates in an immortalized human bronchial epithelial cell line and its tumorigenic derivative. *Oncology* **54**:335–341.

66. Nalbontoglu, J., Phear, G., and Meuth, M. (1987) DNA sequence analysis of spontaneous mutations at the aprt locus of hamster cells. *Mol. Cell Biol.* **7**:1445–1449.

67. Richards, B., Zhang, H., Phear, G., and Meuth, M. (1997) Conditional mutator phenotypes in hMSH2-deficient tumor cells. *Science* **277**:1523–1526.

68. Loeb, L. A. (1997) Transient expression of a mutator phenotype in cancer cells. *Science* **277**:1449–1450.

69. Seshadri, R., Kutlaca, R. J., Trainor, K., Matthews, C., and Morely, A. A. (1987) Mutation rate of normal and malignant lymphocytes. *Cancer Res.* **47**:407–409.

70. Eshleman, J. R., Lang, E. Z., Bowerfield, G. K., Parsons, R., Vogelstein, B., Willson, J. K. V., et al. (1995) Increased mutation rate at the hprt locus accompanies microsatellite instability in colon cancer. *Oncogene* **10**:33–37.

71. Bhattacharyya, N. P., Skandalis, A., Ganesh, A., Groden, J., and Meuth, M. (1994) Mutator phenotypes in human colorectal carcinoma cell lines. *Proc. Natl. Acad. Sci. USA* **91**:6319–6323.

72. Glaab, W. E. and Tindall, K. R. (1997) Mutation rate at the hprt locus in human cancer cell lines with specific mismatch repair-gene defects. *Carcinogenesis* **18**:1–8.

73. Tlsty, T. D., Margolin, B. H., and Lum, K. (1989) Differences in the rates of gene amplification in nontumorigenic and tumorigenic cell lines as measured by Luria-Delbruck fluctuation analysis. *Proc. Natl. Acad. Sci. USA* **86**:9441–9445.

74. Tlsty, T. D. (1990) Normal diploid human and rodent cells lack a detectable frequency of gene amplification. *Proc. Natl. Acad. Sci. USA* **87**:3132–3136.

75. Wright, J. A., Smith, H. S., Watt, F. M., Hancock, M. C., Hudson, D. L., and Stark, G. R. (1990) DNA amplification is rare in normal human cells. *Proc. Natl. Acad. Sci. USA* **87**:1791–1795.

76. Eshleman, J. R. and Markowitz, S. D. (1996) Mismatch repair defects in human carcinogenesis. *Human Mol. Genet.* **5**:1489–1494.

77. Lengauer, C., Kinzler, K. W., and Vogelstein, B. (1997) Genetic instability in colorectal cancers. *Nature* **386**:623–627.

78. Lindor, N. M., Jalal, S. M., van de Walker, T. J., Cunningham, J. M., Dahl, R. J., and Thibodeau, S. N. (1998) Search for chromosome instability in lymphocytes with germ-line mutations in DNA mismatch repair genes. *Cancer Genet. Cytogenet.* **104**:48–51.

79. Eshleman, J. R., Casey, G., Kochera, M. E., Sedwick, W. D., Swinler, S. E., Veigl, M. L., et al. (1998) Chromosome number and structure both are markedly stable in RER colorectal cancers and are not destabilized by mutation of p53. *Oncogene* **17**:719–725.

80. Cahill, D. P., Lengauer, C., Yu, J., Riggins, G. J., Willson, J. K. V., Markowitz, S. D., et al. (1998) Mutations of mitotic checkpoint genes in human cancers. *Nature* **392**:300–303.

81. Baker, S. J., Fearon, E. R., Nigro, J. M., Hamilton, S. R., Preisinger, A. C., Jessup, J. M., et al. (1989) Chromosome 17 deletions and p53 gene mutations in colorectal carcinomas. *Science* **244**:217–221.

82. Bos, J. L. (1989) Ras oncogenes in human cancer: a review. *Cancer Res.* **49**:4682–4689.

83. Dalla Favera, R., Bregni, M., Erikson, J., Patterson, D., Gallo, R. C., and Croce, C. M. (1982) Assignment of the human c-myc oncogene to the region of chromosome 8 which is translocated in Burkitt lymphoma cells. *Proc. Natl. Acad. Sci. USA* **79**:7824–7827.

84. Dalla Favera, R., Martinotti, S., Gallo, R. C., Erikson, J., and Croce, C. M. (1983) Translocation and rearrangements of the c-myc oncogene in human differentiated B cell lymphomas. *Science* **219**:963–967.

85. Rosenberg, S. M., Thulin, C., and Harris, R. S. (1998) Transient and heritable mutators in adaptive evolution in the lab and in nature. *Genetics* **148**:1559–1566.

86. Akiyama, Y., Iwanaga, R., Saitoh, K., Shiba, K., Ushio, K., Ikeda, E., et al. (1997) Transforming growth factor β type II receptor gene mutations in adenomas from hereditary nonpolyposis colorectal cancer. *Gastroenterology* **112**:33–39.

87. Jacoby, R. F., Marshall, D. J., Kailas, S., Schlack, S., Harms, B., and Love, R. (1995) Genetic instability associated with adenoma to carcinoma progression in hereditary nonpolyposis colon cancer. *Gastroenterology* **109**:73–82.

88. Konishi, M., Kikuchi-Yanoshita, R., Tanaka, K., Muraoka, M., Onda, A., Okumura, Y., et al. (1996) Molecular nature of colon tumors in hereditary nonpolyposis colon cancer, familial polyposis, and sporadic colon cancer. *Gastroenterology* **111**:307–317.

89. Aaltonen, L. A., Peltomaki, P., Mecklin, J.-P., Jarvinen, H., Jass, J. R., Green, J. S., et al. (1994) Replication errors in benign and malignant tumors from hereditary nonpolyposis colorectal cancer patients. *Cancer Res.* **54**:1645–1648.

90. Aaltonen, L. A., Peltomaki, P., Leach, F. S., Sistonen, P., Pylkkanen, L., Mecklin, J.-P., et al. (1993) Clues to the pathogenesis of familial colorectal cancer. *Science* **260**:812–816.

91. Jackson, A. L., Chen, R., and Loeb, L. A. (1998) Induction of microsatellite instability by oxidative DNA damage. *Proc. Natl. Acad. Sci. USA* **95**:12468–12473.

92. Beckman, K. B. and Ames, B. N. (1997) Oxidative decay of DNA. *J. Biol. Chem.* **272**:19633–19636.

93. Feig, D. I., Reid, T. M., and Loeb, L. A. (1994) Reactive oxygen specific in tumorigenesis. *Cancer Res.* **54**:1890s–1894s.

94. Cerutti, P. A. (1985) Prooxidant states and tumor promotion. *Science* **227**:375–381.

95. Baba, S. (1997) Recent advances in molecular genetics of colorectal cancer. *World J. Surg.* **21**:678–687.
96. Spitz, M. R. and Bondy, M. L. (1993) Genetic susceptibility to cancer. *Cancer* **72**:991–995.
97. Kastan, M. B. and Kuerbitz, S. J. (1993) Control of G1 arrest after DNA damage. *Environ. Health Perspect. Suppl.* **101**:55–58.
98. Coleman, W. B. and Tsongalis, G. J. (1995) Multiple mechanisms account for genomic instability and molecular mutation in neoplastic transformation. *Clin. Chem.* **41**:644–657.
99. Sancar, A. and Sancar, G. B. (1988) DNA repair enzymes. *Ann. Rev. Biochem.* **57**:29–67.
100. Kaufmann, W. K. (1989) Pathways of human cell postreplication repair. *Carcinogenesis* **10**:1–11.
101. Weeda, G., Hoeijmakers, J. H. J., and Bootsma, D. (1993) Genes controlling nucleotide excision repair in eukaryotic cells. *BioEssays* **15**:249–258.
102. Jiricny, J. (1998) Eukaryotic mismatch repair: an update. *Mutation Res.* **409**:107–121.
103. Jiricny, J. (1998) Replication errors: Cha(lle)nging the genome. *EMBO J.* **17**:6427–6436.
104. Schmutte, C. and Fishel, R. (1999) Genomic instability: first step to carcinogenesis. *Anticancer Res.* **19**:4665–4696.
105. Jiricny, J. (2000) Mediating mismatch repair. *Nature Genet.* **24**:6–8.
106. Fishel, R., Lescoe, M. K., Rao, M. R. S., Copeland, N. G., Jenkins, N. A., Garber, J., et al. (1993) The human mutator gene homolog *MSH2* and its association with hereditary nonpolyposis colon cancer. *Cell* **75**:1027–1038.
107. Cleaver, J. E. and Kraemer, K. H. (1995) Xeroderma pigmentosum and Cockayne syndrome. *In: The Metabolic and Molecular Bases of Inherited Disease,* 7th ed. (Scriver, C. R., Beaudet, A. L., Sly, W. S., and Valle, D., eds.), McGraw-Hill, New York, pp. 4393–4419.
108. Bootsma, D., Kraemer, K. H., Cleaver, J. E., and Hoeijmakers, J. H. J. (1998) Nucleotide excision repair syndromes: Xeroderma pigmentosa, Cockayne syndrome, and trichothiodystrophy. *In: The Genetic Basis of Human Cancer* (Vogelstein, B. and Kinzler, K. W., eds.), McGraw-Hill, New York, pp. 245–274.
109. Boder, E. (1985) Ataxia-telangiectasia: An overview. *In: Ataxia-telangiectasia: Genetics, Neuropathology, and Immunology of a Degenerative Disease of Childhood* (Gatti, R. A. and Swift, M., eds.), Alan R. Liss, New York, pp. 1–63.
110. Gatti, R. A. (1998) Ataxia-telangiectasia. *In: The Genetic Basis of Human Cancer* (Vogelstein, B. and Kinzler, K. W., eds.), McGraw-Hill, New York, pp. 275–300.
111. Swift, M., Morrell, D., Massey, R. B., and Chase, C. L. (1991) Incidence of cancer in 161 families affected by ataxia-telangiectasia. *N. Engl. J. Med.* **325**:1831–1836.
112. Auerbach, A. D., Buchwald, M., and Joenje, H. (1998) Fanconi anemia. *In: The Genetic Basis of Human Cancer* (Vogelstein, B. and Kinzler, K. W., eds.), McGraw-Hill, New York, pp. 317–332.
113. German, J. and Passarge, E. (1989) Bloom's syndrome. XII. Report from the Registry for 1987. *Clin. Genetics* **35**:57–69.
114. German, J. and Ellis, N. A. (1998) Bloom syndrome. *In: The Genetic Basis of Human Cancer* (Vogelstein, B. and Kinzler, K. W., eds.), McGraw-Hill, New York, pp. 301–315.
115. Chaganti, R. S. K., Schonberg, S., and German, J. (1974) A manyfold increase in sister chromatid exchanges in Bloom's syndrome lymphocytes. *Proc. Natl. Acad. Sci. USA* **71**:4508–4512.
116. Langlois, R. G., Bigbee, W. L., Jensen, R. H., and German, J. (1989) Evidence for increased in vivo mutation and somatic recombination in Bloom's syndrome. *Proc. Natl. Acad. Sci. USA* **86**:670–674.
117. Gatti, R. A. (1991) Localizing the genes for ataxia telangiectasia: A human model for inherited cancer susceptibility. *Adv. Cancer Res.* **56**:77–104.
118. Digweed, M. (1993) Human genetic instability syndromes: Single gene defects with increased risk of cancer. *Toxicol. Lett.* **67**:659–681.
119. Ellis, N. A., Groden, J., Ye, T.-Z., Straughen, J., Lennon, D. J., Ciocci, S., et al. (1995) The Bloom's syndrome gene product is homologous to RecQ helicases. *Cell* **83**:655–666.
120. Savitsky, K., Bar-Shira, A., Gilad, S., Rotman, G., Ziv, Y., Vanagaite, L., et al. (1995) A single ataxia telangiectasia gene with a product similar to PI-3 kinase. *Science* **268**:1749–1753.
121. Trichopoulos, D., Petridou, E., Lipworth, L., and Adami, H.-O. (1995) Epidemiology of cancer. *In: The Metabolic and Molecular Bases of Human Disease,* 7th ed. (Scriver, C. R., Beaudet, A. L., Sly, W. S., and Valle, D., eds.), McGraw-Hill, New York, pp. 231–257.
122. Boland, C.R. (1998) Hereditary nonpolyposis colorectal cancer. *In: The Genetic Basis of Human Cancer* (Vogelstein, B. and Kinzler, K. W., eds.), McGraw-Hill, New York, pp. 333–346.
123. Vasen, H. F. A., Offerhaus, G. J. A., den Hartog Jager, F. C. A., Menko, F. H., Nagengast, F. M., Griffioen, G., et al. (1990) The tumour spectrum in hereditary non-polyposis colorectal cancer: A study of 24 kindreds in the Netherlands. *Int. J. Cancer* **46**:31–34.
124. Mecklin, J.-P. and Jarvinen, H. J. (1991) Tumor spectrum in cancer family syndrome (hereditary nonpolyposis colorectal cancer). *Cancer* **68**:1109–1112.
125. Ionov, Y., Peinado, M. A., Malkhosyan, S., Shibata, D., and Perucho, M. (1993) Ubiquitous somatic mutations in simple repeated sequences reveal a new mechanism for colonic carcinogenesis. *Nature* **363**:558–561.
126. Thibodeau, S. N., Bren, G., and Schaid, D. (1993) Microsatellite instability in cancer of the proximal colon. *Science* **260**:816–819.
127. Parsons, R., Li, G.-M., Longley, M., Modrich, P., Liu, B., Berk, T., et al. (1995) Mismatch repair deficiency in phenotypically normal human cells. *Science* **268**:738–740.
128. Fishel, R., Lescoe, M. K., Rao, M. R. S., Copeland, N. G., Jenkins, N. A., Garber, J., et al. (1993) The human mutator gene homolog *MSH2* and its association with hereditary nonpolyposis colon cancer. *Cell* **75**:1027–1038.
129. Leach, F. S., Nicolaides, N. C., Papadopoulos, N., Liu, B., Jen, J., Sistonen, P., et al. (1993) Mutations of a *mutS* homolog in hereditary nonpolyposis colorectal cancer. *Cell* **75**:1215–1225.
130. Bronner, C. E., Baker, S. M., Morrison, P. T., Warren, G., Smith, L. G., Lescoe, M. K., et al. (1994) Mutation in the DNA mismatch repair gene homologue hMLHI is associated with hereditary nonpolyposis colon cancer. *Nature* **368**:258–261.
131. Papadopoulos, N., Nicolaides, N. C., Wei, Y.-F., Ruben, S. M., Carter, K. C., Rosen, C. A., et al. (1994) Mutation of a mutL homolog in hereditary colon cancer. *Science* **263**:1625–1629.
132. Nicolaides, N. C., Papadopoulos, N., Liu, B., Wel, Y.-F., Carter, K. C., Ruben, S. M., et al. (1994) Mutations of two PMS homologues in hereditary nonpolyposis colon cancer. *Nature* **371**:75–80.
133. Schwartz, R. A. and Torre, D. P. (1995) The Muir-Torre syndrome: a 25 year retrospect. *J. Am. Acad. Dermatol.* **33**:90–104.
134. Cohen, P. R., Kohn, S. R., and Kurzrock, S. R. (1991) Association of sebaceous gland tumors and internal malignancy: the Muir-Torre syndrome. *Am. J. Med.* **90**:606–613.
135. Honchel, R., Halling, K. C., Schaid, D. J., Pittelkow, M., and Thibodeau, S. N. (1994) Microsatellite instability in Muir-Torre syndrome. *Cancer Res.* **54**:1159–1163.
136. Turcot, J., Despres, J.-P., and St. Pierre, F. (1959) Malignant tumors of the central nervous system associated with familial polyposis of the colon: report of two cases. *Dis. Colon Rectum* **2**:465–468.
137. Hamilton, S. R., Liu, B., Parsons, R. E., Papadopoulos, N., Jen, J., Powell, S. M., et al. (1995) The molecular basis of Turcot's syndrome. *N. Engl. J. Med.* **332**:839–847.
138. Yunis, J. J. (1983) The chromosomal basis of human neoplasia. *Science* **221**:227–236.
139. Croce, C. M. (1986) Chromosome translocations and human cancer. *Cancer Res.* **46**:6019–6023.
140. Mitelman, F. (1994) *Catalog of Chromosome Aberrations in Cancer,* 5th ed. Wiley-Liss Publishers, New York.
141. Le Beau, M.M. (1997) Molecular biology of cancer: Cytogenetics. *In: Cancer: Principles and Practice of Oncology,* 5th ed. (DeVita, V. T. Jr., Hellman, S., and Rosenberg, S. A., eds.), Lippincott-Raven, Philadelphia, pp. 103–119.
142. Meltzer, P. S. and Trent, J. M. (1998) Chromosome rearrangements in human solid tumors. *In: The Genetic Basis of Human Cancer*

(Vogelstein, B., and Kinzler, K. W., eds.), McGraw-Hill, New York, pp. 143–160.

143. Thrash-Bingham, C. A., Greenberg, R. E., Howard, S., Bruzel, A., Bremer, M., Goll, A., et al. (1995) Comprehensive allelotyping of human renal cell carcinomas using microsatellite DNA probes. *Proc. Natl. Acad. Sci. USA* **92**:2854–2858.

144. Baker, S. J., Peisinger, A. C., Jessup, J. M., Paraskeva, C., Markowitz, S., Willson, J. K. V., et al. (1990) p53 gene mutations and 17p allelic deletions as late events in colorectal tumorigenesis. *Cancer Res.* **50**:7717–7722.

145. Carter, S. L., Negrini, M., Baffa, R., Gillum, D. R., Rosenberg, A. L., Schwartz, G. F., et al. (1994) Loss of heterozygosity at 11q22-q23 in breast cancer. *Cancer Res.* **54**:6270–6274.

146. Ross, J. S. (1996) DNA ploidy and cell cycle analysis in cancer diagnosis and prognosis. *Oncology* **10**:867–82.

147. Cowlen, M. S. (1997) Nucleic acid hybridization and amplification in situ: principles and applications in molecular pathology. In: *Molecular Diagnostics: For the Clinical Laboratorian* (Coleman, W. B. and Tsongalis, G. J., eds.), Humana Press, Totowa NJ, pp. 163–191.

148. Vogelstein, B., Fearon, E. R., Kern, S. E., Hamilton, S. R., Preisinger, A. C., Nakamura, Y., et al. (1989) Allelotype of colorectal carcinomas. *Science* **244**:207–211.

149. Aldaz, C. M., Chen, T., Sahin, A., Cunningham, J., and Bondy, M. (1995) Comparative allelotype of *in situ* and invasive human breast cancer: high frequency of microsatellite instability in lobular breast carcinomas. *Cancer Res.* **55**:3976–3981.

150. Kawanishi, M., Kohno, T., Otsuka, T., Adachi, J., Sone, S., Noguchi, M., et al. (1997) Allelotype and replication error phenotype of small cell lung carcinoma. *Carcinogenesis* **18**:2057–2062.

151. Boige, V., Laurent-Puig, P., Fouchet, P., Flejou, J. F., Monges, G., Bedossa, P., et al. (1997) Concerted nonsyntenic allelic losses in hyperploid hepatocellular carcinoma as determined by a high-resolution allelotype. *Cancer Res.* **57**:1986–1990.

152. Seymour, A. B., Hruban, R. H., Redston, M., Caldas, C., Powell, S. M., Kinzler, K. W., et al. (1994) Allelotype of pancreatic adenocarcinoma. *Cancer Res.* **54**:2761–2764.

153. Radford, D. M., Fair, K. L., Phillips, N. J., Ritter, J. H., Steinbrueck, T., Holt, M. S., et al. (1995) Allelotyping of ductal carcinoma in situ of the breast: deletion of loci on 8p, 13q, 16q, 17p and 17q. *Cancer Res.* **55**:3399–3405.

154. Ghadimi, B. M., Sackett, D. L., Difilippantonio, M. J., Schrock, E., Neumann, T., Jauho, A., et al. (2000) Centrosome amplification and instability occurs exclusively in aneuploid, but not diploid colorectal cancer cell lines, and correlates with numerical chromosomal aberrations. *Genes Chromosomes Cancer* **27**:183–190.

155. Harwood, J., Tachibana, A., Davis, R., Bhattacharyya, N. P., and Meuth, M. (1993) High rate of multilocus deletion in a human tumor cell line. *Human Mol. Genet.* **2**:165–171.

156. Phear, G., Bhattacharyya, N. P., and Meuth, M. (1996) Loss of heterozygosity and base substitution at the APRT locus in mismatch-repair-proficient and -deficient colorectal carcinoma cell lines. *Mol. Cell. Biol.* **16**:6516–6523.

157. Kastan, M. B., Onyekwere, O., Sidransky, D., Vogelstein, B., and Craig, R. W. (1991) Participation of p53 protein in the cellular response to DNA damage. *Cancer Res.* **51**:6304–6311.

158. Filatov, L., Golubovskaya, V., Hurt, J. C., Byrd, L. L., Phillips, J. M., and Kaufmann, W. K. (1998) Chromosomal instability is correlated with telomere erosion and inactivation of G2 checkpoint function in human fibroblasts expressing human papillomavirus type 16 E6 oncoprotein. *Oncogene* **16**:1825–1838.

159. Honma, M., Momose, M., Tanabe, H., Sakamoto, H., Yu, Y., Little, J. B., et al. (2000) Requirement of wild-type p53 protein for maintenance of chromosomal integrity. *Mol. Carcinogenesis* **28**:203–214.

160. Tarapore, P. and Fukasawa, K. (2000) p53 mutation and mitotic infidelity. *Cancer Invest.* **18**:148–155.

161. Rabinovitch, P. S., Dziadon, S., Brentnall, T. A., Emond, M. J., Crispin, D. A., Haggitt, R. C., et al. (1999) Pancolonic chromosomal instability precedes dysplasia and cancer in ulcerative colitis. *Cancer Res.* **59**:5148–5153.

162. Hruban, R. H., Wilentz, R. E., and Kern, S. E. (2000) Genetic progression in the pancreatic ducts. *Am. J. Pathol.* **156**:1821–1825.

163. Doxsey, S. (1998) The centrosome: a tiny organelle with big potential. *Nature Genet.* **20**:104–106.

164. Pihan, G. A., Purohit, A., Wallace, J., Knecht, H., Woda, B. Quesenberry, P., et al. (1998) Centrosome defects and genetic instability in malignant tumors. *Cancer Res.* **58**:3974–3985.

165. Zhou, H., Kuang, J., Zhong, L., Kuo, W. L., Gray, J. W., Sahin, A., et al. (1998) Tumour amplified kinase STK15/BTAK induces centrosome amplification, aneuploidy and transformation. *Nature Genet.* **20**:189–193.

166. Bischoff, J. R., Anderson, L., Zhu, Y., Mossie, K., Ng, L., Souza, B., et al. (1998) A homologue of Drosophila aurora kinase is oncogenic and amplified in human colorectal cancers. *EMBO J.* **17**:3052–3065.

167. Wolf, G., Elez, R., Doermer, A., Holtrich, U., Ackermann, H., Stutte, H. J., et al. (1997) Prognostic significance of polo-like kinase (PLK) expression in non-small cell lung cancer. *Oncogene* **14**:543–549.

168. Tanaka, T., Kimura, M., Matsunaga, K., Fukada, D., Mori, H., Okano, Y. (1999) Centrosomal kinase AIK1 is overexpressed in invasive ductal carcinoma of the breast. *Cancer Res.* **59**:2041–2044.

169. Carroll, P. E., Okuda, M., Horn, H. F., Biddinger, P., Stambrook, P. J., Gleich, L. L., et al. (1999) Centrosome hyperamplification in human cancer: chromosome instability induced by p53 mutation and/or Mdm2 overexpression. *Oncogene* **18**:1935–1944.

170. Tutt, A., Gabriel, A., Bertwistle, D., Connor, F., Paterson, H., Peacock, J., et al. (1999) Absence of BRCA2 causes genome instability by chromosome breakage and loss associated with centrosome amplification. *Curr. Biol.* **9**:1107–1110.

171. Hartwell, L. H. (1992) Defects in cell cycle checkpoint may be responsible for the genomic instability of cancer cells. *Cell* **71**:543–546.

172. Hartwell, L. H. and Kastan, M. B. (1994) Cell cycle control and cancer. *Science* **266**:1821–1828.

173. Hartwell, L. H. and Weinert, T. A. (1989) Checkpoints: Controls that ensure the order of cell cycle events. *Science* **246**:629–634.

174. Cahill, D. P., da Costa, L. T., Carson-Walter, E. B., Kinzler, K. W., Vogelstein, B., and Lengauer, C. (1999) Characterization of MAD2B and other mitotic spindle checkpoint genes. *Genomics* **58**:181–187.

175. Li, Y. and Benezra, R. (1996) Identification of a human mitotic checkpoint gene: hsMAD2. *Science* **274**:246–248.

176. Jaffrey, R. G., Pritchard, S. C., Clark, C., Murray, G. I., Cassidy, J., Kerr, K. M., et al. (2000) Genomic instability at the *BUB1* locus in colorectal cancer, but not in non-small cell lung cancer. *Cancer Res.* **60**:4349–4352.

177. Myrie, K. A., Percy, M. J., Azmin, J. N., Neeley, C. K., and Petty, E. M. (2000) Mutation and expression analysis of human BUB1 and BUB1B in aneuploid breast cancer cell lines. *Cancer Lett.* **152**:193–199.

178. Sato, M., Sekido, Y., Horio, Y., Takahashi, M., Saito, H., Minna, J. D., et al. (2000) Infrequent mutation of the hBUB1 and hBUBR1 genes in human lung cancer. *Japn. J. Cancer Res.* **91**:504–509.

179. Yamaguchi, K., Okami, K., Hibi, K., Wehage, S. L., Jen, J., and Sidransky, D. (1999) Mutation analysis of hBUB1 in aneuploid HNSCC and lung cancer cell lines. *Cancer Lett.* **139**:183–187.

180. Imai, Y., Shiratori, Y., Kato, N., Inoue, T., and Omata, M. (1999) Mutational inactivation of mitotic checkpoint genes, *hsMAD2* and *hBUB1*, is rare in sporadic digestive tract cancers. *Japn. J. Cancer Res.* **90**:837–840.

181. Gualberto, A., Aldape, K., Kozakiewicz, K., and Tlsty, T. D. (1998) An oncogenic form of p53 confers a dominant, gain-of-function phenotype that disrupts spindle checkpoint function. *Proc. Natl. Acad. Sci. USA* **95**:5166–5171.

182. Shigeta, T., Takagi, M., Delia, D., Chessa, L., Iwata, S., Kanke, Y., et al. (1999) Defective control of apoptosis and mitotic spindle

checkpoint in heterozygous carriers of ATM mutations. *Cancer Res.* **59**:2602–2607.

183. Canman, C., Lim, D. S., Cimprich, K. A., Taya, Y., Tamai, K., Sakaguchi, K., et al. (1998) Activation of the ATM kinase by ionizing radiation and phosphorylation of p53. *Science* **281**:1677–1679.

184. Banin, S., Moyal, L., Shieh, S., Taya, Y., Anderson, C. W., Chessa, L., et al. (1998) Enhanced phosphorylation of p53 by ATM in response to DNA damage. *Science* **281**:1674–1677.

185. Zhang, H., Tombline, G., and Weber, B. L. (1998) BRCA1, BRCA2, and DNA damage response: collision or collusion? *Cell* **92**:433–436.

186. Tlsty, T. D., White, A., and Sanchez, J. (1992) Suppression of gene amplification in human cell hybrids. *Science* **255**:1425–1427.

187. Hamlin, J. L., Leu, T.-H., Vaughn, J. P., Ma, C., and Dikwel, P. A. (1991) Amplification of DNA sequences in mammalian cells. *Prog. Nucleic Acid Res.* **41**:203–239.

188. Tlsty, T. D., Briot, A., Gualberto, A., Hall, I., Hess, S., Hixon, M., et al. (1995) Genomic instability and cancer. *Mutation Res.* **337**:1–7.

189. Cooper, G.N. (1995) *Oncogenes,* 2nd ed. Jones and Bartlett, Boston.

190. Livingstone, L. R., White, A., Sprouse, J., Livanos, E., Jacks, T., and Tlsty, T. D. (1992) Altered cell cycle arrest and gene amplification potential accompany loss of wild-type p53. *Cell* **70**:923–935.

191. Yin, Y., Tainsky, M. A., Bischoff, F. Z., Strong, L. C., and Wahl, G. M. (1992) Wild-type p53 restores cell cycle control and inhibits gene amplification in cells with mutant p53 alleles. *Cell* **70**:937–948.

192. Oren, M. (1994) Relationship of p53 to the control of apoptotic cell death. *Semin. Cancer Biol.* **5**:221–227.

193. Nowell, P. C. and Hungerford, D. A. (1960) A minute chromosome in chronic granulocytic leukemia. *Science* **132**:1497.

194. Dubeau, L. (1998) Ovarian cancer. *In: The Genetic Basis of Human Cancer* (Vogelstein, B. and Kinzler, K. W., eds.), McGraw-Hill, New York, pp. 615–620.

195. Nishisho, L., Nakamura, Y., Miyoshi, Y., Miki, Y., Ando, H., Horii, A., et al. (1991) Mutations of chromosome 5q2l genes in FAP and colorectal cancer patients. *Science* **253**:665–669.

196. Groden, J., Thliveris, A., Samowitz, W., Carlson, M., Gelbert, L., Albertson, H., et al. (1991) Identification and characterization of the familial adenomatous polyposis coli gene. *Cell* **66**:589–600.

197. Kinzler, K. W., Nilbert, M. C., Su, L. K., Vogelstein, B., Bryan, T. M., Levy, D. B., et al. (1991) Identification of a chromosome 5q2l gene that is mutated in colorectal cancers. *Science* **251**:1366–1370.

198. Fearon, E. R., Cho, K. R., Nigro, J. M., Kem, S. E., Simons, J. W., Ruppert, J. M., et al. (1990) Identification of a chromosome 18q gene that is altered in colorectal cancers. *Science* **247**:49–56.

199. Sutherland, G. R. and Richards, R. I. (1995) Simple tandem DNA repeats and human genetic disease. *Proc. Natl. Acad. Sci. USA* **92**:3636–3641.

200. Ramel, C. (1997) Mini- and microsatellites. *Environ. Health. Perspect.* **105**:781–789.

201. Peinado, M. A., Malkhosyan, S., Velazquez, A., and Perucho, M. (1992) Isolation and characterization of allelic losses and gains in colorectal tumors by arbitrarily primed polymerase chain reaction. *Proc. Natl. Acad. Sci. USA* **89**:10065–10069.

202. Fujiwara, T., Stolker, J. M., Watanabe, T., Rashid, A., Longo, P., Eshleman, J. R., et al. (1998) Accumulated clonal genetic alterations in familial and sporadic colorectal carcinomas with widespread instability in microsatellite sequences. *Am. J. Pathol.* **153**:1063–1078.

203. Frazier, M. L., Sinicrope, F. A., Amos, C. I., Cleary, K. R., Lynch, P. M., Levin, B., et al. (1999) Loci for efficient detection of microsatellite instability in hereditary non-polyposis colorectal cancer. *Oncol. Rep.* **6**:497–505.

204. Calistri, D., Presciuttini, S., Buonsanti, G., Radice, P., Gazzoli, I., Pensotti, V., et al. (2000) Microsatellite instability in colorectal cancer patients with suspected genetic predisposition. *Int. J. Cancer* **89**:87–91.

205. Lothe, R. A., Peltomaki, P., Meling, G. I., Aaltonen, L. A., Nystrom-Lahti, M., Pylkkanen, L., et al. (1993) Genomic instability in colorectal cancer: Relationship to clinicopathological variables and family history. *Cancer Res.* **53**:5849–5852.

206. Ikeda, M., Orimo, H., Moriyama, H., Nakajima, E., Matsubara, N., Mibu, R., et al. (1998) Close correlation between mutations of E2F4 and hMSH3 genes in colorectal cancers with microsatellite instability. *Cancer Res.* **58**: 594–598.

207. Thibodeau, S. N., French, A. J., Cunningham, J. M., Tester, D., Burgart, L. J., Roche, P. C., et al. (1998) Microsatellite instability in colorectal cancer: Different mutator phenotypes and the principle involvement of hMLH1. *Cancer Res.* **58**:1713–1718.

208. Simms, L. A., Zou, T.-T., Young, J., Shi, Y.-Q., Lei, J., Appel, R., et al. (1997) Apparent protection from instability of repeat sequences in cancer-related genes in replication error positive gastrointestinal cancers. *Oncogene* **14**:2613–2618.

209. Young, J., Leggett, B., Gustafson, C., Ward, M., Searle, J., Thomas, L., et al. (1993) Genomic instability occurs in colorectal carcinomas but not in adenomas. *Human Mutation* **2**:351–354.

210. Peltomaki, P., Lothe, R. A., Aaltonen, L. A., Pylkkanen, L., Nystrom-Lahti, M., Seruca, R., et al. (1993) Microsatellite instability is associated with tumors that characterize the hereditary non-polyposis colorectal cancer syndrome. *Cancer Res.* **53**:5853–5855.

211. Ouyang, H., Shiwaku, H. O., Hagiwara, H., Miura, K., Abe, T., Kato, Y., et al. (1997) The insulin-like growth factor II receptor gene is mutated in genetically unstable cancers of the endometrium, stomach, and colorectum. *Cancer Res.* **57**:1851–1854.

212. Dietmaier, W., Wallinger, S., Bocker, T., Kullmann, F., Fishel, R., and Ruschoff, J. (1997) Diagnostic microsatellite instability: definition and correlation with mismatch repair protein expression. *Cancer Res.* **57**:4749–4756.

213. Hoang, J.-M., Cottu, P. H., Thuille, B., Salmon, R. J., Thomas, G., and Hamelin, R. (1997) BAT-26, an indicator of the replication error phenotype in colorectal cancers and cell lines. *Cancer Res.* **57**:300–303.

214. Bocker, T., Schlegel, J., Kullmann, F., Stumm, G., Zirngibil, H., Epplen, J., et al. (1996) Genomic instability in colorectal carcinomas: comparison of different evaluation methods and their biological significance. *J. Pathol.* **179**:15–19.

215. Canzian, F., Salovaara, R., Hemminki, A., Kristo, P., Chadwick, R. B., Aaltonen, L. A., et al. (1996) Semiautomated assessment of loss of heterozygosity and replication error in tumors. *Cancer Res.* **56**:3331–3337.

216. Iacopetta, B. J., Welch, J., Soong, R., House, A. K., Zhou, X.-P., and Hamelin, R. (1998) Mutation of the transforming growth factor-β type II receptor gene in right-sided colorectal cancer: relationship to clinicopathological features and genetic alterations. *J. Pathol.* **184**:390–395.

217. Liu, B., Farrington, S. M., Petersen, G. M., Hamilton, S. R., Parsons, R., Papadopolous, N., et al. (1995) Genetic instability occurs in the majority of young patients with colorectal cancer. *Nature Med.* **1**:348–352.

218. Zhou, X.-P., Hoang, J.-M., Li, Y.-J., Seruca, R., Carneiro, F., Sobrinho-Simoes, M., et al. (1998) Determination of the replication error phenotype in human tumors without the requirement for matching normal DNA by analysis of mononucleotide repeat microsatellites. *Genes Chromosomes Cancer* **21**:101–107.

219. Kondo, Y., Kanai, Y., Sakamoto, M., Mizokami, M., Ueda, R., and Hirohashi, S. (1999) Microsatellite instability associated with hepatocarcinogenesis. *J. Hepatol.* **31**:529–536.

220. Orimo, H., Nakajima, E., Ikejima, M., Emi, M., and Shimada, T. (1999) Frameshift mutations and a length polymorphism in the hMSH3 gene and spectrum of microsatellite instability in sporadic colon cancer. *Japn. J. Cancer Res.* **90**:1310–1315.

221. Krajinovic, M., Richer, C., Gorska-Flipot, I., Gaboury, L., Novakovic, I., Labuda, D., et al. (1998) Genomic loci susceptible to replication errors in cancer cells. *Br. J. Cancer* **78**:981–985.

222. Ghimenti, C., Tannergard, P., Wahlberg, S., Liu, T., Giulianotti, P. G., Mosca, F., et al. (1999) Microsatellite instability and mismatch repair gene inactivation in sporadic pancreatic and colon tumours. *Br. J. Cancer* **80**:11–16.

223. Komura, K., Masuda, H., and Esumi, M. (1999) Two types of sporadic multiple colorectal cancers with and without HNPCC-like genetic instability. *Hepato-Gastroenterology* **46**:3115–3120.

224. Potocnik, U., Glavac, D., Golouh, R., and Ravnik-Glavac, M. (2000) Evaluation of microsatellite markers markers for efficient assessment of high microsatellite instabile colorectal tumors. *Pflugers Arch Eur. J. Physiol.* **439**:R47–R49.

225. Cravo, M., Lage, P., Albuquerque, C., Chaves, P., Claro, I., Gomes, T., et al. (1999) BAT-26 identifies sporadic colorectal cancers with mutator phenotype: a correlative study with clinico-pathological features and mutations in mismatch repair genes. *J. Pathol.* **188**:252–257.

226. Johannsdottir, J. T., Jonasson, J. G., Bergthorsson, J. T., Amundadottir, L. T., Magnusson, J., Egilsson, V., et al. (2000) The effect of mismatch repair deficiency on tumourigenesis: microsatellite instability affecting genes containing short repeated sequences. *Int. J. Oncol.* **16**:133–139.

227. Stone, J. G., Tomlinson, I. P. M., and Houlston, R. S. (2000) Optimising methods for determining RER status in colorectal cancers. *Cancer Lett.* **149**:15–20.

228. Chao, A., Gilliland, F., Willman, C., Joste, N., Chen, I.-M., Stone, N., et al. (2000) Patient and tumor characteristics of colon cancers with microsatellite instability: A population-based study. *Cancer Epidemiol. Biomarkers Preven.* **9**:539–544.

229. Salahshor, S., Kressner, U., Pahlman, L., Glimelius, B., Lindmark, G., and Lindblom, A. (1999) Colorectal cancer with and without microsatellite instability involves different genes. *Genes Chromosomes Cancer* **26**:247–252.

230. Bapat, B. V., Madlensky, L., Temple, L. K. F., Hiruki, T., Redston, M., Baron, D. L., et al. (1999) Family history characteristics, tumor microsatellite instability and germline MSH2 and MLH1 mutations in hereditary colorectal cancer. *Human Genet.* **104**:167–176.

231. Fleisher, A. S., Esteller, M., Harpaz, N., Leytin, A., Rashid, A., Xu, Y., et al. (2000) Microsatellite instability in inflammatory bowel disease-associated neoplastic lesions is associated with hypermethylation and diminished expression of the DNA mismatch repair gene, hMLH1. *Cancer Res.* **60**:4864–4868.

232. Benachenhou, N., Guiral, S., Gorska-Flipot, I., Michalski, R., Labuda, D., and Sinnett, D. (1998) Allelic losses and DNA methylation at DNA mismatch repair loci in sporadic colorectal cancer. *Carcinogenesis* **19**:1925–1929.

233. Halling, K. C., French, A. J., McDonnell, S. K., Burgart, L. J., Schaid, D. J., Peterson, B. J., et al. (1999) Microsatellite instability and 8p allelic imbalance in stage B2 and C colorectal cancers. *J. Natl. Cancer Inst.* **91**:1295–1303.

234. Pedroni, M., Tamassia, M. G., Percesepe, A., Roncucci, L., Benatti, P., Lanza, G., et al. (1999) Microsatellite instability in multiple colorectal tumors. *Int. J. Cancer* **81**:1–5.

235. Shitoh, K., Konishi, F., Masubuchi, S., Senba, S., Tsukamoto, T., and Kanazawa, K. (1998) Important microsatellite markers in the investigation of replication errors (RER) in colorectal carcinomas. *Japn. J. Clin. Oncol.* **28**:538–541.

236. Gonzalez-Garcia, I., Moreno, V., Navarro, M., Marti-Rague, J., Marcuello, E., Benasco, C., et al. (2000) Standardized approach for microsatellite instability detection in colorectal cancers. *J. Natl. Cancer Inst.* **92**:544–549.

237. Tomita, S., Miyazato, H., Tamai, O., Muto, Y., and Toda, T. (1999) Analyses of microsatellite instability and the transforming growth factor-β receptor type II gene mutation in sporadic human gastrointestinal cancer. *Cancer Genet. Cytogenet.* **115**:23–27.

238. Cravo, M. L., Fidalgo, P. O., Lage, P. A., Albuquerque, C. M., Chaves, P. P., Claro, I., et al. (1999) Validation and simplification of the Bethesda guidelines for identifying apparently sporadic forms of colorectal carcinoma with microsatellite instability. *Cancer* **85**:779–785.

239. Jass, J. R., Do, K.-A., Simms, L. A., Iino, H., Wynter, C., Pillay, S. P., et al. (1998) Morphology of sporadic colorectal cancer with DNA replication errors. *Gut* **42**:673–679.

240. Yao, J., Eu, K. W., Seow-Choen, F., Vijayan, V., and Cheah, P. Y. (1999) Microsatellite instability and aneuploidy rate in young colorectal-cancer patients do not differ significantly from those in older patients. *Int. J. Cancer* **80**:667–670.

241. Calin, G. A., Gafa, R., Tibiletti, M. G., Herlea, V., Becheanu, G., Cavazzini, L., et al. (2000) Genetic progression in microsatellite instability high (MSI-H) colon cancers correlates with clinico-pathological parameters: a study of the TGFβRII, bax, hMSH3, hMSH6, IGFIIR and blm genes. *Int. J. Cancer* **89**:230–235.

242. Georgiades, I. B., Curtis, L. J., Morris, R. M., Bird, C. C., and Wyllie, A. H. (1999) Heterogeneity studies identify a subset of sporadic colorectal cancers without evidence for chromosomal or microsatellite instability. *Oncogene* **18**:7933–7940.

243. Horii, A., Han, H.-J., Shimada, M., Yanagisawa, A., Kato, Y., Ohta, H., et al. (1994) Frequent replication errors at microsatellite loci in tumors of patients with multiple primary cancers. *Cancer Res.* **54**:3373–3375.

244. Mirabelli-Primdahl, L., Gryfe, R., Kim, H., Millar, A., Luceri, C., Dale, D., et al. (1999) β-catenin mutations are specific for colorectal carcinomas with microsatellite instability but occur in endometrial carcinomas irrespective of mutator pathway. *Cancer Res.* **59**:3346–3351.

245. Ottini, L., Palli, D., Falchetti, M., D'Amico, C., Amorosi, A., Saieva, C., et al. (1997) Microsatellite instability in gastric cancer is associated with tumor location and family history in a high-risk population from Tuscany. *Cancer Res.* **57**:4523–4529.

246. Akiyama, Y., Nagasaki, H., Nihei, Z., Iwama, T., Nomizu, T., Utsunomiya, J., et al. (1996) Frequent microsatellite instabilities and analyses of the related genes in familial gastric cancers. *Japn. J. Cancer Res.* **87**:595–601.

247. Nakashima, H., Honda, M., Inoue, H., Shibuta, K., Arinaga, S., Era, S., et al. (1995) Microsatellite instability in multiple gastric cancers. *Int. J. Cancer* **64**:239–242.

248. Paulson, T. G., Wright, F. A., Parker, B. A., Russack, V., and Wahl, G. M. (1996) Microsatellite instability correlates with reduced survival and poor disease prognosis in breast cancer. *Cancer Res.* **56**:4021–4026.

249. Contegiacomo, A., Palmirotta, R., De Marchis, L., Pizzi, C., Mastranzo, P., Delrio, P., et al. (1995) Microsatellite instability and pathological aspects of breast cancer. *Int. J. Cancer* **64**:264–268.

250. De Marchis, L., Contegiacomo, A., D'Amico, C., Palmirotta, R., Pizzi, C., Ottini, L., et al. (1997) Microsatellite instability is correlated with lymph node-positive breast cancer. *Clin. Cancer Res.* **3**:241–248.

251. Caldes, T., Perez-Segura, P., Tosar, A., de la Hoya, M, and Diaz-Rubio, E. (2000) Low frequency of microsatellite instability in sporadic breast cancer. *Int. J. Oncol.* **16**:1235–1242.

252. Imyanitov, E. N., Togo, A. V., Suspitsin, E. N., Grigoriev, M. Y., Pozharisski, K. M., Turkevich, E. A., et al. (2000) Evidence for microsatellite instability in bilateral breast carcinomas. *Cancer Lett.* **154**:9–17.

253. Richard, S. M., Bailliet, G., Paez, G. L., Bianchi, M. S., Peltomaki, P., and Bianchi, N. O. (2000) Nuclear and mitochondrial genome instability in human breast cancer. *Cancer Res.* **60**:4231–4237.

254. Risinger, J. I., Berchuck, A., Kohler, M. F., Watson, P., Lynch, H. T., and Boyd, J. (1993) Genetic instability of microsatellites in endometrial carcinoma. *Cancer Res.* **53**:5100–5103.

255. Katabuchi, H., van Rees, B., Lambers, A. R., Ronnett, B. M., Blazes, M. S., Leach, F. S., et al. (1995) Mutations in DNA mismatch repair genes are not responsible for microsatellite instability in most sporadic endometrial carcinomas. *Cancer Res.* **55**:5556–5560.

256. Myeroff, L. L., Parsons, R., Kim, S.-J., Hedrick, L., Cho, K. R., Orth, K., et al. (1995) A transforming growth factor β receptor type II gene mutation common in colon and gastric but rare in endometrial cancers with microsatellite instability. *Cancer Res.* **55**:5545–5547.

257. Parc, Y. R., Halling, K. C., Burgart, L. J., McDonnell, S. K., Schaid, D. J., Thibodeau, S. N., et al. (2000) Microsatellite instability and hMLH1/hMSH2 expression in young endometrial carcinoma patients: associations with family history and histopathology. *Int. J. Cancer* **86**:60–66.

258. Gurin, C. C., Federici, M. G., Kang, L., and Boyd, J. (1999) Causes and consequences of microsatellite instability in endometrial carcinoma. *Cancer Res.* **59**:462–466.

259. Koul, A., Nilbert, M., and Borg, A. (1999) A somatic BRCA2 mutation in RER⁺ endometrial carcinomas that specifically deletes the amino-terminal transactivation domain. *Genes Chromosomes Cancer* **24**:207–212.

260. Simpkins, S. B., Bocker, T., Swisher, E. M., Mutch, D. G., Gersell, D. J., Kovatich, A. J., et al. (1999) MLH1 promoter methylation and gene silencing is the primary cause of microsatellite instability in sporadic endometrial cancers. *Human Mol. Genet.* **8**:661–666.

261. Sood, A. K., Skilling, J. S., and Buller, R. E. (1997) Ovarian cancer genomic instability correlates with p53 frameshift mutations. *Cancer Res.* **57**:1047–1049.

262. Ogasawara, S., Maesawa, C., Tamura, G., and Satodate, R. (1995) Frequent microsatellite alterations on chromosome 3p in esophageal squamous cell carcinoma. *Cancer Res.* **55**:891–894.

263. Salvucci, M., Lemoine, A., Saffroy, R., Azoulay, D., Lepere, B., Gaillard, S., et al. (1999) Microsatellite instability in European hepatocellular carcinoma. *Oncogene* **18**:181–187.

264. Pifarre, A., Rosell, R., Monzo, M., De Anta, J. M., Moreno, I., Sanchez, J. J., et al. (1997) Prognostic value of replication errors on chromosomes 2p and 3p in non-small-cell lung cancer. *Br. J. Cancer* **75**:184–189.

265. Shridhar, V., Siegfried, J., Hunt, J., del Mar Alonso, M., and Smith, D. I. (1994) Genetic instability of microsatellite sequences in many non-small cell lung carcinomas. *Cancer Res.* **54**:2084–2087.

266. Rosell, R., Pifarre, A., Monzo, M., Astudillo, J., Lopez-Cabrerizo, M. P., Calvo, R., et al. (1997) Reduced survival in patients with stage-I non-small-cell lung cancer associated with DNA replication errors. *Int. J. Cancer* **74**:330–334.

267. Benachenhou, N., Guiral, S., Gorska-Flipot, I., Labuda, D., and Sinnett, D. (1998) High resolution deletion mapping reveals frequent allelic losses at the DNA mismatch repair loci hMLH1 and hMSH3 in non-small cell lung cancer. *Int. J. Cancer* **77**:173–180.

268. Chang, J.-W., Chen, Y.-C., Chen, C.-Y., Chen, J.-T., Chen, S.-K., and Wang, Y.-C. (2000) Correlation of genetic instability with mismatch repair protein expression and p53 mutations in non-small cell lung cancer. *Clin. Cancer Res.* **6**:1639–1646.

269. Kim, C. H., Yoo, C.-G., Han, S. K., Shim, Y.-S., and Kim, Y. W. (1998) Genetic instability of microsatellite sequences in non-small cell lung cancers. *Lung Cancer* **21**:21–25.

270. Uchida, T., Wada, C., Wang, C., Ishida, H., Egawa, S., Yokoyama, E., et al. (1995) Microsatellite instability in prostate cancer. *Oncogene* **10**:1019–1022.

271. Gao, X., Wu, N., Grignon, D., Zacharek, A., Liu, H., Salkowski, A., et al. (1994) High frequency of mutator phenotype in human prostatic adenocarcinoma. *Oncogene* **9**:2999–3003.

272. Dahiya, R., Lee, C., McCarville, J., Hu, W., Kaur, G., and Deng, G. (1997) High frequency of genetic instability of microsatellites in human prostatic adenocarcinoma. *Int. J. Cancer* **72**:762–767.

273. Egawa, S., Uchida, T., Suyama, K., Wang, C., Ohori, M., Irie, S., et al. (1995) Genomic instability of microsatellite repeats in prostate cancer: relationship to clinicopathological variables. *Cancer Res.* **55**:2418–2421.

274. Miet, S. M. D., Neyra, M., Jaques, R., Dubernard, P. M., Revol, A. A. P., and Marcais, C. M. N. (1999) RER+ phenotype in prastate intra-epithelial neoplasia associated with human prostate-carcinoma development. *Int. J. Cancer* **82**:635–639.

275. Fuji, H. and Shimada, T. (1989) Isolation and characterization of cDNA clones derived from the divergently transcribed gene in the region upstream from the dihydrofolate reductase gene. *J. Biol. Chem.* **264**:10057–10064.

276. Palombo, F., Gallihari, P., Iaccrino, I., Lettieri, T., Hughes, M., D'Arrigo, A., et al. (1995) GTBP, a 160-kilodalton protein essen-

tial for mismatch binding activity in human cells. *Science* **268**:1912–1914.

277. Papadopoulos, N., Nicolaides, N. C., Liu, B., Parsons, R., Lengauer, C., Palombo, F., et al. (1995) Mutations of GTBP in genetically unstable cells. *Science* **268**:1915–1917.

278. Lipkin, S. M., Wang, V., Jacoby, R., Banerjee-Basu, S., Baxevanis, A. D., Lynch, H. T., et al. (2000) MLH3: a DNA mismatch repair gene associated with mammalian microsatellite instability. *Nature Genet.* **24**:27–35.

279. Planck, M., Koul, A., Fernebro, E., Borg, A., Kristoffersson, U., Olsson, H., et al. (1999) hMLH1, hMSH2 and hMSH6 mutations in hereditary non-polyposis colorectal cancer families from southern Sweden. *Int. J. Cancer.* **83**:197–202.

280. Loukola, A., Vikki, S., Singh, J., Launonen, V., and Aaltonen, L. A. (2000) Germline and somatic mutation analysis of MLH3 in MSI-positive colorectal cancer. *Am. J. Pathol.* **157**:347–352.

281. Planck, M., Wenngren, E., Borg, A., Olsson, H., and Nilbert, M. (2000) Somatic frameshift alterations in mononucleotide repeat-containing genes in different tumor types from an HNPCC family with germline MSH2 mutation. *Genes Chromosomes Cancer* **29**:33–39.

282. Liu, B., Nicolaides, N. C., Markowitz, S., Willson, J. K. V., Parsons, R. E., Jen, J., et al. (1995) Mismatch repair defects in sporadic colorectal cancers with microsatellite instability. *Nature Genet.* **9**:48–55.

283. Moslein, G., Tester, D. J., Lindor, N. M., Honchel, R., Cunningham, J. M., French, A. J., et al. (1996) Microsatellite instability and mutation analysis of hMSH2 and hMLH1 in patients with sporadic, familial and hereditary colorectal cancer. *Human Mol. Genet.* **5**:1245–1252.

284. Coleman, W. B. and Tsongalis, G. J. (1999) The role of genomic instability in human carcinogenesis. *Anticancer Res.* **19**: 4645–4664.

285. Arzimanoglou, I. I., Gilbert, F., and Barber, H. R. K. (1998) Microsatellite instability in human solid tumors. *Cancer* **82**:1808–1820.

286. Lothe, R. A. (1997) Microsatellite instability in human solid tumors. *Mol. Med. Today* **3**:61–68.

287. Sclotterer, C. and Tautz, D. (1992) Slippage synthesis of simple sequence DNA. *Nucleic Acids Res.* **20**:211–215.

288. Thomas, D. C., Umar, A., and Kunkel, T. A. (1996) Microsatellite instability and mismatch repair defects in cancer cells. *Mutation Res.* **350**:201–205.

289. Lovett, S. T. and Feschenko, V. (1996) Stabilization of diverged tandem repeats by mismatch repair: evidence for deletion formation via a misaligned replication intermediate. *Proc. Natl. Acad. Sci. USA* **93**:7120–7124.

290. Kahn, S. M., Klein, M. G., Jiang, W., Xing, W. Q., Xu, D. B., Perucho, M., et al. (1995) Design of a selectable reporter for the detection of mutations in mammalian simple repeat sequences. *Carcinogenesis* **16**:1223–1228.

291. Farber, R., Petes, T., Dominska, M., Hudgens, S., and Liskay, R. (1994) Instability of simple repeat sequence repeats in a mammalian cell line. *Human Mol. Genet.* **3**:253–256.

292. Boyer, J. C. and Farber, R. A. (1998) Mutation rate of a microsatellite sequence in normal human fibroblasts. *Cancer Res.* **58**:3946–3949.

293. Hanford, M. G., Rushton, B. C., Gowen, L. C., and Farber, R. A. (1998) Microsatellite mutation rates in cancer cell lines deficient or proficient in mismatch repair. *Oncogene* **16**:2389–2393.

294. Mironov, N., Jansen, L. A. M., Zhu, W.-B., Aguelon, A.-M., Reguer, G., and Yamasaki, H. (1999) A novel sensitive method to detect frameshift mutations in exonic repeat sequences of cancer-related genes. *Carcinogenesis* **20**:2189–2192.

295. Umar, A., Koi, M., Risinger, J. I., Glaab, W. E., Tindall, K. R., Kolodner, R. D., et al. (1997) Correction of hypermutability, *N*-methyl-*N*'-nitro-*N*-nitrosoguanidine resistance, and defective mismatch repair by introducing chromosome 2 into human tumor cells with mutations in MSH2 and MSH6. *Cancer Res.* **57**:3949–3955.

296. da Costa, L. T., Lui, B., El-Deiry, W. S., Hamilton, S. R., Kinzler, K. W., Vogelstein, B., et al. (1995) Polymerase δ variants in RER colorectal tumors. *Nature Genet.* **9**:10–11.

297. Ku, J.-L., Yoon, K.-A., Kim, D.-Y., and Park, J.-G. (1999) Mutations in hMSH6 alone are not sufficient to cause the microsatellite instability in colorectal cancer cell lines. *Eur. J. Cancer* **35**:1724–1729.

298. Verma, L., Kane, M. F., Brassett, C., Schmeits, J., Evans, G.R., Kolodner, R. D., et al. (1999) mononucleotide microsatellite instability and germline MSH6 mutation analysis in early onset colorectal cancer. *J. Med. Genet.* **36**:678–682.

299. Parc, Y. R., Halling, K. C., Wang, L., Christensen, E. R., Cunningham, J. M., French, A. J., et al. (2000) hMSH6 alterations in patients with microsatellite instability-low colorectal cancer. *Cancer Res.* **60**:2225–2231.

300. Koi, M., Umar, A., Chauhan, D. P., Cherian, S. P., Carethers, J. M., Kunkel, T. A., et al. (1994) Human chromosome 3 corrects mismatch repair deficiency and microsatellite instability and reduces *N*-methyl-*N*'-nitro-*N*-nitrosoguanidine tolerance in colon tumor cells with homozygous hMLH1 mutation. *Cancer Res.* **54**:4308–4312.

301. Umar, A., Risinger, J. I., Glaab, W. E., Tindall, K. R., Barrett, J. C., and Kunkel, T. A. (1998) Functional overlap in mismatch repair by human MSH3 and MSH6. *Genetics* **148**:1637–1646.

302. Risinger, J. I., Umar, A., Barrett, J. C., Kunkel, T. A. (1995) A hPMS2 mutant cell line is defective in strand-specific mismatch repair. *J. Biol. Chem.* **270**:18183–18186.

303. Risinger, J. I., Umar, A., Glaab, W. E., Tindall, K. R., Kunkel, T. A., and Barrett, J. C. (1998) Single gene complementation of the hPMS2 defect in HEC-1-A endometrial carcinoma cells. *Cancer Res.* **58**:2978–2981.

304. Lettieri, T., Marra, G., Aquilina, G., Gignami, M., Crompton, N. E. A., Palombo, F., et al. (1999) Effect of hMSH6 cDNA expression on the phenotype of mismatch repair-deficit colon cancer line HCT15. *Carcinogenesis* **20**:373–382.

305. Lengauer, C., Kinzler, K. W., and Vogelstein, B. (1997) DNA methylation and genetic instability in colorectal cancer cells. *Proc. Natl. Acad. Sci. USA* **94**:2545–2550.

306. Ahuja, N., Mohan, A. L., Li, Q., Stolker, J. M., Herman, J. G., Hamilton, S. R., et al. (1997) Association between CpG island methylation and microsatellite instability in colorectal cancer. *Cancer Res.* **57**:3370–3374.

307. Kane, M. F., Loda, M., Gaida, G. M., Lipman, J., Mishra, R., Goldman, H., et al. (1997) Methylation of the hMLH1 promoter correlates with lack of expression of hMLH1 in sporadic colon tumors and mismatch repair-defective human tumor cell lines. *Cancer Res.* **57**:808–811.

308. Cunningham, J. M., Christensen, E. R., Tester, D. J., Kim, C.-Y., Roche, P. C., Burgart, L. J., et al. (1998) Hypermethylation of the hMLH1 promoter in colon cancer with microsatellite instability. *Cancer Res.* **58**:3455–3460.

309. Herman, J. G., Umar, A., Polyak, K., Graff, J. R., Ahuja, N., Issa, J.-P. J., et al. (1998) Incidence and functional consequences of hMLH1 promoter hypermethylation in colorectal carcinoma. *Proc. Natl. Acad. Sci. USA* **95**:6870–6875.

310. Deng, G., Chen, A., Hong, J., Chae, H. S., and Kim, Y. S. (1999) Methylation of CpG in a small region of the hMLH1 promoter invariably correlates with the absence of gene expression. *Cancer Res.* **59**:2029–2033.

311. Wheeler, J. M. D., Loukola, A., Aaltonen, L. A., McC Mortensen, N. J., and Bodmer, W. F. (2000) The role of hypermethylation of the hMLH1 promoter region in HNPCC versus MSI+ sporadic colorectal cancers. *J. Med. Genet.* **37**:588–592.

312. Kuismanen, S., Holmberg, M. T., Salovaara, R., Schweizer, P., Aaltonen, L. A., de la Chapelle, A., et al. (1999) Epigenetic phenotypes distinguish microsatellite-stable and –unstable colorectal cancers. *Proc. Natl. Acad. Sci. USA* **96**:12661–12666.

313. Kang, G. H., Shim, Y. H., and Ro, J. Y. (1999) Correlation of methylation of the hMLH1 promoter with lack of expression of hMLH1 in sporadic gastric carcinomas with replication error. *Lab. Invest.* **79**:903–909.

314. Bevilacqua, R. A. U. and Simpson, A. J. G. (2000) Methylation of the hMLH1 promotor but no hMLH1 mutations in sporadic gastric carcinomas with high level microsatellite instability. *Int. J. Cancer* **87**:200–203.

315. Endoh, Y., Tamura, G., Ajioka, Y., Watanabe, H., and Motoyama, T. (2000) Frequent hypermethylation of the hMLH1 gene promoter in differentiated-type tumors of the stomach with the gastric foveolar phenotype. *Am. J. Pathol.* **157**:717–722.

316. Wu, M.-S., Lee, C.-W., Shun, C.-T., Wang, H.-P., Lee, W.-J., Chang, M.-C., et al. (2000) Distinct clinicopathologic and genetic profiles in sporadic gastric cancer with different mutator phenotypes. *Genes Chromosomes Cancer* **27**:403–411.

317. Leung, S. Y., Yuen, S. T., Chung, L. P., Chu, K. M., Chan, A. S. Y., and Ho, J. C. I. (1999) hMLH1 promoter methylation and lack of hMLH1 expression in sporadic gastric carcinomas with high-frequency microsatellite instability. *Cancer Res.* **59**:159–164.

318. Fleisher, A. S., Esteller, M., Wang, S., Tamura, G., Suzuki, H., Yin, J., et al. (1999) Hypermethylation of the hMLH1 gene promoter in human gastric cancers with microsatellite instability. *Cancer Res.* **59**:1090–1095.

319. Honchel, R., Halling, K. C., and Thibodeau, S. N. (1995) Genomic instability in neoplasia. *Semin. Cell Biol.* **6**:45–52.

320. Peltomaki, P. (1997) DNA mismatch repair gene mutations in human cancer. *Environ. Health Perspect.* **105**:775–780.

321. Parsons, R., Myeroff, L. L., Liu, B., Willson, J. K. V., Markowitz, S. D., Kinzler, K. W., et al. (1995) Microsatellite instability and mutations of the transforming growth factor β type II receptor gene in colorectal cancer. *Cancer Res.* **55**:5548–5550.

322. Parsons, R., Li, G.-M., Longley, M. J., Fang, W., Papadopoulos, N., Jen, J., et al. (1993) Hypermutability and mismatch repair deficiency in RER+ tumor cells. *Cell* **75**:1227–1236.

323. Mao, L., Lee, D. J., Tockman, M. S., Erozan, Y. S., Askin, F., and Sidransky, D. (1994) Microsatellite alterations as clonal markers for the detection of human cancer. *Proc. Natl. Acad. Sci. USA* **91**:9871–9875.

324. Risinger, J. I., Umar, A., Boyd, J., Berchuck, A., Kunkel, T. A., and Barrett, J. C. (1996) Mutation of *MSH3* in endometrial cancer and evidence for its functional role in heteroduplex repair. *Nature Genet.* **14**:102–105.

325. Oki, E., Oda, S., Maehara, Y., and Sugimachi, K. (1999) Mutated gene-specific phenotypes of dinucleotide repeat instability in human colorectal carcinoma cell lines deficient in DNA mismatch repair. *Oncogene* **18**:2143–2147.

326. Bocker, T., Diermann, J., Friedl, W., Gebert, J., Holinski-Feder, E., Kamer-Hanusch, J., et al. (1997) Microsatellite instability analysis: a multicenter study for reliability and quality control. *Cancer Res.* **57**:4739–4743.

327. Boland, C. R., Thibodeau, S. N., Hamilton, S. R., Sidransky, D., Eshleman, J. R., Burt, R. W., et al. (1998) A National Cancer Institute workshop on microsatellite instability for cancer detection and familial predisposition: development of international criteria for the determination of microsatellite instability in colorectal cancer. *Cancer Res.* **58**:5248–5257.

328. Siah, S. P., Quinn, D. M., Bennett, G. D., Casey, G., Flower, R. L., Suthers, G., et al. (2000) Microsatellite instability markers in breast cancer: a review and study showing MSI was not detected at BAT25 and BAT26 microsatellite markers in early-onset breast cancer. *Breast Cancer Res. Treat.* **60**:135–142.

329. Lin, H., Wang, X.-F., Ng-Eaton, E., Weinberg, R. A., and Lodish, H. F. (1992) Expression cloning of the TGF-β type II receptor, a functional transmembrane serine/threonine kinase. *Cell* **68**:775–785.

330. Markowitz, S., Wang, J., Myeroff, L., Parsons, R., Sun, L., Lutterbaugh, J., et al. (1995) Inactivation of the type II TGF-β receptor in colon cancer cells with microsatellite instability. *Science* **268**:1336–1338.

331. Yamamoto, H., Sawai, H., Weber, T. K., Rodriguez-Bigas, and Perucho, M. (1998) Somatic frameshift mutations in DNA mis-

match repair and proapoptosis genes in hereditary nonpolyposis colorectal cancer. *Cancer Res.* **58**:997–1003.

332. Duval, A., Gayet, J., Zhou, X.-P., Iacopetta, B., Thomas, G., and Hamelin, R. (1999) Frequent frameshift mutations of the *TCF-4* gene in colorectal cancers with microsatellite instability. *Cancer Res.* **59**:4213–4215.

333. Semba, S., Ouyang, H., Han, S. Y., Kato, Y., and Horii, A. (2000) Analysis of candidate target genes for mutation in microsatellite instability-positive cancers of the colorectum, stomach, and endometrium. *Int. J. Oncol.* **16**:731–737.

334. Percesepe, A., Pedroni, M., Sala, E., Menigatti, M., Borghi, F., Losi, L., et al. (2000) Genomic instability and target gene mutations in colon cancers with different degrees of allelic shifts. *Genes Chromosomes Cancer* **27**:424–429.

335. Oliveria, C., Seruca, R., Seixas, M., and Sobrinho-Simoes, M. (1998) The clinicopathologic features of gastric carcinomas with microsatellite instability may be mediated by mutations in different "target genes": A study of the TGFβRII, IGFIIR, and BAX genes. *Am. J. Pathol.* **153**:1211–1219.

336. Wu, M.-S., Lee, C.-W., Shun, C.-T., Wang, H.-P., Lee, W.-J., Sheu, J.-C., et al. (1998) Clinicopathological significance of altered loci of replication error and microsatellite instability-associated mutations in gastric cancer. *Cancer Res.* **58**:1494–1497.

337. Wang, Y., Shinmura, K., Guo, R. J., Isogaki, J., Wang, D. Y., Kino, I., et al. (1998) Mutational analyses of multiple target genes in histologically heterogenous gastric cancer with microsatellite instability. *Japn. J. Cancer Res.* **89**:1284–1291.

338. Kim, J. J., Baek, M. J., Kim, L., Kim, N. G., Lee, Y. C., Song, S. Y., et al. (1999) Accumulated frameshift mutations at coding nucleotide repeats during the progression of gastric carcinoma with microsatellite instability. *Lab. Invest.* **79**:1113–1120.

339. Shinmura, K., Tani, M., Isogaki, J., Wang, Y., Sugimura, H., and Yokota, J. (1998) RER phenotype and its associated mutations in familial gastric cancer. *Carcinogenesis* **19**:247–251.

340. Duval, A., Iacopetta, B., Ranzani, G. N., Lothe, R. A., Thomas, G., and Hamelin, R. (1999) Variable mutation frequencies in coding repeats of TCF-4 and other target genes in colon, gastric, and endometrial carcinoma showing microsatellite instability. *Oncogene* 18:6806–6809.

341. Guo, R.-J., Wang, Y., Kaneko, E., Wang, D.-Y., Arai, H., Hanai, H., et al. (1998) Analyses of mutation and loss of heterozygosity of coding sequences of the entire transforming growth factor beta type II receptor gene in sporadic human gastric cancer. *Carcinogenesis* **19**:1539–1544.

342. Inoue, K., Kohno, T., Takakura, S., Hayashi, Y., Mizoguchi, H., and Yokota, J. (2000) Frequent microsatellite instability and BAX mutations in T cell acute lymphoblastic leukemia cell lines. *Leukemia Res.* **24**:255–262.

343. Leung, S. Y., Chan, T. L., Chung, L. P., Chan, A. S. Y., Fan, Y. W., Hung, K. N., et al. (1998) Microsatellite instability and mutation of DNA mismatch repair genes in gliomas. *Am. J. Pathol.* **153**:1181–1188.

344. Massague, J. (1990) The transforming growth factor-beta family. *Ann. Rev. Cell Biol.* **6**:597-641.

345. Massague, J., Blain, S. W., and Lo, R. S. (2000) TGFβ signaling in growth control, cancer, and heritable disorders. *Cell* **103**:295–309.

346. Moses, H., Yang, E., and Pietenpol, J. (1990) TGF-β stimulation and inhibition of cell proliferation: new mechanistic insights. *Cell* **63**:245–247.

347. Wang, J., Sun, L., Myeroff, L., Wang, X., Gentry, L. E., Yang, J., et al. (1995) Demonstration that mutation of the type II transforming growth factor β receptor inactivates its tumor suppressor activity in replication error-positive colon carcinoma cells. *J. Biol. Chem.* **270**:22044–22049.

348. Grady, W. M., Rajput, A., Myeroff, L., Liu, D. F., Kwon, K., Willis, J., et al. (1998) Mutation of the type II transforming growth factor-β receptor is coincident with the transformation of human colon adenomas to malignant carcinomas. *Cancer Res.* **58**:3101–3104.

349. Huang, J., Papadopoulos, N., McKinley, A., Farrington, S. M., Curtis, L. J., Wyllie, A. H., et al. (1996) *APC* mutations in colorectal

tumors with mismatch repair deficiency. *Proc. Natl. Acad. Sci. USA* **93**:9049–9054.

350. Yamamoto, H., Sawai, H., and Perucho, M. (1997) Frameshift somatic mutations in gastrointestinal cancer of the microsatellite mutator phenotype. *Cancer Res.* **57**:4420–4426.

351. Malkhosyan, S., Rampino, N., Yamamoto, H., and Perucho, M. (1996) Frameshift mutator mutations. *Nature* **382**:499–500.

352. Yamamoto, H., Itoh, F., Fukushima, H., Adachi, Y., Itoh, H., Hinoda, Y., et al. (1999) Frequent Bax frameshift mutations in gastric cancer with high but not low microsatellite instability. *J. Exp. Clin. Cancer Res.* **18**:103–106.

353. Yoshitaka, T., Matsubara, N., Ikeda, M., Tanino, M., Hanafusa, H., Tanaka, N., et al. (1996) Mutations of E2F-4 trinucleotide repeats in colorectal cancer with microsatellite instability. *Biochem. Biophys. Res. Commun.* **227**:553–557.

354. Souza, R. F., Yin, J., Smolinski, K. N., Zou, T.-T., Wang, S., Shi, Y.-Q., et al. (1997) Frequent mutation of the E2F-4 cell cycle gene in primary human gastrointestinal tumors. *Cancer Res.* **57**:2350–2353.

355. Calin, G., Herlea, V., Barbanti-Brodano, G., and Negrini, M. (1998) The coding region of the Bloom syndrome BLM gene and of the CBL proto-oncogene is mutated in genetically unstable sporadic gastrointestinal tumors. *Cancer Res.* **58**:3777–3781.

356. Capozzi, E., Della Puppa, L., Fornasarig, M., Pedroni, M., Boiocchi, M., and Viel, A. (1999) Evaluation of the replication error phenotype in relation to molecular and clinicopathological features in hereditary and early onset colorectal cancer. *Eur. J. Cancer* **35**:289–295.

357. Schneider, A., Borgnat, S., Lang, H., Regine, O., Lindner, V., Kassem, M., et al. (2000) Evaluation of microsatellite analysis in urine sediment for diagnosis of bladder cancer. *Cancer Res.* **60**:4617–4622.

358. Gonzalez-Zulueta, M., Ruppert, J. M., Tokino, K., Tsai, Y. C., Spruck, C. H., Miyao, N., et al. (1993) Microsatellite instability in bladder cancer. *Cancer Res.* **53**:5620–5623.

359. Orlow, I., Lianes, P., Lacombe, L., Dalbagni, G., Reuter, V. E., and Cordon-Cardo, C. (1994) Chromosome 9 allelic losses and microsatellite alterations in human bladder tumors. *Cancer Res.* **54**:2848–2851.

360. Li, M., Zhang, Z.-F., Reuter, V. E., and Cordon-Cardo, C. (1996) Chromosome 3 allelic losses and microsatellite alterations in transitional cell carcinoma of the urinary bladder. *Am. J. Pathol.* **149**:229–235.

361. Christensen, M., Jensen, M. A., Wolf, H., and Orntoft, T. F. (1998) Pronounced microsatellite instability in transitional cell carcinomas from young patients with bladder cancer. *Int. J. Cancer* **79**:396–401.

362. Bonnal, C., Ravery, V., Toublanc, M., Bertrand, G., Boccon-Gibod, L., Henin, D., et al. (2000) Absence of microsatellite instability in transitional cell carcinoma of the bladder. *Urology* **55**:287–291.

363. Schmitt, F. C., Soares, R., Gobbi, H., Milanezzi, F., Santos-Silva, F., Cirnes, L., et al. (1999) Microsatellite instability in medullary breast carcinomas. *Int. J. Cancer* **82**:644–647.

364. Toyama, T., Iwase, H., Iwata, H., Hara, Y., Omoto, Y., Suchi, M., et al. (1996) Microsatellite instability in *in situ* and invasive sporadic breast cancers of Japanese women. *Cancer Lett.* **108**:205–209.

365. Jonsson, M., Johannsson, O., and Borg, A. (1995) Infrequent occurrence of microsatellite instability in sporadic and familial breast cancer. *Eur. J. Cancer* **31A**:2330–2334.

366. Han, H.-J., Yanagisawa, A., Kato, Y., Park, J.-G., and Nakamura, Y. (1993) Genetic instability in pancreatic cancer and poorly differentiated type of gastric cancer. *Cancer Res.* **53**:5087–5089.

367. Yee, C. J., Roodi, N., Verrier, C. S., and Parl, F. F. (1994) Microsatellite instability and loss of heterozygosity in breast cancer. *Cancer Res.* **54**:1641–1644.

368. Shaw, J. A., Walsh, T., Chappell, S. A., Carey, N., Johnson, K., and Walker, R. A. (1996) Microsatellite instability in early sporadic breast cancer. *Br. J. Cancer* **73**:1393–1397.

369. Wooster, R., Cleton-Jansen, A.-M., Collins, N., Mangion, J., Cornelis, R. S., Cooper, C. S., et al. (1994) Instability of short tandem repeats (microsatellites) in human cancers. *Nature Genet.* **6**:152–156.

370. Minobe, K., Bando, K., Fukino, K., Soma, S., Kasumi, F., Sakamoto, G., et al. (1999) Somatic mutation of the PTEN/MMAC1 gene in breast cancers with microsatellite instability. *Cancer Lett.* **144**:9–16.

371. Karnik, P., Plummer, S., Myles, J., Tubbs, R., Crowe, J., and Williams, B. R. G. (1995) Microsatellite instability at a single locus (D11S988) on chromosome 11p15.5 as a late event in mammary tumorigenesis. *Human Mol. Genet.* **4**:1889–1894.

372. Anbazhagan, R., Fujii, H., and Gabrielson, E. (1999) Microsatellite instability is uncommon in breast cancer. *Clin. Cancer Res.* **5**:839–844.

373. Benachenhou, N., Guiral, S., Gorska-Flipot, I., Labuda, D., and Sinnett, D. (1999) Frequent loss of heterozygosity at the DNA mismatch-repair loci hMLH1 and hMSH3 in sporadic breast cancer. *Br. J. Cancer* **79**:1012–1017.

374. Wheeler, J. M. D., Beck, N. E., Kim, H. C., Tomlinson, I. P. M., Mortensen, N. J. M., and Bodmer, W.F. (1999) Mechanisms of inactivation of mismatch repair genes in human colorectal cancer cell lines: The predominant role of hMLH1. *Proc. Natl. Acad. Sci. USA* **96**:10296–10301.

375. Watatani, M., Yoshida, T., Kuroda, K., Ieda, S., and Yasutomi, M. (1996) Allelic loss of chromosome 17p, mutation of the p53 gene, and microsatellite instability in right- and left-sided colorectal cancer. *Cancer* **77**:1688–1693.

376. Ilyas, M., Tomlinson, I. P. M., Novelli, M. R., Hanby, A., Bodmer, W. F., and Talbot, I. C. (1996) Clinico-pathological features and p53 expression in left-sided sporadic colorectal cancers with and without microsatellite instability. *J. Pathol.* **179**:370–375.

377. Risio, M., Reato, G., di Celle, P. F., Fizzotti, M., Rossini, F. P., and Foa, R. (1996) Microsatellite instability is associated with the histological features of the tumor in nonfamilial colorectal cancer. *Cancer Res.* **56**:5470–5474.

378. Orimo, H., Ikejima, M., Nakajima, E., Emi, M., and Shimada, T. (1998) A novel missense mutation and frameshift mutations in the type II receptor of transforming growth factor-β gene in sporadic colon cancer with microsatellite instability. *Mutation Res.* **382**:115–120.

379. Iino, H., Simms, L., Young, J., Arnold, J., Winship, I. M., Webb, S. I., et al. (2000) DNA microsatellite instability and mismatch repair protein loss in adenomas presenting in hereditary non-polyposis colorectal cancer. *Gut* **47**:37–42.

380. Samowitz, W. S. and Slattery, M. L. (1997) Microsatellite instability in colorectal adenomas. *Gastroenterology* **112**:1515–1519.

381. Caduff, R. F., Johnston, C. M., Svoboda-Newman, S. M., Poy, E. L., Merajver, S. D., and Frank, T. S. (1996) Clinical and pathological significance of microsatellite instability in sporadic endometrial carcinoma. *Am. J. Pathol.* **148**:1671–1678.

382. Mironov, N. M., Aguelon, A.-M., Hollams, E., Lozano, J.-C., and Yamasaki, H. (1995) Microsatellite alterations in human and rat esophageal tumors at selective loci. *Mol. Carcinogenesis* **13**:1–5.

383. Meltzer, S. J., Yin, J., Manin, B., Rhyu, M.-G., Cottrell, J., Hudson, E., et al. (1994) Microsatellite instability occurs frequently and in both diploid and aneuploid cell populations of Barrett's-associated esophageal adenocarcinomas. *Cancer Res.* **54**:3379–3382.

384. Kagawa, Y., Yoshida, K., Hirai, T., Toge, T., Yokozaki, H., Yasui, W., et al. (2000) Microsatellite instability in squamous cell carcinomas and dysplasias of the esophagus. *Anticancer Res.* **20**:213–217.

385. Seruca, R., Santos, N. R., David, L., Constancia, M., Barroca, H., Carneiro, F., et al. (1995) Sporadic gastric carcinomas with microsatellite instability display a particular clinicopathologic profile. *Int. J. Cancer* **64**:32–36.

386. Halling, K. C., Harper, J., Moskaluk, C. A., Thibodeau, S. N., Petroni, G. R., Yustein, A. S., et al. (1999) Origin of microsatellite instability in gastric cancer. *Am. J. Pathol.* **155**:205–211.

387. Rhyu, M.-G., Park, W.-S., and Meltzer, S. J. (1994) Microsatellite instability occurs frequently in human gastric carcinoma. *Oncogene* **9**:29–32.

388. Wu, M.-S., Sheu, J.-C., Shun, C.-T., Lee, W.-J., Wang, J.-T., Wang, T.-H., et al. (1997) Infrequent hMSH2 mutation in sporadic gastric adenocarcinoma with microsatellite instability. *Cancer Lett.* **112**:161–166.

389. Dos Santos, N. R., Seruca, R., Constancia, M., Seixas, M., and Sobrinho-Simoes, M. (1996) Microsatellite instability at multiple loci in gastric carcinoma: clinicopathologic implications and prognosis. *Gastroenterology* **110**:38–44.

390. Semba, S., Yokozaki, H., Yamamoto, S., Yasui, W., and Tahara, E. (1996) Microsatellite instability in precancerous lesions and adenocarcinomas of the stomach. *Cancer* **77**:1620–1627.

391. Kim, H. S., Woo, D. K., Bae, S. I., Kim, Y. I., and Kim, W. H. (2000) Microsatellite instability in the adenoma-carcinoma sequence of the stomach. *Lab. Invest.* **80**:57–64.

392. Suzuki, H., Itoh, F., Yoyota, M., Kikuchi, T., Kakiuchi, H., Hinoda, Y., et al. (1999) Distinct methylation pattern and microsatellite instability in sporadic gastric cancer. *Int. J. Cancer* **83**:309–313.

393. Chung, Y.-J., Song, J.-M., Lee, J.-Y., Jung, Y.-T., Seo, E.-J., Choi, S.-W., et al. (1996) Microsatellite instability-associated mutations associate preferentially with the intestinal type of primary gastric carcinomas in a high-risk population. *Cancer Res.* **56**:4662–4665.

394. Chong, J.-M., Fukayama, M., Hayashi, Y., Takizawa, T., Koike, M., Konishi, M., et al. (1994) Microsatellite instability in the progression of gastric carcinoma. *Cancer Res.* **54**:4595–4597.

395. Mironov, N. M., Aguelon, M. A.-M., Potapova, G. I., Omori, Y., Gorbunov, O. V., Klimenkov, A.A., et al. (1994) Alterations of (CA)ₙ DNA repeats and tumor suppressor genes in human gastric cancer. *Cancer Res.* **54**:41–44.

396. Tamura, G., Sakata, K., Maesawa, C., Suzuki, Y., Terashima, M., Satoh, K., et al. (1995) Microsatellite alterations in adenoma and differentiated adenocarcinoma of the stomach. *Cancer Res.* **55**:1933–1936.

397. Shinmura, K., Sugimura, H., Naito, Y., Shields, P. G., and Kino, I. (1995) Frequent co-occurrence of mutator phenotype in synchronous, independent multiple cancers of the stomach. *Carcinogenesis* **16**:2989–2993.

398. Shiao, Y.-H., Bovo, D., Guido, M., Capella, C., Cassaro, M., Busatto, G., et al. (1999) Microsatellite instability and/or loss of heterozygosity in young gastric cancer patients in Italy. *Int. J. Cancer* **82**:59–62.

399. Izumoto, S., Arita, N., Ohnishi, T., Hiraga, S., Taki, T., Tomita, N., et al. (1997) Microsatellite instability and mutated type II transforming growth factor-β receptor gene in gliomas. *Cancer Lett.* **112**:251–256.

400. Dams, E., Van de Kelft, E. J. Z., Martin, J.-J., Verlooy, J., and Willems, P. J. (1995) Instability of microsatellites in human gliomas. *Cancer Res.* **55**:1547–1549.

401. Kanamori, M., Kon, H., Nobukuni, T., Nomura, S., Sugano, K., Mashiyama, S., et al. (2000) Microsatellite instability and the PTEN1 gene mutation in a subset of early onset gliomas carrying germline mutation or promoter methylation of the hMLH1 gene. *Oncogene* **19**:1564–1571.

402. Amariglio, N., Friedman, E., Mor, O., Stiebel, H., Phelan, C., Collins, P., et al. (1995) Analysis of microsatellite repeats in pediatric brain tumors. *Cancer Genet. Cytogenet.* **84**:56–59.

403. El-Naggar, A.K., Hurr, K., Huff, V., Clayman, G. L., Luna, M. A., and Batsakis, J. G. (1996) Microsatellite instability in preinvasive and invasive head and neck squamous carcinoma. *Am. J. Pathol.* **148**:2067–2072.

404. Mark, Z., Toren, A., Amariglio, N., Schiby, G., Brok-Simoni, F., and Rechavi, G. (1998) Instability of dinucleotide repeats in Hodgkin's disease. *Am. J. Hematol.* **57**:148-152.

405. Ben-Yehuda, D., Krichevsky, S., Caspi, O., Rund, D., Polliack, A., Abeliovich, D., et al. (1996) Microsatellite instability and p53 mutations in therapy-related leukemia suggest mutator phenotype. *Blood* **88**:4296–4303.

406. Zhu, Y.-M., Das-Gupta, E. P., and Russell, N. H. (1999) Microsatellite instability and p53 mutations are associated with abnormal expression of the MSH2 gene in adult acute leukemia. *Blood* **94**:733–740.

407. Wada, C., Shionoya, S., Fujino, Y., Tokuhiro, H., Akahoshi, T., Uchida, T., et al. (1994) Genomic instability of microsatellite repeats and its association with the evolution of chronic myelogenous leukemia. *Blood* **83**:3449–3456.

408. Rimsza, L. M., Kopecky, K. J., Ruschulte, J., Chen, I. M., Slovak, M. L., Karanes, C., et al. (2000) Microsatellite instability is not a defining genetic feature of acute myeloid leukemogenesis in adults: results of a retrospective study of 132 patients and review of the literature. *Leukemia* **14**:1044–1051.

409. Volpe, G., Gamberi, B., Pastore, C., Roetto, A., Pautasso, M., Parvis, G., et al. (1996) Analysis of microsatellite instability in chronic lymphoproliferative disorders. *Ann. Hematol.* **72**:67–71.

410. MacDonald, G. A., Greenson, J. K., Saito, K., Cherian, S. P., Appelman, H. D., and Boland, C.R. (1998) Microsatellite instability and loss of heterozygosity at DNA mismatch repair gene loci occurs during hepatic carcinogenesis. *Hepatology* **28**:90–97.

411. Yamamoto, H., Itoh, F., Fukushima, H., Kaneto, H., Sasaki, S., Ohmura, T., et al. (2000) Infrequent widespread microsatellite instability in hepatocellular carcinomas. *Int. J. Oncol.* **16**:543–547.

412. Caligo, M. A., Ghimenti, C., Marchetti, A., Lonobile, A., Buttitta, F., Pellegrini, S., et al. (1998) Microsatellite alterations and p53, TGFβRII, IGFIIR and BAX mutations in sporadic non-small-cell lung cancer. *Int. J. Cancer* **78**:606–609.

413. Kim, W. S., Park, C., Hong, S. K., Park, B. K., Kim, H. S., and Park, K. (2000) Microsatellite instability (MSI) in non-small cell lung cancer (NSCLC) is highly associated with transforming growth factor-β type II receptor (TGF-βRII) frameshift mutation. *Anticancer Res.* **20**:1499–1502.

414. Miozzo, M., Sozzi, G., Musso, K., Pilotti, S., Incarbone, M., Pastorino, U., et al. (1996) Microsatellite alterations in bronchial and sputum specimens of lung cancer patients. *Cancer Res.* **56**:2285–2288.

415. Fong, K. M., Zimmerman, P. V., and Smith, P. J. (1995) Microsatellite instability and other molecular abnormalities in non-small cell lung cancer. *Cancer Res.* **55**:28–30.

416. Zhou, X., Kemp, B. L., Khuri, F. R., Liu, D., Lee, J. J., Wu, W., et al. (2000) Prognostic implication of microsatellite alteration profiles in early stage non-small cell lung cancer. *Clin. Cancer Res.* **6**:559–565.

417. Gotoh, K., Yatabe, Y., Sugiura, T., Takagi, K., Ogawa, M., Takahashi, T., et al. (1999) Frameshift mutations in TGFβRII, IGFIIR, BAX, hMSH3 and hMSH6 are absent in lung cancers. *Carcinogenesis* **20**:499–502.

418. Merlo, A., Mabry, M., Gabrielson, E., Vollmer, R., Baylin, S. B., and Sidransky, D. (1994) Frequent microsatellite instability in primary small cell lung cancer. *Cancer Res.* **54**:2098–2101.

419. Bedi, G. C., Westra, W. H., Farzadegan, H., Pitha, P. M., and Sidransky, D. (1995) Microsatellite instability in primary neoplasms from HIV+ patients. *Nature Med.* **1**:65–68.

420. Gamberi, B., Gaidano, G., Parsa, N., Carbone, A., Roncella, S., Knowles, D. M., et al. (1997) Microsatellite instability is rare in B-cell non-Hodgkin's lymphomas. *Blood* **89**:975–979.

421. Martinsson, T., Sjoberg, R.-M., Hedborg, F., and Kogner, P. (1995) Deletion of chromosome 1p loci and microsatellite instability in neuroblastomas analyzed with short-tandem repeat polymorphisms. *Cancer Res.* **55**:5681–5686.

422. Hogarty, M. D., White, P. S., Sulman, E. P., and Brodeur, G. M. (1998) Mononucleotide repeat instability is infrequent in neuroblastoma. *Cancer Genet. Cytogenet.* **106**:140–143.

423. Ishwad, C. S., Ferrell, R. E., Rossie, K. M., Appel, B. N., Johnson, J. T., Myers, E. N., et al. (1995) Microsatellite instability in oral cancer. *Int. J. Cancer* **64**:332–335.

424. Tangir, J., Loughridge, N. S., Berkowitz, R. S., Muto, M. G., Bell, D. A., Welch, W. R., et al. (1996) Frequent microsatellite instability in epithelial borderline ovarian tumors. *Cancer Res.* **56**:2501–2505.

425. Brentnall, T. A., Chen, R., Lee, J. G., Kimmey, M. B., Bronner, M. P., Haggitt, R. C., et al. (1995) Microsatellite instability and K-ras mutations associated with pancreatic adenocarcinoma and pancreatitis. *Cancer Res.* **55**:4264–4267.

426. Terrell, R. B., Wille, A. H., Cheville, J. C., Nystuen, A. M., Cohen, M. B., and Sheffield, V. C. (1995) Microsatellite instability in adenocarcinoma of the prostate. *Am. J. Pathol.* **147**:799–805.

427. Perinchery, G., Nojima, D., Goharderakhshan, R., Tanaka, Y., Alonzo, J., and Dahiya, R. (2000) Microsatellite instability of dinucleotide tandem repeat sequences is higher than trinucleotide, tetranucleotide and pentanucleotide repeat sequences in prostate cancer. *Int. J. Oncol.* **16**:1203–1209.

428. Entius, M. M., Keller, J. J., Drillenburg, P., Kuypers, K. C., Giardiello, F. M., and Offerhaus, G. J. A. (2000) Microsatellite instability and expression of hMLH-1 and hMSH-2 in sebaceous gland carcinomas as markers for Muir-Torre syndrome. *Clin. Cancer Res.* **6**:1784–1789.

429. Visser, M., Bras, J., Sijmons, C., Devilee, P., Wijnaendts, L. C. D., van der Liden, J. C., et al. (1996) Microsatellite instability in childhood rhabdomyosarcoma is locus specific and correlates with fractional allelic loss. *Proc. Natl. Acad. Sci. USA* **93**:9172–9176.

430. Murty, V. V. V. S., Li, R.-G., Mathew, S., Reuter, V. E., Bronson, D. L., Bosl, G. J., et al. (1994) Replication error-type genetic instability at 1q42-43 in human male germ cell tumors. *Cancer Res.* **54**:3983–3985.

431. Larson, A. A., Kern, S., Sommers, R. L., Yokota, J., Cavenee, W. K., and Hampton, G. M. (1996) Analysis of replication error (RER+) phenotypes in cervical carcinoma. *Cancer Res.* **56**:1426–1431.

432. Risinger, J. I., Umar, A., Boyer, J. C., Evans, A. C., Berchuck, A., Kunkel, T. A., et al. (1995) Microsatellite instability in gynecologic sarcomas and in hMSH2 mutant uterine sarcoma cell lines defective in mismatch repair activity. *Cancer Res.* **55**:5664–5669.

433. Ottini, L., Falchetti, M., D'Amico, C., Amorosi, A., Saieva, C., Masala, G., et al. (1998) Mutations at coding mononucleotide repeats in gastric cancer with microsatellite mutator phenotype. *Oncogene* **16**:2767–2772.

434. Togo, G., Toda, N., Kanai, F., Kato, N., Shiratori, Y., Kishi, K., et al. (1996) A transforming growth factor β type II receptor gene mutation common in sporadic cecum cancer with microsatellite instability. *Cancer Res.* **56**:5620–5623.

435. Souza, R. F., Lei, J., Yin, J., Appel, R., Zou, T.-T., Zhou, X., et al. (1997) A transforming growth factor β1 receptor type II mutation in ulcerative colitis-associated neoplasms. *Gastroenterology* **112**:40–45.

436. Lu, S.-L., Akiyama, Y., Nagasaki, H., Saitoh, K., and Yuasa, Y. (1995) Mutations of the transforming growth factor-β type II receptor gene and genomic instability in hereditary nonpolyposis colorectal cancer. *Biochem. Biophys. Res. Commun.* **216**:452–457.

437. Ohue, M., Tomita, N., Monden, T., Miyoshi, Y., Ohnishi, T., Izawa, H., et al. (1996) Mutations of the transforming growth factor β type II receptor gene and microsatellite instability in gastric cancer. *Int. J. Cancer* **68**:203–206.

7 Chromosomes and Chromosomal Instability in Human Cancer

TAKASHI SHIMAMOTO, MD AND KAZUMA OHYASHIKI, MD

INTRODUCTION

Many human cancers have chromosomal abnormalities, and frequently specific abnormalities are associated with specific forms of cancer. These findings have emerged gradually over the past 30 years as increasingly better techniques have become available for preparation and analysis of human chromosomes. Because of the ease with which leukemia cells can be obtained and analyzed, most studies of karyotypic abnormalities have been performed on hematopoietic malignancies. Initial studies simply characterized the gross chromosomal abnormalities occurring in different types of cancer cells. More recently, molecular rearrangements that are associated with many chromosomal abnormalities have been characterized in detail. These rearrangements frequently involve cellular proto-oncogenes or tumor-suppressor genes.

It has long been considered that chromosomal instability, an end-point of genomic instability, is an integral component of human cancer. The multiple phenotypes of genomic stability may induce a variety of karyotypic abnormalities, such as chromosomal translocations, inversions, deletions, or amplifications. Mechanisms leading to chromosomal instability have been suggested to involve faulty DNA repair processes, abnormal chromosome telomere maintenance, or aberrant cell-cycle control. Three DNA repair pathways that are essential for genomic homeostasis have been identified and characterized, including 1) nucleotide excision repair, 2) exonucleolytic proofreading by DNA polymerase, and 3) postreplicative mismatch correction. Lesions in each of these DNA repair processes have been observed in specific human cancers. The telomerase enzyme contributes to chromosomal homeostasis by maintenance of chromosome telomeres. In fact, it has been proposed that the immortalization of human cells requires an alteration of chromosome telomere homeostasis involving the reactivation of the telomerase enzyme after a period of telom-

ere shortening. In addition, when regulatory components of a cell-cycle checkpoint are mutated or otherwise inactivated, the probability of a cell sustaining genetic damage during one round of the cell-cycle increases. Therefore, dysfunctional cell-cycle checkpoint controls may contribute to genetic damage and genomic instability, thereby predisposing cells to neoplastic transformation and tumorigenesis.

This chapter describes the common chromosomal abnormalities in hematopoietic malignancies and solid tumors, and then discusses DNA repair defects associated with certain cancers, focusing on the potential roles of DNA excision repair, DNA polymerase enzymes, and mismatch-repair genes in chromosomal instability. We also discuss chromosomal telomeres, the telomerase enzyme, and cell-cycle checkpoints in neoplastic transformation and tumorigenesis.

OVERVIEW OF CHROMOSOMAL ABNORMALITIES IN HUMAN CANCER

Chromosomal abnormalities in human cancers can involve both the number, and more frequently, the structure of chromosomes (1,2). In general, these chromosomal changes fall into three categories (3). The first category is reciprocal translocation, which is an exchange of chromosomal materials between two chromosomes. This rearrangement can result in the abnormal expression of translocated genes as a consequence of their new location in the genome, or it can alter the structure of genes at the site of translocation. The second category involves nonreciprocal exchanges of chromosomal material. These exchanges can result in either deletion or addition of chromosome regions. Although such changes are frequently observed in tumors, the consequences of this type of chromosomal aberration are known in only a few instances (for example, deletions at 17p, 13q, or 11p are associated with loss of the tumor-suppressor genes *p53*, *pRb*, or *WT1*, respectively). The third category involves an increase in the amount of DNA in a specific region of a chromosome. The increased genetic material results in areas on chromosomes referred to as homogeneously staining regions (HSRs). HSRs are associated with extensive gene

From: *The Molecular Basis of Human Cancer* (W. B. Coleman and G. J. Tsongalis, eds.), © Humana Press Inc., Totowa, NJ.

Table 1
Chromosome Abnormalities in Myeloid Leukemias

Type	Affected gene	Disease
t(8;21)(q22;q22)	*AML1* (21q22) + *MTG8* (8q22)	AML(M2)
t(15;17)(q22;q11–21)	*PML* (15q22) + *RARα* (17q11–21)	APL
t(11;17)(q23;q21)	*PLZF* (11q23) + *RARα* (17q11–21)	APL
inv(16)(p13;q22)	*MYH11* (16p13) + *CBFβ* (16q22)	AML(M4Eo)
t(6;9)(p23;q34)	*DEK* (6p23) + *CAN* (9q34)	AML
t(7;11)(p15;p15)	*HOXA9* (7p15) + NUP98 (11p15)	AML
t(4;11)(q21;q23)	*MLL* (11q23) + AF4 (4q21)	ALL/AML
t(9;11)(p22;q23)	*MLL* (11q23) + AF9 (9p22)	ALL/AML
t(11;17)(q23;q21)	*MLL* (11q23) + AF17 (17q21)	AML
t(11;19)(q23;p13)	*MLL* (11q23) + *ENL* (19p13)	ALL/AML
t(9;22)(q34;q11)	ABL (9q34) + *BCR* (22q11)	CML
t(3;21)(q26;q22)	*EVI1* (3q26) + *AML1* (21q22)	CML/MDS
t(5;12)(q33;p13)	*PDGFβ* (5q33) + *TEL* (12p13)	CMML

Abbreviations: AML, acute myeloid leukemia; APL, acute promyelocytic leukemia; ALL, acute lymphoblastic leukemia; CML, chronic myelogenous leukemia; MDS, myelodysplastic syndrome.

amplifications *(4)*. Another form of gene amplification leads to chromosomal abnormalities called double minute chromosomes (DMs). DMs appear as two small dots of dark staining material in a standard metaphase preparation. It is generally believed that DMs represent the first stage in gene amplification and that HSRs result from the integration of DMs into the chromosome (4). Recently, Tanaka et al. *(5)* reported a previously undiscovered cytogenetic mechanism for gene amplification apart from HSRs or DMs. These investigators employed fluorescence *in situ* hybridization (FISH), and found that complex chromosome aberrations with the *ABL* proto-oncogene were partially duplicated in some secondary leukemias. These chromosomal segments translocated onto structurally abnormal chromosomes. This type of translocation has been termed segmental jumping translocation.

Chromosomal abnormalities are designated according to the International System for Human Cytogenetic Nomenclature *(6)*. To describe the karyotype or chromosomal complement of a cell type or tumor, the total chromosome number is listed first, followed by the sex chromosomes, and then a complete list of any chromosomal abnormalities.

CHROMOSOMAL ABNORMALITIES IN MYELOID LEUKEMIAS

CHRONIC MYLOGENOUS LEUKEMIA The first specific chromosome abnormality to be associated with cancer was the Philadelphia chromosome in chronic mylogenous leukemia (CML). The actual cytogenetic defect is a reciprocal translocation between chromosomes 9 and 22 [t(9;22)(q34;q11)] *(7)*. This chromosomal abnormality is present in the leukemic cells of at least 90% of patients with CML. The abnormality is also seen in some patients with acute myeloid leukemia (AML) and acute lymphoid leukemia (ALL) *(8)*. The Philadelphia chromosome occurs in a pluripotential stem cell that gives rise to cells of both lymphoid and myeloid lineages. The genetic consequence of the Philadelphia chromosome is the translocation of the *ABL* proto-oncogene on chromosome 9

to a location on chromosome 22, termed the breakpoint cluster region (or *BCR* locus) (Table 1). Almost all CML patients with a Philadelphia chromosome show this rearrangement, indicating that the translocation involves a limited region on chromosome 22. The most commonly involved segment of chromosome 22 is referred to as the major-*BCR* (M-*BCR*) *(9)*. This fusion creates a 210 kDa protein that possesses high levels of tyrosine kinase activity and is phosphorylated on tyrosine residues *(10)*. In approximately half of the Philadelphia chromosome-positive acute leukemias, molecular analysis has revealed that the translocation does not involve the M-*bcr* region, but involves another segment of chromosome 22 termed the minor-*BCR* (m-*BCR*). The resulting fusion protein has a molecular mass of 190 kDa *(11)*. Recently, a new breakpoint cluster region, referred to as the micro-*BCR* (or μ-*BCR*), has been identified in CML *(12)*. This reciprocal translocation results in a BCR/ABL fusion protein of 230 kDa. CML resulting from p230 BCR/ABL is rare, and it has been associated with the chronic neutrophil leukemia (CNL) variant or with thrombocytosis or both *(12)*.

Most patients with CML entering the blast phase show additional chromosomal abnormalities, most commonly involving the acquisition of an addition chromosome 8, loss of chromosome 7, gain of a second Philadelphia chromosome, or isochromatin for the long arm of chromosome 17, designated i(17q). The i(17q) is related to myeloid blast crisis; no other chromosomal changes are correlated with the phenotype of the blast crisis *(8)*.

ACUTE MYELOID LEUKEMIA With improved techniques for cell culture and chromosome banding, at least 80% of patients with AML have been shown to have gross chromosomal abnormalities *(8)*. Many of the abnormalities that have been described are characteristic of a specific type of leukemia, and some have prognostic significance (Table 1).

In almost all patients with acute promyelocytic leukemia (APL), the leukemic cells have a translocation involving chromosomes 15 and 17, described as t(15;17)(q21;q11–21). This translocation represents a unique abnormality that has not been observed in other type of AMLs, and involves the gene for the retinoic acid α receptor (*RARα*) on chromosome 17. The translocation breakpoint consistently occurs within the *RARα* gene and within a gene designated *PML* on chromosome 15, and this translocation creates the PML/RARα fusion protein *(13,14)*. The fusion protein interferes with normal myeloid cell differentiation, possibly through dominant negative effects against the transcriptional activity of RARα. These observations provide the rationale for the use of all-*trans* retinoic acid to treat patients with APL.

A translocation involving chromosomes 8 and 21, described as t(8;21)(q22;q22), represents the most frequent chromosome abnormality in the myeloid leukemias and is most often found in myeloblasts with evidence of granulocytic differentiation (M2 designation according to the FAB classification). It has been shown that t(8;21) breakpoints on chromosome 21 cluster within a single specific intron of the *AML1* gene. This gene is highly homologous to the *Drosophila* segmentation gene *runt*, which encodes a nuclear protein and regulates the expression of other pair-rule genes. The translocation juxtaposes the *AML1* gene with the *MTG8* on chromosome 8, resulting in the synthesis of an *AML1*/MTG8 fusion transcript *(15)*. The *MTG8* gene is not expressed in normal hematopoietic cells, whereas aml1 is expressed. The chimeric *AML1*/MTG8 transcription factor may contribute to myeloid leukemogenesis through the dominant negative effect on *AML1*.

Inversion of chromosome 16 is a characteristic karyotypic abnormality associated with acute myelomonocytic leukemia and increased bone marrow eosinophils (M4Eo designation according to the FAB classification). This inversion joins the amino-terminal sequences of the *CBFβ* gene to the carboxy-terminus of the smooth muscle myosin heavy-chain (SMMHC) gene (*MYH11*), resulting in the formation of a *CBFβ/MYH11* fusion gene *(16)*. *CBFβ* is known as a subunit of a heterodimeric transcription factor formed with *CBFα*. The repeated coiled-coil of SMMHC may result in dimerization of the CBFβ fusion protein, which would lead to alterations in transcriptional regulation and contribute to leukemic transformation.

The t(6;9)(p23;q34) is associated with a specific subtype of AML. This leukemia is characterized by a poor prognosis, affects young adults, and is classified mostly as M2 or M4 (according to the FAB classification). The breakpoints on chromosome 6 and 9 are situated in the genes named *DEK* and *CAN*, respectively, and this translocation results in the *DEK/CAN* fusion gene. The *DEK/CAN* chimeric protein localizes to cell nuclei, suggesting that the abnormal transcription factor may lead to aberrations in the transcription of various target genes and contribute to leukemogenesis *(17)*.

Recurring cytogenetic abnormalities that involve chromosome band 3q26 including t(3;3), inv(3), or t(3;21), are found in AML or CML blast crisis with the high frequency of platelets and increased number of megakaryocytes in bone marrow findings. The *EVI1* gene is located on chromosome 3q26 and encodes a zinc finger-containing transcription factor. Although normal *EVI1* transcripts are not expressed in normal hematopoietic cells, ectopic expression of *EVI1* is found in leukemic cells with the 3q26 anomaly, suggesting that the abnormal ex-

pression of *EVI1* protein in human hematopoietic cells could contribute to the development of leukemia *(18)*. The *AML1/EVI1* fusion gene has been cloned, characterized, and localized to the t(3;21) translocation *(19)*. It has been clearly demonstrated that this fusion protein has the ability to block differentiation of myeloid cells, and this ability could be due to the dominant-negative effect of the fusion protein over the *AML1* transactivation, which could be important for hematopoietic cell differentiation *(20)*.

Chromosome 11q23 is a frequent site for cytogenetic alterations in a variety of hematopoietic malignancies. Rearrangements of 11q23, including t(4;11)(q21;q23), t(9;11)(p22;q23), t(6;11)(q27;q23), or t(11;19)(q23;p13), are generally observed in pediatric ALL and leukemias with mixed lymphoid-myeloid features. The gene involved in recurring 11q23 translocations codes for *MLL* gene (also called *HRX*, *ALL-1*, and *HTRX*). This gene is a homolog of the *Drosophila trithorax* gene and is involved in homeotic gene regulation *(21,22)*. The *MLL* protein contains two types of DNA-binding motifs consisting of zinc fingers and adenine-thymine AT hook motifs, and 11q23 translocation disrupts the *MLL* gene between these two motifs.

CHROMOSOMAL ABNORMALITIES IN LYMPHOID MALIGNANCIES

ACUTE LYMPHOID LEUKEMIA The correlation of cytogenetic changes with morphology in AML lead to the identification and characterization of specific disease-associated chromosomal abnormalities. However, the correlations established for AML were not useful in ALL (Table 2), with the exception of the t(8;14)(q24;q32) and its variants in B-cell ALL or Burkitt's lymphoma (BL) (L3 designation according to the FAB classification). In BL, translocations invariably involve chromosome 8 and one of the three chromosomes that carry the immunoglobulin light- or heavy-chain genes: chromosome 14 (heavy-chain genes), chromosome 2 (λ light-chain genes), or chromosome 22 (κ light-chain genes). These translocations rearrange one allele of c-*MYC* proto-oncogene on chromosome 8q24, which encodes a transcription factor consisting of a basic region helix-loop-helix-zipper (bHLH) motif, into the immunoglobulin locus carried on one of these chromosomes, resulting in dysregulation of c-*MYC* expression through the strong enhancer of immunoglobulin genes *(23,24)*.

The t(1;19)(q23;p13) chromosome translocation affects approx 25% of pre-B ALLs, and fuses the N-terminal part of the transcription factor E2A, carrying a transcription domain, to the DNA-binding homeodomain of the transcription factor PBX, replacing the bHLH region of E2A *(25,26)*. The E2A/PBX fusion protein is recognized by the homeodomain of PBX, and can strongly activate transcription, whereas PBX cannot. Target genes that bind the PBX homeodomain in the E2A/PBX fusion protein may be activated and initiate leukemogenesis.

T-cell leukemias (T-ALL) have a number of different recurring translocations. Most of these involve putative transcription factors, and are not normally expressed in T cells. An example of this is the *HOX11* gene, located on chromosome 10q24, which is activated by translocations t(10;14)(q24;q11) and t(7;10)(q35;q24) in T-ALL *(27)*. The *HOX11* gene shares homology with other homeobox-containing genes that nor-

Table 2
Chromosome Abnormalities in Lymphoid Malignancies

Type	Affected gene(s)	Disease
t(1;19)(q23;p13)	PBX1 (1q23) + E2A (19p13)	pre-B-ALL
t(17;19)(q22;p13)	HLF (17q22) + E2A (19p13)	pro-B-ALL
t(8;14)(q24;q32)	c-MYC (8q24) + IgH (14q32)	B-ALL(L3)/NHL(Burkitt's)
t(2;8)(p12;q24)	c-MYC (8q24) + Igα (2p12)	B-ALL(L3)/NHL(Burkitt's)
t(8;22)(q24;q11)	c-MYC (8q24) + Igλ (22q11)	B-ALL(L3)/NHL(Burkitt's)
t(5;14)(q31;q32)	IL3 (5q31) + IgH (14q32)	pre-B-ALL
t(12;21)(p13;q22)	TEL (12P13) + AML1 (21q22)	pre-B-ALL
t(11;14)(q13;q32)	BCL1 (11q13) + IgH (14q32)	B-CLL
t(14;19)(q32;q13.1)	BCL3 (19q13.1) + IgH (14q32)	B-CLL
t(14;18)(q32;q21)	BCL2 (18q21) + IgH (14q32)	B-NHL(FL)
t(3;14)(q27;q32)	BCL6 (3q27) + IgH (14q32)	B-NHL
t(10;14)(q24;q32)	LYT-10 (10q24) + IgH (14q32)	B-NHL
t(8;14)(q24;q11)	c-MYC (8q24) + TCRα (14q11)	T-ALL
t(1;7)(p34;q34)	LCK (1p34) + TCRβ (21q22)	T-ALL
t(7;9)(q34;q34)	TAL2 (9q34) + TCRβ (21q22)	T-ALL
t(1;14)(p32;q11)	TAL1 (1p32) + TCRα (14q11)	T-ALL
t(10;14)(q24;q11)	HOX11 (10q24) + TCRα (14q11)	T-ALL
t(7;10)(q35;q24)	HOX11 (10q24) + TCRβ (21q22)	T-ALL
t(9;12)(p24;p13)	JAK2 (9p24) + TEL (12p13)	T-ALL/pre-B-ALL
t(4;16)(q26;p13)	IL2 (4q26) + BCM (16p13)	T-NHL
t(2;5)(p23;q35)	NPM (5q35) + ALK (2p23)	T-NHL(ALCL)

Abbreviations: NHL, non-Hodgkin's lymphoma; FL, follicular lymphoma; ALCL, anaplastic large cell lymphoma.

mally code for sequence-specific DNA-binding proteins. When abnormally expressed, *HOX11* may contribute to T-cell leukemogenesis.

The t(1;14)(p32;q11) chromosome translocation has been observed in 3% of T-ALL patients. This translocation results in the juxtaposition of the *SCL* gene (also called *TAL1*) from chromosome 1p32 with the *TCRα/δ* chain locus on chromosome 14q11 *(28)*. The *SCL* gene encodes DNA-binding protein containing bHLH motif, which can dimerize with protein E47. The chromosomal translocation probably causes ectopic SCL protein expression, activating specific target genes that are normally transcriptionally silent in T cells.

MALIGNANT LYMPHOMA B-cell malignant lymphomas have translocations involving chromosome 14q32, which contains the immunoglobulin heavy chain gene. Two specific translocations involving this locus have been characterized. The chromosomal rearrangements occur at precise locations on chromosomes 11 and 18 at the *BCL1* and *BCL2* loci, respectively. The *bcl1* gene, which is aberrantly expressed as a consequence of the t(11;14)(q13;q32) translocation, encodes cyclin D1 *(29)*. Cyclin D1 forms a complex with a cyclin-dependent kinase (cdk), and functions in cell-cycle regulation. The *BCL2* gene is consistently associated with t(14;18) chromosomal translocation observed in a large percentage of human B-cell follicular lymphomas *(30)*. The *BCL2* gene product is suggested to mediate inhibition of cellular apoptosis. Thus, constitutive activation of the *BCL2* gene may contribute to the formation of follicular lymphomas by blocking programmed cell death *(31,32)*.

Anaplastic large-cell lymphoma (ALCL) is a variant of non-Hodgkin's lymphomas composed of large pleomorphic cells

that usually express the CD30 antigen and is characterized by frequent cutaneous and extranodal involvement. This type of lymphomas frequently exhibits the t(2;5)(p23;q35) chromosomal translocation that fuses the *NPM* gene (for *nucleophosmin*) on chromosome 5q35 to a novel protein kinase gene, *ALK* (for anaplastic lymphoma kinase), on chromosome 2p23 *(33)*. The *ALK/NPM* fusion protein has tyrosine kinase activity, and tumorigenesis may be induced by this fusion protein.

CHRONIC LYMPHOID LEUKEMIA The t(14;19)(q32;q13.1) chromosome translocation is found in some cases of human B-cell chronic lymphocytic leukemia (B-CLL). The translocation results in divergent orientation (head-to-head) of the immunoglobulin heavy-chain gene on chromosome 14 and *bcl3* gene on chromosome 19 *(34)*. The *BCL3* gene is a distinct member of the IκB family, may function as a positive regulator to nucleon factor-κB (NF-κB) activity. Thus, overexpression of *BCL3* gene by the translocation may alter the transcriptional activity of NF-κB.

CHROMOSOMAL ABNORMALITIES IN SOLID TUMORS

EWING'S SARCOMA Sarcomas include soft tissue tumors that often have characteristic translocations (Table 3). Ewing's sarcoma is a tumor of childhood and early adult life. This type of sarcoma exhibits a remarkably consistent reciprocal chromosome translocation, described as t(11;22)(q24;q12) *(35)*. Cloning of the breakpoints of the t(11;22)(q24;q12) has demonstrated that this rearrangement generates two fusion genes involving the *ews* gene, localized in band 22q12, and a member of the *ets* gene family, the *FLI1* gene, localized in band 11q24 *(36,37)*. The normal EWS protein has three glycine-rich seg-

Table 3
Chromosome Abnormalities in Solid Tumors

Type	Affected gene	Disease
t(11;22)(q24;q12)	FLI1 (1q23) + EWS (22p12)	Ewing's sarcoma/PNET
t(21;22)(q22;q12)	ERG (21q22) + EWS (22p12)	Ewing's sarcoma/PNET
t(7;22)(p22;q12)	ETV1 (7p22) + EWS (22p12)	Ewing's sarcoma/PNET
t(12;22)(q13;q12)	ATF1 (12q13) + EWS (22p12)	Clear cell sarcoma (MMSP)
t(11;22)(p13;q12)	WT1 (11p13) + EWS (22p12)	DSRCT
t(12;16)(q13;p11)	CHOP (12q13) + TLS (16p11)	Myxoid liposarcoma
t(2;13)(q35;q14)	PAX3 (2q35) + FKHR (13q14)	Alveolar rhabdomyosarcoma
t(1;13)(p36;q14)	PAX7 (1p36) + FKHR (13q14)	Alveolar rhabdomyosarcoma
t(6;14)(q21;q24)	unknown	Ovarian carcinoma
-22	NF2 (22q12)	Meningioma
del 13q	Rb1 (13q14)	Retinoblastoma
del 11p	WT1 (11p13)	Wilms' tumor
del 5q	APC (5q21-22)	Colon carcinoma

Abbreviations: PNET, peripheral neuroectodermal tumor; MMSP, malignant melanoma of soft parts; DSRCT, desmoplastic small round cell tumor.

ments and an RNA-binding domain *(38)*. The *EWS/FLI1* fusion protein is consistent with the N-terminal domain of EWS and the DNA binding domain of *FLI1*. The evidence suggest that the DNA-binding activity and transcriptional activation of various target genes by the *EWS/FLI1* fusion protein are essential for tumorigenesis leading to Ewing's sarcoma *(39)*.

In Ewing's sarcoma and peripheral neuroepithelioma (termed ES/PNE), a masked t(21;22)(q22;q12) is present instead of the t(11;22). It involves *EWS* and another *ETS* family gene highly homologous to *FLI1*, but located at 21q22, designated *ERG (40)*. The functional consequences of this rearrangement are thought to be analogous to the *EWS/FLI1* fusion, and there is also a similar spectrum of molecular variants.

CLEAR CELL SARCOMA The *EWS* gene also plays a role in other tumors, including clear cell sarcoma (CCS), which typically displays the t(12;22)(q13;q12) translocation *(41)*. CCS is a deep-seated tumor typically arising in young adults. The tumor produces melanin, which supports a neural-crest origin and accounts for its other name, malignant melanoma. The molecular study of the breakpoints of the t(12;22) have demonstrated that the *EWS* gene on chromosome 22 fuses to the *ATF-1* gene on chromosome 12, which encodes a leucine-zipper domain and a basic DNA-binding domain *(42)*. A fusion transcript is thereby produced in which the RNA-binding domain of the ews protein is replaced by the leucine-zipper and DNA-binding domain of the *ATF-1* protein. Thus, the DNA-binding and dimerization capacities of *ATF-1* in the fusion protein probably lead to activation of *ATF-1* targets in this type of sarcoma.

DESMOPLASTIC SMALL ROUND CELL TUMOR The desmoplastic small round cell tumor (DSRCT) is a recognized type of sarcoma characterized by an aggressive clinical course, widespread abdominal involvement, and a peculiar histologic appearance with prominent desmoplasia *(43)*. Cytogenetic analysis revealed a recurring chromosomal translocation in this tumor, described as t(11;22)(p13;q12) *(44)*. This translocation involves the *EWS* gene at 22p12 and the Wilms' tumor gene

(*WT1*) at 11p13. The resulting fusion gene encodes a putative protein in which the RNA-binding domain of the EWS protein is replaced by the three C-terminal zinc fingers of the *WT1* DNA-binding domain *(45)*. *WT1* is an important tumor-suppressor gene when its expression is homozygously inactivated in Wilms' tumor, emphasizing the versatility of transcription factor involvement in embryonal tumors affecting different cell lineages.

MYXOID LIPOSARCOMA Myxoid liposarcomas typically occur in the thigh or retroperitoneum of an adult, and contain the translocation t(12;16)(q13;p11) in at least 75% of cases *(46)*. This translocation results in a fusion of the chop gene in 12q13 and the *FUS* (also designated *TLS*) gene in 16p11 *(47,48)*. The *CHOP* gene encodes a member of the CCAAT/ enhancer binding family, which has a leucine zipper-type dimerization motif and a putative DNA-binding domain. The *CHOP* gene product is suggested to function in a dominant negative manner by dimerizing, binding, and inhibiting other transcription-factor complexes. The *FUS* gene is homologous to the *EWS* gene; the fus gene product contains a glutamine-serine-tyrosine-rich segment, three glycine-rich stretches, and a RNA binding domain. The *FUS* protein domain in the fusion protein provides a transcriptional activation domain related to possible DNA-binding activity of chop, analogous to the *ews* gene fusions.

ALVEOLAR RHABDOMYOSARCOMA About 90% of alveolar rhabdomyosarcoma display the translocation t(2;13)(q35;q14) as a hallmark cytogenetic abnormality *(46)*. This translocation involves the *PAX3* paired box gene on chromosome 2 and the *FKHR*, a member of the forkhead DNA-binding domain family, on chromosome 13 *(49,50)*. The fusion transcript encodes a putative chimeric transcription factor, consisting of the paired box and homeodomain DNA-binding regions of the PAX3 protein joined to the forkhead DNA-binding domain of the *FKHR* protein.

A variant of the t(2;13) translocation, described as t(1;13)(p36;q14), has been shown to involve the same gene at

13q14 (*FKHR*), and another member of the *PAX* gene family, *PAX7* at 1p36 *(51)*. The translocation involving *PAX7* has a similar effect on *PAX3*, suggesting that the two genes are involved in the pathogenesis of rhabdomyosarcoma.

OTHER SOLID TUMORS Ovarian tumors frequently contain the recurring translocation t(6;14)(q21;q24) *(3)*. The significance of this translocation, which has been found in other tumors, is unclear. Almost all meningiomas exhibit hemizygousity for chromosome 22. Loss of chromosome 22 loci, and specifically inactivation of the *NF2* tumor-suppressor gene at 22q12, is considered one of several critical steps in the tumorigenesis of meningioma *(52)*. Almost all forms of retinoblastoma involve abnormalities in chromosome 13q14, and in some cases these involve a deletion 13q14 that can be demonstrated karyotypically. The molecular consequence of the deletion of this chromosomal segment is loss of the *Rb1* tumor-suppressor gene. Recently, deletions in 13q14 have been shown to be involved in the development of other forms of cancer as well *(53)*. Wilms' tumor is a kidney tumor of childhood, showing deletion or mutation of the short arm of chromosome 11. The *WT1* tumor-suppressor gene, located at 11p13, is known to be inactivated in these tumors *(54)*. Inactivation of tumor-suppressor gene *APC* at 5q21-22 represents a critical step in colorectal tumorigenesis *(55)*. In addition to translocations and deletions, tumor cells often show increases in chromosomal materials, namely DMs or HSRs. Human neuroblastomas were the first tumors shown to harbor DMs and HSRs, and in these tumors the gene amplification is likely to involve the *N-MYC* gene *(56)*. Amplification of *N-MYC* is usually seen in advanced tumors (stage III and IV). Some small-cell carcinomas also contain amplified *L-MYC* genes in DMs and HSRs *(57)*. These amplifications are found in the late stages of small-cell carcinoma-tumor progression. Additional evidence of gene amplifications have been described, involving *EGFR*, *c-ERBB2*, or *BCL1* genes in various solid tumors.

OVERVIEW OF DNA-REPAIR AND -REPLICATION PROCESSES

Maintaining genetic stability requires not only an extremely accurate mechanism for replicating the DNA before a cell divides, but also mechanisms for repairing the many accidental lesions that occur in DNA. Most spontaneous changes in DNA are temporary because they are immediately corrected by the various cellular DNA repair processes. There are a variety of repair and replication mechanisms, each catalyzed by a different set of enzymes. DNA repair (including replication-coupled repair mechanisms) involves at least four processes: 1) The altered portion of a damaged DNA strand is recognized and removed by enzymes called DNA-repair nucleases; 2) DNA polymerase binds to the 3'-OH end of the cut DNA strand and fills in the gap by making a complementary copy of the information stored in the residual template strand; 3) During DNA replication, proofreading occurs through the 3'→5' exonuclease activity of the DNA polymerase enzyme; 4) Postreplication or mismatch repair (MMR), removes any replication errors that were missed by the proofreading exonuclease and remain in the newly synthesized DNA. Inactivation of any of these DNA-repair processes can result in a large increase in spontaneous

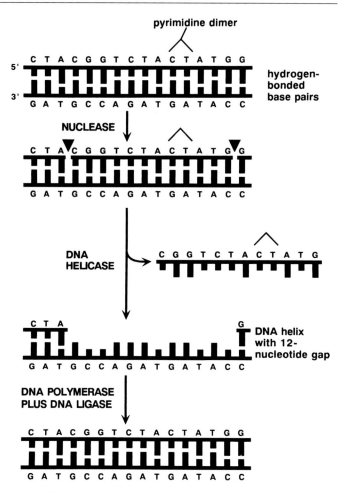

Fig. 1. DNA repair processes that may occur in mammalian cells. Base damage can be recognized by an endonuclease that cuts on either side of the lesion containing 25–30 nucleotides. DNA helicase separates the DNA double strands, and removes damaged nucleotides. DNA polymerase synthesizes new DNA and ligase seals the remaining nick.

mutability, and in the case of humans, predisposition to cancer development.

NUCLEOTIDE EXCISION REPAIR AND CANCER

MECHANISM OF DNA EXCISION REPAIR There are two main mechanisms for excision of DNA damage. These mechanisms are base excision repair (BER) and nucleotide excision repair (NER) *(58)*. In general terms, BER removes an abnormal base from the DNA strand. Release of the damaged base from the DNA is catalyzed by the class of enzymes called DNA glycosylases. Each glycosylase is specific for a particular type or class of DNA lesion. The resulting apurinic or apyrimidinic site is cleaved by an AP endonuclease, DNA polymerase fills the gap, and DNA ligase seals the remaining nick.

Another mode for damaged DNA excision is NER (Figure 1), which involves the removal of the section of DNA containing the lesion, followed by repair synthesis using the remaining intact DNA strand as a template for restoring the gap *(58,59)*. Once a bulky DNA lesion is found, the phosphodiester back-

Table 4
The Polypeptides Required for Excision Repair in Humans

XP protein	ERCC protein	Yeast homolog	Activity	Comments
XPA	—	RAD14	DNA binding	binds damaged DNA
XPB	ERCC3	RAD25	helicase	3' to 5' DNA helicase in TFIIH
XPC	—	RAD4	DNA binding	binds ssDNA
XPD	ERCC2	RAD3	helicase	5' to 3' DNA helicase in TFIIH
XPE		—		binds damaged DNA?
XPF	ERCC4	RAD1	nuclease incision	complex with ERCC1, 5'-
XPG	ERCC5	RAD2	nuclease	3'-incision
—	ERCC1	RAD10	nuclease incision	complex with ERCC4, 3'-

Abbreviations: XP, xeroderma pigmentosum; ERCC, excision repair cross-complementing rodent repair deficiency.

bone of the abnormal strand is cleaved on both sides of the distortion, and the portion of the strand containing the lesion is peeled away from the DNA double helix by a DNA helicase enzyme. The gap produced in the DNA helix is then repaired in the usual manner by DNA polymerase and DNA ligase. The importance of these repair processes is indicated by the large investment that cells make in DNA-repair enzymes. Individuals with the genetic disease xeroderma pigmentosum (XP), for example, are defective in a NER process that can be shown by genetic analysis to require at least seven different gene products (59).

PROTEINS INVOLVED IN NER Most proteins involved in NER have been discovered through analysis of XP (60). These proteins are summarized in Table 4. The damage recognition step involves the DNA-binding proteins XPA and XPE (61,62). Mammalian XPA and XPE proteins show a preference for binding damaged over undamaged DNA. Differential recognition by XPA may be an important factor in determining faster repair. The next step of NER involves the introduction of two incisions into the damaged DNA strand, one on each side of the DNA lesion. The size of the repair patch formed during NER is about 25–30 nucleotides long. Two different nucleases are used to create the dual incisions. In mammalian cells, these are the XPG/ERCC5 protein, which makes the 3'-incision (63), and the complex consisting of XPF/ERCC4 and ERCC1, which makes the 5'-incision (64). The portion of the strand containing the lesion is peeled away from the DNA double helix by a DNA helicase enzyme. These processes combine to remove the damaged segment of DNA, leaving a single-stranded gap in the DNA at the site of the lesion. This gap is subsequently filled through the action of DNA polymerase enzymes.

The multiprotein complex TFIIH participates in both basal transcription and in NER. TFIIH is normally found in the initiation complex at promoters transcribed by RNA polymerase II. Known NER proteins are components of TFIIH (65,66). Human TFIIH contains the XPB (ERCC3) and XPD (ERCC2) proteins. XPB and XPD contain seven conserved helicase domains, and they have 3'→5' and 5'→3' DNA helicase activities, respectively. TFIIH also contains a kinase, composed of cdk7 and cyclin H. TFIIH may regulate transcription initiation by

phosphorylating DNA polymerase II. Recently, Leveillard et al. reported that the p53 tumor-suppressor protein interacts both physically and functionally with the TFIIH complex (67). This interaction might provide an immediate and direct link between p53 and the multiple functions of TFIIH in transcription, DNA repair and possibly the cell cycle.

MUTATIONS OF NER AND CANCER FAMILY SYNDROMES Defective excision repair in humans is associated with some autosomal recessive diseases that strongly predispose to malignant disease (68). XP is caused by an absence or greatly reduced level of excision repair. The disease is hereditary with autosomal recessive inheritance. The clinical manifestations of XP result from DNA damage from exposure to ultraviolet (UV) light that cannot be corrected due to the defective NER in these patients. Cell-fusion studies have identified seven XP complementation groups, XPA through XPG, suggesting that many distinct gene products are involved in NER (69).

Bloom's syndrome (BS) is a rare disorder with autosomal recessive inheritance, and major clinical manifestations are growth deficiency, unusual facies, and sun-sensitive facial erythema (70). Increased sister chromatid exchanges (SCE) and chromosomal instability are typical in vitro findings demonstrable in lymphocyte and fibroblast cultures from BS patients (71). These patients also have an increased susceptibility to cancer (72). The tumor spectrum exhibited by BS patients include various rare tumor types, acute leukemias, and acute lymphomas, when tumor onset occurs during the first two decades of life; whereas various carcinomas predominate when tumor onset occurs after the second decade. The first step in positional cloning effort to isolate the BS gene (*BLM*) was to identify genetic linkages between the *BLM* locus and mapped polymorphic markers (73). BLM protein is a member of a growing subfamily of helicases, including *recQ* in *Escherichia coli*, *RECQL* in humans, *SGS1* in yeast, and the gene product encoded by the Werner syndrome (WS) gene *WRN*. *RecQ* genes are suppressors of illegitimate recombination in *E. coli* and would lead to DNA instability in humans. Gene products of *SGS1* and *WRN* are especially similar to *BLM*, and contain the seven conserved helicase motifs (74). These proteins are likely

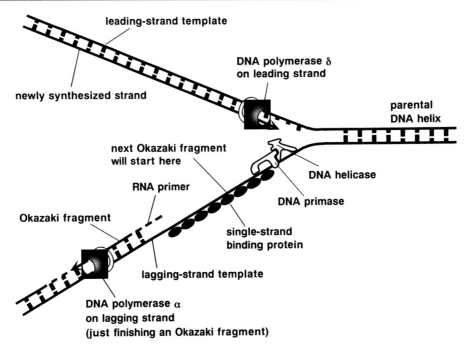

Fig. 2. A mammalian replication fork during DNA replication. The major types of proteins that act at a DNA replication fork are illustrated, showing their positions on the DNA. The replication fork makes use of two DNA polymerase enzymes, one for the leading strand, and one for the lagging strand. The leading-strand polymerase is designed to keep a tight hold on the DNA, whereas that on the lagging-strand must be able to release the template and then rebind each time a new Okazaki fragment is synthesized.

Table 5
Properties of DNA polymerase in eukaryotic cells

Type	Distribution	3' to 5' activity	Function
α	Nuclei	-	Synthesis of Okazaki fragment in lagging strand
ß	Nuclei	-	Base excision repair
γ	Mitochondria	+	Replication of mitochondrial DNA repair Proofreading activity
δ	Nuclei	+	Synthesis of reading strand Joining of Okazaki fragment Proofreading activity
ε	Nuclei	+	Replication? Proofreading?

Exonuclease appears as a label above the Type column.

to play similar roles in DNA metabolism. Because helicase activity is important for the DNA excision-repair process, cancer susceptibility in BS patients may result from abnormality of the DNA-repair system.

REPLICATION ERROR AND CANCER

PROOFREADING AND MMR An overview of DNA replication is illustrated in Fig. 2. Human cells require a high-fidelity DNA-replication and -repair mechanisms to ensure the integrity of the approx 3×10^9 base pairs of DNA contained in the genome. The fidelity of DNA replication is extremely high, with about 1 error made for every 1×10^9 base pairs of DNA replicated. This level of fidelity is much higher than might be expected, given that the standard complementary base pairing (AT and GC) observed in mammalian DNAs are not the only

ones possible. The high fidelity of DNA replication depends on several proofreading and MMR mechanisms that act sequentially to remove errors *(75)*.

One proofreading process depends on special properties of the DNA polymerase enzyme *(76,77)*. Several DNA polymerase enzymes are known in mammalian cells (Table 5). DNA polymerase enzymes are able to correct mismatched nucleotides by means of a separate catalytic subunit that removes unpaired residues at the primer terminus. Excision by this 3'→5' proofreading exonuclease activity continues until enough nucleotides have been removed from the 3'-end to regenerate a base-paired terminus that can prime DNA synthesis. In this way, DNA polymerase functions as a self-correcting enzyme that removes its own polymerization errors as it moves along the DNA.

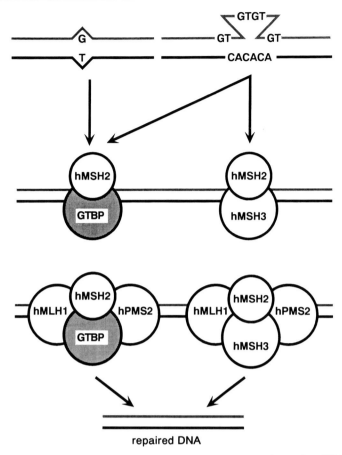

Fig. 3. Model for mismatch repair system in mammalian cells. The heterodimer, consisting of hMSH2 and hMSH6, can recognize a one-base mismatch or one-nucleotide loop. On the other hand, the heterodimer consisting of hMSH2 and hMSH3 can recognize dinucleotide loop or more.

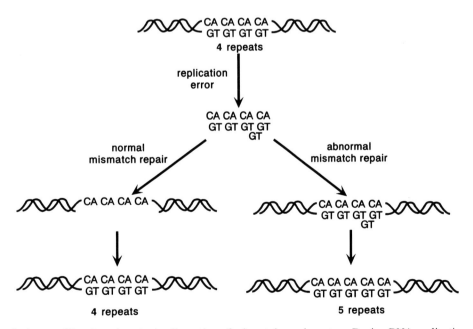

Fig. 4. The principle of microsatellite alterations in the disruption of mismatch repair system. During DNA replication, slippage occurs and CA repeats could be altered and not be removed, if the repair system is damaged.

Another mechanism that removes replication errors missed by the proofreading exonuclease is the MMR system (Fig. 3). In *E. coli*, two MMR genes are well known, namely *MutS* and *MutL*. Interaction of the MutS and MutL proteins with the heteroduplex activates a latent endonuclease associated with MutH protein, which cleaves the unmethylated strand at a d(GATC) site. Although little is known about the reaction responsible for unbiased correction of continuous heteroduplexes, nick-directed MMR in humans has been extensively examined. This type of repair depends on the gene products of *MLH1*, *MSH2*, *MSH3*, *MSH6* (or *GTBP*), *PMS1*, and *PMS2*, implicating these human homolog of *MutS* and *MutL* in the reaction *(78)*. Available evidence suggests that mismatch recognition in human cells is mediated by the MSH2-MSH6 protein heterodimer (designated hMutSα), with the MLH1-PMS2 protein heterodimer (hMutLα) providing MutL function.

MICROSATELLITE INSTABILITY IN HUMAN CANCER
The human genome is punctuated with repetitive nucleotide sequences or microsatellites. These repetitive dinucleotide, trinucleotide, and tetranucleotides are frequently, but not invariably, located between genes and have been classified as junk DNA. Because microsatellites are usually less than 100 bp long and are embedded in DNA with unique sequence, they can be amplified in vitro using the polymerase chain reaction (PCR). Microsatellites are easy to clone and characterize and display considerable polymorphism due to variation in the number of units *(79,80)*. Microsatellite instability (MSI) may reflect replication error (RER), because RER replication error results in accumulation of changes in the length of microsatellite and other short repeat sequences (Fig. 4).

In studies on hereditary nonpolyposis colorectal cancer (HNPCC) and sporadic colorectal-cancer patients, frequent mutations in the microsatellite-repeat sequences were first described *(79,80)*. These mutations are typically tumor-specific and indicative of somatic origin. Since the original description of MSI in HNPCC tumors and sporadic colon cancer, MSI has been described for a significant fraction of sporadic tumors, including colorectal, endometrial, stomach, ovarian, cervical, pancreatic, esophageal, and small-cell lung cancer (SCLC) *(81–83)*. These data suggest that RER followed by MSI could be a common mechanism involved in neoplastic transformation. Moreover, Wada et al. found a frequent occurrence of MSI in the evolution of CML *(84)*, indicating MSI to be a late genetic event in the evolution of CML to blast crisis. On the other hand, Kaneko et al. reported that MSI contributes to the pathogenesis of myelodysplastic syndromes (MDS) in some patients, especially as an early genetic event *(85)*. MSI has also been observed in other hematopoietic malignancies including CLL, Burkitt's lymphoma (BL), and HIV-associated lymphomas *(86–88)*.

MUTATIONS OF MMR GENES IN HUMAN CANCER
The basis of the MSI phenotype has been clarified by genetic analysis of HNPCC families and biochemical assay of tumor cell lines that express MSI. Four genes have been implicated to date in HNPCC: *MSH2*, *MLH1*, *PMS1*, and *PMS2 (89)*. The majority fraction of HNPCC examined to date harbor mutations in *MSH2* or *MLH1*, whereas *PMS1* and *PMS2* mutations appear to be responsible for only a small fraction of HNPCC

patients. These data suggest that MSI in tumors arising in patients with HNPCC is due to the presence of mutations in one of four known (*hMSH2*, *hMLH1*, *hPMS1*, and *hPMS2*) DNA MMR genes. Isolation of hMutSa have implicated MSH6 in mismatch repair, but mutations in the *MSH6* locus have not been identified in HNPCC kindred. However, *MSH6* defects have been identified in several sporadic MSI-positive colorectal cancers *(90)*.

Mutation analysis of these four *MMR* genes in endometrial carcinomas displaying MI revelaed that two of nine tumors contain *hMSH2* mutations, suggesting that mutations in these four *MMR* genes are not responsible for MI in the majority of sporadic endometrial carcinomas *(91)*.

Recently, Hangaeshi et al. examined alterations of hMLH1 gene in a total of 43 human leukemia cell lines by PCR-SSCP *(92)*. Mutations of the *hMLH1* gene were detected in three cell lines from lymphoid leukemias, suggesting that disruption of *MMR* may play an important role in the development of human lymphoid leukemias.

TARGET GENES OF MISMATCH-REPAIR DEFECTS
Markowitz et al. documented a strong correlation between defects in the *type II TGF-β receptor* (*TGFβRII*) gene and expression of MSI in tumor cells. The mutations responsible for defective TGFβRII function in these tumor cells were located in microsatellite-repeat units within the coding sequence of the gene, and consisted of expansion (insertions) mutations in an $(A)_{10}$ repeat in seven cases and a $(GT)_3$ repeat in one case *(91)*. Because the failure to respond to TGF-β growth inhibition is a characteristic of certain cancers, these findings directly link RER and a mutational hot spot in a growth control locus. Other genes that are targets for mutations in MSI-positive cells during the course of carcinogenesis have proven elusive. Ouyang et al. examined mutations of the *insulin-like growth factor-2 receptor* (*IGF2R*) gene in MSI-positive cancers occurring at various primary sites, and found frameshift mutations in some populations of gastric, endometrial, and colorectal cancers that express MSI *(83)*.

MUTATIONS OF DNA POLYMERASE ENZYMES IN HUMAN CANCER
In the hereditary form, mutations of MMR genes are usually responsible for instability, however, in many sporadic tumors, mutations of the known MMR genes are apparently absent. Da Costa et al. have investigated whether defects in the proofreading DNA-repair function of DNA polymerase δ might contribute to the RER phenotype *(92)*. They examined eight MSI-positive colorectal-cancer cell lines with no known MMR gene defects for mutations in the three highly conserved regions thought to be involved in 3'→5' exonuclease activity (exons I-III). A variation in exon III of *polymerase δ* was observed in 3/8 cell lines, suggesting that the RER phenotype might be related to mutations in the exonuclease domain of DNA polymerase enzyme. Some investigators have reported that the abnormalities of DNA polymerase other than DNA polymerase δ might be associated with tumorigenesis. DNA polymerase α expression correlates with the extent of malignancy and survival in non-SCLC patients, and is therefore considered to be a useful prognostic parameter *(93)*. Furthermore, mutations in the gene encoding DNA polymerase β were detected in a high percentage of human colorectal can-

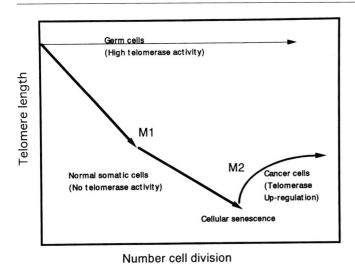

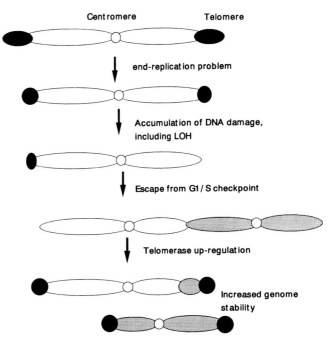

Fig. 5. The telomere/telomerase hypothesis. Telomerase is active in the germ line, maintaining long and stable telomeres, whereas telomerase is repressed in most normal somatic cells. Telomeres progressively shorten during every cell division, leading to an end-replication problem. Transformation events may bypass M1 (the Hayflick limit) point without upregulation of telomerase. When telomere length become critically short on most chromosomes, cells enter M2 crisis. Some of the cells that would otherwise enter M2 crisis escape M2 crisis through telomerase upregulation, and obtain stable chromosomes and maintain active cell division. In hematopoietic cells, low levels of telomerase are detectable but insufficient to protect against telomere shortening completely. Adapted from Harley et al. *(97).*

Fig. 6. Schematic speculative model for telomere dynamics and genome instability in human cancer cells. Telomere shortening leading to an end-replication problem in cells without telomerase activity can induce exposed chromosome ends to be linked DNA damage checkpoint and lead to cell-cycle arrest and/or apoptosis (loss of checkpoint). This process, shortening of telomeres leading to uncapped chromosome ends, may lead to chromosome instability. Some cells may survive due to chromosome end fusion leading to the production of dicentric chromosome. Then telomerase is activated, resulting in restoration of telomere function and induce chromosome stability. Adapted from de Lange *(99).*

cers *(94).* DNA polymerase β gene mutations were also detected in prostate and bladder cancer, although with relatively low frequency *(95).*

TELOMERE AND TELOMERASE IN CANCER

TELOMERES AND TELOMERASE Telomeres, the ends of chromosomes, consist of simple tandem hexameric repeats. In humans, 10–15 kb of TTAGGG repeats are found at the termini of all chromosomes *(96).* Telomeres progressively shorten with age in fibroblasts, peripheral-blood mononuclear cells (PBMCs), and colon mucosa/intestine *(97,98).* In addition, some primary cancer cells also have shortened telomeres *(99).* Thus, the reduction of telomere length in cancer cells and senescent cells is believed to result from active cell division that erodes chromosomal termini *(100,101).* In somatic cells, telomerase—a ribonucleoprotein that compensates for progressive telomere erosion—is not usually detectable *(102).* In some actively proliferative somatic cells, for example, hematopoietic stem cells, intestinal cryptic cells, endothelial cells, endometrium, breast tissue, and basal cells in the epidermis including hair follicles have weak but detectable telomerase activity. Circulating T and B lymphocytes in the peripheral blood also contain telomerase activity. However, the telomerase present in these proliferative cells of renewal tissues is insufficient to completely maintain telomeres throughout life and thus in these somatic cells, as with other somatic cells, telomeres progressively shorten *(100,101)* (Fig. 5).

Characterization of the telomerase enzyme has shown it to consist of an RNA component *(103),* telomerase catalytic component *(104,105),* and TEP1 (TPL1/ILP1) portion *(106).* Al-

though the RNA component binds to telomeric substrate, expression of the RNA component of telomerase ribonucleoprotein itself does not correlate with telomerase activity, and the expression of catalytic protein (named hTERT) is closely associated with telomerase activity *(105).* Moreover, the expression of TRF-1 protein that binds to double strand of telomeric DNA (TTAGGG) is associated with telomere length and negatively regulates telomerase activity *(107,108).* Nevertheless, regulation of reactivation of telomerase activity in cancer cells is not yet fully understood.

TELOMERE/TELOMERASE HYPOTHESIS Normal somatic cells may undergo programmed cell death after a certain number of cell divisions *(109).* The point in time when this normally occurs is operationally defined in cell cultures as M1 (for mortality 1) crisis. To overcome the M1 crisis and continue to proliferate requires certain as yet understood factors to be present. For example, cells infected with certain viruses may acquire immortal cell growth. However, even in immortal cells, proliferation and cell division cease after a fixed number of cell doublings. This point in the natural history of a cell is designated M2 (for mortality 2) crisis. In an experiment of Simian virus 40 (SV40)-infected normal diploid somatic cells, the reactivation of telomerase enzyme activity and the appearance of telomeric chromosomal abnormalities occurred at the M2 crisis point *(110).* This suggests that overcoming growth control of immortal cells after an M2 crisis is correlated with reactivation of telomerase, and critical shortening of telomeres is closely associated with instability of chromosomal termini (Fig. 5). This is why telomerase reactivation is considered as a marker of cancer cells, and telomere shortening is linked to chromosomal instability, typically resulting in DMs and dicentric chromosomes.

TELOMERASE REACTIVATION IN CANCEROUS TISSUE A highly sensitive telomeric repeat amplification protocol (TRAP) assay demonstrated that about 86% of cancer tissues express telomerase activity *(102)*. Induction of telomerase activity is detected in some pre-malignant lesions as well *(111)*. It is hypothesized that telomere shortening triggers reactivation of telomerase activity in neoplastically transforming cells (telomere/telomerase hypothesis) through some unknown mechanism. However, progressive telomere shortening in normal somatic cells does not result in the reactivation of telomerase activity *(100,101)*. Thus, the role of telomere shortening in telomerase reactivation is unclear. The reduction of telomere length is suggested to correlate with downregulation of *TRF-1* expression, allowing speculation that dysregulation of *TRF-1* expression might result in the upregulation of telomerase activity *(107)*. However, the connection between *TRF-1* expression and telomerase activity in cancer cells remains obscure.

TELOMERE DYNAMICS, TELOMERE SHORTENING, AND CHROMOSOME INSTABILITY The evidence suggests that progressive telomere erosion leads to chromosomal instability. Specifically, telomere abnormalities may lead to the appearance of dicentric chromosomes or DMs, because these cytogenetic changes are linked to reconstitution of chromosomal termini (so called telomere-associated chromosome fragments). De Lange *(99)* hypothesized that critical telomere shortening may induce chromosome damage, including damage to chromosome termini, followed by elimination by the G_1/S cell-cycle checkpoint system (Fig. 6). Consistent with this theory, Hiyama et al. reported that 27% of patients with primary lung cancer had telomere-length alterations and 62.5% of them had allelic loss of both the *p53* and *Rb1* genes *(112)*. They concluded that inactivation of both *p53* and *Rb1* gene may promote uncontrolled cell division, resulting in progressive telomere shortening during the development of lung cancer. In other studies, the appearance of dicentric chromosomes was found to be associated with upregulation of telomerase in the YS9;22 human leukemia cell line *(113)*. Moreover, appearance of additional cytogenetic changes, including DMs and dicentric chromosomes, has been correlated with telomerase upregulation in blast-crisis stage CML *(114)*. However, in developing tumors chromosomal changes involving end-to-end chromosome fusion may be eliminated (lost) during the process of karyotypic evolution. This may account for the fact that such chromosomal aberrations are rarely detected in human tumors. In MDS, multiple cytogenetic changes related to chromosome instability are correlated with reduced telomere length *(115)*. Reactivation of telomerase activity is rarely observed in these cases. Therefore, cells exhibiting telomere/telomerase dysregulation, short telomeres, and low levels of telomerase activity, may demonstrate chromosomal instability as well. The

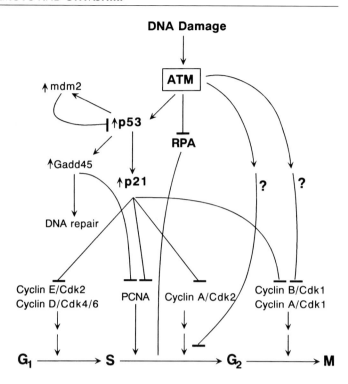

Fig. 7. Involvement of the ATM and p53 proteins in DNA damaged-induced pathways controlling cell-cycle progression. This cascade, which begins with p53 accumulation, is significantly delayed in AT cells following treatment by ionizing radiation, suggesting that the ATM protein acts upstream of p53.

reduction of telomere length in lung cancer is also linked to the frequency of loss of heterozygocity (LOH) and leads us to speculate on a connection between telomere shrinking and genome instability. Although there is no evidence at hand for a relationship between cytogenetic changes and telomere dynamics in solid tumors, there is a possibility that telomere shortening without upregulation of telomerase activity may cause not only genome instability but karyotypic instability.

CELL-CYCLE CHECKPOINTS IN CANCER

CELL-CYCLE CHECKPOINTS AND CHROMOSOMAL INSTABILITY Cell-cycle checkpoint mechanisms ensure that all processes in one phase of the cell cycle are completed before the next phase begins. Such checkpoints are not activated unless an impediment to cell-cycle progression is detected. Therefore, it is not surprising that DNA damage can trigger cell-cycle checkpoint controls, because DNA damage can interfere significantly with cell-cycle processes and diminish their accuracy. For instance, one can imagine that in the presence of DNA double-strand breaks, mitosis would almost certainly result in irreversible chromosome aberrations, and that DNA replication of a damaged template would pose a high risk of mutation. One might therefore intuitively expect that controls would have evolved in cells to delay entry into S and M phases in response to DNA damage, in order to increase the kinetic window of opportunity for DNA repair.

It has been demonstrated that cell-cycle checkpoint abnormalities can lead to the generation of chromosomal aberrations *(116,117)*. For example, a defect in the S/M checkpoint can result in the improper segregation of chromosomes due to the incomplete separation of sister chromatids before DNA replication is successfully completed. Defects in the surveillance of the integrity of DNA can cause chromosomal rearrangements such as deletions, amplifications, and translocations. Defects in spindle surveillance can lead to mitotic nondisjunction, generating whole chromosome gain or loss, whereas defects in the surveillance of the spindle poles can lead to changes in chromosome number (aneuploidy). In such cells with defective checkpoint machinery, the replicated DNA may not be segregated in time into the daughter cells, which may lead to aneuploidy and future chromosomal instability.

p53 GENE Mice deficient in the *p53* gene have a predisposition to cancer in multiple organ systems *(118)*. In humans, tumor cells in the Li-Fraumeni syndrome have defects in both copies of *p53*, whereas the nontumor cells have a defect in only one. Furthermore, more than 50% of sporadic cancer patients are found to exhibit *p53* mutations *(119)*. The gene product of the *p53* tumor-suppressor gene is a checkpoint factor that mediates G_0/G_1 cell-cycle arrest or apoptosis in response to DNA damage (Fig. 7). p53 also harbors an intrinsic exonuclease activity and binds to Rad51 recombinase, a factor that facilitates DNA repair, indicating that p53 is directly involved in the DNA repair mechanism *(120)*. Moreover, p53 seems to be involved in the regulation of centrosome replication and the prevention of DNA replication when a mitotic-spindle inhibitor hampers chromosome replication *(121,122)*. Therefore, the loss of p53 function cause enhanced gene amplification, and chromosomal instability *(123,124)*.

ATM GENE IN ATAXIA TELANGIECTASIA Ataxia telangiectasia (AT) is inherited in autosomal recessive manner with full penetrance. The clinical manifestations of AT include not only ataxia, telangiectasia, and predisposition to cancer, but also abnormalities in the development and function of various tissues, resulting in premature aging, female hypogonadism, growth retardation, and delayed puberty *(125)*. AT patients are highly prone to acute cancer, which mainly involves a range of lymphoid malignancies of B-cell and T-cell origin *(126)*. Cells from AT patients are defective in their responses to certain DNA-damaging agents and display an increased rate of chromosomal breakage. In these cases, the DNA-repair system seems to be normal but G_1/S and G_2/M checkpoints are defective *(126)*.

AT is caused by a single gene mutation involving the *ATM* gene, located at chromosome 11q22-q23. The *ATM* gene encodes a protein of 350 kDa that belongs to an expanding family of protein kinases involved in the checkpoint response to DNA damage such as the budding yeast Mec1 and fission yeast Rad3 *(127,128)*. All of the members of this family harbor a highly conserved domain similar to the catalytic domain of phosphatidylinositol 3-kinase. Some studies show that the accumulation of p53 protein in response to DNA damage is significantly delayed in AT cells following treatment with ionizing radiation. These data indicate that the ATM is involved in the transmission of checkpoint signals via a phosphorylation cascade and acts upstream of p53 in response to DNA damage (Fig. 7). In addition, the *ATM* gene has homology with the *TEL1* gene of yeast, in which mutations lead to shortened telomeres.

Metcalfe et al. showed that *ATM* mutation in the homozygous state confers a predisposition to accelerated telomere shortening *(129)*, and Smilenov et al. demonstrated that the *ATM* gene product is involved in telomere metabolism but not telomerase activity *(130)*.

ACKNOWLEDGMENT

We thank Ayako Hirota for excellent medical figures.

REFERENCES

1. Rowley, J. D. (1982) Identification of the constant chromosome regions involved in human hematologic malignant disease. *Science* **216**:749–755.
2. Yunis, J. J. (1986) Chromosomal rearrangements, genes, and fragile sites in cancer: clinical and biological implications. *In: Important Advances in Oncology* (DeVita, V., Hellman, S., and Rosenberg, S., eds.), Lippincott, Philadelphia, PA, pp. 93–128.
3. Squire, J., and Phillips, R. A. (1992) Genetic basis of cancer. *In*: The Basic Science of Oncology (Tannock, I. F., and Hill, R. P., eds.), McGraw-Hill, New York, NY, pp. 41–60.
4. Weiner, A.M. (1987) Chromosome abnormalities associated with human tumors. *In*: Molecular Biology of the Gene, 4th ed. (Watson, J. D., Hopkins, N. H., Roberts, J. W., Steitz, J. A., and Weiner, A. M., eds.), Benjamin/Cummings, Menlo Park, CA, pp. 1074–1086.
5. Tanaka, K., Arif, M., Eguchi, M., Kyo, T., Dohy, H., and Kamada, N. (1997) Frequent jumping translocations of chromosomal segments involving the ABL oncogene alone or in combination with CD3-MLL genes in secondary leukemias. *Blood* **89**:596–600.
6. ISCN (1991) *Guidelines for Cancer Cytogenetics: Supplement to an International System for Human Cytogenetic Nomenclature VI.* (Mitelman, F., ed.), Karger, Basel, Switzerland.
7. Rowley, J. D. (1973) A new consistent chromosomal abnormality in chronic myelogenous leukemia: myelogenous leukemia identified by quinacrine fluorescence and Giemsa staining. *Nature* **243**:290–293.
8. Rowley, J. D., and Testa, J. R. (1982) Chromosome abnormalities in malignant hematologic diseases. *Adv. Cancer Res.* **36**:103–148.
9. Groffen, J. J., Stephenson, J. R., Heisterkamp, N., de Klein, A., Bartram, C. R., and Grosveld, G. (1984) Philadelphia chromosomal breakpoints are clustered within a limited region, bcr, on chromosome 22. *Cell* **36**:93–99.
10. Dreazen, O., Cannani, E., and Gale, R. P. (1988) Molecular biology of chronic myelogenous leukemia. *Semin. Hematol.* **25**:35–48.
11. Hermans, A., Heisterkamp, N., von Lindern, M., van Baal, S., Meijer, D., van der Plas, D., et al. (1987) Unique fusion of bcr and c-abl genes in Philadelphia chromosome positive acute lymphoblastic leukemia. *Cell* **51**:33–40.
12. Pane, F., Frigeri, F., Sindona, M., Luciano, L., Ferrara, F., Cimino, R., et al. (1996) Neutrophilic-chronic myeloid leukemia: a distinct disease with a specific molecular marker (BCR/ABL with C3/A2 junction). *Blood* **88**:2410–2414.
13. Kakizuka, A., Miller, W. H., Jr., Umesono, K., Warrell, R. P., Jr., Frankel, S. R., Murty, V. V., et al. (1991) Chromosomal translocation t(15;17) in human acute myelocytic leukemia fuses RARα with a novel putative transcription factor, PML. *Cell* **66**:663–674.
14. de The, H., Lavau, C., Marchio, A., Chomienne, C., Degos, L., and Dejean, A. (1991) The PML-RARa fusion mRNA generated by the t(15;17) translocation in acute promyelocytic leukemia encodes a functionally altered RAR. *Cell* **66**:675–684.
15. Miyoshi, H., Kozu, T., Shimizu, K., Enomoto, K., Kaneko, Y., and Kamada, N. (1993) The t(8;21) translocation in acute myeloid leukemia results in production of an AML1-MTG8 fusion transcript. *EMBO J.* **12**:2715–2721.
16. Liu, P., Tarle, S. A., Hajra, A., Claxton, D. F., Marlton, P., Freedman, M., et al. (1993) Fusion between transcription factor CBFβ/PEBP2β and a myosin heavy chain in acute myeloid leukemia. *Science* **261**:1041–1044.

17. von Lindern, M., Fornerod, M., van Baal, S., Jaegle, M., de Wit, T., Buijs, A., et al. (1992) The translocation (6;9), associated with a specific subtype of acute myeloid leukemia, results in the fusion of two genes, dek and can, and the expression of a chimeric, leukemia-specific dek-can mRNA. *Mol. Cell Biol.* **12**:1687–1697.

18. Morishita, K., Parganas, E., Willman, C. L., Whittaker, M. H., Drabkin, H., Oval, J., et al. (1992) Activation of EVI1 gene expression in human acute myelogenous leukemias by translocations spanning 300–400 kilobases on chromosome band 3q26. *Proc. Natl. Acad. Sci. USA* **89**:3937–3941.

19. Mitani, K., Ogawa, S., Tanaka, T. Miyoshi, H., Kurokawa, M., Mano, H., et al. (1994) Generation of the AML1-EVI-1 fusion gene in the t(3;21)(q26;q22) causes blastic crisis in chronic myelocytic leukemia. *EMBO J.* **13**:504–510.

20. Tanaka, T., Tanaka, K., Ogawa, S., Kurokawa, M., Mitani, K., Nishida, J., et al. (1995) An acute myeloid leukemia gene, AML1, regulates hematopoietic myeloid cell differentiation and transcriptional activation antagonistically by two alternative spliced forms. *EMBO J.* **14**:341–350.

21. Tkachuk, D. C., Kohler, S., and Cleary, M. L. (1992) Involvement of a homolog of Drosophila trithorax by 11q23 chromosomal translocations in acute leukemias. *Cell* **71**:691–700.

22. Gu, Y., Nakamura, T., Alder, H., Prasad, R., Canaani, O., Cimino, G., et al. (1992) The t(4;11) chromosome translocation of human acute leukemias fuses the ALL-1 gene, related to Drosophila trithorax, to the AF -4 gene. *Cell* **71**:701–708.

23. Hamlyn, P. H., and Rabbitts, T.H. (1983) Translocation joins c-myc and immunoglobulin gamma-1 genes in a Burkitt lymphoma revealing a third exon in the c-myc oncogene. *Nature* **304**:135–139.

24. Siebenlist, U., Hennighausen, J. Battey, J., and Leder, P. (1984) Chromatin structure and protein binding in the putative regulatory region of the c-myc gene in a Burkitt lymphoma. *Cell* **37**:381–391.

25. Nourse, J., Mellentin, J. D., Galili, N., Wilkinson J., Stanbridge, E., Smith, S. D., et al. (1990) Chromosomal translocation t(1;19) results in synthesis of a homeobox fusion mRNA that codes for a potential chimeric transcription factor. *Cell* **60**:535–545.

26. Kamps, M. P., Murre, C., Sun, X. H., and Baltimore, D. (1990) A new homeobox gene contributes the DNA binding domain of the t(1;19) translocation protein in pre-B ALL. *Cell* **60**:547–555.

27. Hatano, M., Roberts, C. W. M., Minden, M., Crist, W. M., and Korsmeyer, S. J. (1991) Deregulation of a homeobox gene, HOX11, by the t(10;14) in T cell leukemia. *Science* **253**:79–82.

28. Chen, Q., Cheng, J. T., Tsai, L. H., Schneider, N., Buchanan, G., Carroll, A., et al. (1990) The tal gene undergoes chromosome translocation in T cell leukemia and potentially encodes a helix-loop-helix protein. *EMBO J.* **9**:415–424.

29. Motokura, T., Bloom, T., Kim, H. G., Juppner, H., Ruderman, J. V., Kronenberg, H. M., et al. (1991) A novel cyclin encoded by a bcl 1-linked candidate oncogene. *Nature* **350**:512–515.

30. Tsujimoto, Y., Finger, L. R., Yunis, J., Nowell, P. C., and Croce, C. M. (1984) Cloning of the chromosome breakpoint of neoplastic B cells with the t(14;18) chromosome translocation. *Science* **226**:1097–1099.

31. Vaux, D. L., Cory, S., and Adams, J. M. (1988) Bcl-2 gene promotes haematopoietic cell survival and cooperates with c-myc to immortalize pre-B cells. *Nature* **335**:440–442.

32. Strasser, A., Harris, A. W., and Cory, S. (1991) bcl-2 transgene inhibits T cell death and perturbs thymic self-censorship. *Cell* **67**:889–899.

33. Morris, S. W., Kirstein, M. N., Valentine, M. B., Dittmer, K. G., Shapiro, D. N., Saltman, D. L., et al. (1994) Fusion of a kinase gene, ALK, to a nucleolar protein gene, NPM, in non-Hodgkin's lymphoma. *Science* **263**:1281–1284.

34. Ohno, H., Takimoto, G., and McKeithan, T. W. (1990) The candidate proto-oncogene bcl-3 is related to genes implicated in cell lineage determination and cell cycle control. *Cell* **60**:991–997.

35. Turc-Carel, C., Aurias, A., Mugneret, F., Lizard, S., Sidaner, I., Volk, C., et al. (1988) Chromosomes in Ewing's sarcoma. I. An evaluation of 85 cases and remarkable consistency of t(11;22)(q24;q12). *Cancer Genet. Cytogenet.* **32**:229–238.

36. Delattre, O., Zucman, J., Plougastel, B., Desmaze, C., Melot, T., Peter, M., et al. (1992) Gene fusion with an ETS DNA-binding domain caused by chromosome translocation in human tumours. *Nature* **359**:162–165.

37. Zucman, J., Delattre, O., Desmaze, C., Plougastel, B., Joubert, I., Melot, T., et al. (1992) Cloning and characterization of the Ewing's sarcoma and peripheral neuroepithelioma t(11;22) translocation breakpoints. *Genes Chromosomes Cancer* **5**:271–277.

38. Ohno, T., Ouchida, M., Lee, L., Gatalica, Z., Rao, V. N., and Reddy, E. S. P. (1994) The EWS gene, involved in Ewing family tumors, malignant melanoma of soft parts and desmoplastic small round cell tumors, codes for an RNA binding protein with novel regulatory domains. *Oncogene* **9**:3087–3097.

39. Bailly, R. A., Bosselut, R., Zucman, J., Cormier, F., Delattre, O., Roussel, M., et al. (1994) DNA-binding and transcriptional activation properties of the EWS-FLI-1 fusion protein resulting from the t(11;22) translocation in Ewing sarcoma. *Mol. Cell. Biol.* **14**:3230–3241.

40. Sorensen, P. H. B., Lessnick, S. L., Lopez-Terrada, D., Liu, X. F., Triche, T. J., and Denny, C. T. (1994) A second Ewing's sarcoma translocation, t(21;22), fuses the EWS gene to another ETS-family transcription factor, ERG. *Nature Genet.* **6**:146–151.

41. Bridge, J. A., Borek, D. A., Neff, J. R., and Huntrakoon, M. (1990) Chromosomal abnormalities in clear cell sarcoma. Implications for histogenesis. *Am. J. Clin. Pathol.* **93**:26–31.

42. Zucman, J., Delattre, O., Desmaze, C., Epstein, A., Stenman, G., Speleman, F., et al. (1993) EWS and ATF-1 gene fusion induced by t(12;22) translocation in malignant melanoma of soft parts. *Nature Genet.* **4**:341–345.

43. Gerald, W. L., Miller, H. K., Battifora, H., Miettinen, M., Silva, E. G., and Rosai, J. (1991) Intra-abdominal desmoplastic small round-cell tumor. Report of 19 cases of a distinctive type of high-grade polyphenotypic malignancy affecting young individuals. *Am. J. Surg. Pathol.* **15**:499–513.

44. Rodriguez, E., Sreekantaiah, C., Gerald, W., Reuter, V. E., Motzer, R. J., and Chaganti, R. S. K. (1993) A recurring translocation, t(11;22) (p13;q11.2), characterizes intra-abdominal desmoplastic small round-cell tumors. *Cancer Genet. Cytogenet.* **69**:17–21.

45. Gerald, W. L., Rosai, J., and Ladanyi, M. (1995) Characterization of the genomic breakpoint and chimeric transcripts inthe EWS-WT1 gene fusion of desmoplastic small round cell tumor. *Proc. Natl. Acad. Sci. USA* **92**:1028–1032.

46. Sreekantaiah, C., Ladanyi, M., Rodriguez, E., and Chaganti, R. S. K. (1994) Chromosomal aberrations in soft tissue tumors. Relevance to diagnosis, classification, and molecular mechanisms. *Am. J. Pathol.* **144**:1121–1134.

47. Crozat, A., Aman, P., Mandahl, N., and Ron, D. (1993) Fusion of CHOP to a novel RNA-binding protein in human myxoid liposarcoma. *Nature* **363**:640–644.

48. Rabbitts, T. H., Forster, A., Larson, R., and Nathan, P. (1993) Fusion of the dominant negative transcription regulator CHOP with a novel gene FUS by translocation t(12;16) in malignant liposarcoma. *Nature Genet.* **4**:175–180.

49. Galili, N., Davis, R. J., Fredericks, W. J., Mukhopadhyay, S., Rauscher III F. J., Emanuel, B. J., et al. (1993) Fusion of a fork head domain gene to PAX3 in the solid tumour alveolar rhabdomyosarcoma. *Nature Genet.* **5**:230–235.

50. Shapiro, D. N., Sublett, J. E., Li, B., Downing, J. R., and Naeve, C. W. (1993) Fusion of PAX3 to a member of the forkhead family to transcription factors in human alveolar rhabdomyosarcoma. *Cancer Res.* **53**:5108–5112.

51. Davis, R. J., D'Cruz, C. M., Lovell, M. A., Biegel, J. A., and Barr, F. G. (1994) Fusion of PAX7 to FKHR by the variant t(1;13)(p36;q14) translocation in alveolar rhabdomyosarcoma. *Cancer Res.* **54**:2869–2872.

52. Ruttledge, M. H., Sarrazin, J., Rangaratnam, S., Phelan, C. M., Twist, E., Merel, P., et al. (1994) Evidence for the complete inactivation of the NF2 gene in the majority of sporadic meningioma. *Nature Genet.* **6**:180–184.

53. Weinberg, R. A. (1991) Tumor suppressor genes. *Science* **254**:1138–1146.

54. Tadokoro, K., Fujii, H., Ohshima, A., Kakizawa, Y., Shimizu, K., Sakai, A., et al. (1992) Intragenic homozygous deletion of the WT1 gene in Wilms' tumor. *Oncogene* **7**:1215–1221.

55. Powell, S. M., Zilz, N., Beazer-Barclay, Y., Bryan, T. M., Hamilton, S. R., Thibodeau, S. N., et al. (1992) APC mutations occur early during colorectal tumorigenesis. *Nature* **359**:235–237.

56. Schwab, M., Varmus, H. E., Bishop, J. M., Grzeschik, K. H., Naylor, S. L., Sakaguchi, A. Y., et al. (1984) Chromosome localization in normal human cells and neuroblastomas of a gene related to c-myc. *Nature* **308**:288–291.

57. Nau, M. M., Brooks, B. J., Battey, J., Sausville, E., Gazdar A. F., Kirsch, I. R., et al. (1985) L-myc, a new myc-related gene amplified and expressed in human small cell lung cancer. *Nature* **318**:69–73.

58. Friedberg, E. C., Walker, G. C., and Siede, W. (1995) *DNA Repair and Mutagenesis*. ASM Press, Washington, DC.

59. Sancar, A. (1996) DNA excision repair. *Ann. Rev. Biochem.* **65**:43–81.

60. Auerbach, A. D., and Verlander, P. C. (1997) Disorders of DNA replication and repair. *Curr. Opin. Pediatrics* **9**:600–616.

61. Robins, P., Jones, C. J., Biggerstaff, M., Lindahl, T., and Wood, R. D. (1991) Complementation of DNA repair in xeroderma pigmentosum group A cell extracts by a protein with affinity for damaged DNA. *EMBO J.* **10**:3913–3921.

62. Treber, D. K., Chen, Z. H., and Essigmann, J. M. (1992) An ultraviolet light-damaged DNA recognition protein absent in xeroderma pigmentosum group E cells binds selectively to pyrimidine (6-4) pyrimidone photoproducts. *Nucleic Acids Res.* **20**:5805–5810.

63. Scherly, D., Nouspikel, T., Corlet, J., Ucla, C., Bairoch, A., and Clarkson, S. G. (1993) Complementation of the DNA repair defect in xeroderma pigmentosum group G cells by a human cDNA related to yeast RAD2. *Nature* **363**:182–185.

64. O'Donovan, A., Davies, A. A., Moggs, J. G., West, S. C., and Wood, R. D. (1994) XPG endonuclease makes the 3' incision in human DNA nucleotide excision repair. *Nature* **371**:432–435.

65. van Vuuren, A. J., Vermeulen, W., Weeda, G., Appeldoorn, E., Jaspers, N. G. J., van der Eb A. J., et al. (1994) Correlation of xeroderma pigmentosum repair defect by basal transcription factor BTF2 (TFIIH). *EMBO J.* **13**:1645–1653.

66. Drapkin, R., Reardon, J. T., Ansari, A., Huang, J. C., Zawel, L., Ahn, K., et al. (1994) Dual role of TFIIH in DNA excision repair and in transcription by RNA polymerase II. *Nature* **368**:769–772.

67. Leveillard, T., Andera, L., Bissonnette, N., Schaeffer, L., Bracco, L., Egly, J.-M., et al. (1996) Functional interactions between p53 and the TFIIH complex are affected by tumour-associated mutations. *EMBO J.* **15**:1615–1624.

68. Cleaver, J. E. (1968) Defective repair replication of DNA in xeroderma pigmentosum. *Nature* **218**:652–656.

69. Tanaka, K., and Wood, R. D. (1994) Xeroderma Pigmentosum and nucleotide excision repair of DNA. *Trends. Biochem. Sci.* **19**:83–86.

70. German, J. (1993) Bloom syndrome: a mendelian prototype of somatic mutational disease. *Medicine* **72**:393–406.

71. German, J., Ellis, N. A., Proytcheva, M. (1996) Bloom's syndrome: XIX. Cytogenetic and population evidence for genetic heterogeneity. *Clin. Genet.* **49**:223–231.

72. German, J. (1997) Bloom's syndrome: XX. The first 100 cancers. *Cancer Genet. Cytogenet.* **93**:100–106.

73. Ellis, N. A., Groden, J., Ye, T.-Z., Straughen, J., Lennon, D. J., Ciocci, S., et al. (1995) The Bloom's syndrome gene product is homologous to RecQ helicases. *Cell* **83**:655–666.

74. Ellis, N. A., and German, J. (1996) Molecular genetics of Bloom's syndrome. *Human Mol. Genet.* **5**:1457–1463.

75. Alberts, A., Bray, D., Lewis, J., Raff, M., Roberts, K., and Watson, J. D. (1994) *Molecular Biology of the Cell*. Garland, New York, NY.

76. Simon, M., Giot, L., and Faye, G. (1991) The 3' to 5' exonuclease activity located in the DNA polymerase δ subunit of Saccharomyces cerevisiae is required for accurate replication. *EMBO J.* **10**:2165–2170.

77. Morrison, A., Bell, J. B., Kunkel, T. A., and Sugino, A. (1991) Eukaryotic DNA polymerase amino acid sequence required for 3' to 5' exonuclease activity. *Proc. Natl. Acad. Sci. USA* **88**:9473–9477.

78. Palombo, F., Iaccarino, I., Nakajima, E., Ikejima, M., Shimada, T., and Jiricny, J. (1996) hMutSb, a heterodimer of hMSH2 and hMSH3, binds to insertion/deletion loops in DNA. *Curr. Biol.* **6**:1181–1184.

79. Ionov, Y. M., Peinado, A., Malkhosyan, S., Shibata, D., and Perucho, M. (1993) Ubiquitous somatic mutations in simple repeated sequences reveal a new mechanism for colonic carcinogenesis. *Nature* **363**:558–561.

80. Thibodeau, S. N., Bren, G., and Schaid, D. (1993) Microsatellite instability in cancer of the proximal colon. *Science* **260**:816–819.

81. Risinger, J. I., Berchuck, A., Kohler, M. F., Watson, P., Lynch, H. T., and Boyd, J. (1993) Genetic instability of microsatellites in endometrial carcinoma. *Cancer Res.* **53**:5100–5103.

82. Orth, K., Hung, J. Gazdar, A., Bowcock, A., Mathis, J. M., and Sambrook, J. (1994) Genetic instability in human ovarian cancer cell lines. *Proc. Natl. Acad. Sci. USA* **91**:9495–9499.

83. Ouyang, H., Shiwaku, H. O., Hagiwara, H., Miura, K., Abe, T., Kato, Y., et al. (1997) The insulin-like growth factor II receptor gene is mutated in genetically unstable cancers of the endometrium, stomach, and colorectum. *Cancer Res.* **57**:1851–1854.

84. Wada, C., Shionoya, S., Fujino, Y., Tokuhiro, H., Akahoshi, T., Uchida, T., et al. (1994) Genomic instability of microsatellite repeats and its association with the evolution of chronic myelogenous leukemia. *Blood* **83**:3449–3456.

85. Kaneko, H., Horiike, S., Inazawa, J., Nakai, H., Misawa, S. (1995) Microsatellite instability is an early genetic event in myelodysplastic syndrome. *Blood* **86**:1236–1237.

86. Gartenhaus, R., Johns, M. M. III, Wang, P., Rai, K., and Sidransky, D. (1996) Mutant phenotype in a subset of chronic lymphocytic leukemia. *Blood* **87**:38–41.

87. Robledo, M., Martinez, B., Arranz, E., Trujillo, M. J., Gonzalez, A. A., Rivas, C., et al. (1995) Genetic instability of microsatellites in hematologic neoplasms. *Leukemia* **9**:960–964.

88. Bedi, G. C., Westra, W. H., Farzadegan, H., Pitha, P. M., and Sidransky, D. (1995) Microsatellite instability in primary neoplasms from HIV+ patients. *Nature Med.* **1**:65–68.

89. Liu, B., Parsons, R., Papadopoulos, N., Nicolaides, N. C., Lynch, H. T., Watson, P., et al. (1996) Analysis of mismatch repair genes in hereditary non-polyposis colorectal cancer patients. *Nature Med.* **2**:169–174.

90. Papadopoulos, N., Nicolaides, N. C., Liu, B., Parsons, R., Lengauer, C., Palombo, F., et al. (1995) Mutations of GTBP in genetically unstable cells. *Science* **268**:1915–1917.

91. Katabuchi, H., van Rees, B., Lambers, A.R., Ronnett, B.M., Blazes, M.S., Leach, F.S. et al. (1995) Mutations in DNA mismatch repair genes are not responsible for microsatellite instability in most sporadic endometrial carcinomas. *Cancer Res.* **55**:5556–5560.

92. Hangaishi, A., Ogawa, S., Mitani, K., Hosoya, N., Chiba, S., Yazaki, Y., and Hirai, H. (1997) Mutations and loss of expression of a mismatch repair gene, *hMLH1*, in leukemia and lymphoma cell lines. *Blood* **89**:1740–1747.

93. Markowitz, S., Wang, J., Myeroff, L., Parsons, R., Sun, L., Lutterbaugh, J., et al. (1995) Inactivation of the type II TGF-β receptor in colon cancer cells with microsatellite instability. *Science* **268**:1336–1338.

94. da Costa, L. T., Liu, B., el-Deiry, W., Hamilton, S. R., Kinzler, K. W., Vogelstein, B., et al. (1995) Polymerase d variants in RER+ colorectal tumors. *Nature Genet.* **9**:10–11.

95. Tateishi, M., Ishida, T., Hamatake, M., Fukuyama, Y., Kodono, S., Sugimachi, K., et al. (1994) DNA polymerase alpha as an independent prognostic parameter in non-small cell lung cancer: an immunohistochemical study. *Eur. J. Surg. Oncol.* **20**:461–466.

96. Wang, L., Patel, U., Ghosh, L., and Banerjee, S. (1992) DNA polymerase beta mutations in human colorectal cancer. *Cancer Res.* **52**:4824–4827.

97. Dobashi, Y., Shuin, T., Tsuruga, H., Uemura, H., Torigoe, S., and Kubota, Y. (1994) DNA polymerase β gene mutation in human prostate cancer. *Cancer Res.* **54**:2827–2829.

98. Moyzis, R. K., Buckingham, J. M., Cram, L. S., Dani, M., Deaven, L. L., Jones, M. D., et al. (1988) A highly conserved repetitive DNA sequence, (TTAGGG)$_n$, present at the telomeres of human chromosomes. *Proc. Natl. Acad. Sci. USA* **85**:6622–6626.

99. Harley, C. B., Futcher, A. B., and Greider, C. W. (1990) Telomeres shorten during aging of human fibroblasts. *Nature* **345**:458–460.

100. Hastie, N. D., Dempster, M., Dunlop, M. G., Thompson, A. M., Green, D. K., and Allshire, R. C. (1990) Telomere reduction in human colorectal carcinoma and with aging. *Nature* **346**:866–868.

101. de Lange, T. (1995) Telomere dynamics and genome instability in human cancer. *In: Telomeres* (Blackburn, E. H. and Greider, C. W., eds.), Cold Spring Harbor Laboratory Press, Cold Spring Harbor, NY, pp. 265–293.

102. Shay, J. W. (1995) Aging and cancer: are telomeres and telomerase the connection? *Mol. Med. Today* **1**:378–384.

103. Shay, J. W., and Wright, W. E. (1996) Telomerase activity in human cancer. *Curr. Opin. Oncol.* **8**:66–71.

104. Kim, N. W., Piatyszek, M. A., Prowse, K. R., Harley, C. B., West, M. D., Ho, P. L. C., et al. (1994) Specific association of human telomerase activity with immortal cells and cancer. *Science* **266**:2011–2015.

105. Feng, J., Funk, W. D., Wang, S. S., Weinrich, S. L., Avilion, A. A., Chiu, C. P., et al. (1995) The RNA component of human telomerase. *Science* **269**:1236–1241.

106. Nakamura, T. M., Morin, G. B., Chapman, K. B., Weinrich, S. L., Adrews, W. H., Lingner, J., et al. (1997) Telomerase catalytic subunit homologs from fission yeast and human. *Science* **277**:955–959.

107. Meyerson, M., Counter, C. M., Eaton, E. N., Ellisen, L. W., Steiner, P., Caddle, S. D., et al. (1997) hEST2, the putative human telomerase catalytic subunit gene, is up-regulated in tumor cells and during immortalization. *Cell* **90**:785–795.

108. Nakayama, J., Saito, M., Nakamura, H., Matsuura, A., and Ishikawa, F. (1997) TLP1: a gene encoding a protein component of mammalian telomerase is a novel member of WD repeats family. *Cell* **88**:875–884.

109. Broccoli, D., Smogorzewska, A., Chong, L., and de Lange, T. (1997) Human telomeres contain two distinct Myb-related proteins, TRF1 and TRF2. *Nature Genet.* **17**:231–235.

110. van Steensel, B., and de Lange, T. (1997) Control of telomere length by the human telomeric protein TRF1. *Nature* **385**:740–743.

111. Harley, C. B., and Sherwood, S. W. (1997) Telomerase, checkpoints and cancer. *Cancer Surv.* **29**:263–284.

112. Counter, C. M., Avilion, A. A., LeFeuvre, C. E., Stewart, N. G., Grider, C. W., Harley. C. B., et al. (1992) Telomere shortening associated with chromosome instability is arrested in immortal cells with express telomerase activity. *EMBO. J.* **11**:1921–1929.

113. Shay, J. W. and Bacchetti, S. (1997) A survey of telomerase activity in human cancer. *Eur. J. Cancer* **33**:787–91.

114. Hiyama, K., Ishioka, S., Shirotani, Y., Imai, K., Hiyama, E., Murakami, I., et al. (1995) Aleterations in telomric repeat length in lung cancer are associated with loss of heterozygosity in p53 and Rb. *Oncogene* **10**:937–944.

115. Ohyashiki, K., Ohyashiki, J. H., Iwama, H., Hayashi, S., Shay, J. W., and Toyama, K. (1996) Telomerase reactivation in leukemia cells. *Int. J. Oncol.* **8**:417–421.

116. Ohyashiki, K., Ohyashiki, J. H., Iwama, H., Hayashi, S., Shay, J. W., and Toyama, K. (1997) Telomerase activity and cytogenetic changes in chronic myeloid leukemia with disease progression. *Leukemia* **23**:190–194.

117. Ohyashiki, J. H., Ohyashiki, K., Fujimura, T., Kawakubo, K., Shimamoto, T., Iwabuchi, A., et al. (1994) Telomere shortening associated with disease evolution patterns in myelodysplastic syndromes. *Cancer Res.* **54**:3557–3560.

118. Hartwell, L. H. (1992) Defects in a cell cycle checkpoint may be responsible for the genomic instability of cancer cells. *Cell* **71**:543–546.

119. Hartwell, L. H. and Kastan, M. B. (1994) Cell cycle control and cancer. *Science* **266**:1821–1828.

120. Donehower, L. A., Harvey, M., Slagle, B. L., McArthur, M. J., Montgomery Jr, C. A., Butel, J. S., et al. (1992) Mice deficient for p53 are developmentally normal but susceptible to spontaneous tumours. *Nature* **356**:215–221.

121. Levine, A. J., Momand, J., and Finaly, C. A., (1991) The p53 tumor suppressor gene. *Nature* **351**:453–456.

122. Sturzbecher, H. W., Donzelmann, B., Henning, W., Knippschild, U., and Buchhop, S. (1996) p53 is linked directly to homologous recombination processes via RAD51/RecA protein interaction. *EMBO J.* **15**:1992–2002.

123. Cross, S. M., Sanche, C. A., Morgan, C. A., Schimke, M. K., Ramel, S., Idzerda, R. L., et al. (1995) A p53-dependent mouse spindle checkpoint. *Science* **267**:1353–1356.

124. Fukasawa, K., Choi, T., Kuriyama, R., Rulong, S., and van Woude, G. F. (1996) Abnormal centrosome amplification in the absence of p53. *Science* **271**:1744–1747.

125. Livingstone, L. R., White, A., Sprouse, J., Livanos, E., Jacks, T., and Tlsty, T. D. (1992) Altered cell cycle arrest and gene amplification potential accompany loss of wild-type p53. *Cell* **70**:923–935.

126. Yin, Y., Tainsky, M. A., Bischoff, F. Z., Strong, L. C., and Wahl, G. M. (1992) Wild-type p53 restores cell cycle control and inhibits gene amplification in cells with mutant p53 alleles. *Cell* **70**:937–948.

127. Shiloh, Y. (1997) Ataxia-telangiectasia and the Nijmegen breakage syndrome: related disorders but genes apart. *Ann. Rev. Genet.* **31**:635–662.

128. Taylor, A. M. R., Metcalfe, J. A., Thick, J., and Mak, Y.-F. (1996) Leukemia and lymphoma in ataxia telangiectasia. *Blood* **87**:423–438.

129. Savitsky, K., Bar-Shira, A., Gilad, S., Rotman, G., Ziv, Y., Vanagaite, L., et al. (1995) A single ataxia-telangiectasia gene with a product similar to PI-3 kinase. *Science* **268**:1749–1753.

130. Zakian, V. A. (1995) ATM-related genes: what do they tell us about functions of the human gene? *Cell* **82**:685–687.

131. Metcalfe, J. A., Parkhill, J., Campbell, L., Stacey, M., Biggs, P., Byrd, P. J., et al. (1996) Accelerated telomere shortening in ataxia telangiectasia. *Nature Genet.* **13**:350–353.

132. Smilenov, L. B., Morgan, S. E., Mellado, W., Sawant, S. G., Kastan, M. B., and Pandita, T. K. (1997) Influence of ATM function on telomere metabolism. *Oncogene* **15**:2659–2665.

8 Hereditary Cancer

BRUCE M. BOMAN, MD, PHD, LAEL MELCHERT, MS
AND JEREMY Z. FIELDS, PHD

INTRODUCTION

The purpose of this chapter is to provide a clearer understanding of contemporary problems in the field of hereditary cancer, particularly as they relate to mortality, and with the ultimate goals of stimulating needed research and of improving patient care. This will be done both by discussing general principles that apply to all hereditary cancers and by showing specific examples. There are several previous reviews (1–4) to which the reader is referred for detailed descriptions and discussions of specific hereditary-cancer syndromes. However, because the field is changing rapidly, one of the more reliable and comprehensive sources for accurate and current information on specific hereditary-cancer syndromes is the Internet (see the Online Mendelian Inheritance in Man at http://www.hgmp.mrc.ac.uk/omim/index.html).

Hereditary cancers are estimated to account for only 5–10% of all cancers. One of the most common of these is hereditary nonpolyposis colon cancer (HNPCC), which has an estimated frequency of 1 case per 200–300 individuals in the general population. Another common type is hereditary breast cancer (1 per 200 women). Though fewer in number than sporadic cancers, hereditary cancers represent an important health-care problem. These cancers represent over 50,000 new cases each year in the United States, and are just as lethal as sporadic cancers. Moreover, when these cancers are identified, other members of a patient's family can be warned regarding their own high risk for cancer development. Furthermore, affected individuals represent a high-risk group in which implementation of measures for cancer prevention may reduce mortality.

Research on hereditary-cancer syndromes has been remarkably useful in furthering our understanding of the molecular basis of how all cancers arise. For instance, hereditary-cancer families have provided reproducible models in which the consequences of a single inherited mutation can be studied. These

include abnormalities in cell-signaling pathways and in cell biology in general, acquisition of subsequent genetic mutations, and development of malignancies and metastases. One result of such studies has been the discovery that somatic mutations involving the same or a similar group of genes are responsible for initiating and promoting some sporadic cancers. For example, *APC* mutation is frequently found in sporadic colorectal cancer (CRC).

A few definitions will be helpful before discussing hereditary cancer. Cancer is a disease that develops by clonal expansion of a genetically altered cell that exhibits uncontrolled growth and other malignant behaviors (invasion and metastasis). Sporadic cancers represent a class of tumors that are caused by a cumulative series of somatic mutations that are acquired by a cell during the patient's lifetime. In contrast, hereditary cancer represents a class of tumors in which the first mutation in an identical or similar carcinogenic process is inherited. When a mutant allele is inherited, it is found in every cell of the body because it has been transmitted through the germline. Inheritance of a mutated allele of a cancer-susceptibility gene substantially increases an individual's predisposition to develop cancer.

Most hereditary-cancer traits involve an autosomal dominant mode of transmission from parent to child (Table 1). Despite the mutant gene being present in every cell in the body at birth, the newborn's tissues still usually appear histologically normal and most of the cells do not progress toward cancer. Nonetheless, in the majority of offspring who inherit such a trait, the probability is extremely high that at least one cell in the body will eventually acquire the aforementioned cumulative series of somatic genetic changes and become malignant. This carcinogenic process usually occurs in just one specific organ or a few tissue types, and the pattern of tumor types depend on the hereditary cancer syndrome.

In an individual with a germline mutation, the initial condition in all cells is the presence of one wild-type allele and one mutated allele, a state referred to as heterozygosity. During

From: *The Molecular Basis of Human Cancer* (W. B. Coleman and G. J. Tsongalis, eds.), © Humana Press Inc., Totowa, NJ.

Table 1
Summary of Selected Inherited Cancer Syndromes[a]

Syndrome	Primary tumor	Associated cancers or traits	Chromosomal location	Cloned gene	Proposed function of gene product
Dominant inheritance					
Familial Retinoblastoma	Retinoblastoma	Osteosarcoma	13q14.3	Rb1	Cell cycle and transcriptional regulation; E2F binding
Li-Fraumeni Syndrome	Sarcomas, Breast Cancer	Brain Tumors, Leukemia	17p13.1	*p53*	Transcription factor; Response to DNA damage and stress; Apoptosis
Familial Adenomatous Polyposis (FAP)	Colorectal Cancer	Colorectal Adenomas, Duodenal and Gastric Tumors, CHRPE, Jaw Osteomas and Desmoid Tumors (Gardner Syndrome), Medulloblastoma (Turcot Syndrome)	5q21	*APC*	Regulation of β-catenin; Microtubule binding
Hereditary Nonpolyposis Colorectal Cancer (HNPCC)	Colorectal Cancer	Endometrial, Ovarian, Hepatobiliary and Urinary Tract Cancer Glioblastoma (Turcot Syndrome)	*2p16* *3p21* 2q32 7p22	hMSH2 *hMLH1* *hPMS1* *hPMS2*	DNA mismatch repair
Neurofibromatosis Type 1 (NF1)	Neurofibromas	Neurofibrosarcoma, AML, Brain Tumors	17q11.2	*NF1*	GAP for p21 c-ras proteins; Microtubule binding?
Neurofibromatosis Type 2 (NF2)	Acoustic Neuromas Meningiomas	Gliomas, Ependymomas	22q12.2	*NF2*	Links membrane proteins to cytoskeleton?
Wilms Tumor	Wilms Tumor	WAGR (Wilms, Aniridia, Genitourinary Abnormalities, Mental Retardation)	11p13	*WT1*	Transcriptional repressor
Beckwith-Wiedmann Syndrome (BWS)	Wilms Tumor	Organomegaly, Hemi-hypertrophy, Hepatoblastoma, Adrenocortical Cancer	11p15	*p57[KIP2]* Others? Contiguous Gene disorder	Cell cycle regulator
Nevoid Basal Cell Carcinoma Syndrome (NBCCS)	Basal Cell Skin Cancer	Jaw Cysts, Palmar and Plantar Pits, Medullo-blastomas, Ovarian Fibromas	9q22.3	*PTCH*	Transmembrane receptor for hedgehog signaling molecule
Familial Breast Cancer 1	Breast Cancer	Ovarian Cancer	17q21	*BRCA1*	Interacts with Rad51 protein, Repair of double-strand breaks
Familial Breast Cancer 2	Breast Cancer	Male Breast Cancer, Pancreatic Cancer, Others? (Ovarian)	13q12	*BRCA2*	Interacts with Rad51 protein, Repair of double-strand breaks
Von Hippel-Lindau Syndrome (VHL)	Renal Cancer (Clear Cell)	Pheochromocytomas, Retinal Angiomas, Hemangioblastomas	*3q25*	VHL	Regulates transcriptional elongation by RNA polymerase II?
Herediatary Papillary Renal Cancer (HPRC)	Renal Cancer (Papillary Type)	Other Cancers?	7q31	*c-met*	Transmembrane receptor for HGF
Familial Melanoma	Melanoma	Pancreatic Cancer, Dysplastic Nevi, Atypical Moles	9p21 12q13 Others?	*p16[INK4A]* *cdk4*	Inhibitor of cdk4 and cdk6 Cyclin-dependent kinase
Multiple Endocrine Neoplasia Type 1 (MEN1)	Pancreatic Islet Cell Cancer	Parathyroid Hyperplasia Pituitary Adenomas	11q13	*MEN1*	Unknown
Multiple Endocrine Neoplasia Type 2 (MEN2)	Medullary Thyroid Cancer	Type 2A Pheochromocytoma, Parathyroid Hyperplasia Type 2B Pheochromocytoma, Mucosal Hamartoma, Familial Medullary Thyroid Cancer	10q11.2	*c-ret*	Transmembrane receptor tyrosine kinase for GDNF

Table 1 (*Continued*)

Syndrome	Primary tumor	Associated cancers or traits	Chromosomal location	Cloned gene	Proposed function of gene product
Multiple Exostoses	Exostoses (Cartilaginous Protuberances on Bones)	Chondrosarcoma	8q24.1 11p11-p13 19p	EXT1 EXT2 EXT3	Unknown Unknown Unknown
Cowden Disease	Breast Cancer, Thyroid Cancer (Follicular Type)	Intestinal Hamartomous Polyps, Skin Lesions	10q23	PTEN	Dual-specificity phosphatase with similarity to tensin
Hereditary Prostate Cancer	Prostate Cancer	Unknown	1q25 Others?	Unknown	Unknown
Palmoplantar Keratoderma	Esophageal Cancer	Leukoplakia	17q25	Unknown	Unknown
Recessive Inheritance					
Ataxia Telangiectasia	Lymphoma	Cerebellar Ataxia, Immunodeficiency, Breast Cancer in Heterozygotes?	11q22	ATM	DNA Repair, Induction of p53
Bloom Syndrome	Solid Tumors	Immunodeficiency, Small Stature	15q26.1	BLM	DNA helicase?
Xeroderma Pigmentosum	Skin Cancer	Pigmentation Abnormalities Hypogonadism	Multiple Complementation Groups	XPB XPA	DNA repair helicases, XPD nucleotide excision repair
Fanconi Anemia	AML	Pancytopenia, Skeletal Abnormalities	9q22.3 16q24.3 Two Others?	FACC FACA	DNA repair? DNA repair?

[a]Adapted from Fearon (3), with permission from the American Association for the Advancement of Science.

carcinogenesis, the next genetic change acquired by a cell often involves loss of the remaining wild-type allele at that same cancer-susceptibility locus (this is the second step in Knudson's well-known two-hit hypothesis). This loss of heterozygosity (LOH), followed by the acquisition of still other mutations, ultimately leads to the loss of that cell's ability to control its growth and the development of a malignant state. A cancer can then form through clonal expansion (cellular replication) of such a malignant cell and the daughter cells produced will also contain this array of genetic alterations.

When a sporadic cancer develops, a single cell in the body will sequentially acquire all of the carcinogenic mutations including the first (initiating) genetic alteration. A similar process occurs in the development of a hereditary cancer, that is, a single cell acquires additional somatic mutations in the process of becoming malignant. A critical difference in the individual carrying the hereditary-cancer trait is that there is a much higher probability of malignancy, perhaps an order of magnitude or more. Because of the presence of a germline mutation, these patients also exhibit a much higher probability for multiple primary malignancies.

In accordance with the aforementioned theoretical background, real-life diagnosis of a cancer as a hereditary cancer has traditionally been based on a combination of the following: 1) clinical information about the patient (cancer type, age at diagnosis), and 2) a carefully obtained family history showing a pattern of inheritance of tissue-specific cancers that is consistent with Mendelian genetics. Clinical diagnosis of hereditary cancer relies on the fact that the typical cancers in any given hereditary-cancer syndrome involve the same organ sites in multiple individuals, both within a single family, and among different families. Hence, cancer patients that have a family history of a similar cancer phenotype tend to be grouped into a single hereditary-cancer diagnosis. Similarly, individuals whose cancer syndromes exhibit comparable characteristics (premonitory signs, early age of onset) are also assumed to be affected with the same hereditary trait.

With today's advances in molecular genetics, especially DNA sequencing, it has become possible, at least in some cases, to confirm definitively the presence of a hereditary-cancer trait. These molecular diagnoses are based on techniques that identify a specific DNA mutation in the gene that is believed to be the causal cancer-susceptibility gene for the hereditary cancer. A cancer-susceptibility gene refers to a mutated gene that: 1) is transmitted through the germline to offspring in successive generations, 2) causes expression of a mutated gene product (protein), and 3) is the initiating event of a carcinogenic process that results in a malignancy or that renders the individual more susceptible to development of such a malignancy. In contrast, a diagnosis of sporadic cancer is the appropriate clinical conclusion reached when: 1) there is no history of the same site-specific cancer in any two generations involving siblings, offspring, parents, aunts, uncles, or either set of grandparents; 2) there are no other indicators of hereditary cancer (premonitory signs, cancer phenotype, age of onset); and 3) no germline mutation is known or suspected.

Familial cancer is a term used to indicate a type of cancer that is associated with a family history that includes one or more first or second-degree relatives with the same site-specific cancer, but that has not been shown to meet the diagnostic criteria for hereditary cancer. At the molecular level, its origin is unclear. Nevertheless, epidemiologic studies have clearly shown that unaffected individuals (those in whom cancer has not yet developed) in families diagnosed with familial cancer are at substantially increased risk for developing that cancer, and the risk increases as the number of first or second-degree relatives with cancer increases. For example, the lifetime risk for CRC in a family identified as having familial CRC varies between 1.5 and 6-fold depending upon the prevalence of CRC in the family (2).

To accurately identify hereditary cancer, a physician should carefully construct a nuclear pedigree (technically, a modified nuclear pedigree). This is a simple diagram that not only outlines a family tree, but also, includes specific information about the members of that kindred. Important information includes any diagnosis of cancer, cancer type and site, age at cancer diagnosis, age at death, cause of death, presence of bilateral or multiple cancers, and presence of any precursor lesions (e.g., adenomatous polyps). In taking a cancer family history, it is best to obtain at least a three-generation history. For diagnosis, the critical family members include all of the patient's first-degree relatives (siblings, offspring, and parents), second-degree relatives (aunts, uncles, and grandparents), and cousins. Other relatives, especially the second-degree relatives, often provide important genetic information because they are usually older and beyond the age of highest cancer risk. The pedigree is valuable for making medical evaluations and recommendations including: 1) patient and family risk assessment; 2) need for verification of cancer diagnosis in family members by requesting medical records; 3) indications for genetic counseling, testing, surveillance, and management; and 4) eligibility for research protocols.

Unfortunately, during the physician's medical work-up of cancer patients, a family history of cancer is often the most neglected aspect of the history and physical. This is unfortunate because diagnosis of a hereditary cancer usually depends on gathering detailed information about both affected and unaffected relatives. Essential information to obtain about affected relatives includes: type and location of primary cancer, age at diagnosis, the current age or the age at and cause of death, tumor stage, occurrence of synchronous and metachronous cancers, possible environmental exposures, ethnic background, and race. Information to obtain about unaffected relatives includes: current age or age at and cause of death, current and past health problems, and phenotypic signs of cancer syndromes or precursor lesions (such as adenomatous polyps). Information about family members who have not had cancer is helpful when interpreting a pedigree for several reasons: 1) the absence of cancer in an older generation indicates it is less likely that a cancer-predisposing mutation has been transmitted, and 2) any associated physical findings may help diagnosis when a particular hereditary cancer is suspected. For example, mucocutaneous lesions and macrocephaly in a family member may expand a differential diagnosis to include Cowden's disease, a syndrome associated with an increased risk for breast, thyroid, and other cancers.

Although the aforementioned clinical and genetic aspects of cancers provide a useful basis for their classification, important variations can arise. For instance, in any given population of cancer patients, tumors that have a similar phenotype may have acquired a nonidentical series of genetic mutations (genotypic variability). Even in cases of hereditary cancer displaying a similar phenotype, germline mutations may exist at entirely different chromosomal loci. Conversely, in any given population of patients that have an identical genotype, there can still be great variability in the phenotype, including differences in the pattern of expression of the cancer types that occur in a given hereditary-cancer syndrome, and even diversity in whether cancer is expressed at all. This variability is due to a host of genetic, environmental, and other factors that can influence whether any given germline or somatic mutation is eventually expressed in one of the body's tissues as a malignancy. Indeed, this variability complicates the ability of physicians to interpret clinical and research data. However, at the same time it suggests that carcinogenesis is not unchangeable, and that development of novel strategies that modify this pathogenic process should be vigorously pursued.

TYPES OF HEREDITARY CANCER

There are over 20 known hereditary-cancer syndromes (3). The characteristics of several of these syndromes are summarized in Table 1, which includes information about the primary tumor, associated cancers or traits, chromosomal location of the germline mutation, the name of the cloned gene, and the proposed function of the gene product. Identification of an individual, through family history, phenotypic features, and gene tests, as belonging to a hereditary-cancer family provides useful information regarding that person's increased relative risk for that cancer. This identification is important because penetrance is high for most hereditary cancers and this has immediate bearing on the management of the problem by the clinician and on decisions to be made by the patient. It is also important because it provides, as noted, key insights into the molecular etiology of each cancer type and suggests starting points for researchers who are trying to develop treatments based on these insights.

Because identifying a mutation in a cancer-susceptibility gene is so important, a number of strategies have been developed by cancer researchers to successfully isolate and clone cancer-susceptibility genes. Such molecular genetic studies often rely, at least initially, on having well-defined hereditary models (kindreds) for study. Thus, it has been of critical importance to establish clear criteria that allow recognition of families and individuals at risk for a particular inherited-cancer syndrome. For example, in research studies, it is best to find and study large families where multiple members are affected across two or more generations. One confounding factor that can occur, especially when dealing with heritable forms of the more common cancers (colon, breast, lung), is that sporadic cancer can occur in the same organ in some members of a hereditary cancer family.

Table 2
Classification of Inherited Cancer Genes

Class	Gene	Syndrome
Genes involving positive (oncogenes) or negative signaling (tumor-suppressor genes)		
Tumor-suppressor genes	*Rb1*	Hereditary retinoblastoma (Rb)
	p53	Li-Fraumeni syndrome
	APC	Familial Adenomatous Polyposis (FAP)
	NF1	Neurofibromatosis 1 (NF1)
	NF2	Neurofibromatosis 2 (NF2)
	WT1	Wilms tumor
	PTCH	Nevoid basal cell carcinoma
	BRCA1[a]	Hereditary breast cancer 1
	BRCA2[a]	Hereditary breast cancer 2
	VHL	Von Hippel-Lindau (VHL) syndrome
	p16^{INK4A}	Familial melanoma
	MEN1	Multiple endocrine neoplasia type 1 (MEN1)
Proto-oncogenes	c-*met*	Hereditary papillary renal cancer
	c-*ret*	Multiple endocrine neoplasia type 2 (MEN2)
	SMAD4/DPC4	Juvenile polyposis
	PTEN	Cowdon
	STK11/LKB1	Peutz-Jeghans (PJS)
	CDH1	Hereditary diffuse gastric cancer (HDGC)
Genes involved in genetic stability		
DNA mismatch repair	*hMSH2*	Hereditary nonpolyposis colon cancer
	hMLH1	(HNPCC)
	hPMS1	
	hPMS2	
	hMSH6	
Nucleotide excision repair	*XPB*	Xeroderma pigmentosum
	XPD	
	XPA	
Other DNA repair genes	*ATM*	Ataxia telangiectasia (AT)
	BLM	Bloom's syndrome
	FACC,	Fanconi's anemia
	FACA	

[a]*BRCA1* and *BRCA2* may serve in genetic stability as well.

LESSONS LEARNED ABOUT CANCER AND CELL BIOLOGY FROM STUDYING HEREDITARY CANCERS

Research on hereditary cancers has provided a window to further our understanding of the origins (especially the molecular etiology) and mechanisms of carcinogenesis. For example, from studies of hereditary-cancer syndromes we now know much more about cellular signaling pathways that are disrupted by various mutant genes, and we are able to identify members of two classes of cancer-related genes that regulate cell growth, oncogenes, and tumor-suppressor genes. Kinzler and Vogelstein *(4)* call these gatekeeper genes, because they directly regulate the growth of tumors. For example, wild-type (not mutated) tumor-suppressor genes inhibit cell growth or promote apoptosis. Another class of cancer-related genes involves those that maintain the stability and fidelity of replication of the genome. These genes are referred to as caretakers *(4)* because they modify genetic stability. Table 2 lists the currently known genes of each of the aforementioned classes.

A proto-oncogene is a gene that, when its function is activated through mutation, promotes cell growth and/or leads to

cancer. Among the most well-known proto-oncogenes are members of the c-*ras* family and the c-*myc* family of genes. Although most mutations in proto-oncogenes are not inherited, a few proto-oncogenes are responsible for hereditary-cancer syndromes (they can be inherited) and are thus classified as cancer-susceptibility genes. For example, c-*ret* is an oncogene associated with the inherited predisposition to multiple endocrine neoplasia 2 (MEN2), and familial medullary thyroid cancer. c-*met* is a proto-oncogene associated with hereditary papillary renal carcinoma syndrome. Proto-oncogenes are genes that, when mutated, cause a gain-of-function, and it appears that only a single allele of the gene needs to be mutated to gain that function. In contrast, for tumor-suppressor genes, it appears that it is necessary that both wild-type alleles are lost in order for a cancer to develop. Indeed, the protein product of even a single, wild-type tumor-suppressor gene allele is usually sufficient to suppress cell proliferation and inhibit carcinogenesis.

Another class of genes responsible for hereditary cancer that usually requires loss of both wild-type alleles is the class that involves inactivation of proteins associated with maintaining genetic stability. This can lead to genetic instability, additional

Table 3
Genotype/Phenotype Relationships in FAP

Phenotype	Region containing the germline mutation (codon)
Attenuated polyposis (AFAP)	Before 157 or After ~1800
Classical polyposis	169–1606
Profuse polyps (>5000 adenomas)	1255–1467
CHRPE[a]	463–1387
Gardner syndrome (including desmoids)	1403–1578

[a]Congenital hypertrophy of the retinal-pigment epithelium.

mutations, and ultimately tumor development. An example is the family of DNA mismatch-repair (MMR) genes (Table 2). Inherited MMR mutations are thought to be responsible for development of the majority of cases of hereditary CRC. When any one of these genes is inactivated (by mutation of both alleles), genetic instability and promotion of carcinogenesis results.

Studies of hereditary-cancer syndromes have yielded important information about the role of allelic variations and modifier genes in cancer development (3). Familial adenomatous polyposis (FAP) is an example of a hereditary-cancer syndrome in which allelic variations can lead to diversity in the phenotype. This phenotypic variability corresponds to differences in the location of the mutation (different codons) within the *APC* gene (Table 3). In FAP, the vast majority of germline *APC* mutations occur at different sites in the 5′-part of the gene and encode truncated proteins in which varying lengths of the carboxyl-terminal portion are deleted. These mutations invariably result in adenomatous polyps (although polyposis is variant) and subsequently CRC. However, differences in the nature of the DNA mutation within the *APC* gene contribute to variations in the tumor spectrum of extracolonic cancers and in expressions of the polyposis phenotype. For example, individuals with Gardner syndrome not only have polyposis but also tend to have extracolonic lesions, such as desmoid tumors and osteomas. This variant is associated with *APC* mutations that occur between codons 1403 and 1578. Another variant phenotype results from mutations between *APC* codons 463 and 1387, and shows congenital hypertrophy of the retinal-pigment epithelium, a nonmalignant retinal lesion. Yet other variant forms result from mutations upstream of codon 160 and downstream of codon 1800, and these show attenuated forms (flat adenomas or fewer polyps) of polyposis (5–7).

Even when individuals have the same mutation in an *APC* allele, phenotypic differences can occur. For example, identical *APC* germline mutations have been found in three distinct groups of patients, including 1) those with only intestinal polyposis, 2) those with Gardner syndrome, and 3) those with polyposis and medulloblastoma (8). This finding and other evidence (incomplete penetrance) strongly supports the idea that other factors modify the expressivity of hereditary-cancer traits. One such factor is the activity of modifier genes. An example of a modifier gene is *Mom-1*, which stands for "modifier of *Min*." *Min* is a *mouse* genetic model of FAP caused by a germline *APC* mutation. Although different inbred strains of mice all have the same *Min* mutation, the phenotype varies depending on variations in *Mom-1* and one such phenotypic variation is the number of colonic polyps. *Mom-1* has been found to encode a secretory type II phospholipase A2 protein (9–12). Other modifier genes that affect FAP expressivity also code for enzymes (13,14). These findings are consistent with the observation that a single mutation is usually not sufficient for complete carcinogenesis, most cancers require additional genetic changes.

The likelihood that an individual who carries a hereditary-cancer trait will develop the expected cancer for that genotype (the penetrance of the inherited cancer trait) can also vary with environmental, dietary, and lifestyle factors, although these interactions are less well-defined. Because predisposition to HNPCC and other hereditary-cancer syndromes (Tables 1 and 2) has been shown to be associated with genetic instability, it is not unreasonable to think that certain proto-oncogenes and tumor-suppressor genes in HNPCC-affected individuals would be more likely to undergo mutation in response to environmental carcinogens (dietary factors, toxins, pollutants) and would be more likely to remain unrepaired in such repair-deficient cells. In HNPCC, inactivation of an MMR gene (both alleles) is associated with increased mutation rates for other genes by two to three orders of magnitude. Indeed, it has been hypothesized that the multi-step carcinogenic pathway leading to CRC may be promoted by MMR mutations that increase the mutation rate of other genes in the pathway (15). For example, mutations in the *APC* gene and in the TGFβ receptor type II (*TGFβRII*) gene have been found to occur in cancer cells that have MMR defects (16,17). Another example is that in some Japanese hereditary-cancer families, the spectrum of expressed cancers has shifted during the last century from gastric cancers to those cancers (like CRC) occurring frequently in HNPCC (15). Gastric carcinoma in Japan is a disease that is widely thought to be modified by environmental factors, particularly dietary factors. Hence, recent changes toward a more Western type of dietary intake in Japan may be affecting the type of cancer expressed in Japanese hereditary-cancer families. In the instance of an inherited mutation involving another DNA-repair gene, *ATM* (Table 2), there is evidence that individuals with ataxia telangiectasia (AT) are at increased risk of cancer from exposure to ionizing radiation. An estimated 0.5–1% of the general population who are *ATM* heterozygotes have a five-fold increased risk for breast cancer, which may account for 3.8–18% of sporadic breast-cancer cases in the United States (18). A more recent study showed a heterozygous *ATM* mutation in 2/401 (0.5%) women with early onset of breast cancer compared to 2/202 (1%) of healthy controls (19). Because heterozygous *ATM* mutations do not tend to occur in early-onset breast cancer, this suggests that they mainly result in a genetic predisposition for later-onset breast cancer.

Yet another benefit from studying inherited cancer-susceptibility genes is a recognition of the role of mutations and their mutant proteins in sporadic cancers and an increased understanding of the function that the normal protein from the wild-type gene plays in the biology of a given cell type. For example, mutations in the *APC* gene are responsible for initiation of FAP. An added benefit of studies that led to this finding was the realization that *APC* mutations are probably responsible for initiating many or most cases of sporadic CRC as well. Indeed, mutations in the *APC* gene have been found in tumor tissues from most cases (>70%) of sporadic CRC. Moreover, the identification of the *APC* gene as being implicated in CRC has resulted in many studies that have begun to reveal cellular roles for the wild-type APC protein. In particular, the APC protein is now thought to serve a growth-suppressing function in colonocytes. This seems to occur through the interactions of APC with intracellular signaling cascades involving APC binding to β-catenin *(20,21),* microtubules *(22–24),* and other proteins.

Thus, research on hereditary-cancer syndromes has been fruitful in a variety of ways. It has led to the discovery of the functions of genes responsible for hereditary cancers. It has led to insights into sporadic CRC such as the multi-step genetic alterations necessary for development of malignancies. It has taught us that there are striking similarities between sporadic cancers and hereditary cancers with regard to genetic mutations and cellular mechanisms. It has helped us understand variability, due to allelic variations and modifier genes, in the tumor-phenotype spectrum in seemingly identical hereditary-cancer genotypes. And all this has led to a greater appreciation that cancer, both hereditary and sporadic, requires and is modified by a complex spectrum of factors. This complexity indicates that hereditary and sporadic cancer development may be less an inevitable consequence of a relentless (auto-catalytic) process initiated by a single allelic mutation, and more the cumulative breakdown, over time, in the defense and repair systems of the body due to both multiple genetic and multiple environmental/lifestyle factors. Much of modern cancer research is based on the hope that at least some of these factors and their associated processes are modifiable either through treatment or prevention.

DIAGNOSIS AND MANAGEMENT OF HEREDITARY-CANCER SYNDROMES

This section will discuss several general issues in the diagnosis and management of hereditary cancer, including: 1) factors that affect the clinician's ability to diagnosis hereditary cancer (penetrance, expressivity, and the nature of the genetic mutation), 2) gene testing (methods of DNA testing, which hereditary-cancer syndromes should have gene testing, and general principles of gene testing), and 3) principles in the diagnosis and management of hereditary cancer. We will then describe the application of these principles in the diagnosis and management of hereditary cancers using prototype models, drawn from the basic and clinical literature on hereditary CRC (FAP, HNPCC).

FACTORS THAT AFFECT THE ABILITY TO DETECT AND DIAGNOSE HEREDITARY CANCER

Penetrance Penetrance is defined as the fraction of individuals with a given genotype (genetic trait) who manifest the expected phenotype *(25).* When the frequency of manifestation of a phenotype is less than 100%, the trait is said to exhibit reduced penetrance. In an individual who has a genotype that characteristically produces an abnormal phenotype but who is phenotypically normal, the trait is said to be nonpenetrant *(26).* The length of time it takes for expression of the phenotype to occur, or whether expression of the phenotype occurs at all

during the lifetime of an individual who carries the genetic trait, often depends on a variety of factors. First, the inherited mutation is typically a mutation in only one of the two alleles of a given gene. However, theoretical considerations and empirical findings suggest that loss of function of both alleles has to occur. This suggestion is consistent with Knudson's two hit hypothesis *(27,28).* Moreover, in many cancer syndromes, such as ones involving the colon and breast, for cells to develop into malignancies, mutations have to occur in several additional genes *(29,30).* The two-hit hypothesis appears to be more applicable to loss of tumor-suppressor genes than to activation of proto-oncogenes *(31)* where loss of a single allele may suffice. This hypothesis also explains why individuals harboring a cancer-susceptibility gene mutation have a higher cancer risk than those who do not. Thus, if the probability of loss of a single allele in a single cell is 1 in 100,000 (1×10^{-5}), then the probability that both alleles will mutate depends on the probability of two hits occurring in that same cell. This probability is the product of the two individual probabilities: $(1 \times 10^{-5}) \times (1 \times 10^{-5})$ which is (1×10^{-10}). However, in the germline carrier, the first hit already exists in every cell (probability = 1) and the total probability is therefore $(1) \times (10^{-5})$ which is (1×10^{-5}). In other words, the probability that the second hit will occur in carriers of a hereditary-cancer trait is increased 100,000-fold, and it is therefore not surprising that penetrance is high for most hereditary-cancer syndromes.

Incomplete penetrance occurs for a variety of reasons, but the earliest and simplest reason is that a person who has inherited a mutant tumor-suppressor allele fails to acquire a mutation at the second allele. Penetrance would be reduced in a similar fashion if an individual with a germline mutation for a hereditary-cancer syndrome acquires the second hit, but then fails to acquire any of the additional somatic mutations that are needed for the development of a malignant tumor. Reduced penetrance would also be observed if the progression to malignancy was slowed by temporal variations in environmental conditions, especially conditions that influence the carcinogenic process or the survival of transformed cells (chemical carcinogens, radiation, diet, immune modulators, and stressors). Biochemical consequences of these external agents might include increased presence of or reduced detoxification of carcinogens (high animal fat-content diet, slow acetylators), activation of mutagen precursors, and incomplete DNA repair (e.g., MMR defects in HNPCC).

Expressivity Expressivity is a term that refers to the range of phenotypes expressed by individuals with a given genotype under any given set of environmental conditions, or over a range of environmental conditions *(32).* In a germline carrier, a hereditary-cancer trait with highly variable expressivity may range in expression from mild to severe disease *(26),* or the phenotype may vary in terms of the age of onset or in the spectrum of cancers *(25).* Two additional factors that can modulate expressivity are: 1) the status and activity of modifier genes and 2) allelic variations. An example of widely varying expressivity is the FAP syndrome (Table 3).

Nature of the Mutation Several factors relating to the nature of mutations in cancer-predisposing genes affect our ability to diagnose hereditary-cancer patients. First, the num-

Table 4
A Comparison of Two Types of Hereditary Breast Cancer[a]

Characteristic	Hereditary Breast Cancer 1	Hereditary Breast Cancer 2
Germline mutation	BRCA1	BRCA2
Mode of transmission	Autosomal dominant	Autosomal dominant
Gene function	Tumor-suppressor gene[b]	Tumor-suppressor gene[b]
Median age at diagnosis	45–50 yr	55 yr
Penetrance (breast cancer)	36–87%	37–80%
Bilateral breast cancer	Frequent	Frequent
Ovarian cancer	Frequent	Occasional
Male breast cancer	Uncommon	Occasional (6–9%)
Nonmammary cancers showing increased incidence	Colon and prostate cancer	Gastric, prostate, biliary cancers, and melanoma

[a]From Marcus et al. (115), and Garber (133).
[b]BRCA1 and BRCA2 may serve in genetic stability as well.

ber of genes that can give rise to a particular hereditary-cancer trait is important. For example, the only known germline mutation involved in FAP is *APC*. In contrast, in HNPCC, there are five known genes (*hMSH2, hMLH1, hPMS1, hPMS2,* and *hMSH6* (also known as *GTBP*), that each can be responsible for this hereditary syndrome (Table 2). In the case of hereditary breast cancer (Table 4), the *BRCA1* and *BRCA2* genes have been found to be mutated in hereditary breast-cancer families *(33–35)*. Moreover, in hereditary breast cancer and HNPCC there may be other cancer-inducing genes because mutations in the known loci can be found in only 70% of these hereditary-cancer families. For example, germline mutation in the *TGFβRII* has been shown to account for one HNPCC family *(36)*. Indeed, in those syndromes that are initiated by just one inherited cancer susceptibility gene, it is easier to detect germline mutations compared to the syndromes that involve multiple genes.

Other Factors Affect Gene Testing Cancer-susceptibility genes that exhibit mutational hotspots are much more easily screened for germline mutations. Thus, in Li-Fraumeni kindreds, most p53 mutations occur in exons 5–8 with mutational hotspots at codons 175, 245, 248, and 273. Moreover, in certain populations, specific mutations in a cancer-susceptibility gene often occur with high frequency, which facilitates gene testing. The frequent presence of specific mutations in a cancer-susceptibility gene in certain populations likely originates because of a *founder effect*. A founder effect is defined as the occurrence of one or more mutations at increased frequency in a population because of the presence of the mutation (by chance) in the ancestral founders of the population *(37)*. For example, three mutations in hereditary breast cancer, *BRCA1* (185delAG and 5382insC) and *BRCA2* (6174delT) have been found to occur frequently in Ashkenazi Jews. Another example is the frequent occurrence of HNPCC in the Navajo Native American Indian population *(38)* and this was discovered to be due to a founder *hMLH1* mutation (Dr. Henry Lynch, personal communication). Indeed, founder mutations involving *hMLH1* have been identified in Finnish, English, and Korean HNPCC kindreds. Those involving *BRCA1* have been found in Scandinavian, Eastern European, and Russian hereditary breast-cancer kindreds. Clearly, knowing the specific mutation occurring

in certain populations greatly facilitates our ability to screen for cancer-susceptibility genes.

The type of mutation can also make a difference in gene testing. For example, the mutational type in some cancer-susceptibility genes involves a change that generates a new stop codon, resulting in truncation of the gene product. Such mutational types that can cause protein truncation include frame-shifts, nonsense mutations (premature stop signal), and splice-site mutations. These protein-truncation-causing mutations can be readily detected by the protein truncation test (PTT) *(39)* that is also called the in vitro synthesized protein assay (IVSP). Cancer-susceptibility genes in which frequent germline mutations occur that cause protein truncation and that are detectable by the PTT assay include *APC, NF1, NF2, BRCA1, BRCA2, hMSH2, hMLH1, ATM, FACC,* and *FACA (40)*. Other mutation types such as missense mutations (single base-pair substitution) pose a greater diagnostic challenge. In this case, it is often a diagnostic dilemma to determine whether the missense mutation is responsible for the inherited syndrome or if it is simply a normal polymorphism found in the general population. Other mutations can involve genomic rearrangement of the promoter or enhancer regions that alter gene expression, intron/exon splice sites, and those in the polyA tail that influence mRNA stability and that ultimately result in reduction in protein levels.

In order to screen for mutations in these cancer-susceptibility genes, various molecular techniques have been developed. In those hereditary-cancer families that have been shown, through molecular testing, to have a specific mutation in an inherited cancer-susceptibility gene, it becomes relatively easy to test at-risk family members for the same germline mutation. This can provide beneficial information to both those family members who test negative as well as those who test positive.

Genetic tests detect changes in DNA sequence. A causal association between a gene and hereditary trait is based on a positive correlation between the presence of the altered gene and the presence of the phenotype. However, there can be a great deal of normal variation (polymorphism) in the DNA sequence of a given gene in a population. For example, a single missense DNA change in *BRCA1* can be a nondisease-causing polymorphism, or variant of unknown significance, or a highly penetrant cancer-susceptibility mutation. Therefore, these variations in DNA sequence should not be considered to be mutations unless they are associated with negative consequences (such as loss of function or a disease phenotype). Thus, the notion of a normal (wild-type) gene should be afforded a wider definition than that of a single (fixed) DNA sequence. A gene (allele) must also be considered in the context of the diploid nature of cells with each allele being composed of two potentially different DNA sequences, each of which codes for a similar yet variable protein and resultant phenotype. Moreover, a given base pair sequence does not necessarily predict the way a trait will be manifested. For example, individuals with the same DNA sequence can have different clinical manifestations, or none at all (variable penetrance), and even a given individual can have different constellations of clinical signs at different times. For example, there is a T→A substitution at nucleotide 3920 in the *APC* gene, the I1307K polymorphism, which appears to create a hypermutable region resulting in a familial colon cancer syndrome. In a study by Laken et al. *(41)*, the I1307K allele was present in 28% of Ashkenazi Jewish individuals with a family history of colorectal cancer, and was present in 6% of all Ashkenazi Jews. This substitution creates an 8 nucleotide polyA tract in place of the AAATAAAA sequence that is normally present. The polymorphism does not directly affect the function of the *APC* gene, but may render the DNA susceptible to errors in replication, thereby creating new mutations that can lead to loss of gene function. Therefore, individuals who carry the I1307K polymorphism may develop cancer at a slightly higher rate than those with normal *APC* genes. More recent studies have reported conflicting findings with some supporting the hypothesis that the I1307K mutation increases CRC risk (42–46), whereas the observations from other studies (47–50) have not supported this role for I1307K.

GENE TESTING

Identification and Isolation of Cancer-Susceptibility Genes
For an updated list of cloned human genes, the reader is referred to the NIH database on the Internet at http://www.ncbi.nlm.nih.gov/dbEST/dbEST_genes. Two key steps that have led to the identification of cancer susceptibility genes and the nature of genetic alterations in these genes are: 1) mapping of a cancer susceptibility gene to a particular chromosome, and 2) cloning the gene and determining its precise sequence in order to identify both the location of the mutations within the gene and the type of mutations (e.g. substitution, deletion). A technique that has been used for chromosome localization for quite some time is linkage analysis. This is best accomplished using large, multi-generation families and it works well for mapping rare alleles that cause highly penetrant Mendelian cancer syndromes. The goal is to show statistically that a given genetic marker (polymorphism) located on a particular chromosome co-segregates with a particular disease phenotype, such as cancer. Limitations of linkage analysis *(3)* include variable penetrance, phenocopies, genetic heterogeneity, and other pitfalls. Karyotypic aberrations and allelic LOH can also yield clues regarding the possible chromosome localization of hereditary cancer genes *(51–57)*.

Several strategies have been used for isolating cancer-susceptibility genes. One technique is representational difference analysis, which is a combination of subtraction hybridization and cloning methods to isolate a specific DNA deletion. To date, this technology has aided in the cloning of inherited cancer genes such as the hereditary breast-cancer gene (*BRCA2*) at chromosome 13q12 *(34)*. A second technique, positional candidate gene cloning, has also been used based on strategies aiming to locate the position of a disease-causing gene. For example, the major susceptibility genes for MEN2 (c-*ret*), and hereditary papillary renal carcinoma (c-*met*) were characterized by classical positional cloning techniques *(58–63)*. A third technique, comparative genomic hybridization (CGH) was employed in studies aimed at the localization of the *STK11/LKB1* gene responsible for Peutz-Jeghers syndrome *(64–66)*. Functional approaches have proven useful in isolation of the genes responsible for HNPCC *(3,67,68)*. In this case, the human homologs of known bacteria and yeast genes (*mutL* and *mutS*), which have a role in DNA mismatch repair, were found to be the inherited mutated genes responsible for HNPCC.

General Principles of Gene Testing Currently accepted indications for gene testing are based on clinical criteria that identify those individuals who are at increased risk for hereditary cancer (enhanced likelihood of carrying a mutation in a cancer-susceptibility gene). Two clinical situations today commonly trigger the decision to conduct gene testing. One situation occurs when a patient with cancer is tested in order to determine whether he or she has a hereditary cancer. In this case, the clinical indications for testing usually rely on a positive family history, clinical information such as young age at cancer diagnosis, or presence of clinical signs suggesting hereditary cancer. Cancer patients can benefit from a cancer-susceptibility gene test if a positive or negative result will change their medical management or reduce risk for additional primary cancers through preventive approaches. The other situation involves testing individuals who have not been diagnosed with cancer, but may be predisposed to develop cancer if they carry a mutation in a cancer-susceptibility gene in their germline. In this case, the clinical indications for testing are usually based on being an at-risk member in a known hereditary-cancer family or having premonitory clinical signs (e.g. polyposis in FAP) suggesting hereditary cancer. Ideally, in either of the aforementioned situations, the initial testing in the family should begin with an affected member because if a mutation is identified in someone who is affected (has cancer or a premonitory sign), then testing will be more informative for other family members. This is particularly important in the presymptomatic identification of individuals who have a cancer susceptibility gene mutation and will benefit by preventive measures to reduce their risk for cancer. Currently, gene testing is not practical for broad-based screening specific populations in which cancer-susceptibility gene mutations occur in high frequency. However, when gene testing becomes inexpensive, reliable, and valid, it may become practical to screen populations to diagnose those individuals who carry a cancer-susceptibility gene mutation that occurs with a relatively high frequency, like in hereditary breast-cancer mutations among Ashkenazi Jews.

Identification of individuals carrying frequently occurring founder mutations could have tremendous health-care benefits in certain populations. Studies have indicated that three spe-

Table 5
Methods for Detecting Mutations in Cancer-Susceptibility Genes[a]

Approach	Assay
Deletion of known mutations	Allele specific oligonucleotide analysis
	Allele-specific amplification (including gel-shift assay)
	Ligation detection
	Single base pair primer extension
	Introduction of new restriction sites
Detection of unknown mutations	
Indirect gene tracking	Linkage analysis
Screening techniques	Single-strand conformation polymorphism (SSCP)
	Denaturing gradient-gel electrophoresis (DGGE)
	Heteroduplex analysis
	RNAse/chemical cleavage
	Carbodiimide modification (CDI)
	Monoallelic mutation analysis (MAMA)
	In vitro synthesized protein assay (IVSP) or Protein truncation test (PTT)
	Functional assays
	Microsatellite instability test (MSI)
	Southern blot analysis
	Immunoassay for gene product
Direct gene analysis	Direct gene sequencing

[a]Information based upon published literature (4,75–78).

cific founder mutations in *BRCA1/2* occur with increased frequency in Ashkenazi Jews, both with and without a strong family history of cancer. The carrier frequency for these three founder mutations is about 1 in 40 as compared to the frequency of all *BRCA1* mutations in non-Jewish populations being between 1 in 500 to 1 in 833 (http://www.nhgri.nih.gov/intramural_research/lab_transfer/bic) (69–72). Moreover, between 20–30% of breast cancer diagnoses in Jewish patients under 40 yr of age, and 40–60% of Jewish women with ovarian cancer carry one of the three founder mutations regardless of their family history. Therefore, for an individual of Ashkenazi Jewish descent, even having one family member with early-onset breast cancer is associated with a reasonable probability of finding a *BRCA1* or *BRCA2* mutation. Although this indicates that population-based screening would be beneficial, potential pitfalls exist. For example, although the founder mutations appear to account for the majority of identifiable *BRCA1* and *BRCA2* mutations in Ashkenazi Jewish individuals, novel disease-conferring mutations not previously described in this population have also been identified in these genes. This means that a negative result for the founder mutations does not rule out the possibility of a mutation elsewhere in *BRCA1* or *BRCA2*. Therefore, if population-based screening becomes feasible for Ashkenazi women, those women who have a high risk for hereditary breast cancer, but test negative for the three common founder mutations, should still subsequently have full sequencing of *BRCA1* and *BRCA2* (73).

Age at Which Gene Testing is Recommended The primary factors that determine the age at which gene testing is recommended for at-risk family members in hereditary-cancer kindreds include: 1) the childhood and adolescent ages during which psychological development occurs, 2) the age at which symptoms develop from premalignant lesions in a given at-risk individual, and 3) the earliest age at which the cancer risk begins for a given hereditary-cancer syndrome based on genetic

epidemiology studies, 4) the youngest age-at-cancer-diagnosis that occurs in the particular family that is undergoing gene testing of its at-risk members, and 5) parents' request for gene testing in family planning. In general, the time when gene testing is recommended to be done for at-risk individuals is 18 yr or older. Genetic testing for children should be performed only if the test is for childhood-onset hereditary-cancer disorders for which there are effective interventions and the test can be adequately interpreted.

Generally, gene testing is not recommended for children unless there is a medical benefit to the child. Thus, if the medical benefits from a gene test will not be realized in childhood, testing should be postponed until children reach adulthood and they can make their own (autonomous) informed decision to pursue testing.

In some instances, gene testing of children is justified because the hereditary cancer affects children. Examples of hereditary-cancer syndromes for which testing of children would be considered appropriate include MEN2a and MEN2b, FAP, VHL, and Rb. In such situations, medical benefit can be gained through screening and/or prophylactic surgery. In situations where medical and legal factors warrant gene testing for children, genetic counseling should be provided that is tailored to the child's age level and that incorporates certain aspects of counseling that address ramifications on psychological development. Usually the appropriate time when gene testing is recommended to be done for at-risk individuals is five yr before the cancer risk begins in a given hereditary-cancer syndrome. However, if an individual in a particular family is diagnosed with cancer at an age that is younger than the generally recommended testing age, then gene testing of at-risk members in such a family should begin at least five yr before the youngest age-at-cancer-diagnosis in the family.

In those syndromes that have premonitory signs, such as polyposis in FAP, early testing is indicated if symptoms develop (hematochezia in FAP at-risk children) to clarify the genotype of the affected individual. Another situation for gene testing can involve requests for prenatal diagnosis by an affected person who is considering abortion to avoid birth of cancer-predisposed offspring. In the latter two situations, many variables need to be considered in performing gene testing including sensitivity and specificity of testing, effectiveness of preventive measures (prophylactic surgery), legal and ethical ramifications, and psychological issues. Overall, the appropriate age at which gene testing is recommended in hereditary-cancer families is at the latest age when a positive test result would still permit the greatest beneficial outcome *(74).*

Use of Gene Testing by Clinicians Most analyses for genetic alterations in oncology began as research-based molecular technologies used to identify cancer-susceptibility gene mutations and to determine the nature of mutations occurring in hereditary as well as sporadic cancers. Recently, however, such assays have been incorporated into gene-testing services used in the clinical diagnosis and management of patients. This has been done despite the fact that there are few studies available to practitioners that provide information on the sensitivity, specificity, and positive predictive value (PPV) of genetic tests in a clinical setting. Sensitivity of a test is defined as the proportion of individuals with the disease who test positive. Specificity is the proportion of individuals without the disease who test negative. Positive predictive value is the proportion of individuals who test positive and actually have the disease. Until this statistical information becomes available, clinicians will need to evaluate the available options for diagnosing hereditary cancer on a case-by-case basis. Moreover, quality control and other problems exist with clinical use of gene testing. Currently, uniform international and national regulatory policies and procedures are lacking which guarantee quality of testing in terms of validity, standardization, and reliability. In addition, the availability of gene testing for clinical purposes is restricted to select academic centers and some commercial laboratories. Most molecular technologies used in gene testing are too complex to be adapted to routine assays or automated systems that are widely utilized in clinical laboratories or in community hospitals.

Indeed, few physicians, including oncologists and pathologists, are qualified to assess and interpret results from gene testing, or understand the potential implications of the test results. The integration of clinical criteria with gene testing adds further complexity to clinical diagnostic approaches for hereditary cancer that will need to be evaluated in terms of efficiency (measure of the proportion of individuals correctly diagnosed) and cost-effectiveness. Future guidelines for diagnosis will likely be based on a combination of clinical criteria and gene testing that provides an optimal balance between sensitivity and specificity.

Methods for Gene Testing The currently used laboratory methods for gene testing are listed in Table 5. Several reviews have been published on these methods for detection of mutations in hereditary cancer *(4, 75–78).* The ability to detect mutations in at-risk individuals who are members of families having known germline mutations is technologically much easier to achieve than detection of unknown mutations. Labora-

tory methods used to diagnose known germline mutations in at-risk individuals usually involve polymerase-chain reaction (PCR)-based techniques designed to detect alterations in nucleic acid sequences that can differ by as little as a single base. These include allele-specific oligonucleotide analysis, allele-specific amplification including band-shift assay, ligation detection, single-base primer extension, and introduction of new restriction sites (Table 5). These methods may also be used to detect individuals with specific (founder) mutations that frequently occur in certain populations (*BRCA1* or *BRCA2* mutations in Ashkenazi Jews).

Laboratory methods used to detect unknown mutations (Table 5) include single-strand conformational polymorphism (SSCP) analysis, denaturing gradient-gel electrophoresis (DGGE), heteroduplex analysis, RNAse or chemical-cleavage method, carbodiimide modification (CDI), monoallelic mutation analysis (MAMA), PTT, functional assays, southern plots, immuno-assays and sequencing. Linkage analysis has also been used in the past to test whether a gene marker cosegregates with a given phenotype in an extended kindred with an unknown mutation. However, with the emergence of newer, more sophisticated technologies, linkage analysis is now mainly used as a method to identify the chromosomal location of new genes in research studies rather than to detect affected members in hereditary cancer families (by indirectly tracking the inheritance of a cancer-susceptibility gene). One exception is the use of polymorphic markers within the *Rb1* gene for linkage-type of analysis (for allelotype) to screen presymptomatically for retinoblastoma in families with this hereditary disorder *(37).* This molecular approach is sometimes taken because the *Rb1* gene is very large (27 exons and 180 kb of genomic DNA) and mutation detection can be difficult.

Nonetheless, even with the availability of newer methods, detection of unknown mutations is still often problematic. Methods such as DGGE, SSCP, heteroduplex, RNAse/chemical cleavage, CDI, MAMA, PTT, and functional assays lack specificity in terms of being able to identify the specific type of mutation and its location. Therefore, once the test shows positivity, DNA sequencing is required pinpoint the mutation. Consequently, tests like DGGE have become a common way to screen for the presence of unknown mutations in genes like *BRCA1, hMSH2, hMLH1*, and others. In addition, testing for microsatellite instability (MSI) in tumors can be used to screen for possible HNPCC cases. Although sequencing is very specific (and sensitive), it is laborious and expensive. Some of the limitations associated with sequencing someday may be overcome by technological development of a computer-based "sequencing" chip that has enhanced throughput and lowered cost. Another limiting factor with screening tests is decreased sensitivity. Methods, such as DGGE, SSCP, heteroduplex, and CDI are more proficient at detecting large mutations (insertions or deletions of >4 bp) as compared to point mutations. PTT is unable to detect mutations (missense) that do not cause protein truncation. The sensitivity of these screening methods for detection of mutations is variable, but it is usually 70% or greater. However, the ability to detect unknown mutations should improve significantly with future technological advances.

Table 6
Comparison of Two Types of Hereditary Colorectal Cancer[a]

Characteristic	FAP	HNPCC
Frequency of the trait	1 in every 5,000–10,000 individuals	1 in every 200–400 individuals
Germline mutation	*APC*	*hMLH1, hMSH2, hPMS1, hPMS2, hMSH6,* and *TGFBRII*
Mode of transmission	Autosomal dominant	Autosomal dominant
Gene function	Tumor suppressor (growth inhibitor)	DNA mismatch repair[b]
Penetrance	100%	90% (80% lifetime CRC risk)
Predominant location of CRCs	Distal (left) colon	Proximal (right) colon
Median age at CRC diagnosis	39 yr	43 yr
Multiple 1° (synchronous and metachronous) CRCs	Frequent	Frequent
Adenomas (polyps)	Adenomatous polyposis coli (hundreds to thousands of polyps). Usually polyposis develops during adolescence (median age of onset is 16 yr).	Discrete adenomas with anatomic distribution and number similar to the general population. Adenomas are often large and villous with high-grade dysplasia. Adenoma to carcinoma interval is accelerated (2–3 yr).
Extracolonic features	Epidermoid cysts, desmoid tumors, fibromas, osteomas, abnormal dentition, gastric and duodenal polyps, and congenital hypertrophy of the retinal pigment epithelium. Increased risk for other tumors including thyroid, duodenal, pancreatic and ovarian carcinomas, hepatoblastoma, and medulloblastoma	Increased risk for other tumors including endometrial (lifetime risk = 20–43%), ovarian (RR = 3.5), gastric (RR = 4.1), small bowel (RR = 25.0), hepatobiliary (RR = 4.9), ureteral (RR = 22.0), and renal (RR = 3.2) carcinomas.

[a]See (82)
[b]Except for TGFβRII.

Which Hereditary-Cancer Syndromes Should Have Gene Testing? Because gene testing for hereditary-susceptibility genes has medical value, namely for reducing cancer mortality by screening and early intervention in affected individuals, several professional medical organizations have now established policy statements regarding their use. For example, the American Society of Clinical Oncology (ASCO) has recently issued their position statement on indications for cancer predisposition testing (79). Genetic tests that may be utilized as part of the standard management of hereditary-cancer families include *APC*, c-*ret*, *Rb1*, *VHL*, *BLM*, *NF1*, and *NF2*, because test results in these syndromes will change medical care or prenatal management. The medical benefit of other gene tests, including *hMSH2*, *hMLH1*, *hPMS1*, *hPMS2*, *BRCA1*, *BRCA2*, *p53*, *p16INK4A*, *CDKY*, is presumed but not established. Tests for individuals without a family history of cancer (in whom significance of diagnosis of a germline mutation is not clear) and tests for hereditary syndromes in which germline mutations are uncommon or medical benefit is not established include *ATM* and *PTCH*. Because new gene-testing approaches are still being translated from basic research (e.g. isolation and characterization of new cancer susceptibility genes) to clinical diagnostics, the ASCO statement strongly endorses the incorporation of gene testing into the context of ongoing trials. The American College of Medical Genetics is another organization that has issued policy statements on genetic testing, some of which are directly related to cancer genetics. These statements can be found at http://www.faseb.org/genetics/acmg.

PROTOTYPE MODELS FOR DIAGNOSIS AND MANAGEMENT OF HEREDITARY CANCER

FAP Although the classical approach to the diagnosis of FAP was based on an individual's phenotype, diagnosis can now be confirmed by determination of the patient's genotype in most cases. The primary phenotypic finding provides the basis of the main clinical criterion for FAP (Table 6): colonic and rectal expression of hundreds to thousands of adenomatous polyps at a young age, where classically ≥ 100 to clinically make the diagnosis. Most individuals who carry gene mutations for FAP develop adenomatous polyps during adolescence, while almost all affected individuals exhibit polyposis by the age of 35 (15% of affected individuals develop polyps by 10 yr of age, 75% by 20 yr, and 90% by 30 yr). The median age of onset of CRC is 39 yr, and cancer is inevitable if the colon is not removed. Clinical documentation of polyposis is an indication for prophylactic total colectomy as the lifetime risk of colorectal cancer is nearly 100%. Hence, the penetrance of the *APC* mutation is nearly 100%.

Several extracolonic manifestations are associated with FAP (Table 6). One such feature, congenital hypertrophy of the retinal pigment epithelium is present in about 70% of patients. These are pigmented lesions of the retina that can be detected by ophthalmologic examination of the fundus, and this is a

Table 7
Genetic Testing for FAP

Candidates for genetic testing

FAP proband or another FAP-affected member in the family. At-risk members in those FAP families having a known segregating *APC* mutation.

Strategy for genetic testing in FAP families in which the germline mutation is unknown

Attempt to identify the specific *APC* mutation in an FAP-affected individual (one having the polyposis phenotype). If a germline *APC* mutation is detected, then at-risk relatives can be tested to determine their genotype. Individuals with positive test results for *APC* mutations should be managed according to the guidelines shown in Table 8.

If the *APC* mutation is not identified in an FAP-affected individual (one having the polyposis phenotype), this should be considered a false negative result for the genetic test. In such a case, the FAP patient and at-risk family members should be screened and managed according to Table 8.

Strategy for genetic testing in FAP families in which the germline mutation is known

In families where the specific germline *APC* mutation is known, those at-risk relatives who test negative (do not have the mutation) do not need annual screening. However, such individuals who test negative are still recommended to have colon screening by flexible colonoscopy at least twice before age 35 yr followed by conventional CRC guidelines for the general population *(80,108)*.

Table 8
Surveillance and Management Options for FAP Families[a]

At-risk family member (genotype not known)

Annual flexible sigmoidoscopy beginning at age 10 yr[b], unless symptoms (such as hematochezia) develop, then surveillance should begin immediately regardless of age.

Exam should also involve search for extracolonic manifestations including CHRPE.

Other tumors that need to be screened for include gastro duodenal polyps and periampullary carcinomas as well as those other cancer types found in the pedigree.

Proven germline gene carrier (based on polyposis phenotype or known genotype)

Prophylactic colectomy recommended (usually after adenomas develop).

[a]From Lynch et al. *(1,82)*.
[b]Or 5 yr earlier than the age of the youngest CRC patient in a given family, if this would yield an age less than 20–25 yr.

---

fairly reliable marker for the disease in some families. Other extracolonic features include gastric and duodenal polyps, periampullary carcinomas, osteomas (particularly involving the mandible and long bones), epidermoid cysts, abnormal dentition (missing or extra-numerary teeth), desmoid tumors, thyroid cancer, brain tumors, and infrequently, hepatoblastoma. A variant of FAP is the attenuated familial adenomatous polyposis (AFAP) syndrome, previously known as the hereditary flat-adenoma syndrome. This attenuated variant is characterized by a different polyp phenotype wherein the adenomas are flatter, fewer in number, and occur predominantly on the right side of the colon. The risk to develop CRC remains high, and the average age of diagnosis is 55 yr. Congenital hypertrophy of the retinal-pigment epithelium does not appear to be associated with AFAP, but upper gastrointestinal lesions do occur and may be as common as in classic FAP. Attenuated FAP also arises from *APC* mutations, but the mutations tend to be located at the 5′ and 3′ ends of the gene (Table 3). It is currently being investigated why these mutations lead to an attenuated form of FAP. An unfortunate aspect of the natural history of FAP and AFAP is that diagnosis of many cases occurs after CRC has already developed, thus precluding some otherwise effective preventive strategies. This occurs, in part, because ≥ 30% of cases are associated with *de novo* mutations, wherein affected individuals have no family history of the disease.

The strategy for gene testing in FAP *(80)* is outlined in Table 7. Gene testing services for the detection of FAP are available commercially. The purpose of gene testing in FAP is to confirm the diagnosis in an individual who has the polyposis phenotype (with or without CRC), to identify an *APC* mutation in the pedigree, or to provide presymptomatic diagnosis of affected members in FAP families that have a known *APC* mutation. *APC* gene sequencing, however, is difficult due to the large size of the gene and the wide spectrum of mutations that have been identified (>700). A variety of methodologies for detection of *APC* mutations have been used. However, PTT is the most common method, because the majority of mutations result in a truncated protein. Once a mutation is identified in an affected individual, testing has close to 100% accuracy in its ability to classify other at-risk family members as either carriers or noncarriers of the mutation. Nevertheless, the PTT assay does not identify mutations in all cases. Using this method, mutations are detectable in approx 70–85% of cases of classical FAP, and are even less for attenuated FAP. Additional methodologies, such as direct DNA sequencing may be subsequently performed to increase detection.

The surveillance and management options for FAP *(1,81–83)* are outlined in Table 8. The recommended clinical screening approach for FAP involves sigmoidoscopy, which is usually sufficient for identifying the polyposis phenotype in FAP. Surveillance for at-risk family members in FAP is generally recommended to begin at age 10–12. If sigmoidoscopy is negative, repeat screening for FAP should be performed routinely on an annual basis until age 40. Further surveillance is recommended for extracolonic tumors as indicated in Table 8. All FAP patients should have baseline upper gastrointestinal endoscopy at age 20–25. Recommendations for repeating endoscopic surveillance of the upper GI tract depends on the severity of gastroduodenal premalignant disease. Patients with severe dysplasia should be followed with endoscopy every 6 months and a prophylactic gastroduodencectomy should be considered. Surgical management of patients diagnosed with FAP involves a colectomy *(1,81)*. Recommendation for prophylactic surgery depends on several variables including number of rectal polyps, APC genotype, history of desmoids in the family, presence

Table 9
Clinical Criteria for Identification of HNPCC

Amsterdam Criteria (ACI)[a]
- Histologically confirmed CRC in at least three relatives, one of whom is a first-degree relative of the other two.
- Occurrence of the disease in at least two successive generations.
- Age at CRC diagnosis below 50 yr of age in at least one patient.
- Exclusion (zero evidence) of FAP

Modified Amsterdam Criteria (ACII)[b]
- There should be at least three relatives with an HNPCC-associated cancer (CRC, cancer of the endometrium, small bowel, ureter, or renal pelvis). One should be a first-degree relative of the other two.
- At least two successive generations should be affected.
- At least one should be diagnosed before the age of 50.
- Exclusion (zero evidence) of FAP

Bethesda Criteria[c]
- Individuals with cancer in families that meet the Amsterdam Criteria.
- Individuals with two HNPCC-related cancers, including synchronous and metasynchronous CRCs or associated extracolonic cancers.
- Individuals with CRC and a first-degree relative with CRC and/or HNPCC-related extracolonic cancer and/or colorectal adenoma; one of the cancers diagnosed at <45 yr of age, and the adenoma diagnosed at <40 yr of age.
- Individuals with CRC or endometrial cancer diagnosed at <45 yr of age.
- Individuals with right-sided CRC with an undifferentiated pattern (solid/cribiform) on histopathology diagnosed at <45 yr of age.
- Individuals with signet-ring cell-type CRC diagnosed at <45 yr of age.
- Individuals with adenomas diagnosed at <40 yr of age.

[a]See Vasen et al. (84).
[b]See Vasen et al. (86).
[c]See Rodriguez-Bigas et al. (87).

Table 10
Genes Responsible for HNPCC

Gene	Frequency (%) among HNPCC families
hMSH2	~ 30%
hMLH1	~ 30%
hPMS1	Rare
hPMS2	Rare
hMSH6 (GTBP)	Uncommon
TGFβRII	Rare
Undetermined locus	~ 30%

associated with an increased incidence of carcinoma of the endometrium and ovary and of other digestive-tract cancers. Genetic diagnostic criteria for HNPCC were established in August 1990 by the International Collaborative Group on HNPCC who met in Amsterdam, The Netherlands. This was done in response to the need to develop minimum clinical criteria for the identification of HNPCC, and to provide a basis for uniformly identifying this entity among research studies. These criteria for diagnosis of HNPCC, known as the Amsterdam Criteria (84,85), are outlined in Table 9. Limitations of the Amsterdam Criteria in their ability to identify HNPCC families were recognized, and at subsequent meetings two other sets of criteria (Table 9) were established including the Modified Amsterdam Criteria (ACII) (86) and the Bethesda Criteria (87).

Confirmation of the presence of the HNPCC hereditary-cancer trait is obtained from gene testing for mutations in DNA MMR genes. This family of genes includes hMLH1, hMSH2, hPMS1, hMSH6, hPMS2, and TGFβRII and accounts for about 70% of HNPCC cases (Table 10). As can be seen in Table 10, the majority (about 60%) of HNPCC families having identifiable DNA mismatch repair gene mutations involve hMSH2 and hMLH1. However, some studies show that the frequency of detectable hMSH2 and hMLH1 mutations in HNPCC families is less than reported in earlier studies (88,89). A much smaller proportion of HNPCC families have mutations in hPMS1, hMSH6, hPMS2, or TGFβRII. Therefore, genetic analysis of hMSH2 and hMLH1 should be done first and, if negative, then the less commonly involved genes should be considered. It is known that functional inactivation of MSH2 or MLH2 leads to the accumulation of DNA replication errors. The functional consequence of such MMR alterations is variation in the size of simple repetitive DNA sequences (microsatellites) (90), which has been termed MSI or replication error (RER) (91) (Table 11). MSI is found in the majority (90–100%) of HNPCC tumors (92) as well as in some (10–20%) sporadic cases of CRC (93,94). This suggests that MMR defects can also be acquired as somatic mutations and can lead to the development of sporadic CRC. This is not totally surprising because it is well-known that the second carcinogenic event in a cell with a germline MMR mutation involves an acquired somatic mutation in the remaining wild-type allele. The function of MMR genes involves repair of base-pair mismatches that occur during normal DNA replication. For a heterozygous cell, a cell with one wild-type and one mutant germline MMR allele, a mutation in the wild-type allele often involves LOH and defec-

of cancer, psycholsocial issues, perception of risk and family experiences. If these is a paucity of rectal adenomas or if there is a family history of desmoids, an ileorectal anastomososis is often considered. When the rectum is involved with multiple polyhposis, an ileal pouch anal anastomosis is often considered. And, if the patient has already developed rectal cancer, a totoproctocolectomy with ileostomy is usually performed. Post-operatively it is important to continue endoscopic screening of rectal segment or the ileal anal anastomosis including polypectomies. For those individuals at risk for AFAP, annual colonoscopy and upper endoscopy is recommended beginning at age 20. AFAP patients are usually managed surgically by prophylactic colectomy, particularly if too many polyps are present to manage by polypectomy. Chemopreventive treatment with sulindac may also be considered to prevent adenomae, but this does not substitute for prophylactic surgery.

HNPCC Because there is no known premonitory sign for HNPCC, the classical diagnosis of HNPCC is based on the individual's phenotype (Table 6), which is CRC in conjunction with a positive family history. HNPCC is the most common inherited form of CRC and, like FAP, is associated with an early age of disease onset (mean of 44 yr). HNPCC is also

Table 11
Current Criteria for Identifying Microsatellite
Instability (MSI)[a]

Degree of MSI	Number of Markers Affected[b]
High MSI	$\geq$ 2 (out of 5 loci tested)
Low MSI	1 (out of 5 loci tested)
No MSI	0 (out of 5 loci tested)

[a]From National Cancer Institute workshop on microsatellite instability for cancer detection and familial predisposition (91).

[b]The recommended panel of markers includes BAT25, BAT26, D2S123, Mfd15 (D17S250), APC (D5S346). It is also recommended that immunohistochemistry for MMR protein expression is performed.

tive DNA repair, and it will increase the susceptibility of all genetic material to mutation. Consequently, many unrepaired base-pair mismatches in the DNA will occur, and these errors will then remain permanently in the genome of that cell. This is the mechanism whereby defects in DNA can lead to widespread genetic instability. If the error is in a genomic DNA region that encodes a functional, growth-regulating gene such as *APC* or another tumor-suppressor gene, that error can alter a cell's ability to regulate its growth. This mechanism is thought to lead to promotion of human cancers.

Although all cells in an HNPCC-affected individual contain one mutant MMR allele, carcinogenesis is thought to start when a second hit occurs in a cell, a hit that renders dysfunctional the remaining wild type allele in that cell. In HNPCC, this apparently occurs most often in colon cells although some extracolonic cancers also occur, albeit less frequently. MSI is typically diagnosed in biopsied tumor tissues surgical specimens through DNA analysis (Table 11).

Commercial gene testing is now available for the identification of HNPCC. Table 12 outlines the strategies for gene testing in HNPCC. To diagnose HNPCC, tests for a germline mutation in any of several MMR genes should be conducted (Table 10). Because each MMR mutation can be at a different locus, searches can be time-consuming and genetic sequencing can be expensive. An alternative test that avoids these problems is one of the screening tests such as the DGGE assay. HNPCC scanning can also be done using immunohistochemistry for MMR proteins or MSI testimony for errors in repeat DNA sequences. Tumors showing abnormality usually indicate defects in germline MMR genes and suggests the possibility of HNPCC. However, false-positive MSI will be given by about 10–20% of those individuals who have sporadic CRC but lack the germline mutation. For example in a recent Finnish study involving 509 consecutive patients with CRC (95), 12% (63 patients) had tumors that tested positively for MSI. Of this MSI-positive subgroup, 10 patients (2% of the total group) were found to have germline mutations involving *hMSH2* or *hMLH1*. In the 10 patients with germline mutations, 9 had first degree relatives with endometrial cancer or CRC, 7 were younger (<50 yr of age), and 4 had a prior history of CRC or endometrial cancer.

The purpose of gene testing in HNPCC is to confirm the diagnosis of HNPCC in CRC-affected patients who meet the Amsterdam Criteria (ACI & ACII), Bethesda Criteria, or who are considered at-risk based on early age at CRC diagnosis. It

Table 12
Genetic Testing for HNPCC

Candidates for genetic testing

HNPCC probands or other HNPCC-affected individual in families that meet the Amsterdam Criteria (ACI or ACII) (Table 9).

CRC patients who meet the Bethesda Criteria (Table 9) or who are diagnosed at a young age (<55yr).[a]

At-risk members of HNPCC families having a known MMR mutation.

Strategy for genetic testing in HNPCC families in which germline mutation is unknown

In a CRC-affected individual, test for a germline MMR mutation (Fig. 1).

When MMR mutation is identified, then test at-risk relatives. Screen and manage according to Table 13.

When MMR mutation is not identified in a family meeting the ACI or ACII, assume the test result to be a false-negative. Screen and manage according to Table 13 (same as proven germline carrier).

Strategy for genetic testing in HNPCC families in which germline mutation is known

At-risk relatives who truly test positive, screen and manage according to Table 13.

At-risk relatives who test negative should:
1. Discontinue annual screening.
2. Follow conventional CRC screening guidelines for the general population.

[a]Described in text (98,103,134).

is important to begin testing an affected member of the family for HNPCC (one with CRC) in order to identify an MMR mutation in the pedigree. Once an MMR mutation is detected in an HNPCC family, testing can be offered to all members at risk (with and without cancer) for detecting a germline mutation. In those HNPCC families having known MMR mutations, it becomes possible to presymptomatically diagnose individuals who carry the mutation before they develop cancer. Consequently, because conclusive results can be obtained whether a family member has (positive test) or does not have (negative test) the mutation, this provides information for making surveillance and management decisions by HNPCC family members.

Table 13 outlines the surveillance and management measures for HNPCC families (1,82,83). Because colon tumors tend to occur mainly proximal in location in HNPCC, colonoscopy (as opposed to sigmoidoscopy in classic FAP) is the preferred screening method for HNPCC. Surveillance is generally recommended to begin at 20–25 yr of age. If endoscopy is negative, repeat screening should be performed every 2–3 yr for HNPCC. There is insufficient evidence for or against prophylactic colectomy for CRC prevention in individuals who are presymptomatically diagnosed with the HNPCC trait (germline carriers). Prophylactic subtotal colectomy is usually not accepted by the patient in view of the survival benefits with aggressive screening alone coupled with polypectomies (discussed below). Surveillance should also be recommended for extracolonic tumors as indicated in Table 13.

Table 13
Surveillance and Management Options for HNPCC Families[a]

At-risk family member (genotype not known)

Colonoscopy every 2–3 yr beginning at age 20–25 yr.[b]
If adenomas are found, screen annually.
For females: annual gynecologic exam from age 30–35 yr onward.
Screening for other tumors,[c] according to other cancer types found
    in the pedigree.

Proven gene carrier (genotype known)

Same as management for at-risk family member, except
    colonoscopies recommended every 1–2 yr.
For affected females:
    Screening for endometrial cancer by endometrial curettage;
        initiated at age 25 and annually thereafter.
    Screening for ovarian cancer using vaginal probe ultrasound,
        Doppler color flow imagery of ovaries and CA-125 tumor
        marker beginning at age 25 and annually thereafter.
Consider prophylactic hysterectomy and oophorectomy.

---

*HNPCC patient with colon cancer (regardless whether genotype is
known)*

Subtotal colectomy.
For females, consider prophylactic hysterectomy and
    oophorectomy.
Screening for other tumors,[c] according to other cancer types found
    in the pedigree.

---

[a]From Lynch et al. *(1, 82)* and Liu et al. *(83)*.
[b]Or 5 yr earlier than the age of the youngest patient in a given family,
if this would yield an age less than 20–25 yr.
[c]If screening for that tumor type is feasible.

The overall approaches to surgical management and risk assessment for patients newly diagnosed with CRC are illustrated in Fig. 1. The initial assessment is based on the clinical criteria for HNPCC and FAP. The management of those CRC patients diagnosed with HNPCC should include a subtotal colectomy. In HNPCC, affected female patients should also consider prophylactic bilateral oophorectomy and hysterectomy, especially if the patient is postmenopausal or is no longer considering childbearing.

Screening Recommendations for Nonhereditary CRC If an at-risk person who is a member of an HNPCC kindred with a known mutation truly tests negative, then such individuals should be screened according to the American Cancer Society guidelines for the general population. Screening in individuals considered average risk should begin at age 50 with an annual fecal occult blood test plus either sigmoidoscopy (every 5 yr) or a total colon exam by colonoscopy (every 10 yr) or by double-contrast barium enema (every 5–10 yr). Digital rectal exam should be performed at the time of the sigmoidoscopy or the total colon exam. Screening of individuals with moderate risk (persons diagnosed with discrete adenomatous polyps) should involve a colonoscopy at the time of adenoma diagnosis and total colon exam within three yr of polyp removal. If the colon exam is normal, then the patient is considered as being at average risk.

ROADBLOCKS TO REDUCING MORTALITY IN HEREDITARY CANCERS

A significant portion of individuals affected with hereditary cancer traits will not be identified as such due to two underlying problems: 1) the detection of affected individuals using clinical criteria has low sensitivity so that many with the trait will fail to be diagnosed, and 2) molecular gene testing for germline mutations has its limitations and pitfalls. These problems present roadblocks to reducing mortality in hereditary cancers.

Overall changes in mortality due to cancer have been carefully tracked during the past several decades by the National Cancer Institute (NCI). The U.S. Cancer Mortality rate, age-adjusted to 1970 figures, increased by an estimated 0.3% annually from 1975 through 1993. This steady rise in mortality rates occurred despite the dramatic increase in cancer-research efforts and advances in cancer treatment. However, the mortality rate from colorectal cancer decreased dramatically, perhaps partly due to earlier detection. Whether improved treatment approaches do not appear to have contributed much to the decline in colorectal-cancer deaths is uncertain. According to Bailar and Gornik *(96)*, decline in the mortality rates of some cancers (cervix, uterus, colon, rectum, stomach) is clearly the result of a reduced incidence of disease or early detection in the population. Increased mortality from lung carcinoma can be attributed, for the most part, to changes in smoking patterns. The high mortality from breast cancer, especially in older women, continues in spite of more effective treatment, and thus probably reflects a rising incidence of disease. Overall, it appears that trends in cancer mortality are largely due to changing cancer incidence or earlier cancer detection rather than improvements in therapy.

Among the challenges we must address to overcome these increasing mortality rates *(96)*, Bailar and Gornik list the following: 1) the means to prevent most cancers has not yet been clearly recognized or defined, adequately tested, or shown to be effective or feasible; and 2) the research needed on prevention of cancer will require as much time and commitment as we have given in the study of cancer treatment. It seems reasonable that the population of hereditary-cancer patients, because of their extremely high risk for cancer, would be an important group on which to focus our cancer prevention efforts in order to reduce their mortality.

DIAGNOSTIC CRITERIA HAVE LIMITED SENSITIVITY: HEREDITARY CRC AS A MODEL

Accuracy of Clinical Criteria: The HNPCC Model The recognition of HNPCC as a hereditary disorder, distinct from either sporadic CRC or FAP, has relied on a combination of clinical data and a family history. Thus, unless the family history clearly shows a pattern of genetic transmission consistent with an autosomal-dominant hereditary trait, it will not often permit a definitive identification of HNPCC. The major reason for this limitation is that the phenotypic expression of HNPCC is not specific enough in the individual patient to allow the physician to unambiguously distinguish HNPCC from sporadic CRC.

Although the Amsterdam Criteria were established to provide a uniform definition of the disorder for use in cooperative

DIAGNOSIS OF COLORECTAL CANCER

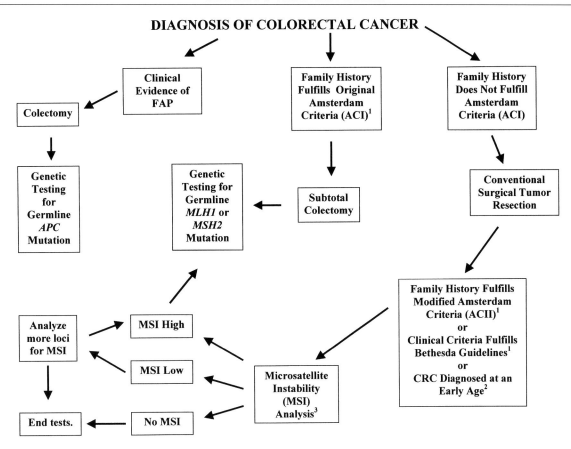

Fig. 1. Approaches to surgical management and risk assessment for patients newly diagnosed with CRC[a]. The Amsterdam Criteria and the Bethesda Criteria are described in the text (84, 86, 87) and are given in Table 9[b]. Early age at CRC diagnosis is described in the text (98, 103, 134)[c]. In testing CRC patients who are AC positive, some genetic laboratories recommend pre-testing using DGGE, MSI and immunostaining for MLH1 and MSH2 prior to performance of gene sequencing.

and other research studies, they have now been adopted by the practicing clinician and geneticist for every day diagnosing of HNPCC families. However, their accuracy in detecting HNPCC when used in the clinical setting is not known and may be unacceptably low. For example, in a study done by Genuardi and coworkers (97), a series of 32 Italian putative HNPCC individuals was investigated. Patients were selected according to clinical criteria suggestive of HNPCC but not meeting the Amsterdam Criteria. This included one of the following criteria: 1) family history of CRC and/or other extracolonic tumors; 2) early-onset CRC; and/or 3) presence of multiple primary malignancies in the same individual. Gene testing showed pathogenetic truncating MMR mutations in 4 (12.5%) cases, and 2 (6.25%) missense *hMLH1* variants of uncertain significance. All pathogenetic mutations were associated with early age (<40 yr) at onset and proximal CRC location. These data confirm that the Amsterdam Criteria have limited sensitivity because nearly 20% of the patients not meeting the Amsterdam criteria had germline mutations identified.

Influence of Family Size Because many HNPCC-affected individuals in the general population may not have a family history that is positive for HNPCC, the Amsterdam Criteria will have limited sensitivity. Although a positive family history is the basis of the Amsterdam Criteria, significant underestimation of HNPCC in a population can arise when family size is small. Boman and Watson (98) used computer-generated pedi-

grees to determine the maximum possible sensitivity of the Amsterdam Criteria in accurately diagnosing HNPCC in families carrying an autosomal dominant trait and other clinical criteria must be considered. The results showed that, based on family size, the proportion of such families that are capable of being diagnosed (maximum possible sensitivity) depends significantly on the family size. The sensitivity is likely to decrease when confounding factors such as reduced penetrance, variable age of manifestation, inadequate screening, and inaccurate family histories are taken into account.

Others have confirmed the seriousness of these underestimates. In one recent study (99), a total of 1052 patients with CRC were classified as HNPCC or non-HNPCC according to the Amsterdam Criteria. Linear discriminant analysis revealed that diagnosis of HNPCC was most likely to occur when first-degree pedigrees had more than seven relatives. These data show that diagnostic guidelines (Amsterdam Criteria) proposed by the International Collaborative Group (ICG) on HNPCC are often too stringent for use with small families. Thus, if possible, small pedigrees must be expanded to reliably exclude HNPCC.

Age at CRC Diagnosis in the Individual Patient Because many HNPCC patients in the general population do not have a family history that is positive for HNPCC, the age at CRC diagnosis may have important value as a criterion for the identification of individual HNPCC patients because the median age at CRC diagnosis is 44 yr in HNPCC (compared to 62 yr in

Table 14
Characteristics of FAP Probands vs HNPCC Probands

Characteristic	FAP	HNPCC
Diagnosis of proband	Based on premonitory signs such as adenomatous polyposis coli and extracolonic signs such as CHRPE	No premonitory signs known. Diagnosis based on Amsterdam Criteria requiring at least three family members that are CRC-affected
Percentage of probands who have cancer at diagnosis.	66.6%	100% (In addition, at least two other family members will have CRC at time of diagnosis of an HNPCC proband)
Percentage of families that have only one affected individual (isolated cases).	40%	Unknown.
Ten-yr survival	40%	60%

the general CRC population). Hall et al. showed that when CRC arises prior to age 45, the possibility of HNPCC has higher likelihood and family members of the affected individual have increased relative risk for HNPCC, as much as five-fold or higher *(100)*. Liu et al. demonstrated that MSI occurs frequently in young patients (58% of those under 35 yr) *(101)*. Many (42%) of these young patients with MSI-positive CRC will have a detectable germline mutation in known DNA MMR genes. In another study, the clinical features were described for three groups of CRC patients (in a population-based registry) in whom the disease occurred at a relatively early age of onset (group I: <40 yr; group II: 41–50 yr; group III: 51–55 yr). Hereditary CRC (HNPCC and FAP), and suspected HNPCC accounted for 38.4% of group I patients, 17.1% of group II, 10.2% of group III, and only 3.5% of individuals older than 55 *(p = 0.001) (102)*. These studies suggest that age-at-diagnosis as a criterion may have predictive value for identification of individual HNPCC patients.

Another question is whether age-at-diagnosis of the other extracolonic cancers that frequently occur in HNPCC has predictive value in individual patients in the population. In a Finnish study, the age at diagnosis of other integral cancers occurring in HNPCC was evaluated *(104)*. These other cancers (including gastric, biliary tract, urinary tract, and ovarian tumors) occurred at approximately the same age in HNPCC patients as do those same cancer types in the general population. Endometrial carcinomas occurred at a somewhat earlier age. Thus, although the age at CRC diagnosis may have value as a diagnostic criterion for the individual with HNPCC, the age at diagnosis of most other integral cancers would be predicted to not have similar diagnostic value.

Existence of Probands Because of the problem of small family size, the challenge is to diagnose HNPCC-affected individuals without a family history, and to identify these probands with the hereditary CRC trait before CRC develops. A proband for a disease is the original person presenting with, or likely to be subject to, a mental or physical disorder and whose case serves as the stimulus for a hereditary or genetic study. Hereditary-cancer probands are patients: 1) who are newly diagnosed to have the cancer or premonitory sign, and 2) who have no known antecedent family history of the disease. Diagnosis of a proband often leads to detection of this heredi-

tary disease in their family, although up to 40–50% have been reported to be isolated cases (negative family history) in disorders such as FAP (*APC*), neurofibromatosis (*NF1* and *NF2*), and medullary thyroid cancer (*MEN2B*) *(105–112)*. This is presumably due to a *de novo* germ-line mutation in the cancer-susceptibility genes of the affected individuals. Because an estimated 40–50% of probands are isolated cases, they are not in identified hereditary-cancer families.

In contrast, the recent development of clinical criteria for diagnosing hereditary-cancer syndromes and the emergence of specific molecular gene testing makes it possible to determine which individuals within many hereditary-cancer families are affected (have the germline mutation). Thus, strategies for cancer prevention and early detection (before metastasis) can be effectively implemented in these affected family members. However, other carriers of a germline mutation (probands) may not be identified as being affected with a hereditary-cancer trait for a variety of reasons. Thus, for these other carriers, it is difficult to identify them as having hereditary-cancer traits before the actual cancer develops. And without that early identification, it is not possible to institute interventions that lead to cancer prevention and/or early detection of tumors. This difficulty might be overcome if there were premonitory indicators of the cancer syndrome that were quantitative, accurate, reliable, practical, and affordable, and that could form the basis of a diagnostic criterion. Indeed, some hereditary-cancer syndromes have physical findings that may serve as premonitory signs. These include FAP, Cowden's syndrome, Fanconi anemia, Muir-Torre syndrome, MEN2b, Peutz-Jeghers syndrome, Turcot syndrome, and WAGR syndrome (Table 1) *(37)*. In contrast and unfortunately, there are no well-established clinical or physical premonitory signs for HNPCC and most other major hereditary-cancer syndromes.

FAP Probands Unfortunately a significant proportion of probands will already have developed cancer by the time that they are diagnosed. One estimate of this proportion comes from a consideration of FAP (Table 14). In this hereditary cancer, the multiple polyposis phenotype allows the clinician to unambiguously diagnose the hereditary-cancer trait. Theoretically, the FAP phenotype should provide a clinical sign that is sufficient for premonitory diagnosis and this should lead to cancer prevention. Yet, modern clinical experience is that approx two-thirds of FAP probands will have already developed CRC prior to diagnosis of FAP *(105–107)*. Surgery at this point is therapeutic rather than prophylactic and the prognosis is much less favorable compared to prophylactic surgical call-up cases. The cumulative 10-yr survival rate in FAP proband patients is only about 40% despite the fact that this is a relatively young patient population with a median age of 39, with many productive years of life ahead. Therefore, even if there is a premonitory sign to detect affected people, because of high cancer incidence in probands screening and management only partially reduces mortality rate. Thus, despite the fact that CRC can theoretically be prevented in FAP-afflicted individuals in families where this hereditary disease has already been identified (call-up cases), this uncommon hereditary disease is still estimated to account for as many as 1% of all newly diagnosed cases of CRC. Indeed, many (if not most) FAP patients with diagnosed CRC are FAP probands *(108)*.

Obviously, the challenge faced by the health-care system is to identify and diagnose FAP probands before they develop CRC so that prophylactic measures (colectomy) can be taken for them and for members of their extended family that also might be affected by FAP. An even greater challenge is to detect probands in all other hereditary-cancer types because premonitory clinical signs for most of them are not known. Indeed, HNPCC is much more common (20–30 times) than FAP.

HNPCC Probands Like most other hereditary cancer patients, HNPCC individuals lack a known premalignant phenotype that makes proband detection extremely difficult (Table 14). Based on our experience with FAP and on their being several genes that can undergo *de novo* mutation in HNPCC, the frequency of HNPCC probands among HNPCC families might be predicted to be 40–50% or greater. Thus, we should explore whether possible clinical features might serve as criteria to distinguish CRC in the individual carrying the HNPCC trait from sporadic (non-HNPCC) CRC. Age at diagnosis should be considered as a possible screening criterion in HNPCC. Other possible criteria might include early-onset discrete adenomas or other clinical features that characterize HNPCC.

GENE TESTING HAS LIMITATIONS AND PITFALLS
Molecular testing has limitations because current approaches will not detect most individuals affected with a hereditary-cancer trait before they develop cancer. For example, MSI analysis is usually performed on cancer tissue and therefore does not detect possible hereditary-cancer traits prior to tumor development. Moreover, MSI does not directly detect germline mutations, and acquired MMR mutations will also be cause MSI. Additionally, detecting germline mutations will not detect probands because current gene-testing methods cannot practically and efficiently be used for broad-based screening purposes. Unless the mutation in a family is known, current tests for germline mutations are cumbersome, expensive, and not widely available (Table 5). Even those molecular screening tests that are available for detecting germline mutations have limitations, such as limited sensitivity.

Another limiting factor related to gene testing is that health-care systems are not geared to provide wide-scale clinical genetic services. This includes insufficient training, experience, and expertise of physicians, financial reimbursement being inadequate or lacking for clinical genetic services, and limited number of cancer genetic centers for routine referral of identified families for further diagnosis, management, and counseling. Even in situations where gene testing can be sufficiently provided in a clinical setting, there can be many pitfalls, such as mutations that escape detection, misinterpretation of results, and an inability to accurately predict and calculate risk for disease *(112)*. A main question that should be posed when considering genetic testing is whether it is beneficial for the patient to know that he or she carries a gene mutation. Certainly genetic tests can be helpful under the right circumstances, such as when the results affect clinical decisions that can reduce mortality. However, gene testing also has problems that stem from interpreting the significance of gene test results (either positive or negative). One problem in interpreting the significance of gene test results reflects the current lack of information regarding the risks associated with a positive result. Genetic factors (or genetic risks) are often used to explain the causes of ill health and unwanted behavior. However, it is often difficult to say with absolute certainty that the presence of a single germline (allelic) mutation in a person will cause a complex disorder such as cancer. Even when evidence for such an association is compelling, the vast majority of cells in the patient's body will never become malignant. These difficulties can create dilemmas and problems for advocates of gene testing *(113)*.

A major pitfall of genetic testing involves the inability to predict cancer risk. Even in cases where a known cancer-susceptibility gene mutation is detected, accurate prediction that a given individual will develop cancer is still not possible. Indeed, calculation of risk inevitably has the variable of time entered into estimation of the probability of developing cancer. Moreover, there are other variables, such as modifying genes, lifestyle, and environmental factors that can affect risk associated with a cancer-susceptibility gene. Because we do not know how to account for, or even identify, all of these variable factors, determining one's risk for cancer when a mutation is present in the germline can be inaccurate. Thus, even in the case of classical Mendelian inheritance, the relationship between the gene's DNA sequence and the phenotype is not simple, further complicating interpretation and management. One example involves the DNA sequences of *BRCA1* in association with hereditary breast-ovarian cancer syndrome *(33–35,114)*. Table 4 shows a comparison of the genotypic and phenotypic features of these two types of hereditary breast cancer. Although over 100 variants of the *BRCA1* sequence have already been identified, only a few of them have been shown to be deleterious. These cases have mostly been found: 1) in families with an unusually high incidence of ovarian and/or breast cancer, and/or 2) where these cancers occur at a young age (the patient selection skews the population toward higher risk). Over 90% of women in the general population with breast cancer or ovarian cancer do not fall into these categories, calling into question the relevance of these genetic tests for most women. Moreover, even if a woman from a cancer-prone family tests positive for one of the cancer-linked genes, it does not automatically mean that a tumor will develop, even though her lifetime risk is considerably greater than in the general popula-

Table 15
Surveillance and Management Options for Hereditary Breast Cancer Patients[a]

Proven gene carrier (BRCA1 or BRCA2 Positive)

Screening for breast cancer using annual mammography beginning at age 25–35, clinical breast exam every 6–12 mo beginning at age 25–35, and breast self-examination monthly.

Screening for ovarian cancer using vaginal probe ultrasound, Doppler color flow imagery of ovaries and CA-125 tumor marker every 6–12 mo beginning at age 25–35.

Screening for colon cancer and prostate cancer according to average-risk population guidelines

Prophylactic mastectomy and oophorectomy or cehmoprevention should be considered in order to reduce risk for breast and ovarian cancer *(134a–e)*.

Hereditary breast cancer patient with breast cancer

Mastectomy with consideration of prophylactic mastectomy of the opposite breast

Hereditary breast cancer patient with ovarian cancer

Conventional surgical or other treatment

[a]From Burke et al. *(116)*.

tion. Indeed, the confidence limits on risk associated with *BRCA1* and *BRCA2* mutations are large, suggesting that other factors must be involved.

Another potential pitfall involves interpretation of a negative test result. In gene testing, a negative test result does not always mean that the individual has no risk. For instance, the failure to find a mutation in a hereditary-cancer family that does not have a known segregating germline mutation may incorrectly be interpreted as a lack of risk and members at-risk may wrongly fail to comply with proper screening recommendations. When the mutation is unknown in a family, negativity means that the test results are inconclusive or uninformative due to limitations in the testing technology such that a mutation cannot be ruled out. In such circumstances, at-risk family members should still follow screening guidelines for hereditary cancer (and not guidelines for the general population). For example, if a woman in a family having known *BRCA1* or *BRCA2* mutations tests negative for the mutation, it does not indicate that she will not develop breast cancer; it only indicates that her risk is reduced to the value seen in women in the general population.

Another uncertainty is the problem of what to do if a woman tests positive, because prophylactic surgery (mastectomy and oophorectomy) is considered quite drastic by the patient. The surveillance and management options *(116)* for hereditary breast-cancer patients are outlined in Table 15. In proven gene carriers (*BRCA1*- or *BRCA2*-positive), recent evidence indicates that prophylactic mastectomy or oophorectomy or chemoprevention may be beneficial in order to reduce risk for developing breast or ovarian cancer *(114a–e)*.

Other pitfalls and limitations in gene testing include the following: 1) gene testing might be offered by health-care professions who are inadequately educated or experienced in he-

reditary cancers and/or who do not provide proper patient information, education, or genetic counseling; 2) there are numerous psychological, social, and ethical issues in gene testing *(117)*; 3) national and international health-care systems are often insufficiently developed to provide care for hereditary-cancer patients and to establish testing algorithms and cost-effective management strategies. Certainly, since the emergence of commercially available genetic tests, many health-care professionals have not kept abreast of the policies and recommendations for patient education and genetic counseling. Patient counseling is an essential part of determining cancer risk by gene-testing services. This also has relevance to issues of privacy and discrimination, especially in regard to concerns involving employment and insurance.

HOW DO WE REDUCE MORTALITY FROM HEREDITARY CANCER?

The key to reducing mortality from hereditary cancer is to identify hereditary-trait carriers before cancer develops. The needs are: 1) to improve the identification of families with the hereditary-cancer trait, 2) to identify probands (40–50% of cases) before they get cancer, and 3) to more effectively manage individuals affected with hereditary-cancer traits.

TO IMPROVE THE IDENTIFICATION OF FAMILIES WITH HEREDITARY-CANCER TRAITS To increase the number of hereditary-cancer kindreds that are accurately diagnosed, it is important to utilize clinical criteria that have higher sensitivity. For example, for diagnosing HNPCC families, we recommend using Modified Amsterdam Criteria (Table 9), as follows: 1) reported cases of CRC should be verified so that they can be included as diagnostic of affected individuals in families; 2) verified cases of other HNPCC-associated cancers should be included; 3) three sibling clusters (including CRC and/or endometrial cancers) should be accepted as long as there is a second-degree affected relative in the preceding or succeeding generation. Although these modified criteria are predicted to have higher sensitivity, they may also have decreased positive predictive value (PPV), which represents the proportion of people who meet the positive criterion who actually have the disease. Hopefully, lower PPV can be overcome by adding to the total clinical genetic-testing regime a second test that has a high PPV. This can generally be accomplished by adding molecular (DNA) testing to determine from the genotype whether there is a hereditary-cancer trait. This integration of clinical and gene testing will allow such false-positives from the first screen to be identified.

IDENTIFYING PROBANDS BEFORE THE ONSET OF CANCER Another way to increase survival of hereditary-cancer patients is through identification of individuals with hereditary-cancer traits before they develop cancer. FAP can be used as a benchmark to illustrate the effectiveness that presymptomatic diagnosis can have on reducing mortality in hereditary cancer families. In FAP, individuals who are affected but left untreated have a very high frequency of CRC, the lifetime probability being very close to 100%. In contrast, cancer-prevention programs can often increase survival in families in which FAP has already been identified. Once the first case of FAP has been identified in a family, these prevention programs include:

1) early screening of other family members at risk, 2) prophylactic surgical treatment (colectomy) of those FAP family members found to be affected (call-up cases), and 3) regular postoperative examinations. The result has been a much-reduced frequency of CRC (3–9%) in postsurgical call-up cases *(105–107)*. This success has been somewhat tempered by the observation that some surgically treated FAP patients remain predisposed to develop other life-threatening problems including intra-abdominal fibromas and desmoids, cancer in retained rectal segments, and extracolonic malignancies such as periampullary carcinomas. Thus, the risk of death remains from other FAP-related problems. This is exemplified by a study of FAP call-up cases (n = 222), who were treated with prophylactic colectomy, that showed the risk of dying prematurely was still significantly greater (relative risk = 3.35) than the age- and sex-matched general population *(118)*. However, this is significantly improved over the risk (100% for CRC) if FAP patients are left untreated.

HNPCC can also be used to demonstrate the effectiveness in reducing mortality when family members in known HNPCC kindreds are screened. Once a patient is identified to be at risk in an HNPCC-affected family, surveillance consisting of colonoscopy or barium enema plus sigmoidoscopy has been shown to significantly reduce the rate of tumor development and increase survival for these patients. For example, a recent Finnish study *(119)* evaluated the occurrence of CRC and mortality rate in a series of about 251 members of HNPCC families (individuals who were at 50% risk for HNPCC) according to whether or not they received screening. In one subgroup, subjects (n = 133) were screened at three-yr intervals; another subgroup consisted of subjects (n = 119) who refused screening and who were simply followed. CRC developed in 19 controls (16%) vs. 8 in the screened group (6%) —a 62% reduction in CRC. There were 9 deaths due to CRC in the controls vs. no deaths in the screened group. Moreover, the ten-yr survival was significantly improved in the subgroup that underwent screening compared to the control group. Overall, the results indicate that three-yr interval screening significantly reduces the occurrence of CRC and improves survival of HNPCC patients. The results also indicate that the adenomas in HNPCC, where it is known that there is genetic instability due to MMR mutations *(92)*, are more likely to become malignant than sporadic adenomas in individuals in the general population. It can be calculated that one cancer was prevented for every 2.8 polypectomies performed on HNPCC-at-risk individuals in the surveillance group compared to one cancer prevented for every 41 to 119 polypectomies performed during screening in the general population *(120–122)*. Therefore, to reduce mortality in FAP and HNPCC probands, the challenge is to identify probands before CRC develops. Identifying probands in FAP before they develop cancer may require exploring the potential value of identifying extracolonic manifestations such as congenital hypertrophy of the retinal pigment epithelium. Some FAP affected individuals could be identified during ophthalmologic exams performed on adolescents for prescribing corrective lenses (perhaps even as part of a professionally supported education program for opthalmologists).

To identify probands in HNPCC, two developments would be very useful: 1) inexpensive, practical, easy, widely available test for carriers of the hereditary trait (germline mutations); 2) clinical criteria that have predictive value for presymptomatic HNPCC diagnosis. Age at diagnosis of discrete adenomas may be useful because the age distribution of adenomas occurs about two to three yr before CRC develops. Therefore, in HNPCC, the median age of adenomas is predicted to be 41–42 yr of age. The histopathology of the adenoma may also carry predictive value because HNPCC adenomas tend to be large and have a high villous component reflecting increased risk for malignant transformation. In comparison, although CRC in HNPCC is usually proximally located, the location of the adenoma is not helpful because adenomas in HNPCC families have the same anatomic distribution (proximal vs distal) as do sporadic adenomas. MSI may have predictive value because early studies suggest that adenomas from HNPCC patients exhibit alterations in their microsatellite sequences *(92)*. If any of these features of adenomas were found to be predictive of HNPCC, it may be possible to identify HNPCC probands before they develop cancer. In this approach, it might become feasible to target individuals in the existing health-care system who have premalignant adenomas. Gastroenterologists and other physicians could play an important role in this effort.

TOWARDS A MORE EFFECTIVE MANAGEMENT OF INDIVIDUALS AFFECTED WITH HEREDITARY-CANCER TRAITS, PARTICULARLY THOSE WHO ARE IDENTIFIED BEFORE CANCER DEVELOPS To succeed at reducing mortality from hereditary cancer, it will be necessary that practitioners provide effective clinical management of individuals in known hereditary-cancer families and offer equally effective clinical management for affected probands. Obviously, physicians need to take more responsibility for obtaining accurate family histories from their patients and for screening and following up on family members. For an updated listing of clinical genetics programs/laboratories, the GeneTests Internet directory can be contacted at *http://www.genetests.org*. A directory of genetic counseling services listed by state and city can be contacted at http://www.nsgc.org/resource_link.html.

In addition to knowing where to refer patients for genetics services, physicians must become more knowledgeable as to the basic facts and principles of inherited cancers. This includes learning how to accurately interpret the results of genetic tests and how to appropriately manage and counsel patients with hereditary disorders. Unfortunately, one recent study on interpretation of FAP molecular testing results shows that many physicians are lacking in these clinical genetic skills *(123)*. Nearly one-third of physicians who received results on *APC* gene testing for FAP misinterpreted the findings. Moreover, only a small percentage of patients received genetic counseling (19%) or provided written informed consent before the genetic test was performed (17%). These findings suggest that many physicians do not appreciate the possible consequences of having the test performed, including the emotional burden and employment or insurance discrimination.

A recent report on "What physicians need to know about genetics" has been established by a working group convened by the National Center for Genome Research (NCGR), Santa Fe, NM. It is recommended that practicing physicians become knowledgeable about the following points *(124)*: 1) identifying genetic abnormalities; 2) accessing genetic services; 3) interpreting risk factors; 4) understanding the science of genetic testing; and 5) incorporating patient advocacy issues into genetic testing. Physicians should be able to identify those patients under their care who would benefit from genetic services. Physicians should know how to access genetic services after a risk factor for a gene-related disease is identified. Physicians should be able to interpret risk information provided in genetic test reports and to explain the information (and options for further management) to patients. Physicians should have the basic fund of knowledge needed to read and interpret the medical literature and to answer patient questions about gene testing, gene therapy, and prognosis for genetic-related conditions. Physicians should be knowledgeable about patient-advocacy issues, such as informed consent, patient autonomy, confidentiality, privacy requirements, and the potential for discrimination and stigmatization resulting from genetic test results. This will facilitate important discussions on relevant ethical, legal, social, cultural, and financial issues with patients *(117)*.

Finally, it will be important to enhance our health-care system so that we can more effectively deal with hereditary cancer families; for example, the NCI has set up the National Cancer Genetics Network for this purpose. Such a system should provide more effective management of affected individuals. This could also provide a mechanism to develop awareness campaigns among those practitioners who may be involved in gene testing. Such educational efforts are vitally important because much of the burden will probably fall on primary-care practitioners (family practice, surgeons, internists, physician assistants, and nursing assistants). In addition, some specialists will probably have responsibility in this field. For example, awareness campaigns on gene testing for hereditary CRC might be focused on gastroenterologists and colorectal surgeons. Indeed, similar targeted efforts have already succeeded, such as widespread screening for CRC using occult blood testing of stool samples. In addition, efforts to establish a national cancer genetic system now provides a means to develop research protocols to investigate the integration of clinical and molecular approaches for diagnosing hereditary cancer including optimal integration, practicality, and cost-effectiveness. A national system would also deal with several other issues on genetic test development including quality control, certification of diagnostic laboratories, principles for patient consent, policies on privacy and discrimination, guidelines for distribution of genetic tests to the medical community, and recommendations for professional education.

GENETIC COUNSELING

Genetic knowledge can identify individuals who will benefit from preventive practices and early detection of cancer. But when a genetic test is ordered, a clinician sets in motion a chain of events that potentially can have profound medical, psychological, and ethical consequences. Physicians who offer testing to families, and the genetic counselors, nurses, psychologists, and other health-care providers who participate in

this process will be expected to be knowledgeable of the potential consequences. We need to ensure that our interpretations of genetic tests are accurate, that our assessments of cancer risk are appropriate, and that our mode of conveying information is not counterproductive. Therefore, it is important to remember that genetic-susceptibility testing is just one part of the overall cancer risk-assessment program *(125–127)*. Moreover, genetic predisposition testing is a multi-step process involving the following six procedures *(128)*: 1) identify at-risk patients; 2) provide pre-test counseling; 3) provide informed consent; 4) Select and offer a test; 5) carry out the test and disclose results; 6) provide post-test counseling and follow-up. Because genetic testing raises many medical, social, psychological, and ethical issues for individuals and their families, genetic counseling is integral to the overall testing process before a test is ordered. Genetic counseling is provided to assess cancer risk, provide patient education, and discuss the medical and psychosocial implications of testing. Whether provided by a genetic counselor, nurse, or physician, the content of cancer genetic counseling should remain uniform. Risk assessment involves evaluating an individual's actual and perceived cancer risk. Patient education should include information about cancer etiology, current information about known or suspected risk factors, basics of genes and cancer risk, and the basics of inheritance. Before deciding to be tested, patients should have ample opportunity to discuss the risks, benefits, and limitation of testing and to have their questions answered. Basic information about the test procedure, such as turnaround time and accuracy of the testing and alternatives to testing should also be provided. Potential outcomes should be explored with patients who are considering genetic testing and how possible results, whether positive, negative, or indeterminate, may influence medical management before a choice is made to proceed with testing. The health-care professional who opts to take on the responsibility of this genetic counseling must provide the depth of content and time required to ensure that the patient who does proceed with testing has made a fully informed choice after having weighed the risks, benefits and limitations.

Genetic counselors are health-care professionals, who usually hold a master's degree and have comprehensive training in clinical and molecular genetics, risk assessment, and the psychosocial aspects of hereditary cancer. Therefore, genetic counselors and other cancer genetics professionals can provide services at all levels of the multi-step process of genetic testing including documenting and interpreting pedigrees, estimating cancer risk, and distinguishing families with true hereditary predisposition from those associated with environmental exposure or a clustering of sporadic cancers due to chance. Genetic counselors also help individuals and families comprehend medical/scientific facts, explain how heredity contributes to cancer risk, explain options for dealing with the risk of disease, assist in choosing an appropriate course of action according to a family's belief system, assist in making the best possible adjustment to a diagnosis or risk status, and help patients understand the psychosocial aspects of genetic testing.

GENERAL ASSESSMENT Some patients may seek genetic testing because they perceive their cancer risk to be higher than it actually is. The extent to which risk perception contributes to

Table 16.
Potential Consequences of Gene Testing for Hereditary Cancer[a]

If a test shows presence of a cancer susceptibility gene:

Positive consequences
- Removal of uncertainty and doubt.
- More focused approaches toward cancer prevention and early detection.
- Ability to appropriately plan and prepare emotionally for the future (e.g., family).
- Increased compliance with surveillance recommendations.
- Clearer information on cancer-risk that can be used in considering prophylactic surgical options.

Negative consequences
- Denial, anger, dejection, chronic anxiety.
- Concern about possible rejection and stigmatization by family or friends
- Apprehension about death.
- Potential for employment discrimination or interference with education.
- Worry about offspring regarding possible gene transmission.
- Potential for insurance discrimination.
- Fear about surgery and possible changes in lifestyle.

If test shows absence of an cancer susceptibility gene:

Positive consequences
- Relief from uncertainty and anxiety.
- Ability to make more desirable life choices including career plans.
- Assurance that offspring are not affected.
- Reduced medical expenses.
- Better chance to receive insurance.

Negative consequences
- Survivor guilt from negative test result while other family members are affected.
- Potential false interpretation that cancer risk is zero.

If test gives indeterminate result:

Positive consequences
- Additional information has often been acquired about family history.
- Hereditary cancer risk has often been made based on clinical information.
- Professional relationships established with genetic counselor.
- Screening and management recommendations can still often be made based on clinical information.
- Research protocols or molecular studies may become available.

Negative consequences
- Anger over lack of a definitive result.
- Potential false interpretation that cancer risk is equivalent to that in the general population.
- Continued anxiety over cancer risk.

[a] Adapted from Petersen and Brensinger (130).

a patient's motivation for genetic testing should be assessed before testing. The education process should be sensitive to patient-specific concerns and tailored to the individual's educational level and ability to grasp complex issues. First, the physicians should assess personal and family medical history, risk perception, and motivation for testing (129). Second, clinicians should educate the patient about basic genetics, inheritance, cancer genetics, and risk. Third, a discussion should be conducted regarding risks, benefits and limitations of testing, test procedures, alternatives to testing, and management options.

PRE-TEST COUNSELING Because of the potential consequences, it is essential to explain several important issues to the patient before ordering the test. These include: 1) how test results will be disclosed; 2) that patient confidentiality and privacy will be maintained; 3) that a patient is welcome to bring a support person; 4) that the results will be disclosed in person and not by other means; 5) that the psychological impact of disclosing the results will be explored and addressed; and 6) that follow-up measures will be discussed.

INFORMED CONSENT Basic elements of an informed consent for germline DNA testing include the following (130): 1) the patient should be given information, in an understandable manner, on the specific test being performed; 2) the physicians should point out the implications of a positive and a negative test result; 3) it should be pointed out that there is a possibility that the test will not be informative (not all mutations are detectable); 4) options for risk estimation without gene testing should be evaluated; 5) risk of passing a mutation to offspring should be considered. 6) technical accuracy of the test should be discussed, including sensitivity, specificity, and PPV of the test to be performed.

POST-TEST COUNSELING The post-test genetic counseling should include assessing the patient response to the disclosure of the results, reviewing the meaning of the results, discussing the patient's plans for sharing results with family members, and discussing medical follow-up plans.

LIMITATIONS OF GENETIC TESTING Genetic testing is not fool-proof. The limitations should be made clear to the patient. For example, not all mutations are detectable. Also, there is uncertain significance attached to the presence of some mutations (e.g. missense mutations). A negative result is informative only if the mutation has been identified in the family. Test results indicate probability, not certainty, of developing cancer, and the efficacy of most interventions is unproven.

ETHICS AND IMPLICATIONS OF GENE TESTING The potential consequences (from both positive and negative results) of gene testing for hereditary cancer are outlined in Table 16 (130).

MEDICAL LEGAL ISSUES Two court cases have resulted in the ruling that physicians have a duty to warn other family members that they may be at risk for cancer: Pate vs Threlkel (Florida, 1995) and Safer vs Pack (New Jersey, 1996). It is recommended by the American Cancer Society (131) that the physician/provider assume the following duties. All physicians should take a family history. Providers should have guidelines for recognizing at-risk individuals, and responsibility for family reporting. Guidelines for referral for genetic counseling and testing services are needed. Gag rules employed by managed-care providers and similar entities, particularly as they apply to predisposition testing and clinical surveillance, are inappropriate.

A PHILOSOPHICAL PERSPECTIVE ON GENE TESTING AND SURVIVAL

The main goal in Oncology is to increase survival for cancer patients. One might view this goal from a philosophical perspective in relation to survival of humans over the ages. To quote from R.A. Ruden *(132)* on survival:

We are here because we survived. We each survived because we made it through gestation and the birth canal into the care of people who, whatever their strengths and weaknesses or shortcomings, managed to feed and protect us. We survived because, as a group, science and society collaborated to shield us from disease that a century ago would have killed us before we emerged from childhood. We survived as individuals by being fortunate enough to avoid both the natural and unnatural disasters that threaten us as we navigate the minefield that is life.

In a broader sense, we are survivors because our parents survived, and theirs and theirs. We are survivors because our primate and reptilian ancestors survived, as did even our most ancient ancestors - insentient creatures, unaware of their own existence. We are survivors because Nature, the embodiment and force behind biology, endowed them all with traits and tools and miraculous mechanisms to make sure they got done what living creatures must do to perpetuate their species: survive.

As we move into the next millennium, science and technology may provide additional means to help us survive. For example, from the explosive growth in information about the human genome, and from new molecular tests for hereditary-cancer traits, we may soon be able to predict many of the diseases that an individual is particularly susceptible to develop. Among the important questions and issues for future research will be: 1) how accurately and effectively can we make these predictions; 2) can they be made (via gene testing) on a significant number of individuals in the general population, with high sensitivity and low cost; and 3) once an individual is predicted to have a high probability to develop a disease, can preventive measures and/or lifestyle changes improve survival for this person? Thus, from a philosophical perspective, predicting who will get which disease based on gene testing and then preventing those diseases can perhaps best be viewed as a new survival technique.

ACKNOWLEDGMENTS

We would like to thank the following individuals for their support and assistance in the preparation of this manuscript: Gretchen M. Matika, Sandy Ehrlich, Marcia Lewis, Karen Simpson, Catherine M. Boman, Joan B. Fields, Mayo Alumni Association (1998 Delegation to Malaysia), and Bobbi Fuxa. This work was supported in part by funding from CA*TX Biotechnology Inc. (Gladwyne, PA), Chiron Corporation, NIH (5R21CA71531), and The Storz Foundation. Supported, in part, by Senior (F33) Fellowship (AG05735) to JZF.

REFERENCES

1. Lynch, H. T., Boman, B. M., and Lynch, J. F. (1993) Familial predisposition on malignancy. *In: Medical Oncology* (Calabresi, P. and Schein, P., eds.), McGraw-Hill, New York, pp 121–142.

2. Burt, R. W. (1996) Familial risk and colorectal cancer. *Gastroenterol. Clin. North Am.* **25**:793–803.

3. Fearon, E. R. (1997) Human cancer syndromes: ´clues to the origin and nature of cancer. *Science* **278**:1043–1050.

4. Kinzler, K. W. and Vogelstein, B. (1998) *The Genetic Basis of Human Cancer* (Kinzler, K. W., and Vogelstein, B., eds.), McGraw-Hill, New York, pp. 241–242.

5. Spirio, L., Olschwang, S., Groden, J., Robertson, M., Samowitz, W., Joslyn, G., et al. (1993) Alleles of the *APC* Gene: an attenuated form of familial polyposis. *Cell* **75**:951–957.

6. van der Luijt, R. B., Meera Khan, P., Vasen, H. F., Breukel, C., Tops, C. M., Scott, R. J., et al. (1996) Germline mutations in the 3´ part of APC exon 15 do not result in truncated proteins and are associated with attenuated adenomatous polyposis coli. *Human Genet.* **98**:727–734.

7. Soravia, C., Berk, T., Madlensky, L., Mitri, A., Cheng, H., Gallinger, S., et al. (1998) Genotype-Phenotype correlations in attenuated adenomatous polyposis coli. *Am. J. Human Genet.* **62**:1290–1301.

8. Kinzler, K. W. and Vogelstein, B. (1998) Colorectal tumors. *In: The Genetic Basis of Human Cancer* (Kinzler, K. W., and Vogelstein, B., eds.), McGraw-Hill, New York, pp. 565–587.

9. Dietrich, W. F., Lander, E. S., Smith, J. S., Moser, A. R., Gould, K. A., Luongo, C., et al. (1993) Genetic identification of Mom-1, a major modifier locus affecting Min-induced intestinal neoplasia in the mouse. *Cell* **75**:631–639.

10. MacPhee, M. Chepnik, K. P., Liddell, R. A., Nelson, K. K., Siracusa, L. D., and Buchberg, A. M. (1995) The secretory phospholipase A2 gene is a candidate for the Mom-1 locus, a major modifier of APCMin-induced intestinal neoplasia. *Cell* **81**:957–966.

11. Cormier, R. T., Hong, K. H., Halberg, R. B., Hawkins, T. L., Richardson, P., Mulherkar, R., et al. (1997) Secretory phospholipase Pla2g2a confers resistance to intestinal tumorigenesis. *Nature Genet.* **17**:88–89.

12. Dragani, T. A. and Maneti, G. (1997) Mom-1 leads the pack. *Nature Genet.* **17**:7–8.

13. Laird, P. W., Jackson-Grusby, L., Fazeli, A., Dickinson, S. L., Jung, W. E., Li, B., et al. (1995) Suppression of intestinal neoplasia by DNA hypomethylation. *Cell* **81**:197–205.

14. Oshima, M., Dinchuk, J. E., Kargman, S. L., Oshima, H., Hancock, B., Kwong, E., et al. (1996) Suppression of intestinal polyposis in APC delta716 knockout mice by inhibition of cyclooxygenase 2 (COX-2). *Cell* **87**:803–809.

15. Huang, J., Papadopoulos, N., McKinley, A. J., Farrington, S. M., Curtis, L. J., Wyllie, A. H., et al. (1996) *APC* mutations in colorectal tumors with mismatch repair deficiency. *Proc. Natl. Acad. Sci. USA* **93**:9049–9054.

16. Markowitz, S., Wang, J., Myeroff, L., Parsons, R., Sun, L., Lutterbaugh, J., et al. (1995) Inactivation of the type II TGF-beta receptor in colon cancer cells with microsatellite instability. *Science* **268**:1336–1338.

17. Holtzman, N. A. (1996) Are we ready to screen for inherited susceptibility to cancer? *Oncology* **10**:57–67.

18. Swift, M., Morrell, D., Massey, R. B., and Chase, C. L. (1991) Incidence of cancer in 161 families affected by ataxia telangiectasia. *N. Engl. J. Med.* **325**:1831–1836.

19. FitzGerald, M. G., Bean, J. M., Hegde, S. R., Unsal, H., MacDonald, J., Harkin, P. D., et al. (1997) Heterozygous ATM mutations do not contribute to early onset of breast cancer. *Nature Genet.* **15**:307–310.

20. Miyoshi, Y., Nagase, H., Ando, H., Horii, A., Ichii, S., Nakatsuru, S., et al. (1993) Association of the APC tumor suppressor protein with catenins. *Science* **262**:1734–1737.

21. Rubinfeld, B., Souza, B., Albert, I., Muller, O., Chamberlain, S., Masiarz, F., et al. (1993) Association of the APC gene product with β-catenin. *Science* **262**:1731–1734.

22. Munemitsu, S., Souza, B., Muller, O., Albert, I., Rubinfeld, B., Polakis, P. (1994) The APC gene product associates with microtu-

bules in vivo and promotes their assembly in vitro. *Cancer Res.* **54**:3676–3681.

23. Smith, K. J., Levy, D. B., Maupin, P., Pollard, T. D., Vogelstein, B., Kinzler, K. W. (1994) Wild-type but not mutant APC associates with the microtubule cytoskeleton. *Cancer Res.* **54**:3672–3675.

24. Gao, Z. Q., Gao, Z. P., Bhattacharya, G., Wang, L. J., Wu, J. M., and Boman, B. M. (1998) APC's basic domain in its carboxyl region mediates tubulin polymerization in vitro. *Proc. Am. Assoc. Cancer Res.* **39**:616a.

25. Lynch, H. T. (1996) Glossary of key terms. *Oncology* **10**:39–40.

26. Thompson, J. S. and Thompson, M. W. (1973) *Genetics in Medicine,* 2nd ed. W.B. Saunders & Co., Philadelphia, PA.

27. Knudson, A. G. (1971) Mutation and cancer: statistical study of retinoblastoma. *Proc. Natl. Acad. Sci. USA* **68**:820–823.

28. Knudson, A. G. (1978) Retinoblastoma: a prototypic hereditary neoplasm. *Semin. Oncol.* **5**:57–60.

29. Fearon, E. R. and Vogelstein, B. (1990) A genetic model for colorectal tumorigenesis. *Cell* **61**:759–767.

30. Smith, H. D., Lu, Y., Deng, G., Martinez, O., Krams, S., Ljung, B. M., et al. (1993) Molecular aspects of early stages of breast cancer progression. *J. Cell. Biochem.* **17G**:144–152.

31. Knudson, A. G. (1993) All in the (cancer) family. *Nature Genet.* **5**:103–104.

32. King, R. C. and Standsfield, W. D. (1997) *A Dictionary of Genetics,* 5th ed. Oxford University Press, New York, NY.

33. Miki, Y., Swensow, J., Shattuck-Eidens, D., Futreal, A., Harshman, K., Tavtigian, S., et. al. (1994) A strong candidate for the breast and ovarian cancer susceptibility gene BRCA1. *Science* **266**:66–71.

34. Wooster, R., Bignell, G., Lancaster, J., Swift, S., Seal, S., Mangion, J., et al. (1995) Identification of the breast cancer susceptibility gene BRCA2. *Nature* **378**:789–792.

35. Tavtigian, S. V., Simard, J., Romens, J., Couch, F., Shattuck-Eidens, D., Neuhausen, S., et al. (1996) The complete BRCA2 gene and mutations in chromosome 13q-linked kindreds *Nature Genet.* **12**:333–337.

36. Lu, S.-L., Kawabata, M., Imamura, T., Akiyama, Y., Nomizu, T., Miyazono, K., et al. (1998) HNPCC associated with germline mutation in the TGF-beta type II receptor gene. *Nature Genetics* **19**:17–18.

37. Offit, K. (1998) Hereditary and acquired risks for cancer. *In: Clinical Cancer Genetics: Risk Counseling & Management.* Wiley-Liss, New York, NY.

38. Lynch, H. T., Drouhard, T., Vasen, H. F. A., Cavalieri, J., Lynch, J., Nord, S., et al. (1996) Genetic counseling in a Navajo Hereditary nonpolyposis colorectal cancer kindred. *Cancer* **77**:30–35.

39. Powell, S. M., Petersen, G. M., Krush, A. J., Booker, S., Jen, J., Giardiello, F. M., et al. (1993) Molecular diagnosis of familial adenomatous polyposis. *N. Engl. J. Med.* **329**:1982–1987.

40. Hogervorst, F. B. L. (1997) The Protein Truncation Test (PTT). *Promega Notes* **62**:7–10.

41. Laken, S. J., Petersen, G. M., Gruber, S. B., Oddoux, C., Ostrer, H., Giardiello, F. M., et al. (1997) Familial colorectal cancer in Ashkenazim due to a hypermutable tract in APC. *Nature Genet.* **17**:79–83.

42. Rozen, P., Shomrat, R., Strul, H., Naiman, T., Karminsky, N., Legum, C., et al. (1999) Prevalence of the I1307K APC gene variant in Israeli Jews of differing ethnic origin and risk for colorectal cancer. *Gastroenterology* **116**:54–57.

43. Prior, T. W., Chadwick, R. B., Papp, C., Arcot, A. N., Isa, A. M., Pearl, D. K., et al. (1999) The I1307K polymorphism of the APC gene in colorectal cancer. *Gastroenterology* **116**:58–63.

44. Gryfe, R., DiNicola, N., Gallinger, S., and Redston, M. (1998) Somatic instability of the APC I1307K allele in colorectal neoplasia. *Cancer Res.* **58**:4040–4043.

45. Petersen, G. M., Parmigiani, G., and Thomas, D. (1998) Missense mutations in disease genes: A Bayesian approach to evaluate causality. *Am. J. Human Genet.* **62**:1516–1524.

46. Redston, M., Nathanson, K. L., Yuan, Z. Q., Neuhausen, S. L., Satagopan, J., Wong, N., et al. (1998) The APC I1307K allele and breast cancer risk. *Nature Genet.* **20**:13–14.

47. Woodage, T., King, S. M., Wacholder, S., Hartge, P., Struewing, J. P., McAdams, M., et al. (1998) The APC I1307K allele and cancer risk in a community-based study of Ashkenazi Jews. *Nature Genet.* **20**:62–65.

48. Abrahamson, J., Mosiehi, R., Vesprini, D., Karlan, B., Fishman, D., Smotkin, D., et al. (1998) No association of the I1307K APC allele with ovarian cancer risk in Ashkenazi Jews. *Cancer Res.* **58**:2919–2922.

49. Petrukhin, L., Dangel, J., Vanderveer, L., Costalas, J., Bellacosa, A., Grana, G., et al. (1997) The I1307K APC mutation does not predispose to colorectal cancer in Jewish Ashkenazi breast and breast-ovarian kindreds. *Cancer Res.* **57**:5840–5484.

50. Lothe, R. A., Hektoen, M., Johnsen, H., Meling, G. I., Andersen, T. I., Rognum, T. O., et al. (1998) The APC gene I1307K variant is rare in Norwegian patients with familial and sporadic colorectal or breast cancer. *Cancer Res.* **58**:2923–2924.

51. Francke, U., Holmes, L. B., Atkins, L., and Riccardi, V. M. (1979) Aniridia-Wilms' tumor association: Evidence for specific deletion of 11p13. *Cytogenet. Cell Genet.* **24**:185–192.

52. Riccardi, V. M., Wheeler, T. M., Pickard, L. R. and King, B. (1980) The pathophysiology of neurofibromatosis. II. Angiosarcoma as a complication. *Cancer Genet. Cytogenetics* **2**:275–280.

53. Herrera, L., Kakati, S., Gibas, L., Pietrzak, E., and Sandberg, A. (1986) Gardner syndrome in a man with an interstitial deletion of 5q. *Am. J. Med. Genet.* **25**:473–476.

54. Fountain, J. W., Wallace, M. R., Bruce, M. A., Seizinger, B. R., Menon, A. G., Gusella, J. F., et al. (1989) Physical mapping of a translocation breakpoint in neurofibromatosis. *Science* **244**:1085–1087.

55. O'Connell, P., Leach, R., Cawthon, R. M., Culver, M., Stevens, J., Viskochil, D., et al. (1989) Two NF1 translocations map within a 600-kilobase segment of 17q11.2. *Science* **244**:1087–1088.

56. Wildrick, D. M. and Boman, B. M. (1988) Chromosome 5 allele loss at the glucocorticoid receptor locus in human colorectal carcinomas. *Biochem. Biophys. Res. Commun.* **150**:591–598.

57. Solomon, E., Voss, R., Hall, V., Bodmer, W. F., Jass, J. R., Jeffreys, A. J., et al. (1987) Chromosome 5 allele loss in human colorectal carcinomas. *Nature* **328**:616–619.

58. Mulligan, L. M., Kwok, J. B., Healey C. S., Elsdon, M. J., Eng, C., Gardner, E., et al. (1993) Germ-line mutations of the RET proto-oncogene in multiple endocrine neoplasia. *Nature* **363**:458–460.

59. Mulligan, L. M., Eng, C., Healey, C. S., Clayton, D., Kwok, J. B., Gardner, E., et al. (1994) Specific mutations of the RET proto-oncogene are related to disease phenotype in MEN 2A and FMTC. *Nature Genet.* **6**:70–74.

60. van Heyningen, V. (1994) Genetics. One gene—four syndromes *Nature* **367**:319–320.

61. Eng, C. (1996) The RET proto-oncogene in multiple endocrine neoplasia type 2 and Hirschsprung's disease. *N. Engl. J. Med.* **335**:943–951.

62. Eng, C. and Mulligan, L. M., (1997) Mutations of the RET proto-oncogene in the multiple endocrine neoplasia type 2 syndromes, related sporadic tumours, and Hirschprung disease. *Human Mutat.* **9**:97–109.

63. Schmidt, L., Duh, F. M., Chen, F., Kishida, T., Glenn, G., Choyke, P., et al. (1997), Germline and somatic mutations in the tyrosine kinase domain of the MET proto-oncogene in papillary renal carcinomas. *Nature Genet.* **16**, 68–73.

64. Hemminki, A., Tomlinson, I., Markie, D., Jarvinen, H., Sistonen, P., Bjorkqvist, A. M., et al. (1997) Localization of a susceptibility locus for Peutz-Jeghers syndrome to 19p using comparative genomic hybridization and targeted linkage analysis. *Nature Genet.* **15**:87–90.

65. Hemminki, A., Markie, D., Tomlinson, I., Avizienyte, E., Roth, S., Loukola, A., et al. (1998) A serine/threonine kinase gene defective in Peutz-Jeghers syndrome. *Nature* **391**:184–187.

66. Jenne, D. E., Reimann, H., Nezu, J., Friedel, W., Loff, S., Jeschke, R., et al. (1998) Peutz-Jeghers syndrome is caused by mutations in a novel serine threonine kinase. *Nature Genet.* **18**:38-43.

67. Marra, G. and Boland, C. R. (1995) Hereditary nonpolyposis colorectal cancer: the syndrome, the genes, and historical perspectives. *J. Natl. Cancer Inst.* **87**:1114–1125.

68. Kinzler, K. W. and Vogelstein, B. (1996) Lessons from hereditary colorectal cancer. *Cell* **87**:159–170.

69. Muto, M. G., Cramer, D. W., Tangir, J., eBerkowitz, R., and Mok, S. (1996) Frequency of the BRCA1 del185Ag mutation among Jewish women with OVCA and matched populations controls. *Cancer Res.* **56**:1250–1252.

70. Abeliovich, D., Kaduri, L., Lerer, I., Weinberg, N., Amir, G., Sagi, M., et al. (1997) Founder mutations 185delAG and 5382insC in BRCA1 and 6174delT in BRCA2 appear in 60% of Ovarian cancer and 30% of early-onset breast cancer patients among Ashkenazi Jewish women. *Am. J. Human Genet.* **60**:505–514.

71. Struewing, J. P., Hartge, P., Wacholder, S., Baker, S. M., Berlin, M., McAdams, M., et al. (1997) The risk of cancer associated with specific mutations of BRCA1 and BRCA2 amongst Ashkenazi Jews. *N. Engl. J. Med.* **336**:1401–1408.

72. FitzGerald, M. G., MacDonald, D. J., Krainer, M., Hoover, I., O'Neil, E., Unsal, H., et al. (1996) Germ-line BRCA1 mutations in Jewish and non-Jewish women with early onset breast cancer. *N. Engl. J. Med.* **334**:143–149.

73. Frank, T. S., Manley, S. A., and Olufunmilayo, O. I., (1998) Sequence analysis of BRCA1 and BRCA2: Correlation of mutations with family history and ovarian cancer risk. *J. Clin. Oncol.* **16**:2417–2425.

74. Wertz, D. C. (1994) Genetic testing for children and adolescents: Who decides? *JAMA* **272**:875–881.

75. Cotton, R. (1993) Current methods of mutation detection. *Mutation Res.* **285**:125–144.

76. Cotton, R. G. H. (1996) Detection of unknown mutations in DNA: a catch-22. *Am. J. Human Genet.* **59**:289–291.

77. Dianzani, I., Camaschella, C., Ponzone, A., and Cotton, R. G. H. (1993) Dilemmas and progress in mutation detection. *Trends Genet.* **9**:403–405.

78. Forrest, S., Cotton, R., Landegren, U. and Southern, E. (1996) How to find all those mutations. *Nature Genet.* **10**:375–376.

79. Anonymous (1996) Statement of the American Society of Clinical Oncology: genetic testing for cancer susceptibility. *J. Clin. Oncol.* **14**:1730–1739.

80. Giardiello, F. M. (1997) Genetic testing in hereditary colorectal cancer. *JAMA* **278**:1278–1281.

81. Boman, B. M. and Levin, B. (1986) Familial polyposis. *Hosp. Pract.* **21**:155–170.

82. Lynch, H. T., Watson, P., Smyrk, T. C., Lanspa, S. J., Boman, B. M., Boland, C. R., et al.. (1992) Colon cancer genetics. *Cancer* **70**:1300–1312.

83. Liu, B., Farrington, S. M., Petersen, G. M., Hamilton, S. R., Parsons, R., Papdopoulos, N., et al. (1995) Genetic instability occurs in the majority of young patients with colorectal cancer. *Nature Med.* **1**:348–352.

84. Vasen, H. F. A., Mecklin, J. P. l., Meera Khan, P., and Lynch, H. T. (1991) The International Collaborative Group on Hereditary Nonpolyposis Colorectal Cancer. *Dis. Colon Rectum* **34**:424–425.

85. Vasen, H. F. A., Mecklin, J. P., Meera Khan, P., and Lynch, H. T. (1994) The International Collaborative Group on Hereditary Nonpolyposis Colorectal Cancer. *Anticancer Res.* **14**:1661–1664.

86. Vasen, H. F., Watson, P., Mecklin, J. P., and Lynch, H. T. (1999) New clinical criteria for hereditary nonpolyposis colorectal cancer (HNPCC, Lynch syndrome) proposed by the International Collaborative Group on HNPCC. *Gastroenterology* **116**:1453–1456.

87. Rodriguez-Bigas, M. A., Boland, C. R., Hamilton, S. R., Henson, D. E., Jass, J. R., Khan, P. M., et al. (1997) A national cancer institute workshop on hereditary nonpolyposis colorectal cancer syndrome: Meeting highlights and Bethesda guidelines. *J. Natl. Cancer Inst.* **89**:1758–1762.

88. Wijnen, J., Khan, M. P., Vasen, H., van der Klift, H., Mulder, A., van Leeuwen-Coornelisse, I., et al. (1997) Hereditary nonpolyposis colorectal cancer families not complying with the Amsterdam criteria show high frequency of mismatch-repair-gene mutations. *Am. J. Human Genet.* **61**:329–335.

89. Lynch, H. T., Watson, P. A., Franklin, A., Smith, S., Tinley, S., Lynch, J., et al. (1998) Molecular genetics and genetic counseling in HNPCC (Lynch syndromes). *Proc. Am. Soc. Clin. Oncol.* **17**:547a.

90. Dietmaier, W., Wallinger, S., Bocker, T., Jullmann, F., Fishel, R., and Rüschoff, J. (1997) Diagnostic microsatellite instability: Definition and correlation with mismatch repair protein expression. *Cancer Res.* **57**:4749–4756.

91. Boland, C. R., Thibodeau, S. N., Hamilton, S. R., Sidransky, D., Eshleman, J. R., Burt, R. W., et al. (1998) National Cancer Institute workshop on microsatellite instability for cancer detection and familial predisposition: development of international criteria for the determination of microsatellite instability in colorectal cancer. *Cancer Res.* **71**:5248–5257.

92. Konishi, M., Kikuchi-Yanoshita, R., Tanaka, K., Muraoka, M., Onda, A., Okumura, Y., et al. (1996) Molecular nature of colon tumors in hereditary nonpolyposis colon cancer, familial polyposis, and sporadic colon cancer. *Gastroenterology* **111**:307–317.

93. Bocker, T., Diermann, J., Friedl, W., Gebert, J., Holinski-Feder, E., Karner-Hanusch, J., et al. (1997) Microsatellite instability analysis: a multicenter study for reliability and quality control. *Cancer Res.* **57**:4739–4743.

94. Boland C. R. (1998) Hereditary nonpolyposis colorectal cancer. *In: The Genetic Basis of Human Cancer* (Kinzler, K. W. and Vogelstein, B., eds.), McGraw-Hill, New York, NY, pp. 333–346.

95. Aaltonen, L. A., Salovaara, R., Kristo, P., Canzian, F., Hemminki, A., Peltomaki, P., et al. (1998) Incidence of hereditary nonpolyposis colorectal cancer and the feasibility of molecular screening for the disease. *N. Engl. J. Med.* **338**:1481–1487.

96. Bailar, III, J. C. and Gornik, H. L. (1997) Cancer undefeated. *N. Engl. J. Med.* **336**:1569–1574.

97. Genuardi, M., Anti, M., Capozzi, E., Leonardi, F., Fornasarig, M., Novella, E., et al. (1998) *MLH1* and *MSH2* constitutional mutations in colorectal cancer families not meeting the standard criteria for hereditary nonpolyposis colorectal cancer. *Int. J. Cancer.* **75**:835–839.

98. Boman, B. M., Fant, G., Fields, J. Z., Lynch, H. T., Watson, P. A. (1998) Improving the detection of hereditary nonpolyposis cancer. *Proc. Am. Soc. Clin. Oncol.* **17**:561a.

99. Percesepe, A., Anti, M., Roncucci, L., Armelao, F., Marra, G., Pahor, M., et al. (1995) The effect of family size on estimates of the frequency of hereditary non-polyposis colorectal cancer. *Br. J. Cancer* **72**:1320–1323.

100. Hall, N. R., Finan, P. J., Ward, B., Turner, G., and Bishop, D. T. (1994) Genetic susceptibility to colorectal cancer in patients under 45 years of age. *Br. J. Surg.* **81**:1485–1489.

101. Liu, B., Nicolaides, N. C., Markowitz, S., Willson, J. K., Parsons, R. E., Jen, J., et al. (1995) Mismatch repair gene defects in sporadic colorectal cancers with microsatellite instability. *Nature Genet.* **9**:48-55.

102. Fante, R., Bennatti, P., di Gregorio, C., De Pietri, S., Pedroni, M., Tamassia, M. G., et al. (1997) Colorectal carcinoma in different age groups: a population-based investigation. *Am. J. Gastroenterol.* **92**:1505–1509.

103. Syngal, S., Fox, E. A., Li, C., Dovidio, M., Eng, C., Kolodner, R. D., et al. (1999) Interpretation of genetic test results for hereditary nonpolyposis colorectal cancer: Implications for clinical predisposition testing. *JAMA* **282**:247–253.

104. Aarino, M., Mecklin, J. P., Aaltonen, L. A., et al. (1995) Lifetime risk of different cancers in hereditary nonpolyposis colon cancer (HNPCC) syndrome. *Int. J. Cancer* **64**:430–433.

105. Bulow, S. (1987) Familial polyposis coli. *Dan. Med. Bull.* **34**:1–15.

106. Alm, T. and Licznerski, G. (1973) The intestinal polyposis. *Clin. Gastroenterol.* **2**:577–602.

107. Bussey, H. J. R. (1975) *Familial Polyposis Coli.* The John Hopkins University Press, Baltimore, MD.

108. Arvantis M. L., Jagelman, D. G., Fazio, V. W., Lavery, I. C. and McGannon, E. (1990) Mortality in patients with familial adenomatous polyposis. *Dis. Colon Rectum.* **33**:639–642.

109. Gutmann, D. H. and Collins F. S. (1998) Neurofibromatosis type 1. *In: The Genetic Basis of Human Cancer* (Kinzler, K. W., and Vogelstein, B., eds.), McGraw-Hill, New York, pp. 423–442.

110. MacCollin, M. and Gusella, J. (1998) Neurofibromatosis type 2. *In: The Genetic Basis of Human Cancer* (Kinzler, K. W., and Vogelstein, B., eds.), McGraw-Hill, New York, pp. 443–453.

111. Carlson, K. M., Bracamontes, J., Jackson, C. E., Clark, R., Lacroix, A., Wells, S. A., et al. (1994) Parent-of-origin effects in multiple endocrine neoplasia type 2B. *Am. J. Human Genet.* **55**:1076–1082.

112. Ponder, B. (1997) Genetic testing for cancer risk. *Science* **278**:1050–1054.

113. Hubbard, R. and Lewontin, R. C. (1996) Pitfalls of genetic testing. *N. Engl. J. Med.* **334**:1192–1193.

114. Shattuck-Eidens, D. S., Oliphant, A., McClure, M., McBride, C., Gupte, J., Rubano, T., et al. (1997) *BRCA1* sequence analysis in women at high risk for susceptibility mutations: Risk factor analysis and implications for genetic testing. *JAMA* **278**:1242–1250.

114a. Schrag, D., Kuntz, K.M., Garber, J.E. and Wecki, J.C. (2000) Life expectancy gains from cancer prevention strategies for women with breast cancer and BRCA1 or BRCA2 mutations. *JAMA* **283**: 617–624.

114b. Hartman, L.C., Schaid, D.J., Woods, J.E., Crotty, T.P., Myers, J.L., Arnold, P.G., Petty, P.M., Sellers, T.A., Johnson, J.L., McDonnell, S.K., Frost, M.H. and Jenkins, R.B. (1999) Efficacy of bilateral prophylactic mastectomy in women with a family history of breast cancer. *N. Engl. J. Med.* **340**: 77–84.

114c. Rebbeck, T.R., Levin, A.M., Eisen, A., Snyder, C., Watson, P., Cannon-Albright, L., Isaacs, C., Olopade, O., Garber. J.E., Godwin, A.K., Oaly, M.B., Narod, S.A., Neuhausen, S.L., Lynch, H.T. and Weber, B.L. (1999) Breast cancer risk after bilateral prophylactic oophorectomy in BRCA1 mutation carriers. *J. Natl. Cancer Inst.* **91**:1475–1479.

114d. Grann, V.R., Jocobsen, J.S., Whang, W., Hershman, D., Heitjen, D.F., Antman, K.H. and Neugut, A.I. (2000) Prevention with tamoxifen or other hormones versus prophylactic surgery in BRCA1/2 positive women: A decision analysis. *Cancer J. Sci. Am.* **6**:13–20.

114e. Lynch, H.T. and Casey, M.J. (2001) Current status of prophylactic surgery for hereditary breast and gynecologic cancers. *Curr. Opin. Obstet. Gynecol.* **13**:25–30.

115. Marcus, J. N., Page, D. L., Watson, P., Narod, S. A., Lenoir, G. M. and Lynch, H. T. (1997) *BRCA1* and *BRCA2* hereditary breast carcinoma phenotypes. *Cancer* **80**:543–556.

116. Burke W., Daly, M., Garber, J., Botkin, J., Kahn, M. J., Lynch, P., et al. (1997) Recommendations for follow-up care of individuals with an inherited predisposition to cancer. II. BRCA1 and BRCA2. Cancer genetics Studies Consortium. *JAMA* **277**:997–1003.

117. Lerman, C. and Croyle, R. T. (1996) Emotional and behavioral responses to genetic testing for susceptibility to cancer. *Oncology* **10**:191–199.

118. Spigelman, A. D. and Thomson, J. P. S. (1994) Introduction, history and registries. *In: Familial Adenomatous Polyposis and Other Polyposis Syndromes* (Phillips, R. K. S., ed.), Arnold, London, UK, pp. 3–14.

119. Järvinen, H. J., Aarino, M., Mustonen, H., Aktan-Collab, K., Aaltonen, L.A., Peltonaki, P., de la Chapelle, A., Mecklin, J.P. (2000) Controlled 15-year trial on screening for colorectal cancer in families with hereditary nonpolyposis colorectal cancer. Gastroenterology 118: 829–834.

120. Winawer, S., Zauber, A. G., O'Brien, M. J., Ho, M. N., Gottlieb, L., Sternberg, S. S., et al. (1993) National Polyp Study Workgroup. Randomized comparison of surveillance intervals after colonoscopic removal of newly diagnosed adenomatous polyps. *N. Engl. J. Med.* **328**:901–906.

121. Vasen, H. F. A., den Hartog Jager, F. C. A., Menko, F. H., and Nagengast, F. M. (1989) Screening for hereditary non-polyposis colorectal cancer: a study of 22 kindreds in The Netherlands. *Am. J. Med.* **86**:278–281.

122. Lynch, H. T. and Smyrk, T. (1996) Hereditary nonpolyposis colorectal cancer (Lynch Syndrome). *Cancer* **78**:1149–1167.

123. Giardiello, F. M., Brensinger, J. D., Petersen, G. M., Luce, M. D., Hylind, L. M., Bacon, J. A., et al. (1997) The use and interpretation of commercial *APC* gene testing for familial adenomatous polyposis. *N. Engl. J. Med.* **336**:823–827.

124. Stephenson, J. (1998) Group drafts core curriculum for 'What docs need to know about genetics.' *JAMA* **279**:735–736.

125. Lemon, S. J., Tinley, S. T., Fusaro, R. M., and Lynch, H. T. (1997) Cancer risk assessment in a hereditary cancer prevention clinic and its first year's experience. *Cancer* **80**:606–613.

126. Lynch, H. T. and Lynch, J. (1996) Genetic counseling for hereditary cancer. *Oncology* **10**:27–34.

127. Menko, F. H., Wijnen, J. T., Khan, P. M., Vasen, H. F. A., and Oosterwijk, M. H. (1996) Genetic counseling in hereditary nonpolyposis colorectal cancer. *Oncology* **10**:71–82.

128. American Society of Clinical Oncology (1998) Cancer Genetics Satellite Symposium on The Role of Genetics in Clinical Cancer Care, 34th Annual Meeting, Los Angeles CA, May 15, 1998.

129. Peters, J. A. and Stopfer, J. E. (1996) Role of the genetic counselor in familial cancer. *Oncology* **10**:159–175.

130. Petersen, G. M. and Brensinger, J. D. (1996) Genetic testing and counseling in familial adenomatous polyposis. *Oncology* **10**:89–98.

131. Lynch, P., Severin, M., Mills, A., Bosserman, L. Carson, D., Chamber, D. C., et al. (1997) Medical/legal issues in genetic testing: Workshop no. 3. *Cancer* **80**:630–631.

132. Ruden, R. A. and Byalick, M. (1997) *The Craving Brain.* HarperCollins, New York, NY.

133. Garber, J. (1999) A 40-year old woman with a strong family history of breast cancer. *JAMA* **282**:1953–1960.

134. Weber, T. K., Chin, H. M., Rodriguez-Bigas, M., Keitz, B., Gillagan, R., O'Malley, L., et al. (1999) Novel hMLH1 and hMSH2 germline mutations in African Americans with colorectal cancer. *JAMA* **281**:2316–2320.

ETIOLOGY OF   V
HUMAN CANCERS

9 Evolution of Research in Cancer Etiology

Lorenzo Tomatis, MD and James Huff, PhD

INTRODUCTION

In this chapter, we briefly review the evolution of approaches, methods, and changing fashions in etiological research, and make an attempt to analyze whether and to what extent these factors have affected priorities in cancer control and prevention.

For a long period in history, cancer (like other disease specters) was believed to be equivalent to a curse of God, and cancer etiology was therefore part of the concept of divine punishment. Thus, the only possible protection from cancer was pious obedient behavior, while recognition of one's sins and repentance opened the only available path to God's forgiveness. Traces of such belief are still with us, not only as remainders of old superstitions but also as components of today's attribution of a prominent role in the origin of disease to individual behavior, habits, and lifestyles. Individual behaviors and lifestyle certainly play important roles, but today individuals tend to be considered not only responsible for their disease, but also guilty of causing it, a situation very close to suffering the curse of God. It has been proposed that all financial coverage for the treatment of so-called self-inflicted diseases be withdrawn *(1),* in order to guarantee that guilty patients are not a burden on society. The spectrum of diseases considered to be self-inflicted is wide, ranging from those related to the use of tobacco to those related to excess alcohol consumption, excess nutrition, and lack of exercise. Apart from the fact that certain individuals may be genetically predisposed to some conditions, the commonly used term life-style does not distinguish the various causes of habitual behavior, like smoking, alcohol drinking, unhealthy dietary habits, and lack of daily exercise *(2).* The assumption that all behavioral choices are free choices does not reflect the actual situation. Social pressures and ubiquitous advertising are possibly the most relevant environmental factors that could be addressed in implementing efficient primary prevention. Only a minority of inner-directed, strong-willed people can resist such pressures and make fully autonomous choices.

In ancient times, cancer was never considered to be transmissible. However, between the seventeenth and eighteenth centuries, cancer was believed to be a contagious disease. As a consequence, special hospitals were built in certain European countries to isolate patients with cancer, almost in the same way as was done for patients with leprosy *(3,4).* This period did not last long and the conviction that cancer was not contagious again prevailed. Such conviction was strengthened during the apogee of microbiology by the inability to identify a germ or bacterium that could be related to cancer. This may at least partly explain the little attention paid to the experiments of Rous *(5)* at the beginning of this century on the role of viruses in the origin of tumors. The hypothesis of a parasitic origin of cancer had a period of celebrity in 1926, when the Danish scientist Fibiger received the Nobel Prize for showing that gastric cancer in rats was caused by a nematode. Fibiger's results were not reproducible. He died shortly after the attribution of the Prize, thereby sparing himself and the Nobel Committee some perhaps embarrassing explanations *(6).* The hypothesis of a viral origin for human cancer never completely disappeared. In the first half of this century, this theory gained the support of great scientists such as Oberling in France and Zilber in the then Soviet Union *(4).* It was a favorite hypothesis at the time of President Nixon's war against cancer and has recently returned to the stage with renewed strength.

The rivalry between proponents of chemical and viral carcinogenesis was based in part on different schools of thought but was also related to competition for research funds. In general, scientists in the field of viral carcinogenesis, and later of molecular biology, considered that the scientists involved in chemical carcinogenesis were old-fashioned and not particularly brilliant *(7–9),* while those working in chemical carcinogenesis looked with suspicion at the viral oncologists. Chemical carcinogenesis prevailed, in terms of funding and popularity, until the mid-1960s and early 1970s. Then came President

From: *The Molecular Basis of Human Cancer* (W. B. Coleman and G. J. Tsongalis, eds.), © Humana Press Inc., Totowa, NJ.

Nixon's declaration of war against cancer. The dread disease had to be conquered with the kind of concerted effort that had split the atom and taken humans to the moon. The search for a viral etiology of human cancer was launched as a glorious challenge, and viral carcinogenesis obtained a considerable increase in funding.

Besides the hypothesis of an infectious (parasitic or viral) etiology, the main theories of the origins of cancer have included the cell-irritation theory, proposed by Virchow, and the embryonic-rest theory, proposed by Cohnheim (3,10–12). It is of some interest that the 1905 report of the Huntington Cancer Research Fund noted the unsuccessful attempts made to identify the cause of cancer and stated that: "It has therefore seemed advisable, instead of treading the ordinary beaten track, to branch out into new methods, and attempt to investigate, not so much the cause of cancer as the conditions under which it may arise" with the "hope that by collecting a number of data a deeper insight into the question may ultimately be obtained, and a nearer approach be made to a conception of the nature of the processes involved" (11). In spite of the obviously different levels of knowledge, the predominant trend in cancer research today could be described in similar words.

EARLY REPORTS

The reports of Agricola (circa 1494–1555) and Paracelsus (circa 1493–1541), who described the disease of Schneeberg miners, are sometimes quoted as the first etiological observations on human cancer. They were probably the first to provide an accurate description of an occupational disease, but they did not actually mention the words cancer or tumor. It was only in the middle of the last century that the miners' disease was actually considered to be neoplastic. Described initially as lymphosarcoma, it was finally diagnosed as bronchogenic carcinoma by Harting and Hesse in 1869 (4). The causal relationship between pulmonary cancer and occupational exposure of miners to high concentrations of radon was firmly established in the early 1940s (13).

The first reports that environmental agents were causative factors in human cancer were those of John Hill, who reported that nasal tumors were associated with the use of tobacco snuff (14), and of Percival Pott, who noted the causality of scrotal cancer in chimney sweeps (15). Thus, tobacco and soot became the first of two leading categories of risk factors for human cancer, one related to a personal habit and the other related to occupation. The next reports of human cancers associated with environmental factors came about a century later and concerned the occurrence of skin cancer after therapeutic use of arsenic in Fowler's solution (16) and the high incidence of urinary bladder tumors in aniline dye workers (17). The International Labour Office (ILO) published a report in 1921 in which certain aromatic amines were labeled as carcinogenic to exposed workers (18). Several industrial production processes were subsequently identified as sources of exposure to carcinogens, and numerous chemicals and chemical mixtures were recognized as causative agents of human cancer (2,19–22).

Ionizing radiation may have been the first carcinogen encountered by the human species. However, Roentgen was the first to introduce it into medical practice and scientific research in 1895 (23). Ionizing radiation, which is clearly of natural origin, was recognized as a cause of human tumors seven yr after initiation of its artificial use (24,25). That is an exceptionally short delay in comparison with the much longer periods—in certain instances several decades—before which certain chemicals that had been introduced into the environment were recognized as human carcinogens. Evidence for its carcinogenicity did not prevent the spread of use of ionizing radiation, often in the absence of even the most elementary precautions. Over 40 years passed before the natural radioactivity present in uranium mines was accepted as carcinogenic (13). Several additional decades passed before it was accepted that natural radioactivity at concentrations lower than those found in the mines also represented a carcinogenic risk (26). The case of ionizing radiation is a pertinent example of the lengthy, stepwise progression from scientific evidence for the carcinogenicity of an environmental agent to the official recognition of a cancer risk to humans at both high and low levels of exposure.

ENDOGENOUS AND EXOGENOUS CAUSES OF CANCER

The causes of cancer can be divided roughly into two broad categories: exogenous (or environmental), and endogenous (or genetic). However, an inherited genetic alteration is sufficient in only a limited number of cases to cause tumors. In most instances, an inherited increase in susceptibility becomes manifest only after a series of environmental insults. Inherited polymorphisms of a variety of genes (e.g. those responsible for the activation and detoxification of carcinogens or for DNA repair) may affect responses to environmental risk factors and substantially weaken any attempt to establish practical exposure thresholds in risk assessment. Increased susceptibility or predisposition to cancer may be related to uncontrollable spontaneous replication errors in germ cells or to germ-cell alterations caused by exposure of preceding generations to damaging agents. The classification of cancer causes into these two broad categories has been operationally useful, as it favored the concentration and funding of those research efforts that on the basis of the technology and methods available at the time offered the greatest possibility of success. For a long time, this meant that the prevailing area of research focused on the identification of exogenous environmental causes of human cancer. Expansion of research on environmental causes of cancer also coincided with and possibly contributed to growing awareness of the relationships between socioeconomic conditions and health and to a tendency toward greater equity in health care and services. Research on the endogenous component of carcinogenesis gained importance and gradually took over when methods of molecular biology were applied to cancer research. The strong impetus given to research on viruses played an indirect but important role in this shift of interest. Cancer virology received a generous share of the funds made available by the Nixon administration and became fashionable and highly advertised. Unfortunately it did not produce the hoped-for solution to the cancer riddle. However, it did contribute to the development of scientists with new skills and interests, who became essential to the rapid development of molecular biology and molecular genetics. This was probably one the best (albeit unintended) results from Nixon's war on cancer. Even the strongest traditional disciplines, such as biochemistry and pathology (and more recently epidemiology), are now becoming molecular. In parallel with the growing role of research on the endogenous/genetic causes of cancer and on mechanisms underlying the carcinogenesis process, interest in the role of socioeconomic factors and public health as a whole has decreased.

OLD AND NEW CARCINOGENS

Large sections of the world's population have enjoyed the advantages of a society characterized by rapid expansion of chemical and manufacturing industries. At the same time, they have not escaped the disadvantages of a situation that contains the basis for growing morbidity among older people. The clear advantages of modern industrialized society are a reduction in childhood mortality and in mortality from infectious disease at all ages and an extension of life expectancy. The main disadvantage is the increased frequency of chronic, degenerative diseases including cancer. Therefore, the extension of the duration of life does not necessarily translate into an actual gain of years of active life. The increase in the frequency of diseases, like cancer, cerebrovascular diseases and neurological disorders coincide with increases in the number and concentration of toxic and carcinogenic agents in the environment.

Increased exposure to old carcinogens occurred while new carcinogens were being introduced into our environment. These increases were also not immediately accompanied by improvements in certain basic resources, including food, which, even if not necessarily insufficient in quantity, was often dietetically unbalanced. Among the old carcinogens are ionizing and non-ionizing radiation, mycotoxins, certain combustion products, and certain viruses and parasites. To this short list should perhaps be added certain hormones that are formed endogenously but are also under partial exogenous influence. It is uncertain how many other natural chemicals, polemically depicted as more numerous and also potentially more dangerous than synthetic chemicals (27), should be considered suitable candidates for addition to the aforementioned list. The new carcinogens are agents to which humans have been exposed for a relatively short time. They include chemicals synthesized *de novo* by the chemical industry and natural substances that entered our environment in large quantities only after massive exploitation of their natural reservoirs. This is the case for asbestos and certain metals, such as nickel, chromium, cadmium, and arsenic. Mining, refining, manufacture, and use of products of which these substances are important components developed explosively in the second part of the 19th century, which resulted in high exposures to metals and to asbestos in the workplace and in their widespread presence in the general environment.

This is also the case for the tobacco plant and its leaves, which are, by definition natural, old products. However, cigarettes and the tobacco smoke consequently inhaled could hardly be described as natural products. Industrial production of cigarettes and progressive expansion of the habit of smoking began in the middle of the 19th century in parallel with the development of the chemical and manufacturing industry. The first industrial production of cigarettes was set up in Havana, Cuba,

in 1853. Subsequently, production of cigarettes was initiated in London during 1856 and in Virginia around 1860 (28). In fact, the tobacco industry is itself a chemical manufacturing industry.

PREDOMINANCE OF EXPERIMENTAL CHEMICAL CARCINOGENESIS

The epidemiological approach to cancer etiology has been characterized mainly by descriptions of 1) variations in cancer incidence and mortality, 2) cancer types in different populations, and 3) consequences of relatively long exposures in relatively well-defined populations. By definition, epidemiology can contribute to primary prevention only after hazardous exposures have exerted their effects for quite some time. The experimental approach has as one of its principal characteristics the capacity, or at least the potential, to predict adverse effects in humans before they occur. In terms of primary prevention, this obviously represents a remarkable advantage over the retrospective epidemiological approach. The predictive capacity of experimental results was highly regarded by a considerable proportion of scientists and regulators during the period in which the origin of most cases of cancer was considered to be related mainly to exposure to environmental (mostly industrial) chemicals. Although the roots of experimental carcinogenesis can be traced to the second half of the nineteenth century, experimental carcinogenesis in modern terms was triggered by the successful experiment of Yamagiwa and Ichikawa in Japan (29). They were the first to induce skin tumors, by painting coal-tar onto the inner side of rabbits' ears. Three years later, a pupil of Ichikawa's, Tsutsui (30), developed a method for the induction of skin tumors in mice. In 1922, using the method described by Tsutsui (30), Passey (31) succeeded in inducing malignant skin tumors with soot extracts in mice. Passey's results in mice were considered to represent the final confirmation of the observations of Pott made a century-and-a-half previously of an excess incidence of scrotal cancer among chimney sweeps (15). This sequence of events seems to imply that clinical observations had to be confirmed experimentally in order to be accepted. It also marks the beginning of the golden age of experimental carcinogenesis. The findings of Murphy and Sturm (32) and of Sasaki and Yoshida (33) that carcinogens can exert their effects distant from the site of their entry into the body further strengthened its role.

The first chemical carcinogen was identified in 1930. Initially believed to be 1,2,7,8-dibenzanthracene, it was eventually identified as 1,2,5,6-dibenzanthracene. Additional compounds were then isolated from coal-tar, and several were synthesized *de novo* (34,35). The observation that polycyclic hydrocarbons produce different pathological changes in different species suggested two metabolic pathways: one toward more active pathogenic substances, and one toward detoxification by conversion into less harmful or harmless compounds (36). Boyland and Horning pointed out that a proximate carcinogen is not the compound as applied but one of its metabolites (37), which "acts by forming complexes with DNA" (38). The terms proximate and ultimate carcinogen were proposed by Elisabeth and James Miller to identify stages in the metabolic activation of carcinogenic aromatic amines. When they reported the results of their studies with 4-dimethylaminobenzene and benzo[a]pyrene, they produced evidence, and remained firmly convinced, that the main targets of carcinogens were proteins (39,40).

Evidence that chemicals have similar carcinogenic effects in different species reinforced the conviction that exogenous agents are at the origin of most cases of cancer. The reasoning was in fact pushed further: the experimental induction of tumors not only confirmed clinical and epidemiological observations, and also predicted them, but could even largely replace them. The strength of the argument lay in the fact that experimental evidence for the carcinogenicity of many agents shown to be carcinogenic to humans actually preceded the epidemiological observations and thereby predicted the effects in humans. This was the case for 4-aminobiphenyl, diethylstilbestrol, vinyl chloride, aflatoxin (41,42), and 1,3-butadiene (43).

Implementation of primary prevention of occupational cancers was delayed in several instances by a sort of seesaw between the degree of relevance that was alternatively attributed to experimental and epidemiological results. For instance, in the cases of the aromatic amines and of bischloromethyl ether the greatest importance was given to that part of the evidence that was missing. It follows that when epidemiological evidence appeared weak, it was imperative to strengthen it, and when epidemiological evidence was available, it was imperative to obtain experimental confirmation. Further, when epidemiological evidence was available, it was deemed necessary to obtain further confirmation by the same route of administration or the same target organ(s) in both humans and animals (44). This unavoidably resulted in delays in the implementation of primary prevention.

The credibility of experimental results as effective predictors of human risk was systematically questioned by industry, which was concerned that evaluation of certain of their products as potentially carcinogenic to humans would impose costly investments and jeopardize profits and production rentability. In industrial terms, a reduction of profit is always described as a severe loss. Numerous scientists supported industry point of view, either because they worked in or for industry or industrial laboratories or because, in good faith, they wanted greater degree of certitude that the available methods could not provide. Regulatory agencies and health authorities wanted to be reassured that the findings of experimental studies were truly predictive of probable outcomes in humans. As a consequence, doubtful or inadequate negative epidemiological observations were sometimes inappropriately considered as more convincing than positive experimental results (45).

LIMITS OF THE EXPERIMENTAL APPROACH AND THE RISING STAR OF EPIDEMIOLOGY

A significant contribution of experimental carcinogenesis to understanding of mechanisms of malignant transformation was the hypothesis that carcinogenesis is a multi-step multifactorial process (46–48). However, the development of this brilliant, convincing hypothesis was not followed by the development of adequate methods for identifying the various actors in the carcinogenesis process nor for evaluating their respective roles. This is an important limitation of the experimental approach to the identification of human carcinogens,

which has contributed to the general attitude of many scientists and regulators to accept the hypothesis of the multifactorial origin of most tumors, while continuing to behave as though they could be attributed to a single factor (49).

The inability to reproduce in the laboratory and confirm the evidence for the carcinogenicity of tobacco smoke provided by epidemiological studies in the 1950s (50,51) undermined the credibility of the traditional experimental approach of predicting human risks. In 1964, a group of scientists met at World Health Organization (WHO) Headquarters in Geneva to prepare a document on cancer prevention (52). The document amply stressed the convincing epidemiological evidence for the carcinogenicity of tobacco smoke in humans but still recommended that experimental studies be continued, as though experimental studies were to have the final word. However, in those same years statisticians and epidemiologists developed criteria for assessing the causation of chronic diseases, which took into consideration biological plausibility but were based primarily if not entirely on epidemiological evidence (53).

After it was proposed and then accepted that epidemiological results could alone prove causation, a further step was taken in the early 1970s. In that period, the view that only the epidemiological approach could provide acceptable evidence for a causal relationship between an exposure and human cancer began openly to prevail. Experimental results, in particular those of long-term bioassays, then began to be considered of secondary importance. Moreover, it was also claimed that long-term bioassays were too expensive and were consuming funds that could be more fruitfully used to support basic and clinical research. In the last few decades, epidemiology has played the most important role in the identification of agents or exposures that are carcinogenic to humans. The criteria for inclusion of an agent or exposure within Group 1 (agents or exposures definitely carcinogenic to humans) of the International Agency for Research on Cancer (IARC) Program on the Evaluation of Carcinogenic Risks to Humans required that there be sufficient evidence of a causal relationship provided by convincing epidemiological data (54). After much debate and intense scientific discussions, IARC decided to amend this stringent rule (55,56). Beginning in 1992, the criteria for inclusion of a compound within Group 1 is as follows: "This category is used when there is sufficient evidence of carcinogenicity in humans. Exceptionally, an agent (mixture) may be placed in this category when evidence in humans is less than sufficient but there is sufficient evidence of carcinogenicity in experimental animals and strong evidence in exposed humans that the agent (mixture) acts through a relevant mechanism of carcinogenesis." The change in the criteria for admission into Group 1 implies that experimental results can play a more significant role in the evaluation of risk. It does not necessarily indicate that risk would be evaluated by criteria that are more closely oriented toward the protection of public health. Experimental data may in fact be used to provide additional evidence for placing an agent or exposure in Group 1, even if the epidemiological evidence is less than sufficient. This was the case, for instance, for ethylene oxide and 2,3,7,8-TCDD. However, these criteria may be used to claim that "the mechanism of carcinogenicity in experimental animals does not operate in humans" in spite of sufficient experimental evidence of carcinogenicity *(56)*. Thus, agents or exposures presently classified in Group 2B (possibly carcinogenic to humans), and even in Group 2A (probably carcinogenic to humans), could be brought down to Group 3 (not classifiable as to its carcinogenicity to humans). This was the case for di(2-ethylhexyl) phthalate and sacaharine.

According to the evaluations made by IARC, 225 chemicals, chemical mixtures, or exposure circumstances have been assigned to Group 2B of the IARC classification (agents that are possibly carcinogenic to humans). For these agents, there is usually sufficient experimental evidence of carcinogenicity, humans are or may be exposed to most of them, but epidemiological data are not available or are considered inadequate. There are various possible explanations for the lack of epidemiological data *(57)*: 1) the chemical or chemical mixture entered the environment too recently to produce any measurable effect; 2) the number of individuals exposed is too small and/or the level of production is too low to allow measurement of any increase in risk; 3) difficulties in tracing exposed individuals, in particular because exposed workers left a company or because there was a change in ownership of a company; 4) it was believed or stated *a priori* that those chemicals could not represent a hazard,; or 5) nobody wished to perform a study for which it might have been hard to find financial support and that, if focused on an industrial product, did not encourage support from industry. In such cases, absent or inadequate epidemiological data cannot be considered equivalent to a negative finding and cannot be considered more relevant for public health than positive experimental findings. As it is unlikely that most such chemicals will ever become the object of an epidemiological study, results of experimental tests are and will remain the only information on which to base regulatory decisions and preventive measures.

The relevance of results obtained in long-term animal tests has been questioned by the U.S. Environmental Protection Agency (EPA) *(58)*. On the basis of generalized mechanistic considerations, the EPA proposed that the induction of tumors in rodents at the following sites be discounted when evaluating carcinogenicity: kidney and urinary bladder in the male rat, thyroid (follicular cell) in the rat, forestomach by gavage in rat and mouse, lung following inhalation of particles in rat and mouse, and liver in mouse. If this proposal were adopted, a considerable number of chemicals would no longer be considered carcinogens, and the level of certainty of carcinogenicity for an additional number of chemicals would be reduced *(59)*. Thus, the evidence for the carcinogenicity of chemicals and mixtures such as trichlorethylene, tetrachloroethylene, chlordane, heptachlor, ethylene thiourea, and whole diesel exhaust would be considered insignificant. As mentioned, there is a paucity of epidemiological data and a low probability that new epidemiological data will become available in the near future. An indiscriminate downgrading of the experimental data would therefore result in the elimination of the only indication of potential hazard for humans from a considerable number of environmental chemicals and chemical mixtures.

Within the IARC Monographs Program for the Evaluation of the Carcinogenic Risk to Humans, there has been a recent tendency to use data on mechanisms to discredit the results of long-term bioassays, rather than to assess objectively their capacity to predict similar effects in humans. However, the IARC has not dropped the recommendation that appears in the Preamble to each Monograph volume that: "in the absence of adequate data on humans, it is biologically plausible and prudent to regard agents and mixtures for which there is sufficient evidence of carcinogenicity in experimental animals as if they presented a carcinogenic risk to humans." The criteria used by the U.S. National Toxicology Program (NTP) *(60)* to list substances that may present a potential hazard to human health and to prepare its Report on Carcinogens are similar, although not identical, to those of IARC *(60a)*. The NTP list of carcinogens consists of two groups: Group 1, which contains substances known to be human carcinogens, and Group 2, which contains substances reasonably anticipated to be a human carcinogens. Substances in Group 1 are those for which "there is sufficient evidence of carcinogenicity from studies in humans which indicate a causal relationship between exposure to the agent, substance or mixture, and human cancer." As for IARC until 1992, the definitive recognition of human carcinogenicity by the NTP has relied entirely and exclusively on epidemiological data.

The NTP, like IARC and in tune with the proposal of EPA, is also planing to make more use of data on mechanisms to verify whether some of the chemicals included in its lists of carcinogens should be deleted. If it could be demonstrated that sufficient evidence of carcinogenicity is based on the induction of tumors by mechanisms that do not apply to the human situation, then the finding would lose all significance. On the basis of this reasoning and on that of an inadequate negative experimental study, it has been proposed to delete saccharin from Group 2 of the NTP list of carcinogens. Ethyl acrylate is also being considered for removal from the list, despite evidence of genotoxicty, carcinogenicity in rats and mice, and limited evidence of carcinogenicity in humans.

THE TWO-STAGE HYPOTHESIS

Several scientists have contributed to the development of the two-stage hypothesis. Rous and Kidd *(61)* were probably the first to report an enhancing effect of turpentine on the induction of skin papillomas after tar painting. A few years later, Rous repeated the experiments with methylcholanthrene and benzo[*a*]pyrene instead of tar and laid down the basis for the two-stage theory by proposing the concept of an initiating and a promoting process *(46,62)*. Charles and Luce-Clausen in that same period *(63)* provided one of the first observations of the mutational events that characterize the formation of papillomas after painting of benzpyrene. In evaluating the kinetics of papilloma formation, they proposed that the first step in neoplastic growth is the mutation "of some particular gene which is essential to normal differentiation of new skin cells." Cells with only one mutated allele can still give rise to normal descendants, neoplastic growth starts when the second allele also mutates.

The two-stages hypothesis, which was developed by Berenblum *(47,62)*, and Berenblum and Shubik *(48)*, remained for many years the dominating mechanistic hypothesis. Initially unsuccessful attempts to extend the experimental model beyond mouse skin and difficulty in identifying promoters other that croton oil and TPA, most likely contributed to the delay in the general acceptance of carcinogenesis as a multi-step process. With a better (albeit incomplete) understanding of the different steps involved, it became clear that the transition from normal to neoplastic tissue, interpreted in evolutionary terms as a Darwinian combination of variation plus natural selection (8), was a much more complicated process than the two-stage model of initiation and promotion (64). The steps that were once grouped under the term "promotion" have generally been interpreted as a nongenetic series of events mainly characterized by the proliferation of mutated clones of cells. However, nuclear alterations are conspicuously present in the proliferating clones, and additional chromosomal abnormalities are seen in the final phase of the process (progression). Thus, the border between genetic and nongenetic or epigenetic events is rather blurred.

HOW MANY CARCINOGENS ARE MUTAGENS?

The hypothesis underlying the widespread use of short-term tests for mutagenicity was that most carcinogens are also mutagens, implying that the mechanism of action of most carcinogens is based on a mutational event. The somatic mutation hypothesis for carcinogenesis is generally attributed to Theodor Boveri, but it was only after the discovery of the structure of DNA as the genetic material in cells by Watson and Crick (65) that the mechanisms of mutation could be studied. The initial change, or first stage (initiation), of the carcinogenesis process, assumed to be irreversible, was then attributed to mutations in nuclear DNA caused by a carcinogen. Boveri, who was working on worms and sea-urchin eggs, considered that the atypical groups of cells that originated from cells with chromosomal abnormalities were analogous to cancer, because he found that cancer cells often have abnormal numbers of chromosomes. He had the brilliant intuition that the irreparable defects in cancer were in the nucleus and not in the cytoplasm. However, the gross and numerical chromosomal anomalies he observed can hardly be considered as those that initiate the neoplastic process (4,8,66,67).

In the 1970s, environmental hazards were still of great concern to the general public and many scientists. There was a widely held belief that measures must be taken urgently to control environmental hazards. It seemed justified therefore to propose that: "the Salmonella/microsome test be used for the screening of food additives, drugs and chemicals to which humans are exposed and for the routine testing of all new chemicals under development that are potential sources of human exposure" (68). There is little doubt that the Salmonella or Ames test, has contributed to the identification of mutagenic carcinogens already present in our environment (68–70). It has also been very useful for screening new chemicals before their commercial production and introduction into the environment. Results of the first set of Salmonella/microsome mutagenicity assays were suggested to provide evidence that most carcinogens are mutagens (71). Shortly thereafter, the sensitivity of the assay or its capacity to identify carcinogens was suggested to be 90%, and its specificity or the power to discriminate between carcinogens and noncarcinogens to be 87% (69). A sensitivity of 76% and a specificity of 57% were reported a few

years later (72), and even lower values were reported subsequently (73). It is clear that the rates of specificity and sensitivity for this assay depend heavily on the selection of carcinogens investigated. In addition, other studies confirmed that the relationship between mutagenic potency in the Salmonella test and carcinogenic potency in rodents is weak or nonexistent (73).

The conviction that most if not all carcinogens are mutagens and that their mechanism of action necessarily involves an alteration in nuclear DNA is widely supported. The exponential increase with age in the incidence of tumors in adults suggests a sequence of events, "each rendered more likely by the occurrence of a previous event" (74). Tumor progression has been defined as a stepwise acquisition of malignant characteristics (75), requiring many genomic changes that are greatly favored by increased genomic instability (76,77). The increasing evidence for multiple genetic alterations in common human tumors provides additional evidence for a stepwise process in which cells acquire their malignant behavior, up to invasiveness and capacity to metastasize (78). Mutations in at least four or five genes are required for a malignant tumor to grow. The mutations need not occur in a fixed sequence, because it is the accumulation of changes that is important (79).

CAUSES WITHOUT MECHANISMS AND MECHANISMS WITHOUT CAUSES

The rehabilitation of experimental cancer research began in parallel with the expanding role of molecular biology, accompanied by considerable changes in the goals and priorities of experimental research and in its relevance to disease etiology. Among these changes was the beheading, perhaps temporary but certainly preoccupying, of the concept of etiopathogenesis: by concentrating almost exclusively on the pathogenesis of cancer, the etiological component is often left aside. Mortality from certain cancers could be reduced if it were possible to interrupt the sequence of events that lead to invasiveness and metastasis. This will require a better understanding of the mechanisms underlying the various steps in the process of carcinogenesis. However, the events leading to a malignant growth have causes, and a preventive action aimed at avoiding exposure to such causes remains a very efficient way to reduce morbidity and mortality. For instance, despite the progress made in the understanding of the mechanisms involved in the progression to malignancy, it is not yet possible to plan an efficient primary prevention of colorectal cancer because little is known about its etiology. Advances in molecular characterization of colorectal cancers may help in predicting cancer risks in relatives of HNPCC patients, favoring an early diagnosis of the disease (80). It is instead conceivable, that mortality for colorectal cancer could be reduced if the understanding of the mechanisms enabled the clinician to stop the progression of the process before it leads to invasion and metastases. However, understanding of the mechanisms governing tumor progression does not clarify the causes of germline mutations that are at the basis of the increased risk in these patients.

In the case of hepatocellular carcinoma (HCA), an efficient primary prevention is possible by vaccination against Hepatitis B virus (HBV) of children soon after birth in regions of the world where HBV infection is highly prevalent (81,82). This is a plausible strategy in spite of the fact that the mechanism(s) by which chronic HBV infection increases the risk of liver cancer are not understood. In addition, it is possible to reduce the risk of liver cancer by drastically reducing exposure to aflatoxin in areas where exposure is common. A specific mutation of the p53 gene is particularly frequent in HCAs occurring in regions of the world where exposure to aflatoxin is high (83). There is good evidence that this mutation is an early event that may be related to exposure to aflatoxin beginning during the prenatal period (84).

UNATTAINABILITY OF ABSOLUTE CERTAINTY

The absolute certainty that an agent or exposure is the cause of a particular cancer is difficult to obtain, but a reasonable certainty is generally what we accept as proof of causality. This also applies to the tubercle bacillus whose association with tuberculosis was at the origin of the Henle-Koch postulates and was the basis of the germ theory. According to the Henle-Koch postulates, to establish that a microorganism can be considered a causal agent of the disease, three basic requirements must be satisfied: 1) the organism must be found in all cases of the disease in question; 2) it must be isolated from patients with the disease and grown in pure culture; 3) when the pure culture is inoculated into susceptible animals or humans, it should reproduce the disease. Given these requirements a microorganism must be a necessary factor for the disease, but does not need to be a sufficient cause of it. In fact not all carriers of the mycobacterium develop the disease. For noninfectious diseases such as cancer, which are likely to have multiple causal agents, each causal factor is thought to produce a change at the cellular or subcellular level that becomes (one of) the necessary precondition of the disease. Within the multifactorial hypothesis the various factors involved in the induction of cancer can act independently or in a cumulative way, and each of the factors is necessary, but none taken individually is sufficient (85). A sufficient cause, by definition, implies the inevitability of the effect; that is, that cancer will always occur after exposure to a given agent. The agents that are identified as human carcinogens may commonly be called sufficient causes but they are actually components of sufficient causes. They do not imply the inevitable occurrence of the effect, but an increased probability of the effect (86). A cause of cancer may therefore be defined as a factor that increases the probability that cancer will develop in an individual. An operational definition of cause used in epidemiology and public health is: a factor, the elimination of which decreases the occurrence of a disease in a population (87). Similarly a risk factor has been defined as "an attribute or exposure that increases the probability of the disease" (88). The hypothesis of multiple causes is presently extended also to infectious diseases. For instance, tubercle bacillus is considered an agent acting in cooperation with several other causes, such as poor nutrition, low socioeconomic status, family exposure, and genetic susceptibility (89). Very rarely is the exposure to an agent, even extended over a long period of time and at high concentrations, associated with the occurrence of cancer in 100% of the individuals exposed. Not all heavy smokers develop lung cancer, nor do all individuals infected with HBV and exposed to aflatoxin develop liver can-

cer. The occurrence of bladder cancer in all components of a group of workers exposed to aromatic amines (90,91) remains an exceptional event that on the one side provides evidence for extremely poor working conditions, and on the other that exposure to high concentrations of carcinogens overwhelms any possible genetically determined resistance.

The unattainability of absolute certainty in establishing a causal relationship should not generate a level of distrust in the data that will interfere with the efforts to prevent disease. An association should not be evaluated as noncausal merely because error is possible. The first and main goal of etiologic research is to find out whether a particular agent or risk factor can cause cancer, a goal that is eminently qualitative. The criteria for establishing causality for cancer are very demanding and stringent (53,92), and this has helped to reduce the risk for epidemiologists of falling into the trap of false-positive results. However, the criteria were not originally intended to be interpreted rigidly. As the absolute proof of a causal association is unattainable, a certain degree of uncertainty is inevitable. The experience of the past teaches us that "the greatest lesson from the history of public health [.....] is that we do not have to establish causality to prevent disease" (93). Although we hope to do better in the future, the lesson of the past is also that preventive measures have been efficiently implemented independently from how much was known of the specific etiologic agent involved or of the mechanism(s) underlying the origin of the neoplastic growth.

WHAT IS A CARCINOGEN?

The difficulties in defining a cause-effect relationship between exposure to a given agent or risk factor and the occurrence of cancer and the widely accepted hypothesis of the multi-factorial origin of most cancers largely explain why the definitions of carcinogen have remained rather vague and generic, or eminently operational. There is actually not much difference in depth between the definitions given in dictionaries and those appearing in the scientific literature. The Merriam Webster Dictionary (94) very synthetically defines a carcinogen as: "a substance or agent producing or inciting cancer." The Encyclopedia Britannica (95) gives the following definition: "Any of a number of agents that can cause cancer, including chemicals, radiation, and viruses. Exposure to such agents, singly or in combination, can initiate cancer under conditions not wholly understood." Definitions proposed by scientists do not necessarily convey much more insight, but provide some more information. Hueper and Conway (96) very reasonably write: "Carcinogens may be defined as chemical, physical, and parasitic agents of natural and man-made origin, which are capable, under proper conditions of exposure, of producing cancers in animals, including man, in one or several organs and tissues, regardless of the route of exposure and the dose and physical state of the agent used. Such cancers would not have occurred without the intervention of these agents." The IARC provided an indirect operational definition of carcinogen at the inception of its Program on the Evaluation of Carcinogenic Risks to Humans: "For present practical purposes, no distinction is made between the induction of tumours and the enhancement of tumour incidence, although it is noted that there may be fundamental differences in mechanisms that will eventually be elucidated. The response to a carcinogen in experimental animals may be observed in several forms: (i) as a significant increase in the frequency of one or several types of neoplasms, as compared with zero frequency in control animals; (ii) as the occurrence of neoplasms not observed in control animals; (iii) as a decreased latent period as compared to control animals; (iv) as a combination of (i) and (iii)." *(54).* This indirect definition of a carcinogen was reproduced, with minor changes, in all volumes of the IARC Monographs between 1972 and 1987. Another indirect way of defining a carcinogen was through the definition of chemical carcinogenesis: "The widely accepted meaning of the term chemical carcinogenesis, and that used in these [IARC] monographs, is the induction by chemicals of neoplasms that are not usually observed, the earlier induction by chemicals of neoplasms that are usually observed, and/or the induction by chemicals of more neoplasms that are usually found—although fundamentally different mechanisms may be involved in these three situations. Etymologically the term carcinogenesis means the induction of cancer, that is, of malignant neoplasms; however, the commonly accepted meaning is the induction of various types of neoplasms or of a combination of malignant and benign tumours". In 1987 the definition of carcinogen in the Preamble to the IARC Monographs appears considerably shortened: "The term 'carcinogen' is used in these monographs to denote an agent that is capable of increasing the incidence of malignant neoplasms; the induction of benign neoplasms may in some circumstances contribute to the judgement that an agent is carcinogenic" *(54).* A definition of what is a carcinogen is not given in the comprehensive report on "Mechanisms of Carcinogenesis in Risk Identification" issued by IARC as a result of a week-long workshop of experts to evaluate whether carcinogens could be classified according to their mechanisms of action. Likewise, no definition of carcinogen appears in the NTP "Report on Carcinogens" *(60).*

HOW MANY CARCINOGENS?

Individual scientists, scientific agencies, and health authorities have proposed lists of human carcinogens. Among the best known was the list prepared by Hueper and Conway *(96),* which included 17 agents or groups of agents that they considered definitely carcinogenic to humans (Table 1). Most of these agents were identified in the working environment, but Hueper and Conway considered that for at least six of them there was also evidence of a risk for the general population, namely arsenic, coal tar and pitch, mustard gas, soot, ionizing radiation, and UV light. The WHO Technical report entitled "Prevention of Cancer" *(52)* was published in that same year, from which can be extracted a list of 16 agents carcinogenic to humans. Of some interest is that atmospheric pollution was considered an important cause of lung cancer, while commercial benzol was mentioned as a suspected human carcinogen.

The systematic approach adopted by IARC in the evaluation of carcinogenic risks to humans has made the IARC evaluations one of the most authoritative sources for preparing a list of human carcinogens. The agents or complex exposures included in Group 1 of the IARC classification (definitely carcinogenic to humans) were 18 in 1979, 53 in 1989, 75 in 1998,

Table 1
Chemicals and Groups of Chemicals
With Carcinogenic Potential in Humans[a]

Chemicals
4-Aminophenyl
Arsenic
Asbestos
Asphalt
Auramine
Benzidine
Benzol (benzene)
Chromium
Mustard gas
2-Naphtylamine
Nickel

Groups of Chemicals
Anthracene oil
Carbon black
Coke
Creosote oil
Crude paraffin oil
Diesel oil
Isopropyl oil
Lampblack
Lubricating oil and greases
Petrolium fuel oil
Shale oil and paraffin oil
Synthetic hydrogenated coal
oil and tar
tar oil

Others
Clonorchis sinensis
Schistosoma haematobium
Ionizing radiation
Ultraviolet radiation

[1] Adapted from Hueper and Conway *(96).*

and may be grouped in five broad categories (Table 2). The first two categories made up of chemicals or complex exposures related to the working environment represent half (37/75 or 50%) of the recognized human carcinogens. Medical drugs have increased considerably in the last 20 yr and are now second in frequency (19/75 or 25%). A remarkable increase was also that of biological agents, reflecting the growing interest and the availability of adequate research tools. The mixed category environmental agents/life habits includes tobacco smoke that is estimated to be by itself at the origin of a conspicuous proportion of human cancers. Due to the lack of adequate data that could satisfy the rigorous criteria of evaluation adopted by IARC, dietary factors, in spite of their widely advertised role in increasing/decreasing cancer risks, have not yet been included in the evaluation program.

The list of substances known to be human carcinogens that the NTP prepared for the "First Report on Carcinogens" *(97)* included 26 agents (of which 17 related to the working environment) and was largely based on the evaluations made by IARC in its first 16 Monographs. At that time the principle was endorsed "that positive, well-conducted studies on laboratory animals provide strong presumptive evidence of human carci-

Table 2
Numbers of Agents and Complex Exposures With Carcinogenic Potential to Humans[a]

Type of exposure	Year		
	1979	1989	1997
Industrial processes/occupational exposures	4	12	13
Chemicals or chemical mixtures[b]	12	16	24
Medical drugs	2	17	19
Biological agents	-	2	10
Environmental agents/life habits	-	6	9
Total	18	53	75

[a]From IARC data.
[b]Chemicals identified mainly in occupational settings.

nogenicity. Furthermore epidemiological evidence—that is statistical studies of human populations—can be used to confirm carcinogenicity in man" *(97)*. The preparation of the biannual Report on Carcinogens has undergone several important changes adopting slightly different criteria for carcinogen evaluation since this program was initiated. The 8th Report on Carcinogens *(60)* carries a list of 29 chemicals, of which 12 are related to the working environment and 13 are medical drugs.

The IARC and NTP lists include most of the important occupational carcinogens, the most obvious carcinogenic medical drugs, most of the biological agents that can today be suspected to enhance the risk of cancer, and the most obvious environmental factors or life habits, first of all tobacco smoke. It is hard to foresee how many more agents will eventually be identified as human carcinogens. The IARC has evaluated 59 chemicals or complex exposures as probably carcinogenic to humans (IARC Group 2A) and 225 chemicals or complex mixtures as possibly carcinogenic to humans (IARC Group 2B) while the NTP in its 8th Report on Carcinogens *(60)* lists 169 substances "reasonably anticipated to be a human carcinogen." It is not possible, at present, to predict how many of these agents will eventually be proven to be human carcinogens. It is of concern that 1,3-butadiene has not been evaluated by IARC as a human carcinogen, and was included into Group 2A in spite of the experimental, epidemiological, and mechanistic data, all pointing to its carcinogenicity in humans. NTP has categorized 1,3-butadiene as "known to be carcinogenic to humans" (Ninth Report on Carcinogens, National Health Service, NTP, Research Triangle park, NC 27709-2510, 2000.

It can be anticipated that the number of medical drugs found to be carcinogenic will increase over time. These agents represent prime candidates for epidemiological investigations into cancer induction given the ease in measuring their exposure levels (doses) and in identifying and following up the exposed individuals. Clearly, a strict surveillance on the mutagenicity/carcinogenicity of drugs before their introduction to the market will substantially decrease the probability that new drugs reveal carcinogenic effects after long-term usage. Unfortunately there are examples indicating that certain drugs are allowed for long-term treatments without previous adequate testing for possible long-term adverse effects *(98)*. The role of dietary/nutritional factors cannot at present be accurately measured,

but one can assume that the outcome of several ongoing large studies may permit in the future the identification of agents that enhance or increase cancer risks.

ETIOLOGY AND PREVENTION: SUMMARY AND CONCLUSION

Primary prevention of cancer has evolved through time, in close relation to progress in the understanding and interpretation of cancer etiology. In ancient times, etiology and prevention were entirely included within the concept of disease being equivalent to a divine punishment. The only conceivable prevention of cancer was therefore a pious and obedient behavior. Following a brief period between the seventeenth and eighteenth centuries during which cancer was believed to be contagious and cancer patients were isolated to prevent the transmission of the disease, environmental agents were identified as being causally related to human cancer. The first environmental agents to be identified as human carcinogens were tobacco snuff (related to habitual consumption), and chimney soot (related to occupational exposure). They were followed a century later by arsenic used in therapy, aromatic amines, ionizing radiation, and a long series of chemicals or chemical mixtures that were found to be human carcinogens in the working environment. All these agents were identified on the basis of clinical observations, case reports, or epidemiological studies. Those that had been identified in the working environment were called occupational carcinogens, a term that seemed to imply that their carcinogenicity was not only directly related, but also limited, to the occupational setting. Because most human carcinogens that have been identified within the first half of this century were occupational carcinogens, prevention of human cancer became focused on eliminating or reducing to a minimum occupational exposures to identified human carcinogens. During that same period results from long-term animal tests provided evidence for the carcinogenicity of an additional large number of industrial chemicals, and attempts were made to deal with these carcinogenic agents as if they were *de facto* human carcinogens. The IARC recommended that: "…in the absence of adequate data on humans, it is biologically plausible and prudent to regard agents and mixtures for which there is sufficient evidence of carcinogenicity in experimental animals as if they presented a carcinogenic risk to humans" *(54)*. However, primary prevention of even the most obvious carcinogenic hazards has encountered serious obstacles and unjustifiable delays. Aromatic amines were shown to be carcinogenic in exposed workers at the end of last century *(17)*, the ILO officially declared benzidine and 2-naphthylamine human carcinogens in 1921 *(18)*, but the first official action toward phasing out of these aromatic amines was not taken until the late 1960s. The first report of an increased risk for lung cancer in workers exposed to bis-chloromethylether is dated 1962, but no action was taken by regulators until 1975 *(41)*.

Legislation prohibiting the manufacture of a limited number of chemicals identified as human carcinogens was introduced in the late 1960s in certain industrialized countries, but did not cover the same chemical carcinogens in each country. Moreover, the criteria to determine which chemicals may be hazardous to humans on the basis of the experimental evidence of carcinogenicity varied considerably from country to country and were in general overly exclusive *(99,100)*. In most industrialized countries the number of occupational cancers has decreased considerably due to the combined effect of banning or severely reducing exposure to certain carcinogens, the modernization of most industrial productions, the overall reduction of the number of industrial workers, and the transfer of hazardous industries in developing countries. Therefore, occupational cancers are becoming a very serious problem in developing countries where industrialization is a rather recent phenomenon and where exposure levels to hazardous chemicals generally exceed the regulatory levels in industrialized countries *(101)*.

The epidemiological evidence for the carcinogenicity of tobacco smoke provided by studies in the 1950s *(50,51)* marked the beginning of a campaign for prevention focused on personal habits or life-styles. Tobacco smoke and dietary factors are suggested to account for a large proportion (perhaps up to 75%) of all human cancers *(102,103)*. The percentage of cancers attributable to so-called occupational carcinogens and man-made chemicals in the general environment has been estimated to be between 1% and 3%. The percentage of cases attributable to occupational carcinogens, however, may rise up to 40% in workers exposed in certain occupations. The role of multiple chemical carcinogens at low concentrations and of their possible additive or synergistic interaction has been suggested to be minimal, but this is largely due to the difficulty in accurately quantifying risks derived by multiple exposures, rather than to convincing scientific evidence. Strong evidence for a causal association is in this case considered a necessary requirement, whereas the evidence concerning the widely recognized role of dietary factors is mostly circumstantial and often very weak.

The possibility of actively combating the effects of carcinogens to which people may be almost constantly exposed is very attractive and can incite understandable, but perhaps excessive, enthusiasm. A new approach to prevention, called chemoprevention, has been tested in several trials. However, the results of two large trials with alpha-tocopherol (vitamin E) and beta-carotene did not produce any evidence of a beneficial effect; on the contrary they showed some adverse effects *(104,105)*. These results do not exclude the possibility that beta-carotene and vitamin E could exert a protective effect at different doses, after longer periods of administration, or in respect of other variables, but serve to underline a most important requirement in the planning of clinical trials. When planning trials, it is essential to understand the mechanisms of action of the compounds employed. In chemoprevention, this may be more important because this type of active intervention may occur in the context of continued exposure to a carcinogen or a carcinogenic mixture.

For many decades primary prevention of cancer was implemented on the basis of evidence for a causal relationship between an exposure and human cancer that took into consideration biological plausibility, but was independent from the degree of understanding of the underlying mechanisms. One of the credos of public health has been that prevention can be implemented before having established causality or before reaching a complete understanding of mechanisms. The rapid development and expansion of molecular biology and molecular genetics has provided methods and tools that permit investigations of the finest details of the carcinogenic process. A deeper knowledge of mechanisms may allow future interventions aimed at stopping the sequence of events leading to invasiveness and metastases and may substantially improve therapeutic interventions. However, at present the emphasis on research into the pathogenesis of cancer seems to have encouraged an almost complete elimination of research on etiology.

From a period in which cancer causes, or components of causes, were identified with little understanding of the underlying mechanisms, we have entered a period in which the understanding of mechanisms progresses rapidly without yet contributing to the identification of new carcinogenic agents or the definition of primary prevention strategies. In this context a most urgent and complicated issue is development of a better understanding of the role of low-level exposures to multiple risk factors and of the extent and nature of their possible interaction.

The most reasonable and socially acceptable development of prevention should be the blending of the population approach; that is, the shifting of the distribution of risk factors across an entire population in a favorable direction, with the high-risk approach, as has been discussed in depth with regard to cardiovascular diseases *(106)*. Interventions aimed at reducing or eliminating genetically determined weaknesses in the interaction with the environment will, therefore, not make in any way obsolete or redundant interventions aimed at eliminating or reducing exposure to environmental carcinogens and at improving socioeconomic conditions.

REFERENCES

1. Hacker, A. (1997) The medicine in our future. *NY Rev. Books* **46**:26–31.
2. Tomatis, L., Agthe, C., Bartsch, H., Huff, J., Montesano, R., Saracci, R., et al. (1978) Evaluation of the carcinogenicity of chemicals: a review of the monograph program of the International Agency for Research on Cancer. *Cancer Res.* **38**:877–885.
3. Ackerknecht, E. H. (1965) *History and Geography of the Most Important Diseases.* Hafner Publishing Co., New York.
4. Shimkin, M. B. (1979) *Contrary to Nature.* DHEW publication No. (NIH) 79-720, Washington, DC.

5. Rous, P. (1911) A sarcoma of the fowl transmissible by an agent separable from the tumor cells. *J. Exp. Med.* **13**:397–411.

6. Hixson, J. (1976) *The Patchwork Mouse.* Anchor Press, Garden City, NY.

7. Weinberg, R. (1996) *Racing to the Beginning of the Road.* Harmony Book, New York.

8. Cairns, J. (1997) *Matters of Life and Death.* Princeton University Press, Princeton, NJ.

9. Jacob, F. (1997) *La Souris, la Mouche et l'Homme.* Editions Odile Jacob, Paris.

10. Conheim, J. (1889) *Lectures on General Pathology. A Handbook for Practicians and Students.* The New Sydenham Society, London.

11. Triolo, V. A. (1964) Nineteenth century foundations of cancer research. Origins of experimental research. *Cancer Res.* **24**:4–27.

12. Triolo, V. A. (1965) Nineteenth century foundations of cancer research. Advances in tumor pathology, nomenclature, and theories of oncogenesis. *Cancer Res.* **25**:75–106.

13. Schuttmann, W. (1993) Schneeberg lung disease and uranium mining in the Saxon Ore Mountain (Erzgebirge). *Am. J. Ind. Med.* **23**:355–368.

14. Hill, J. (1761) *Cautions Against the Immoderate Use of Snuff.* R. Baldwin and J. Jackson, London.

15. Pott, P. (1775) *Chirurgical Observations Relative to the Cataract, the Polypus of the Nose, the Cancer of the Scrotum, the Different Kinds of Ruptures and the Mortifications of the Toes and Feet.* Hawes, Clarke, and Collins, London.

16. Hutchinson, J. (1988) On some examples of arsenic-keratosis of the skin and of arsenic-cancer. *Trans. Path. Soc. London* **39**:352–363.

17. Rehn, L. (1895) Bladder tumours in fuchsin workers. *Arch. Fur Klin. Chirurgie* **50**:588–600.

18. International Labour Office (1921) *Cancer of the Bladder Among Workers in Aniline Factories.* Studies and Reports, Series F, No. 1, ILO, Geneva.

19. Tomatis, L., Ai tio, A., Wilbourn, J., and Shuker, L. (1989) Human carcinogens so far identified. *Jpn. J. Cancer Res.* **80**:795–807.

20. Vainio, H., Wilbourn, J., and Tomatis, L. (1994) Identification of environmental carcinogens: The first step in risk assessment. *In: The Identification and Control of Environmental and Occupational Diseases: Hazard and Risks of Chemicals in the Oil Refining Industry* (Mehlman, F. and Upton, A., eds.), Princeton Scientific Publishing Co., Princeton, NJ, pp. 1–19.

21. Huff, J. (1994) Chemicals causally associated with cancers in humans and in laboratory animals: a perfect concordance. *In: Carcinogenesis* (Waalkes, M. P. and Ward, J. P., eds.), Raven Press, New York, pp 25–37.

22. Huff, J. (1998) Carcinogenicity results in animals predict cancer risks to humans. *In: Public Heath & Preventive Medicine* (. Wallace, R. B, ed.), Appleton & Lange, Stamford, CT, pp. 543–569.

23. Roentgen, W. C. (1895) Ueber eine neue Art von Strahlen. *Sitzungsber. Phys. Med. Gesellsch. Wurtzb.* 132–141.

24. Frieben, A. (1902) Demonstration eines Cancroid der rechten Handruckens, das sich nach langdauernder Einwirkung von Rontgenstrahlen entwickelt hat. *Fortschr. Roentgenstr.* **6**:106–111.

25. Sick, H. (1902) Karzinom der Haut das auf dem Boden eines Roentgenulcus entstanden ist. *Muench. Med. Wochenschr.* **50**:1445.

26. International Agency for Research on Cancer (1988) *Man-Made Mineral Fibers and Radon.* IARC Monograph on the Evaluation of Carcinogenic Risk to Humans, Vol. 43, IARC, Lyon.

27. Ames, B. N., Profet, M., and Gold, L. S. (1990) Nature's chemicals and synthetic chemicals: comparative toxicology. *Proc. Natl. Acad. Sci. USA* **87**:7782–7786.

28. International Agency for Research on Cancer (1985) *Tobacco Smoking.* IARC Monograph on the Evaluation of Carcinogenic Risk to Humans, Vol. 38, IARC, Lyon.

29. Yamagiwa, K. and Ichikawa, K. (1915) Experimentelle Studie ueber die Pathogenese der Epithelialgeschwuelste. *Mitt. Med. Ges.* **15**:295–344.

30. Tsutsui, H. (1918) Ueber das kuenstlich erzeugte Cancroid bei der Maus. *Gann* **12**:17–21.

31. Passey, R. D. (1922) Experimental soot cancer. *Br. Med. J.* **ii**:1112–1113.

32. Murphy, J. B. and Sturm, E. (1925) Primary lung tumors in mice following the cutaneous application of coal tar. *J. Exp. Med.* **42**:693–700.

33. Sasaki, T. and Yoshida T. (1935) Experimentlle erzeugung des Leberkarzinom durch Futterung mit o-Amidoazotoluol. *Virchows Arch. Path. Anat.* **295**:175–200.

34. Kennaway, E. L. and Hieger, I. (1930) Carcinogenic substances and their fluorescence spectra. *Br. Med. J.* **1**:1044–1046.

35. Cook, J. W., Hieger, I., Kennaway, L., and Mayneord, W. V. (1932) The production of cancer by pure hydrocarbons. Part I. *Proc. Royal Soc. Part B* **111**:455–84.

36. Boyland, E. and Levi A. A. (1935) Metabolism of polycyclic compounds. I. Production of dihydroxydihydro-anthracene from anthracene. *Biochem. J.* **29**:2679–2683.

37. Boyland, E. and Horning, E. S. (1949) The induction of tumours with nitrogen mustards. *Br. J. Cancer* **3**:118–123.

38. Boyland, E. and Weigert, F. (1947) Metabolism of carcinogenic compounds. *Br. Med. Bull.* **4**:354–359.

39. Miller, E. C. and Miller, J. A. (1947) The presence and significance of bound aminoazo dyes in the livers of rats fed *p*-dimethylaminoazobenzene. *Cancer Res.* **7**:468–480.

40. Miller, E. C. and Miller, J. A. (1952) In vivo combinations between carcinogens and tissue constituents and their possible role in carcinogenesis. *Cancer Res.* **12**:547–556.

41. Tomatis, L. (1977) The value of long-term testing for the implementation of primary prevention. *In: Origins of Human Cancer* (Hiatt, H. H., Watson, J. D., and Winsten, J. A., eds.), Cold Spring Harbor Laboratory Press, Cold Spring Harbor, NY, pp. 1339–1357.

42. Huff, J. (1993) Chemicals and cancer in humans: first evidence in experimental animals. *Environ. Health Perspect.* **100**:201–210.

43. Melnick, R. (1995) Mechanistic data indicate that 1,3-butadiene is a human carcinogen. *Carcinogenesis* **16**:157–163

44. Tomatis, L. (1979) The predictive value of rodent carcinogenicity tests in the evaluation of human risk. *Ann. Rev. Pharmacol. Toxicol.* **19**:511–530.

45. International Agency for Research on Cancer (1985) *Interpretation of Negative Epidemiological Evidence for Carcinogenesis* (Wald, N. J. and Doll, R., eds.), IARC Scientific Publication No. 65, IARC, Lyon.

46. Friedewald, W. F. and Rous, P. (1944) The initiating and promoting elements in tumor production. *J. Exp. Med.* **80**:101–126.

47. Berenblum, I. (1941) The mechanism of carcinogenesis: a study of the significance of carcinogenic action and related phenomena. *Cancer Res.* **1**:897–814.

48. Berenblum, I. and Shubik, P. (1947) A new quantitative approach to the study of the stages of chemical carcinogenesis in the mouse's skin. *Br. J. Cancer* **1**:383–391.

49. Tomatis, L., Huff, J., Hertz-Picciotto, I., Sandler, D. ., Bucher, J., Boffetta, P., et al. (1997) Avoided and avoidable risks of cancer. *Carcinogenesis* **18**:97–105.

50. Doll, R., and Hill, B. A. (1950) Smoking and carcinoma of the lung. *Br. Med. J.* **2**:739–748.

51. Wynder, E. L. and Graham, F. A. (1950) Tobacco smoking as a possible etiologic factor in bronchiogenic carcinoma. A study of six hundred and eighty-four proved cases. *JAMA* **143**:329–336.

52. World Health Organization (1964) *Prevention of Cancer.* WHO Tech. Rep. No. 276, Geneva, Switzerland.

53. Bradford Hill, A. (1971) *Principles of Medical Statistics.* The Lancet Ltd., London.

54. International Agency for Research on Cancer (1987) *Overall Evaluation of Carcinogenicity: An Updating of IARC Monographs Volumes 1 to 42.* IARC Monographs on the Evaluation of Carcinogenic Risks to Humans, Supplement 7, IARC, Lyon, 1987.

55. International Agency for Research on Cancer (1983) *Approaches to Classifying Chemical Carcinogens According to Mechanism of Action.* IARC Intern. Tech. Rep. No. 83/001, IARC, Lyon.

56. International Agency for Research on Cancer (1992) *Mechanisms of Carcinogenesis in Risk Identification* (Vainio, H., Magee , P.,

McGregor, D., and McMichael, A. J., eds.), IARC Scientific Publication No. 116, IARC, Lyon.

57. Karstadt, M., Bobal, R., and Selikoff, I. J. (1981) A survey of availability of epidemiologic data on humans exposed to animal carcinogens. *In: Quantification of Occupational Cancer* (Peto, R. and Schneiderman, M., eds.), Banbury Report No. 9, Cold Spring Harbor Laboratory Press, Cold Spring Harbor, NY, pp. 223–245.

58. Environmental Protection Agency (1996) Proposed guidelines for carcinogen risk assessment, notice of availability and opportunity to comment on proposed guidelines for carcinogen risk assessment. *Fed. Reg.* **61**:17959–18011.

59. Karstadt, M., and Haseman, J. K. (1997) Effect of discontinuing certain tumor types/sites on evaluations of carcinogenicity in laboratory animals. *Am. J. Ind. Med.* **31**:485–494.

60. National Toxicology Program (2000): *9th Report on Carcinogens.* National Institute for Environmental Health Sciences, Research Triangle Park, NC.

60a. Huff, J. (1998) NTP report on carcinogens-history, concepts, procedure, processes. *Eur. J. Oncol.* **3**:343–355.

61. Rous, P. and Kidd, J. C. (1941) Conditional neoplasms and sub-threshold neoplastic states: A study of the tar tumors in the rabbit. *J. Exp. Med.* **1**:383–391.

62. Berenblum, I. (1974) *Carcinogenesis as a Biological Problem.* American Elsevier Publishing Co., New York.

63. Charles, D. R. and Luce-Clausen, M. L. (1942) The kinetics of papilloma formation in benzpyrene-treated mice. *Cancer Res.* **2**:261–263.

64. Barrett, J. C. (1992) Mechanisms of action of known human carcinogens. *In: Mechanisms of Carcinogenesis in Risk Identification* (Vanio, H., Magee, P. N.,. McGegor, D. B, and McMichael, A. J., eds.), IARC, Lyon, pp. 115–134.

65. Watson, J. D and Crick, F. H. C. (1953) Molecular structure of nucleic acid. A structure of deoxiribose nuclei acid. *Nature* **171**:737–738.

66. Burdette, W. J. (1955) The significance of mutation in relation to the origin of tumors: a review. *Cancer Res.* **15**:201–226.

67. Lawley, P. D. (1994) Historical origins of current concepts of carcinogenesis. *Adv. Cancer Res.* **65**:17–111.

68. Ames, B. N. and McCann, J. (1976) Carcinogens are mutagens:a simple test system. *In: Screening Tests in Chemical Carcinogenesis* (Montesano, R., Bartsch, H., Tomatis, L., eds.), IARC Scientific Publication No. 12, IARC, Lyon, pp.493–501.

69. McCann, J., Choi, E., Yamasaki, E., and Ames, B. N. (1975) Detection of carcinogens as mutagens in the Salmonella/microsome test: assay of 300 chemicals. *Proc. Natl. Acad. Sci. USA* **72**:5135–5139.

70. Sugimura, T., Nagao, M. ,Kawachi, M., Honda, M., Yahagi, T., Seino, Y., et al. (1977) Mutagens-carcinogens in food, with special reference to highly mutagenic pyrolytic products in broiled foods. *In: Origins of Human Cancer* (Hiatt, H. H., Watson, J. D., and Winsten, J. A., eds.), Cold Spring Harbor Laboratory Press, Cold Spring Harbor, NY, pp. 1561–1577.

71. Ames, B. N., Durston, W. E., Yamasaki, E., and Lee, F. D. (1973) Carcinogens are mutagens: a simple test system combining liver homogenates for activation and bacteria for detection. *Proc. Natl. Acad. Sci. USA* **70**:2281–2285.

72. Bartsch, H., Malaveille, C., Camus, A. M., Martel-Planche, G., Brun, G., Hautefeuille, A., et al. (1980) Bacterial and mammalian mutagenicity tests: validation and comparative studies on 180 chemicals. *In: Molecular and Cellular Aspects of Carcinogen Screening Tests* (Montesano, R., Bartsch, H., and Tomatis, L., eds.), IARC Scientific Publication No. 27, IARC, Lyon.

73. Fetterman, B. A, Kim, B. S., Margolin, B. H., Scildcrout, J. S., Smith, M. G., Wagner, S. M., et al. (1997) Predicting rodent carcinogenicity from mutagenic potency measured in the Ames salmonella assay. *Environ. Mol. Mut.* **29**:312–322.

74. Armitage, P. and Doll, R. (1954) The age distribution of cancer and a multi-stage theory of carcinogenesis. *Br. J. Cancer* **8**:1–12.

75. Foulds, L. (1969) *Neoplastic Development.* Academic Press, New York.

76. Nowell, P. (1976) The clonal evolution of tumor cell populations. *Science* **194**:23–28.

77. Cheng, K. C. and Loeb, L. A. (1993) Genomic instability and tumor progression: mechanistic consideration. *Adv. Cancer Res.* **60**:121–156.

78. Vogelstein, B., Fearon, E. R., Hamilton, S. R., Kern, S. E., Presinger, A. C., Leppert, M., et al. (1988) Genetic alterations during colorectal-tumor development. *N. Eng. J. Med.* **319**:525–532.

79. Fearon, E. R. and Vogelstein, B. (1990) A genetic model for colorectal tumorigenesis. *Cell* **61**:759–776.

80. Wijnen, J. T., Vasen, H. F. A., Meera Kahn, P., Zwinderman, A. H., van de Klift, H., Mulder, A., et al. (1998) Clinical findings with implications for genetic testing in families with clustering of colorectal cancer. *N. Engl. J. Med.* **339**:511–518.

81. Inskip, H. M., Hall, A. J., Chotard, J., Loik, F., and Whittle, H. (1991) Hepatitis B vaccine in the Gambian Expanded Programme on Immunization: factors influencing antibody release. *Int. J. Epidemiol.* **20**:764–769.

82. Fortuin, M., Chotard, J., Jack, A. D., Maine, N. P., Mendy, M, Hall, A. J., et al. (1993) Efficacy of hepatitis B vaccine in the Gambian expanded programme on immunization. *Lancet* **341**:1129–1131.

83. Montesano, R., Hainaut, P., and Wild, C. P. (1997) Hepatocellular carcinoma: from gene to public health. *J. Natl. Cancer Inst.* **89**:1844–1851.

84. Wild, C. P., Rasheed, P. N., Jawis, M. F., Hall, A. J., and Montesano, R. (1991) In utero exposure to aflatoxin in west Africa. *Lancet* **337**:1602.

85. Lilienfeld, A. M. and Lilienfeld, D. E. (1980) *Foundation of Epidemiology.* Oxford University Press, New York, pp. 292–295.

86. Rothman, K. J. (1982) Causation and causal inference. *In: Cancer Epidemiology and Prevention* (Schottenfeld, D. and Fraumeni, J., eds.), W.B. Saunders Co., Philadelphia, pp. 15–22.

87. Tomatis, L., Aitio, A., Day, N. E., Heseltine, E. ,Kaldor, J., Miller, A. B., et al. (1990) *Cancer: Causes, Occurrence and Control.* IARC Scientific Publication No. 100, IARC, Lyon.

88. Last, J. (1988) *A Dictionary of Epidemiology.* Oxford University Press, New York, London.

89. Susser, M. (1988) Falsification, verification and causal inference in epidemiology: Reconsiderations in the light of Sir Karl Popper's philosophy. *In: Causal Inference* (Rothman, K.J., ed.), Epidemiology Resources Inc., Chestnut Hill, MA, pp. 33–57.

90. Case, R. A. M., Hosker, M. E., Mcdonald, D. B., and Pearson, J. T. (1954) Tumours of the urinary bladder in workmen engaged in the manufacture and use of certain dyestuff intermediates in the British chemical industry. I. The role of aniline, benzidine, alpha-naphthylamine and beta-naphthylamine. *Br. J. Industr. Med.* **11**:75–94.

91. Williams, M. H. C. (1958) Occupational tumours of the bladder. *Cancer* **3**:337–342.

92. Rothman, K .J. (ed.) (1988) *Causal Inference.* Epidemiology Resources Inc., Chestnut Hill, MA.

93. Lanes, S. F. (1988) Error and uncertainty in causal inference. *In: Causal Inference* (Rothman, K. J., ed.), Epidemiology Resources Inc., Chestnut Hill, MA, pp.173–188.

94. Merriam-Webster's Collegiate Dictionary, Merriam-Webster Inc., Springfield, MA, 1997.

95. Encyclopedia Britannica, 1995.

96. Hueper, W. C. and Conway, W. D. (1964) *Chemical Carcinogenesis and Cancers.* Charles C. Thomas Publisher, Springfield, IL.

97. National Toxicology Program (1980) *First Report on Carcinogens.* National Institute for Environmental Health Sciences, Research Triangle Park, NC.

98. Olivero, O. A., Anderson, L. M., Diwan, B. A., Haines, D. C., Harbaugh, S. W., Moskal, T. J., et al. (1997) Transplacental effects of 3′-azido-2′,3′-dideothymidine (AZT): tumorigenicity in mice and genotoxicity in mice and monkeys. *Int. J. Cancer* **89**:1602–1608.

99. Montesano, R. and Tomatis, L. (1977) Legislation concerning chemical carcinogens in several industrialized countries. *Cancer Res.* **37**:310–316.

100. Carnevale, F., Montesano, R., Partensky, C., and Tomatis, L. (1987) Comparisons of regulations on occupational carcinogens in several industrialized countries. *Am. J. Ind. Med.* **12**:453–473.

101. Pearce, N., Matos, E., Vainio, H., Boffetta, P., and Kogevinas, M. (eds.) (1994) *Occupational Cancer in Developing Countries.* IARC Scientific Publication No. 129, IARC, Lyon.

102. Doll, R. and Peto, R. (1981) The causes of cancer: Quantitative estimates of avoidable risks of cancer in the United States today. *J. Natl. Cancer Inst.* **66**:1191–1308.

103. Ames, B. N., Gold, L. S., and Willett, W. C. (1995) The causes and prevention of cancer. *Proc. Natl. Acad. Sci. USA* **92**:5258–5265.

104. Alpha-Tocoferol, Beta Carotene Cancer Prevention Study Group (1994) The effect of vitamin E and beta carotene on the incidence of lung cancer and other cancers in male smokers. *N. Engl. J. Med.* **330**:1029–1035.

105. Omenn, G. S., Goodman, G. E., Thorquist, M. D., Balmes, J., Cullen, M. R., Glass, A., et al. (1994) Effects of a combination of beta carotene and vitamin A on lung cancer and cardiovascular disease. *N. Engl. J. Med.* **334**:1150–1155.

106. Rose, G. (1992) *The Strategy of Preventive Medicine.* Oxford University Press, New York.

10 Cellular Responses to Chemical Carcinogens

EDWARD L. LOECHLER, PhD, BRYAN HENRY, PhD,
AND KWANG-YOUNG SEO, PhD

INTRODUCTION

Cancer is the second leading cause of death in the United States. It is estimated that approximately a third of all Americans will develop cancer in their lifetime. The American Cancer Society estimated that 1,220,000 new cases of cancer and 550,000 deaths occurred in 2000 (*see* www.cancer.org). Agents that can cause cancer are called carcinogens. Carcinogens can be classified into agents that are chemical, viral, or physical (radiation such as untraviolet [UV] light, X-rays, and gamma rays). Approximately 60–90% of all cancers are now generally believed to be due to these environmental factors to which humans are exposed in food, water, or air. It is important to mention that the term environmental factors includes both natural and human-made agents.

Chemicals can contribute to tumor formation in at least three ways: 1) as genotoxins, 2) as co-carcinogens, and 3) as tumor promoters. The nomenclature in this regard is phenomenological. The term carcinogen refers to any substance that can contribute to the process of tumor formation. However, it is most often associated with substances that are genotoxic, and can initiate the process of carcinogenesis by causing a mutation (as mutagens), which is defined as any heritable change in the primary sequence of DNA. It is sensible that mutagens are carcinogens, given that cancer cells grow in an unregulated fashion because they have mutations in particular genes whose function it is to provide proper growth control for the cell. A variety of endogenous processes, which occur spontaneously inside cells, can also contribute to mutagenesis and carcinogenesis, including spontaneous DNA damage, such as hydrolysis of or oxidative damage to the DNA bases, as well as polymerase errors. A co-carcinogen is a substance that by itself does not cause a tumor to form, but, when present at the same time as a genotoxin, enhances the potency of that genotoxin. A tumor promoter is a substance that by itself does not cause a

tumor, but enhances tumor formation when it is given (usually repeatedly) after exposure to a genotoxin.

This chapter will focus on chemical agents that are genotoxic, and these agents will be generally referred to as carcinogens. In addition, the roles of co-carcinogens and tumor promoters will be discussed. It is important to mention that there are other ways of classifying carcinogens, such as genetic vs epigenetic carcinogens. All cells, from bacteria to human, face similar kinds of problems when dealing with damage to their genomes. For example, often both mutational patterns and DNA repair are similar in most cells. Based on this premise, the discussion will not be limited to how human cells respond to chemical carcinogens, but will also draw on what is known from a variety of other systems, including bacteria. There are a number of excellent books and book chapters that comprehensively discuss classical aspects of chemical carcinogenesis *(1–8)*, including an extraordinary two-volume treatise edited by Charles Searle *(1)*. Although these topics are not ignored herein, they will be treated more lightly, and the focus will be on relatively new topics concerning biological responses to chemical carcinogens, including apoptosis, cell-cycle effects, double-strand break (dsb) repair, nucleotide-excision repair (NER) in humans, and transcription-coupled repair.

HISTORICAL BREAKTHROUGHS IN OUR UNDERSTANDING OF THE RELATIONSHIP BETWEEN EXPOSURE TO CHEMICAL CARCINOGENS AND HUMAN CANCER

The notion that human cancer might be caused by environmental factors, in particular chemicals, began in 1761 when John Hill *(9)* noted the development of nasal cancer as a consequence of excessive use of tobacco snuff, and was followed in 1775 by Percival Pott *(10)*, who noted the unusually high incidence of scrotal cancer among chimney sweeps exposed to chimney soots. However, such associations were not definitive and required verification, notably in experimental systems. In 1915 Yamagiwa and Ichikawa *(11)* first showed experimentally that chemicals (a mixture of coal tars) caused skin cancer

From: *The Molecular Basis of Human Cancer* (W. B. Coleman and G. J. Tsongalis, eds.), © Humana Press Inc., Totowa, NJ.

Table 1
Carcinogenicity to Humans for Selected Substances from the IARC Monograph Database

Chemical family	Category[a]
PAHs	
TCDD (dioxin)	1
2,3,7,8-tetrachlorodibenzo-p-dioxin benzo[a]pyrene	2A
Benzo[a]anthracene	2A
PCBs (polychlorinated biphenyls)	2A
Benzo[b]fluoranthene	2B
AAs	
4-aminobiphenyl	1
Benzidine	1
IQ (2-amino-3-methylimidazo[4,5-f]quinoline)	2A
MeIQ (2-amino-3,4-dimethylimidazo[4,5-f]quinoline)	2B
PhIP (2-amino-1-methy-6-phenylimidazo[4,5-b]pyridine)	2B
4-nitropyrene	2B
Alkylating Agents	
Sulfur mustard	1
DMS, DES, ENU	2A
EDB (ethylene dibromide)	2A
NNK (4-(N-nitrosomethylamino)-1-(3-pyridyl)-1-butanone)	2B
Many nitrosamines	2B
DMN (N-nitrosodimethylamine)	2A
Mycotoxins	
Aflatoxins (naturally occurring)	1
Aflatoxin M1	2B
Sterigmatocystin	2B
Metals (as compounds)	
Nickel	1
Chromium	1
Cadmium	1
Arsenic	1
Beryllium	1
Cobalt	2B
Fibers	
Silica (asbestos)	1
Wood dust	1
Ceramic fibers	2B
Glasswool	2B
Acrylic fibers	3
Others	
Vinyl chloride	1
Tobacco smoke	1
Tobacco products	1
Cyclophosphamide	1
Sulfur mustard	1
Nitrogen mustard	1
Formaldehyde	2A
Cisplatin	2A
Methylene chloride	2B
Hydrazine	2B
Hydrogen peroxide	3
Ethylene	3

[a]Categorization by Group based on the following criteria of evaluation for agents as stated in the Preamble to the IARC Monographs. Group 1, The agent is carcinogenic to humans. This category is used when there is sufficient evidence of carcinogenicity in humans. Group 2, This category includes agents for which, at one extreme, the degree of evidence of carcinogenicity in humans is almost sufficient, as well as those for which, at the other extreme, there are no human data but for which there is evidence of carcinogenicity in experimental animals. Agents are assigned to either group 2A (probably carcinogenic to humans) or group 2B (possibly carcinogenic to humans). Group 3, The agent is not classifiable as to its carcinogenicity to humans. This category is used most commonly for agents, mixtures, and exposure circumstances for which the evidence of carcinogenicity is inadequate in humans and inadequate or limited in experimental animals. Group 4, The agent (mixture) is probably not carcinogenic to humans.

when painted on the ears of rabbits. The first pure, synthetic compound that demonstrated carcinogenicity was dibenz[a,h]anthracene *(12)*, and the first compound isolated from a complex mixture (coal tar) shown to be carcinogenic was benzo[a]pyrene *(13)*. These chemicals are examples of the large class of compounds called polycyclic aromatic hydrocarbons (PAHs). Wilhelm Hueper wrote the first comprehensive book about exposures to chemical carcinogens and cancer *(14)*, which began as an outgrowth of his pioneering work in the 1930s showing that certain aniline dyes caused bladder cancer in dogs *(15)*. His work was initiated because of concern about the observation, first made by Rehn *(16)* that workers in the aniline dye industry developed bladder cancer at an alarmingly high rate *(16–21)*. The pursuit of the observation of an acute hepatotoxic disease in turkeys (turkey "X" disease), resulted in the isolation of the mycotoxins (aflatoxin B_1) by Gerald Wogan and colleagues *(22)*, which eventually led to the realization that these agents (produced by molds that grow on improperly stored foods [peanuts]) also cause liver cancer *(23)*.

The association between exposure to a chemical (or chemical mixtures) and human cancer has been established in numerous epidemiological studies, most significantly the role of smoking in lung cancer. The first report of this association appeared in 1939 *(24)*, but subsequent reports were more definitive, with the most influential studies being published by Hill and Peto *(25–27)*. The first report of an association between exposure to asbestos and cancer appeared in 1942 *(28)*, although it took the monumental work of Irving Selikoff to build the definitive case for this association *(29)*. The ability of chemicals to cause human cancer was clearly, dramatically, and regrettably demonstrated in the case of occupational exposures to a number of chemicals, such as *bis*-chloromethylether (lung cancer), and vinyl chloride (hepatic angiosarcoma) *(30)*. The notion that 60–90% of all human cancers are likely to be due to environmental factors was first apparent from the work of Higginson *(31)*, who showed that cancer incidence varied between countries, probably because of differences in environmental factors. This conclusion was reinforced by Haenszel and his collaborators *(32,33)*, who showed that immigrants and their descendants tended to adopt the cancer risks of the country to which they immigrated.

On the biological side, the hypothesis that cancer might develop from mutations in the genetic substance of cells was first proposed by Theodor Boveri in 1914 *(34)*. The link between damage to the genetic substance (later recognized to be DNA) and mutations was provided in the pioneering work by H.J. Muller showing that X-irradiation caused mutations in *Drosophila (35)*. While suspected for many years, the strongest support showing that carcinogens are mutagens emerged from the work of Bruce Ames, who developed the so-called Ames test, which utilizes a bacteria that has been engineered to be extraordinarily sensitive to the induction of mutations *(4–6,36)*. The correlation between mutagens and carcinogens in the Ames test has generally been found to be quite high (~80%). The role of mutations in human cancer was further substantiated when a number of investigators, notably Robert Weinberg *(37)*, Mariano Barbacid *(38)*, and Michael Weigler *(39)*, showed that the 12th codon of the c-H-*ras* gene derived from the cells of a

human bladder cancer was changed from 5'-GGC to 5'-GTC, which resulted in an amino acid substitution at that position from glycine to valine.

Perhaps the clearest example of a role for a specific etiological agents in the cause of human cancer comes from the findings that the mutations in the p53 tumor-suppressor gene show patterns that seem to give a clue about the etiological agent responsible *(40–42)*. This has been referred to as a mutagenic fingerprint *(40)*.

CLASSES OF CARCINOGENS

The International Agency for Research on Cancer (IARC) maintains a registry of human carcinogens and suspected human carcinogens, which has been developed based on a careful examination of epidemiological studies on humans, animal model studies and the use of a variety of short-term tests, such as the Ames test. There are 850 compounds that have been evaluated to date, and these are discussed in a series called the *IARC Monographs*, which currently includes Monographs 1–76, along with eight Supplements. A complete listing of the chemicals evaluated and the carcinogenic hazard they pose can be found at the IARC website at www.iarc.fr by pursuing the IARC Monographs Database. Some information from this data base is given in Table 1. In addition, the National Toxicology Program (NTP) conducts animal assays for long-term cancer studies of suspected hazardous chemicals. The chemicals studied have been chosen based on human exposure, level of production, and chemical structure. Information on the compounds studied can be found in the Abstracts of NTP Long-Term Cancer Studies or at The NTP website at ntp-server.niehs.nih.gov.

The number of compounds that is or may be carcinogens is extensive. However, these chemicals can be subdivided into different classes (Table 1), including PAHs, heterocyclic amines (HAs) or aromatic amines, alkylating agents, mycotoxins, metals and fibers (notably asbestos), as well as other chemicals and mixtures, such as tobacco smoke, certain anticancer drugs (cyclophosphamide and cisplatin), warfare agents (sulfur mustard), and oxidizing agents (hydrogen peroxide). In each of these classes, there are typically one or two chemicals that have emerged as representatives and are the most studied, and some of these are shown in Fig. 1.

THE STEPS IN CHEMICAL CARCINOGENESIS

The impact of chemical carcinogens on biological systems is exceedingly complex, but can be subdivided into a number of steps to simplify its presentation. While the details vary depending on the carcinogen, the paradigm shown in Fig. 2, which utilizes one particularly well-studied chemical carcinogen, benzo[a]pyrene, illustrates many of the principles. Steps in the horizontal direction lead toward carcinogenicity, and include: 1) metabolic activation, 2) reaction with DNA (adduction), 3) adduct mutagenesis, and 4) tumorigenesis. Steps in the vertical direction lead to diminished carcinogenicity, and include: 1) metabolic detoxification, 2) carcinogen deactivation and DNA repair, 3) cell-cycle delay, and 4) apoptosis.

CARCINOGEN METABOLISM Most potent carcinogenic substances, such as the PAHs, HAs, and aflatoxins are hydrophobic, have an affinity for lipid-rich areas of the body (1-8),

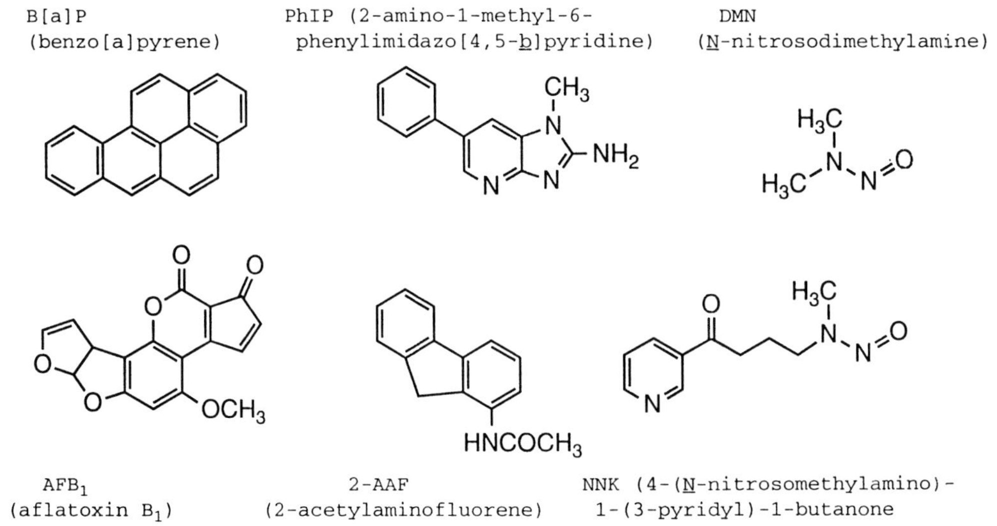

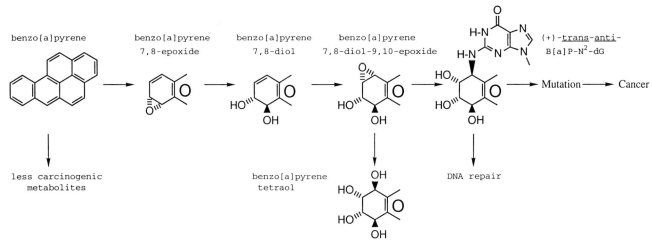

B[a]P
(benzo[a]pyrene)

PhIP (2-amino-1-methyl-6-
phenylimidazo[4,5-<u>b</u>]pyridine)

DMN
(<u>N</u>-nitrosodimethylamine)

AFB₁
(aflatoxin B₁)

2-AAF
(2-acetylaminofluorene)

NNK (4-(<u>N</u>-nitrosomethylamino)-
1-(3-pyridyl)-1-butanone

Fig. 1. Structures of chemical carcinogens. The structures of several chemical carcinogens discussed in the text are shown, including a PAH (benzo[a]pyrene), a mycotoxin (AFB₁), two HAs (PhIP and 2-AAF), and two alkylating agents (DMN and NNK).

Fig. 2. The carcinogenesis paradigm. In this example the paradigm is applied using benzo[*a*]pyrene. The horizonal arrows lead toward greater toxicity (in particular cancer), while the vertical arrows lead toward lesser toxicity.

and their accumulation can cause toxicity if not removed (43–47). Thus, organisms have evolved mechanisms to rid themselves of these xenobiotic, toxic substances. Most metabolism leads to the formation of less toxic or less carcinogenic substances, which are eventually excreted from the body. However, in some circumstances, metabolism produces metabolites (which are sometimes called ultimate carcinogens) that are more carcinogenic than the parent compound. The first studies in this regard were conducted by Elizabeth Miller and James Miller (48), who established the principle that many chemical carcinogens are not inherently cancer-causing without being covalently modified (metabolized) by cellular enzymes (43–47). Metabolism is classified as being phase I, involving the metabolic oxidation (hydroxylation), reduction, or hydrolytic modification of xenobiotics, or phase II, involving metabolic conjugation of xenobiotics (45–47).

Phase I Metabolism of Xenobiotics One of the principal strategies for metabolizing xenobiotics involves hydroxylation, which increases polarity and water solubility, facilitating clear-

ance of the toxic compound (45–47). Metabolism occurs in most tissues of the body, but is most extensive in the liver. Hydroxylation is usually by the mixed function oxidases (P450s), which are ubiquitous. Organisms have many P450s with varying substrate specificities. A recent review (49) lists 481 P450s that are classified into 74 gene families, of which 20 have been found in humans. Individual isozymes are designated using a nomenclature where the first Arabic number denotes the family, the letter the subfamily, and the final number the individual member within that subfamily (P450 1A1). The corresponding gene is designated, *CYP1A1*. A particular P450 usually metabolizes multiple substrates (most PAHs are metabolized by P450 1A1), and often a particular chemical can be metabolized by multiple P450s (PAHs are also metabolized by P450 1B1). Additional information about P450s (inducibility, substrates, and inhibitors) has been reviewed (50). Human P450s responsible for the activation of a variety of carcinogens have been categorized (51) as follows: P450 1A1 metabolizes multi-ring PAHs; P450 1A2 metabolizes HAs; P450 3A4 metabolizes mycotoxins; and P450 2A6 metabolizes nitrosamines, single-ring PAHs, and chlorinated hydrocarbons.

Although P450 enzymes usually generate less toxic, hydroxylated species, they also form reactive intermediates, notably epoxides, such as the 7,8-epoxide of benzo[a]pyrene *(8,52–54)*. These epoxides are very reactive and spontaneously hydrolyze to the corresponding diols, in a reaction that is also catalyzed by the enzyme epoxide hydrolase. A second epoxidation of the 7,8-diol leads to the formation of the 7,8-diol-9,10-epoxide, which is the ultimate carcinogen of benzo[a]pyrene in part because it is not a good substrate for epoxide hydrolase. Mycotoxins (like aflatoxin B$_1$) are also activated to epoxides, which react directly with DNA *(23)*.

P450s activate carcinogens in other ways as well. For example, dimethylnitrosamine activation involves initial α-hydroxylation, which leads to demethylation (via loss of formaldehyde), and following several chemical rearrangements results in the formation of the methyl diazonium ion, which ultimately reacts with DNA *(55)*. In general, nitrosamines, which can be formed by the reaction of secondary amines with nitrite under acidic conditions (notably, in the stomach), are activated via α-hydroxylation *(55,56)*. Nitrosamines are found ubiquitously in the environment *(56)*, and are an interesting group of carcinogens because they cause tumors in a wide array of organs depending on the exact structure of the nitrosamine *(55,56)*. 4-(N-nitrosomethylamino)-1-(3-pyridyl)-1-butanone or NNK (Fig. 1) is of particular interest, because there is some evidence that it may be the most important carcinogen in cigarette smoke *(27)*.

A number of genes encoding P450 enzymes are inducible *(57)*, such as *CYP1A1* and *CYP1B1*, which metabolize PAHs. Induction involves the binding of the PAH (or other compounds such as TCDD or PCBs) to the cytosolic arylhydrocarbon receptor (AhR), which then dissociates from HSP90 and translocates to the nucleus, where it heterodimerizes with a protein called ARNT (arylhydrocarbon receptor nuclear translocator protein). This complex binds in enhancers of a battery of genes containing the xenobiotic-response elements (XREs: 5'-[T/G]nGCGTG-3') and activates the expression of these genes (like *CYP1A1*).

Phase II Metabolism of Xenobiotics

Phase II metabolism of carcinogens is also important *(8,52–54,58,59)*. Enzymes that participate in phase II metabolism of chemicals include glutathione-S-transferases (GSTs), UDP-glucuronosyltransferases (UGTs), sulfotransferases, and acetyltransferases (NATs).

Glutathione-S-transferases GSTs catalyze the attack of glutathione on a variety of xenobiotics. There are a large number of GST isozymes with broad substrate specificities. These enzymes are present in high concentrations in various subcellular fractions including the microsomes, the outer mitochondrial membrane, the nuclear membrane, and the cytosol. The broad substrate specificities and cellular localization of the GSTs make them the most versatile form of protection for cells against damaging electrophiles, such as carcinogenic epoxides. GST levels are highest in liver, but also are found in the intestines, adrenal gland, testes, and thymus. A variety of reviews have appeared on GSTs *(60–62)*.

UDP-glucuronosyltransferases UGTs are located in the endoplasmic reticulum and nuclear membrane of hepatocytes, and at lower levels in intestine, kidney, and olfactory epithelium. UGTs catalyze the conjugation of UDP-glucuronic acid to a variety of acceptor xenobiotic by nucleophilic attack at C1 of UDP-glucuronic acid displacing the UDP moiety. A number of reviews have appeared that discuss the structure, mechanism, biochemistry, and molecular biology of this class of enzymes *(63–65)*.

Sulfotransferases Sulfotransferases are typically cytosolic and form sulfate monoesters between substrates with hydroxyl groups and 3'-phosphoadenosine 5'-phosphosulfate (PAPS). These derivatives are less reactive, more water-soluble, avidly bound by plasma proteins, and ultimately excreted via the bile and urine. Recent reviews describe the sulfotransferase genes *(66)*, substrates and inhibitors *(67)*, and metabolism of a wide array of xenobiotics *(68,69)*.

Acetyltransferases NATs are hepatic cytosolic enzymes that catalyze N-acetyltransfers, O-acetyltransfers, and N,O-acetyltransfers from acetyl CoA to a variety of xenobiotics. Several reviews have appeared that discuss the enzymology and bioactivation of NATs *(70)*, including carcinogenicity of HAs *(71)*, and polymorphisms of human NAT genes *(72)*.

The Role of Phase II Enzymes in Toxification Reactions

In some cases phase II reactions are involved in toxification of chemicals. For example, ethylene dibromide (EDB) binds to DNA following the GST-catalyzed formation of an episulfonium ion between glutathione and the ethylene group *(73,74)*, and this conjugation is likely involved in the ability of this chemical to effect neoplastic transformation of cells. Likewise, the action of sulfotransferases and/or NATs on N-hydroxylated HAs can enhance carcinogenesis. Activation of HAs to species that react with DNA can be quite complicated, but initially involves P450-catalyzed N-hydroxylation to give a hydroxylamine, which can react with DNA directly, or which can be conjugated with an acyl or sulfate group by phase II enzymes to give species that also can react with DNA. HAs may be responsible for a variety of cancers, but are most clearly associated with bladder cancer, and the process by which HAs form adducts in the bladder is exceedingly complex *(75–80)*. HAs are N-oxidized in the liver and then converted to N-glucuronides, which are transported by circulation to the kidneys where they are excreted into the urinary bladder lumen. However, the lower pH of urine results in these relatively labile glucuronides hydrolyzing back to their aromatic hydroxylamines, which are then capable of forming DNA adducts in the bladder. In terms of human cancer, much attention has been focused on the HAs formed as pyrolysis products during cooking of meat and fish, such as 2-amino-1-methy-6-phenylimidazo[4,5-<u>b</u>]pyridine, 2-amino-3-methylimidazo[4,5-<u>f</u>]quinoline, and 2-amino-3,4-dimethylimidazo[4,5-<u>f</u>]quinoline (Table 1). These compounds are very likely to contribute to a variety of human cancers *(81–84)*.

Polymorphisms in the Genes Responsible for Xenobiotic Metabolism

It appears that humans can be differentially susceptible to carcinogenic insults depending on polymorphisms in a variety of these xenobiotic metabolizing enzymes. About 10% of Caucasians have a highly inducible form of *CYP1A1*, which is genetically linked to an isoleucine/Ævaline polymorphism that makes this P450 1A1 more active. One or both of these markers seem to increase PAH adduct formation resulting in an increased risk to lung cancer from smoking, with the effect being most dramatic in light smokers. PAHs are conjugated by GSTM1, which is deleted in ~50% of Caucasians, leading to an increased risk of smoking-related (and possibly other) lung and bladder cancers. HAs are acetylated by NAT2, which detoxifies them, and ~50% of Caucasians have a NAT2 that is relatively less active. These individuals are called slow acetylators, and this has been associated (although not universally so) with enhanced risk to bladder cancer. Finally, there are clear differences in xenobiotic metabolism based on race, age and gender, all of which may affect cancer outcome.

ADDUCTION

PAHs While the majority of the benzo[a]pyrene diol epoxide (Fig. 2) reacts with water to give the corresponding benzo[*a*]pyrene tetraol, a significant fraction can covalently react with DNA, which principally occurs at the N^2-position of the guanine base in DNA to give the adduct (+)-*trans-anti*-B[a]P-N^2-dG (Fig. 2) *(8,52–54,85)*. PAHs typically react with DNA following metabolic activation to epoxides and almost universally react at exocyclic nitrogen atoms, most extensively at N^2-dG and N^6-dA *(8,52–54,85)*. There is an interesting trend that has been noted in this regard; PAHs that show a relatively higher ratio of N^6-dA/N^2-dG adducts tend to be more potent carcinogens *(86)*.

Reactive PAH epoxides retain an aromatic region, and evidence suggests that this planar portion readily intercalates between the base pairs in DNA *(87)*. In fact, it has been argued that adduction at exocyclic amino groups in DNA (like N^2-dG) can only occur following carcinogen intercalation, since this is the only way for the electrophilic epoxide to gain access to the nucleophilic orbital of an exocyclic amino group, which is sp^2 hybridized, perpendicular to the plane of the dG and in conjugation with the rest of the aromatic system *(88)*.

Once adduction occurs, PAH adducts usually do not remain intercalated, but rather have a tendency to rearrange for reasons that have been discussed *(88)*. There is an enormous number of conformations that PAH adducts appear to be able to adopt in DNA, but they can be divided into four basic categories *(89)*. In the first category, the dG moiety of an N^2-dG adduct continues to base pair with its complementary cytosine, and the PAH moiety of the adduct lies in the minor groove, either pointing toward the base on the 5'-side or 3'-side of the adduct. A base-paired N^6-dA adduct has the PAH moiety in the major groove. In the second category, there are examples where the dG moiety of the adduct has undergone an anti/Æsyn base rotation, resulting in a Hoogsten base pair between the dG moiety of the adduct and its complementary base, and the PAH is then in the major groove. In the third category, the adducts are called base-displaced because the PAH moiety of the adduct stacks with the surrounding base pairs and the dG moiety is displaced into either the major or the minor groove. In the fourth category, PAH adducts continue to be intercalated after adduction (for instance with some N^6-dA adducts).

It is important to mention that there appears to be a second important pathway of PAH metabolism *(90–94)*. P450s also activate PAHs (like B[*a*]P) via one-electron oxidation, to give a radical cation that then reacts with DNA. In this case adduction appears to occur principally at N7-dG and N7-dA. These adducts are inherently unstable and evidence suggests they breakdown quickly with the loss of the DNA base, leaving the deoxyribose with no base attached, which is called an apurinic site. If unrepaired, apurinic sites are very mutagenic when bypassed by a DNA polymerase since there is no coding information. There is some evidence to suggest that the radical cation pathway may be very important to PAH carcinogenesis *(92)*.

HAs HAs (via *N*-hydroxylamines or their acetylated or sulfated derivatives) preferentially form adducts at C8-dG, although N2-dG, O6-dG, and C8-dA adducts may also form *(75,76)*. The best studied aromatic amine is 2-acetylaminofluorene, which predominantly forms C8-dG adducts (95% in cells, with 15% being acetylated and 80% deacetylated), the rest being formed at N^2-dG (5%) *(75)*. HAs are unique in their preference for reaction with a nonheteroatom (carbon) in DNA, which probably involves C8-dG attack on an electrophilic nitrenium ion to give a C-N adduct bond. There is some evidence for N7-attack at a carbon atom in the aromatic amine followed by rearrangement to C8-dG *(95)*. The interesting observation in this regard is that when the electrophilic site in the carcinogen is a carbon (for instance, the epoxides of PAHs such as B[a]P, Fig. 1), then the nucleophilic site in DNA is a heteroatom, but when the electrophilic site in the carcinogen is a heteroatom (nitrogen in the case of the nitrenium ions of various activated HAs) then the nucleophilic site in DNA is a carbon. Thus, there is a strong preference for carbon-heteroatom adduct bonds compared to carbon-carbon or heteroatom-heteroatom bonds. This reflects the well-known principle that covalent bonds are stronger between atoms of differing electronegativity. HAs probably also react with DNA following intercalation *(88)*. As with PAH adducts, once the adduct is formed, there are a myriad of possible conformations that can form, including the same four broad categories as described previously for the PAHs *(96)*. In addition, C8-dG adducts have a tendency to induce B/ÆZ-DNA conformational changes, at least in DNA sequences prone to Z-DNA formation (sequences with repetitive, alternating 5'-GC-3' base pairs) *(8,96,97)*.

Alkylating Agents Alkylating agents react at virtually all of the heteroatoms in DNA *(8)*. Although adducts at nitrogen atoms in DNA are quantitatively more important, adducts at oxygen, notably O^6-dG, O^4-dT, and O^2-dC, are most important for mutagenesis and carcinogenesis. In fact, the fraction of adduction at oxygen vs nitrogen atoms in DNA depends on the reactivity of the alkylating agent; highly reactive alkylating agents give a higher ratio of O/N adducts *(98)*. This has been rationalized as being due to a difference in reaction pathway; S_N1 for more reactive and S_N2 for less reactive agents *(99)*. However, a recent analysis suggests that all of these agents react with DNA via an S_N2 mechanism, and the explanation lies in a violation of the Swain-Scott principle, although the underlying reason for this is unclear *(98)*.

The adducts of alkylating agents do not show great conformational complexity, although there are two rotamers possible in the case of alk6G and alk4T adducts *(100)*. The *syn* and *anti* conformations have the alkyl group at O^6 pointing toward N1-

dG and N7-dG, respectively, and both conformations have been observed experimentally *(100)*. Although it is unclear what the biological consequences of each is, it is noteworthy that m6G exists in two states (probably conformations), one capable of blocking DNA polymerization in vitro while the other allows bypass *(101)*.

Aflatoxins Aflatoxins react principally at N7-dG *(102,103)*. This appears to be dictated by the fact that the coumerin ring of aflatoxins is flat and planar, and intercalates nicely into DNA orienting the epoxide of the AFB_1-oxide for reaction at N7-dG *(104)*. Unlike the PAHs and HAs, the intercalated conformation for AFB_1-N7-dG is not strained and dominates in duplex DNA *(105)*.

DNA REPAIR Cells have evolved elaborate systems to remove DNA adducts and restore the genetic integrity of their DNA. A complete review of this topic is beyond the scope of this chapter. A comprehensive treatment of this topic has appeared *(106)*, and a discussion of DNA repair in light of different kinds of DNA damage can be found in Chaney and Sancar *(107)*. Cells have developed a relatively small number of strategies to identify and repair DNA adducts, but there is considerable complexity within each of these strategies.

Nucleotide Excision Repair The NER apparatus consists of numerous proteins, and the basic strategy for repair involves nicking on both sides of the DNA damage in the same strand *(106)*. The resulting short oligonucleotide containing the lesion is displaced and the resulting single-stranded gap is resynthesized by a DNA polymerase. NER repairs a multitude of DNA lesions of varying structure, including those formed by PAHs, HAs, aflatoxins, UV light, and even less bulky, alkyl lesions. It remains to be elucidated how the NER complex is able to recognize such a broad spectrum of DNA damage, but it is generally assumed that the lesions either cause some kind of common deformation of DNA (such as a bend), or affect (decrease) the stability of the DNA duplex, which is then detected by the NER apparatus. The mechanisms for NER in yeast and mice are fairly well-understood *(106,109)*. Nonetheless, this discussion will be limited to NER in *Escherichia coli* and human cells.

NER in *E. coli (106)* begins with the binding to DNA of two subunits of UvrA, followed by one subunit of UvrB, and this $UvrA_2B$ complex, which has helicase activity, scans DNA for lesions. Once a lesion is encountered, UvrA dissociates and the endonuclease UvrC binds and nicks ~7–8 nucleotides and ~3–4 nucleotides on the 5'-side and 3'-side of the lesion, respectively. Thereafter, UvrB/C dissociates, and the lesion-containing oligonucleotide (~12-mer) is displaced by the action of UvrD (a helicase), and DNA polymerase I resynthesizes the DNA to fill the short gap.

NER in human cells *(106,108,109)* requires the factors, XPA, RPA, XPC, TFIIH, XPG, and ERCC1-XPF. XPA and RPA together bind to damaged DNA, a process that requires ATP hydrolysis. The XP designation associated with many of these names is derived from a genetic disease called xeroderma pigmentosum (XP), which results from defects in different aspects of NER. XPA is a 30 kDa protein monomer. Replication protein A (RPA) is a heterotrimer single-strand binding protein, first isolated as being required for DNA replication in

vitro, that consists of Rpa1 (70 kDa), Rpa2 (34 kDa), and Rpa 3 (13 kDa). TFIIH is part of the basal-transcription apparatus, and is made up of CAK (cyclin activating kinase) and TFIIH-core. NER requires TFIIH-core, which includes the XPB and XPD helicases, as well as p62, p52, p44, and p34. XPG and ERCC1-XPF are structure-specific DNA nucleases that cleave on the 3'-side (2–9 nucleotides from the lesion) and 5'-side (16–25 nucleotides from the lesion), which liberates a damage-containing oligonucleotide that is 26–27 nucleotides long. The precise role for XPC (which associates with HHR23B) is unknown, and with some lesions it appears to be dispensable. NER may also require XPE, which is a heterodimer composed of 38 kDa and 128 kDa protein subunits. DNA polymerases δ and ε holoenzymes resynthesize DNA *(110)*, and repair is completed following the action of a DNA ligase. Additional factors may be involved in NER, such as IF7, CAF-1 (a chromatin assembly factor), and even the p53 tumor-suppressor protein. Recently, it has been shown that the human mismatch repair proteins, hMSH2 and hMSH6, can bind to certain kinds of DNA damage that are known to be repaired by NER *(108)*. However, these proteins do not seem to affect the ability of the human NER complex to function in vitro. The significance of this observation remains unclear.

Transcription Coupled Repair RNA polymerases are blocked by DNA damage, and this can trigger a special kind of DNA repair for lesions in the transcribed strand called transcription coupled repair (TCR) *(111,112)*. TCR is needed both because a blocked RNA polymerase hides DNA damage from repair, and because concentrating repair on the transcribed strand insures that essential transcription resumes in cells as quickly as possible. In human cells, TCR appears to require CS-A (44 kDa) and CS-B (168 kDa), which may in fact be the coupling factors, although this has not been established definitively *(112)*. The CS designation is derived from another genetic disease called Cockayne Syndrome. *E. coli* also has TCR and the coupling factor is the Mfd protein *(112)*. It has also been shown that mismatch repair (MMR) proteins are involved in TCR in *E. coli* and human cells *(112)*, although their exact role is not clear.

Base Excision Repair Relevant to chemically damaged DNA, base excision repair (BER) mechanisms function to repair a number of lesions formed by alkylating agents, notably, those at 3A, 3G, 2C, and 2T *(106,108,110,113–116)*. BER is more extensively involved in the repair of lesions that arise via several spontaneous hydrolytic reactions of DNA (depurination, and deamination of cytosine and m5C), and lesions formed when DNA is damaged by oxidizing agents. BER involves lesion recognition by a DNA glycosylase, which breaks the glycosylic bond leaving an apurinic or apyrimidinic site in DNA, which is subsequently removed by the endonucleolytic action of an AP endonuclease on the 5'-side (exonuclease III or endonuclease IV in *E. coli* and APE in human cells), and a DNA deoxyribophosphodiesterase (dRpase) on the 3'-side (RecJ in *E. coli* and DNA polymerase β in human cells). This leaves a one-base gap, which is filled in by a DNA polymerase (DNA polymerase I in *E. coli* and DNA polymerase β in human cells) and the nick is sealed by a DNA ligase (*E. coli* DNA ligase and the DNA ligase III/XRCC1 heterodimer in humans). BER can also be coupled to transcription *(112)*.

There are a multitude of DNA glycosylases, which can either have a fairly selective substrate specificity (for instance the Tag protein removes principally 3-methyladenine in *E. coli*) or have a broad substrate specificity (the AlkA protein in *E. coli* has the largest substrate specificity, and removes most alkylated purines and pyrimidines with positive charges or weakened glycosylic bonds) *(113)*. Evidence suggests that glycosylases flip the altered base out of the DNA helix into the enzyme active site where hydrolysis of the glycosylic bond of the damaged base occurs *(115,116)*.

Recently, a second BER pathway has been found in human cells that differs in that ~7 nucleotides are removed *(114)*. This BER pathway requires FEN1, and may itself have several variations (such as a PCNA-stimulated polymerase β-directed pathway, and a PCNA-dependent, polymerase δ/ε-directed pathway).

Alkylguanine Alkyltranferases Alkylguanine alkyltranferases are responsible for the repair of the alkylation lesions most relevant to mutagenesis and carcinogenesis, alk6G *(106)*. *E. coli* has two such proteins (termed Ada and Ogt), whereas human cells seem to have only one (MGT). Repair involves S_N2 attack of the thiolate of an active-site cysteine on the alkyl group, which directly reverses the adduction step and restores the integrity of the base in DNA. Ada also repairs alk4T and some phosphotriesters, although human MGT does not. Interestingly, the alkyl group is irreversibly bound to the active site thiol, and, thus, each protein is only able to repair one lesion per active site *(106)*.

In *E. coli*, alkylated Ada serves a second role in that it binds to Ada boxes upstream of several genes involved in the repair of alkyl DNA damage (notably, Ada itself and 3-methyladenine DNA glycosylase II), and acts as an inducer of their gene expression *(106)*. This is called the adaptive response and serves to protect *E. coli* from both the toxic and mutagenic effects of alkylating agents.

Damage Avoidance DNA Repair Pathways In addition to pathways that repair DNA damage, cells have a variety of mechanisms for avoiding the detrimental effects of DNA damage without actually removing the damage. These damage avoidance pathways involve either recombination or DNA polymerase bypass of lesions.

Recombinational Repair Two pathways of homologous recombination can be involved in DNA repair as exemplified by the RecF pathway and the RecBCD pathway in *E. coli*. Much is known about recombinational repair in yeast as well *(106,117,118)*.

The RecF pathway is initiated by single-stranded gaps in DNA (ssDNA), particularly, those that are formed when a DNA polymerase is blocked by a lesion *(106)*. In the current model, single-strand binding protein (SSB) coats this ssDNA, and then a complex involving RecF, RecO, and RecR removes SSB and allows RecA to bind to ssDNA *(119)*. RecA is the protein that does homology searches and performs the actual cross-over event during recombinational repair and recombination. RecA catalyzes the filling of the gap from a lesion-free, homologous sister chromosome. The gap created on the sister chromosome

is filled in by a DNA polymerase. The RecF pathway also requires RecJ, RecN, and RecQ, whose exact functions are unknown.

The RecBCD pathway *(120)* is initiated by dsbs in DNA, which result from various insults to the genome, including ionizing radiation. The RecBCD complex binds a double-stranded DNA (dsDNA) end and degrades one strand in a 3'→5' direction through the nuclease function of RecD. Degradation continues until a χ-site (5'-GCTGGTGG-3') is encountered, whereupon RecD is released and DNA degradation stops. RecBC continues in the 3'→5' direction acting as a helicase, and the 3'-end generated is used by RecA to initiate recombination.

RecA does homology searches by coating DNA and creating a fibrous network in which the searching occurs *(106)*. RecA has three binding sites, each for one strand of DNA, and each monomer covers approx three bases on each strand, respectively. When RecA finds homology, it creates a Holliday junction, which is the name for the three-stranded or four-stranded cross-over structure. After RecA creates a Holliday junction, RuvA and RuvB bind and translate the Holliday junction in order to increase the size of the heteroduplex region of DNA *(121–123)*. *E. coli* expresses another protein (RecG) that performs this function. Finally, the Holliday junction is resolved back to two duplexes by the nucleolytic action of the RuvC protein *(124)*.

Lesion–Bypass DNA Polymerases The RecF pathway is initiated by the presence of single-stranded gaps in DNA that result from the DNA polymerase becoming stalled at sites of DNA damage. In some cases bypass by recombinational repair is impossible, such as when the homologous chromosome cannot donate DNA because it also contains DNA damage. In these cases, a newly recognized class of so-called "lesion-bypass DNA polymerases" are required to bypass the DNA damage *259–261)*. *E. Coli* has at least three lesion-bypass DNA polymerases: DNA polymerases II *(polB)*, IV *(dinB)* and V *(umuD/C)*, and it is likely that each has a different bypass specificity. They are inducible as part of the SOS response to DNA damage *(106)*. The UVM pathway (associated with bypass of exocyclic adducts) is also DNA damage inducible, but in an SOS-independent fashion *(125,126)*. Human cells have at least four lesion bypas DNA polymerases zeta, eta, DinB1 (or kappa or theta), and iota *(259–261)*. (Note: new DNA polymerases are emerging so quickly that there is confusion over their naming.) Humans with the genetic disease xeroderma pigmentosum in complementation group V (for "variant") are skin cancer-prone when exposed to UV light, because they have a mutation in the hRAD30 gene, which encodes DNA polymerase eta. Eta has been shown to bypass thymine dimers (the major UV lesion) relatively accurately *(262)*. These (and other) results suggest that eta is the lesion-bypass DNA polymerase responsible for bypassing UV damage and minimizing mutagenesis. DNA insertases can also be involved in mutagenesis, the best understood being yeast REV1 and its human counterpart hREV1 *(263)*.

Double-Strand Break Repair Although *E. coli* principally repairs dbs by homologous recombination (via the RecBCD pathway), higher eukaryotes (notably, rodents and humans) seem to repair them principally via a nonhomologous, end-joining process, which is called dsb repair (108). Although this process has been best studied in the case of ionizing radiation-induced dbs, it probably is important in the case of all DNA-damaging agents. A number of excellent reviews describing different aspects of dsb repair have appeared (128–133), including dsb in yeast (134). Dsb repair is initiated by DNA-dependent protein kinase (DNA-PK). DNA-PK is a complex comprised of a regulatory complex called Ku (a heterodimer of 70 kDa and 86 kDa protein subunits) that binds to DNA ends and recruits DNA-PKcs, which is the massive, catalytic subunit (460 kDa). DNA-PK is also involved in the rejoining step in V(D)J recombination associated with antibody diversity. DNA-PK probably initiates end-joining by bringing double-stranded ends together and then mediates subsequent steps by phosphorylating other dsb repair proteins.

At least five other proteins are likely to be involved in dsb repair, including hMre11 and hRAD50 (135,136), which were identified based on homology with their yeast counterpart (137). hMre11 (81 kDa) and hRAD50 (153 kDa) are part of a large complex (~2,000 kDa) that includes at least three other proteins (of ~350 kDa, 200 kDa, and 95 kDa). This complex appears to be assembled in large nuclear foci (136). Although the function of this complex is unknown, hMre11 is homologous to known ATP-dependent double-stranded exonucleases and hRAD50 shows some homology to myosin, suggesting a possible role as part of a contractile system.

Recently, it has been recognized that not all cells exposed to DNA-damaging agents (like alkylating agents and ionizing radiation) respond similarly (138,139). In fact, a subpopulation of cells appear to acquire a persistent global genomic instability, a property that is more typically associated with tumor cells (140,141). The features of this instability include increased spontaneous mutagenesis (142) and chromosomal rearrangements that are continuously evolving (143–145). This state persists for many generations after the initial exposure to DNA damaging agents, and is unlikely to be due to residual DNA damage. This genomic instability is likely to be due to a persistent genetic or epigenetic change (such as in the regulation at cell-cycle check points) that increases the incidence or tolerance for chromosomal breakage and reunion events. Although the underlying mechanism is unknown, it seems sensible to imagine that this state has something to do with the cellular loss or misregulation of its dsb repair apparatus.

DNA DAMAGE LEADING TO CELL-CYCLE ARREST AND APOPTOSIS In addition to repairing DNA damage, eukaryotic cells try to avoid the adverse affects of damage by at least two other mechanisms, cell-cycle arrest and apoptosis.

Cell-Cycle Arrest To avoid the adverse effects of DNA damage, cells appear to have mechanisms by which they assess the integrity of their genome, and delay both the onset of DNA synthesis, as well as chromosomal segregation, if their DNA is significantly damaged. It is thought that this permits the cell more time to conduct DNA repair to remove the deleterious damage.

Actively dividing cells go through four phases in their cell cycle, G_1 (gap 1), S (DNA synthesis), G_2 (gap 2), and M (mitosis). Quiescent cells are in a different phase called G_0. Cells become committed to traverse from G_1 to S at a point called the G_1/S checkpoint, which is very close temporally to the onset of DNA synthesis (146). There has been considerable interest in knowing exactly how the onset of DNA synthesis is controlled at the G_1/S checkpoint, how DNA damage is detected, and how this damage alters the normal signaling pathway (147,148).

Proteins called cyclins are the master switches that control progression of the cell through the phases of the cell cycle. Each cyclin is transcribed for a brief crucial period during the cell cycle (following mitogen stimulation). However, they and their mRNAs are very labile, which results in a transient spike of protein activity. Increases in the levels of cyclin D family members (D1-D3) lead to binding to and activation of cyclin-dependent kinases (cdk4 and/or cdk6) (149). In this complex the cdk phosphorylates the retinoblastoma protein family (pRb, p107 and p130), which is in a complex with E2F family members (E2F1-E2F5) (150–152). This releases E2F and it binds DP family members (DP1-DP4), which leads to the activation of two other cyclin/cdk complexes, cyclin E/cdk2 (and/or cdk4) and cyclin A/cdk2. This triggers the onset of S phase (153–155).

Transcription factor p53 clearly can play a key role in the control of cell-cycle arrest prior to DNA synthesis in response to DNA damage. p53 has been comprehensively reviewed (156). Most studies on the blocking of entry into S-phase by DNA damage have been done with UV and ionizing radiation, which leads to increased levels of p53. p53 levels are normally quite low due to its extreme lability ($t_{1/2}$ ~20 min). DNA damage increases both the $t_{1/2}$ of p53 protein and translational efficiency of p53 mRNA by poorly understood mechanisms, although the ATM (ataxia telangiectasia) gene product may play a role in this control with some types of DNA damage, such as X-rays. p53 enhances the expression of a number of genes, notably the cdk-inhibitor family (including, $p15^{INK4B}$, $p16^{INK4A}$, $p18^{INK4C}$, $p19^{INK4D}$, $p21^{WAF1/CIP1}$, $p27^{KIP1}$, and $p57^{KIP2}$) as well as GADD45 (directly involved in DNA repair), mdm2 (autoregulator of p53 levels), and bax. Importantly, $p21^{WAF1/CIP1}$ and PCNA interact with a number of cyclin/CDK complexes (like cyclin D1/cdk4, cyclin E/cdk2, and cyclin A/cdk2). It appears that one molecule of $p21^{WAF1/CIP1}$ in this complex is required for cdk kinase activity, but two molecules of $p21^{WAF1/CIP1}$ inhibit the kinase function of the complex. Formation of a complex between PCNA and $p21^{WAF1/CIP1}$ results in the inhibition of PCNA function in DNA replication, although its role in DNA repair is unaffected.

Emerging evidence suggests that arrest of the cell cycle by chemical carcinogen-induced DNA damage may be fundamentally different than arrest induced by radiation. Although B[a]P treatment appears to increase p53 levels, including in cells in vivo (157), in some cases this does not lead to an increase in p21 levels (158). In addition, there is one study indicating that p53 is not required for B[a]P-induced G_1/S arrest (159), which implies that different kinds of DNA damage may signal the cell cycle by different mechanisms.

Apoptosis Apoptosis is a physiological and pathological process of cell deletion that functions as an essential mechanism to maintain normal tissue stasis, and operates during development when a cell type must be eliminated. However, apoptosis also occurs when cells are exposed to excessive genotoxic and nongenotoxic insults. A number of reviews of various aspects of apoptosis have appeared *(160–169)*.

At the cellular level, apoptosis is a regulated, orderly process; it was first described in 1972 by Kerr, Wylie, and Currie *(170)*, that includes cytoplasmic vacuolization, plasma-membrane blebbing, chromatin condensation, and fragmentation of nuclear DNA. Cleavage of nuclear DNA occurs between the nucleosomes to yield a characteristic ladder that is readily detectable when DNA from cells undergoing apoptosis is separated in an agarose gel. Eventually, the apoptotic cell is engulfed and degraded by phagocytic macrophages.

Apoptosis can be induced in many ways. The best-studied physiological signals are Fas ligand and tumor necrosis factor (TNF) *(161,162,166,167)*. It is clear that the generation of reactive oxygen species (ROS) can initiate apoptosis, although the actual trigger could be DNA damage, protein damage, and/or direct oxidation of fatty-acid peroxides *(161,166,169,171)*. Chemical agents that damage DNA also induce apoptosis, although it is unclear exactly how *(161,165,166,169)*.

Many studies of apoptosis have focused on the bcl2 family of proteins (homologous to the *Caenhorhabditis elegans* Ced-9 protein), of which bcl2, bcl_{xL}, bcl_w, and mcl1 appear to inhibit apoptosis, whereas bax, bik, bak, bad, and bcl_{xs} appear to activate apoptosis *(167,168)*. Most of these family members can form homodimers and heterodimers, and the ratio of specific dimers determines whether or not a cell will undergo apoptosis. The only structural information available about these proteins is for bcl_{xL}, which resembles pore-forming bacteria toxins (such as colicons and diptheria toxin) *(172)*, suggesting that it probably is involved in transport *(162,173)*.

Bcl2 family members are located in the outer mitochondrial membrane, the endoplasmic reticulum, and the nuclear envelope. It appears that when bcl2 (or a family member) receives an apoptotic signal, it causes a change or discontinuity of the outer mitochondrial membrane (or perhaps a change in ion flux or potential) *(174)*, and this leads cytochrome C to become redistributed from the mitochondria to the cytosol *(160)*. Once in the cytosol, cytochrome C appears to activate one or a number of cysteine-containing, aspartate-specific proteases, called caspases *(160,162,163,168,175)*. Caspase activation appears to require proteins in addition to cytochrome C, which itself does not have to be redox-active *(176,177)*. There are a large number of cytosolic caspases, which are activated during apoptosis, and there may be a caspase (protease) cascade *(160,162,163,168,175)*. Considerable attention has been focused on caspase-3 (also called, CPP32, Tama, apopain, and CED-3), which recognizes and cleaves proteins at DXXD sequences *(160,162,163,168,175)*. Caspase-3 can be activated by a variety of lethal stimuli, and it cleaves a variety of substrates, such as lamin B, which unpins the nuclear envelope, as well as gelosin, actin, and intermediate filaments. These cleavages probably result in the changes in cell shapes and movement associated with apoptosis.

The crucial apoptotic DNA nuclease has been identified *(164)*, and is called CAD (caspase-activated DNase). CAD forms a heterodimer with ICAD, which is a strongly acidic protein that stabilizes and inhibits CAD. CAD becomes active when caspase-3 cleaves ICAD. Caspase-3 also cleaves DNA-PK, which is involved in dbs repair, and this is likely to insure that CAD cleavages of DNA are not reversed. Finally, caspase-3 cleaves poly(ADP-ribose) polymerase, which probably inhibits other aspects of DNA repair that might interfere with apoptotic-related DNA damage.

p53 also plays a role in apoptosis *(156,165–167,171,178)*. Although the details are not clear, DNA damage leads to increased levels of p53, which enhances the expression of a number of genes, notably bax in the context of apoptosis. The increase in bax levels shifts the equilibrium toward bax/bcl2 heterodimers, which inhibits the anti-apoptotic activity of bcl2. Increased p53 expression also leads to activation of IGF-BP3, which is thought to have a pro-apoptotic effect. It is clear that this process is complex and involves a number of other proteins with which p53 interacts directly *(178)* and indirectly *(179)*.

MUTAGENESIS If a chemical-carcinogen adduct is not repaired, then a DNA polymerase may attempt to read past this adduct (for instance (+)-*trans-anti*-B[a]P-N^2-dG; Fig. 2), in which case it has a much greater chance of incorporating the wrong base. For example, dA is frequently inserted opposite dG adducts of bulky carcinogens, which will result in a GCÆTA mutation when dT is incorporated opposite this dA in the next round of replication *(180)*.

There are three general types of mutations: 1) a base substitution involves the exchange of one base pair for another, for instance GCÆTA; 2) a deletion or insertion involves the loss or gain, respectively, of one or more base pairs from a DNA sequence; 3) frameshift mutations are simply the insertion or deletion of (3n + 1) or (3n + 2) base pairs in the coding region of a gene.

Several terms are often used in mutagenesis. Regarding quantitative effects, mutations are never randomly distributed, an effect that has led to the term mutational hotspot, which refers to sites where more mutations are found than would be expected based on a random distribution. Although the cutoff for a mutational hotspot is somewhat arbitrary and must be evaluated statistically, sites with more than 5–15% of the total mutations are usually considered hotspots. A mutational hotspot can be caused by: 1) a hotspot for adduction; 2) a coldspot for DNA repair; and/or 3) a hotspot during mutagenic processing, notably during replicative bypass of lesions. Regarding qualitative effects, two terms are sometimes used. Mutagenic specificity refers to the quantitative amount of mutations found in each of the different categories of mutations; for instance, GCÆAT (15%), GCÆTA (10%), and so on. Mutagenesis results are also often presented pictorially with each base pair in a mutational target sequence of DNA presented horizontally and with the number of mutations at each site indicated vertically; this presentation is called a mutational spectrum *(181)*.

Considerable effort has been devoted to trying to understand what kinds of mutations chemical carcinogens cause and why. Perhaps one of the most remarkable findings is that in broad outline the mutagenic specificity of a particular agent is remarkably similar in cells as disparate as *E. coli* and human. In fact, DNA-repair strategies and mechanisms are often very similar as well. This probably reflects the fact that the same adducts are generated in DNA from a particular mutagen, and, thus, all cells face similar problems.

PAHs While potent, bulky mutagens are identified with a propensity to induce GCÆTA mutations, the PAHs (such as (+)-*anti*-B[a]PDE) also induce a significant fraction of GCÆAT and GCÆCG mutations as well *(182–188)*. In certain cell systems, especially with certain PAHs that form a significant fraction of dA adducts, ATÆTA mutations are also prevalent, as well as ATÆGC and ATÆCG mutations, as best demonstrated in a fine study of four enantiomers of the diol epoxides of benzo[c]phenanthrene *(188)*. PAHs are also able to induce a large fraction of insertions and deletions *(182–188)*. One remarkable finding was obtained when (+)-*anti*-B[a]PDE mutagenesis was studied in the HPRT gene of V-79 cells. In this study, the fraction of mutations at GC (vs AT) base pairs increased in a dose-dependent manner *(184–187)*. Recent work suggests that this effect dissipates in NER-deficient cells *(189)*, perhaps reflecting a lower affinity for adenine adducts by NER complexes. This result shows that, although our earlier statement that mutagenesis is remarkably similar in all types of cells is generally true, there are numerous nuances and subtleties.

The mechanism(s) by which PAHs are able to induce such a broad spectrum of mutations is just beginning to emerge. This effort has been problematic because when a particular carcinogen reacts with DNA, it usually forms adducts at many sites on the DNA bases, which has made it difficult to know what mutation is associated with what adduct and why. This problem was overcome by the development of techniques called site-directed, site-specific, or adduct site-specific mutagenesis, which has permitted the study of mutagenesis by individual DNA adducts *(190–191)*. Adduct site-specific mutagenesis involves the synthesis of an oligonucleotide that contains an adduct of known structure at a defined position, and the use of recombinant DNA techniques to incorporate this modified oliogonucleotide into an autonomously replicating plasmid-based or viral-based vector. This vector can be studied in vitro or placed in cells, where biological processing occurs, the nature of which can be deduced from an analysis of the progeny vectors.

A variety of studies have shown that mutations induced by (+)-*anti*-B[a]PDE are principally due to its major adduct [+ta]-B[a]P-N²-dG, which has been shown to be fully capable of inducing GÆT, GÆA, and GÆC mutations *(192–196)*. This fact raises the question: how can a single adduct induce different kinds of mutations? The most reasonable hypothesis is that an adduct can adopt multiple conformations in DNA, and that each of these conformations can induce a different type of mutation. In fact, there is also evidence for there being relatively nonmutagenic conformations of carcinogen DNA adducts *(183,196)*. In addition, conformation (and mutagenesis) can be influenced by factors, such as the DNA sequence context surrounding the adduct. For example, [+ta]-B[a]P-N²-dG induces principally (~95%) GÆT mutations in a 5'-T<u>G</u>C-3' sequence context *(192)*, but principally (~80%) GÆA mutations in a 5'-C<u>G</u>T-3' sequence context *(194)*. Although it is unknown currently which conformation is responsible for which mutation (and why), my laboratory has recently generated a hypothesis that a particular base-displaced conformation with the guanine moiety of the adduct in the major groove induces GÆT mutations, whereas a particular base displaced conformation with the adduct in the minor groove induces GÆA mutations. This notion is a hypothesis and not a conclusion, but it gives a sense of the horizons for this area of research.

HAs Carcinogenic HAs are also able to induce a varied spectra of mutations. One frequently noted observation is that activated 2-aminofluorene (2-AF) induces principally base-substitution mutations (GCÆTA), while 2-acetylaminofluorene (2-AAF) induces primarily -1 and -2 deletions. A review of this topic has appeared recently *(97)*. The major 2-AF adduct (AF-C8-dG) was shown to induce GÆT mutations (which correlates with what was observed for 2-AF), although this has only been studied in a single DNA sequence context *(197,198)*. Activated 2-AAF induces -2 frameshifts in so-called Nar I sequences (5'-G₁G₂CG₃CC-3') *(97)*. Fuchs and coworkers have shown that these mutations are the result of efficient mutagenesis during replication of 2-AAF-C8-dG situated at G₃ position, but not G₁ or G₂ positions *(199)*, and have nothing to do with G₃ position being a hotspot for adduction *(197)* or a coldspot for DNA repair *(200,201)*. This work is probably the most definitive on this subject, and serves as a model for how the question of hotspot mutagenesis should be investigated.

Some very interesting studies have been done on -1 frameshift mutations induced by 2-AAF-C8-dG in runs of three or four consecutive G:C base pairs *(202,203)*. The mutation frequency increased dramatically as the adduct was moved from the 5'-most to the 3'-most dG in the run. A Streisinger slippage-type event in the lesion-containing strand is envisioned and it appears that the correct base must have been incorporated opposite the lesion (that is at the dCMP opposite 2-AAF-C8-dG) prior to the slippage event in the mutagenic pathway.

Unrepaired lesions in DNA can either be bypassed by a DNA polymerase, which Fuchs and Colleagues termed trans-lesion synthesis (TLS) or subjected to damage-avoidance mechanisms, notably, recombinational repair. Fuchs finds that TLS is <1% with AAF-C8-dG, which increases to ~13% following SOS induction, whereas it is ~70% (and unaffected by SOS induction) for AF-C8-dG *(204)*. Interestingly, although SOS induction leads to enhanced TLS, the fraction of mutational events per TLS is SOS-independent.

Alkylating Agents As mentioned earlier, alkylating agents form adducts at many sites in DNA. It appears that adducts at a number of sites (7G and triesters) are not very mutagenic *(8,205)*. All evidence suggests that GCÆAT mutations, which predominate in most cases, are induced by alk6G *(190)*. The mechanism for this is unclear, but probably involves the formation of an alk6G:T mispair when the alkyl group is in a particular conformation (*anti*) that permits pairing with dT. Interestingly, both the *anti* and *syn* conformations of the alkyl group at 6G are similar in energy *(100)*, and each may be processed differently by a DNA polymerase *(101)*.

Current evidence indicates that ATÆGC mutations are induced by alk4T adducts *(190)*, which shares many structural similarities (and probably mutagenic mechanism) with alk6G lesions. The fraction of ATÆTA mutations frequently increases when the size of the alkyl group increases from methyl to ethyl, which correlates with an increased relative fraction of alkyl adduct formation at 2T, and ethyl-2T has been shown to be paired with dT by several purified DNA polymerases *(206)*, suggesting that ethyl-2T is likely to be the lesion responsible for AT$\rightarrow$TA mutations induced by ethylating agents.

Aflatoxin B1 AFB$_1$ is generally regarded to induce a preponderance of G$\rightarrow$T mutations, although in certain cases it has been shown to induce a significant fraction of G$\rightarrow$A mutations as well *(180)*. AFB$_1$-N7-dG has a somewhat unstable glycosylic bond, whose breakage leads to the formation of AP sites, which are known to be highly mutagenic *(207,208)*. An adduct site-specific study has shown that AFB$_1$-N7-dG is directly capable of inducing G$\rightarrow$T mutations, and that an AP site is not an obligate intermediate in its mutagenesis *(209)*, although this still leaves open the question as to whether this adduct or an AP site is responsible for mutagenesis in circumstances when the adduct is not replicated immediately.

DNA Polymerase No discussion of mutagenesis would be complete without some information about DNA polymerase mechanism, because most mutagenic events occur when a carcinogen-DNA adduct is encountered by a DNA polymerase. Although polymerase bypass of carcinogen adducts has been studied *(191)*, virtually nothing is known about the details of the mechanism. In contrast, some detailed information is emerging about how a DNA polymerase incorporates a correct base during replication. The following discussion is based on a recent evaluation *(210)* of what is known in this regard.

The best-understood polymerase is probably human DNA polymeraseβ, which is involved in BER. It appears that the single strand–double strand junction of a primer/template is severely kinked ($\sim$90∞), because the next base to be copied is initially complexed with a histidine (His34) that keeps it from being in a position to base pair with an incoming dNTP. Subsequently, a conformational change occurs during translocation and prior to polymerization with the C-terminal domain moving dramatically to generate an active site poised for catalysis. Critically, this movement allows Arg283 to interact with either the O^2-position of a pyrimidine or the N3-position of a purine in the template strand (these hydrogen-bond acceptor sites are in the same position in the minor groove of DNA). This leads to the formation of a pocket that tightly accommodates a canonical Watson-Crick base pair, but would not accommodate an incorrect base pair. Evidence suggests that polymerase fidelity depends critically on the geometric shape of the base pair in the active site, which includes more than just hydrogen bonding. It is unknown whether the steps outlinedearlier for DNA polymerase β are fundamentally similar for true replicative polymerases as well, although recent evidence suggests that coliphage T7 DNA polymerase has a fundamentally similar mechanism *(210)*.

TUMORIGENESIS

In most cases, cells in an organism are in a state of stasis, and new cells are only produced (by cell division) to replace old cells that have been discarded for one reason or another. There are numerous cases when this is not completely true, notably, during development. Cell division is tightly regulated and is overseen by the protein products of a set of growth-control genes. If these genes become mutated, then the cell loses the

checks and balances necessary to insure that it only divides when appropriate. Normal cells have so-called tumor-suppressor genes, which permit cell division to occur only when a cell receives a proper growth signal (to repair damaged tissue). The loss of a tumor-suppressor gene by mutation may contribute to uncontrolled cell growth (cancer). A second class of genes called proto-oncogenes are active in the signaling pathways for cell growth; if these genes are mutated to their oncogenic form, then they can potentially send their signals to grow continually rather than only when it is proper *(211)*.

The best-understood tumor-suppressor gene and proto-oncogene are *p53* and c-*ras*, respectively, and each has been found to be mutated in $\sim$ 50% *(41,42,156)* and $\sim$20% *(211)* of all human tumors, respectively. Human tumors are also associated with mutations in genes that encode proteins involved in DNA repair.

Mutations in *p53* are so prevalent in human cancer that a large number have been sequenced from a variety of human tumors. This has lead to the development of a data base that is managed by the IARC *(42)*, and can be accessed through the IARC's website at www.iarc.fr by pursuing the IARC *p53* Database. Mutations in *p53* and *APC* associated with human colon tumors are principally GC$\rightarrow$AT mutations in 5'-CG-3' sequences, which are known to be modified to contain 5-methylcytosine *(40–42,212,213)*. Although the detailed pathway of mutagenesis has not been determined for these tumors, it has the hallmarks of the pathway that begins with the spontaneous deamination of 5-methylcytosine to T, which was first described in *E. coli* approx 20 yr ago *(214,215)*, and is a hotspot for spontaneous mutagenesis in *E. coli (214–217)*. In certain kinds of skin cancer, GC$\rightarrow$AT mutations predominate in 5'-PyC-3' sequences *(218–221)*, which is exactly what is expected based on studies of UV-light mutagenesis, as observed in cells from *E. coli* to human *(218–225)*.

Liver cancer is high in certain human populations exposed to aflatoxins, and a very high fraction of these tumors contain G$\rightarrow$T mutations in codon 249 (A<u>G</u>G) of p53 *(40–42)*. The specificity for this single codon is remarkable. Although the G$\rightarrow$T mutation is certainly consistent with what is commonly believed to be the mutagenic specificity for AFB$_1$, it may be more apparent than real, because a G$\rightarrow$A mutation at this wobble position is phenotypically silent and would not have been detected *(180)*.

In the case of lung cancer, which is mostly attributable to cigarette smoking, G$\rightarrow$T mutations predominate and hotspots are found at a number of sites, notably three 5'-CG-3' sites *(41,42)*. Recently, it was shown that (+)-*anti*-B[a]PDE preferentially reacts and is also repaired more slowly at these same three CpGs *(226,227)*, raising the intriguing possibility that in fact B[a]P itself, which is known to be one of the major PAHs in cigarette smoke *(27)*, may be responsible for mutations induced by cigarette smoking. There are a number of caveats that must be mentioned in this regard. For example, if the comparisons between (+)-*anti*-B[a]PDE reactivity hotspots and *p53* mutational hotspots are expanded beyond these three CpG sites, then in a number of cases the correlation does not hold. Although this raises some doubts, it does not rule out (+)-*anti*-

B[a]PDE as the causative agent, because other factors (differential adduct repair or mutagenesis during adduct bypass) may occur in the sites that do not correlate. A second caveat is that other agents may also show a preference for reaction at the three 5-methylcytosine-containing 5'-CG-3' sites. To underscore the latter concern, it has also been noted that the pattern of mutations in p53 from human breast tumors also correlates with (+)-anti-B[a]PDE reactivity hotspots (227). However, there is some evidence that smoking-related breast cancer may correlate with the slow acetylator polymorphism, which is more consistent with the involvement of HAs (228).

METALS AND ASBESTOS

The effects of metals on biological systems, including effects on the processes involved with carcinogenesis, are vexing on at least three levels (229). First, while a variety of metals can be toxic, they are often also essential for life. For example, dietary chromium is required for insulin secretion, and glucose and fat metabolism, but it is also carcinogenic. Iron is important in countless biochemical processes, and yet is also a catalyst that generates the hydroxyl radical, which is thought to be the major ROS that damages DNA. Selenium can protect cells against oxidative damage, which is beneficial, and yet selenium may also pose a cancer risk. Second, metal carcinogenesis is also complicated by the fact that metals can shuttle between various redox states, each with a different biological effect; this can be further modulated (and confused) by the nature of the ligands. Third, metals can affect DNA and its replication in a myriad of ways. Metals can bind directly to DNA to give adducts, can bind to DNA polymerases or repair proteins and adversely affect their action, and/or they can participate in redox reactions that can lead to DNA damage indirectly. For all of these reasons, metals have proven to be one of the hardest category of carcinogens to study.

Metals can be divided into three groups (229). The first includes Ni, Cr, As, Be, and Cd, which are classified as human carcinogens, and probably directly contribute to the carcinogenesis process. Cu and Fe are required for metabolism, but become toxic and potentially carcinogenic when present in excess, and are probably active via their ability to generates ROS. Finally, some metals, such as Zn, are not highly toxic.

CHROMIUM Chromium is carcinogenic (229–231), and principally gives bronchial carcinomas, and lung and nasal tumors. Chromium is mutagenic and causes a variety of different kinds of mutations. Cr(VI) is generally regarded to be the most toxic redox state, although it can be reduced inside cells, and Cr(III) forms DNA adducts, including DNA-DNA and DNA-protein cross-links. Chromium can redox cycle, catalyzing the conversion of H_2O_2 to the hydroxyl radical (Fenton reaction), which oxidizes the DNA bases (G$Æ$8oxoG) and leads to single-strand breaks. Chromium can also inhibit DNA repair. Finally, chromium can alter cellular physiology by activating stress-response pathways, which can affect carcinogenesis. Stress-response proteins induced by chromium (and other) metals, include the heat-shock proteins HSP70 and HSP90, heme oxygenases (HSP23), multidrug resistance (MDR) genes, c-fos, and ubiquitin.

ARSENIC Arsenic (229,231) causes cancer of the skin, lung, and bladder. Arsenic induces chromosomal aberrations, as well as gene amplification, and inhibits DNA repair. The prevailing view is that arsenic is not a mutagen, and is most likely to be a co-carcinogen or tumor promoter. Arsenic also induces oxidative-stress enzymes, although the significance and mechanism are not clear. As(III) is probably most important.

NICKEL Nickel (229,231,232) is an essential nutrient in animals and principally exists as Ni(II). Nickel is a recognized human carcinogen, causing cancer of the lungs and oral cavity, as well as a lower risk for cancers of the larynx, prostate, and kidney. Nickel is also a potent carcinogen in rats and mice, although it is a very weak mutagen (at best). Nickel is known to generate ROS and give 8oxoG and strand breaks. However, the most intriguing potential role for nickel in carcinogenesis may be its ability to induce DNA hypermethylation (formation of m5C in 5'-CG-3' sequences), which is one cellular mechanism for turning off gene expression and could possibly lead to the silencing of tumor-suppressor genes.

ASBESTOS Arguably, asbestos (229,233) has posed (and poses) the greatest environmental and occupational risk for cancer. Asbestos causes pleural mesothelioma, and various bronchogenic carcinomas. The three most plausible mechanisms for asbestos tumorigenesis involve its potential to causes oxidative damage to DNA. Following inhalation, asbestos fibers remain embedded in the lung. Although asbestos is a silicate fiber, it generally contains high amounts of metals (crocidolite asbestos contains as much as 27% iron), which may serve as catalysts leading to the formation of ROS, which can cause local DNA damage, ultimately leading to cancer. In addition, asbestos-related ROS can affect gene expression; notably, the activation of the transcription factor nuclear factor-κB (NF-κB), and the activation of MAPK (mitogen-activated protein kinase), the latter ultimately leading to regulation of AP-1. This response is reminiscent of the properties of tumor promoters, which could be asbestos' role in tumorigenesis. Finally, there is also evidence that these lodged, inert asbestos fibers may be attacked by phagocytes and alveolar macrophages leading to the chronic and continuous generation of a significant amount of ROS. Evidence for ROS-based DNA damage is the observation that asbestos exposure leads to the formation of 8oxoG in DNA. In addition, there may also be a role for nitric oxide (NO) or one of its byproducts in asbestos carcinogenesis.

TUMOR PROMOTERS AND CO-CARCINOGENS

Beginning with the early work of Boutwell (234), the process of tumor formation has been operationally divided into the so-called three-stage carcinogenesis model, involving initiation, promotion, and progression (234–236). Initiation is the result of genotoxic DNA damage and mutagenesis, whereas promotion is brought about by tumor promoters, which are regarded as being nongenotoxic substances that enhance the carcinogenicity of initiating, genotoxic carcinogens when administered after the genotoxin, but which are not carcinogenic in their own right (234,235). In fact, some tumor promoters cause DNA damage although this DNA damage probably contributes to promotion via its affect on gene expression and not via genotoxicity. The classic tumor promoters are the phorbol esters, and the one most extensively studied is 12-*O*-tetradecanoylphorbol-13-acetate (TPA).

Tumor promoters are capable of causing a variety of changes in cells, making it difficult to be certain which are important, although evidence is mounting that the mechanism includes signal-transduction pathways involving the transcription factor AP-1. Tumor promoters fall into two classes *(238,239)*, those that bind a protein and activate a signal-transduction pathway directly, and those that cause cellular damage, which in turn affects signal transduction. For example, the phorbol esters, indole alkaloids, and polyacetates act by binding to protein kinase C (PKC), which activates a phosphorylation cascade. There can be other protein targets for tumor promoters. In contrast, tumor promoters, such as the peroxides, benzo[e]pyrene, and chrysarobin seem to act through a free radical or pro-oxidant mechanism. Regardless of the exact pathway, the effects of tumor promoters seem to converge, in that they all lead to the activation of the transcription factor AP-1, which is a so-called immediate early-response gene *(211)*. This causes specific expansion of cells, notably those that are initiated *(238)*. There is a good correlation between the abilities of tumor promoters to induce sustained hyperplasia and their tumor-promoting activities.

TPA binds to and activates PKC *(211,240)*, which is a serine/threonine kinase that is normally activated by calcium and/or diacylglycerol *(211)*. Thereafter, there is some evidence *(241,242)* that the pathway involves PKC activation of c-raf, either directly (by phosphorylation) or indirectly by activating c-ras, which activates c-raf. Activated c-raf phosphorylates mitogen-activated protein kinase kinase (MEK1), which in turn phosphorylates (and activates) ERK. Activated ERK phosphorylates (and activates) transcription factors, notably members of the AP-1 family, importantly the heterodimer between c-jun and c-fos. However, whatever the pathway between PKC and AP-1, there is good evidence that AP-1 activation is mechanistically important to tumor-promoting activity of TPA *(243–245)*. Activated AP-1 binds to so-called TPA response elements (TREs: 5'-TGAGTCA-3') in the promoter region of a variety of genes (like those encoding collagenase and ornithine decarboxylase) to activate gene expression *(211,246)*. In detail this can be quite complex, because there are many members of the AP-1 family (c-jun, junB, junD, c-fos, fosB, fra-1, and fra-2), whose levels vary throughout the cell cycle, and some activate transcription (like c-jun/fos), while others seem to repress transcription (like c-jun/fra-1). It is unclear how the activation of these AP-1-dependent genes contributes to tumor promotion, but generally speaking the effect is to increase cellular proliferative capacity.

Another potent tumor promoter, palytoxin, binds to a Na$^+$/K$^+$-ATPase and affects sodium ion transport *(242,247)*, which leads to activation (by phosphorylation) of SEK1, which in turn phosphorylates and activates JNK, finally, resulting in phosphorylation and activation AP-1 family members. Okadaic acid is a polyether compound that acts as a tumor promoter *(248)* by binding to and activity of several serine/threonine phosphatases

(types 1 and 2A) *(249)*, which also leads to enhanced protein phosphorylation and ultimately to AP-1 activation *(250,251)*.

Skin-tumor promoters such as benzoyl peroxide, t-butyl hydroperoxide, cumene hydroperoxide, and dicumyl peroxide undergo metal-dependent activation to form alkoxyl, alkyl, and aryl radicals that lead to lipid, protein, and DNA damage (probably via ROS), which mediate their cytotoxic and mitogenic effects *(239)*. Although these peroxide tumor promoters are in fact genotoxic, they probably do not work by causing mutations, but rather they lead to the induction of the immediate early-response genes, such as c-*jun*. Thus, this class of tumor promoters, whose initial mechanism of action is very different than the receptor-mediated tumor promoters, converges on the same molecular-signaling pathways.

It is clear that agents that are usually considered genotoxins can also act as promoters. This has been most extensively studied for UV irradiation, and it appears that UVA (320–400 nm) acts almost entirely as a tumor promoter, whereas both UVB (280–320 nm) and UVC (200–280 nm) appear to be initiators and promoters *(252,253)*. This also involves AP-1 activation *(254,255)*.

Finally, co-carcinogens can in principle work by a variety of mechanisms. In a number of cases, co-carcinogens result in a net increase in adduct levels *(256–258)*, which can be the result of increased metabolism *(257)* or even due to the formation of novel genotoxins between the carcinogen and co-carcinogen *(258)*.

ACKNOWLEDGMENTS

The authors gratefully acknowledge the helpful suggestions of Bruce Demple, Thomas Gilmore, Thomas Kunkel, Isabelle Mellon, Elizabeth Snow, Steven Tannenbaum, Cyrus Vaziri, David Waxman, and Richard Wood. This work was completed while E.L.L. was supported by grants from the N.I.H. (ES03775, ES03926).

REFERENCES

1. Searle, C. E. (ed.) (1984) *Chemical Carcinogens*, 2nd ed. (ACS Monograph 182), American Chemical Society, Washington DC.
2. Politzer, P. and Martin, F. J. (eds.) (1988) *Chemical Carcinogens.* (Bioactive Molecules, vol. 5), Elsevier, New York.
3. Bowman, M.C. (ed.) (1982) *Handbook of Carcinogens and Hazardous Substances.* Marcel Dekker, Inc., New York.
4. Bartsch, H., Hemminli, K., and O'Neill, I. K. (eds.) (1988) *Methods for Detecting DNA Damaging Agents in Humans: Applications in Cancer Epidemiology and Prevention.* International Agency for Research on Cancer, Lyon, France.
5. Milman, H. A. and Weisburger, E. K. (eds.) (1985) *Handbook of Carcinogen Testing.* Noyes Publications, Park Ridge, NJ.
6. Montesano, R., Bartsch, H., Vainio, H., Wilbourn, J., and Yamasaki, H. (eds.) (1986) *Long-term and Short-term Assays for Carcinogens: A Critical Appraisal.* International Agency for Research on Cancer, Lyon, France.
7. Harvey, R. G. (1997) *Polycyclic Aromatic Hydrocarbons: Chemistry and Cancer.* Wiley-VCH, Inc., New York, New York.
8. Singer, B. and Grunberger, D. (1983) *Molecular Biology of Mutagens and Carcinogens.* Plenum Press, New York.
9. Redmond, D. E., Jr. (1970) Tobacco and Cancer: the first clinical report, 1761. *N. Engl. J. Med.* **282**:18–23.
10. Pott, P. (1963) Chirurgical observations relative to the cancer of the scrotum. London, 1775. *Natl. Cancer Inst. Monograph* **10**:7–13.

11. Yamagiwa, K. and Ichikawa, K. (1915) *Verh. Japn. Path. Ges.* **5**:142–148.

12. Kennaway, E. L. and Hieger, I. (1930) Carcinogenic substances and their fluorescent spectra. *BMJ* **ii**:1044–1046.

13. Cook, J. W., Hewett, C. L., and Hieger, I. (1933) The isolation of a cancer-producing hydrocarbon from coal tar, Parts I–III. *J. Chem. Soc.* 395–405.

14. Hueper, W. C. (1942) *Occupational Tumors and Allied Diseases.* Thomas Co., Springfield IL.

15. Hueper, W. C., Wiley, F. H., and Wolfe, H. D. (1938) Experimental production of bladder tumors in dogs by administration of beta-naphthylamine. *J. Ind. Hyg. Toxicol.* **20**:46–84.

16. Rehn, L. (1895) Blasengeschwulste bei fuchsinarbeitern. *Arch. Klin. Chir.* **50**:588–600.

17. Case, R. A. M., Hosker, M. W., McDonald, D. B., and Pearson, J. T. (1954) Tumors of the urinary bladder in workmen engaged in the manufacture and use of certain dyestuff intermediates in the British chemical inductry. *Br. J. Ind. Med.* **11**:75–104.

18. Doll, R. and Peto, R. (1981) *The Causes of Cancer.* Oxford Press, New York.

19. Schulte, P. A., Ward, E., Boeniger, M., and Hills, B. (1988) Occupational exposure to N-substituted aryl compounds. *In: Carcinogenic and Mutagenic Responces to Aromatic Amines and Nitroarenes* (King, C. M., Romano, L. J. and Schuetzle, D., eds.), Elsevier Science, New York, pp. 23–35.

20. Guerin, M. R. and Buchanan, M. V. (1988) Environmental exposure to N-substituted aryl compounds. *In: Carcinogenic and Mutagenic Responces to Aromatic Amines and Nitroarenes* (King, C. M., Romano, L. J. and Schuetzle, D., eds.), Elsevier Science, New York, pp. 37–45.

21. Ross, R. K., Paganini-Hill, A. and Henderson, B. E. (1988) Epidemeology of bladder cancer. *In: Diagnosis and Management of Genitourinary Cancer* (Skinner, D. G. and Lieshovsky, G., eds.), W.B. Saunders Co., Philadephia, pp. 23–31.

22. Asao, T., Buchi, G., Abdel-Kader, M. M., Chang, S. B., Wick, E. L., and Wogan, G. N. (1963) Aflatoxins B and G. *J. Am. Chem. Soc.* **85**:1706–1707.

23. Eaton, D. L. and Groopman, J. D. (eds.) (1994) *The Toxicology of Aflatoxins.* Academic Press, New York.

24. Muller, F. H. (1939) Tobacco abuse and carcinoma of the lung. *Z. Krebsforsch.* **49**:57–85.

25. Doll, R. and Hill, A. B. (1950) Smoking and carcinoma of the lung. *Br. Med. J.* **ii**:739–748.

26. Peto, R. (1986) Tobacco: an overview of health effects. *In: Tobacco: A Major International Health Hazard* (Zaridze, D. G. and Peto, R., eds.), International Agency for Research on Cancer, Lyon, France, pp. 12–22.

27. Hoffmann, D. and Hoffmann, I. (1997) The changing cigarette, 1950–1995. *J. Toxicol. Environ. Health* **50**:307–364

28. Holleb, H. B. and Angrist, A. (1942) Bronchiogenic carcinoma in association with pulmonary asbestosis. *Am. J. Pathol.* **xviii**:123.

29. Selikoff, I. and Hammond, E. C. (1978) Asbestos-associated diseases in the United States shipyards. *Cancer* **28**:67–99.

30. Blair, A. and Kazerouni, N. (1997) Reactive chemicals and cancer. *Cancer Causes Control* **8**:473–490.

31. Higginson, J. (1969) Present trends in cancer epidemiology. *Canadian Cancer Conf.* **8**:40–75.

32. Haenszel, W. and Kurihara, M. (1968) Studies of Japanese migrants. I. Mortality from cancer and other diseases among Japanese in the United States. *J. Natl. Cancer Inst.* **40**:43–68.

33. Haenszel, W. (1975) Migrant studies. *In: Persons at High Risk of Cancer. An approach to Cancer Etiology and Control.* (Fraumeni Jr., J. F., ed.), Academic Press, New York, pp. 361–371.

34. Boveri, T. (1914) Zur frage der entstehung maligner tumoren. Gustave Fischer Verlag, Jena, Germany.

35. Crow, J. F. and Abrahamson S. (1997) Seventy years ago: mutation becomes experimental. *Genetics* **147**:1491–1496.

36. McCann, J., Choi, E., Yamasaki, E., and Ames, B. N. (1975) Detection of carcinogens as mutagens in the Salmonella/microsome test: assay of 300 chemicals. *Proc. Natl. Acad. Sci. USA* **72**:5135–5139.

37. Tabin, C. J., Bradley, S. M., Bargmann, C. I., Weinberg, R. A., Papageorge, A. G., Scolnick, E. M., et al. (1982) Mechanism of activation of a human oncogene. *Nature* **300**:143–149.

38. Reddy, E. P., Reynolds, R. K., Santos, E., and Barbacid, M. (1982) A point mutation is responsible for the acquisition of transforming properties by the T24 human bladder carcinoma oncogene. *Nature* **300**:149–152.

39. Taparowsky, E., Suard, Y., Fasano, O., Shimizu, K., Goldfarb, M., and Wigler, M. (1982) Activation of the T24 bladder carcinoma transforming gene is linked to a single amino acid change. *Nature* **300**:762–765.

40. Vogelstein, B., and Kinzler, K. W. (1992) Carcinogens leave fingerprints. *Nature* **355**:209–210.

41. Greenblatt, M. S., Bennett, W. P., Hollstein, M., and Harris, C. C. (1994) Perspectives in Cancer Research: Mutations in the p53 tumor suppressor gene: clues to cancer etiology and molecular pathogenesis. *Cancer Res.* **54**:4855–4878.

42. Hainaut, P., Hernandez, T., Robinson, A., Rodriguez-Tome, P., Flores, T., Hollstein, M., et al. (1998) IARC database of p53 gene mutations in human tumors and cell lines: updated compilation, revised formats and new visualisation tools. *Nucleic Acids Res.* **26**:205–213.

43. Ortiz de Montellano, P. R. (ed.) (1995) *Cytochrome P450: Structure, Mechanism, and Biochemistry*, 2nd ed., Plenum Press, New York.

44. Schenkman, J. B. and Greim, H. (eds.) (1993) *Cytochrome P450.* Springer-Verlag, New York.

45. Jakoby, W. B., Bend, J. R., and Caldwell, J. (eds.) (1982) *Metabolic Basis of Detoxification: Metabolism of Functional Groups.* Academic Press, New York.

46. Caldwell, J. and Jakoby, W. B. (eds.) (1983) *Metabolic Basis of Detoxification.* Academic Press, New York.

47. Jakoby, W. B. (ed.) (1980) *Enzymatic Basis of Detoxification.* Academic Press, New York.

48. Miller, E. C. (1978) Some current perspectives on chemical carcinogenesis in humans and experimental animals: presidential address. *Cancer Res.* **38**:1479–1496.

49. Nelson, D. R., Koymans, L., Kamataki, T., Stegemann, J. J., Feyereisen, R., Waxman, D. J., et al. (1996) P450 superfamily: update on new sequences, gene mapping, accession numbers and nomeclature. *Pharmacogenetics* **6**:1–42.

50. Correia, M. A. (1995) Rat and human liver cytochrome P450. Substrate and inhibitor specificities and functional markers. *In: Cytochrome P450: Structure, Mechanism, and Biochemistry.* (Ortiz de Montellano, P. R., ed.), Plenum Press, New York, pp. 607–630.

51. Guengerich, F. P. (1995) Human cytochrome P450 enzymes. *In: Cytochrome P450: Structure, Mechanism, and Biochemistry.* (Ortiz de Montellano, P. R., ed.), Plenum Press, New York, pp. 473–535.

52. Harvey, R. G. (1991) *Polycyclic Aromatic Hydrocarbons: Chemistry and Cancer*, Cambridge University Press, Cambridge, UK.

53. Phillips, D. H. (1983) Fifty years of benzo[a]pyrene. *Nature* **303**:468–472.

54. Conney, A. H. (1982) Induction of microsomal enzymes by foreign chemicals and carcinogens by polycyclic aromatic hydrocarbons. *Cancer Res.* **42**:4875–4917.

55. Preussmann, R. and Stewart, B. W. (1984) N-nitroso carcinogens. *In: Chemical Carcinogens*, 2nd ed. (ACS Monograph 182), (Searle, C. E., ed.), American Chemical Society, Washington DC, pp. 643–828.

56. Preussmann, R. and Eisenbrand, G. (1984) N-nitroso carcinogens in the environment. *In: Chemical Carcinogens*, 2nd ed. (ACS Monograph 182), (Searle, C. E., ed.), American Chemical Society, Washington DC, pp. 829–868.

57. Whitlock, J. P., Jr. and Denison, M. S. (1995) Induction of cytochrome P450 enzymes that metabolize xenobiotics. *In: Cytochrome P450: Structure, Mechanism, and Biochemistry* (Ortiz de Montellano, P.R., ed.), Plenum Press, New York, pp. 367–390.

58. Jakoby, W. B. and Ziegler, D. M. (1990) The enymes of detoxification. *J. Biol. Chem.* **265**:20715–20718.

59. Miller, J. A. and Surh, Y.-J. (1994) Historical perspectives on conjugate-dependent bioactivation of foreign compounds. *Adv. Pharmacol.* **27**:1–16.

60. Andersson, C., Mosialou, E., Weinander, R., and Morgenstern, R. (1994) Enzymology of microsomal glutathione S-transferase. *Adv. Pharmacol.* **27**:19–35.

61. Ketterer, B. and Christodoulides, L. G. (1994) Enzymology of cytosolic glutathione S-transferase. *Adv. Pharmacol.* **27**:37–51.

62. Commandeur, J. N. M., Stijntjes, G. J., and Vermeulen, N. P. E. (1995) Enzymes and transport systems involved in the formation and disposition of glutathione S-conjugates. *Pharmacol. Rev.* **47**:271–330.

63. Zia-Amirhosseini, P., Spahn-Langguth, H., and Benet, L. Z. (1994) Bioactivation by glucuronide-conjugate formation. *Adv. Pharmacol.* **27**:385–397.

64. Bock, K. W. (1994) UDP-glucuronosyltransferases and their role in metabolism and disposition of carcinogens. *Adv. Pharmacol.* **27**:367–383.

65. Tephly, T. R. and Burchell, B. (1990) UDP-glucuronosyltransferases: a family of detoxifying enzymes. *Trends Pharmacol. Sci.* **11**:276–279.

66. Coughtrie, M. W. H., Bamforth, K. J., Sharp, S., Jones, A. L., Borthwick, E. B., Barker, E. V., et al. (1994) Sulfation of endogenous compounds and xenobiotics: interactions and function in health and disease. *Chem. Biol. Interactions* **92**:247–256.

67. Matsui, M. and Homma H. (1994) Biochemistry and molecular biology of drug-metabolizing sulfotransferase. *Int. J. Biochem.* **26**:1237–1247.

68. Falany, C. N. and Wilborn, T. W. (1994) Biochemistry of cytosolic sulfotransferases involved in bioactivation. *Adv. Pharmacol.* **27**:301–330.

69. Machejda, C. J. and Koepke, M. B. K. (1994) Carcinogen activation by sulfate conjugate formation. *Adv. Pharmacol.* **27**:331–362.

70. Hanna, P. E. (1995) N-acetyltransferases, O-acetyltransferases, and N,O-acetyltransferases: enzymology and bioactivation. *Pharmacol. Rev.* **47**:401–430.

71. King, C. M., Land, S. J., Jones, R. F., Debiec-Rychter, M., Lee, M.-S., and Wang, C. Y. (1997) Role of acetyltransferases in the metabolism and carcinogenicity of aromatic amines. *Mut. Res.* **376**:123–128.

72. Grant, D. M., Hughes, N. C., Janezic, S. A., Goodfellow, G. H., Chen, H. J., Gaedigk, A., et al. (1997) Human acetyltransferase polymorphisms. *Mut. Res.* **376**:61–70.

73. Ozawa, N. and Geungerich, F. P. (1983) Evidence for formation of an S-[2-(N7-guanyl)ethyl]glutathione adduct in glutathione-mediated binding of the carcinogen 1,2-dibromoethane to DNA. *Proc. Natl. Acad. Sci. USA* **80**:5266–5270.

74. Kim, M. S. and Guengerich, F. P. (1997) Synthesis of oligonucleotides containing the ethylene dibromide DNA adducts S-[2-(N7-guanyl)ethyl]glutathione, S-[2-(N²-guanyl)ethyl]glutathione, and S-[2-(O⁶-guanyl)ethyl]glutathione at a single site. *Chem. Res. Toxicol.* **10**:1133–1143.

75. Beland, F. A. and Kadlubar, F. F. (1985) Formation and persistence of arylamine DNA adducts *in vivo. Environ. Health Perspectives* **62**:19–30.

76. Kadlubar, F. F. and Beland, F. A. (1985) Chemical properties of ultimate carcinogenic metabolites of arylamine and arylamides. *In:* Polycyclic Hydrocarbons and Carcinogenesis (Harvey, R. G., ed.), American Chemical Society, Washington, DC, pp. 341–370.

77. Kadlubar, F. F. (1994) DNA adducts of carcinogenic aromatic amines. *IARC Sci. Publ.* **125**:199–216.

78. Kadlubar, F. F., Miller, J. A., and Miller, E. C. (1994) Hepatic microsomal N-glucuronidation and nucleic acid binding of N-hydroxy arylamines in relation to urinary bladder carcinogenesis. *Cancer Res.* **37**:805–814.

79. Wise, R. W., Zenser, T. V., Kadlubar, F. F., and Davis, B. B. (1984) Metabolic activation of carcinogenic aromatic amines by dog bladder and kidney prostaglandin H synthase. *Cancer Res.* **44**:1893–1897.

80. King, C. M., Romano, L. J. and Schuetzle, D. (eds.) (1988) *Carcinogenic and Mutagenic Responses to Aromatic Amines and Nitroarenes.* Elsevier Science, New York.

81. Nagao, M., Wakabayashi, N. M., Ushijima, T., Toyota, M., Totsuka, Y., and Sugimura, T. (1996) Human exposure to carcinogenic heterocyclic amines and their mutationmal fingerprints in experimental animals. *Environ. Health Perspectives* **104**:497–501.

82. Gooderham, N. J., Murray, S., Lynch, A. M., Edwards, R. J., Yadollahi-Farsani, M., Bratt, C., et al. (1996) Heterocyclic amines: evaluation of their role in diet associated human cancer. *Br. J. Pharmacol.* **42**:91–98.

83. Layton, D. W., Bogen, K. T., Knize, M. G., Hatch, F. T., Johnson, V. M., and Felton, J. S. (1995) Cancer risk of heterocyclic amines in cooked foods: an analysis and implications for research. *Carcinogenesis* **16**:39–52.

84. Perera, F. (1997) Environment and cancer: who are susceptible? *Science* **278**:1068–1073.

85. Dipple, A., Moschel, R. C., and Bigger, A. H. (1984) Polynuclear aromatic carcinogens. *In: Chemical Carcinogens,* 2nd ed. (ACS Monograph 182) (Searle, C. E., ed.), American Chemical Society, Washington DC, pp. 41-164.

86. Agarwal, R., Canella, K. A., Yagi, H., Jerina, D. M., and Dipple, A. (1996) Benzo[c]phenthrene-DNA adducts in mouse epidermis in relation to the tumorigenicities of four configurationally isomeric 3,4-dihydrodiol 1,2-epoxides. *Chem. Res. Toxicol.* **9**:586–592.

87. Geacintov, N. E. (1986) Is intercalation a critical factor in the covalent binding of mutagenic and tumorigenic polycyclic aromatic diol epoxides to DNA? *Carcinogenesis* **7**:759–766.

88. Loechler, E. L. (1991) Molecular modeling in mutagenesis and carcinogenesis. *Methods Enzymol.* **203**:458–476.

89. Geacintov, N. E., Cosman, M., Hingerty, B. E., Amin, S., Broyde, S., and Patel, D. J. (1997) NMR solution structures of stereoisomeric polycyclic aromatic carcinogen-DNA adducts: Principles, patterns and diversity. *Chem. Res. Toxicol.* **10**:111–131.

90. Cavalieri, E. L., Rogan, E. G., Devanesan, P. D., Cremonesi, P., Cerny, R.L., Gross, M. L., et al. (1990) Binding of benzo[a]pyrene to DNA by cytochrome P-450 catalyzed one-electron oxidation in rat liver microsomes and nuclei. *Biochemistry* **29**:4820–4827.

91. Devanesan, P. D., RamaKrishna, N. V. S., Todorovic, R., Rogan, E. G., Cavalieri, E. L., Jeong, H., et al. (1992) Identification and quantitation of benzo[a]pyrene-DNA adducts formed by rat liver microsomes in vitro. *Chem. Res. Toxicol.* **5**:302–309.

92. Chakravarti, D., Pelling, J., Cavalieri, E. L., and Rogan, E. G. (1995) Relating aromatic hydrocarbon-induced DNA adducts and the c-H-ras mutations in mouse skin papillomas: The role of apurinic sites. *Proc. Natl. Acad. Sci. USA* **92**:10422–10426.

93. Chen, L., Devanesan, R., Higginbotham, S., Ariese, F., Jankowiak, R., Small, G. J., et al. (1996) Expanded analysis of benzo[a]pyrene-DNA adducts formed in vitro and in mouse skin: their significance in tumor initiation. *Chem. Res. Toxicol.* **9**:897–903.

94. Todorovic, R., Ariese, F. Devanesan, R., Jankowiak, R., Small, G. J., Rogan, E. G., et al. (1997) Determination of benzo[a]pyrene- and 7,12-dimethylbenz[a]anthracene-DNA adducts formed in rat mammary glands. *Chem. Res. Toxicol.* **10**:941–947.

95. Humphreys, W. G., Kadlubar, F. F., and Guengerich, F. P. (1992) Mechanism of C8 alkylation of guanine residues by activated arylamines: evidence for initial adduct formation at the N7 position. *Proc. Natl. Acad. Sci. USA* **89**:8278–8282.

96. Patel, D. J., Mao, B., Gu, Z., Hingerty, B. E., Gorin, A., Basu, A. K., et al. (1998) Nuclear magnetic resonance solution structures of covalent aromatic amine-DNA adducts and their mutagenic relevance. *Chem. Res. Toxicol.* **11**:391–407.

97. Hoffmann, G. R. and Fuchs, R. P. (1997) Mechanisms of frameshift mutations: Insights from aromatic amines. *Chem. Res. Toxicol.* **10**:347–359.

98. Loechler, E. L. (1994) A violation of the Swain-Scott principle and not S_N1 vs. S_N2 reaction mechanisms, explains why carcinogenic alkylating agents can form different proportions of adducts at oxygen vs. nitrogen in DNA. *Chem. Res. Toxicol.* **7**:277–280.

99. Lawley, P. D. (1984) carcinogenesis of alkylating agents. *In: Chemical Carcinogens,* 2nd ed., (ACS Monograph 182), (Searle, C. E., ed.), American Chemical Society, Washington DC, pp. 325–484.

100. Loechler, E. L. (1991) Rotation about the C6-O^6 Bond in O^6-methylguanine: the *syn* and *anti*-conformers can be of similar energies in duplex DNA as estimated by molecular modeling techniques. *Carcinogenesis* 12:1693–1699.

101. Dosanjh, M. K., Loechler, E. L., and Singer, B. (1993) Evidence from in vitro replication that O^6-methylguanine can adopt multiple conformations. *Proc. Natl. Acad. Sci. USA* 90:3983–3987.

102. Essigmann, J. M., Croy, R. G., Nadzan, A. M., Busby, W. F., Reinhold, V. N., Buchi, G., et al. (1977) Structural identification of the major DNA adducts formed by aflatoxin B₁ in vitro. *Proc. Natl. Acad. Sci. USA* 74:1870–1974.

103. Baiuley, G. S. (1994) Role of aflatoxin B1 adducts in the cancer process. *In: The Toxicology of Aflatoxins* (Eaton, D. L. and Groopman, J. D., eds.), Academic Press, New York, pp. 137–148.

104. Gopalakrishnan, S., Byrd, S., Stone, M. P., and Harris, T. M. (1989) Carcinogen-nucleic acid interactions: Equilibrium binding studies of aflatoxin B₁ with the oligonucleotide d(ATGCAT)₂ and with plasmid pBR322 support intercalative association with the B-DNA helix. *Biochemistry* 28:726–734.

105. Gopalakrishnan, S., Harris, T. M., and Stone, M. P. (1990) Intercalation of afaltoxin B₁ in two oligodeoxynucleotide adducts: Comparative ¹H NMR analysis of d(ATC^{AFB}GAT):d(ATCGAT) and d(AT^{AFB}GCAT)₂. *Biochemistry* 29:10438–10448.

106. Friedberg, E. C. Walker, G. W., and Seide, W. (1995) *DNA Repair and Mutagenesis.* ASM Press,Washington, DC.

107. Chaney, S. G. and Sancar, A. (1996) DNA repair: enzymatic mechanisms and relevance to drug response. *J. Natl. Cancer Inst.* 88:1346–1360.

108. Wood, R. D. (1997) Nucleotide excision repair in mammalian cells. *J. Biol. Chem.* 272:23465–23468.

109. Wood, R. D. and Shivji, M. K. K. (1997) Which DNA polymerases are used for DNA repair in eukaryotes? *Carcinogenesis* 18:605–610.

110. Hanawalt, P. C. (1994) Transcription-coupled repair and human disease. *Science* 266:1957–1958.

111. Lindahl, T., Karran, P., and Wood, R. D. (1997) DNA excision repair pathways. *Curr. Opin. Genet. Dev.* 7:158–169.

112. Scicchitano, D. A. and Mellon, I. (1997) Transcription and DNA damage: A link to a kink. *Environ. Health Perspectives* 105:145–153.

113. Krokan, H. E., Standal, R., and Slupphaug, G. (1997) DNA glycosylases in the base excision repair of DNA. *Biochem. J.* 325:1–25.

114. Wilson, D. M., III and Thompson, L. H. (1997) Life without DNA repair. *Proc. Natl. Acad. Sci. USA* 95:12754–12757.

115. Kunkel, T. A. and Wilson, S. H. (1996) Push and pull of base flipping. *Nature* 384:25–26.

116. Roberts, R. (1995) On base flipping. *Cell* 82:9–12.

117. Camerini-Otero, R. D. and Hseih, P. (1995) Homologous recombination proteins in prokaryotes and eukaryotes. *Ann. Rev. Genet.* 29:509–552.

118. Kanaar, R. and Hoeijmakers (1998) From competition to collaboration. *Nature* 391:335–336.

119. Hegde, S. P., Qin, M.-H., Li, X.-H., Atkinson, M. A. L., Clark, A. J., Rajagopalan, M., et al. (1996) Interactions of RecF protein with RecO, RecR, and single-stranded DNA binding proteins reveals roles for the RecF-RecO-RecR complex in DNA repair and recombination. *Proc. Natl. Acad. Sci. USA* 93:14468–14473.

120. Dixon, D. A. and Kowalczykowski, S. C. (1993) The recombination hotspot χ is a regulatory sequence that acts by attentuating the nuclease activity of the *E. coli* RecBCD enzyme. *Cell* 73:87–96.

121. West, S. C. (1997) Processing of recombination intermediates by the RuvABC proteins. *Ann. Rev. Genet.* 31:213–244.

122. Parsons, C. A., Stasiak, A., Bennett, R. J., and West, S. C. (1995) Structure of a multisubunit complex that promotes DNA branch migration. *Nature* 374:375–378.

123. Rafferty, J. B., Sedelnikova, S. E., Hargreaves, D., Artymiuk, P. J., Baker, P. J., Sharples, G. J., et al. (1996) Crystal structure of DNA recombination protein RuvA and a model for its binding to the Holliday junction. *Science* 274:415–421.

124. Ariyoshi, M., Vassylyev, D. G., Iwasaki, H., Nakamura, H., Shinagawa, H., and Morikawa, K. (1994) Atomic resolution of the RuvC resolvase: a Holliday junction-specfic endonuclease from E. coli. *Cell* 78:1063–1072.

125. Wang, G., Rahman, W. S., and Humayun, M. Z. (1997) Replication of M13 single-stranded viral DNA bearing single site-specfic adducts by *Escherichia coli* cell extracts: differential efficiency of translesion DNA synthesis for SOS-dependent and SOS-independent lesions. *Biochemistry* 36:9486–9492.

126. Palewala, V. A., Pandya, G. A., Bhanot, O. S., Solomon, J. J., Murphy, H. S., Dunman, P. M., et al. (1994) UVM, an ultraviolet-inducible RecA-independent mutagenic phenomenon in *Escherichia coli. J. Biol. Chem.* 269:27433–27440.

127. Napolitano, R. L., Lambert, I. B., and Fuchs, R. P. (1997) SOS factors involved in translesion synthesis. *Proc. Natl. Acad. Sci. USA* 94:5733–5738.

128. Dynan, W. S. and Yoo, S. (1998) Interaction of Ku protein and DNA-dependent protein kinase catalytic subunit with nucleic acids. *Nucleic Acids Res.* 26:1551–1559.

129. Jin, S., Inoue, S., and Weaver, D. T. (1997) Functions of the DNA dependent protein kinase. *Cancer Surv.* 29:221–261.

130. Jeggo, P. A. (1997) DNA-PK at the cross-roads of biochemistry and genetics. *Mut. Res.* 384:1–14.

131. Jackson, S. P. (1997) DNA-dependent protein kinase. *Int. J. Biochem. Cell Biol.* 29:935–938.

132. Lieber, M. R., Grawunder, U., Wu, X., and Yaneva, M. (1997) Tying up loose ends: roles for Ku and DNA-dependent protein kinase in the repair of double-strand breaks. *Curr. Opin. Genet, Dev.* 7:99–104.

133. Hendrickson, E. A. (1997) Cell-cycle regulation of mammalian DNA double-strand-break repair. *Am. J. Human Genet.* 61:795–800.

134. Stahl, F. (1996) Meiotic recombination in yeast: Coronation of the double-strand-break repair model. *Cell* 87:965–968.

135. Dolganov, G. M., Maser, R. S., Novikov, A., Tosto, L., Chong, S., Brtessan, D. A., et al. (1996) Human Rad50 is physically associated with human Mre11: identification of a conserved multiprotein complex implicated in recombinational repair. *Mol. Cell Biol.* 16:4832–4841.

136. Maser, R. S., Monsen, K. J., Nelms, B. E., and Petrini, J. H. (1997) hMre11 and hRad50 nuclear foci are induced during the normal cellular response to DNA double-strand breaks. *Mol. Cell Biol.* 17:6087–6096.

137. Johzhuka, K. and Ogawa, H. (1995) Interaction of Mre11 and Rad50: two proteins required for DNA repair and meiosis-specific double-srand break formation in Saccharamoyces cerevisiae. *Genetics* 139:1521–1532.

138. Murane, J. P. (1996) Role of induced genetic instability in the mutagenic effects of chemicals and radiation. *Mut. Res.* 367:11–23.

139. Kronenberg, A. (1994) Radiation-induced genomic instability. *Int. J. Rad. Biol.* 66:603–609.

140. Solomon, E., Borrow, J., and Goddard, A. D. (1991) Chromosome aberrations and cancer. *Science* 254:1153–1160.

141. Rabbitts, T. H. (1994) Chromosomal translocations in human cancer. *Nature* 372:143–149.

142. Chang, W. P. and Little, J. B. (1992) Persitently elevated frequency of spontaneous mutations in progeny of CHO cells surviving X-irradiation: association with delayed reproductive death phenotype. *Mut. Res.* 270:191–199.

143. Grosovsky, A. J., Parks, K. K., Giver, C. R., and Nelson, S. L. (1996) Clonal analysis of delayed karyotypic abnormalities and gene mutations in radiation-induced genetic instability. *Mol. Cell Biol.* 16:6252–6262.

144. Holmberg, K., Meijer, A. E., Auer, G., and Lambert, B. O. (1995) Delayed chromosomal instability in human T-lymphocyte clones exposed to ionizing radiation. *Int. J. Rad. Biol.* 68:245–255.

145. Holmberg, K., Falt, S., Johansson, A., and Lambert, B. (1993) Clonal chromosomal aberrations and genomic instability in X-irradiated human T-lymphocyte cultures. *Mut. Res.* **286**:321–330.

146. Pardee, A. B. (1989) G1 events and regulation of cell proliferation. *Science* **240**:603–608.

147. Hartwell, L. H. and Kastan, M. B. (1994) Cell cycle control and cancer. *Science* **266**:1821–1828.

148. Paulovich, A. G., Toczyski, D. P., and Hartwell, L. H. (1997) When checkpoints fail. *Cell* **88**:315–321.

149. Sherr, C. J. (1993) Mammalian G1 cyclins. *Cell* **73**:1059–1065.

150. Weinberg, R. A. (1995) The retinoblastoma protein and cell cycle control. *Cell* **81**:323–330.

151. Weinberg, R. A. (1996) E2F and cell proliferation: a world turned upside down. *Cell* **85**:457–459.

152. Herwig, S. and Strauss, M. (1997) The Rb protein: a master regulator of cell cycle, differentiation and apoptosis. *Eur. J. Biochem.* **246**:581–601.

153. Hunter, T. (1997) Oncoprotein networks. *Cell* **88**:333–346.

154. Collins, K., Jacks, T., and Pavletich, N. P. (1997) The cell cycle and cancer. *Proc. Natl. Acad. Sci. USA* **94**:2776–2778.

155. Elledge, S. J. (1996) Cell cycle checkpoints: preventing an idenitity crisis. *Science* **274**:1664–1672.

156. Levine, A. J. (1997) p53, the cellular gatekeeper for growth and division. *Cell* **88**:323–331.

157. Bjelogrlic, N. M., Mäkinen, M., Stenbäck, and Vähäkangas, K. (1994) Benzo[a]pyrene-7,8-diol-9,10-epoxide-DNA adducts and increased p53 protein in mouse skin. *Carcinogenesis* **15**:771–774.

158. Khan, Q. A., Vousden, K. H., and Dipple, A. (1997) Cellular response to DNA damage from a potent carcinogen involves stabilization of p53 without induction of p21 (waf1/cip1). *Carcinogenesis* **18**:2313–2318.

159. Vaziri, C. and Faller, D. V. (1997) A benzo[a]pyrene-induced cell cycle checkpoint resulting in p53-independent G1 arrest in 3T3 fibroblasts. *J. Biol. Chem.* **272**:2762–2769.

160. Hengartner, M. O. (1998) Death cycle and Swiss army knives. *Nature* **391**:441–442.

161. Wertz, I. E. and Hanley, M. R. (1996) Diverse molecular provocation of programmed cell death. *Trends Biol. Res.* **21**:359–364.

162. Nagata, S. (1997) Apoptosis by death factor. *Cell* **88**:355–365.

163. Cohen, G. M. (1997) Caspases: the executioners of apoptosis. *Biochem. J.* **326**:1–16.

164. Wyllie, A. (1998) An endonuclease at last. *Nature* **391**:20–21.

165. Vuax, D. L. and Strasser, A. (1996) The molecular biology of apoptosis. *Proc. Natl. Acad. Sci. USA* **93**:2239–2244.

166. Hale, A. J., Smith, C. A., Sutherland, L. C., Stoneman, V. E. A., Longhorn, V. L., Culhane, A. C., et al. (1996) Apoptosis: molecular regulation of cell death. *Eur. J. Biochem.* **236**:1–26.

167. White, E. (1996) Life, death, and the pursuit of apoptosis. *Genes Develop.* **10**:1–15.

168. Peter, M. E., Heufelder, A. E., and Hengartner, M. O. (1997) Advances in apoptosis research. *Proc. Natl. Acad. Sci. USA* **94**:12736–12737.

169. Kerr, A. H., Wylie, J. F., and Currie, A. R. (1972) Apoptosis: a basic biological phenomenon with wide-ranging implications in tissue kinetics. *Br. J. Cancer* **26**:239–257.

170. Jacobson, M. D. (1996) Reactive oxygen species and programmed cell death. *Trends Biol. Res.* **21**:83–86.

171. Kinzler, K. W. and Vogelstein, B. (1996) Life (and death) in a malignant tumor. *Nature* **379**:19–20.

172. Muchmore, S. W., Sattlet, M., Liang, H., Meadows, R. P., Harlan, J. E., Yoon, H. S., et al. (1996) X-ray and NMR structure of human Bcl-xL an inhibitor of programmed cell death. *Nature* **381**:335–341.

173. Zamzami, N., Susin, S. A., Marchetti, P., Hirsch, T., Gomez-Monterrey, I., Castedo, M., et al. (1996) Mitochondrial control of nuclear apoptosis. *J. Exp. Med.* **183**:1533–1544.

174. Vander Heiden, V., Chandel, N. S., Williamson, E. K., Schumacker, P. T. and Thompson, C. B. (1997) Bcl-xL regulates the membrane potential and volume homeostasis of mitochondria. *Cell* **91**:627–637.

175. Salvesen, G. S. and Dixit, V. M. (1997) Caspases: intracellular signaling by proteolysis. *Cell* **91**:443–446.

176. Hampton, M. B., Zhivotsky, B., Slater, A. F. G., Burgess, D. H., and Orrenius, S. (1998) Importance of the redox state of cytochrome C during caspase activation in cytosolic extracts. *Biochem. J.* **329**:95–99.

177. Kluck, R. M., Martin, S. J., Hoffman, B. M., Zhou, J. S., Green, D. R., and Newmeyer, D. D. (1997) Cytochrome c activation of CPP32-like proteolysis plays a critical role in a Xenopus cell-free apoptosis system. *EMBO J.* **16**:4639–3649.

178. Oren, M. (1998) Teaming up to restrain cancer. *Nature* **391**:233–234.

179. Yin, Y., Terauchi, Y., Solomon, G. S., Aizawa, S., Rangarajan, P. N., Yazaki, Y., et al. (1998) Involvement of p85 in p53-dependent apoptotic response to oxidative stress. *Nature* **391**:707–710.

180. Loechler, E. L. (1994) Mechanism by which aflatoxins and other bulky carcinogens induce mutations. In: *The Toxicology of Aflatoxins: Human Health, Veterinary, and Agricultural Significance* (Eaton, D. L. and Groopman, J.D., eds.), Academic Press, Orlando, FL, pp. 149–178.

181. Miller, J. H. (1983) Mutational specificity in bacteria. *Ann. Rev. Genet.* **17**:215-238.

182. Rodriguez, H. and Loechler, E. L. (1993) Mutational spectra of the (+)-*anti*-diol epoxide of benzo[a]pyrene in a *supF* gene of an *Escherichia coli* plasmid: DNA sequence context influences hotspots, mutational specficity and the extent of SOS enhancement of mutagenesis. *Carcinogenesis* **14**:373–383.

183. Rodriguez, H. and Loechler, E. L. (1993) Mutagenesis by the (+)-*anti*-diol epoxide of benzo[a]pyrene: What controls mutagenic specificity? *Biochemistry* **32**:373–383.

184. Wei, S.-J. C., Chang, R. L., Wong, C.-Q., Bhachech, N., Cui, X. X., Hennig, E., et al. (1991) Dose-dependent differences in the profile of mutations induced by an ultimate carcinogen from benzo[a]pyrene. *Proc. Natl. Acad. Sci. USA* **88**:11227–11230.

185. Wei, S.-J. C., Chang, R. L., Bhachech, N., Cui, X. X., Merkler, K. A., Wong, C. Q., et al. (1993) Dose-dependent differences in the profile of mutations induced (+)-7R,8S-dihydroxy-9S,10R-epoxy-7,8,9,10-tetrahydrobenzo[a]pyrene in the coding region of the hypoxanthine (guanine) phosphoribosyltransferase gene in Chinese hamster V79 cells. *Cancer Res.* **53**:3294–3301.

186. Wei, S.-J. C., Chang, R. L., Hennig, E., Cui, X. X., Merkler, K. A., Wong, C.-Q., et al. (1994) Mutagenic selectivity at the HPRT locus in V-79 cells: comparison of mutations caused by bay-region benzo[a]pyrene 7,8-diol-9,10-epoxide enantiomers with high and low carcinogenic activity. *Carcinogenesis* **15**:1729–1735.

187. Wei, S.-J. C., Chang, R. L., Cui, X. X., Merkler, K. A., Wong, C.-Q., Yagi, H., et al. (1996) Dose-dependent differences in the mutational profiles of (-)-(1R,2S,3S,4R)-3,4-dihydroxy-1,2-epoxy-1,2,3,4-tetrahydrobenzo[c]phenanthrene and its less carcinogenic enantiomer. *Cancer Res.* **56**:3695–3703.

188. Bigger, C. A. H., St. John, J., Yagi, H., Jerina, D. M., and Dipple, A. (1992) Mutagenic specificities of four stereoisomeric benzo[c]phenanthrene dihydrodiol epoxides. *Proc. Natl. Acad. Sci. USA* **89**:368–372.

189. D'Ayala, M., Cui, X. X., Merkler, K. A., Wong, C.-Q., Yagi, H., Jerina, D. M., et al. (1998) Lack of dose dependence in mutation profile induced by (+)-7R,8S-dihydroxy-9S,10R-epoxy-7,8,9,10-tetrahydrobenzo[a]pyrene [(+)-BPDE] at the *hprt* gene in repair deficient Chinese hamster V-H1 cells. *Proc. Am. Assoc. Cancer Res.* **39**:639a.

190. Singer, B. and Essigmann J. M. (1991) Site-specific mutagenesis: retrospective and prospective. *Carcinogenesis* **12**:949–955.

191. Loechler, E. L. (1996) Commentary: The role of adduct site-specific mutagenesis in understanding how carcinogen DNA adducts cause mutations: perspective, prospects and problems. *Carcinogenesis* **17**:895–902.

192. Mackay, W., Benasutti, M., Drouin, E., and Loechler, E. L.(1992) Mutagenesis by the major adduct of activated benzo[a]pyrene, (+)-*anti*-BP-N2-Gua, when studied in an *Escherichia coli* plasmid using site-directed methods. *Carcinogenesis* **13**:1415–1425.

193. Jelinsky, S. A., Mao, B., Geacintov, N. E., and Loechler, E. L. (1995) The major, N^2-Gua adduct of the (+)-*anti*-benzo[a]pyrene diol epoxide is capable of inducing GÆA and GÆC, in addition to GÆT, mutations. *Biochemistry* **34**:13545–13553.

194. Shukla, R., Liu, Y., Geacintov, N., and Loechler, E. L. (1997) The major, N^2-dG adduct of (+)-*anti*-B[a]PDE shows a dramatically different mutagenic specificity (predominantly, GÆA) in a 5'-CGT-3' sequence context. *Biochemistry* **36**:10256–10261.

195. Shukla, R, Jelinsky, S., Liu T., Geacintov, N. E., and Loechler, E. L. (1997) How stereochemistry affects mutagenesis by N^2-dG adducts of B[a]PDE: configuration of the adduct bond is more important than of the hydroxyl groups. *Biochemistry* **36**:13263–13269.

196. Moriya, M., Spiegel, S., Fernandes, A., Amin, S., Liu, T.-M., Geacintov, N. E., et al. (1996) Fidelity of translesion synthesis past benzo[a]pyrene diol epoxide-2'-deoxyguanosine DNA adducts: marked effects of host cell, sequence context, and chirality. *Biochemistry* **35**:16646–16651.

197. Fuchs, R. P. P. (1985) DNA binding spectrum of the carcinogen N-acetoxy-N-2-acetylaminofluorene significantly differs from the mutation spectrum. *J. Mol. Biol.* **177**:173–180.

198. Reid, T. M., Lee, M.-S., and King, C. M. (1990) Mutagenesis by site-specific arylamine adducts in plasmid DNA: enhancing replication of the adducted strand alters mutation frequency. *Biochemistry* **29**:6153–6161.

199. Burnouf, D., Koehl, P., and Fuchs, R. P. P. (1989) Single adduct mutagenesis: Strong effect of the position of a single acetylaminofluorene adduct within a mutation hot spot. *Proc. Natl. Acad. Sci. USA* **86**:4147–4151.

200. Seeberg, E. and Fuchs, R. P. P. (1990) Acetylaminofluorene bound to different guanines of the sequence -GGCGCC- is excised with different efficiencies by the UvrABC exicision nuclease in a pattern not correlated to the potency of mutation induction. *Proc. Natl. Acad. Sci. USA* **87**:191–194.

201. Delagoutte, E., Bertrand-Burggraf, E., Dunand, J., and Fuchs, R. P. (1997) Sequence-dependent modulation of nucleotide excision repair: the efficiency of the incision reaction correlated with the stability of the pre-incision UvrB-DNA complex. *J. Mol. Biol.* **266**:703–710.

202. Lambert, I. B., Napolitano, R. L., and Fuchs, R. P. P. (1992) Carcinogen-induced frameshift mutagenesis in repetitive equences. *Proc. Natl. Acad. Sci. USA* **89**:1310–1314.

203. Napolitano, R. L., Lambert, I. B., and Fuchs, R. P. P. (1994) DNA sequence determinants of carcinogen-induced frameshift mutagenesis. *Biochemistry* **33**:1311–1315.

204. Koffel-Schwartz, N., Coin, F., Veaute, X., and Fuchs, R. P. (1996) Cellular strategies for accomodating replication-hindering adducts in DNA: control by the SOS response in *Escherichia coli*. *Proc. Natl. Acad. Sci. USA* **93**:7805–7810.

205. Ezaz-Nikpay, K. and Verdine, G. L. (1994) The effects of N7-methylguanine on duplex DNA structure. *Chem. Biol.* **1**:235–240.

206. Bhanot, O. P., Grevatt, P. C., Donahue, J. M., Gabrielides, C. N., and Solomon, J. J. (1992) In vitro DNA replication implicates O^2-ethyldeoxythymidine in transversion mutagenesis by ethylating agents. *Nucleic Acids Res.* **20**:587–594.

207. Kunkel, T. A. (1984) Mutational specificity of depurination. *Proc. Natl. Acad. Sci. USA* **81**:1494–1498.

208. Lawrence, C. W., Borden, A., Banerjee, S. K., and LeClerc, J. E. (1990) Mutation frequency and spectrum resulting from a single abasic site in a single-stranded vector. *Nucleic Acids Res.* **18**:2153–2157.

209. Bailey, E. A., Iyer, R. S., Stone, M. P., Harris, T. M., and Essigmann, J. M. (1996) Mutational properties of the primary aflatoxin B_1-DNA adduct. *Proc. Natl. Acad. Sci. USA* **93**:1535–1539.

210. Kunkel, T. A. and Wilson, S. H. (1998) DNA polymerases on the move. *Nature Struct. Biol.* **5**:95–103.

211. Cooper, G. M. (1995) *Oncogenes,* 2nd ed. Jones and Bartlett, London.

212. Cooper, D. N. and Krawczak, M. (1993) *Human Gene Mutations.* BIOS Scientific Publishers Limited, London UK.

213. Nagase, H. and Nakamura, Y. (1993) Mutations of the APC (Adenomatous Polyposis Coli) gene. *Human Mut.* **2**:425–434.

214. Coulondre, C., Miller, J. H., Farabaugh, P. J., and Gilbert, W. (1978) Molecular basis of base substitution hotspots in *Escherichia coli*. *Nature* **278**:775–780.

215. Duncan, B. K. and Miller, J. H. (1980) Mutagenic deamination of cytosine residues in DNA. *Nature* **287**:560–565.

216. Schaaper, R. M. and Dunn, R. L. (1987) Spectra of spontaneous mutations in *Escherichia coli* strains defective in mismatch corrections: the nature of in vivo DNA replication errors. *Proc. Natl. Acad. Sci. USA* **84**:6220–6224.

217. Schaaper, R. M. and Dunn, R. L. (1991) Spontaneous mutation in the Escherichia coli strains lacI gene. *Genetics* **129**:317–326.

218. Brash, D. E., Rudolph, J. A., Simon, J. A., Lin, A., McKenna, G. J., Baden, H. P., et al. (1991) A role for sunlight in skin cancer: UV-induced p53 mutations in squamous cell carcinoma. *Proc. Natl. Acad. Sci. USA* **88**:10124–10128.

219. Dumaz, N., Stary, A., Soussi, T., Daya-Grosjean, L., and Sarasin, A. (1994) Can we predict solar ultraviolet radiation as the causal event in human tumors by analyzing the mutation spectra of the p53 gene? *Mut. Res.* **307**:375–386.

220. Daya-Grosjean, L. Dumaz, N., and Sarasin, A. (1995) The specificity of p53 mutation spectra in sunlight induced human cancers. *J. Photochem. Photobiol.* **28**:115–124.

221. D'errico, M., Calcagnile, A., and Dogliotti, E. (1996) Genetic alterations in skin cancer. *Ann. Ist. Super. Sanita* **32**:53–63.

222. Miller, J. H. and Reznikoff, W. S., eds. (1980) *The Operon,* 2nd ed., Cold Spring Harbor Press, Cold Spring Harbor, NY.

223. Miller, J. H. (1983) Mutagenic specificity in bacteria. *Ann. Rev. Genet.* **17**:215–238.

224. Miller, J. H. (1985) Mutagenic specificity of ultraviolet light. *J. Mol. Biol.* **182**:45–65.

225. Hsia, H. C., Lebkowski, J. S., Leong, P. M., Calos, M. P., and Miller, J. H. (1989) Comparison of ultraviolet irradiation-induced mutagenesis of the *lacI* gene in *Escherichia coli* and in human 293 cells. *J. Mol. Biol.* **205**:103–113.

226. Denissenko, M. F., Pao, A., Tang, M., and Pfeifer, G. P. (1996) Preferential formation of benzo[a]pyrene adducts at lung cancer mutational hotspots in p53. *Science* **274**:430–432.

227. Denissenko, M. F., Pao, A., Pfeifer, G. P., and Tang, M.-S. (1998) Slow repair of bulky DNA adducts along thre nontranscribed strand of the human p53 gene may explain the strand bias of transversion mutations in cancers. *Oncogene* **16**:1241–1247.

228. El-Bayoumy, K. (1992) Environmental carcinogens that may be involved in human breast cancer etiology. *Chem. Res. Toxicol.* **5**:585–590.

229. Klein, C. B., Snow, E. T., and Frenkel, K. (1998) Molecular mechanisms in metal carcinogenesis: Role of oxidative stress. *In: Molecular Biology of Free Radicals in Human Diseases* (Aruoma, O. I. and Halliwell, B., eds.), OICA International, Santa Lucia, West Indies, pp. 80–137.

230. Klein, C. B. (1996) Carcinogenicity and genotoxicity of chromium. *In: Toxicology of Metal* (Magos, L. and Suzuki, T., eds.), CRC Press, Boca Raton, FL.

231. Snow, E. T. (1992) Metal carcinogenesis: mechanistic implications. *Pharmacol. Ther.* **53**:31–65.

232. Snow, E.. and Costa, M. (1998) Nickel toxicity and carcinogenesis. *In: Environmental and Occupational Medicine,* 3rd ed. (Rom, W.N., ed.), Lippincott-Raven, Philadelphia, PA.

233. Mossman, B. T., Faux, S., Janssen, Y., Jimenez, L. A., Timblin, C., Zanella, C., et al. (1997) Cell signalling pathways elicited by asbestos. *Environ. Health Perspect.* **105**:1121–1125.

234. Boutwell, R. K. (1964) Some biological aspects of skin carcinogenesis. *Prog. Exp. Tumor Res.* **4**:207–250.

235. Boutwell, R. K. (1974) The function and mechanism of promoters of carcinogens. *CRC Crit. Rev. Toxicol.* **2**:419–443.

236. Boutwell, R. K. (1985) Tumor promoters in human carcinogenesis. *Important. Adv. Oncol.* **1985**:16–27.

237. Slaga, T. J. and DiGiovanni, J. (1984) *In: Chemical Carcinogens,* 2nd ed. (ACS Monograph 182), (Searle, C. E., ed.), American Chemical Society, Washington DC, pp. 1279–1321.

238. Slaga, T. J., DiGiovanni, J., Winberg, L. D., and Budunova, I. V. (1995) Skin carcinogenesis: characteristics, mechanisms, and prevention. *Prog. Clin. Biol. Res.* **391**:1–20.

239. Kensler, T., Guyton, K., Egner, P., McCarthy, T., Lesko, S., and Akman, S. (1995) Role of reactive intermediates in tumor promotion and progression. *Prog. Clin. Biol. Res.* **391**:103–116.

240. Nishizuki, Y. (1984) The role of protein kinase C in cell surface signal transduction and tumor promotion. *Nature* **308**:693–698.

241. El-Shemerly, M. Y., Besser, D., Nagasawa, M., and Nagamine, Y. (1997) 12-O-tetradecanoylphorbol-13-acetate activates the Ras/extracellular signal-regulated kinase (ERK) signaling pathway upstream of SOS involving serine phosphorylation of Shc in NIH3T3 cells. *J. Biol. Chem.* **272**:30599–30602.

242. Kuroki, D. W., Bignami, G. S., and Wattenberg, E. V. (1996) Activation of stress-activated protein kinase/c-Jun N-terminal kinase by the non-TPA-type tumor promoter palytoxin. *Cancer Res.* **56**:637–644.

243. Dong, Z., Crawford, H. C., Lavrovsky, V., Taub, D., Watts, R., Matrisian, L. M., and Colburn, N. H. (1997) A dominant negative mutant of jun blocking 12-O-tetradecanoylphorbol-13-acetate-induced invasion in mouse keratinocytes. *Mol. Carcinogenesis* **19**:204–212.

244. Dong, Z., Lavrovsky, V., and Colburn, N. H. (1995) Transversion reversion induced in JB6 RT101 cells by AP-1 inhibitors. *Carcinogenesis* **16**:749–756.

245. Bernstein, L. R. and Colburn, N. H. (1989) AP-1/jun function is differentially induced in promotion-sensitive and resistant JB6 cells. *Science* **244**:566–569.

246. Ransome, L .J. and Verma, I. M. (1990) Nuclear proto-oncogenes FOS and JUN. *Ann. Rev. Cell Biol.* **6**:539–557.

247. Kuroki, D. W., Minden, A., Sanchez, I., and Wattenberg, E. V. (1997) Regulation of a c-Jun amino-terminal kinase/stress-activated protein kinase cascade by a sodium-dependent signal transduction pathway. *J. Biol. Chem.* **272**:23905–23911.

248. Suganuma, M., Fujiki, H., Suguri, H., Yoshizawa, S., Hirota, M., Nakayasu, M., et al. (1988) Okadaic acid: An additional non-phorbol-12-tetradecanoate-13-acetate-type tumor promoter. *Proc. Natl. Acad. Sci. USA* **85**:1768–1771.

249. Nagao, M., Sakai, R., Kitagawa, Y., Ikeda, I., Sasaki, K., Shima, H., et al. (1989) Role of protein phosphatases in malignant transformation. *Princess Takamatsu Symp.* **20**:177–184.

250. Schonthal, A., Tsukitani, Y., and Feramisco, J. R. (1991) Transcriptional and post-translational regulation of c-fos expression by the tumor promoter okadaic acid. *Oncogene* **6**:423–430.

251. Peng, J., Bowden, G. T., and Domann, F. E. (1997) Activation of AP-1 by okadaic acid in mouse keratinocytes associated with hyperphorphorylation of c-jun. *Mol. Carcinogenesis* **18**:37–43.

252. Willis, I., Menter, J. M., and Whyte, H. J. (1981) The rapid induction of cancers in the hairless mouse utlizing the principle of photoaugmentation. *J. Invest. Dermatol.* **76**:404–408.

253. Strickland, P. T. (1986) Photocarcinogenesis by near-ultraviolet (UVA) radiation in Sancar mice. *J. Invest. Dermatol.* **87**:272–278.

254. Ronai, Z. A., Lambert, M. E., and Weinstein, I. B. (1990) Inducible cellular responses to ultraviolet irradiation and other mediators of DNA damage in mammalian cells. *Cell Biol. Toxicol.* **6**:105–126.

255. Angel, P. (1995) The role and regulation of the Jun proteins in response to phorbol esters and UV light. *In: Inducible Gene Expression*, (Baeuerle, P. A., ed.), Birkhauser, Boston, pp. 62-92.

256. Melikian, A. A., Leszczynska, J. M., Hecht, S. S., and Hoffmann, D. (1986) Effects of the co-carcinogen catechol on benzo[a]pyrene metabolism and DNA adduct formation in mouse skin. *Carcinogenesis* **7**:9–15.

257. Lau, H. H. and Baird, W. M. (1992) The co-carcinogen benzo[e]pyrene increases the binding of a low dose of the carcinogen benzo[a]pyrene to DNA in Sencar mouse epidermis. *Cancer Lett.* **63**:229–236.

258. Reed, G.A. and Jones, B.C. (1996) Enhancement of benzo[a]pyrene diol epoxide mutagenicity by sulfite in a mammalian test system. *Carcinogenesis* **17**:1063–1068.

259. Friedberg, E.C., Feaver, W.J. and Gerlach, V.L. (2000) The many faces of DNA polymerases: strategies for mutagenesis and for mutational avoidance. *Proc. Natl. Acad. Sci USA*, **97**:5681–5683.

260. Johnson, R.E., Washington, M.T., Prakash, S. and Prakash, L. (1999) Bridging the gap: a family of novel DNA polymerases that replicate faulty DNA. *Proc. Natl. Acad. Sci. USA,* **96**:12224–12226.

261. Goodman, M.F. and Tippin, B. (2000) Sloppier copier DNA polymerases involved in genome repair. *Curr. Opin. Genet. Dev.* **10**:162–168.

262. Yu, S.L., Johnson, R.E., Prakash, S. and Prakash, L. (2001) Requirement of DNa polymerase eta for error-free bypass of UV-inuduced CC and TC photoproducts *Mol. Cell. Biol.* **21**:185–188.

263. Gibbs, P.E., Wang, X.D., Li, Z., McManus, T.P., McGregor, W.G., Lawrence, C.W. and Maher, V.M. (2000) The function of the human homolog of Sccharomyces cerevisiae REV1 is required for mutagenesis induced by UV light. *Proc. Natl. Acad. Sci. USA* **97**:4186–4191.

11 Physical Agents in Human Carcinogenesis

CYNTHIA R. TIMBLIN, PHD, YVONNE JANSSEN-HEININGER, PHD,
AND BROOKE T. MOSSMAN, PHD

INTRODUCTION

Since the original observations of Brand and Stanton *(1)* in which plastics and other solid materials implanted under the skin of rodents induced sarcomas, the concept of foreign body carcinogenesis has been viable and intriguing. The development of human lung cancers and mesotheliomas after exposure to insoluble particulates such as asbestos fibers has strengthened the argument that physical carcinogenesis is of importance in occupational and environmental settings. Crystalline silica has recently been classified as a carcinogen in humans *(2)*. However, despite intense research efforts, diverse theories on mechanisms of physical carcinogenesis exist, and the molecular basis for these malignancies is slowly being unraveled. In this chapter, we will focus on the physical agents asbestos and silica, first addressing the epidemiology of these inhaled pollutants, and secondly emphasizing recent cellular and molecular data from our laboratory and others. Lastly, we will discuss how this information has contributed to an understanding of the pathogenesis of lung cancer and mesothelioma and the design of potential therapeutic strategies.

THE COMPLEXITY OF ASBESTOS AND SILICA

There are important physical and chemical differences between asbestos fibers (defined by United States regulatory agencies as having a greater than 3:1 length to diameter ratio) and nonfibrous particles such as silica. Fig. 1 shows the geometry of long (>10 μm) crocidolite asbestos fibers in comparison to antigorite (a nonfibrous analog of chrysotile asbestos) particles of <2 μm. Crystalline silica is morphologically similar to antigorite, occurring in blocky, plate-like, or spherical particle agglomerates. In addition, the size and chemistry of asbestos and silica differ vastly according to mineral type, industrial application, and subclassification. These properties may dictate the respirability, clearance patterns, solubility, and toxicity of these inhaled materials.

Asbestos is a family of naturally occurring minerals of six subtypes, which vary in their geographical distribution. Chrysotile [$Mg_6Si_4O_{10}(OH)_8$], the type of asbestos that is most prevalent in buildings and past industrial settings of the United States, is a curly fiber which tends to occur in bundles (fibrils) and breaks down in the lung over time due to leaching of magnesium from the fiber surface and fragmentation *(3)*. On the other hand, amphibole types of asbestos including crocidolite ($Na_2(Fe^{3+})_2(Fe^{2+})_3Si_8O_{22}(OH)_2$), amosite [$(Fe,Mg)_7Si_8O_{22}(OH)_2$], tremolite [$Ca_2Mg_5Si_8O_{22}(OH)_2$], anthophyllite [$(Mg,Fe)_7Si_8O_{22}(OH)_2$], and actinolite [$Ca_2(Mg,Fe)_5Si_8O_{22}(OH)_2$] are more durable and needle-like fibers. The persistence of amphibole fibers, such as crocidolite and amosite, in human lungs, may be one factor accounting for their increased pathogenicity, in comparison to chrysotile, in malignant mesothelioma *(4)*. Often deposits of one type of asbestos can be found in association with another type, such as the situation in Canada where chrysotile can be mined in the presence of tremolite fibers *(5)*.

Crystalline silica (SiO_2) also occurs as many polymorphs, the most common being quartz, tridymite, and cristobalite. Quartz is a major mineral component of sands accounting for 12% of the earth's crust by weight and like asbestos, has been used in a myriad of industrial applications. Several billion metric tons of crushed stone, sand, and gravel are used yearly in highway construction and cement in the United States.

Although asbestos and silica are the most widely studied physical agents affecting the lung, a number of other naturally occurring and synthetic fibers are being scrutinized in the toxicology and regulatory arenas because of their ability to cause lung cancers in rodents after inhalation or intratracheal instillation. However, epidemiological studies thus far fail to provide a compelling association between workplace exposures and the development of lung cancers and mesotheliomas. A notable exception is the zeolite fiber, erionite, which is associated with

From: *The Molecular Basis of Human Cancer* (W. B. Coleman and G. J. Tsongalis, eds.), © Humana Press Inc., Totowa, NJ.

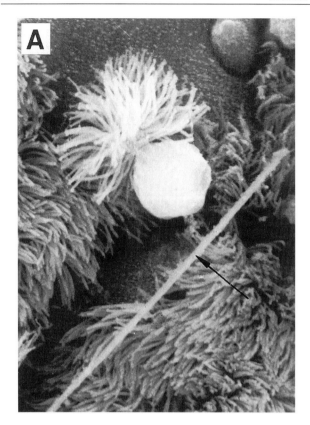 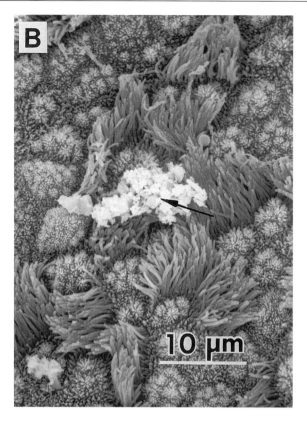

Fig. 1. Physical features of fibers and particles as illustrated by scanning electron microscopy. **(A)** shows a long (>10 μm) fiber (arrow) of crocidolite asbestos on the tracheal epithelial surface. Note the sloughing ciliated cell. **(B)** shows small particles (arrow) of antigorite, the nonfibrous chemically similar analog of chrysotile asbestos, on the surface of a ciliated cell.

the development of mesotheliomas and lung tumors in areas of Turkey, where it is used in construction of homes *(4,6)*.

EPIDEMIOLOGY AND INTERACTIONS OF ASBESTOS AND SILICA WITH COMPONENTS OF CIGARETTE SMOKE

The epidemiology of asbestos-induced lung cancers and mesotheliomas has been described comprehensively elsewhere *(6–9)*. These reports show conclusively that lung cancers and mesotheliomas are associated with inhalation of excessive quantities of respirable asbestos fibers in the past workplace, although differences exist among fiber types. Whether or not exposures to chrysotile asbestos induce human mesotheliomas is still a subject of controversy *(8,10)*. Lung cancers have been documented in both chrysotile and other asbestos-exposed cohorts, but almost exclusively in smokers. However, the risk of lung cancer is increased synergistically in asbestos workers who smoke in comparison to the risk of lung cancer in smokers in the general population *(11)*. Thus, much work experimentally has focused on possible interactions between asbestos fibers and components of cigarette smoke. In contrast, the development of mesotheliomas in humans is not associated with smoking histories, suggesting that asbestos fibers are unique etiologic agents in the causation of this disease.

Whether or not silica in the absence of smoking is an occupational carcinogen in the causation of human lung cancer is unclear, as epidemiological studies are confounded by smoking influences and risks are less striking than those previously

reported in workers exposed to asbestos *(2,12)*. Moreover, exposure to silica particles has not been associated with the development of mesothelioma in humans or rodents, and silica particles are not genotoxic in a number of cell models *(2)*. However, tumors have been reported in one species of rodent, the rat, after inhalation or intratracheal injection of silica *(2)*. Whether these results are at all relevant to the prediction of tumor induction in humans is unclear because rats develop histologically distinct tumors from humans, which are observed in response to inhalation of overload quantities of a number of insoluble materials including carbon black, diesel-exhaust particles, and coal dust, which are not carcinogenic in humans *(2)*.

Because of the strong links between smoking and inhalation of asbestos fibers in the causation of lung cancer, a number of research investigators have focused on possible mechanisms of synergism. Fig. 2 shows a hypothetical series of events that occur when components of cigarette smoke and asbestos fibers are inhaled together, i.e., as co-carcinogens. It has been known for many years that polycyclic aromatic hydrocarbons (PAH) and other carcinogenic components of cigarette smoke can be metabolized by epithelial cells of the lung and interact to form DNA adducts. This contrasts with the lack of effects of asbestos fibers on the induction of aneuploidy and chromosomal aberrations in human bronchial cells *(13)* and their inability to induce DNA breakage in hamster tracheal epithelial (HTE) cells *(14)*. However, if the PAH, benzo(a)pyrene (B[a]P), is coated on asbestos fibers rather than added directly to monolayers of HTE cells, increased uptake of B[a]P and DNA alkylation oc-

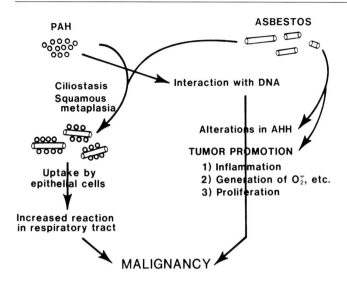

Fig. 2. Hypothetical schema of interactions between polycylic hydrocarbons (PAH) and asbestos fibers in tumor promotion and carcinogenesis. In contrast to asbestos, PAH are metabolized by cells and form adducts with DNA. Adsorption of PAH to asbestos fibers increases cell uptake, metabolism by the aryl hydrocarbon hydroxylase system (AHH), and DNA adduct formation. Moreover, smoking impairs clearance of asbestos fibers from the lung due to ciliostasis and the induction of squamous metaplasia. In addition, asbestos fibers act as classical tumor promoters in mouse skin by eliciting inflammation, generation of oxidants, and proliferation of tracheobronchial epithelial cells.

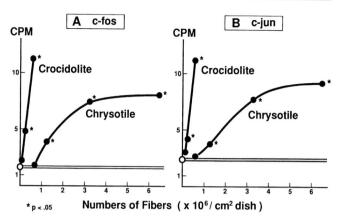

Fig. 3. Expression of *c-fos* and *c-jun* following asbestos treatment of rat pleural mesothelial cells. Quantitation of Northern-blot analyses showing increases in steady-state levels of c-*fos* and c-*jun* in rat pleural mesothelial (RPM) cells 8 h after addition of crocidolite or chrysotile asbestos *(20)*. Results have been graphed to indicate the numbers of fibers added to dishes (cpm = counts per minute). Reprinted with permission from Janssen et al. *(81).*

curs *(15).* Increased uptake of PAH or asbestos in the lung may also occur because both PAH and asbestos fibers impair normal lung clearance and induce ciliostasis, epithelial cell sloughing, and the induction of squamous metaplasia, a precancerous, but sometimes reversible lesion where normal mucociliary cells are converted to a flattened keratinizing epithelium *(16).* In addition to affecting the uptake and clearance of PAH directly, asbestos fibers also cause alterations in the aryl hydrocarbon hydroxylase (AHH) enzyme system responsible for detoxification and/or increased metabolism of PAH to carcinogenic forms.

Other documented properties of asbestos fibers after inhalation may be related to their capacity to act as tumor promoters, agents which may not initiate DNA lesions or carcinogenesis, but promote cancers after DNA mutations by PAH and other carcinogens. For example, inhalation or intratracheal instillation of asbestos causes inflammation, a process generating cytokines, chemokines, and reactive oxygen (ROS) and reactive nitrogen species (RNS) *(5).* These changes are typically observed after application of classical tumor promoters, such as 12-O-tetradecanoylphorbol 13-acetate (TPA) to mouse skin. In addition, asbestos fibers stimulate cell proliferation and a number of cell-signaling pathways related to induction of early-response genes and polyamine biosynthesis. These increases in cell proliferation may be critical to the promotion of lung carcinomas. The induction of squamous metaplasia by long asbestos fibers also occurs with increases in uptake of tritiated thymidine by basal cells of the tracheobronchial epithelium. Thus, fibers may stimulate proliferation of cells previously transformed by PAH *(17,18).* Co-exposures to asbestos and

cigarette smoke also cause more marked increases in squamous metaplasia and increased numbers of tracheal epithelial cells incorporating tritiated thymidine *(19).* This may represent a repair process after initial epithelial cell injury as sloughing epithelial-cells are noted within hours after exposure to fibers.

EARLY RESPONSE PROTO-ONCOGENES AND ASBESTOS-INDUCED PROLIFERATION AND APOPTOSIS

In attempting to identify how asbestos fibers induce cells to proliferate, we used progenitor cell types of mesothelioma and lung cancers, respectively, including isolates of rat pleural mesothelial cells (RPM), HTE cells, and a rat alveolar type II epithelial cell line (RLE). In brief, we addressed the hypothesis that interaction of asbestos fibers with the cell surface would initiate signaling cascades resulting in changes in early-response gene expression. Experiments showed dose-dependent increases in c-*fos* and c-*jun* steady state mRNA levels by both crocidolite and chrysotile asbestos in RPM cells, which were more protracted in time (first appearing at 8 and 24 h after exposure), in comparison to the more rapid changes (2 h or less) observed after addition of TPA (a positive control for gene expression changes) to the medium *(20).* Fig. 3 shows the quantitation of Northern-blot analyses by phosphorimaging in these experiments as a function of fiber number. The sharp dose response at lower concentrations of crocidolite asbestos indicates that this is a more potent type of asbestos in proto-oncogene induction. Results here also correlate with epidemiological evidence suggesting increased pathogenicity of crocidolite in the induction of human malignant mesothelioma *(4,6,8,10,11).*

Subsequent studies indicate that crocidolite exposure causes increases in c-*myc* expression *(21).* Moreover, a variety of nonfibrous analogs of asbestos and nonpathogenic particles, including latex and glass beads, do not induce increases in proto-oncogene expression in epithelial or mesothelial cells *(22).* The fact that carcinogenic fibers selectively stimulate early-response gene expression also was indicated by positive results with erionite fibers, which are more mesotheliomagenic than crocidolite asbestos fibers after inhalation by rodents or humans (23). In our studies, Na-erionite fibers caused significantly increased levels of c-*jun* mRNA at lower mass concentrations than crocidolite asbestos in RPM cells (24).

Members of the *Fos* and *Jun* protein family form heterodimers and homodimers that comprise the AP-1 transcription factor, which is associated with activation of a variety of intermediate-response genes. Accordingly, increased c-*fos* and c-*jun* expression in RPM and HTE cells occurs with increases in AP-1 binding to DNA and activation of AP-1-dependent gene expression (20,25). One AP-1 regulated gene is *odc* (ornithine decarboxylase), which encodes a rate-limiting enzyme in the biosynthesis of polyamines. These growth-regulatory molecules have been linked to proliferation, malignant transformation, and tumor promotion (26,27). Experiments with HTE cells indicate that *odc* mRNA levels and enzyme activity are increased in a dose-dependent fashion at time periods and concentrations of fibers when proliferation is observed (28,29). These changes are not observed with nonfibrous chemically similar analogs of asbestos, indicating the importance of fiber geometry. Increases in c-*jun* and *odc* mRNA levels are also observed in the lungs of rats inhaling crocidolite asbestos (30), verifying the relevance of our in vitro results in an animal model where proliferation of bronchiolar epithelial and mesothelial cells has been established (31). Our observation that overexpression of c-*jun* is associated with increased cell proliferation and morphologic transformation of tracheal epithelial cells further supports the role of this proto-oncogene in tumor promotion by asbestos (25).

Increased expression of early response proto-oncogenes is also linked to the development of apoptosis in a number of cell types. We recently demonstrated that apoptosis and cell proliferation, as measured by incorporation of 5'-bromodeoxyuridine (BrdU), occur simultaneously in mesothelial cells exposed to crocidolite asbestos (32,33). It is likely that the balance between cell proliferation and apoptosis is critical in the responses of the lung to mineral dusts and whether or not repair or disease occurs. For example, mesothelial cells exhibit proliferation but not apoptosis at comparable concentrations of erionite, a more pathogenic fiber than even crocidolite asbestos (24). Apoptosis has been documented in alveolar macrophages after exposure to silica (34), but it is unclear whether this occurs in vivo.

EXPRESSION OF PROTO-ONCOGENES AND TUMOR-SUPPRESSOR GENES IN ASBESTOS-ASSOCIATED LUNG CANCERS AND MESOTHELIOMAS

Activation of proto-oncogenes and/or inactivation of tumor-suppressor genes undoubtedly occur during the long period of development of asbestos-induced malignancies. However, there are no candidate proto-oncogenes nor tumor-suppressor genes clearly linked to the establishment of lung cancers or mesotheliomas. For example, lung tumors in smokers with and without occupational exposure to asbestos showed a high frequency (57%) of c-K-*ras* mutations in adenocarcinomas, which were significantly associated with lifetime smoking, but not

with occupational exposure to asbestos *per se* (35,36). Several laboratories have examined mutations in the tumor suppressor genes *p53*, *Rb1*, *WT1*, and the *NF2* gene. Unlike c-K-*ras* mutations, which appear to arise late in lung-tumor development, mutations of the *p53* gene are observed in preinvasive lesions of human bronchi and may be related to loss of cell cycle control (36). *p53* mutations have been observed in some human mesotheliomas (37,38), but pRb protein expression in these tumors is comparable to that occurring in normal human mesothelial lines (39). Immmunostaining for p53 proteins and the frequency of *p53* mutations in mesotheliomas do not appear to be linked to asbestos exposures (40).

Recurrent deletions of specific chromosomal segments on 1p, 3p, 6q, and 9p have been documented in human mesotheliomas, suggesting that these regions may reveal the locations of other tumor-suppressor genes whose loss or inactivation may play a role in the development of mesothelioma (41). Homozygous deletions of the *p16* gene has been observed in approx 22% of primary mesotheliomas (42), and two laboratories have identified somatic mutations of the *NF2* gene in mesotheliomas, but not lung cancers (43,44). How these *NF2* mutations contribute to the induction of mesothelioma or other tumors is unclear. Moreover, why mesothelioma is not an outcome of the hereditary disease related to *NF2* is another unanswered question.

CELL-SIGNALING PATHWAYS LEADING TO ASBESTOS-INDUCED PROLIFERATION AND APOPTOSIS

Activity of transcription factors is regulated by a number of signaling cascades involving phosphorylation and dephosphorylation of protein kinases. One pathway linked to early-response genes, proliferation, and apoptosis is the mitogen-activated protein kinase (MAPK) cascade, which includes the extracellular signal-related kinases (ERKs); the Jun amino-terminal kinases (JNKs), which are also called stress-activated protein kinases (SAPKs), and p38 (45). These pathways are activated in response to a number of growth factors and other stimuli and transduce signals received at the cell surface to the nucleus. In RPM cells, both crocidolite and chrysotile asbestos cause dose-related increases in ERK phosphorylation and activity in the absence of JNK and p38 activation. These increases, which are not observed with a variety of nonpathogenic fibers and particles, are observed prior to elevations in c-*fos* and c-*jun* mRNA levels.

In an attempt to determine upstream events, including whether asbestos fibers interact with growth-factor receptors on the cell surface to trigger ERK activation, we added growth factors to cultures of RPM cells to determine whether we could induce ERK activation. Epidermal growth factor (EGF) and transforming growth factor-α (TGF-α) induced ERK activity in these cells (46). However, other growth factors, including insulin-like growth factor (IGF) and platelet-derived growth factor (PDGF) did not activate ERK (46). Both EGF and TGF-α bind to the epidermal growth factor receptor (EGFR). Asbestos-induced ERK activity was also abolished when RPM cells were pretreated with suramin, an agent inducing internalization of growth-factor receptors, or the tyrphostin, AG1478, a

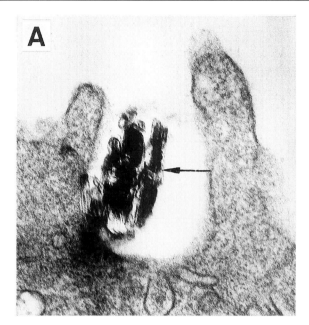
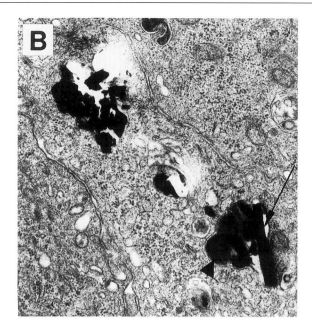

Fig. 4. Phagocytosis of asbestos fibers by tracheal epithelial cells in organ cultures. Transmission electron micrographs indicating uptake and phagocytosis of crocidolite asbestos fibers (arrows) in tracheal epithelial organ cultures. **(A)** shows uptake of fibers by a superficial epithelial cell. **(B)** indicates asbestos fibers in phagolysosomes stained for acid phosphatase (arrowhead).

specific inhibitor of the EGFR tyrosine kinase *(46)*. Subsequent studies have revealed that crocidolite asbestos stimulates autophosphorylation of the EGFR *(46)* and inhibits binding of EGF to the EGFR *(48)*. Moreover, fibers stimulate EGFR biosynthesis as documented by elevations in *EGFR* mRNA and protein levels *(48)*. To determine whether phosphorylation of the EGFR by asbestos was related to increases in c-*fos* and c-*jun* mRNA levels and apoptosis, AG1478 was used in comparative studies with the nonspecific tyrphostin (A10) *(48)*. Although asbestos-associated increases in c-*fos* mRNA levels could be diminished after pretreatment of RPM cells with AG1478, but not A10, c-*jun* levels were unaffected. AG1478 also significantly inhibited apoptosis. These results support our previously published studies showing that PD98059, an inhibitor of mitogen-activated protein kinase kinase (MEK1), an upstream regulator of ERK activity, inhibited apoptosis by asbestos *(47)*. Our data are unusual in that ERK activation by EGF and other stimuli are linked in most other cell types with proliferation, whereas JNK activation has been associated causally with apoptosis *(49,50)*. However, inhibition of EGFR activity using antisense approaches ameliorates cisplatin-induced apoptosis *(51)*, suggesting that pathways of apoptosis by other toxic agents involve EGFR-modulated signaling cascades. Whether AG1478 and transfection with dominant negative mutants of EGFR affect asbestos-induced proliferation of RPM cells is presently under investigation. It is likely that long asbestos fibers interact directly with the EGFR receptor on the cell surface as accumulation of the external domain of the EGFR protein is observed at sites of contact and internalization of crocidolite fibers >50 µm in length *(52)*. In contrast, glass fibers and shorter crocidolite asbestos fibers do not cause this clustering. The nuclear factor-κB (NF-κB) pathway represents another signaling cascade activated by asbestos fibers and may be related causally to cell survival *(53)* and/or inflammation *(54)*.

As summarized in a recent review *(5)*, asbestos activates a number of chemokines and cytokines that are key to the development of inflammation and pulmonary fibrosis. Because lung cancers develop in patients often exhibiting asbestosis, these lesions may promote or provide a favorable environment for tumor growth.

Work from our laboratory has demonstrated that crocidolite asbestos fibers activate NF-κB in RPM and HTE cells as evaluated by electrophoretic gel-mobility shift analyses and promoter reporter assays *(21,55)*. Moreover, we have shown increased localization of p65, the major transactivating component of NF-κB, in rat lungs after inhalation of asbestos *(55)*. Striking increases in p65 immunofluorescence are seen in bronchoalveolar epithelial cells at 5 d after inhalation of crocidolite or chrysotile asbestos. After 20 d, increased immunoreactivity of p65 is observed in fibrotic and inflammatory lesions. The functional ramifications of these changes are currently being explored using transgenic mice models.

ARE EFFECTS OF ASBESTOS FIBERS PHYSICAL OR MEDIATED BY REACTIVE OXYGEN AND NITROGEN SPECIES?

The more protracted effects of asbestos on cell signaling and induction of early-response gene expression in comparison to soluble agents such as TPA or EGF in vitro may be reflective of the time necessary for fibers to precipitate onto the cell surface and/or be phagocytized by cells. Early studies with tracheal organ cultures indicated that short fibers were phagocytized effectively by differentiated epithelial cells and incorporated in membrane-bound phagolysosomes *(56)* (Fig. 4). This occurs in lung after inhalation of fibers which in time are transported through intracellular or extracellular pathways to cells of the interstitium *(5)*. In contrast, long fibers (>10 µm in length) are cleared less effectively and can be encompassed

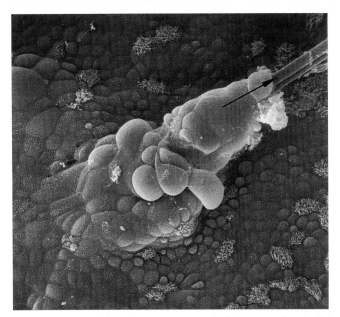

Fig. 5. Asbestos-induced squamous metaplasia in tracheal epithelial organ cultures. Scanning electron micrograph indicating the development of squamous metaplasia in a tracheal epithelial organ culture in response to long (>10 μm) asbestos fibers (arrow). Note how the squamous epithelial cells surround the fibers that are imbedded in the epithelium.

by proliferating epithelial cells (Fig. 5). Under these conditions, the epithelial cells undergo squamous metaplasia and increased uptake of tritiated thymidine *(17,18)*, suggesting that long fibers serve as physical matrices to support cell growth. These observations are consistent with data showing that long asbestos fibers preferentially induce cell transformation, proliferation of bronchoalveolar epithelial cells, lung tumors, and mesotheliomas in rodents *(57–59)*. Long fibers are also more fibrogenic in these animal models *(5)*.

The discovery that antioxidants ameliorated the toxicity of asbestos fibers in tracheal epithelial cells and mesothelial cells *(60,61)* suggested that oxidants played a key role in asbestos-associated biologic effects, a hypothesis confirmed by a number of laboratories. These free radical species can be catalyzed by redox reactions on the fiber surface *(62)* or released by cells after frustrated phagocytosis of longer fibers *(63)*. For example, iron on the surface of crocidolite fibers can drive the formation of hydroxyl radical, an extremely deleterious species initiating lipid peroxidation and DNA damage, from superoxide and hydrogen peroxide via the Haber-Weiss or Fenton reaction *(62)*. Pretreatment of crocidolite fibers with iron chelators modifies their toxicity *(60,61)* and ability to initiate the ERK cascade *(47)*. The demonstration that crocidolite asbestos induces oxidative DNA damage and repair in RPM cells *(64,65)*, and lipid peroxidation in lung after inhalation *(66)*, lends further support to the theory that ROS mediate the acute effects of asbestos. Moreover, studies showing amelioration of asbestos-induced inflammation and pulmonary fibrosis in rats after implantation of mini-pumps containing polyethylene-glycol (PEG) conjugated catalase support a direct role of ROS in lung disease *(67)*.

Both crocidolite and chrysotile asbestos also stimulate production of RNS from alveolar macrophages *in vitro* and after inhalation *(68)*, a phenomenon correlating temporally with increased inflammation. Fig. 6 shows a hypothetical sequence of early events in the respiratory tract ,which may occur after inhalation of asbestos or silica and trigger the production of chemokines such as macrophage inflammatory proteins (MIP-1, MIP-2), inflammatory mediators TNF-α, and the interleukins. These agents also induce oxidative stress, perpetuate the inflammatory process *(5)*, and induce mitogenesis of lung epithelial cells (unpublished data). Although silica has not been shown to induce oxidative DNA damage in cells or genotoxicity *(2)*, freshly fractured dust may generate oxidants that elicit the cascades depicted in Fig. 6 *(69)*.

The fact that antioxidant status is important in signal-transduction cascades elicited by asbestos is supported by studies showing amelioration of c-*fos* and c-*jun* expression after pretreatment of RPM cells with N-acetylcysteine (NAC) *(70)*. Increases in binding to the NF-κB DNA sequence by crocidolite asbestos was also abolished in these studies indicating that the redox status of the cell is also important in this signaling pathway *(21)*. Recent work by other laboratories have also revealed the importance of the hydroxyl radical and lipid peroxidation in NF-κB activation by asbestos and silica *(71–75)*. Understanding the relationship of these asbestos-associated signaling pathways to the development of lung cancer and mesothelioma will be critical in designing therapeutic strategies for these tumors.

THERAPEUTIC APPROACHES TO MESOTHELIOMA

Asbestos is one of several etiologic agents associated with the development of lung cancers. However, the majority of mesotheliomas are associated with occupational exposures to asbestos and are unique neoplasms in this regard. Unfortunately, the prognosis for mesothelioma is poor *(6)*. However, recent reports indicate some success in reducing the progression of early stage tumors after injection of recombinant human interferon-γ (IFN-γ) into the pleural cavity of patients *(76,77)*. In addition to its immunomodulatory effects, IFN-γ causes growth inhibition of some mesothelioma cell lines *(78)*. In lines in which IFN-γ inhibited proliferation, the janus kinase 2 (JAK2) and signal transducer and activator of transcription 1 (STAT1) were phosphorylated and accompanied by STAT1 binding to DNA, suggesting that the effects of IFN-γ on proliferation were mediated through activation of JAK/STAT signaling cascades *(78)*.

Another promising treatment strategy for mesothelioma is gene therapy. In this regimen, the herpes simplex virus thymidine kinase (HSV-*tk*) gene confers drug sensitivity to cells through enzymatic phosphorylation of the antiviral agent, acyclovir, and its derivative, ganciclovir. The HSV-*tk* gene is delivered to cells with an adenoviral vector and appears successful in causing mesothelioma cell death and increased survival in an animal model of mesothelioma *(79)*. A cell-based HSV-*tk* gene delivery approach using gene-modified tumor cells also appears to be promising in killing mesothelioma cells

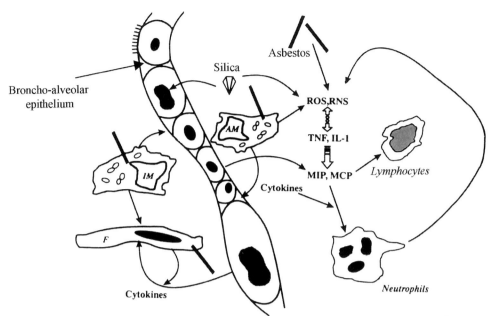

Fig. 6. Early events occurring in the lung after inhalation of asbestos fibers or freshly fractured silica. These minerals generate reactive oxygen/ reactive nitrogen species (ROS/RNS), which then cause increased production of TNF-α and IL-1 from cells leading to increased elaboration of chemokines (MIP, MCP, and others), cytokines, and an inflammatory response. Note that fibers and particles are cycled in the lung and interact with a variety of lung cells, including alveolar macrophages (AM), interstitial macrophages (IM), and fibroblasts (F). Adapted with permission from Mossman and Churg (5).

in vitro and in prolonging survival of mice with malignant mesothelioma (80).

SUMMARY AND CONCLUSIONS

Physical agents including the heterogeneous minerals, asbestos and crystalline silica, are insoluble in lung and not metabolized by cells. However, silicic acid and other chemical components of these particulates, such as magnesium, a major component of chrysotile asbestos, can be leached from fibers over time, leading to their fragmentation in lung tissue. The chemical composition of these minerals and iron-driven redox reactions on the surface of asbestos fibers, particularly the most pathogenic forms, crocidolite and amosite, can also lead to oxidant generation. Experiments from a number of laboratories indicate that ROS and RNS may mediate the toxic, fibrogenic, and carcinogenic effects of asbestos. Although less emphasis has been placed on silica, this mineral can generate ROS when freshly fractured, and the early inflammatory and fibrogenic events in lung may be similar mechanistically to those observed after inhalation of asbestos (Fig. 6). In this regard, chemokines and cytokines released by cells of the immune system, epithelial cells, and fibroblasts in response to these agents may be crucial to the establishment of cell proliferation and fibrogenesis. Whether or not asbestos or silica is a carcinogen in human lung cancers in the absence of smoking is questionable, especially for the latter mineral, which is not genotoxic in a variety of bioassays (2). However, crocidolite and amosite asbestos induce mesotheliomas in man, and the amphibole asbestos tremolite, which contaminates many chrysotile ores, may be the causal agent in mesotheliomas associated with exposure to chrysotile (4,6–11). Because the durability of crocidolite, amosite, and tremolite asbestos fibers far exceeds that of

chrysotile, the physical persistence of these fibers in human lungs may explain, in part, their carcinogenic potential (3).

The molecular basis of asbestos-induced lung cancers and mesotheliomas is complex and poorly defined. As discussed earlier, conventional proto-oncogenes and alterations in tumor-suppressor genes are not observed in the majority of these tumors. Both crocidolite and chrysotile asbestos are genotoxic in rodent cells, but human cells have yielded disparate results (4,6,13). An alternative scenario to direct damage of DNA by asbestos is that fibers either generate ROS and/or interact directly with growth factor receptors, causing phosphorylation of these and other proteins at the cell surface. These events then trigger a number of signaling cascades that regulate transcription of early response proto-oncogenes and other genes that may play a role in initiating or promoting carcinogenesis. Two morphologic features that are causally related to asbestos-associated stimulation of c-*jun* and c-*fos* by asbestos are proliferation and apoptosis, respectively. The knowledge that asbestos fibers induce oxidative stress and initiate signaling pathways with phenotypic endpoints that are blocked using antioxidants and other pharmacologic agents may be valuable in designing preventive and therapeutic approaches to lung cancers and mesotheliomas.

ACKNOWLEDGMENTS

We thank Laurie Sabens for assistance with typing, Michael Jung and Andrew Cummins for illustrative materials, and Dr. Raymond Robledo for proofreading and editorial suggestions. Research in the Environmental Pathology Program and Dr. Mossman's laboratory is supported by R01s and a T32 grant from the National Institute of Environmental Health Sciences and grants from the National Heart, Lung and Blood Institute.

REFERENCES

1. Maroudas, N. G., O'Neill, C. H., and Stanton, M. F. (1973) Fibroblast anchorage in carcinogenesis by fibers. *Lancet* **1**:807–809.

2. IARC. Silica, some silicates, coal dust and para-aramid fibrils. (1997) IARC Monographs on the Evaluation of Carcinogenic Risks to Humans, vol. 68, Lyon, France.

3. Guthrie, G. D., Jr., and Mossman, B. T. (eds.) (1993) *Health Effects of Mineral Dusts, Reviews in Mineralogy*, vol. 28 (Ribbe, P. H., ed.), Mineralogical Society of America, Washington, DC.

4. Mossman, B. T., Bignon, J., Corn, M., Seaton, A., and Gee, J. B. L. (1990) Asbestos: scientific developments and implications for public policy. *Science* **247**:294–301.

5. Mossman, B. T. and Churg, A. (1998) State-of-the-Art: mechanisms in the pathogenesis of asbestosis and silicosis. *Am. J. Respir. Crit. Care Med.* **157**:1666–1680.

6. Mossman, B. T., Kamp, D. W., and Weitzman, S. A. (1996) Mechanisms of carcinogenesis and clinical features of asbestos-associated cancers. *Cancer Invest.* **14**:466–480.

7. Price, B. (1997) Analysis of current trends in United States mesothelioma incidence. *Am. J. Epidemiol.* **145**:211–218.

8. McDonald, J. C. and McDonald, A. D. (1996) The epidemiology of mesothelioma in historical context. *Eur. Respir. J.* **9**:1932–1942.

9. Camus, M, Siemiatycki, J., and Meek, B. (1998) Nonoccupational exposure to chrysotile asbestos and the risk of lung cancer. *N. Engl. J. Med.* **338**:1565–1571.

10. Churg, A. (1988) Chrysotile, tremolite, and malignant mesothelioma in man. *Chest* **93**:621–628.

11. Mossman, B. T. and Gee, J. B. L. (1989) Medical progress. Asbestos-related diseases. *N. Engl. J. Med.* **320**:1721–1730.

12. Weill, H. and McDonald, J. C. (1996) Exposure to crystalline silica and risk of lung cancer: the epidemiological evidence. *Thorax* **51**:97–102.

13. Kodama, Y., Boreiko, C. J., Maness, S. C., and Hesterberg, T. W. (1993) Cytotoxic and cytogenetic effects of asbestos on human bronchial epithelial cells in culture. *Carcinogenesis* **14**:691–697.

14. Mossman, B. T., Eastman, A., Landesman, J. M., and Bresnick, E. (1983) Effects of crocidolite and chrysotile asbestos on cellular uptake, metabolism and DNA after exposure of hamster tracheal epithelial cells to benzo(a)pyrene. *Environ. Health Perspect.* **51**:331–335.

15. Eastman, A., Mossman, B. T., and Bresnick, E. (1983) Influence of asbestos on the uptake and benzo(a)pyrene and DNA alkylation in hamster tracheal epithelial cells. *Cancer Res.* **43**:1251–1255.

16. McFadden, D., Wright, J. L., Wiggs, B., and Churg, A. (1986) Smoking inhibits asbestos clearance. *Am. Rev. Respir. Dis.* **133**:372–374.

17. Mossman, B. T., Craighead, J. E., and MacPherson, B. V. (1980) Asbestos-induced epithelial changes in organ cultures of hamster trachea: Inhibition by retinyl methyl ether. *Science* **207**:311–313.

18. Woodworth, C. D., Mossman, B. T., and Craighead, J. E. (1983) Induction of squamous metaplasia in organ cultures of hamster trachea by naturally occurring and synthetic fibers. *Cancer Res.* **43**:4906–4912.

19. Mossman, B. T., Eastman, A., and Bresnick, E. (1984) Asbestos and benzo[a]pyrene act synergistically to induce squamous metaplasia and incorporation of [3H]thymidine in hamster tracheal epithelium. *Carcinogenesis* **5**:1401–1404.

20. Heintz, N. H., Janssen, Y. M. W., and Mossman, B. T. (1993) Persistent induction of c-*fos* and c-*jun* expression by asbestos. *Proc. Natl. Acad. Sci. USA* **90**:3299–3303.

21. Janssen, Y. M. W., Barchowsky, A., Treadwell, M., Driscoll, K. E., and Mossman, B. T. (1995) Asbestos induces nuclear factor κB (NF-κB) DNA-binding activity and NF-κB-dependent gene expression in tracheal epithelial cells. *Proc. Natl. Acad. Sci. USA* **92**:8458–8462.

22. Janssen, Y. M. W., Heintz, N. H., Marsh, J. P., Borm, P. J. A., and Mossman, B. T. (1994) Induction of c-*fos* and c-*jun* protooncogenes in target cells of the lung and pleura by carcinogenic fibers. *Am. J. Respir. Cell Mol. Biol.* **11**:522–530.

23. Wagner, J. C., Skidmore, J. W., Hill, R. J., and Griffiths, D. M. (1985) Erionite exposure and mesothelioma in rats. *Br. J. Cancer* **51**:727–730.

24. Timblin, C. R., Guthrie, G. D., Janssen, Y. M. W., Walsh, E. S., Vacek, P., and Mossman, B. T. (1998) Patterns of c-*fos* and c-*jun* proto-oncogene expression, apoptosis, and proliferation in rat pleural mesothelial cells exposed to erionite or asbestos fibers. *Toxicol. Appl. Pharmacol.* **151**:88–97.

25. Timblin, C. R., Janssen, Y. M. W., and Mossman, B. T. (1995) Transcriptional activation of the proto-oncogene c-*jun*, by asbestos and H_2O_2 is directly related to increased proliferation and transformation of tracheal epithelial cells. *Cancer Res.* **55**:2723–2726.

26. Auvinen, M., Paasinen, A., Andersson, L. C., and Holtta, E. (1992) Ornithine decarboxylase activity is critical for cell transformation. *Nature* **360**:355–358.

27. Soler, A. P., Gilliard, G., Megosh, L., George, K., and O'Brien, T. G. (1998) Polyamines regulate expression of the neoplastic phenotype in mouse skin. *Cancer Res.* **58**:1654–1659.

28. Marsh, J. P. and Mossman, B. T. (1988) Mechanisms of induction of ornithine decarboxylase activity in tracheal epithelial cells by asbestiform minerals. *Cancer Res.* **48**:709–714.

29. Marsh, J. P. and Mossman, B. T. (1991) Role of asbestos and active oxygen species in activation and expression of ornithine decarboxylase in hamster tracheal epithelial cells. *Cancer Res.* **51**:167–173.

30. Quinlan, T. R., Marsh, J. P., Janssen, Y. M. W., Leslie, K. O., Hemenway, D., Vacek, P., et al. (1994) Dose responsive increases in pulmonary fibrosis after inhalation of asbestos. *Am. J. Respir. Crit. Care Med.* **150**:200–206.

31. BeruBe, K. A., Quinlan, T. R., Moulton, G., Hemenway, D., O'Shaughnessy, P., Vacek, P., et al. (1996) Comparative proliferative and histopathologic changes in rat lungs after inhalation of chrysotile or crocidolite asbestos. *Toxicol. Appl. Pharmacol.* **137**:67–74.

32. BeruBe, K. A., Quinlan, T. R., Fung, H., Magae, J., Vacek, P., Taatjes, D. J., et al. (1996). Apoptosis is observed in mesothelial cells after exposure to crocidolite asbestos. *Am. J. Respir. Cell Mol. Biol.* **15**:141–147.

33. Goldberg, J. L., Zanella, C. L., Janssen, Y. M. W., Timblin, C. R., Jimenez, L. A., Vacek, P., et al. (1997) Novel cell imaging approaches show induction of apoptosis and proliferation in mesothelial cells by asbestos. *Am. J. Respir. Cell Mol. Biol.* **17**:265–271.

34. Iyer, R. Hamilton, R. F., Li, L., and Holian, A. (1996) Silica-induced apoptosis mediated via scavenger receptor in human alveolar macrophages. *Toxicol. Appl. Pharmacol.* **141**:84–92.

35. Husgafvel-Pursiainen, K., Hackman, P., Ridanpaa, M., Anttila, S., Karjalainen, A., Partanen, T., et al. (1993) K-ras mutations in human adenocarcinoma of the lung: association with smoking and occupational exposure to asbestos. *Int. J. Cancer* **53**:250–256.

36. Sundaresan, V., Ganly, P., Hasleton, P., Rudd, R., Sinha, G., Bleehen, N. M., et al. (1992) p53 and chromosome 3 abnormalities, characteristic of malignant lung tumors, are detectable in preinvasive lesions of the bronchus. *Oncogene* **7**:1989–1997.

37. Cote, R. J., Jhanwar, S. C., Novick, S., and Pellicer, A. (1991) Genetic alterations of the p53 gene are a feature of malignant mesotheliomas. *Cancer Res.* **51**:5410–5416.

38. Metcalf, R. A., Welsh, J. A., Bennett, W. P., Seddon, W. B., Lehman, T. A., Pelin, K., et al. (1991) p53 and Kirsten-ras mutations in human mesothelioma cell lines. *Cancer Res.* **52**:2610–2615.

39. Van der Meeren, A., Seddon, M. B., Kispert, J., Harris, C. C., and Gerwin, B. I. (1993) Lack of expression of the retinoblasoma gene is not frequently involved in the genesis of human mesothelioma. *Eur. Respir. Rev.* **3**:177–179.

40. Mayall, F. G., Goddard, H., and Gibbs, A. R. (1993) The frequency of p53 immunostaining in asbestos-associated mesotheliomas and non-asbestos-associated mesotheliomas. *Histopathol.* **22**:383–386.

41. Taguchi, T., Jhanwar, S. C., Siegfried, J. M., Keller, S. M., and Testa, J. R. (1993) Recurrent deletions of specific chromosomal sites in 1p, 3p, 6q, and 9p in human malignant mesothelioma. *Cancer Res.* **53**:4349–4355.

42. Cheng, J. Q., Jhanwar, S. C., Klein, W. M., Bell, D. W., Lee, W. C., Altomare, D. A., et al. (1994) p16 alterations and deletion mapping of 9p21-p22 in malignant mesothelioma. *Cancer Res.* **54**:5547–5551.
43. Sekido, Y., Pass, H. I., Bader, S., Mew, D. Y., Christman, M. F., Gazdar, A. F., et al. (1995) Neurofibromatosis type 2 (NF2) gene is somatically mutated in mesothelioma but not in lung cancer. *Cancer Res.* **55**:1227–1231.
44. Bianchi, A. B., Mitsunaga, S. I., Cheng, J. Q., Klein, W. M., Jhanwar, S. C., Seizinger, B., et al. (1995) High frequency of inactivating mutations in the neurofibromatosis type 2 gene (NF2) in primary malignant mesotheliomas. *Proc. Natl. Acad. Sci. USA* **92**:10854–10858.
45. Su, B. and Karin, M. (1996) Mitogen-activated protein kinase cascades and regulation of gene expression. *Curr. Opin. Immunol.* **8**:402–411.
46. Zanella, C. L., Posada, J., Tritton, T. R., and Mossman, B. T. (1996) Asbestos causes stimulation of the ERK-1 mitogen-activated protein kinase cascade after phosphorylation of the epidermal growth factor receptor. *Cancer Res.* **56**:5334–5338.
47. Jimenez, L. A., Zanella, C., Fung, H., Janssen, Y. M. W., Vacek, P., Charland, C., et al. (1997) Role of extracellular signal-regulated protein kinases in apoptosis by asbestos and H₂O₂. *Am. J. Physiol.* **273**:L1029–L1035.
48. Zanella, C. L., Timblin, C. R., Cummins, A., Jung, M., Goldberg, J., Raabe, R., et al. (1999) Asbestos-induced phosphorylation and biosynthesis of the epidermal growth factor receptor (EGF-R) is linked causally to c-fos expression and apoptosis in mesothelial cells. *Am. J. Physiol.* **277**:L684–L693.
49. Xia, Z., Dickens, M., Raingeaud, J., Davis, R. J., and Greenberg, M. E. (1995) Opposing effects of ERK and JNK-p38 MAP kinases on apoptosis. *Science* **270**:1326–1331.
50. Chen, Y. R., Meyer, C. F., and Tan, T. H. (1996) Persistent activation of c-Jun N-terminal kinase 1 (JNK1) in γ radiation-induced apoptosis. *J. Biol. Chem.* **271**:631–634.
51. Dixit, M., Yang, J., Poirier, M. C., Price, J. O., Andrews, P. A., and Arteaga, C. L. (1997) Abrogation of cisplatin-induced programmed cell death in human breast cancer cells by epidermal growth factor antisense RNA. *J. Natl. Cancer Inst.* **89**:365–373.
52. Pache, J. C., Janssen, Y. M. W., Walsh, E. S., Quinlan, T. R., Zanella, C. L., Low, R. B., et al. (1998) Increased epidermal growth factor-receptor protein in a human mesothelial cell line in response to long asbestos fibers. *Am. J. Pathol.* **152**:333–340.
53. Beg, A. A. and Baltimore, D. (1996) An essential role for NF-κB in preventing TNF-α-induced cell death. *Science* **274**:782–784.
54. Blackwell, T. S., Holden, E. P., Blackwell, T. R., DeLarco, J. E., and Christman, J. W. (1994) Cytokine-induced neutrophil chemoattractant mediates neutrophilic alveolitis in rats: association with nuclear factor κ B activation. *Am. J. Respir. Cell Mol. Biol.* **11**:464–472.
55. Janssen, Y. M. W., Driscoll, K. E., Howard, B., Quinlan, T. R., Treadwell, M., Barchowsky, A., et al. (1997) Asbestos causes translocation of p65 protein and increases NF-κB DNA binding activity in rat lung epithelial and pleural mesothelial cells. *Am. J. Pathol.* **151**:389–401.
56. Mossman, B. T., Kessler, J. B., Ley, B. W., and Craighead, J. E. (1977) Interaction of crocidolite asbestos with hamster respiratory mucosa in organ culture. *Lab. Invest.* **36**:131–139.
57. Adamson, I. Y. and Bowden, D. H. (1987) Response of mouse lung to crocidolite asbestos. 1. Minimal fibrotic reaction to short fibres. *J. Pathol.* **152**:99–107.
58. Oshimura, M., Hesterberg, T. W., Tsutsui, T., and Barrett, J. C. (1984) Correlation of asbestos-induced cytogenetic effects with cell transformation of Syrian hamster embryo cells in culture. *Cancer Res.* **44**:5017–5022.
59. Stanton, M. F., Layard, M., Tegeris, A., Miller, E., May, M., Morgan, E., et al. (1981) Relation of particle dimension to carcinogenicity in amphibole asbestoses and other fibrous minerals. *J. Natl. Cancer Inst.* **67**:965–975.
60. Mossman, B. T., Marsh, J. P., and Shatos, M. A. (1986) Alteration of superoxide dismutase (SOD) activity in tracheal epithelial cells by asbestos and inhibition of cytotoxicity by antioxidants. *Lab. Invest.* **54**:204–212.
61. Goodglick, L. A. and Kane, A. B. (1990) Cytotoxicity of long and short crocidolite asbestos fibers in vitro and in vivo. *Cancer Res.* **50**:5153–5163.
62. Weitzman, S. A. and Graceffa, P. (1984) Asbestos catalyzes hydroxyl and superoxide radical generation from hydrogen peroxide. *Arch. Biochem. Biophys.* **228**:373–376.
63. Hansen, K. and Mossman, B. T. (1987) Generation of superoxide (O⁻₂) from alveolar macrophages exposed to asbestiform and nonfibrous particles. *Cancer Res.* **47**:1681–1686.
64. Fung, H., Kow, Y. W., Van Houten, B., and Mossman, B. T. (1997) Patterns of 8-hydroxydeoxyguanosine (8OHdG) formation in DNA and indications of oxidative stress in rat and human pleural mesothelial cells after exposure to crocidolite asbestos. *Carcinogenesis* **18**:101–108.
65. Fung, H., Quinlan, T. R., Janssen, Y. M. W., Timblin, C. R., Marsh, J. P., Heintz, N. H., et al. (1997) Inhibition of protein kinase C (PKC) prevents asbestos-induced c-fos and c-jun protooncogene expression in mesothelial cells. *Cancer Res.* **57**:3101–3105.
66. Petruska, J. M., Wong, S. H., Sunderman, F. W., and Mossman, B. T. (1990) Detection of lipid peroxidation in lung and in bronchoalveolar lavage cells and fluid. *Free Rad. Biol. Med.* **9**:51–58.
67. Mossman, B. T., Marsh, J. P., Sesko, A., Hill, S., Shatos, M. A., Doherty, J., et al. (1990) Inhibition of lung injury, inflammation and interstitial pulmonary fibrosis by polyethylene glycol-conjugated catalase in a rapid inhalation model of asbestosis. *Am. Rev. Respir. Dis.* **141**:1266–1271.
68. Quinlan, T. R., Hacker, M. P., Taatjes, D., Timblin, C., Goldberg, J., Kimberley, P., et al. (1998) Mechanisms of asbestos-induced nitric oxide production by rat alveolar macrophages in inhalation and in vitro models. *Free Radic. Biol. Med.* **24**:778–788.
69. Vallyathan, V., Shi, X., Dalal, N. S., Irr, W., and Castranova, V. (1988) Generation of free radicals from freshly fractured silica dust: potential role in acute silica-induced lung injury. *Am. Rev. Respir. Dis.* **138**:1213–1219.
70. Janssen, Y. M., Heintz, N. H., and Mossman, B. T. (1995) Induction of c-fos and c-jun proto-oncogene expression by asbestos is ameliorated by N-acetyl-L-cysteine in mesothelial cells. *Cancer Res.* **55**:2085–2089.
71. Gilmour, P. S., Brown, D. M., Beswick, P. H., MacNee, W., Rahman, I., and Donaldson, K. (1997) Free radical activity of industrial fibers: role of iron in oxidative stress and activation of transcription factors. *Environ. Health Perspect.* **105**:1313–1317.
72. Chen, F., Lu, Y., Demers, L. M., Rojanasakul, Y., Shi, X., Vallyathan, V., et al. (1998) Role of hydroxyl radical in silica-induced NF-κB activation in macrophages. *Ann. Clin. Lab. Sci.* **28**:1–13.
73. Faux, S. P. and Howden, P. J. (1997) Possible role of lipid peroxidation in the induction of NF-κB and AP-1 in RFL-6 cells by crocidolite asbestos: evidence following protection by vitamin E. *Environ. Health Perspect.* **105**:1127–1130.
74. Simeonova, P. P., Toriumi, W., Kommineni, C., Erkan, M., Munson, A. E., Rom, W. N., et al. (1997). Molecular regulation of IL-6 activation by asbestos in lung epithelial cells. Role of reactive oxygen species. *J. Immunol.* **159**:3921–3928.
75. Simeonova, P. P. and Luster, M. I. (1996) Asbestos induction of nuclear transcription factors and interleukin 8 gene regulation. *Am. J. Respir. Cell Mol. Biol.* **15**:787–795.
76. Boutin, C., Viallat, J. R., Van Zandwijk, N., Douillard, J. Y., Paillard, J. C., Guerin, J. C., et al. (1991) Activity of intrapleural recombinant α-interferon in malignant mesothelioma. *Cancer* **67**:2033–2037.
77. Boutin, C., Nussbaum, E., Monnet, I., Bignon, J., Vanderschueren, R., Guerin, J. C., et al. (1994) Intrapleural treatment with recombinant α-interferon in early stage malignant pleural mesothelioma. *Cancer* **74**:2460–2467.

78. Buard, A., Vivo, C., Monnet, I., Boutin, C., Pilatte, Y., and Jaurand, M. C. (1998) Human malignant mesothelioma cell growth: activation of janis kinase 2 and signal transducer and activator of transcription 1α for inhibition by interferon-γ. *Cancer Res.* **58**, 840–847.

79. Elshami, A. A., Kucharczuk, J. C., Zhang, H. B., Smythe, W. R., Hwang, H. C., Litzky, L. A., et al. (1996) Treatment of pleural mesothelioma in an immunocompetent rat model utilizing adenoviral transfer of the herpes simplex virus thymidine kinase gene. *Hum. Gene Ther.* **7**:141–148.

80. Schwarzenberger, P., Lei, D., Freeman, S. M., Ye, P., Weinacker, A., Theodossiou, C., et al. (1998) Antitumor activity with the HSV-tk-gene-modified cell line PA-1-STK in malignant mesothelioma. *Am. J. Respir. Cell Mol. Biol.* **19**:333–337.

81. Janssen, Y., Marsh, J., Quinlan, T., Timblin, C., Berube, K., Jimenez, L., et al. (1994) Activation of early cellular responses by asbestos: Induction of c-*fos* and c-*jun* protooncogene expression in rat pleural mesothelial cells. *In: Cellular and Molecular Effects of Mineral and Synthetic Dusts and Fibres* (Davis, J. M. G. and Jaurand, M. C., eds.), NATO-ASI Series, Springer-Verlag, Berlin, pp. 205–213.

12 Viral Mechanisms of Human Carcinogenesis

Felix Hoppe-Seyler, MD and Karin Butz, PhD

INTRODUCTION

Within the last two decades of cancer research, it has become increasingly clear that viruses play an important role in the development of a significant percentage of human cancers. At present, it is recognized that viral infections are linked to at least 15% of all malignant tumors in humans and thus represent the second most common identified risk factor for cancer, exceeded only by tobacco smoking *(1)*. Cancer-associated viruses are found in several virus families and encompass both DNA and RNA viruses (Table 1). In the past few years, significant progress has been made towards elucidation of the molecular mechanisms through which viruses contribute to cell transformation. Different tumor viruses target common cellular pathways for growth control, but also exhibit unique (virus-specific) properties that contribute to oncogenesis.

HUMAN PAPILLOMAVIRUSES

Human papillomaviruses (HPV) are small, nonenveloped DNA viruses with a circular double-stranded genome of approx 8 kb. They are highly species-specific and strictly epitheliotropic. Based on sequence differences within the L1 open reading frame (ORF) (which codes for a structural viral protein), more than 140 different HPV types have been classified to date *(2,3)*. Research on HPV biology has been hampered for a long time by the lack of an appropriate tissue-culture system for virus propagation. However, tissue-culture systems have been recently developed, allowing productive replication of several HPV types *in vitro* (4,5).

HPVs are causative agents for benign proliferative lesions, including skin warts (e.g. types HPV2 and HPV4) and genital warts (e.g. types HPV6 and HPV11). Other, high-risk HPV types (in particular HPV16 and HPV18) are strongly associated with the development of human cancers *(2)*. Most notable is their association with the development of cervical cancer, which represents the second most common cancer in females worldwide, with more than 400,000 new cases diagnosed annually and over 200,000 deaths per year *(6)*.

Most cervical carcinomas develop in the transformation zone of the cervix, located between the columnar cells of the endocervix and the squamous epithelium of the vagina. Typically, there is a long latency period between initial infection and cancer development, usually within the range of several decades. Histologically, cervical cancer is usually preceeded by dysplastic lesions, including low-grade and high-grade squamous intraepithelial lesions (SIL), or cervical intraepithelial neoplasia (CIN) grades 1–3. These dysplastic lesions can either regress, persist, or progress to cancer, which occurs in a minority of cases. The cytological detection of dysplastic cells (Pap smear) in screening programs has dramatically reduced the incidence of cervical cancer in the Western world, as it facilitates the early clinical management of lesions with potential for neoplastic progression.

Case-control and prospective epidemiological studies have shown that HPV infection preceedes high-grade dysplasia and invasive cancer, and represents the strongest independent risk factor for the development of cervical cancer *(7–9)*. Analyses of cervical cancers on the molecular level also emphazise that HPV plays a key role in cervical carcinogenesis. More than 90% of cervical-cancer biopsies contain DNA sequences of high-risk HPV types. Within these biopsies, the viral DNA is present in every tumor cell and is also found in metastases derived from these tumors. Most HPV-associated cervical cancers carry the viral DNA integrated into the cellular chromosomes at one or multiple loci *(2,3)*. There is strong evidence that the transforming activities of HPVs are dependent on the expression of two viral early genes, designated E6 and E7. This can be deduced from several observations: 1) although the viral integrants can show substantial rearrangements or deletions within their genomes, the E6 and E7 genes are always retained and intact within HPV-positive tumors; 2) the E6/E7 genes are regularly expressed both in HPV-positive tumors and in de-

From: *The Molecular Basis of Human Cancer* (W. B. Coleman and G. J. Tsongalis, eds.), © Humana Press Inc., Totowa, NJ.

Table 1
Human Tumor Viruses

Virus	Virus family	Genome type	Genome characteristics	Associated human cancers
Human Papilloma Virus (HPV)	Papovaviridae	DNA	~8 kb Circular double-stranded	Anogenital, skin, and oral cancers, others?
Hepatitis B Virus (HBV)	Hepadnaviridae	DNA	3.2 kb Circular partial double-stranded	Hepatocellular carcinoma
Hepatitis C Virus (HCV)	Flaviviridae	RNA	9.4 kb Linear single-stranded	Hepatocellular carcinoma
Epstein-Barr Virus (EBV)	Herpesviridae	DNA	~172 kb Linear double-stranded	Nasopharyngeal carcinoma Burkitts lymphoma Hodgkins lymphoma B-cell and T-cell lymphomas Stomach cancer (?)
Human Herpesvirus 8 (HHV8)	Herpesviridae	DNA	~160–170 kb Linear double-stranded	Kaposi's Sarcoma Body-cavity lymphoma Multiple myeloma (?)
Human T Cell Lymphotropic Virus-1 (HTLV-1)	Retroviridae	RNA	9 kb Linear single-stranded (2 molecules)	Adult T-cell leukemia

rived cell lines, such as the well-known HeLa cervical carcinoma cell line *(10)*; 3) both E6 and E7 possess transforming potential in various experimental settings *(2,3)*; and 4) experimental inhibition of E6/E7 expression using sequence-specific anti-sense constructs has been shown to result in the loss of the tumorigenic phenotype of cervical cancer cell lines *(11)*.

Transcription of the HPV E6/E7 oncogenes initiates from a common promoter and is controlled by a variety of host-cell transcription factors, which bind to the viral transcriptional control region *(12)*. Interestingly, *in situ* hybridization studies have revealed that only very low amounts of viral E6/E7 transcripts (if any at all) can be detected in the proliferating basal cells of early dysplastic lesions. However, in later stages of dysplasia and invasive cancers E6/E7 transcripts are clearly detectable in the proliferative cells of the lesion *(13)*. Thus, loss of host-cell control of viral E6/E7 transcription, which normally restricts E6/E7 expression levels in basal cells, could result in the deregulated expression of the viral oncogenes and may be an important step during progression of HPV-associated carcinogenesis *(2)*. In addition, the integration event could also contribute to increased viral E6/E7 expression. Usually, HPV integration results in the disruption of the viral E2 gene, which codes for a transcriptional repressor of the HPV16 and HPV18 *E6/E7* promoter *(14)*. Thus, the lack of this negative regulator may result in increased *E6/E7* expression. Moreover, the integration event can lead to the stabilization of the *E6/E7* mRNA by removing negative regulatory elements from its 3′-terminus *(15)*.

Much progress has been recently made in understanding the transforming activities of the E6 and E7 oncoproteins on the molecular level *(16–18)*. Mediated by a cellular protein, called E6AP (for E6-associated protein), the E6 protein of high-risk HPVs forms a complex with the p53 tumor-suppressor protein and can induce the degradation of p53 via ubiquitin-mediated proteolysis *(19)*. The p53 protein is thought to play an important role for the maintenance of the genomic stability in the cell

(20–22). Following DNA damage, the endogenous p53 levels of a normal cell increase (Fig. 1). By activating transcription of cellular target genes, such as $p21^{WAF1}$ *(23)*, p53 can induce cell-cycle arrest in G_1. This provides the cell with enough time to efficiently correct the acquired DNA lesion, before it is converted to a mutation during DNA replication in the following S-phase. Alternatively, the p53-mediated response to DNA damage can result in apoptotic cell death. DNA damage-induced apoptosis may involve p53-mediated transcriptional activation of the *bax* gene *(24)* as well as p53-transactivation-independent pathways *(25)*. Thus, p53 is thought to prevent the emergence of genetically altered cells by allowing efficient repair of DNA lesions or by eliminating genetically altered cells via apoptosis *(20,22)*.

By its ability to degrade p53 and inhibit its function, the interaction of E6 with wild-type p53 may have the same effect as the functional inactivation of p53 by somatic mutation. Indeed, in experimental cell systems, co-expression of high-risk E6 can result in the inhibition of p53-mediated transactivation *(26,27)*, as well as in the loss of p53-associated responses to genotoxic stress *(28)* and in genetic instability *(29)*. In line with the interpretation that the expression of E6 functionally corresponds to a *p53* mutation, cervical-cancer cell lines were found to contain either HPVs or *p53* mutations *(30)*. It should be noted, however, that this correlation may not be as strict in primary tumors *(31)*. The issue is further complicated by the observation that HPV-positive cancer-cell lines, which express the *E6* gene from viral integrates, retain some p53 activity, and can, in principle, induce certain p53-associated responses to genotoxic stress *(32,33)*. Nevertheless, taken together, available evidence strongly suggests that the inactivation of p53 by the viral E6 oncoprotein plays an important role in HPV-associated cell transformation. In this context, it is also noteworthy that the ability of E6 to efficiently induce degradation of p53 is limited only to the high-risk HPV types and thus correlates with the transformation potential of individual HPV types *(19)*.

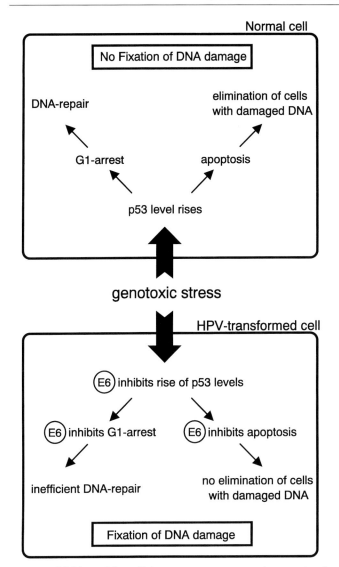

Fig. 1. Inhibition of the cellular response to genotoxic stress by the HPV E6 oncoprotein. Upper panel, Within a normal cell, genotoxic stress results in increased p53 protein levels. By transcriptionally activating the *p21*^WAF1 gene, p53 can induce cell-cycle arrest in G₁, presumably enabling the cell to correct the acquired DNA lesion before entry into S phase. Alternatively, p53 can induce apoptosis through transcriptional activation of the *bax* gene. In addition, there is also evidence for p53-dependent apoptosis not involving the transcriptional activation function of p53 protein. Lower panel, High-risk E6 protein can interfere with the normal cellular response to DNA damage on several levels. It inhibits or reduces the increase of p53 protein levels and it interferes with p53-mediated transactivation of *p21*^WAF1 or *bax*, thus blocking G₁ arrest (and subsequent DNA repair) and apoptosis induction. Moreover, E6 can also inhibit apoptosis by p53-independent mechanisms. Overall, expression of *E6* results in genetic instability.

Studies of mutant E6 proteins that were no longer able to complex p53 indicated that the E6 oncoprotein possesses transforming properties that are independent of targeting p53 *(34,35)*. Activities contributing to this p53-independent transformation potential may include the ability of E6 to transcriptionally modulate heterologous promoters *(36,37)*, to inhibit apoptosis *(38)*, to activate telomerase *(39)*, and to associate with various other cellular proteins besides p53, including the calcium-binding protein ERC55 *(40,41)*.

The E7 oncoprotein binds to the product of the retinoblastoma gene, pRb, and thus also targets a cellular tumor suppressor protein. It is noteworthy that the affinity of high-risk E7 proteins to pRb usually is several-fold higher than that of low-risk E7 proteins *(42)*. pRb plays an important role in cell-cycle control by coordinating entry of cells from G₁ into S phase *(43)*. In a simplistic model, unphosphorylated pRb binds cellular proteins, such as members of the E2F family of transcription factors *(44)*, in early G₁ (Fig. 2). E2F proteins are believed to transcriptionally activate genes involved in the stimulation of cell proliferation and DNA replication. By binding to E2F, pRb inhibits E2F-mediated transcriptional activation and thus blocks cell-cycle progression from G₁ to S. This block is relieved by phosphorylation of pRb through the action of the cyclin-dependent kinases (cdks), resulting in the dissociation of the E2F/pRb complex. Free E2F is then able to transactivate its cell cycle-promoting target genes, ultimately resulting in progression into S phase *(43,44)*. The E7 oncoprotein can disrupt pRb-mediated control of the cell cycle through at least three different mechanisms, resulting in free E2F and unscheduled activation of E2F target genes. These mechanisms include: 1) the direct binding of E7 to pRb, which results in a competitive interference with pRb/E2F complex formation *(45)*; 2) E7-induced degradation of pRb *(46,47)*; and 3) E7-mediated interference with regulatory pathways upstream of pRb, such as blocking the activity of the p21^WAF1 cdk inhibitor *(48,49)*. On the cellular level, these activities of E7 may contribute to the disruption of signals that would normally prevent DNA synthesis and cellular proliferation in the differentiated epithelial cells located above the proliferating basal layer *(48–50)*.

Experimental evidence suggest that interaction with pRb is not the only activity through which E7 can contribute to cell transformation. Analyses of mutant E7 proteins indicated that their transformation potential does not necessarily correlate with their ability to bind pRb *(51–53)*. E7 interacts with the pRb-related proteins p107 and p130 *(54)*, and has been found in complexes with the cell-cycle regulatory proteins cyclin A, cyclin E, p21^WAF1, and p27^KIP1 *(55–57)*. Disturbances in molecular pathways associated with these cell-cycle regulatory proteins may further contribute to the dysregulation of cell growth by E7. The E7 protein has been shown to interfere with the cellular response to DNA damage by overriding p53-mediated growth arrest *(58–61)*, possibly contributing to genetic instability *(29)*. It is noteworthy that by targeting p21^WAF1, E7 could affect other regulatory pathways associated with this cellular factor. For example, E7 may disturb p21^WAF1-mediated regulation of DNA-methylation *(62)* or interfere with the negative effect of p21^WAF1 on DNA replication *(63)*. Furthermore, E7 has transcriptional modulatory activities. Besides activating E2F-regulated promoters, including the b-*myb*, *cyclin E*, and *cyclin A* promoters *(64,65)*, E7 can influence transcription of cellular genes in an E2F-independent fashion by interacting with proteins of the AP1 family of transcription factors *(66)* or with general transcription factors, such as TATA-binding protein (TBP) *(67)*.

The transforming potential of E6 and E7 are strongly enhanced when these factors are co-expressed *(68,69)*. A possible molecular explanation for this cooperativity could be provided

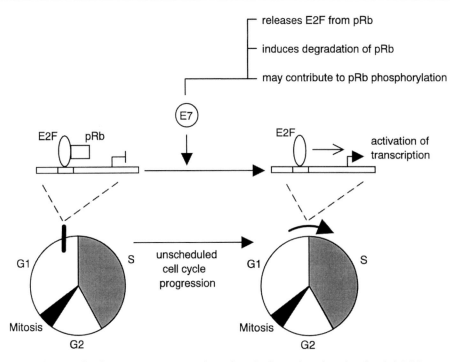

Fig. 2. Interference with pRb function by the HPV E7 oncoprotein. In late G_1, hypophosphorylated pRb inhibits progression into S phase by complexing cellular factors, such as the transcription factor E2F. Expression of HPV E7 protein can release E2F by competitively binding to pRb, by inducing degradation of pRb, and possibly by contributing to pRb phosphorylation (through targeting the p21^{WAF1} protein). Unbound E2F is able to transcriptionally activate its cell cycle promoting target genes, resulting in unscheduled cell cycle progression and loss of normal cellular growth control.

by the observation that normal cells can react to growth-deregulating influences by inducing apoptosis *(38,70)*. This process eliminates cells that receive inappropriate growth-stimulatory signals. However, this safeguard mechanism is impaired by expression of E6 protein, which can interfere with apoptosis induction through p53-dependent and p53-independent pathways. The coordinated induction of cell proliferation and inhibition of apoptosis results in the outgrowth of cells with deregulated growth behavior. In addition, cells emerging through the functional cooperativity between E6 and E7 may accumulate mutations in the cellular genome, due to genetic destabilization and induction of chromosomal aberrations associated with the expression of these viral factors.

Besides their association with cervical carcinomas, HPVs are also linked to additional human cancers, both within and outside the anogenital region. Cancers of the vulva, vagina, penis, and anus contain HPV DNA in more than 50% of cases *(2)*. Furthermore, HPVs have been linked to skin cancers. Classically, HPVs are associated with squamous-cell carcinomas arising in sun-exposed areas in individuals suffering from the rare hereditary disease *Epidermodysplasia verruciformis*. These tumors usually contain HPV5 or HPV8 DNA in an episomal state *(71)*. In addition, HPVs may also play a role in the development of skin cancers in both immunosuppressed and immunocompetent patients. This suggestion is based on the observation that certain HPV types (including previously undescribed types) are present in a substantial proportion of basal- and squamous-cell carcinomas of the skin *(72)*. Oral and laryngeal cancers are estimated to be HPV-positive in 10–20%

of cases, although the detection rate varies considerably between studies *(2)*. Sporadic reports linking HPVs to a number of additional malignancies, such as esophageal, colon, bladder, ovarian, and prostate cancer, await further investigation.

HEPATITIS B VIRUS

Hepatitis B virus (HBV) is an enveloped DNA virus with a strong tropism for hepatocytes. It belongs to the family of *Hepadnaviridae* and contains a small, partially double-stranded genome of 3.2 kb with 4 ORFs. These ORFs include: 1) the preS/S gene, which encodes proteins forming the viral envelope; 2) the C gene, which encodes the nucleocapsid (or core) protein; 3) the P gene, which encodes the viral polymerase/reverse transcriptase, and 4) the X gene, whose role in HBV biology is poorly understood *(73,74)*.

HBV infection leads to an acute hepatitis, which usually resolves after elimination of the virus. However, in certain instances, and for yet largely unknown reasons, HBV infection can become chronic. Persistant infections are most common after transmission of the virus at birth, with an incidence of 70–90% in neonates born to mothers that are positive for HBeAg (a cryptic antigenic determinant of the Hepatitis B core antigen). This contrasts acute HBV infections in adults, which lead to persistant infections in only 1–8% of affected individuals *(75)*. Persistent HBV infection is linked to the development of hepatocellular cancer (HCC). There are more than 200 million chronic carriers worldwide, and geographic areas with a high proportion of chronically HBV-infected individuals in the population (such as Southeast Asia and sub-Saharan Africa) exhibit a high prevalence of HCC. Based on prospective epidemiological studies, chronically HBV-infected individuals exhibit an 100-fold increased risk for HCC development *(76)*, which typically arises several decades following initial infection. It is estimated that approx 60–80% of all HCCs are linked to chronic HBV infection *(73,77)*. On a worldwide scale, more than 300,000 of new cases of HCC arise per year and with over 300,000 annual deaths, liver cancer represents the fourth most common cause of cancer death in humans *(6)*.

HBV-positive HCCs typically contain the viral DNA integrated at apparently random chromosomal sites and individual tumors are monoclonal with respect to the integration pattern. Integration often leads to rearrangements and deletions within the viral DNA, which can abrogate the expression of viral genes and, in general, HBV is no longer replicated in the tumor cells *(73,74)*. No HBV ORF is consistently retained and expressed in HCC, in contrast, for example, to the HPV *E6/E7* oncogenes in cervical cancer.

It appears that both direct and indirect effects of the virus can contribute to HCC development. Among the viral factors possibly directly involved in hepatocyte transformation, much interest has focussed on the viral X-protein (HBX). Experimentally, HBX has transforming potential in certain cell lines *(78,79)* and transgenic mice expressing *HBX* from the authentic HBV promoter develop HCC *(80)*. On the molecular level, HBX can transcriptionally activate a broad array of cellular and viral promoters (including cellular protooncogenes, such as c-*myc* and c-*jun*). Because HBX does not directly bind to DNA, HBX-mediated transcriptional modulation may occur through the interaction with cellular transcription factors in the nucleus, through post-transcriptional modulation of their activities, or through affecting signal-transduction cascades in the cytoplasm *(73,81,82)*. These activities of HBX could result in the deregulation of cellular genes involved in normal growth control and contribute to cellular transformation. Moreover, it has been observed that HBX can bind to the p53 protein *(83)*, inhibiting p53-mediated transcriptional transactivation *(84)* and induction of apoptosis *(85)*. Thus, HBX may have similar biological effects as the HPV E6 protein. A close correlation has been observed between the HBX-p53 interaction and the development of HCC in a transgenic mouse model *(86)*. However, at least in this experimental setting, the mechanism by which HBV inhibits p53 is apparently different from that observed in HPV-infected cervical cancer cells. In transgenic mice, p53 is sequestered by HBX in the cytoplasm of hepatocytes. Similarly, ectopic expression of the *HBX* gene in human hepatoma cell lines resulted in cytoplasmic retention of wild-type and mutant p53 *(87)*. Thus, HBX may interfere with p53 function by blocking the entry of p53 into the nuclear compartment, thereby blocking p53-mediated transcriptional activation of cellular target genes. However, more work is required to relate these observations to human hepatocarcinogenesis, because there is little evidence for a predominant cytoplasmic localization of p53 in human hepatomas and the subcellular localization of the HBX protein itself is still a matter of debate *(74)*. The issue could be further complicated by the observation of variant *HBX* transcripts (often detected in chronically infected liver), which may encode truncated HBX proteins differing in their biologi-

cal potential *(88)*. Moreover, it should be noted that many HBV-positive HCCs do not appear to express HBX at all *(73)*, indicating that the factor is either not essential for HBV-associated cell transformation or that its tumorigenic effect is transient and dispensable for the maintenance of the transformed phenotype.

The HBV integration event in some hepatomas can result in the deletion of the 3′-end of the HBV preS/S gene. This leads to the synthesis of a truncated preS/S-protein, which exhibits transactivation potential for a wide range of viral and cellular promoters *(89)*. In addition, besides affecting the activities of cellular genes in *trans*, the virus may also exert *cis*-effects by the integration event into the host genome. For example, in rare instances, it has been observed that integration can disrupt or alter growth-regulatory genes, such as the *retinoic acid receptor-β* gene *(90)* or the *cyclin A* gene *(91)*. Moreover, it is possible that transcriptional control elements of the virus (enhancers) may affect neighboring cellular genes in *cis*.

In contrast to these viral *trans*- and *cis*-activities, one could also envision an indirect role for HBV during hepatocarcinogenesis. In this scenario, cell transformation is not due to direct effects of the virus but rather is the result of the host response to the viral infection. In particular, the chronic proliferation, regeneration, and inflammation during persistent HBV infection of the liver may be associated with a higher risk to acquire mutations in the cellular DNA. The accumulation of mutations (potentially affecting proto-oncogenes and tumor-suppressor genes) may result in hepatocytes with tumorigenic growth behavior. Indeed, chronic liver injury, for example during alcoholic cirrhosis, is also associated with an increased risk for the development of HCC *(92)*. Furthermore, transgenic mouse models show that continuous mitogenic stimulation of hepatocytes by overexpressed transforming growth factor-a (TGF-a) results in the development of liver cancer *(93)*.

HEPATITIS C VIRUS

Hepatitis C virus (HCV) is a spherical enveloped RNA virus and represents a separate genus of the virus family *Flaviviridae*. Its genome of 9.5 kb contains a single large ORF coding for at least three structural and six nonstructural proteins. These proteins are generated by specific cleavage from a large polyprotein precursor of approx 3,000 amino acids. Due to genetic heterogeneity, HCVs can be subdivided into 6 major genotypes (HCV types 1 to type 6) and more than 50 subtypes. Individual virus isolates consist of closely related, yet heterogenous populations of virus genomes (quasispecies) *(94,95)*.

After cloning of HCV by recombinant DNA techniques *(96)*, it soon was realized that the virus represents the primary infectious agent causing post-transfusion non-A, non-B hepatitis. HCV-infection becomes chronic in over 80% of cases, with 20–30% progressing to cirrhosis, and development of HCC in a subset of these *(97)*. The ability of the virus to mutate rapidly and the coordinate emergence of virus quasispecies may contribute to the high percentage of chronic infections by facilitating escape from immune surveillance. Furthermore, it may explain the apparent lack of lasting immunity against HCV infections, as indicated by the observation that repeated exposure can lead to re-infection. The genetic heterogeneity of HCVs could have important clinical implications and may influence the clinical course or the therapeutic response. Further, it may represent a major obstacle in generating effective anti-HCV vaccines *(95,98,99)*.

A substantial percentage of HCC-patients worldwide exhibit HCV antibodies and HCV RNA in the serum. This is observed in certain countries in Southern Europe (Italy, Spain) and in Japan, where more than 50% of HCC cases are associated with HCV *(100)*. Seroepidemiological studies defined HCV as a clear risk factor for liver cancer, and the risk of chronically HCV-infected persons to develop HCC is estimated to be in the range of 2–7% after 20 yr of infection *(100)*. Although the HCV core protein has been reported to possess some transforming potential in vitro *(101)*, an indirect role for the virus during hepatocarcinogenesis is currently favored. Similarly, as postulated for the indirect oncogenic effects of HBV, HCV-associated HCCs may result from virally induced chronic inflammation and cirrhosis. Indeed, cirrhosis is found in 97% of HCC-patients with HCV markers *(102)*.

EPSTEIN-BARR VIRUS

Epstein-Barr virus (EBV) is a member of the human herpesvirus subfamily *Gammaherpesviridae*. EBVs are enveloped viruses with a double-stranded DNA genome of 172 kb, encompassing more than 100 ORFs. Based on sequence variations within the EBNA (Epstein-Barr-virus nuclear antigen) genes, EBV isolates can be grouped in either EBV1 (or type A), or EBV2 (or type B) *(103)*.

EBV is a ubiquitous virus, infecting more than 90% of the human population *(104)*. Primary infection with EBV usually occurs in childhood. In most cases, the clinical course is inapparent. However, in a subset of infected persons, primary EBV infection can result in infectious mononucleosis, a self-limited lymphoproliferative disease, particularly when primary infection is delayed into adolescence. At current, it is a matter of debate whether EBV primarily infects the oropharyngeal epithelia and secondarily B-cells, which circulate through the mucosa-associated lymphoid tissue, or whether B-cells also represent the main target site for primary EBV infection *(105)*. After binding to the CD21 molecule (the cellular receptor for EBV) and internalization, EBV causes a latent infection in lymphoid cells, which persists for life in a small subpopulation of B-lymphocytes *(104)*. Although EBV has a very high transforming potential *in vitro*, it rarely causes tumors in humans, suggesting that EBV-infected cells are subject to continous surveillence by cytotoxic T-cells. This is in line with the observation that T-cell immunosuppression can lead to the development of malignant lymphomas. However, EBVs are also closely associated with the development of lymphoid and epithelial malignancies in apparently immunocompetent hosts.

A number of EBV genes that are expressed in EBV-associated malignancies have activities that may contribute to the deregulation of normal cell growth and oncogenesis. In this respect, much work has concentrated on the latent membrane protein 1 (*LMP1*) gene, which encodes an integral membrane protein of 386 amino acids. *LMP1* has properties of an proto-oncogene in rodent cell lines *(106,107)* and can morphologically transform human epithelial cells *(108,109)*. Experimentally, expression of *LMP1* has multiple effects, which include increased expression of cellular-adhesion molecules, upregulation of lymphocyte-activation antigens, activation of the antiapoptotic *bcl2* gene (in some cell types), and induction of the activity of transcription factors, such as AP1 and nuclear factor kB (NF-kB) *(103,110)*. It has been found that, although not homologous on the protein level, LMP1 can act like a ligand-independent, constitutively activated, TNF-receptor-type molecule and exhibits similar effects as activated CD40 *(111)*. Thus, *LMP1* expression may enable EBVs to activate latently infected B-cells, abrogating the need for contacting CD40-ligand expressing T-cells. In this scenario, the oncogenic potential of LMP1 is related to its ability to mimick TNF-receptor signaling and may be closely linked to its ability to constitutively activate signal-transduction pathways normally used by B-cell growth factors *(111)*.

Proteins of the EBNA group (such as EBNA1, EBNA2, EBNA3C, and EBNA-LP) may contribute to EBV-associated cell transformation and oncogenesis. The EBNA1 protein is the only protein consistently expressed in all EBV-positive malignancies and can induce B-cell lymphomas in transgenic mouse models *(112)*. EBNA1 is a DNA binding protein which is necessary for maintenance and replication of the EBV genome in mammalian cells. EBNA1 also acts as a transcriptional activator inducing expression of the cellular recombinase-activating genes *RAG1* and *RAG2* in vitro *(113)*. The EBNA2 protein also functions as a transcriptional activator, with the capacity to induce cellular genes, including *CD23* and *CD21* (encoding the cellular EBV receptor), the tyrosine kinase c-*fgr*, *cyclin D2* (in concert with EBNA-LP), as well as latent viral genes, such as *LMP1*, *LMP2a*, and *LMP2b* *(103,110)*. EBNA2 exerts its transcriptional activity indirectly through intermediate DNA transcription factors, such as RBP-Jk or CBF1 *(114,115)*, the human homolog of *Drosophila* suppressor of hairless, or PU.1 *(116)*. It also has been found that EBNA2 can induce B-cell proliferation by overriding different restriction points of the cell cycle *(117)*. In this respect, it bears similarities to the EBNA3C protein, which antagonizes cell-cycle regulatory pathways. EBNA3C has been reported to exhibit transforming potential in experimental systems, to bind to pRb in vitro, and to override the antiproliferative effects of pRb in vivo *(118)*. Moreover, another EBNA protein, namely EBNA-LP, has also been suggested to complex with pRb in vitro, and to interact with p53 *(119)*. The in vivo significance of this latter finding is not clear and immortalization of human B-cells by EBV was not detectably linked to functional impairment of p53 *(120)*.

It is important to note that only a subset of EBV genes are expressed in EBV-associated tumors and this subset varies between different tumor types. Commonly, three types of latency are distinguished: 1) latency pattern type 1, in which EBNA1 appears to be the only viral protein expressed; 2) latency pattern type 2, in which, in addition to EBNA1, the latent membrane proteins LMP1, LMP2a, LMP2b are expressed; and 3) latency pattern type 3, where at least 9 proteins (the 6 nuclear proteins EBNA1, EBNA2, EBNA3A, EBNA3B, EBNA3C, EBNA-LP, and the three membrane proteins LMP1, LMP2a, LMP2b) are expressed. In all three latency patterns, the noncoding *EBER1/2* transcripts of unknown function, and the *BARF0* gene with uncertain coding capacity are also expressed

(104). It should, however, be noted that, under certain circumstances, this separation is not strictly applicable and intermediate expression patterns can be observed. Moreover, tumor cells within the same lymphoma can also show some heterogeneity with respect to the expression pattern of EBV genes *(121)*.

The human malignancy classically associated with EBV infection is Burkitt's lymphoma (BL) *(122)*. This, often multifocal tumor is composed of monoclonal proliferations of B-cells. On a worldwide scale, BL is a low-incidence tumor. However, its prevalence shows striking geographic variations. BL occurs in an endemic form (eBL) in equatorial Africa, where it can represent the most common childhood tumor. Interestingly, these regions also exhibit a high incidence of malarial infection, which may act as a cofactor for eBL development *(123,124)*. Although the exact mechanisms by which EBVs contribute to eBL are still unknown, several observations indicate that EBV may play a causal role. For example, BL-patients have an increased antibody titer against the viral capsid antigen (VCA) and prospective seroepidemiological investigations indicated that children from an endemic area exhibited significantly elevated anti-VCA titers before clinical tumor development *(125)*. Furthermore, EBV DNA is found in more than 95% of eBL tumors, where it is present in a monoclonal form in every tumor cell. Because the structure of EBV genomes can vary between latently infected cells due to variations in the number of terminal repeats *(103)*, the detection of a single form of the EBV genome in all tumor cells strongly suggests that they are derived from a single EBV-infected progenitor cell. Moreover, the viral DNA is transcriptionally active, typically exhibiting latency pattern 1 expression (restricted to EBNA1) *(126)*. It is noteworthy that EBNA1 can evade immune recognition through an internal protein region interfering with antigen processing *(127)* and may allow escape of EBV-positive BL-cells from the cytotoxic T-cell response. In further support for a causal role for EBV in BL development, there is experimental data showing that EBV can induce lymphoma-like diseases in primates and the malignant phenotype of a BL cell line was reported to be dependent on the presence of EBV *(128)*.

Strikingly, in addition to EBV, eBLs typically contain specific chromosomal translocations, which are balanced and reciprocal. They involve regulatory sequences of the immunoglobulin genes on chromosome 14q32 (76% of cases), 22q11 (16% of cases), or 2p11 (8% of cases), which are joined to the c-*myc* proto-oncogene on 8q24 *(124,129)*. These translocation events can result in the deregulation of c-*myc* expression and may thereby contribute to oncogenicity. Indeed, there is experimental evidence indicating that c-*myc* activation can render the proliferation of EBV-transformed cells independent of *LMP1* and *EBNA2* expression *(130)*. The observation that EBNA1 has the potential to induce the recombination-activating genes *RAG1* and *RAG2*, may provide a direct link between EBV and the translocation events observed in BL. However, neglecting a formally possible hit and run mechanism, it appears that EBV infection is not a necessary prerequisite for BL-development and rearrangement of the c-*myc* locus. This can be deduced from the rare eBLs that are EBV-negative and from sporadic cases of BL (sBL), which, although of low prevalence, represent the most common form of BL in developed countries.

This latter form of BL also contains the typical c-*myc* translocations but appears to be EBV-positive in only 15–20% of cases. However, recent evidence indicates that the actual percentage of EBV-positive sBL may be higher, because EBV fragments have been detected in sBL tumor cells, which would have been undetectable by previous screening techniques *(131)*.

Of particular clinical importance is the association of EBV with the development of B-cell lymphomas in immunocompromised patients *(132,133)*. Immunosuppression in these patients may be congenital (X-linked lymphoproliferative syndrome) *(134)*, or in the majority of cases may be the result of an HIV-infection or of drug-induced immunosuppression following organ transplantation. The incidence of B-cell lymphoma is elevated approx 50-fold in organ recipients under immunosuppression *(132)* and the total number strongly increased in recent years with the use of more profound immunosuppressive therapy. Typically, the EBV genomes contained in these tumors exhibit latency type 3 gene expression, which in immunocompetent hosts would be highly immunogenic. Interestingly, reduction of immunosuppression can induce regression of the lymphomas *(135)*. These often multifocal tumors can arise both from host or donor lymphocytes *(136)* and are histologically categorized as high-grade immunoblastic lymphomas. They appear to initiate as polyclonal or oligoclonal proliferations, but eventually are composed of only one predominating clone within individual foci *(104)*. In AIDS patients, two histological forms of B-cell lymphomas are recognized, namely Burkitt's-like lymphomas, which typically appear during progression to AIDS, and immunoblastic lymphomas at later stage, concomitantly with severe immunosuppression *(137)*.

Other EBV-associated lymphomas include certain types of T-cell lymphoma (such as nasal T-cell lymphoma) *(138,139)* and Hodgkin's disease (HD) *(138,140,141)*. An infectious nature for HD was initially suspected from seroepidemiological evidence, which suggested that HD is the result of a delayed exposure to a relatively common infectious agent *(142)*. A connection between EBV and HD can be deduced from several observations: 1) persons with a history of infectious mononucleosis have a two-fold to four-fold increased risk of developing HD; 2) retrospective serological studies reveal significantly raised antibody titers against EBV VCA before development of HD; and 3) monoclonal EBV genomes are present in the pathognomic Reed-Sternberg (RS) cells in up to 50% of HD cases in the Western world *(104,138,141)*. Interestingly, the detection rate of EBV in the tumors shows a correlation with the histological subtype. Although EBV is rarely detectable in the lymphocyte-predominant type, it is present in 30% of the nodular-sclerosis type, and in up to 90% in the mixed cellularity and lymphocyte-depleted subtypes. The EBV genomes within RS cells are present at all involved anatomical sites and are transcriptionally active, typically exhibiting latency type 2 gene expression.

EBV can infect epithelial cells (the exact route of infection is not known) and contribute to the development of epithelial cancers, such as undifferentiated nasopharyngeal carcinoma (NPC) *(143,144)*. Undifferentiated NPC accounts for up to 80% of all NPC cases and occurs with high prevalence in certain areas of East Asia, such as in Southern China. The reason for the clustering of this tumor in these specific geographical areas is not known, but a combination of genetic and lifestyle factors may play a role. IgG antibodies against EBV antigens can be used as marker for tumor progression and remission of NPC *(145)*. Moreover, detection of IgA antibodies against EBV VCA (rarely found in the normal population) has been successfully employed as a marker for increased tumor risk in screening programs in high-incidence areas *(146)*. NPC tumor cells contain EBV DNA *(143)* in a monoclonal form in every tumor cell and usually exhibit latency type 2 gene expression, including expression of *LMP1*, which can interfere with normal epithelial differentiation. LMP1 protein is detected in up to 65% of cases using standard methods, but its transcript is detectable in virtually all cases by polymerase chain reaction (PCR) analysis *(144)*.

Another nonlymphoid malignancy possibly associated with EBV is gastric carcinoma, where the viral DNA is found in approx 90% of the rare gastric lymphepithelioma-like carcinomas and in approx 10% of the very common gastric adenocarcinomas *(147)*. EBV is present in the malignant epithelial cells, which represent clonal proliferations of EBV-infected cells and regularly express *EBNA1*, but not other *EBNA* genes or *LMP1*.

HUMAN HERPESVIRUS 8

Significant research efforts are currently focused on a second, recently identified herpesvirus that could be a human tumor virus, namely herpesvirus 8 (HHV8). It has been isolated from Kaposi's sarcoma (KS) tissue by an elegant technique allowing the isolation of exogeneous DNA (representational difference analysis) *(148)*, and is therefore alternatively called Kaposi's sarcoma-associated herpesvirus (KSHV).

HHV8 DNA is lost after only a few cell-culture passages from short-term cultures derived from KS lesions, probably through a cytopathic effect of the virus under in vitro growth conditions. However, the virus can be propagated in cell lines from primary effusion lymphoma, resulting in the generation of infective viral particles *(149)*. The encapsidated viral DNA produced in BCL-cell lines is approx 160–170 kb in length. Complete sequencing of the HHV8 genome revealed a 140.5 kb coding region with an estimated 81 ORFs, flanked by repetitive terminal repeats *(150)*. Phylogenetically, HHV8 is a gamma 2 herpesvirus (genus *Rhadinovirus*), showing sequence homologies to EBV and to herpesvirus saimiri, a squirrel-monkey virus capable of transforming human T-cells *(151)*.

Although EBV is the most closely related human virus, HHV8 does not carry ORFs with sequence homology to the EBV *EBNA* or *LMP* genes. In fact, several HHV8 ORFs have significant sequence similarities to human genes *(150,152)*, suggesting that the virus has captured cellular genes during evolution. Among others, viral homologs ressemble cellular genes involved in growth control, cell-cycle regulation, and cytokine signaling. HHV8 contains a gene homologous to the *bcl-2* gene that functions to inhibit apoptosis *(153)* and for an analog of the cellular *cyclin D* gene, whose protein product phosphorylates pRb *(154,155)*. The viral vMIP-I and vMIP-II factors exhibit homology to the cellular chemokine MIP1-α. Interestingly, vMIP-I and v-MIP-II were found to possess strong angiogenic potential and may thereby contribute to the

marked vascularization of KS *(156)*. In addition, the virus also expresses a third chemokine that is more distantly related to MIP1-a. Viral ORF 74 codes for a homolog of cellular chemokine receptors, bearing similarity to the IL-8-receptor (150,152). The viral variant has been found to be constitutively active *(157)* and to possess oncogenic and angiogenic potential *(158)*. Furthermore, the virus encodes a homolog of the cellular interleukin 6 (IL-6) protein, a possible growth factor for KS cells, and for a protein related to the cellular interferon-regulatory factor 1 (150,152). Based on the observation that KS growth appears to be strongly supported by a variety of cytokines, it is intruiging that HHV8 codes for genes homologous to cellular cytokines and cytokine receptors. Thus, HHV8 may directly encode growth factors crucial for the proliferation of KS cells. The cellular genes activated by the EBV EBNA and LMP proteins include *IL-6, cyclin D*, the *IL-8-receptor*, and *bcl-2 (152)*. Therefore, the transforming strategies of EBV and HHV8 may ultimately converge to target similar biochemical pathways involved in the control of cellular proliferation and apoptosis.

KS can be grouped into several clinical classifications: 1) classical KS, a rare tumor of elderly Mediterranean individuals, occuring predominantly in men, with usually a mild clinical course; 2) endemic KS, developing in HIV-negative persons in particular regions of equatorial Africa; 3) iatrogenic KS, occuring in transplant recipients under immunosuppression; and 4) AIDS-epidemic KS, representing the most common tumor in individuals with AIDS. KS lesions exhibit a complex morphology and contain a variety of cell types, including the so-called spindle cells, which are believed to be the tumor cells of KS *(159)*. Furthermore, KS biopsies contain high local levels of various cytokines, such as IL-6, γ-interferon (IFN-γ), basic fibroblast growth factor (bFGF), tumor necrosis factor-γ (TNF-γ), and vascular epithelial growth factor (VEGF). It has been reported that the growth of KS sarcoma cells in vitro is enhanced when cytokines, such as IL-1, IL-6, or the HIV Tat protein are added into the medium *(160)*. These observations suggest that the local dysregulation of cytokines plays an important role in the development of KS lesions.

The contribution of an infectious agent to KS development had already been suspected before HHV8 was isolated from the tumor tissue. The risk of developing KS was found to be 20,000-fold higher in HIV-patients than in the uninfected population *(161)*, which raised the possibility that HIV contributes to KS development. Indeed, HIV appears to promote indirectly KS development through immunosuppression and KS-lesions often regress following aggressive antiretroviral therapy in HIV-positive patients *(162)*. Furthermore, experimental data indicate that HIV may directly contribute to KS-development. For example, HIV-infected lymphocytes and monocytes release various cytokines that have been shown to induce proliferation of spindle cells *(160)*, and HIV-1 Tat protein released from HIV-infected cells stimulates the growth of AIDS-KS cells in vitro *(163)*. However, despite this possible direct contributory role for HIV, the occurance of KS in HIV-negative patients indicates that HIV cannot be solely responsible for KS development. Moreover, it was found that, among HIV-positive individuals, homosexuals were at much higher risk (7-fold to

15-fold) for KS than patients that had acquired the virus by nonsexual routes *(164),* pointing at another sexually transmitted agent as a critical determinant for KS development.

Several recent observations indicate that HHV8 may be this sought-after infectious agent *(152,164,165).* Its DNA is present in virtually all tumor specimens of the four KS subtypes, but not in most control tissues of the same patients. It is noteworthy that herpesvirus particles were observed in KS tissue more than two decades ago by electron microscopy, which may well have represented HHV8 virions *(166). In situ* hybridization studies show that spindle cells of KS lesions are infected by HHV8. Moreover, in concordance with the prevalence of HHV8 DNA, serological studies also hint at a causative role for HHV8 for KS development. KS patients exhibit high titers of anti-HHV8 antibodies, higher than normal controls. In addition, HHV8 infection precedes KS development. In contrast to many other human herpesviruses (like EBV, HSV, VZV), HHV8 infection is not ubiquitous and appears to be present in less than 10% of the normal population. However, these numbers are not undisputed *(167)* and may change with improved serological detection assays. There is also evidence indicating that KS is not the sole proliferative disease associated with HHV8. For example, HHV8 DNA was also found in Castleman's disease, a benign atypical lymphoid hyperplasia *(168),* and in a rare B-cell lymphoma, called body cavity lymphoma (BCL) or primary effusion lymphoma (PEL) *(169).* Moreover, HHV8 has been linked to the development of multiple myeloma. Interestingly, in this latter case, the virus is not present in the tumor cells but may stimulate their growth by producing IL-6 in adjacent macrophage-derived dendritic cells in the bone marrow *(170).*

HUMAN T-CELL LYMPHOTROPIC VIRUS TYPE I AND II

Approximately 10–20 million people worldwide are infected with human T-cell lymphotropic virus (HTLV-I), a human retrovirus that can cause tropic spastic paraparesis (TSP) and is linked to chronic inflammatory arthropathy and uveitis *(171).* HTLV-I infection is endemic in Japan (where more than one million people are infected), other areas of Asia (like Taiwan), the Carribean, and central Africa. Most HTLV-I carrier are asymptomatic but they have a risk of approx 1% for the development of adult T-cell leukemia (ATL) during their lifetime, typically decades after infection *(172).* ATL is an aggressive tumor almost always of the CD4+ type, and infected cells typically exhibit activation markers, such as increased expression of several cytokines. A relative of HTLV-I, HTLV-II, is associated with leukemias, such as atypical hairy-cell leukemia *(173).* However, a definitive role for HTLV-II for the development of human cancers has not yet been demonstrated.

Several observations indicate that HTLV-I plays an etiological role for ATL development. Seroepidemiological evidence links the prevalence of HTLV-I infection to ATL frequency. Experimentally, the virus can immortalize T-cells of various species, including human T-cells *(174,175).* In ATL cells, the HTLV-I provirus is typically integrated into the host chromosome in a randomized manner *(176)* and the clonality of ATL tumor cells correlates with the pattern of viral integration. This clonality of the tumor cells may be the result of a selection

of a malignant cell clone from a pool of polyclonal HTLV-I-positive cells. In line with this interpretation is the long latency before ATL development and the observation of additional genetic defects in HTLV-I positive tumor cells.

Unlike transforming animal retroviruses, HTLV-I does not contain an oncogene. However, the viral *tax* gene has been implicated in contributing to HTLV-I-associated cell transformation *(177),* because its coding region is always retained in tumor cells despite frequent deletion of other viral genes. Moreover, *tax* can immortalize human T-cells *(178)* and transgenic mice with an HTLV-I *tax* gene develop mesenchymal tumors *(179).* The *tax* gene codes for a promiscuous transcriptional activator of cellular and viral genes. On the molecular level, the tax protein transactivates by interacting with cellular transcription factors rather than through direct binding to DNA. These transcription factors include CREB, CREM, CBP, SRF, NF-κB, as well as basic transcription factors, such as the TATA binding protein, TBP *(177).* In addition, there is evidence that the *tax* gene product may also be involved in the suppression of particular genes, such as DNA polymerase β *(180).* Thus, it is possible that tax protein deregulates the expression of cellular genes controlling T-cell proliferation. Interestingly, the tax protein can activate the IL-2 and IL-2-receptor-α genes, which can both stimulate growth of T-cells *(181,182).* In this way, tax could lead to autocrine stimulation of T-cell growth. It should be noted, however, that not all HTLV-I transformed T-cells express IL-2 *(183).*

Furthermore, tax protein can bind to the cellular p16^{INK4A} protein, an inhibitor of cyclin-dependent kinases. This results in the activation of cdk4, an upstream regulator of pRb, and cell-cycle progression *(184).* Thus, during growth deregulation of T-cells, expression of *tax* may be able to substitute for a somatic mutation of p16^{INK4A}. This interpretation is supported by a limited analysis of T-cell lines showing that T-cell lines not infected by HTLV-I contained homozygous deletions of the p16^{INK4A} gene, while HTLV-infected T-cell lines retained wild-type p16^{INK4A} genes *(184).* However, more work is required to investigate this correlation in primary ATLs. Besides targeting pRb-associated pathways, tax protein may also affect p53 function. Although there is no evidence for a direct interaction between tax and p53, tax has been reported in experimental studies to stabilize the p53 protein and to inhibit p53-mediated transactivation *(185).* This is in line with the observation that ATL cells often exhibit elevated p53 levels *(186)* and that the p53-mediated response to ionizing radiation is impaired in some HTLV-I transformed T-cells *(187).*

While these investigations of ATL cell lines point at a possible role for *tax* during HTLV-I associated cell transformation, it is noteworthy that tax protein could not be detected in tumor cells by immunohistochemistry. Moreover, PCR analysis indicates that the majority of tumor cells do not express any viral DNA *(188).* Nevertheless, several scenarios have been proposed to support a role for tax during oncogenesis. For instance, tax protein function may be required transiently during tumor establishment but not for the maintenance of the tumorigenic phenotype. Alternatively, it is possible that only the minority of infected cells that express *tax* accelerate cell growth *(177).*

PERSPECTIVES

Much progress has been made in recent years to elucidate the molecular mechanisms by which viruses contribute to oncogenesis. At present, this is particularly well-characterized for high-risk HPVs where the viral E6 and E7 proteins form complexes with p53 and pRb, respectively, and target these cellular tumor-suppressor proteins for inactivation. Interestingly, other small DNA tumor viruses, which have transforming potential in animal systems (such as SV40, polyomaviruses, and certain types of adenoviruses) also code for factors that bind to and inactivate p53 and pRb. Thus, the picture emerges that different DNA tumor viruses follow a similar strategy ultimately leading to cell transformation *(189)*. To some extent, this strategy may also be shared by other human tumor viruses, such as HBV, EBV, HHV8, and HTLV-I, which also appear to target p53- and/or pRb-associated pathways. It is plausible that these activities evolved to support viral replication within the normal life-cycle of these viruses, for example, to recruit host factors for viral DNA synthesis or to counteract apoptosis of infected cells. However, under certain circumstances, following the deregulation of viral gene expression or in combination with additional genetic alterations of the host cell, these activities may contribute to oncogenesis by leading to uncontrolled cell proliferation, inducing genetic instability, and counteracting the apoptotic elimination of growth-deregulated and genetically altered cells.

The progress in defining the molecular pathways contributing to virus-induced cell transformation opens new possibilities for future therapeutic interventions. For example, because there is experimental evidence that the malignant phenotype of HPV-associated cancers is dependent on the continuous expression of the viral *E6* and *E7* genes, it could be attempted to block their activities. This could be theoretically achieved on several levels, such as on the transcriptional level (through inhibitors of the viral *E6/E7* promoter), on the level of RNA translation (through antisense-constructs and ribozymes), or on the protein level (through identifying small molecules that can inhibit the interaction between the viral oncoproteins and their cellular binding partners) *(16)*. Such virus-specific therapeutic approaches may also gain importance in the treatment of virus-associated preneoplastic lesions (HPV-associated dysplasias).

Clearly, however, although a causative role of tumor viruses for the evolution of a significant proportion of human cancers is strongly supported by epidemiological and experimental data, it appears that in most cases infection with a tumor virus is not sufficient for malignant transformation. This can be deduced from the observations that only a small percentage of infected individuals eventually develop a tumor, that there is typically a long latency period (in the range of decades) between initial viral infection and tumor development, and that tumors are usually monoclonal. These obervations indicate that additional alterations of the host cell are required for oncogenic transformation. It is clearly a major task for future research in tumor virology to find out what determines whether infection with a tumor virus results in malignancy or not. This risk could be influenced by multiple parameters, including the patient's immunological status, the nature of additional genetic alterations within the host cell, the viral integration event, or the possibility that certain virus variants are associated with a higher transforming potential. From the aforementioned considerations, it is also apparent that the sole detection of a tumor virus cannot substitute for conventional cytological and histological cancer diagnosis, but rather may supplement such approaches. For example, the detection of a high-risk HPV type in a low-grade dysplastic lesion of the cervix uteri may identify these women that require a more stringent observation, because it appears that these lesions exhibit a higher potential for progression *(190)*.

It also will be important in the future to sort out if there are other viruses associated with human malignancies and which other malignancies are possibly associated with viral infections. Indeed, several other viruses have been linked to human cancer, such as SV40, to which many millions of people worldwide were exposed in the late 1950s and early 1960s by contaminated poliomyelitis and adenovirus vaccines. SV40 can cause tumors in rodents and transforms human cells in vitro *(191)*. On this background, much concern has been raised about a possible contribution of SV40 to human oncogenesis. However, many studies indicate that there is no significant increase in detectable cancers in vaccinees even decades after exposure to the virus and general consent at an international conference at the NIH in 1997 concluded that SV40 in the polio vaccines is not a public-health threat. There are also sporadic reports of detection of SV40 in mesothelioma and choroid plexus tumors, ependymomas, osteosarcomas, and sarcomas, which are disputed by others *(191)*. Even if these reports are substantiated, it should be kept in mind that the mere presence of these viruses in tumors does not prove a cause-effect relationship. Sequences of human polyomaviruses JC or BK have also been detected in several human tumors, particularly of the central nervous system (CNS) *(192)*. However, a causative role for these viruses for human carcinogenesis is also disputed and BK and JC virus DNA appears to be present also in many normal tissues. Moreover, seroconversion rates of almost 100% by the age of 20 yr indicate that JC or BK virus infections are not necessarily related with an increased risk for the development of cancer *(192)*.

Among the tumors with a possible viral etiology, childhood leukemia appears to be of particular clinical importance. Indeed, certain geographic and socioeconomic settings point at the contribution of an infectious agent for the development of these cancers. A model has been proposed, in which a viral infection of children with absent established immunity, in concert with fetally acquired B-cell mutations, may contribute to the development of leukemia *(193)*.

Strong efforts are also currently being undertaken to generate effective therapeutic and prophylactic vaccines against human tumor viruses. Prophylactic HPV vaccines *(194,195)* are currently being moved into clinical testing, an effective anti-HBV vaccine is already available. Because virus-associated cancers typically evolve decades following infection, it is apparent that a strong decline of their incidence can be expected only after decades following vaccination of a population at risk on a broad basis. First results of a nationwide universal HBV-vaccination program in Taiwan indicated that the incidence of liver cancer in children declined *(196)*, supporting the idea that prophylactic vaccination against human tumor viruses is a promising approach to fight human cancer.

REFERENCES

1. zur Hausen, H. (1991) Viruses in human cancers. *Science* **254**:1167–1173.
2. zur Hausen, H. (1996) Papillomavirus infections: a major cause of human cancers. *Biochim. Biophys. Acta* **1288**:F55–F78.
3. Howley, P. (1996) Papillomavirinae: the viruses and their replication. *In: Fields Virology* (Fields, B. N., Knipe, D. M., Howley, P. M., eds.), Lippincott-Raven, Philadelphia, pp. 2045–2076.
4. Dollard, S. C., Wilson, J. L., Demeter, L. M., Bonnez, W., Reichman, R. C., Borker, T. R., et al. (1992) Production of human papillomavirus and modulation of the infectious program in epithelial raft cultures. *Genes Dev.* **6**:1131–1142.
5. Meyers, C., Frattini, M. G., Hudson, J. B., and Laimins, L. A. (1992) Biosynthesis of human papillomavirus from a continuous cell line upon epithelial differentiation. *Science* **257**:971–973.
6. Pisani, P., Parkin, D. M., and Ferlay, J. (1993) Estimates of the worldwide mortality from eighteen major cancers in 1985. Implications for prevention and projections of future burden. *Int. J. Cancer* **54**:594–606.
7. Bosch, F. X., Munoz, N., de Sanjosé, S., Izarzugaza, I., Gili, M., Viladiu, P., et al. (1992) Risk factors for cervical cancer in Columbia and Spain. *Int. J. Cancer* **52**:750–758.
8. Koutsky, L. A., Holmes, K. K., Critchlow, C. W., Stevens, C. E., Paavonen, J., Beckmann, A. M., et al. (1992) A cohort study of the risk of cervical intraepithelial neoplasia grade 2 or 3 in relation to papillomavirus infection. *N. Engl. J. Med.* **327**:1271–1278.
9. Dillner, J., Lehtinen, M., Björge, T., Luostarinen, T., Youngman, L., Jellum, E., et al. (1997) Prospective seroepidemiologic study of human papillomavirus infections as a risk factor for invasive cervical cancer. *J. Natl. Cancer Inst.* **89**:1293–1299.
10. Schwarz, E., Freese, U. K., Gissmann, L., Mayer, W., Roggenbuck, B., Stremlau, A., et al. (1985) Structure and transcription of human papillomavirus sequences in cervical carcinoma cells. *Nature* **31**:111–114.
11. von Knebel Doeberitz, M. (1992) Papillomaviruses in human disease: Part II. Molecular biology and immunology of papillomavirus infections and carcinogenesis. *Eur. J. Med.* **1**:485–491.
12. Hoppe-Seyler, F. and Butz, K. (1994) Cellular control of human papillomavirus oncogene transcription. *Mol. Carcinogenesis* **10**:134–141.
13. Dürst, M., Glitz, D., Schneider, A., and zur Hausen, H. (1992) Human papillomavirus type 16 (HPV16) gene expression and DNA replication in cervical neoplasia: analysis by in situ hybridization. *Virology* **189**:132–140.
14. Thierry, F. and Yaniv, M. (1987) The BPV 1-E2-trans-acting protein can be either an activator or a repressor of the HPV 18 regulatory region. *EMBO J.* **6**:3391–3397.
15. Jeon, S. and Lambert, P. F. (1995) Integration of HPV 16 DNA into the human genome leads to increased stability of E6/E7 mRNAs: implications for cervical carcinogenesis. *Proc. Natl. Acad. Sci. USA* **92**:1654–1658.
16. Hoppe-Seyler, F. and Scheffner, M. (1997) E6 protein. *In: Papillomaviruses in Human Cancer: The Role of the E6 and E7 Oncoproteins* (Tommassino, M., ed.), Landes Bioscience, Austin, TX, pp. 71–102.
17. Jones, D. L. and Münger, K. (1996). Interactions of the human papillomavirus E7 protein with cell cycle regulators. *Semin. Cancer Biol.* **7**:327–337.
18. Kubbutat, M. H. G. and Vousden. K. H. (1996) Role of the E6 and E7 oncoproteins in HPV-induced anogenital malignancies. *Semin. Virol.* **7**:295–304.
19. Scheffner, M., Werness, B. A., Huibregtse, J. M., Levine, A. J., and Howley, P. M. (1990) The E6 oncoprotein encoded by human papillomavirus types 16 and 18 promotes the degradation of p53. *Cell* **63**:1129–1136.
20. Lane, D. P. (1992) p53, guardian of the genome. *Nature* **358**:15–16.
21. Fritsche, M., Haessler, C., and Brandner, G. (1993) Induction of nuclear accumulation of the tumor-suppressor protein p53 by DNA-damaging agents. *Oncogene* **8**:307–318.
22. Levine, A. J. (1997) p53, the cellular gatekeeper for growth and division. *Cell* **88**:323–331.
23. El-Deiry, W. S., Tokino, T., Velculescu, V. E., Levy, D. B., Parsons, R., Trent, J. M., et al. (1993) WAF-1, a potential mediator or p53 tumor suppression. *Cell* **75**:817–825.
24. Miyashita, T. and Reed, J. C. (1995) Tumor suppressor p53 is a direct transcriptional activator of the human bax gene. *Cell* **80**:293–299.
25. Caelles, C., Helmberg, A., and Karin, M. (1994) p53-dependent apoptosis in the absence of transcriptional activation of p53-target genes. *Nature* **370**:220–223.
26. Mietz, J. A., Unger, T., Huibregtse, J. M., and Howley, P. M. (1992) The transcriptional transactivation function of wild-type p53 is inhibited by SV40 large T-antigen and by HPV-16 E6 oncoprotein. *EMBO J.* **11**:5013–5020.
27. Hoppe-Seyler, F. and Butz, K. (1993) Repression of endogenous p53 transactivation function in HeLa cervical carcinoma cells by human papillomavirus type 16 E6, human mdm-2, and mutant p53. *J. Virol.* **67**:3111–3117.
28. Kessis, T. D., Slebos, R. J., Nelson, W. G., Kastan, M. B., Plunkett, B. S., Han, S. M., et al. (1993) Human papillomavirus 16 E6 expression disrupts the p53-mediated cellular response to DNA damage. *Proc. Natl. Acad. Sci. USA* **90**:3988–3992.
29. White A. E,. Livanos, E. M., and Tlsty, T. (1994) Differential disruption of genomic integrity and cell cycle regulation in normal human fibroblasts by the HPV oncoproteins. *Genes Dev.* **8**:666–677.
30. Scheffner, M., Münger, K., Byrne, J. C., and Howley, P. M. (1991) The state of the p53 and retinoblastoma genes in human cervical carcinoma cell lines. *Proc. Natl. Acad. Sci. USA* **88**:5523–5527.
31. Park, D. J., Wilczynski, S. P., Paquette, R. L., Miller, C. W., and Koeffler, H. P. (1994) p53 mutations in HPV-negative cervical carcinoma. *Oncogene* **9**:205–210.
32. Butz, K., Shahabeddin, L., Geisen, C., Spitkovsky, D., Ullmann, A., and Hoppe-Seyler, F. (1995) Functional p53 protein in human papillomavirus-positive cancer cells. *Oncogene* **10**:927–936.
33. Butz, K., Geisen. C., Ullmann, A., Spitkovsky, D., and Hoppe-Seyler, F. (1996) Cellular responses of HPV-positive cancer cells to genotoxic anti-cancer agents: repression of E6/E7-oncogene expression and induction of apoptosis. *Int. J. Cancer* **68**:506–513.
34. Pim, D., Storey, A., Thomas, M., Massimi, P., and Banks, L. (1994) Mutational analysis of HPV18-E6 identifies domains required for p53 degradation in vitro, abolition of p53 transactivation in vivo and immortalisation of primary BMK cells. *Oncogene* **9**: 1869–1876.
35. Spitkovsky, D., Aengeneyndt, F., Braspenning, J., and von Knebel Doeberitz, M. (1996) p53-independent growth regulation of cervical cancer cells by the papillomavirus E6 oncogene. *Oncogene* **13**:1027–1035.
36. Lamberti, C., Morrissey, L. C., Grossman, S. R., and Androphy, E. J. (1990) Transcriptional transactivation by the human papillomavirus E6 zinc finger protein. *EMBO J.* **9**:1907–1913.
37. Sedman, S. A., Barbosa, M. S., Vass, W. C., Hubbert, N. L., Haas, J. A., Lowy, D. R., et al. (1991) The full length E6 protein of human papillomavirus type 16 has transforming and trans-activating activities and cooperates with E7 to immortalize keratinocytes in culture. *J. Virol.* **65**:4860–4866.
38. Pan, H. and Griep, A. E. (1995) Temporally distinct patterns of p53-dependent and p53-independent apoptosis during mouse lens development. *Genes Dev.* **9**:2157–2169.
39. Klingelhutz, A. J., Foster, S. A., and McDougall, J. K. (1996) Telomerase activation by the E6 gene product of human papillomavirus type 16. *Nature* **380**:79–82.
40. Keen, N., Elston, R., and Crawford L. (1994) Interaction of the E6 protein of human papillomavirus with cellular proteins. *Oncogene* **9**:1493–1499.
41. Chen, J. J., Reid, C. E., Band, V., and Androphy, E. J. (1995) Interaction of papillomavirus E6 oncoproteins with a putative calcium-binding protein. *Science* **269**:529–531.

42. Münger, K. and Phelps, W. C. (1993) The human papillomavirus E7 protein as a transforming and transactivating factor. *Biochim. Biophys. Acta* **1155**:111–123.

43. Weinberg, R. A. (1995) The retinoblastoma protein and cell cycle control. *Cell* **81**:323–330.

44. LaThangue, N. B. (1994) DRTF1/E2F: an expanding family of heterodimeric transcription factors implicated in cell cycle control. *Trends Biochem. Sci.* **19**:108–114.

45. Huang, P. S., Patrick, D. R., Edwards, G., Goodhart, P. J., Huber, H. E., Miles, L., et al. (1993) Protein domains governing interactions between E2F, the retinoblastoma gene product, and human papillomavirus type 16 E7 protein. *Mol. Cell. Biol.* **13**:953–960.

46. Boyer, S. N., Wazer, D. E., and Band, A. (1996) E7 protein of human papilloma virus-16 induces degradation of retinoblastoma protein through the ubiquitin-proteasome pathway. *Cancer Res.* **56**:4620–4624.

47. Jones, D. L., Thompson, D. A., and Münger, K. (1997) Destabilization of the RB tumor suppressor protein and stabilization of p53 contribute to HPV Type 16 E7-induced apoptosis. *Virology* **239**:97–107.

48. Funk, J. O., Waga, S., Harry, J. B., Espling, E., Stillman, B., and Galloway, D. A. (1997) Inhibition of cdk activity and PCNA-dependent DNA replication by p21 is blocked by interaction with the HPV-16 E7 oncoprotein. *Genes Dev.* **11**:2090–2100.

49. Jones, D. L., Alani, R. M., and Münger, K. (1997) The human papillomavirus E7 oncoprotein can uncouple cellular differentiation and proliferation in human keratinocytes by abrogating p21^{CIP1}-mediated inhibition of cdk2. *Genes Dev.* **11**:2101–2111.

50. Cheng, S., Schmidt-Grimminger, D.-C., Murant, T., Broker, T. R., and Chow, L. T. (1995) Differentiation-dependent up-regulation of the human papillomavirus E7 gene reactivates cellular DNA replication in suprabasal differentiated keratinocytes. *Genes Dev.* **9**:2335–2349.

51. Edmonds, C. and Vousden, K. H. (1989) A point mutational analysis of human papillomavirus type 16 E7 protein. *J. Virol.* **63**:2650–2656.

52. Banks, L., Edmonds, C., and Vousden, K. (1990) Ability of HPV16 E7 protein to bind RB and induce DNA synthesis is not sufficient for efficient transforming activity in NIH 3T3 cells. *Oncogene* **5**:1383–1389.

53. Phelps, W. C., Münger, K., Lee, C. L., Barnes, J. A., and Howley, P. M. (1992) Structure-function analysis of the human papillomavirus type 16 E7 protein. *J. Virol.* **66**:2418–2427.

54. Dyson, N., Guida, P., Münger, K., and Harlow, E. (1992) Homologous sequences in adenovirus E1A and human papillomavirus E7 proteins mediate interaction with the same set of proteins. *J. Virol.* **66**:6893–6902.

55. Tommasino, M., Adamczewski, J. P., Carlotti, F., Barth, C. F., Manetti, R., Contorni, M., et al. (1993) HPV16 E7 protein associates with the protein kinase p33CDK2 and cyclin A. *Oncogene* **8**:195–202.

56. McIntyre, M. C., Ruesch, M. N., and Laimins, L. A. (1996) Human papillomavirus E7 oncoproteins bind a single form of cyclin E in a complex with cdk2 and p107. *Virology* **215**:73–82.

57. Zerfass-Thome, K., Zwerschke, W., Mannhardt, B., Tindle, R., Botz, J. W., and Jansen-Dürr, P. (1996) Inactivation of the cdk inhibitor p27^{KIP1} by the human papillomavirus type 16 E7 oncoprotein. *Oncogene* **13**:2323–2330.

58. Vousden, K. H., Vojtesek, B., Fisher, C., and Lane, D. (1993) HPV16-E7 or adenovirus E1A can overcome the growth arrest of cells immortalized with a temperature-sensitive p53. *Oncogene* **8**:1697–1702.

59. Demers, G. W., Foster, S. A., Halbert, C. L., and Galloway, D. A. (1994) Growth arrest by induction of p53 in DNA-damaged keratinocytes is bypassed by human papillomavirus 16 E7. *Proc. Natl. Acad. Sci. USA* **91**:4382–4386.

60. Hickman, E. S., Picksley, S. M., and Vousden, K. H. (1994) Cells expressing HPV16 E7 continue cell cycle progression following DNA damage induced p53 activation. *Oncogene* **9**:2177–2181.

61. Slebos, R. J. C., Lee, M. H., Plunkett, B. S., Kessis, T. D., Williams, B. O., Jacks, T., Hedrick, L., et al. (1994) p53-dependent G1-arrest involves pRb-related proteins and is disrupted by the human

papillomavirus E7 oncoprotein. *Proc. Natl. Acad. Sci. USA* **91**:5320–5324.

62. Chuang, L. S.-H., Ian, H.-I., Koh, T.-W., Ng, H.-H., Xu, G., and Li, B. F. L. (1997). Human DNA-(cytosine-5) methyltransferase-PCNA complex as a target for p21WAF1. *Science* **277**:1996–2000.

63. Waga, S., Hannon, G. J., Beach, D., and Stillman, B. (1994) The p21 inhibitor of cyclin-dependent kinases controls DNA replication by interaction with PCNA. *Nature* **369**:547–578.

64. Lam E. W.-F., Morris, J. D. H., Davies, R., Crook, T., Watson, R. J., and Vousden, K. H. (1994) HPV16 E7 oncoprotein deregulates B-myb expression: correlation with targeting of p107/E2F complexes. *EMBO J.* **13**:871–878.

65. Zerfass, K., Schulze, A., Spitkovsky, D., Friedman, V., Henglein, B., and Jansen-Dürr, P. (1995) Sequential activation of cyclin E and cyclin A gene expression by human papillomavirus type 16 E7 through sequences necessary for transformation. *J. Virol.* **69**:6389–6399.

66. Antinore, M. J., Birrer, M. J., Patel, D., Nader, L., and McCance, D. J. (1996) The human papillomavirus type 16 E7 gene product interacts with and trans-activates the AP1 family of transcription factors. *EMBO J.* **15**:1950–1960.

67. Massimi, P., Pim, D., Storey, A., and Banks, L. (1996) HPV-16 E7 and adenovirus E1a complex formation with TATA box binding protein is enhanced by casein kinase II phosphorylation. *Oncogene* **12**:2325–2330.

68. Hawley-Nelson, P., Vousden, K. H., Hubbert, N. L., Lowy, D. R., and Schiller, J. T. (1989) HPV16 E6 and E7 proteins cooperate to immortalise human foreskin keratinocytes. *EMBO J.* **8**:3905–3910.

69. Münger, K., Phelps, W. C., Bubb, V., Howley, P. M., and Schlegel, R. (1989) The E6 and E7 genes of the human papillomavirus type 16 together are necessary and sufficient for transformation of primary human keratinocytes. *J. Virol.* **63**:4417–4421.

70. Puthenveettil, J. A., Frederickson, S. M., and Reznikoff, C. A. (1996) Apoptosis in human papillomavirus16 E7- but not E6-immortalized uroepithelial cells. *Oncogene* **13**:1123–1131.

71. Jablonska, S. and Majewski, S. (1994) Epidermodysplasia verruciformis: immunological and clinical aspects. *Curr. Topics Microbiol. Immunol.* **186**:157–175.

72. Shahamanin, V., zur Hausen, H., Lavergne, D., Proby, C. M., Leigh, I. M., Neumann, C., et al. (1996) Human papillomavirus infections in non-melanoma skin cancers from renal transplant recipients and nonimmunosuppressed patients. *J. Natl. Cancer Inst.* **88**:802–811.

73. Robinson, W. S. (1994) Molecular events in the pathogenesis of hepadnavirus-associated hepatocellular carcinoma. *Ann. Rev. Med.* **45**:297–323.

74. Ganem, D. (1996) Hepadnaviridae and their replication. *In: Fields Virology* (Fields, B. N., Knipe, D. M., and Howley, P. M., ed.), Lippincott-Raven, Philadelphia, pp. 2703–2737.

75. Hollinger, F. B. (1996) Hepatits B virus. *In: Fields Virology* (Fields, B. N., Knipe, D. M., and Howley, P. M., ed.), Lippincott-Raven, Philadelphia, pp. 2739–2807.

76. Beasley, R. P. (1988) Hepatitis B virus. The major etiology of hepatocellular carcinoma. *Cancer* **61**:1942–1956.

77. Pisani, P., Parkin, D. M., Munoz, N., and Ferlay, J. (1997) Cancer and infection: estimates of the attributable fraction in 1990. *Cancer Epidemiol. Biomark. Prevent.* **6**:387–400.

78. Shirakata, Y., Kawada, M., Fujiki, Y., Sano, H., Kobayashi, M., and Koike, K. (1989) The X gene of hepatitis B virus induced growth stimulation and tumorigenic transformation of mouse NIH 3T3 cells. *Jpn. J. Cancer Res.* **80**:617–621.

79. Höhne, M., Schäfer, S., Seifer, M., Feitelson, M. A., Paul, D., and Gerlich, W. H. (1990) Malignant transformation of immortalised transgenic hepatocytes after transfection with hepatitis B virus DNA. *EMBO J.* **9**:1137–1145.

80. Kim, S., Koike, K., Saito, I., Myamura, F., and Ray, G. (1991) HBx gene of hepatitis B virus induces liver cancer in transgenic mice. *Nature* **351**:317–320.

81. Doria, M., Klein, N., Lucito, R., and Schneider, R. J. (1995) The hepatitis B virus Hbx protein is a dual specificity cytoplasmic activator of Ras and nuclear activator of transcription factors. *EMBO J.* **14**:4747–4757.

82. Koike, K. and Takada, S. (1995) Biochemistry and functions of hepatitis B virus X protein. *Intervirology* **38**:89–99.

83. Feitelson, M. A., Zhu, M., Duan, X.-L., and London, W. T. (1993) Hepatitis X-antigen and p53 are associated in vitro and in liver tissues from patients with primary hepatocellular carcinoma. *Oncogene* **8**:1109–1117.

84. Wang, X. W., Forrester, K., Yeh, H., Feitelson, M. A., Gu, J.-R., and Harris, C. C. (1994) Hepatitis B virus X protein inhibits p53 sequence-specific DNA binding, transcriptional activity, and association with transcription factor ERCC3. *Proc. Natl. Acad. Sci. USA* **91**:2230–2234.

85. Wang, X. W., Tgibson. M. K., Vermeulen, W., Yeh, H., Forrester, K., Stürzbecher, H.-W., et al. (1995) Abrogation of p53-induced apoptosis by the hepatitis B virus X gene. *Cancer Res.* **55**:6012–6016.

86. Ueda, H., Ullrich, S. J., Gangemi, J. D., Kappel, C. A., Ngo, L., Feitelson, M. A., et al (1995) Functional inactivation but not structural mutation of p53 causes liver cancer. *Nature Genet.* **9**:41–47.

87. Takada, S., Kaneniwa, N., Tsuchida, N., and Koike, K. (1997). Cytoplasmic retention of the p53 tumor suppressor gene product is observed in the hepatitis B virus X gene-transfected cells. *Oncogene* **15**:1895–1901.

88. Hilger, C., Velhagen, I., Zentgraf, H., and Schröder, C. H. (1991) Diversity of hepatitis B virus X gene-related transcripts in hepatocellular carcinoma: a novel polyadenylation site on viral DNA. *J. Virol.* **65**:4284–4291.

89. Hildt, E., Hofschneider, P. H., and Urban, S. (1996) The role of hepatitis B virus (HBV) in the development of hepatocellular carcinoma. *Semin. Virol.* **7**:333–347.

90. Dejean, A., Bouguerelet, L., Grzeschik, K. H., and Tiollais, P. (1986) Hepatitis B virus DNA integration in a sequence homologous to v-erb-A and steroid receptor genes in a hepatocellular carcinoma. *Nature* **322**:70–72.

91. Wang, J., Cenivesse, X., Henglein, B., and Brechot, C. (1990) Hepatitis B virus integration in a cyclin A gene in a hepatocellular carcinoma. *Nature* **343**:555–557.

92. Lieber, C. S., Garro, A., Leo, M. A., Mak, K. M., and Worner, T. (1986) Alcohol and cancer. *Hepatology* **6**:1005–1009.

93. Jhappan, C., Stahle, C., Harjins, R. N., Fausto, N., Smith, G. H., and Merlino, G. T. (1990) TGF-α overexpression in transgenic mice induces liver neoplasia and abnormal development of the mammary gland and pancreas. *Cell* **61**:1137–1146.

94. Houghton, M. (1996) Hepatitis C viruses. *In: Fields Virology* (Fields, B. N., Knipe, D. M., and Howley, P. M., eds.), Lippincott-Raven, Philadelphia, pp. 1035–1058.

95. Purcell, R. (1997). The hepatitis C virus: Overview. *Hepatology* **26**:11S–14S.

96. Choo, Q.-L., Kuo, G., Weiner, A. J., Overby, L. R., Bradley, D. W. and Houghton, M. (1989) Isolation of a cDNA clone derived from a blood-borne non-A, non-B viral hepatitis genome. *Science* **244**:359–362.

97. Hoofnagle, J. H. (1997) Hepatitis C: the clinical spectrum of disease. *Hepatology* **26**:15S–20S.

98. Farci, P., Alter, H. J., Govindarajan, S., Wong, D. C., Engle, R., Lesniewski, R. R., et al. (1992) Lack of protective immunity against reinfection with hepatitis C virus. *Science* **258**:135–140.

99. National Institutes of Health consensus development conference panel statement: management of hepatitis C. (1997) *Hepatology* **26**:2S–10S.

100. Di Bisceglie, A. M. (1997) Hepatitis C and hepatocellular carcinoma. *Hepatology* **26**:34S–38S.

101. Ray, R. B., Lagging, L. M., Meyer, K., and Ray, R. (1996) Hepatitis C virus core protein cooperates with ras and transforms primary rat embryo fibroblasts to tumorigenic phenotype. *J. Virol.* **70**:4438–4443.

102. Bhandari, B. N. and Wright, T. L. (1995) Hepatitis C: an overview. *Ann. Rev. Med.* **46**:309–317.

103. Kieff, E. (1996) Epstein-Barr virus and its replication. *In: Fields Virology* (Fields, B. N., Knipe, D. M., and Howley, P. M., eds.), Lippincott-Raven Publishers, Philadelphia, pp. 2343–2396.

104. Rickinson, A. B. and Kieff, E. (1996) Epstein Barr virus. *In: Fields Virology* (Fields, B. N., Knipe, D. M., and Howley, P. M., eds.), Lippincott-Raven, Philadelphia, pp. 2397–2446.

105. Niedobitek, G. and Young, L. S. (1994) Epstein-Barr virus persistance and virus-associated tumors. *Lancet* **343**:333–335.

106. Wang, D., Liebowitz, D., and Kieff, E. (1985) An EBV membrane protein expressed in immortalized lymphocytes transforms established rodent cells. *Cell* **43**:831–840.

107. Baichwal, V. R. and Sugden, B. (1988) Transformation of BALB 3T3 cells by the BNLF-1 gene of Epstein-Barr virus. *Oncogene* **2**:461–467.

108. Dawson, C. W., Rickinson, A. B., and Young, L. S. (1990) Epstein-Barr virus latent membrane protein inhibits human epithelial cell differentiation. *Nature* **344**:777–780.

109. Fahraeus, R., Rymo, L., Rhim, J. S., and Klein, G. (1990) Morphological transformation of human keratinocytes expressing the LMP gene of Epstein-Barr virus. *Nature* **345**:447–449.

110. Knecht, H., Berger, C., Al-Homsi, A. S., McQuain, C., and Brousset, P. (1997) Epstein-Barr virus oncogenesis. *Crit. Rev. Oncol. Hematol.* **26**:117–135.

111. Gires, O., Zimber-Strobl, U., Gonnella, R., Ueffing, M., Marschall, G., Zeidler, R., et al. (1997) Latent membrane protein 1 of Epstein-Barr virus mimics a constitutively active receptor molecule. *EMBO J.* **16**:6131–6140.

112. Wilson, J. B. and Levine, A. J. (1992) The oncogenic potential of Epstein-Barr virus nuclear antigen 1 in transgenic mice. *Curr. Top. Microbiol. Immunol.* **182**:375–384.

113. Srinivas, S. K. and Sixbey, J. W. (1995) Epstein-Barr virus induction of recombinase-activating genes RAG1 and RAG2. *J. Virol.* **69**:8155–8158.

114. Henkel, T., Liang, P. D., Hayward, S. D., and Peterson, M. G. (1994) Mediation of Epstein-Barr virus EBNA2 transactivation by recombination signal-binding protein J kappa. *Science* **265**:92–95.

115. Zimber-Strobl, U., Strobl, L. J., Meitinger, C., Hinrichs, R., Sakai, T., Furukawa, T., et al. (1994) Epstein-Barr virus nuclear antigen 2 exerts its transactivating function through interaction with recombination signal binding protein RBP-J kappa, the homologue of Drosophila suppressor of hairless. *EMBO J.* **13**:4973–4982.

116. Laux, G., Adam,. B., Strobl. L. J., and Moreau-Gachelin, F. (1994) The Spi/PU.1 and Spi-B ets family transcription factors and the recombination signal binding protein RBP-J kappa interact with an Epstein-Barr virus nuclear antigen 2 responsive cis-element. *EMBO J.* **13**:5624–5632.

117. Kempkes, B., Spitkovsky, D., Jansen-Dürr, P., Ellwart, J. W., Kremmer, E., Delecluse, H.-J., et al. (1995). B-cell proliferation and induction of early G1-regulating proteins by Epstein-Barr virus mutants conditional for EBNA2. *EMBO J.* **14**:88–96.

118. Parker, G. A., Crook, T., Bain, M., Sara, E. A., Farrell, P. J., and Allday, M. J. (1996) Epstein-Barr virus nuclear antigen (EBNA)3C is an immortalizing oncoprotein with similar properties to adenovirus E1A and papillomavirus E7. *Oncogene* **13**:2541–2549.

119. Szekely, L., Selivanova, G., Magnusson, K. P., Klein, G., and Wiman, K. G. (1993) EBNA-5, an Epstein-Barr virus-encoded nuclear antigen, binds to the retinoblastoma and p53 proteins. *Proc. Natl. Acad. Sci. USA* **90**:5455–5459.

120. Allday, M. J., Sinclair, A., Parker, G., Crawford, D. H., and Farrell, P. J. (1995) Epstein-Barr virus efficiently immortalizes human B cells without neutralizing the function of p53. *EMBO J.* **7**:1382–1391.

121. Oujedans, J. J., Jiwa, N. M., van den Brule, A. J. C., Gräser, F. A., Horstman, A., Vos, W., et al. (1995) Detection of heterogeneous Epstein-Barr virus gene expression patterns within individual posttransplantation lymphoproliferative disorders. *Am. J. Pathol.* **147**:923–933.

122. Magrath, I. (1990) The pathogenesis of Burkitt's lymphoma. *Adv. Cancer Res.* **55**:133–269.

123. Klein, G. and Klein, E. (1985) Evolution of tumors and the impact of molecular oncology. *Nature* **315**:190–195.

124. Lenoir, G. and Bornkamm, G. W. (1986) Burkitt's lymphoma: a human cancer model for the study of the multistep development of

cancer: proposal for a new scenario. *In:* Advances in Viral Oncology, vol. 7 (Klein, G., ed.), Raven Press, New York, pp. 173–206.

125. Geser, A., de The, G., Lenoir, G., Day, N. E., and Williams, E. H. (1982) Final case reporting from the Ugandian prospective study of the relationship between EBV and Burkitt's lymphoma. *Int. J. Cancer* **29**:397–400.

126. Rowe, M., Rowe, D. T., Gregory, C. D., Young, L. S., Farrell, P. J., Rupani, H., et al. (1987) Differences in B-cell growth phenotype reflect novel patterns of Epstein-Barr virus latent gene expression in Burkitt's lymphoma cells. *EMBO J.* **6**:2743–2751.

127. Levitskaya, J., Coram, M., Levitsky, V., Imreh, S., Steigerwald-Mullen, P. M., Klein, G., et al. (1995) Inhibition of antigen processing by the internal repeat region of the Epstein-Barr virus nuclear antigen-1. *Nature* **375**:685–688.

128. Simuzu, N., Tanabe-Kochikura, A., Kuroiwa, Y., and Takada, K. (1994) Isolation of Epstein-Barr virus (EBV)-negative cell clones from the EBV-positive Burkitt's lymphoma BL line Akata: Malignant phenotypes of BL cells are dependent on EBV. *J. Virol.* **68**:6069–6073.

129. Lam, K. M. C. and Crawford, D. H. (1991) The oncogenic potential of Epstein-Barr virus. *Crit. Rev. Oncogenesis* **2**:229–245.

130. Polack, A., Hortnagel, K., Pajic, A., Baier, B., Falk, M., Mautner, J., et al. (1996) c-myc activation renders proliferation of Epstein-Barr virus (EBV)-transformed cells independent of EBV nuclear antigen 2 and latent membrane protein. *Proc. Natl. Acad. Sci. USA* **93**:10411–10416.

131. Razzouk, B. I., Srinivas, S., Sample, C. E., Singh, V., and Sixbey, J. W. (1996) Epstein-Barr virus DNA recombination and loss in sporadic Burkitt's lymphoma. *J. Infect. Dis.* **173**:529–535.

132. List, A. F., Greco, F. A., and Vogler, L. B. (1987) Lymphoproliferative diseases in immunocompromised hosts: the role of Epstein-Barr virus. *J. Clin. Oncol.* **5**:1673–1689.

133. Oudejans, J. J., Jiwa, N. M., van den Brule, A. J. C., and Meijer, C. J. L. M. (1997). Epstein-Barr virus and its possible role in the pathogenesis of B-cell lymphomas. *Crit. Rev. Oncol. Hematol.* **25**:127–138.

134. Sullivan, J. L. and Woda, B. A. (1989) X-linked lymphoproliferative syndrome. *Immunodeficiency Rev.* **1**:325–347.

135. Starzl, T. E., Nalesnik, M. A., Porter, K. A., Ho, M., Iwatsuki, S., Griffith, B. P., et al. (1984) Reversibility of lymphomas and lymphoproliferative lesions developing under cyclosporin-steroid therapy. *Lancet* **1**:583–587.

136. Larson, R. S., Scott, M. A., McCurley, T. L., and Vnencak-Jones, C. L. (1996) Microsatellite analysis of posttransplant lymphoproliferative disorders: determination of donor/recipient origin and identification of putative lymphomagenic mechanism. *Cancer Res.* **56**:4378–4381.

137. Hamilton-Dutoit, S. J., Pallesen, G., Franzmann, M. B., Karkov, J., Black, F., Skinhoj, P., and Pedersen, C. (1991) AIDS-related lymphoma: Histopathology, immunophenotype, and association with Epstein-Barr virus as demonstrated by in situ nucleic acid hybridization. *Am. J. Pathol.* **138**:149–163.

138. Pallesen, G., Hamilton-Dutoit, S. J., and Shou, X. (1993) The association of Epstein-Barr virus (EBV) with T-cell lymphoproliferation and Hodgkin's disease: two new developments in the EBV field. *Adv. Cancer Res.* **62**:179–239.

139. Meijer, C. J. L. M., Jiwa, N. M., Dukers, D. F., Oudejans, J. J., de Bruin, P. C., Walboomers, J. M. M., et al. (1996) Epstein-Barr virus and human T-cell lymphomas. *Semin. Cancer Biol.* **7**:191–196.

140. Wolf, J. and Diehl, V. (1994) Is Hodgkin's disease an infectious disease? *Ann. Oncol.* **5**:S105–S111.

141. Herbst, H. (1996) Epstein-Barr virus in Hodgkin's disease. *Semin. Cancer Biol.* **7**:183-189.

142. Gutensohn, N. M. and Cole, P. (1980) Epidemiology of Hodgkin's disease. *Semin. Oncol.* **7**:92–102.

143. zur Hausen, H., Schulte-Holthausen, H., Klein, G., Henle, W., Henle, G., Clifford, P., and Santesson, L. (1970) EBV DNA in biopsies of Burkitt tumours and anaplastic carcinomas of the nasopharynx. *Nature* **228**:1056–1058.

144. Niedobitek, G., Agathanggelou, A., and Nicholls, J. M. (1996) Epstein-Barr virus infection and the pathogenesis of nasopharyngeal carcinoma: viral gene expression, tumour cell phenotype, and the role of the lymphoid stroma. *Semin. Cancer Biol.* **7**:165–174.

145. Henle, W., Ho, J. H. C., Henle, G., Chau, J. C. W., and Kwan, H. C. (1977) Nasopharyngeal carcinoma: significance of changes in Epstein-Barr virus-related antibody patterns following therapy. *Int. J. Cancer* **20**:663–672.

146. de The, G. and Zeng, Y. (1986) Population screening for EBV markers: towards improvement of nasopharyngeal carcinoma control. *In: The Epstein-Barr Virus* (Epstein, M. A. and Achog, B. G., eds.), John Wiley & Sons, New York, pp. 237–248.

147. Osato, T. and Imai, S. (1996) Epstein-Barr virus and gastric carcinoma. *Semin. Cancer Biol.* **7**:175–182.

148. Chang, Y., Cesarman, E., Pessin, M. S., Lee, F., Culpepper, C., Knowles, D. M., et al. (1994) Identification of herpesvirus-like sequences in AIDS-associated Kaposi's sarcoma. *Science* **266**:1865–1869.

149. Renne, R., Zhong, W., Herndier, B., McGrath, M., Kedes, D., and Ganem, D. (1996) Lytic growth of Kaposi's sarcoma-associated herpesvirus (human herpesvirus 8) in a cultured B-cell lymphoma line. *Nature Med.* **2**:342–346.

150. Russo, J. J., Bohenzky, R. A., Cheien, M. C., Chen, J., Yan. M., Maddalena, D., et al. (1996) Nucleotide sequence of the Kaposi's sarcoma-associated herpesvirus (HHV8). *Proc. Natl. Acad. Sci. USA* **93**:14862–14867.

151. Biesinger, B., Müller-Fleckenstein, I., Simmer, B., Lang, G., Wittmann, S., Platzer, E., et al. (1992) Stable growth transformation of human T-lymphocytes by herpesvirus saimiri. *Proc. Natl. Acad. Sci. USA* **89**:3116–3119.

152. Neipel, F., Albrecht, J.-C., and Fleckenstein, B. (1997) Cell homologous genes in the Kaposi's sarcoma-associated rhadinovirus human herpesvirus type 8: determinants of its pathogenicity? *J. Virol.* **71**:4187–4192.

153. Cheng, E. H. Y., Nicholas, J., Bellows, D., Hayward, G. S., Guo, H. G., Reitz, M. S., et al. (1997) A Bcl-2 homolog encoded by Kaposi's sarcoma-associated virus, human herpesvirus 8, inhibits apoptosis but does not heterodimerize with Bax or Bak. *Proc. Natl. Acad. Sci. USA* **94**:690–694.

154. Chang, Y., Moore, P. S., Talbot, S. J., Boshoff, C. H., Zarkowska, T., Godden-Kent, D., et al. (1996) Cyclin encoded by KS herpesvirus. *Nature* **382**:410.

155. Swanton, C., Mann, D. J., Fleckenstein, B., Neipel, F., Peters, G., and Jones, N. (1997) Herpes viral cyclin/Cdk6 complexes evade inhibition by CDK inhibitor proteins. *Nature* **390**:184–187.

156. Boshoff, C., Endo, Y., Collins, P. D., Takeuchi, Y., Reeves, J. D., Schweickart, V. L., et al. (1997) Angiogenic and HIV-inhibitory functions of KSHV-encoded chemokines. *Science* **278**:290–294.

157. Arvanitakis, L., Geras-Raaka, E., Varma, A., Gerhengorn, M. C., and Cesarman, E. (1997) Human herpesvirus KSHV encodes a constitutively active G-protein-coupled receptor linked to cell proliferation. *Nature* **385**:347–350.

158. Bais, C., Santomasso, B., Coso, O., Arvanitakis, L., Raaka, E. G., Gutkind, J. S., et al. (1998) G-protein-coupled receptor of Kaposi's sarcoma-associated herpesvirus is a viral oncogene and angiogenesis activator. *Nature* **391**:86–89.

159. Roth, W. K., Brandstetter, H., and Sturzl, M. (1992) Cellular and molecular features of HIV-associated Kaposi's sarcoma. *AIDS* **6**:895–913.

160. Ensoli, B., Barillari, G., and Gallo, R. C. (1992) Cytokines and growth factors in the pathogenesis of AIDS-associated Kaposi's sarcoma. *Immunol. Rev.* **127**:147–155.

161. Beral, V., Peterman, T. A., Berkelman, R. L., and Jaffe, H. W. (1990) Kaposi's sarcoma among patients with AIDS: a sexually transmitted infection? *Lancet* **335**:123–128.

162. Ganem, D. (1996) Human herpesvirus 8 and the biology of Kaposi's sarcoma. *Semin. Virol.* **7**:325–332.

163. Ensoli, B., Barillari, G., Salahuddin, S. Z., Gallo, R. C., and Wong-Staal, F. (1990) Tat protein of HIV-1 stimulates growth of cells derived from Kaposi's sarcoma lesions of AIDS patients. *Nature* **345**:84–86.

164. Ganem, D. (1997) KSHV and Kaposi's sarcoma: the end of the beginning? *Cell* **91**:157–160.

165. Gillison, M. L. and Ambinder, R. F. (1997) Human herpesvirus-8. *Curr. Opin. Oncol.* **9**:440–449.

166. Geraldo, G., Beth, E., and Haguenau, F. (1972) Herpes-type virus particles in tissue culture of Kaposi's sarcoma from different geographic regions. *J. Natl. Cancer Inst.* **49**:1509–1513.

167. Lennette, E. T., Blackbourn, D. J., and Levy, J. A. (1996) Antibodies to human herpesvirus type 8 in the general population and in Kaposi's sarcoma patients. *Lancet* **348**:858–861.

168. Soulier, J., Grollet, L., Oksenhendler, E., Cacoub, P., Cazals-Hatem, D., Babinet, P., et al. (1995) Kaposi's sarcoma-associated herpesvirus-like DNA sequences in multicentric Castleman's disease. *Blood* **86**:1276–1280.

169. Cesarman, E., Chang, Y., Moore, P. S., Said, J. W., and Knowles, D. M. (1995) Kaposi's sarcoma-associated herpesvirus-like DNA sequences in AIDS-related body-cavity-based lymphomas. *N. Engl. J. Med.* **322**:1186–1191.

170. Rettig, M. B., Ma, H. J., Vescio, R. A., Pold, M., Schiller, G., Belson, D., et al. (1997). Kaposi's sarcoma-associated herpesvirus infection of bone-marrow dendritic cells from multiple myeloma patients. *Science* **276**:1851–1854.

171. Cann, A. J. and Chen, I. S. Y. (1996) Human T-cell leukemia virus types I and II. *In: Fields Virology* (Fields, B. N., Knipe, D. M., and Howley, P. M., eds.), Lippincott-Raven, Philadelphia, pp. 1849–1880.

172. Kondo, T., Kono, H., Nonaka, H., Yoshida, R., Bando, F., Inoue, H., et al. (1987) Risk of adult T-cell leukemia lymphoma in HTLV-I carriers. *Lancet* **2**:159.

173. Rosenblatt, J. D., Golde, D. W., Wachsman, W., Giorgi, J. V., Jacobs, A., Schmidt. G. M., et al. (1986) A second isolate of HTLV-II associated with atypical hairy-cell leukemia. *N. Engl. J. Med.* **315**:372–377.

174. Yamamoto, N., Okada, M., Koyanagi, Y., Kannagi, Y., and Hinuma, Y. (1982) Transformation of human leukocytes by cocultivation with an adult T-cell leukemia virus producer cell line. *Science* **217**:737–739.

175. Popovic, M., Lange-Wantzin, G., Sarin, P. S., Mann, D., and Gallo, R. C. (1983) Transformation of human umbilical cord blood T cells by human T cell leukemia/lymphoma virus. *Proc. Natl. Acad. Sci. USA* **80**:5402–5406.

176. Seiki, M., Eddy, R., Shows, T. B., and Yoshida, M. (1984) Nonspecific integration of the HTLV provirus genome into adult T-cell leukaemia cells. *Nature* **309**:640–642.

177. Yoshida, M. (1996) Multiple targets of HTLV-I for dysregulation of host cells. *Semin. Virol.* **7**:349–160.

178. Grassmann, R., Dengler, C., Müller-Fleckenstein, I., Fleckenstein, B., McGuire, K., Dokhlear, M., et al. (1989) Transformation to continuous growth of primary human T-lymphocytes by human T cell leukemia virus type I X-region genes transduced by a herpesvirus saimiri vector. *Proc. Natl. Acad. Sci. USA* **86**:3351–3355.

179. Nerenberg, M., Hinrichs, S. H., Reynolds, R. K., Khoury, G., and Jay, G. (1987) The tat gene of human T lymphotropic virus type I induces mesenchymal tumors in transgenic mice. *Science* **237**:1324–1329.

180. Jeang, K. T., Widen, S. G., Semmes IV, O. J., and Wilson, S. H. (1990) HTLV-I trans-activator protein, Tax, is a trans-repressor of the human beta-polymerase gene. *Science* **247**:1082–1084.

181. Greene, W. C., Leonard, W. J., Wano, Y., Svetlik, P. B., Peffer, N. J., Sodrosky, J. G., et al. (1986) Trans-activator gene of HTLV II induces IL-2 receptor and IL-2 cellular gene expression. *Science* **232**:877–881.

182. Maruyama, M., Shibuya, H., Harada, H., Hatakeyama, M., Seiki, M., Fujita, T., et al. (1987) Evidence for aberrant activation of the interleukin-2 autocrine loop by HTLV-I-encoded p40x and T3/Ti complex triggering. *Cell* **48**:343–350.

183. Kimata, J. T. and Ratner, L. (1991) Temporal regulation of viral and cellular gene expression during human T-lymphotropic virus type I-mediated lymphocyte immortalization. *J. Virol.* **65**:4398–4407.

184. Suzuki, T., Kitao, S., Matsushime, H., and Yaoshida, M. (1996) HTLV-I Tax protein interacts with cyclin-dependent kinase inhibitor p16^{INK4A} and counteracts its inhibitory activity towards cdk4. *EMBO J.* **15**:1607–1614.

185. Pise-Masison, C. A., Choi, K.-S., Radonovich., M., Dittmer, J., Kim, S.-J., and Brady, J. N. (1998) Inhibition of p53 transactivation function by the human T-cell lymphotropic virus type 1 tax protein. *J. Virol.* **72**:1165–1170.

186. Reid, R. L., Lindholm, P. F., Mireskandari, A., Dittmer, J., and Brady, J. N. (1993) Stabilization of wild-type p53 in human T-lymphocytes transformed by HTLV-I. *Oncogene* **8**:3029–3036.

187. Cereseto, A., Diella, F., Mulloy, J. C., Cara, A., Michieli, P., Grassmann, R., et al. (1996) p53 functional impairment and high p21$^{WAF1/CIP1}$ expression in human T-cell lymphotropic/leukemia virus type I-transformed T cells. *Blood* **88**:1551–1560.

188. Kinoshita, T., Shimoyama, M., Tobinai, K., Ito, M., Ito, S., Ikeda, S., et al. (1989) Detection of mRNA for the tax$_1$/rex$_1$ gene of human T cell leukemia virus type I in fresh peripheral blood mononuclear cells of adult T-cell leukemia patients and viral carriers by using the polymerase chain reaction. *Proc. Natl. Acad. Sci. USA* **86**:5620–5624.

189. Hoppe-Seyler, F. and Butz, K. (1995) Molecular mechanisms of virus-induced carcinogenesis: the interaction of viral factors with cellular tumor suppressor proteins. *J. Mol. Med.* **73**:529–538.

190. Walboomers, J. M. M., de Roda Husman, A.-M., van den Brule, A. J. C., Snijders, P. J. F., and Meijer, C. J. L. M. (1994) Detection of genital human papillomavirus infections: critical review of methods and prevalence studies in relation to cervical cancer. *In: Cervical Cancer* (Stern, P., ed.), Oxford University Press, pp. 41–71.

191. Carbone, M., Rizzo, P., and Pass, H. I. (1997) Simian virus 40, poliovaccines and human tumors: a review of recent developments. *Oncogene* **15**:1877–1888.

192. Dörries, K. (1997) New aspects in the pathogenesis of polyomavirus-induced disease. *Adv. Virus Res.* **48**:205–261.

193. Greaves, M. F. and Alexander, F. E. (1993) An infectious etiology for common acute lymphoblastic leukemia in childhood? *Leukemia* **7**:349–360.

194. Schiller, J. T. and Lowy, D. R. (1996) Papillomavirus-like particles and HPV vaccine development. *Semin. Cancer Biol.* **7**:373–382.

195. Tindle, R. W. (1996) Human papillomavirus vaccines for cervical cancer. *Curr. Opin. Immunol.* **8**:643–650.

196. Chang, M. H., Chen, C. J., Lai, M. S., Hsu, H. M., Wu, T. C., Kong, M. S., et al. (1997) Universal hepatitis B vaccination in Taiwan and the incidence of hepatocellular carcinoma in children. Taiwan childhood hepatoma study group. *N. Engl. J. Med.* **336**:1855–1859.

HUMAN TUMOR SYSTEMS   VI

13 The Molecular Biology of Colorectal Carcinoma

Importance of the Wg/Wnt Signal Transduction Pathway

J. MILBURN JESSUP MD, GARY GALLICK PHD, AND BO LIU PHD

INTRODUCTION

Colorectal cancer is the third leading cause of cancer-related death. Although a recent trend indicates the beginning of a decline in the death rate *(1)*, this decline may be owing more to aggressive screening with fetal occult blood tests and flexible sigmoidoscopy *(2)* than to better therapeutic treatments. Better surgical techniques and adjuvant therapy are also undoubtedly responsible for the declining death rate owing to colon cancer. However, it is clear that too many patients still have either synchronous clinical metastases or develop a recurrence or metastasis within several years of resection of the primary cancer. Thus, a better understanding of the biology of neoplastic transformation and progression of tumor cells of the colon and rectum is needed so that novel and more useful therapeutic approaches can be designed. One of the more interesting developments in research on this disease is the tremendous explosion in the knowledge about the basic molecular and cellular biology of the development of colorectal carcinoma. This progress has resulted in the elucidation of molecular events that lead to large-bowel malignancy, and the molecular mechanisms of colorectal carcinogenesis serve as a paradigm for neoplastic development and progression of other solid tumors. The purpose of this chapter is to review the molecular pathways that are involved in colorectal carcinogenesis with an emphasis on their clinical importance. This review will assess the pathologic steps in neoplastic transformation, the signal-transduction pathways that are involved in neoplastic transformation, and the types of genetic alterations that produce neoplastic transformation. A full review of the events involved in the neoplastic progression to metastasis is beyond the scope of this chapter. For a complete review of metastatic progression, the reader is referred to recent reviews *(3,4)*. Furthermore, this review will not address the therapeutic implications of neoplastic transformation. Rather, it will emphasize how the primary genetic alterations

in colorectal carcinoma lead to changes in signal transduction pathways that are responsible for altered growth regulation.

THE BIOLOGY OF FAMILIAL AND SPORADIC COLORECTAL CARCINOMA

The pioneering work of Muto et al. *(5)* revealed that the majority of colorectal carcinomas develop from adenomatous polyps. The polyp-to-carcinoma sequence is based on several descriptive but supportive findings: 1) adenomatous polyps have a similar distribution to cancers that arise in the large bowel *(5,6)*; 2) the distribution of the mean age of developing polyps in the bowel is 5 yr earlier than the mean age of onset of large-bowel cancer *(5,7)*; 3) many large-bowel cancers display remnants of the polyp adjacent to the primary cancer; 4) serial biopsy of polyps that have not been resected reveal a slow process of transformation to an invasive cancer *(5,8)*; 5) endoscopic removal of adenomatous polyps decreases the risk of developing bowel cancer by 76–90% *(2)*; and 6) natural history studies of small unresected polyps reveal that some polyps less than 0.5 cm in diameter may regress, while others either remain unchanged or slowly progress to a larger more dysplastic phenotype *(9)*. Cannon-Albright et al. *(10)* have estimated that 19% of the general population develop adenomatous polyps and are at risk to develop colorectal carcinoma. Recent data also suggest that the general population continues to be at risk for developing adenomatous polyps as they age *(11)*. It is clear that the more adenomas that a patient develops, even without a familial history, the more likely he or she is to develop a colorectal carcinoma *(11)*.

Three recent findings have markedly advanced our understanding of the relationship between the formation of adenomatous polyps and invasive carcinomas. First, the lesion that precedes the development of a polyp is an aberrant crypt focus (ACF) that becomes a microadenoma. The ACF begins as an outpouching of an epithelium-lined sac from the side of the crypt of Lieberkuhn, which then expands and eventually develops into a separate broad-mouthed crypt *(12)*. Microadenomas are identified by methylene blue-dye staining at

From: *The Molecular Basis of Human Cancer* (W. B. Coleman and G. J. Tsongalis, eds.), © Humana Press Inc., Totowa, NJ.

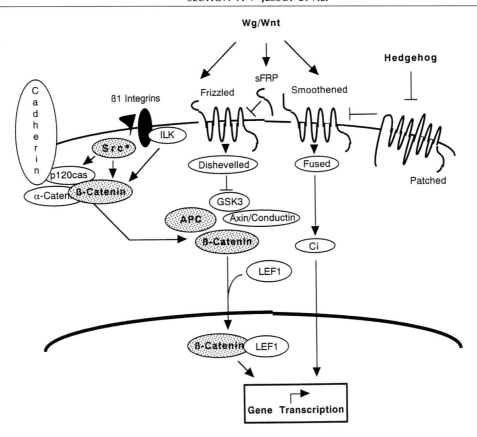

Fig. 1. The Wg/Wnt signal transduction pathway.

colonoscopy or in the pathology specimen because their crypt openings to the lumen of the bowel are several times larger than the normal crypt opening *(13)*. Roncucci et al. *(13)* have reported that microadenomas may be dysplastic, whereas others have shown that loss of tumor-suppressor genes and activation of proto-oncogenes occurs with frequencies similar to those in polypoid adenomas *(14,15)* or in carcinomas *(16–18)*. ACF and microadenomas are important because these lesions develop into adenomas and carcinomas in animal models of carcinogenesis *(19)*. However, the evidence that ACF develop into adenomatous polyps is circumstantial: patients with familial adenomatous polyposis (FAP) have an increased number of ACF compared to the number of ACF in patients with sporadic colorectal carcinomas, which also have more ACF than controls without cancer *(20)*. Recent observations indicate that ACF containing mutations in the adenomatous polyposis coli gene *(APC)* also display microsatellite instability (21), which is another molecular change associated with colorectal carcinogenesis. Thus, clinical detection of ACF may be an important tool for the diagnosis of patients with colorectal cancer.

The second recent finding is that not all adenomas are exophytic, but instead may be flat and difficult to detect on colonoscopy. Japanese investigators have focused on the flat adenoma *(22–25)* as a precursor lesion to carcinomas, many of which are ulcerated lesions that may be more aggressive than exophytic cancers *(26)*. These lesions have also been appreciated in European patients *(27)*. Further, flat adenomas may be precursors to the cancers that develop in hereditary nonpolyposis colorectal cancer (HNPCC) because they display

the microsatellite instability (MSI) that is observed in HNPCC as well as having a proximal large bowel distribution *(25)*. Lynch and his associates have identified several kindreds of patients who display the hereditary flat adenoma syndrome (HFAS) in which colon cancers develop at a later age than in FAP patients, have a proximal colon distribution, and arise in association with flat adenomas *(28)*. However, genetic-linkage studies suggest that these kindreds are linked to deletions on chromosome 5q and may be variants of FAP rather than altered presentations of HNPCC, which has prompted the use of the term attenuated familial adenomatous polyposis (AFAP) for this syndrome *(29)*.

The third observation is that a fraction of bowel cancers appear to arise without an antecedent polyp. Several reports suggested that adenocarcinomas of the bowel may arise without polypoid remnants or altered adjacent mucosa *(30,31)*. Bedenne et al. *(32)* demonstrated that ulcerated, infiltrating cancers in the right colon were less likely to be associated with an adenomatous polyp. These and other results suggested to Jass *(33)* that 10–30% of colorectal cancers may not develop from an antecedent adenomatous polyp, but arise *de novo* from mucosa that appears otherwise normal or has microadenomas. This finding is important because the current technology for diagnosis in asymptomatic individuals requires that a polyp be removed in order to prevent bowel cancer. As a result, under the present screening guidelines, somewhere between 70 and 90% of large-bowel cancers may be identified and removed before they become frankly invasive. However, under the best of circumstances 10–30% of large-bowel cancers may not develop from a benign polyp and may not be detectable and/or treatable until the lesion is frankly invasive.

WG/WNT SIGNAL TRANSDUCTION IS THE PRIMARY PATHWAY FOR THE DEVELOPMENT OF COLORECTAL CARCINOMA

The embryonic development of lower organisms has contributed greatly to defining the molecular interactions in human neoplastic transformation because molecular structure has been highly conserved during evolution. Because these organisms are relatively easy to manipulate genetically, they are useful in defining molecular pathways relevant to human diseases. The most important pathway for the development of colon carcinoma involves the Wingless/Wnt Gene (Wg/Wnt) signal-transduction pathway. However, elements of this pathway are involved in the etiology of other human cancers such as melanoma. Wnt1 is a secreted factor that was originally identified within mouse mammary cancers by its activation upon integration into the mouse mammary tumor virus (MMTV) gene (34). This protein is homologous to the Wingless (Wg) protein of Drosophila that is an important determinant of dorsal-ventral segmentation and regulates the formation of fly imaginal discs. Wg/Wnt control cell fates and both stimulate proliferation as well as induce cell death (35). Although Wnt1 is normally expressed only in the central nervous system (CNS) of vertebrates, there are at least 13 family members, some of which are expressed in mammary, intestinal, and other tissues. The Wnt proteins are ligands for a family of seven transmembrane domain receptor proteins related to Frizzled, a Drosophila polarity gene product required for the normal development of epidermal tissue polarity (36,37). The events downstream of Frizzled are being elucidated fairly quickly. In the normal cell, Wnt stimulates Frizzled to activate Disshevelled and glycogen synthase kinase 3β (GSK3β), which promotes the degradation of β-catenin after complexing with the adenomatous polyposis coli protein (APC) (Fig. 1). If GSK3β or APC activity is decreased, then β-catenin accumulates in the cytoplasm, binds the T-cell factor lymphocyte excitation factor (TCF/LEF) family of transcription factors, and translocates to the nucleus to induce gene transcription (38,39). Wg also induces the expression of a transcriptional repressor Engrailed, a transforming growth factor-β (TGF-β) family member Decapentaplegic, and the cytokine Hedgehog in Drosophila (35). Thus, β-catenin complexed with LEF1 may induce homologs of these genes in vertebrates that block cellular differentiation and facilitate neoplastic transformation.

β-catenin is also important because it binds α-catenin and E-cadherin, which are involved in intercellular adhesion (Fig. 1). Decreased β-catenin disrupts homotypic-cell adhesion and contributes to cellular motility and invasiveness (35), whereas increased β-catenin expression provides signals in Xenopus that are similar to the original Wg/Wnt signal (40). Cadherins mediate intracellular signaling by activation of the c-src family of protein tyrosine kinases, which phosphorylate catenins on tyrosine (41). The viral v-src homolog of the cellular protein tyrosine kinase c-src phosphorylates both β-catenin and a catenin-related protein, p120cas, which does not bind to APC but is phosphorylated in response to growth-factor stimulation

and v-src (42). When phosphorylated, these proteins decrease their binding to E-cadherin and β-catenin. This loss of binding promotes loss of cell adhesion and the accumulation of β-catenin within the cytoplasm. As a result, the cadherin-related proteins also effect the relative amounts of free β-catenin and serve as an example of the interaction between cell adhesion and the regulation of cell growth. In colon cancer c-src is also activated, such that its enzymatic activity is similar to v-src. Therefore, alterations induced by v-src in model systems are of relevance to development and progression of colon cancer.

Because Frizzled has membrane topology that is similar to that of the GTP-binding protein (G-protein)-coupled receptors, it may be involved in these pathways. However, the data are not conclusive for this connection to G-proteins. Wg/Wnt ligation by Frizzled leads to activation of Disshevelled, which in turn inhibits GSK3β (Fig. 1). GSK3β binds Disshevelled (43), β-catenin, and APC. GSK3β appears to inhibit the Wg/Wnt pathway by not only inhibiting Disshevelled but also by decreasing the levels of free β-catenin in the cytoplasm. GSK3β phophorylates APC and increases the binding of APC to β-catenin (44). β-catenin is targeted for degradation after it complexes with GSK3β and APC. Mutation in APC, β-catenin itself, or modulation of GSK3β kinase activity prevents the breakdown of β-catenin and leads to the accumulation of free β-catenin in the cytoplasm. Recent developments suggest that there are secreted homologs of Frizzled. These secreted Frizzled-related proteins (or sFRPs) (45,46) bind Wnt family members and block the Wg/Wnt pathway through competitive inhibition of Frizzled. Melkonyan et al. (47) have identified several similar if not identical sFRPs that differentially regulate the response to pro-apoptotic stimuli in human and murine cells. Lin et al. (48) observed that the cysteine-rich N-terminal domain of Frizzled is sufficient to bind and block the accumulation of β-catenin induced by Wnt. In addition, Sakanaka et al. (49) have reported that axin is a co-factor that binds both β-catenin and GSK3β and may inhibit the transcriptional activation by TcF/LEF-1 upon overexpression in human colon-carcinoma cells even when APC is inactivated by mutation. Similar findings by Behrens et al. (50) have identified a homolog of axin, conductin, that also promotes the degradation of β-catenin in colorectal-carcinoma cell lines. Interestingly, mutation in conductin was associated with accumulation of β-catenin in the cytoplasm with increased LEF/TCF transcriptional activation. In contrast, Novak et al. (51) identified an integrin-linked kinase (ILK) that contains ankyrin-like repeats in a serine-threonine kinase that binds β-1 and β-3 integrin cytoplasmic domains. Overexpression of this protein in intestinal epithelial cells is associated with decreased cell-cell interactions, gain of anchorage-independent growth, and tumorigenicity in athymic nude mice. These actions are associated with a decrease in E-cadherin expression, increased β-catenin translocation to the nucleus and increased transcription of LEF1. These results suggest that the modulation of β-catenin by intercellular adhesion may be quite complex with both positive and negative regulation of LEF1 transcription.

The Notch and Hedgehog pathways in Drosophila and Xenopus also modulate the Wg/Wnt signal-transduction pathway. Wg-mediated activation of Frizzled leads to increased Hedge-

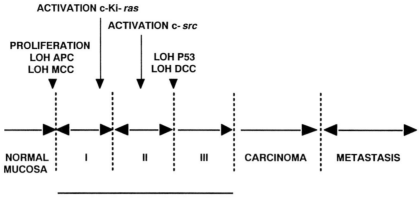

Fig. 2. The FAP pathway. Genetic alterations that occur during the development of colorectal carcinomas either in patients with FAP or sporadically. Right-directed arrows indicate progression from one state to the next. Left-directed arrows indicate that regression from a higher state to a lower may occur.

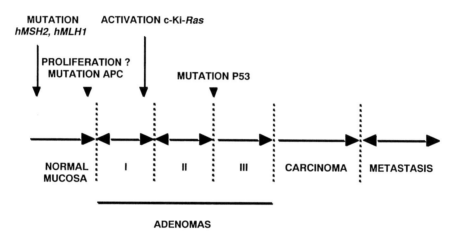

Fig. 3. The HNPCC pathway. Genetic alterations during the development of colorectal carcinomas in patients with HNPCC or that occur sporadically in association with MSI. Right-directed arrows indicate progression from one state to the next. Left-directed arrows indicate that regression from a higher state to a lower may occur.

hog production in neighboring cells. Increased Hedgehog in turn leads to further stimulation of Wg production by either inhibiting Patched or stimulating Smoothened that induces the Cubitus inductus zinc-finger protein to transcriptionally activate Wg *(52,53)*. In contrast, Notch is a family of at least four receptor proteins that are involved with regulation of neighboring cell fates *(54)*. Another of the Notch proteins is also involved in the Wg/Wnt pathway because Notch-4 *(55)* is Int-3 that can also be activated by integration into MMTV as occurs with Wnt-1. Mutations in *APC* and/or β-catenin appear to be essential for the causation of approx 90% of large-bowel carcinomas. Although mutational inactivation of *APC* leads to increased levels of β-catenin and downstream signaling through LEF, mutation in *APC* also directly effects other molecular pathways that involve cell motility and invasiveness as well as response to pro-apoptotic stimuli. Vogelstein and colleagues demonstrated that approx 75% of sporadic colorectal carcinomas contain a somatic mutation in *APC (56)*. However, more recently Morin et al. *(57)* and Sparks et al. *(58)* have found that approx 50% of the colorectal carcinomas that lacked an *APC* mutation have a mutation in β-*catenin* that increases β-catenin protein stability and ability to transcriptionally activate *LEF1*.

In addition, mutations have not been found in *GSK3β*. The general importance of the Wg/Wnt pathway is further underscored by the finding that a significant proportion of human melanomas also contain mutations in β-*catenin (59)*. Thus, modification of the Wg/Wnt signal-transduction pathway is only the beginning of the transformation for bowel epithelium. It also remains to be seen whether mutation in other members of the Wg/Wnt and adjacent signal transduction pathways may also be involved in colorectal carcinogenesis.

THE MOLECULAR PATHWAYS FOR COLORECTAL CARCINOMAS: DIFFERENT CAUSES FOR GENETIC INSTABILITY

Current evidence indicates that colorectal carcinoma develops through as many as three related, but slightly different, alterations of the Wg/Wnt signal-transduction pathway. The first and best described modification involves mutation in the *APC* gene. This germline mutation causes the appearance of hundreds to thousands of adenomatous polyps in the large bowel and is the cause of the autosomally dominantly inherited FAP and related syndromes *(60)*. The molecular alterations that occur in this pathway largely involve deletions of alleles of

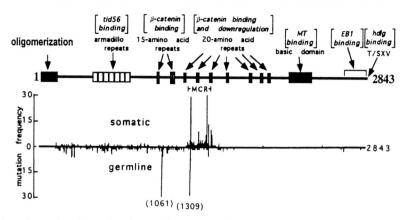

Fig. 4. Frequency and location of mutations in APC. Scheme of APC gene with functional domains identified as well as the profile of the known mutations within the gene. Adapted from Polakis *(84)*.

tumor-suppressor genes, including loss of heterozygosity (LOH) for *APC, p53,* and *DCC* (for Deleted in Colorectal Cancer) *(56)*, combined with mutational activation of proto-oncogenes, especially c-K-*ras (61,62)* (Fig. 2). In contrast, mutation of the human homologs of the bacterial *mutHLS* complex (*hMSH2, hMLH1, hPMS1,* and *hPMS2*) produces the DNA mismatch repair (MMR) defects that appear to cause the HNPCC *(63–68)*. The mutations in DNA MMR enzymes lead to genetic instability that represents errors in the accurate replication of the repetitive mononucleotide, dinucleotide, trinucleotide, and tetranucleotide repeats that are scattered throughout the genome *(69–72)*. As a result, the genomic instability identified in HNPCC is commonly referred to as either replication error positive (RER+) or, because microsatellite regions in the genome contain the nucleotide repeats, as microsatellite instability (originally referred to as MIN but now preferred as MSI). Although these replication errors produce mutations in many of the same tumor-suppressor genes and proto-oncogenes that are involved in the FAP pathway, there is a significant lower frequency of LOH in the HNPCC pathway *(70)* (Fig. 3).

As suggested by Kinzler and Vogelstein *(62)*, both the FAP and HNPCC pathways lead to genomic instability. The FAP pathway is associated with gains or losses of portions or entire chromosomes. This leads to aneuploidy, which has been associated with a poor prognosis in colorectal carcinoma *(73)*. In contrast, tumors in the HNPCC pathway with MSI have instability only in short segments within genes and generally are diploid on cytogenetic analysis. Tomlinson et al. *(74)* demonstrated difficulty in measuring the effect of mutation rate in the HNPCC pathway on the accumulation of errors in genes and suggested that in MSI, the selection of malignant cells is more important than the overall rate of mutation, although mutations in specific target genes may occur at a high rate. In contrast, Lengauer et al. *(75)* observed that genetic instability is very high in tumors arising in the FAP pathway. This suggests that there are two fundamental genetic etiologies in colorectal cancer. The first is the segregator pathway that involves a defect in chromosome segregation in FAP-associated tumors and leads to LOH. The second is the so called mutator pathway, which

involves selection of cells with specific mutations generated by MSI.

Finally, although many sporadic carcinomas appear to follow either the segregator or mutator pathway, colorectal carcinomas that arise *de novo* seem to have a slightly different pattern of molecular alterations that may suggest a third, yet-to-be-defined molecular pathway. *De novo* carcinomas may have similar rates of mutation in the *p53* gene *(76)* as carcinomas that arise in association with adenomatous polyps, but do not appear to contain c-K-*ras* mutations *(77)*. Interestingly, the expression of the intestinal *mucin* gene product MUC2 seems to be lost in *de novo* carcinomas while it is retained in both mucinous cancers and carcinomas arising from polyps *(78)*. These studies with *de novo* colorectal carcinomas need to be better developed before the *de novo* carcinoma is accepted as another molecular pathway for neoplastic transformation. However, it is possible that another, as-yet-undefined set of mutations may be associated with the environmental and dietary causes of carcinoma that epidemiologic studies suggest should be associated with bowel carcinoma.

FAMILIAL ADENOMATOUS POLYPOSIS SYNDROMES AND THE *APC* GENE

Cytogenetic analyses demonstrate a frequent loss of material on chromosome 5q in patients with FAP *(79)* that is associated with loss of *APC*, a tumor-suppressor gene that resides at 5q21 *(60)*. More recent work has demonstrated that the *APC* gene is unambiguously the target of these chromosomal deletions *(80–82)*. The affected gene is the earliest identified primary genetic change in the development of adenomas and is present in adenomatous polyps of 5-mm diameter *(83)*. Somatic mutations occur in 75% of sporadic tumors (56), and other familial syndromes, like Gardner's syndrome *(80)*. The wild-type gene contains 15 exons, which encode a protein of 2843 amino acids *(84)* (Fig. 4). The gene has several regions whose function has been identified. The amino-terminal portion of the protein is involved with oligomerization through homophilic binding *(85,86)*. Then there are two types of binding sites for β-catenin *(87,88)* and GSK3β *(44)*, followed by a site for attachment to microtubules *(89,90)*, the EB1 protein

(91) and the human discs large protein (hdlg) *(92)* (Fig. 4). Interestingly, upon activation of the T-cell receptor T lymphocytes upregulate the expression of *RP1*, an *EB1* homolog, as proliferation and transcription increases *(93)*. Because RP1 binds to wild-type but not mutant APC, APC may be involved in the proliferation of normal lymphocytes and possibly other cell types. Sequence homology also exists between APC and structural proteins like myosin and keratin *(82)*, and the GTPase-activating protein (GAP), which regulates the c-K-*ras* gene product, suggesting a potential role for this gene in signal-transduction processes that are important for cellular proliferation *(83)*.

In addition to the active regions of the molecule the location of a protein within the cell provides clues to its function. Neufeld and White *(94)* have shown that APC is not only in the cytoplasm but also may be present in the nucleus as well, where it is localized primarily within nucleoli. This finding prompted the speculation that APC may be involved with ribosomal RNA (rRNA) function, especially because mutated APC does not enter the nucleus. Neufeld and White *(94)* also demonstrated that cytoplasmic APC was concentrated at the leading edge of cells, possibly in association with areas rich in microtubules *(89,90)*. Because purified APC proteins promote the polymerization of tubulin in vitro to form microtubules *(90)*, Trzepacz et al. *(95)* assessed whether APC may be involved in cell-cycle events, especially during mitosis when changes in microtubule structure are required for the cell to complete division. These investigators found that wild-type APC binds to and is phosphorylated by p34^cdc2 alone as well as active p34^cdc2-cyclin B complexes. Mutant APC does not undergo this phosphorylation nor does it appear to be involved in mitosis. Thus, wild-type APC may promote progression through mitosis. When wild-type *APC* is re-introduced into cells containing mutant *APC*, apoptosis may occur *(96)* and tumorigenicity may be suppressed *(97)*. The role of APC in cell death is controversial not only because the previous studies did not demonstrate a specific segment of APC to be involved in apoptosis, but also because Brown et al. (98) demonstrated that APC expression was lost as a human colonic adenoma-cell line underwent apoptosis during detachment from a substratum. This suggests that loss of attachment causes degradation of APC, which is associated with apoptosis. As a result, the role of APC in apoptosis is complex and must be considered in the context of intercellular and cell/substrate interactions. In addition, at least one human colorectal carcinoma cell line (SW480 that expresses mutant *APC*) has the ability to downregulate expression of wild-type *APC* when it is re-expressed by transfection *(97,99)*. Although this result may be a nonspecific response to the expression of a wild-type protein, it still supports a role for APC in a signal-transduction pathway that is involved in determining cell fate during embryogenesis.

In summary, APC has many roles within the cell that are only now beginning to be understood. APC appears to oligomerize, a finding that suggests that a mutant, truncated protein may alter the function of a wild-type normal APC protein. APC appears to be involved in cell division, invasion, adhesion, and rRNA processing either directly or indirectly.

With so many functions, it is possible specific mutations in functional domains may alter the biological behavior of the malignant cells. Furthermore, it is not surprising that different mutations in APC have different biologic consequences.

MUTATIONAL ANALYSIS OF APC: GENOTYPE-PHENOTYPE ASSOCIATIONS

Mutations of *APC* are generally either point mutations or insertions of mobile genetic elements that lead to chain termination and production of truncated proteins *(100,101)*. Progress has been made in understanding the significance of the different locations of germline and somatic mutations in APC on the biology of colorectal carcinoma, but much remains to be clarified. For example, the location of the mutation may influence the number of adenomatous polyps produced with shorter proteins associated with fewer polyps than longer proteins *(29,102–107)*. Germline mutations at either the 5'-end of the gene (in the oligomerization region) or in the 3'-end in the hdlg region cause an attenuated form of FAP in which there are relatively few adenomatous polyps (usually 5–10, but less than 50) and late onset of polyposis. Van der Luijt et al. *(108)* demonstrated in two kindreds that germline mutations in the 3'-part of exon 15 in *APC* (codons 1862 and 1987) resulted in the creation of termination signals with an attenuated phenotype in that truncated protein was not detected, polyp frequency was generally 10 or less per patient, and cancer development was delayed for 15 yr on average. Spirio et al. *(106)* reported that germline mutations in exons 3 and 4 in the oligomerization region were associated with production of truncated proteins that represented termination signals in codons 83–156 and an attenuated phenotype for polyp production similar to that described by van der Luijt et al. *(108)*. However, other exon 4 mutations involving codon 157 *(109)*, in codon 168 *(110)*, and codons 169–170 *(111)* result in the classic FAP phenotype with hundreds to thousands of adenomatous polyps in the colon and rectum. Thus, there appears to be a very sharp boundary for phenotype that modulates the number of polyps with germline mutations that are located only a few codons apart. This has led Lynch and others *(29)* to propose that there is an AFAP syndrome, which is a variant of FAP even though patients have few polyps and are easily confused with HNPCC. However, the germline mutation, the absence of MSI or mutations in DNA MMR genes, and the left-sided location of the carcinomas supports an association with FAP.

Germline mutations in other regions of the *APC* gene are also associated with specific phenotypes. Olschwang et al. *(112)* observed that congenital hypertrophy of the retinal pigment epithelium (CHRPE) was associated with mutations that were 3' to the alternative splice site in exon 9 or distal to codon 438. Bunyan et al. *(102)* confirmed that CHRPE was associated with mutations distal to exon 9. Profuse polyposis appears to be associated with mutations between codons 1250 and 1464 *(105)*, which also includes the region of most frequent mutation, the mutation cluster region. Mutations outside of this region are generally associated with less severe polyposis. Mutations 3' to codon 1403 are more likely to be associated with the extracolonic tumors that occur in Gardner's syndrome, the variant of FAP that includes desmoids, osteomas, duodenal, and gastric neoplasms *(113)*. Miyoshi et al. *(114)* demonstrated that somatic mutations were even more prevalent in the mutation cluster region.

Deficiencies in the enzymes that repair DNA mismatches is the hallmark of HNPCC. Interestingly, *APC* is as frequently mutated in tumors with MSI but the spectrum of mutations is different *(115)*. Tumors with MSI were more likely to have mutations in mononucleotide or dinucleotide-repeat regions than tumors that did not have MSI *(115)*. Although the regions of mutations were generally similar in MSI-negative and MSI-positive tumors, the types of mutations and amino acid substitutions were different. Because MSI-positive tumors have a better outcome than MSI-negative tumors *(71)*, it is highly likely that the type of somatic mutation may be associated with outcome.

It is also clear that the site of germline mutation in the APC gene is not the only determinant of the resultant phenotype. Other genes appear to modulate the phenotype. This was first identified in mice where mutation in the *APC* gene (Min mice) led to the appearance of polyps in the distal small bowel, as well as the colon *(116)*. Interestingly, expression of polyps was strain-specific and appeared to be related to an adjacent locus named modulator of Min or MOM. Subsequent work demonstrated that in mice the locus appears to be the secreted form of phospholipase A2 *(117,118)*. However, the role of this locus in modulating the phenotype of FAP in humans is controversial *(119,120)*. It should be noted that the creation of other mutant *APC* genes in mice also induces colon polyps and even adenocarcinomas that are restricted to the colon and rectum *(121,122)*. Finally, Laken et al. *(123)* have recently demonstrated that Ashkenazim have a predilection for a single nucleotide transition from T to A at position 3920, which creates a hypermutable site that may lead to increased susceptibility to further mutation. The impact of this mutation is controversial. Clearly, much remains to be elucidated about specific sites of mutations in *APC*, either germline or somatic, and the resultant phenotype or biological aggressiveness of colorectal cancer.

HNPCC

HNPCC is a common autosomal dominant disorder characterized with an early onset of cancers in colon, rectum, endometrium, ovary, and several other organs *(124,125)*. The term HNPCC is used to distinguish this syndrome from FAP, because HNPCC patients do not often present with polyposis. HNPCC was first described by Aldred Warthin about 100 years ago *(126)*. The clinical importance of the disorder was recognized in 1966 when Henry Lynch described two families with an autosomal dominant inheritance pattern of nonpolyposis colorectal cancer and endometrial cancer *(127)*. Patients with HNPCC develop colorectal carcinoma often in the absence of adenomatous polyps and have an early age of onset, frequently before or during their fourth decade of life. Tumors in HNPCC have certain clinical features, such as proximal bowel location and the development of multiple primary-bowel carcinomas that is defined as the Lynch syndrome I, while the development of cancers in endometrium, ovary, and other organs is the Lynch syndrome II *(128)*. The International Collaborative Group (ICG) on HNPCC has defined an HNPCC kindred as meeting the following three minimal criteria (ICG criteria or Amsterdam Criteria): 1) there should be at least three family members with colorectal cancer, two of whom are first-degree relatives; 2) there should be at least two generations represented; 3) at least one individual should be less than 50 yr of age at the time of diagnosis *(129)*. Based on the ICG criteria, it is estimated HNPCC may account for about 6% of total colorectal cancer *(125,130–131)*.

The gene for HNPCC was mapped to chromosome 2p16 or 3p21 by linkage analysis *(69,132)*. It was initially suspected that HNPCC was caused by mutations in a tumor-suppressor gene. According to Knudson's hypothesis for tumor-suppressor genes, an individual with a genetic predisposition to cancer inherits one normal and one defective tumor-suppressor gene *(133)*. A tumor is more likely to occur in such an individual because only the remaining normal gene needs to be inactivated, often through loss of chromosomal regions containing the tumor-suppressor gene. Nevertheless, totally unexpected results were obtained when microsatellite markers tightly linked to the disease locus were used to search for allelic loss. The search did not find any chromosome loss at the 2p16 loci; instead, it identified an unusual genetic-instability phenotype associated with tumors arising from HNPCC patients *(70)*. The instability phenotype was characterized by widespread somatic alterations in genomic microsatellite sequences. These microsatellite sequences are the short tandem-repeat DNA scattered throughout the human genome, and seem particularly prone to insertions or deletions in HNPCC tumors. Interestingly, the same type of MSI found in HNPCC tumors was initially identified in about 15% of sporadic colorectal cancers *(71,72)*.

The discovery of the MSI phenotype in HNPCC tumors suggested that the disease might be caused by mutation in a novel gene associated with replication errors. Investigators studying DNA-replication fidelity in unicellular organisms recognized that the MSI phenotypes observed in HNPCC tumors were similar to those in the mutant yeast lacking a functional DNA MMR system *(134)*. MMR normally functions as a caretaker to correct errors arising from DNA replication, genetic recombination, and chemical modification of DNA. A cell that is defective in MMR accumulates mutations rapidly, especially in the microsatellite-repeat sequences where strand slippage occurs frequently during DNA replication. MMR was first described in bacteria, later in yeast *(135)*. Based on the knowledge learned from the bacterial and yeast MMR systems, it was hypothesized that defective MMR genes might be the cause of HNPCC *(134)*. Direct genetic evidence demonstrating human MMR genes as the cause of HNPCC was provided by the discovery of germline mutation of *hMSH2*, a *mutS* homolog, in HNPCC kindreds linked to chromosome 2p16 *(63,64)*. Subsequently, germline mutations of *hMLH1*, a *mutL* homolog, were found in the other HNPCC kindreds linked to 3p21 *(65,66)*. Six human MMR genes have now been identified. These are the *mutS* homologs, *hMSH2, hMSH3, hMSH6*, and *mutL* homologs, *hMLH1, hPMS1*, and *hPMS2*. Considerable advances have been made in understanding the biological function of human MMR. Biochemical studies of the human MMR proteins show that they are evolutionary conserved and the

Single base mispairs or displaced base   Larger mismatches or displaced loop of 2 to 4 bases

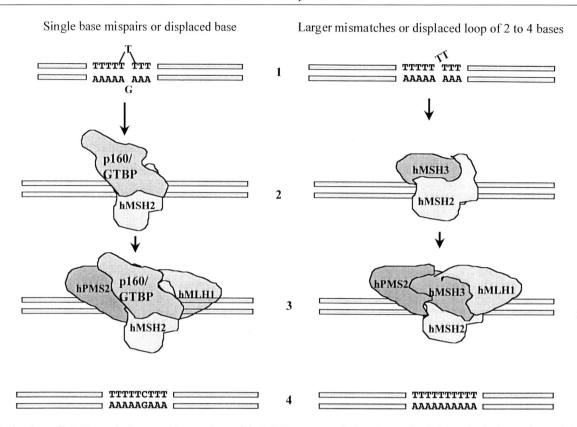

Fig. 5. Mechanism of MMR repair. Proposed interactions of the MMR enzymes during the repair of either single-base mismatch (mispair or displaced base) or multiple-base mismatch or displaced loop of 2–4 bases.

proteins function similarly in mammalian cells, yeast, and bacteria *(136–140)*. Genetic and functional complementation experiments have defined *hMSH2, hMSH3, hMSH6, hMLH1, hPMS1,* and *hPMS2* as the essential components required for the human MMR system *(67,68,141)*. Mutation in any one of these six genes will result in a defective cellular MMR and can lead to the development of the MSI phenotype *(63–65,70,142–146)*. Human MMR is initiated by the binding of a MutS protein complex to the mismatched site in a newly synthesized DNA strand, resulting in the formation of a MutS-DNA complex. The formation of a MutS-DNA complex recruits hMLH1, hPMS1, and hPMS2 proteins to interact with the mismatched DNA. The DNA-MutS-MutL complex initiates the excision and correction of the erroneous DNA strand much as it does in the bacterial and yeast MMR pathways. Biochemical studies using recombinant *hMSH2, hMSH3,* and *hMSH6* indicate that hMSH3 or hMSH6 forms heterodimeric MutS complexes with hMSH2. Whereas the hMSH2:hMSH3 only functions in repairing mismatched sequences arising from insertion or deletion of several nucleotides, the hMSH2:hMSH6 complex recognizes both single-base mismatched DNA and mismatched sequences caused by smaller insertion or deletion of 2–4 nucleotides (Fig. 5) *(147–152)*. In addition to correction of base-pair mismatches and slippage errors arising during DNA replication, MMR also participates in avoiding mutations in DNA recombination and in chemical-induced DNA mismatch *(142,152)*. MMR proteins are expressed in all proliferating cells. However, HNPCC patients carrying germline MMR

mutations develop tumors in a few organs, which are mostly restricted to the proximal colon, endometrium, and less commonly ovary and breast *(153,154)*. In rare instances, patients with HNPCC also develop Muir-Torre syndrome or Turcott syndrome *(155,156)*. The basis for these clinical variations has not been established.

Analysis of HNPCC tumors indicates that about 90% of the HNPCC develop tumors with MSI *(155,156)*. Because the MSI phenotype is the result of homozygous inactivation of a cellular MMR, it is believed that 90% of these HNPCC patients with the MSI phenotype have an inherited mutant MMR gene allele. The remaining 10% of the HNPCC individuals whose tumors lack MSI are likely predisposed to mutations in other unknown genes not involved in cellular MMR. Mutational analysis of MMR genes in HNPCC shows that defective *hMSH2* and *hMLH1* are the major cause of the disease, accounting for more than 95% of the identified germline mutations, whereas mutation of *hPMS1* and *hPMS2* in HNPCC account for less than 5% of total germline mutations (Table 1). One case of germline mutation in *hMSH6* was found in a familial colorectal carcinoma without meeting HNPCC criteria *(158)*. Nevertheless, germline mutations in *hMSH6* and *hMSH3* have not been reported in the classic HNPCC. Depending on the penetrance, it is estimated that germline mutation carriers of a defective mutant MMR gene carriers have a 60–70% lifetime risk for developing colorectal cancer *(159)*. Somatic cells in the great majority of affected HNPCC members have normal MMR function because the wild-type allele functions normally and must

Table 1
Human Mismatch Repair Genes in HNPCC

MMR genes	Chromosome location	Number of kindreds with germline mutation[a]
hMSH2	2p16	21% (10/48 kindreds)
hMSH3	5q11-q13	-
hMSH6	2p16	-
hMLH1	3p21	25% (12/48 kindreds)
hPMS1	2q32	2% (1/48 kindreds)
hPMS2	7p22	2% (1/48 kindreds)

[a]Number of mutations based on the analysis of 48 HNPCC kindreds.

be inactivated by a second-hit before the MSI phenotype develops. However, in several cases a dominant germline MMR mutation has been observed to inhibit the MMR function of the wild-type allele *(160,161)*.

Recent studies indicate that HNPCC tumorigenesis arises from the accumulation of mutations in genes containing simple repeat sequences by mutations in *APC, TGFβRII,* and *bax (115,162–166)*. Mutations in c-K-*ras,* and *p53* genes may not be as frequently associated with tumors arising from HNPCC individuals *(167–169)*. Mutations in *APC, TGFβRII,* and *bax* are clearly caused by a defective MMR-associated carcinogenesis in which the mononucleotide repeat located in the coding region of these genes is specifically targeted for insertions and deletions. Since both *TGFβRII* and *bax* genes are potent inhibitors of cell proliferation, mutations in these genes may lead to transformation of normal colonic epithelial cells into a malignant tumor. The mechanism of defective MMR-associated carcinogenesis seems to extend Knudson's hypothesis for tumor-suppressor genes. Based on Knudson's hypothesis, HNPCC carcinomas with the MSI phenotype arise in patients with one inherited mutant MMR allele and one wild-type allele. However, during tumorigenesis, the remaining wild-type MMR allele is inactivated by somatic mutations. Inactivation of both MMR alleles results in the rapid accumulation of MSI during each round of DNA replication in colon epithelium cells. The importance of MMR in multi-stage carcinogenesis is that it may increase the mutation rate within specific genes without producing widespread defects in chromosome structure *(74)*. Although microsatellite-repeat sequences seem to be the primary targets of the MSI, simple and short polyA or polyG tracks in the gene coding region also become mutable by MSI in cells defective in MMR. A rapid accumulation of MSI in genes critical for controlling cellular proliferation results in the acceleration of tumor progression. Thus, HNPCC patients with a germline mutation in an MMR gene develop colon cancer at a very early age.

HNPCC is preventable if it is diagnosed early. A major clinical implication in understanding the molecular basis of HNPCC is the ability to improve the early diagnosis of the disease through genetic testing. One of the potential problems in the molecular diagnosis of HNPCC is the lack of an effective method to detect germline mutations. In one of the earlier stud-

ies, a cohort of 48 highly selected HNPCC kindreds were analyzed for germline mutation in *hMSH2, hMLH1, hPMS1, hPMS2,* and *hMSH6*. All kindreds had MSI tumors, indicating a defective germline MMR mutation in these kindreds. However, germline mutations were detected in only half of the 48 kindreds *(154)*. Several recent mutational studies have further illustrated the point that germline mutation in an MMR gene could not be effectively detected using current DNA based technologies *(170,171)*. Furthermore, there are six human MMR genes whose exact roles in HNPCC are not fully understood. If a germline mutation is not found in one of the two major MMR genes, *hMSH2* or *hMLH1*, should the other four genes be analyzed? Because mutations in these genes encompass a large spectrum of the coding regions, often the entire coding region for each MMR gene needs to be analyzed to be able to determine if mutations have occurred. Because all the known mutations seem to be heterozygous and few hot spots are evident, the entire coding region for each of the MMR genes has to be analyzed. As a result, a tremendous amount of work is required to identify a single germline mutation in a HNPCC kindred. This makes screening for a single germline mutation in a HNPCC kindred a large effort in both labor and cost.

ALTERATIONS IN EXPRESSION OF CELL-SURFACE AND EXTRACELLULAR-MATRIX PROTEINS IN THE DEVELOPMENT OF COLON CANCER

In colon-tumor cells, many changes follow the original mutations in *APC* that directly affect the proteins of the extracellular matrix (ECM), which in turn alters fundamental growth control. Indeed, recent studies have implicated the ECM as an important mediator of many signaling-transduction processes, including cell adhesion, migration, mitosis, and apoptosis. Cell-cell and cell-ECM interactions are central processes in organogenesis and tissue remodeling, and represent dynamic processes regulating cell proliferation, as dividing cells must transiently detach from the ECM to complete cell division. Loss of contact inhibition is a classic hallmark of many types of tumor cells, leading to unregulated proliferation and inhibition of apoptosis. Long before genetic alterations in colon cancer had been well-characterized, a myriad of changes in cell surface and ECM proteins between normal colonic epithelial cells and colon-tumor cells had been documented *(172)*. Although these changes have been thought to represent potential markers for diagnosis and prognosis, until recently, their ability to directly regulate critical signal transduction pathways had not been appreciated. As of yet, the mechanisms are not firmly established by which APC mutations lead to changes in signaling through the extracellular matrix. However, as stated earlier, alterations in APC/β-catenin-mediated signaling pathways lead to activation of protein tyrosine kinases (PTKs), such as c-src. Among the many functions of c-src is phosphorylation of proteins critical to cytoskeletal organization and communication between colonic epithelial cells and their substratum. As this communication is critical for normal growth regulation, signal-transduction pathways mediated by the ECM will be outlined briefly, and the alterations occurring in these pathways in colon tumor cells will be discussed.

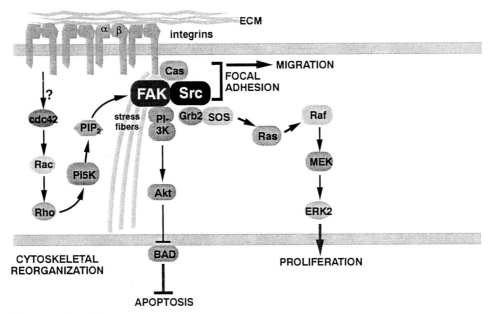

Fig. 6. Protein complexes associated with the cytoskeleton regulate distinct biologic events. In colon tumor cells, multiple changes in tumor suppressor genes, integrin expression, and other ECM and cytoskeletal proteins result in constitutive formation of signaling complexes. Deregulation of the protein tyrosine kinases FAK and c-src in these complexes may be important in colon tumorigenesis.

INTEGRINS AND GROWTH REGULATION

Integrins support cell-cell and cell-ECM interactions. However, considerable amount of recent work has demonstrated that integrins play direct roles in signal-transduction pathways. For a full discussion of integrin-mediated signaling, the reader is referred to many recent reviews (173–177). Several signaling mechanisms mediated by integrins are under investigation. Recently, ILK, a broadly expressed serine/threonine protein kinase was identified through its ability to stably associate with the cytoplasmic domain of β1 integrins (178). Although the role of this kinase is currently not well-understood, it may regulate adhesiveness. Overexpression of ILK in intestinal epithelial cells leads to reduced adherence to the matrix as well as the ability of cells to grow in soft agar. As of yet, no studies have addressed the potential role of this kinase in colon tumorigenesis. A second mechanism by which integrins signal is by inducing complexes of well-described signaling proteins. A simplified view of the basic signaling pathways currently implicated in integrin-mediated signaling is illustrated in Fig. 6. Signaling commences by an initiation event leading to integrin clustering. This initiating event may result from such seemingly diverse signals as cell-ECM interactions, or a mitogen binding a PTK growth-factor receptor. As shown in Fig. 6, integrin aggregation leads directly to the formation of large complexes of proteins in focal adhesions. These complexes contain several signaling proteins, such as c-src, focal adhesion kinase (FAK), and protein tyrosine phosphatase 1B, and structural proteins such as p130^{Cas}, paxillin, tensin, and Grb-2, among others. Signals emanating from this complex intersect major signal-transduction pathways (Fig. 6). Thus, signals that can promote cell survival, inhibit apoptosis, augment proliferation, and alter cytoskeletal organization can be regulated in a coordinated manner. Specifically, integrin-mediated signal transduction has the potential to alter cytoskeletal organiza-

tion, primarily through members of the c-ras superfamily, augment the proliferative response through the canonical c-ras pathway; affect the cells' ability to undergo apoptosis through a PI-3 kinase-mediated pathway; and alter cellular migration, through a pathway requiring FAK, c-src, and p130^{Cas}. In colon-tumor cells, major changes in regulation of these signaling complexes have been identified. As a result of direct interaction with integrins, FAK becomes autophosphorylated, increasing the specific activity of the enzyme and creating a binding site for the tyrosine kinase c-src (179,180). When bound to FAK, the tyrosine kinase activity of c-src increases, and it is able to phosphorylate its substrates, including FAK at a site distinct from the autophosphorylation site. The c-src protein also acts as an adaptor molecule that recruits other proteins to the complex. As a result, FAK and c-src are important for the recruitment of other proteins involved in the complex (Fig. 6).

If signaling complexes derived from integrin-mediated events are critical in normal growth regulation of colonic epithelial cells, alterations in the expression and function of proteins in the complex would be expected to play significant roles in tumorigenicity and tumor progression. Many such alterations have indeed been identified, and evidence that they contribute to the tumorigenic phenotype is increasing. In colon-tumor cells, changes in the expression of integrins and FAK, and the expression and activity of c-src are common.

ALTERATIONS OF INTEGRINS IN COLON CANCER

Alterations of integrin profiles in colon (181,182) and many other tumors (183), are thought to play a role in the ability of tumor cells to escape apoptosis (175). Most commonly, integrins are lost during tumor progression. Recently, experimental strategies to restore integrins have demonstrated the significance of the loss to ECM-mediated events. HT29 adenocarcinoma cells do not express the fibronectin receptor ($\alpha_5\beta_1$ integrins) and cannot attach to fibronectin-coated plates. Additionally, the cells have constitutively high expression and activity of FAK and c-src. Recently, Schmidt et al. *(184)* re-expressed the fibronectin receptor in HT29 by a transfection strategy. The result of this expression was that cells regained some of the normal phenotype. For example, HT29 cells expressing the fibronectin receptor regained the ability to attach to fibronectin-coated plates. Further, this ability was associated with alterations in critical components of focal-adhesion signaling complexes. The kinase activity of c-src is decreased in log-phase cells after re-expression of the fibronectin receptor, but activity transiently increased after attachment of cells to fibronectin-coated plates. These results demonstrate that specific downstream signaling pathways are affected by alterations in the ability of cells to be regulated by the ECM. As shown in Fig. 6, two enzymes are central in mediating these signal-transduction pathways, FAK and c-src. Alterations in both of these enzymes have been observed in colon tumors.

FOCAL ADHESION KINASE

FAK, a 125 kDa nonreceptor PTK, was first identified as a substrate of the viral form of c-src *(185)*. FAK is unusual in that it lacks SH2 and SH3 domains *(180)*. However, FAK possesses a focal adhesion targeting (FAT) domain that contains regions allowing interaction with cytoskleletal proteins, such as paxillin *(186)* and talin *(187,188)*. Near the amino terminus of the protein is a region that allows the in vitro association with the β_1 subunit of integrins *(180)*. As described earlier, aggregation of integrins leads to phosphorylation of FAK. Cells derived from *FAK⁻/⁻* mice maintain the ability to form focal adhesions *(189)*, but have apparent differences in cytoskeletal turnover and cell motility. These results suggest that altered expression of *FAK* in tumor cells might be important to invasiveness and metastasis. In accord with this possibility, *FAK* expression is increased in many tumors, including colorectal carcinomas *(190)*. Further, increased *FAK* expression correlates with increased malignant behavior *(190)*. As of yet, few experiments have assessed directly the effects of FAK overexpression on growth regulation. As illustrated in Fig. 6, the key mediator of FAK signaling is c-src, the PTK activity that is commonly activated in human colon tumors.

THE C-SRC FAMILY OF PTK

The c-*src* gene, first discovered in altered form as the transforming oncogene of Rous Sarcoma Virus *(191)* is the prototype of a closely related gene family, currently comprised of 9 members that encode gene products of molecular weight 55–62 kDa. Each protein in the family has common structural features. The tyrosine kinase domain (src homology 1, or SH1) is highly conserved among all PTKs *(192)*. The c-*src* family gene products each contain other specific homology domains, SH2 and SH3, which are likely involved in regulating the PTK activity and enhancing interactions with specific phosphotyrosine-containing proteins *(193)*. More recently, a SH4 domain has been described that regulates membrane association, partially by directing esterification of myristate and/or palmitate *(194)*. The domains of c-src family members determine their

substrate specificity, and allow interaction with other signaling and structural proteins. The c-src protein (and related family members) phosphorylate a variety of proteins including signaling kinases (such as FAK, kinase C, and cdc2 kinase), and structural proteins such as the cadherins and catenins. Further, as shown in Fig. 1, one of the interactions between c-src and FAK leads to the recruitment of other proteins in this signaling complex.

REGULATION OF C-*SRC* AND C-*YES* IN COLONIC EPITHELIAL CELLS

The c-*src* family of tyrosine kinases appear tightly regulated during colonic stem cell renewal and differentiation. In normal chick intestinal tissue, c-src PTK activity is greater in cells obtained in the rapidly dividing crypts, and the enzyme(s) are primarily associated with the cytoskeleton *(195)*. In contrast, in cells from the villus, the specific activity of c-src is reduced, and the enzyme is primarily associated with the plasma membrane *(195)*. Crude fractionation of human crypt cells has revealed similar results, with higher c-src kinase activity and increased phosphotyrosine in fractions containing primarily crypt cells *(196)*. In tumor cell lines differentiated toward a mature absorptive cell-like phenotype, c-src activity decreases *(197)*, and in specimens obtained from normal mucosa, activity is relatively low. Although fewer studies have examined the activity of the c-yes protein in these processes, current data suggests that its regulation is similar to that of c-src *(198)*, although in HT29 cells, differences in the regulation of c-src and c-yes during the cell cycle have been noted *(199)*.

ACTIVATION OF C-SRC IN COLON TUMORS

In the past few years, evidence has mounted that increased c-src activity is associated with critical stages of colon tumorigenesis and progression. Increases in the specific activity of c-src are observed in polyps of high malignant potential relative to more benign polyps *(200–202)*, in ulcerative colitis as compared to inflammation *(203)*, and in most primary tumors relative to adjacent normal colonic mucosa *(201,202,204)*. Immunohistochemical studies with an antibody that detects the active form of c-src only *(205)* provide further evidence that c-src exists in an activated state in colon tumors. The c-yes protein has also been demonstrated to be activated in polyps and in primary tumors *(206,207)*. In metastases from colon tumors, further increases in expression and activity of c-src have been observed *(201,202,208,209)*. However, the specific activity, but not the expression of c-yes decreases in many metastases *(207)*. Nevertheless, in rare instances when c-yes activation occurs in metastases, the prognosis of the patients is poorer *(207)*. These data demonstrate that the regulation of the two enzymes during tumor progression is not identical, and suggest that activation of c-src and c-yes may have different roles in tumor progression, possibly by phosphorylating unique substrates, or by interacting with different partners in signaling complexes.

To determine if c-src activation affected the growth of colon-tumor cells, we chose an approach based on anti-sense technology. Taking advantage of differences in the DNA sequence at the translation start sites of c-src and c-yes, we were able to identify oligonucleotides that, after addition to the culture media of colon-tumor cells, resulted in inhibition of c-src activity, but not c-yes in the treated cells. We further succeeded in constructing expression vectors based on these sequences. In stable cell lines transfected with this expression vector, tumorigenicity was decreased proportionately to reduction in c-*src* expression *(210)*. In these cell lines, c-*yes* expression was unchanged or minimally increased. These studies demonstrate that c-src inhibition alone is important to tumorigenic growth of HT29 cells. Further studies with these cell lines have demonstrated that decreasing c-src expression decreases the constitutive levels of vascular endothelial growth factor (VEGF), an angiogenic factor important to neovascularization of growing tumors *(211,212)*. Further, the ability of hypoxia to induce VEGF is abolished *(212)*. These results suggest that at least one role for c-src activation in colon-tumor cells is to promote VEGF expression.

IMPLICATIONS OF FAK AND C-SRC IN COLON TUMORIGENESIS

We hypothesize that the ability of c-src to constitutively associate with FAK is critical for the tumorigenic effects of c-src in colon-cancer cells, by deregulating pathways important to cell survival. Normal colonic epithelial cells undergo apoptosis at the tips of the crypt through a process that is mediated by the ECM. In many normal cells, detachment from the ECM leads to a form of apoptosis termed anoikis (Greek for homelessness). Recent experiments have demonstrated an important role for FAK in this process. Detachment of normal epithelial cells from the ECM results in rapid FAK degradation *(213)*, likely an early event in the anoikis pathway, as recent experiments have demonstrated that FAK can be cleaved by caspases *(214)*. Expression of a constitutively activated form of FAK is sufficient to block this process *(215)*. Decreasing the expression of FAK by antisense oligonucleotides *(216)* triggers apoptosis in several different established tumor-cell lines, and microinjection of a FAK antibody induces apoptosis in fibroblasts *(217)*.

Whether the ability of FAK to promote or inhibit apoptosis requires association with c-src is unknown, but our experiments with colon-tumor cells support this possibility. We have demonstrated that constitutive c-src/FAK complexes are found in colon-tumor cells (as opposed to normal cells in which these complexes are labile to detachment from the ECM). Further, decreasing the expression of c-src decreases the expression of FAK, and decreases the survival of cells upon detachment from tissue-culture plastic. These results support signaling from c-src/FAK complexes as critical to one of the biologic effects of activated c-src in colon-tumor cells. Alternatively, FAK and c-src may exert independent functions in colon-tumor cells. Additional studies are in progress to clarify these issues.

C-SRC/FAK COMPLEXES MAY COORDINATELY DEREGULATE VEGF EXPRESSION AND APOPTOSIS INHIBITION

Considerable recent evidence supports a specific signal-transduction pathway for cell survival that implicates integrin engagement leading to FAK autophosphorylation, resulting in PI-3 kinase and akt activation, and phosphorylation of the protein BAD which blocks apoptosis *(173)*. In epithelial cells, expression of constitutively activated forms of either PI-3 kinase or akt are unable to undergo apoptosis *(218)*. Specific inhibitors of PI-3 kinase enhance anoikis *(218)*. Thus, these two multi-functional kinases play important roles in this (and other) survival pathways. Furthermore, although VEGF expression may result from activation of several distinct pathways, at least one inducer of VEGF expression, hypoxia, also requires PI-3 kinase and akt activation *(219)*. Therefore, the major biologic consequences occurring as a result of c-src activation may be due to deregulation of common pathways, as illustrated in Fig. 6. Importantly, proteins that interact with APC-signaling pathways, such as the catenin-related protein p120^{cas}, are also found in c-src/FAK-signaling complexes. Thus, β-catenin/cadherin signaling events, altered as a result of APC mutations, may both mediate and respond to signaling by c-src/FAK complexes.

Mutations in APC may directly regulate transcriptional programs important to growth regulation, but may also be equally important in deregulating pathways resulting from altered association with substrates critical to cell-cell adhesion and cell-ECM interactions. Understanding these processes may provide important leads into the development of novel therapeutic agents for colon-cancer therapy. For example, considerable work is being devoted to developing specific inhibitors for c-src. Such inhibitors may hold promise in the treatment of colon cancer.

REFERENCES

1. Landis, S. H., Wingo, P. A., Bolden, S., and Murray, T. (1998) Cancer statistics, 1998. *CA Cancer J. Clin.* **48**:6–29.
2. Winawer, S. J., Zauber, A. G., Ho, M. N., O'Brien, M. J., Gottlieb, L. S., Sternberg, S. S., et al. (1993) Prevention of colorectal cancer by colonoscopic polypectomy. The National Polyp Study Workgroup. *N. Engl. J. Med.* **329**:1977–1981.
3. Rak, J., Filmus, J., and Kerbel, R. S. (1996) Reciprocal paracrine interactions between tumour cells and endothelial cells: the "Angiogenesis Progression" hypothesis. *Eur. J. Cancer* **32A**:2438–2450.
4. Hanahan, D. and Folkman, J. (1996) Patterns and emerging mechanisms of the angiogenic switch during tumorigenesis. *Cell* **86**:353–364.
5. Muto, T., Bussey, H. J. R., and Morson, B. C. (1975) The evolution of cancer of the colon and rectum. *Cancer* **36**:2251–2276.
6. O'Brien, M. J., Winawer, S. J., Zauber, A. G., Gottlieb, L. S., Sternberg, S. S., Diaz, B., et al. (1990) The National Polyp Study: patient and polyp characteristics associated with high-grade dysplasia in colorectal adenomas. *Gastroenterology* **98**:371–379.
7. Blatt, L. J. (1961) Polyps of the colon and rectum: incidence and distribution. *Dis. Colon Rectum* **4**:277–82.
8. Whitehead, R. (1975) Rectal polyps and their relationship to cancer. *Clin. Gastroenterol.* **4**:545–561.
9. Hoff, G., Foerster, A., Vatn, M. H., Sauar, J., and Larsen, S. (1986) Epidemiology of polyps in the rectum and colon. Recovery and evaluation of unresected polyps 2 years after detection. *Scand. J. Gastroenterol.* **21**:853–862.
10. Cannon-Albright, L. A., Skolnick, M. H., Bishop, D. T., Lee, R. G., and Burt, R. W. (1988) Common inheritance of susceptibility to colonic adenomatous polyps and associated colorectal cancers. *N. Engl. J. Med.* **319**:533–537.

11. Winawer, S. J., Mayer, R. J., Marciniak, D. A., Brown-Davis, C., Van Antwerp, R., Sisk, J. E., et al. (1997) Colorectal cancer screening: clinical guidelines and rationale. *Gastroenterology* **112**:594–642.

12. Nakamura, S. and Kino, I. (1984) Morphogenesis of minute adenomas in familial polyposis coli. *J. Natl. Cancer Inst.* **73**:41–49.

13. Roncucci, L. (1992) Early events in human colorectal carcinogenesis. Aberrant crypts and microadenoma. *Ital. J. Gastroenterol.* **24**:498–501.

14. Yamashita, N., Minamoto, T., Ochiai, A., Onda, M., Esumi, H. (1995) Frequent and characteristic K-ras activation and absence of p53 protein accumulation in aberrant crypt foci of the colon. *Gastroenterology* **108**:434–440.

15. Pretlow, T. P., Brasitus, T. A., Fulton, N. C., Cheyer, C., and Kaplan, E. L. (1993) K-ras mutations in putative preneoplastic lesions in human colon. *J. Natl. Cancer Inst.* **85**:2004–2007.

16. Smith, A. J., Stern, H. S., Penner, M., Hay, K., Mitri, A., Bapat, B. V., et al. (1994) Somatic APC and K-ras codon 12 mutations in aberrant crypt foci from human colons. *Cancer Res.* **54**:5527–5530.

17. Shivapurkar, N., Huang, L., Ruggeri, B., Swalsky, P. A., Bakker, A., Finkelstein, S., et al. (1997) K-ras and p53 mutations in aberrant crypt foci and colonic tumors from colon cancer patients. *Cancer Lett.* **115**:39–46.

18. Losi, L., Roncucci, L., di Gregorio, C., de Leon, M. P., and Benhattar, J. (1996) K-ras and p53 mutations in human colorectal aberrant crypt foci. *J. Pathol.* **178**:259–263.

19. Archer, M. C., Bruce, W. R., Chan, C. C., Corpet, D. E., Medline, A., Roncucci, L., et al. (1992) Aberrant crypt foci and microadenoma as markers for colon cancer. *Environ. Health Persp.* **98**:195–197.

20. Roncucci, L., Stamp, D., Medline, A., Cullen, J. B., and Bruce, W. R. (1991) Identification and quantification of aberrant crypt foci and microadenomas in the human colon. *Human Pathol.* **22**:287–294.

21. Heinen, C. D., Shivapurkar, N., Tang, Z., Groden, J., and Alabaster, O. (1996) Microsatellite instability in aberrant crypt foci from human colons. *Cancer Res.* **56**:5339–5341.

22. Muto, T., Kamiya, J., Sawada, T., Konishi, F., Sugihara, K., Kubota, Y., et al. (1985) Small flat adenoma of the large bowel with special reference to its clinicopathological features. *Dis. Colon Rectum* **28**:847.

23. Minamoto, T., Sawaguchi, K., Ohta, T., Itoh, T., and Mai, M. (1994) Superficial-type adenomas and adenocarcinomas of the colon and rectum: a comparative morphological study. *Gastroenterology* **106**:1436–1443.

24. Kuramoto, S., Ihara, O., Sakai, S., Shimazu, R., Kaminishi, M., and Oohara, T. (1990) Depressed adenoma in the large intestine. Endoscopic features. *Dis. Colon Rectum* **33**:108–113.

25. Watanabe, T., Muto, T., Sawada, T., and Miyaki, M. (1996) Flat adenoma as a precursor of colorectal carcinoma in hereditary nonpolyposis colorectal carcinoma. *Cancer* **77**:627–634.

26. Cohen, A. M., Wood, W. C., Gunderson, L. L., and Shinnar, M. (1980) Pathological studies in rectal cancer. *Cancer* **45**:2965–2968.

27. Stolte, M. and Bethke, B. (1995) Colorectal mini-de novo carcinoma: a reality in Germany too. *Endoscopy* **27**:286–290.

28. Lanspa, S. J., Rouse, J., Smyrk, T., Watson, P., Jenkins, J., and Lynch, H. T. (1992) Epidemiologic characteristics of the flat adenoma of Muto. A prospective study. *Dis. Colon Rectum* **35**:543–546.

29. Lynch, H. T., Smyrk, T. C., McGinn, T., Lanspa, S., Cavalieri, J., Lynch, J. (1995) Attenuated familial adenomatous polyposis (AFAP). A phenotypically and genotypically distinctive variant of FAP. *Cancer* **76**:2427–2433.

30. Desigan, G., Wang, M., Alberti-Flor, J., Dunn, G. D., Halter, S., and Vaughan, S. (1985) De novo carcinoma of the rectum: a case report. *Am. J. Gastroenterol.* **80**:553–556.

31. Shamsuddin, A. M., Kato, Y., Kunishima, N., Sugano, H., and Trump, B. F. (1985) Carcinoma in situ in nonpolypoid mucosa of the large intestine. *Cancer* **56**:2849–2854.

32. Bedenne, L., Faivre, J., Boutron, M.C., Piard, F., Cauvin, J. M., and Hillon, P. (1992) Adenoma: carcinoma sequence or "de novo" carcinogenesis? A study of adenomatous remnants in a population-based series of large bowel cancers. *Cancer* **69**:883–888.

33. Jass, J. R. (1989) Do all colorectal carcinomas arise in preexisting adenomas? *World J. Surg.* **13**:45–51.

34. Nusse, R. (1991) Insertional mutagenesis in mouse mammary tumorigenesis. *Curr. Topics Microbiol. Immunol.* **171**:43–65.

35. Hunter, T. (1997) Oncoprotein networks. *Cell* **88**:333–346.

36. Bhanot, P., Brink, M., Samos, C. H., Hsieh, J. C., Wang, Y., Macke, J. P., et al. (1996) A new member of the *frizzled* family from Drosophila functions as a wingless receptor. *Nature* **382**:225–230.

37. Yang-Snyder, J., Miller, J. R., Brown, J. D., Lai, C.-J., and Moon, R. T. (1996) A frizzled homologue functions in a vertebrate *Wnt* signaling pathway. *Curr. Biol.* **6**:1302–1306.

38. Behrens, J., von Kries, J. P., Kuhl, M., Bruhn, L., Wedlich, D., Grosschedl, R., and Birchmeier, W. (1996) Functional interaction of beta-catenin with the transcription factor LEF-1. *Nature* **382**:638–642.

39. Molenaar, M., van de Wetering, M., Oosterwegel, M., Peterson-Maduro, J., Godsave, S., Korinek, V., et al. (1996) XTcf-3 transcription factor mediates beta-catenin-induced axis formation in Xenopus embryos. *Cell* **86**:391–399.

40. Guger, K. A. and Gumbiner, B. M. (1995) Beta-Catenin has Wnt-like activity and mimics the Nieuwkoop signaling center in Xenopus dorsal-ventral patterning. *Dev. Biol.* **172**:115–125.

41. Fagotto, F., Funayama, N., Gluck, U., and Gumbiner, B. M. (1996) Binding to cadherins antagonizes the signaling activity of beta-catenin during axis formation in Xenopus. *J. Cell Biol.* **132**:1105–1114.

42. Reynolds, A. B., Daniel, J., McCrea, P. D., Wheelock, M. J., Wu, J., and Zhang, Z. (1994) Identification of a new catenin: the tyrosine kinase substrate p120cas associates with E-cadherin complexes. *Mol. Cell Biol.* **14**:8333–8342.

43. Cook, D., Fry, M. J., Hughes, K., Sumathipala, R., Woodgett, J. R., and Dale, T. C. (1996) Wingless inactivates glycogen synthase kinase-3 via an intracellular signaling pathway which involves a protein kinase C. *EMBO J.* **15**:4526–4536.

44. Rubinfeld, B., Albert, I., Porfiri, E., Fiol, C., Munemitsu, S., and Polakis, P. (1996) Binding of GSK3beta to the APC-beta-catenin complex and regulation of complex assembly. *Science* **272**:1023–1026.

45. Rattner, A., Hsieh, J.-C., and Smallwood, P. M. (1997) A family of secreted proteins contains homology to the cysteine-rich ligand-binding domain of frizzled receptors. *Proc. Natl. Acad. Sci. USA* **94**:2859–2863.

46. Finch, P. W., He, X., Kelley, M. J., Üren, A., Schaudies, R. P., Popescu, N. C., et al. (1997) Purification and molecular cloning of a secreted, Frizzled-related antagonist of Wnt action. *Proc. Natl. Acad. Sci. USA* **94**:6770–6775.

47. Melkonyan, H. S., Chang, W. C., Shapiro, J. P., Mahadevappa, M., Fitzpatrick, P. A., Kiefer, M. C., et al. (1997) SARPs: A family of secreted apoptosis-related proteins. *Proc. Natl. Acad. Sci. USA* **94**:13636–13641.

48. Lin, K., Wang, S., Julius, M. A., Kitajewski, J., Moos, M. Jr., and Luyten, F. P. (1997) The cysteine-rich frizzled domain of Frzb-1 is required and sufficient for modulation of Wnt signaling. *Proc. Natl. Acad. Sci. USA* **94**:11196–11200.

49. Sakanaka, C., Weiss, J. B., and Williams, L. T. (1998) Bridging of β-catenin and glycogen synthase kinase-3β by Axin and inhibition of β-catenin-mediated transcription. *Proc. Natl. Acad. Sci. USA* **95**:3020–3023.

50. Behrens, J., Jerchow, B.-A., Wurtele, M., Grimm, J., Asbrand, C., Wirtz, R., et al. (1998) Functional interaction of an axin homolog, conductin, with β-catenin, APC, and GSK3β. *Science* **280**:596–599.

51. Novak, A., Hsu, S.-C., Leung-Hagesteijn, C., Radeva, G., Papkoff, J., Montesano, R., et al. (1998) Cell adhesion and the integrin-linked kinase regulate the LEF-1 and β-catenin signaling pathways. *Proc. Natl. Acad. Sci. USA* **95**:4374–4379.

52. Therond, P. P., Knight, J. D., Kornberg, T. B., and Bishop, J. M. (1996) Phosphorylation of the fused protein kinase in response to signaling from hedgehog. *Proc. Natl. Acad. Sci. USA* **93**:4224–4228.

53. von Ohlen, T., Lessing, D., Nusse, R., and Hooper, J. E. (1997) Hedgehog signaling regulates transcription through cubitus interruptus, a sequence-specific DNA binding protein. *Proc. Natl. Acad. Sci. USA* **94**:2404–2409.

54. Artavanis-Tsakonas, S., Matsuno, K., and Fortini, M. E. (1995) Notch signaling. *Science* **268**:225–232.

55. Jhappan, C., Gallahan, D., Stahle, C., Eugene, C., Smith, G. H., Merlino, G., et al. (1992) Expression of an activatged notch-related int-3 transgene interferes with cell differentiation and induces neoplastic transformation in mammary and salivary glands. *Genes Dev.* **6**:345–355.

56. Vogelstein, B., Fearon, E. R., Hamilton, S. R., Kern, S. E., Leppert, M., Nakamura, Y., et al. (1988) Genetic alterations during colorectal-tumor development. *N. Engl. J. Med.* **319**:525–532.

57. Morin, P. J., Sparks, A. B., Korinek, V., Barker, N., Clevers, H., Vogelstein, B., et al. (1997) Activation of β-catenin-Tcf signaling in colon cancer by mutations in β-catenin or APC. *Science* **275**:1787–1790.

58. Sparks, A. B., Morin, P. J., Vogelstein, B., and Kinzler, K. W. (1998) Mutational analysis of the APC/β-catenin/Tcf pathway in colorectal cancer. *Cancer Res.* **58**:1130–1134.

59. Rubinfeld, B., Robbins, P., El-Gamil, M., Albert, I., Porfiri, E., and Polakis, P. (1997) Stabilization β-catenin by genetic defects in melanoma cell lines. *Science* **275**:1790–1792.

60. Bodmer, W. F., Bailey, C. J., Bodmer, J., Bussey, H. J., Ellis, A., Gorman, P., et al. (1987) Localization of the gene for familial adenomatous polyposis on chromosome 5. *Nature* **328**:614–616.

61. Fearon, E. R. and Vogelstein, B. (1990) A genetic model for colorectal tumorigenesis. *Cell* **61**:759–767.

62. Kinzler, K. W. and Vogelstein, B. (1996) Lessons from hereditary colorectal cancer. *Cell* **87**:159–170.

63. Fishel, R., Lescoe, M. K., Rao, M. R. S., Copeland, N. G., Jenkins, N. A., Garber, J., et al. (1993) The human mutator gene homolog *MSH2* and its association with hereditary nonpolyposis colon cancer. *Cell* **75**:1027–1038.

64. Leach, F. S., Nicolaides, N. C., Papadopoulos, N., Liu, B., Jen, J., Sistonen, P., et al. (1993) Mutations of a *mutS* homolog in hereditary nonpolyposis colorectal cancer. *Cell* **75**:1215–1225.

65. Bronner, C. E., Baker, S. M., Morrison, P. T., Warren, G., Smith, L. G., Lescoe, M. K., et al. (1994) Mutation in the DNA mismatch repair gene homolog *hMLH1* is associated with hereditary nonpolyposis colon cancer. *Nature* **368**:258–261.

66. Papadopoulos, N., Nicolaides, N. C., Wei, Y. F., Ruben, S. M., Carter, K. C., Rosen, C. A., et al. (1994) Mutation of a *mutL* homolog in hereditary colon cancer. *Science* **263**:1625–1629.

67. Nicolaides, N. C., Papadopoulos, N., Liu, B., Wel, Y.-F., Carter, K. C., Ruben, S. M., et al. (1994) Mutations of two PMS homologues in hereditary nonpolyposis colon cancer. *Nature* **371**:75–80.

68. Palombo, F., Gallinari, P., Iaccarino, I., Lettieri, T., Hughes, M., D'Arrigo, A., et al. (1995) GTBP, a 160-kilodalton protein essential for mismatch-binding activity in human cells. *Science* **268**:1912–1914.

69. Peltomaki, P., Aaltonen, L. A., Sistonen, P., Pykkanen, L., Mecklin, J. P., Jarvinen, H., et al. (1993) Genetic mapping of a locus predisposing to human colorectal cancer. *Science* **260**:810–812.

70. Aaltonen, L. A., Peltomaki, P., Leach, F. S., Sistonen, P., Pylkkanen, L., Mecklin, J.-P., et al. (1993) Clues to the pathogenesis of familial colorectal cancer. *Science* **260**:812–816.

71. Thibodeau, S. N., Bren, G., and Schaid, D. (1993) Microsatellite instability in cancer of the proximal colon. *Science* **260**:816–819

72. Ionov, Y., Peinado, M. A., Malkhosyan, S., Shibata, D., and Perucho, M. (1993) Ubiquitous somatic mutations in simple repeated sequences reveal a new mechanism for colonic carcinogenesis. *Nature* **363**:558–561.

73. Witzig, T. E., Moertel, C. G., Paulsen, J. K., Katzmann, J. A., Wieand, H. S., Cha, S. S., et al. (1991) DNA ploidy and cell kinetic measurements as predictors of recurrence and survival in stages B2 and C colorectal adenocarcinoma. *Cancer* **68**:879–888.

74. Tomlinson, I. P. M., Novelli, M. R., and Bodmer, W. F. (1996) The mutation rate and cancer. *Proc. Natl. Acad. Sci. USA* **93**:14800–14803.

75. Langauer, C., Kinzler, K. W., and Vogelstein, B. (1997) Genetic instability in colorectal cancers. *Nature* **386**:623–627.

76. Hanski, C., Bornhoeft, G., Shimoda, T., Hanski, M.L., Lane, D. P., Stein, H., et al. (1992) Expression of p53 protein in invasive colorectal carcinomas of different histologic types. *Cancer* **70**:2772–2777.

77. Aoki, T., Takeda, S., Yanagisawa, A., Kato, Y., Ajioka, Y., Watanabe, H., et al. (1994) APC and p53 mutations in de novo colorectal adenocarcinomas. *Human Mutat.* **3**:342–346.

78. Blank, M., Klussmann, E., Kruger-Krasagakes, S., Schmitt-Graff, A., Stolte, M., Bornhoeft, G., et al. (1994) Expression of MUC2-mucin in colorectal adenomas and carcinomas of different histological types. *Int. J. Cancer* **59**:301–306.

79. Herrera, L., Kakati, S., Gibas, L., Pietrzak, E., and Sandberg, A. A. (1986) Brief clinical report: Gardner syndrome in a man with interstitial deletion of 5q. *Am. J. Med. Genet.* **25**:473–476.

80. Nishisho, I., Nakamura, Y., Miyoshi, Y., Miki, Y., Ando, H., Horii, A., et al. (1991) Mutations of chromosome 5q21 genes in FAP and colorectal cancer patients. *Science* **253**:665–669.

81. Kinzler, K. W., Nilbert, M. C., Su, L.-K., Vogelstein, B., Bryan, T. M., Levy, D.B., et al. (1991) Identification of FAP locus genes from chromosome 5q21. *Science* **253**:661–665.

82. Groden, J., Thliveris, A., Samowitz, W., Carlson, M., Gelbert, L., Albertson, H., et al. (1991) Identification and characterization of the familial adenomatous polyposis coli gene. *Cell* **66**:589–600.

83. Powell, S. M., Zilz, N., Beazer-Barclay, Y., Bryan, T. M., Hamilton, S. R., Thibodeau, S. N., et al. (1992) *APC* mutations occur in early colorectal tumorigenesis. *Nature* **359**:235–237.

84. Polakis, P. (1997) The adenomatous polyposis coli (APC) tumor suppressor. *Biochim. Biophys. Acta* **1332**:F127–F147.

85. Joslyn, G., Richardson, D. S., White, R., and Alber, T. (1993) Dimer formation by an N-terminal coiled coil in the APC protein. *Proc. Natl. Acad. Sci. USA* **90**:11109–11113.

86. Su, L. K., Johnson, K. A., Smith, K. J., Hill, D. E., Vogelstein, B., and Kinzler, K. W. (1993) Association between wild type and mutant APC gene products. *Cancer Res.* **53**:2728–2731.

87. Rubinfeld, B., Souza, B., Albert, I., Muller, O., Chamberlain, S. C., Masiarz, F., et al. (1993) Association of the APC gene product with β-catenin. *Science* **262**:1731–1734.

88. Su, L. K., Vogelstein, B., and Kinzler, K. W. (1993) Association of the tumor-suppressor protein with catenins. *Science* **262**: 1734–1737.

89. Smith, K. J., Levy, D. B., Maupin, P., Pollard, T. D., Vogelstein, B., and Kinzler, K. W. (1994) Wild-type but not mutant APC associates with microtubule cytoskeleton. *Cancer Res.* **54**:3672–3675.

90. Munemitsu, S., Souza, B., Muller, O., Albert, I., Rubinfeld, B., and Polakis, P. (1994) The APC gene product associates with microtubules in vivo and promotes their assembly in vitro. *Cancer Res.* **54**:3676–3681.

91. Su, L. K., Burrell, M., Hill, D. E., Gyuris, J., Brent, R., Wiltshire, R., et al. (1995) APC binds to the novel protein EB1. *Cancer Res.* **55**:2972–2977.

92. Matsumine, A., Ogai, A., Senda, T., Okumura, N., Satoh, K., Baeg, G. H., et al. (1996) Binding of APC to the human homolog of the Drosophila disc large tumor suppressor protein. *Science* **272**:1020–1023.

93. Renner, C., Pfreundschuh, M., Bauer, S., Sahin, U., Ohnesorge, S., Held, G., et al. (1997) RP1, a new member of the adenomatous polyposis coli-binding EB1-like gene family, is differentially expressed in activated T cells. *J. Immunol.* **159**:1276–1283.

94. Neufeld, K. L. and White, R. (1997) Nuclear and cytoplasmic localizations of the adenomatous polyposis coli protein. *Proc. Natl. Acad. Sci. USA* **94**:3034–3039.

95. Trzepacz, C., Lowy, A. M., Kordich, J. J., and Groden, J. (1997) Phosphorylation of the tumor suppressor adenomatous polyposis coli (APC) by the cyclin-dependent kinase p34cdc2. *J. Biol. Chem.* **272**:21681–21684.

96. Morin, P. J., Vogelstein, B., and Kinzler, K. W. (1996) Apoptosis and APC in colorectal tumorigenesis. *Proc. Natl. Acad. Sci. USA* **93**:7950–7954.

97. Groden, J. A., Joslyn, G., Samowitz, W., Jones, D., Bhattachuzya, N., Spirio, L., et al. (1995) Response of colon cancer cell lines to the introduction of APC, a colon-specific tumor suppressor gene. *Cancer Res.* **55**:1531–1539.

98. Browne, S. J., Williams, A. C., Hague, A., Butt, A. J., and Paraskeva, C. (1994) Loss of APC protein expressed by human colonic epithelial cells and the appearance of a specific low-molecular weight form is associated with apoptosis *in vitro*. *Int. J. Cancer* **59**:56–64.

99. Hargest, R. and Williamson, R. (1995) Expression of the APC gene after transfection into a colonic cancer cell line. *Gut* **37**:826–829.

100. Miki, M., Nishisho, I., Horii, A., Miyoshi, Y., Utsunomiya, J., Kinzler, K. W., et al. (1992) Disruption of the APC gene by a retrotransposal insertion of L1 sequence in a colon cancer. *Cancer Res.* **52**:643–645.

101. Powell, S. M., Petersen, G. M., Krush, A. J., Booker, S., Jen, J., Giardiello, F. M., et al. (1993) Molecular diagnosis of familial adenomatosis polyposis. *N. Engl. J. Med.* **329**:1982–1987.

102. Bunyan, D. J., Shea-Simonds, J., Reck, A. C., Finnis, D., and Eccles, D. M. (1995) Genotype-phenotype correlations of new causative APC gene mutations in patients with familial adenomatous polyposis. *J. Med. Genetics* **32**:728–731.

103. Paul, P., Letteboer, T., Gelbert, L., Groden, J., White, R., and Coppes, M. J. (1993) Identical APC exon 15 mutations results in a variable phenotype in familial adenomatous polyposis. *Human Mol. Genet.* **2**:25–31.

104. Caspari, R., Friedl, W., Mandl, M., Moslein, G., Kodmon, M., Knapp, M., et al. (1994) Familial adenomatous polyposis: mutation at codon 1309 and early onset of colon cancer. *Lancet* **343**:629–632.

105. Nagase, H., Miyoshi, Y., Horii, A., Aoki, T., Ogawa, M., Utsunomiya, J., et al. (1992) Correlation between the location of germ-line mutations in the APC gene and the number of colorectal polyps in familial adenomatous polyposis patients. *Cancer Res.* **52**:4055–4057.

106. Spirio, L., Olschwang, S., Groden, J., Robertson, M., Samowitz, W., Joslyn, G., et al. (1993) Alleles of the APC gene: an attenuated form of familial polyposis. *Cell* **75**:951–957.

107. Gayther, S. A., Wells, D., Sen Gupta, S. B., Chapman, P., Neale, K., Tsioupra, K., et al. (1994) Regionally clustered APC mutations are associated with a severe phenotype and occur at a high frequency rate in new mutation cases of adenomatous polyposis coli. *Human Mol. Genet.* **3**:53–56.

108. van der Luijt, R. B., Khan, P. M., Vasen, H. F. A., Breukel, C., Tops, C. M. J., Scott, R. J., et al. (1996) Germline mutations in the 3′ part of exon 15 do not results in truncated proteins and are associated with attenuated adenomatous polyposis coli. *Human Genet.* **98**:727–734.

109. Walon, C., Verellen-Dumoulin, C., Mertens, G., Ngounou, P., Lannoy, N., Smaers, M., et al. (1997) Novel germline mutations in the APC gene and their phenotypic spectrum in familial adenomatous polyposis kindreds. *Human Genet.* **100**:601–605.

110. Olschwang, S., Laant-Puig, P., Groden, J., White, R., and Thomas, G. (1993) Germline mutations in the first fourteen exons of the APC gene. *Am. J. Human Genet.* **52**:273–279.

111. Fodde, R., van der Luijt, R., Wijnen, J., Tops, C., van der Klift, H., van Leeuwen-Cornelisse, I., et al. (1992) Eight novel inactivating germ line mutations in the APC gene identified by denaturing gradient gel electrophoresis. *Genomics* **13**:1162–1168.

112. Olschwang, S., Tiret, A., Laurent-Puig, P., Muluis, M., Parc, R., and Thomas, G. (1993) Restriction of ocular fundus lesions to a specific subgroup of APC mutations in adenomatous polyposis coli patients. *Cell* **75**:959–968.

113. Dobbie, Z., Spycher, M., Mary, J.-L., Haner, M., Guldenschuh, I., Hurliman, R., et al. (1996) Correlation between the development of extracolonic manifestations in FAP patients and mutations beyond codon 1403 in the APC gene. *J. Med. Genet.* **33**:274–280.

114. Miyoshi, Y., Nagase, H., Hori, A., Ichii, S., Nakatsuru, S., Aoki, T., et al. (1992) Somatic mutations of the APC gene in colorectal tumors: mutation cluster region in the APC gene. *Human Mol. Genet.* **1**:229–233.

115. Huang, J., Papadopoulos, N., McKinley, A. J., Farrington, S. M., Curtis, L. J., Wyllie, A. H., et al. (1996) APC mutations in colorectal tumors with mismatch repair deficiency. *Proc. Natl. Acad. Sci. USA* **93**:9049–9054.

116. Gould, K. A. and Dove, W. F. (1996) Action of Min and MOM1 on neoplasia in ectopic intestinal grafts. *Cell Growth Diff.* **7**:1361–1368.

117. MacPhee, M., Chepenik, K. P., Liddell, R. A., Nelson, K. K., Siracusa, L. D., and Buchberg, A. M. (1995) The secretory phospholipase A2 gene is a candidate for the Mom1 locus, a major modifier of Apc^Min-induced intestinal neoplasia. *Cell* **81**:957–966.

118. Dietrich, W. F., Lander, E. S., Smith, J. S., Moser, A. R., Gould, K. A., Luongo, C., et al. (1993) Genetic identification of Mom-1, a major modifier locus affecting Min-induced intestinal neoplasia in the mouse. *Cell* **75**:631–639.

119. Dobbie, Z., Heinimann, K., Bishop, D. T., Muller, H., and Scott, R. J. (1997) Identifiaction of a modifier gene locus on chromosome 1p35-36 in familial adenomatous polyposis. *Human Genet.* **99**:653–657.

120. Tomlinson, I. P. M., Neale, K., Talbot, I. C., Spegelman, A. D., Williams, C. B., Phillips, R. K. S., et al. (1996) A modifying locus for familial adenomatous polyposis may be present on chromosome 1p35-p36. *J. Med. Genet.* **33**:268–273.

121. Oshima, H., Taketo, M. M., Tsutsumi, M., Kobayashi, M., Oshima, M. (1997) Morphological and molecular processes of polyp formation in Apc(delta716) knockout mice. *Cancer Res.* **57**:1644–1649.

122. Yang, K., Lipkin, M., Kucherlapati, R., Khan, P. M., Fodde, R., Kolli, V. R., et al. (1997) A mouse model of human familial adenomatous polyposis. *J. Exp. Zool.* **277**:245–254.

123. Laken, S. J., Vogelstein, B., Kinzler, K. W., Luce, M. C., Offit, K., Winawer, S., et al. (1997) Familial colorectal cancer in Ashkenazim due to a hypermutable tract in APC. *Nature Genetics* **17**:79–83.

124. Boland, C. R. (1983) Familial colonic cancer syndromes. *West. J. Med.* **139**:351–359.

125. Lynch, H. T., Smyrk, T. C., Watson, P., Lanspa, S. J., Lynch, J. F., Lynch, P. M., et al. (1993) Genetics, natural history, tumor spectrum, and pathology of hereditary nonpolyposis colorectal cancer: an updated review. *Gastroenterology* **104**:1535–1549.

126. Warthin, A. S. (1913) Heredity with reference to carcinoma: As shown by the study of the cases examined in the pathological laboratory of the University of Michigan, 1895–1913. *Arch. Int. Med.* **12**:546–555.

127. Lynch, H. T., Shaw, M. W., Magnuson, C. W., Larsen, A. L., and Krush, A. J. (1966) Hereditary factors in cancer. Study of two large midwestern kindreds. *Arch. Int. Med.* **117**:206–212.

128. Lynch, H. T., Lanspa, S. J., Boman, B. M., Smyrk, T., Watson, P., Lynch, J. F., et al. (1988) Hereditary nonpolyposis colorectal cancer: Lynch syndromes I and II. *Gastroenterol. Clin. North Am.* **17**:679–712.

129. Vasen, H. F., Mecklin, J. P., Meera Khan, P., and Lynch, H. T. (1991) The international collaborative group on hereditary nonpolyposis colorectal cancer (ICG-HNPCC). *Dis. Colon Rectum* **34**:424–425.

130. Stephenson, B. M., Finan, P. J., Gascoyne, J., Garbett, F., Murday, V. A., and Bishop, D. T. (1991) Frequency of familial colorectal cancer. *Br. J. Surg.* **78**:1162–1166.

131. Fuchs, C. S., Giovannucci, E. L., Colditz, G. A., Hunter, D. J., Speizer, F. E., and Willett, W. C. (1994) A prospective study of family history and the risk of colorectal cancer. *N. Engl. J. Med.* **331**:1669–1674.

132. Lindblom, A., Tannergard, P., Werelius, B., and Nordenskjold, M. (1993) Genetic mapping of a second locus predisposing to hereditary non-polyposis colon cancer. *Nature Genet.* **5**:279–282.

133. Knudson, A. G. (1985) Hereditary cancer, oncogenes, and antioncogenes. *Cancer Res.* **45**:1437–1443.

134. Strand, M., Prolla, T. A,. Liskay, R. M., and Petes, T. D. (1993) Destabilization of tracts of simple repetitive DNA in yeast by mutations affecting DNA mismatch repair. *Nature* **365**:274–276.

135. Modrich, P. (1991) Mechanisms and biological effects of mismatch repair. *Ann. Rev. Genet.* **25**:229–253.

136. Fishel, R., Ewel, A., Lee, S., Lescoe, M. K., and Griffith, J. (1994) Binding of mismatched microsatellite DNA sequences by the human MSH2 protein. *Science* **266**:1403–1405.

137. Stephenson, C. and Karran, P. (1989) Selective binding to DNA base pair mismatches by proteins from human cells. *J. Biol. Chem.* **264**:21177–21182.

138. Holmes, J., Jr., Clark, S., and Modrich, P. (1990) Strand-specific mismatch correction in nuclear extracts of human and Drosophila melanogaster cell lines. *Proc. Natl. Acad. Sci. USA* **87**:5837–5841.

139. Thomas, D. C., Roberts, J. D., and Kunkel, T. A. (1991) Heteroduplex repair in extracts of human HeLa cells. *J. Biol. Chem.* **266**:3744–3751.

140. Fang, W. H. and Modrich, P. (1993) Human strand-specific mismatch repair occurs by a bidirectional mechanism similar to that of the bacterial reaction. *J. Biol. Chem.* **268**:11838–11844.

141. Modrich, P. and Lahue, R. (1996) Mismatch repair in replication fidelity, genetic recombination, and cancer biology. *Ann. Rev. Biochem.* **65**:101–133.

142. Umar, A., Boyer, J. C., Thomas, D. C., Nguyen, D. C,. Risinger, J. I., Boyd, J., et al. (1994) Defective mismatch repair in extracts of colorectal and endometrial cancer cell lines exhibiting microsatellite instability. *J. Biol. Chem.* **269**:14367–14370.

143. Li, G.-M. and Modrich, P. (1995) Restoration of mismatch repair to nuclear extracts of H6 colorectal tumor cells by a heterodimer of human MutL homologous. *Proc. Natl. Acad. Sci. USA* **92**:1950–1954.

144. Drummond, J. T., Li, G. M., Longley, M. J., and Modrich, P. (1995) Isolation of an *hMSH2*-p160 herterodimer that restores DNA mismatch repair to tumor cells. *Science* **268**:1909–1912.

145. Risinger, J. I., Umar, A., Boyd, J., Berchuck, A., Kunkel, T. A. and Barrett, J. C. (1996) Mutation of MSH3 in endometrial cancer and evidence for its functional role in heteroduplex repair. *Nature Genet.* **14**:102–105.

146. Risinger, J. I., Umar, A., Barrett, J. C., and Kunkel, T. A. (1995) A hPMS2 mutant cell line is defective in strand-specific mismatch repair. *J. Biol. Chem.* **270**:18183–18186.

147. Drummond, J. T., Genschel, J., Wolf, E., and Modrich, P. (1997) DHFR/MSH3 amplification in methotrexate-resistant cells alters the hMutSalpha/hMutSbeta ratio and reduces the efficiency of base-base mismatch repair. *Proc. Natl. Acad. Sci. USA* **94**:10144–10149.

148. Acharya, S., Wilson, T., Gradia, S., Kane, M. F., Guerrette, S., Marsischky, G. T., et al. (1996) hMSH2 forms specific mispair-binding complexes with hMSH3 and hMSH6. *Proc. Natl. Acad. Sci. USA* **93**:13629–13634.

149. Gradia, S., Acharya, S., and Fishel, R. (1997) The human mismatch recognition complex hMSH2-hMSH6 functions as a novel molecular switch. *Cell* **91**:995–1005.

150. Iaccarino, I., Marra, G., Palombo, F., and Jiricny, J. (1998) hMSH2 and hMSH6 play distinct roles in mismatch binding and contribute differently to the ATPase activity of hMutS alpha. *EMBO J.* **17**:2677–2686.

151. Umar, A., Risinger, J. I., Glaab, W. E., Tindall, K. R., Barrett, J. C., and Kunkel, T. A. Functional overlap in mismatch repair by human MSH3 and MSH6. *Genetics* **148**:1637–1646.

152. Ross-Macdonald, P. and Roeder, G. S. (1994) Mutation of a meiosis-specific MutS homolog decreases crossing over but not mismatch correction. *Cell* **79**:1069–1080.

153. Liu, B., Parsons, R. E., Hamilton, S. R., Petersen, G. M., Lynch, H. T., Watson, P., et al. *hMSH2* mutations in hereditary nonpolyposis colorectal cancer kindreds. *Cancer Res.* **54**:4590–4594.

154. Liu, B., Papadopoulos, N., Nicolaides, N. C., Parsons, R., Lynch, H. T., Watson, P., et al. (1996) Analysis of mismatch repair genes in hereditary non-polyposis colorectal cancer patients. *Nature Med.* **2**:169–714.

155. Hamilton, S. R., Liu, B., Parsons, R. E., Papadopoulos, N., Jen, J., Powell, S., et al. (1995) The molecular basis of Turcot's Syndrome. *N. Engl. J. Med.* **332**:839–847.

156. Nystrom-Lahti, M., Wu, Y., Moisio, A-L., Hofstra, R. M. W., Osinga, J., Mecklin, J. P., et al. (1996) DNA mismatch repair gene mutations in 55 kindreds with verified or putive hereditary nonpolyposis colorectal cancer. *Human Mol. Genet.* **5**:763–769.

157. Peltomaki, P., Vasen, H. F. A., and The International Collaborative Group on Hereditary Nonpolyposis Colorectal Cancer (1997) Mutations predisposing to hereditary nonpolyposis colorectal cancer: database and results of a collaborative study. *Gastroenterology* **113**:1146–1158.

158. Akiyama, Y., Sato, H., Yamada, T., Nagasaki, H., Tsuchiya, A., Abe, R., and Yuasa, Y. (1997) Germ-line mutation of the hMSH6/GTBP gene in an atypical hereditary nonpolyposis colorectal cancer kindred. *Cancer Res.* **57**:3920–3923.

159. Dunlop, M., Farrington, S., Carothers, A., Wyllie, A., Sharp, L., Bum, J., et al. (1997) Cancer risk associated with germline DNA mismatch repair gene mutations. *Human Mol. Genet.* **6**:105–110.

160. Parsons, R., Li, G. M., Longley, M., Modrich, P., Liu, B., Berk, T., et al. (1995) Mismatch repair deficiency in phenotypically normal human cells. *Science* **268**:738–740.

161. Nicolaides, N. C., Littman, S. J., Modrich, P., Kinzler, K. W., and Vogelstein, B. (1998) A naturally occurring hPMS2 mutation can confer a dominant negative mutator phenotype. *Mol. Cell. Biol.* **18**:1635–1641.

162. Markowitz, S., Wang, J., Myeroff, L., Parsons, R., Sun, L., Lutterbaugh, J., et al. (1995) Inactivation of the type II TGF-beta receptor in colon cancer cells with microsatellite instability. *Science* **268**:1336–1338.

163. Parsons, R., Myeroff, L. L., Liu, B., Willson, J. K., Markowitz, S. D., Kinzler, K. W., et al. (1995) Microsatellite instability and mutations of the transforming growth factor beta type II receptor gene in colorectal cancer. *Cancer Res.* **55**:5548–5550.

164. Reitmair, A. H., Cai, J. C., Bjerknes, M., Redston, M., Cheng, H., Pind, M. T., et al. (1996) MSH2 deficiency contributes to accelerated APC-mediated intestinal tumorigenesis. *Cancer Res.* **56**:2922–2926

165. Rampino, N., Yamamoto, H., Ionov, Y., Li, Y., Sawai, H., Reed, J. C., et al. (1997) Somatic frameshift mutations in the BAX gene in colon cancers of the microsatellite mutator phenotype. *Science* **275**:967–969.

166. Konishi, M., Kikuchi-Yanoshita, R., Tanaka, K., Muraoka, M., Onda, A., Okumura, Y., et al. (1996) Molecular nature of colon tumors in hereditary nonpolyposis colon cancer, familial polyposis, and sporadic colon cancer. *Gastroenterology* **111**:307–317.

167. Aarnio, M., Salovaara, R., Aaltonen, L. A., Mecklin, J. P., and Jarvinen, H. J. (1997) Features of gastric cancer in hereditary nonpolyposis colorectal cancer syndrome. *Int. J. Cancer* **74**:551–555.

168. Losi, L., Ponz de Leon, M., Jiricny, J., Di Gregorio, C., Benatti, P., Percesepe, A., et al. (1997) K-ras and p53 mutations in hereditary non-polyposis colorectal cancers. *Int. J. Cancer* **74**:94–96.

169. Olschwang, S., Hamelin, R., Laurent-Puig, P., Thuille, B., De Rycke, Y., Li, Y. J., et al. (1997) Alternative genetic pathways in colorectal carcinogenesis. *Proc. Natl. Acad. Sci. USA* **94**:12122–12127.

170. Weber, T. K., Conlon, W., Petrelli, N. J., Rodriguez-Bigas, M., Keitz, B., Pazik, J., et al. (1997) Genomic DNA-based hMSH2 and hMLH1 mutation screening in 32 Eastern United States hereditary nonpolyposis colorectal cancer pedigrees. *Cancer Res.* **57**:3798–3803.

171. Beck, N. E., Tomlinson, I. P., Homfray, T., Frayling, I., Hodgson, S. V., Harocopos, C., et al. (1997) Use of SSCP analysis to identify germline mutations in HNPCC families fulfilling the Amsterdam criteria. *Human Genet.* **99**:219–224.

172. Jessup, J. M. and Gallick, G. E. (1992) The biology of colorectal cancer. *Curr. Prob. Cancer* **16**:261–328.

173. Howe, A., Aplin, A. E., Alahari, S. K., and Juliano, R. L. (1998) Integrin signaling and cell growth control. *Curr. Opin. Cell Biol.* **10**:220–231.

174. Shyy, J. Y.-J. and Chien, S. (1997) Role of integrins in cellular responses to mechanical stress and adhesion. *Curr. Opin. Cell Biol.* **9**:707–713.

175. Frisch, S. M. and Ruoslahti, E. (1997) Integrins and anoikis. *Curr. Opin. Cell Biol.* **9**:701–706.

176. Giancotti, F. G. (1997) Integrin signaling: specificity and control of cell survival and cell cycle progression. *Curr. Opin. Cell Biol.* **9**:691–700.

177. Barth, A. I. M., Nathke, I. S., and Nelson, W. J. (1997) Cadherins, catenins and APC protein: interplay between cytoskeletal complexes and signaling pathways. *Curr. Opin. Cell Biol.* **9**:683–690.

178. Hannigan, G. E., Leung-Hagesteijn, C., Fitz-Gibbon, L., Coppolino, M. G., Radeva, G., Filmus, J., et al. (1996) Regulation of cell adhesion and anchorage-independent growth by a new beta 1-integrin-linked protein kinase. *Nature* **379**:91–96.

179. Calalb, M. B., Polte, T. R., and Hanks, S. K. (1995) Tyrosine phosphorylation of focal adhesion kinase at sites in the catalytic domain regulates kinase activity: a role for Src family kinases. *Mol. Cell Biol.* **15**:954–963.

180. Schaller, M. D., Borgman, C. L., Cobb, B. S., Vines, R. R., Reynolds, A. B., and Parsons, J. T. (1992) pp125FAK, a structurally distinctive focal adhesion kinase associated with focal adhesions. *Proc. Natl. Acad. Sci. USA* **89**:5192–5196.

181. Schreiner, C., Bauer, J., Margolis, M., and Juliano, R. L. (1991) Expression and role of integrins in adhesion of human colonic carcinoma cells to extracellular matrix components. *Clin. Exp. Metastasis* **9**:163–178.

182. Stallmach, A., von Lampe, B., Matthes, H., Bornhoft, G., and Riecken, E. O. (1992) Diminished expression of integrin adhesion molecules on human colonic epithelial cells during benign to malignant transformation. *Gut* **33**:342–346.

183. Juliano, R. L. and Varner, J. A. (1993) Adhesion molecules in cancer: the role of integrins. *Curr. Opin. Cell Biol.* **5**:812–818.

184. Schmidt, R., Streit, M., Herzberg, F., Schirner, M., Schramm, K., Kaufmann, C., et al. (1998) *De novo* expression of the $\alpha5\beta1$-fibronectin receptor in HT29 colon-cancer cells reduces activity of c-Src. Increase of c-Src activity by attachment to fibronectin. *Int. J. Cancer* **76**:91–98.

185. Kanner, S. B., Reynolds, A. B., Vines, R. R., and Parsons, J. T. (1990) Monoclonal antibodies to individual tyrosine-phosphorylated protein substrates of oncogene-encoded tyrosine kinases. *Proc. Natl. Acad. Sci. USA* **87**:3328–3332.

186. Schaller, M. D., Otey, C. A., Hildebrand, J. D., and Parsons, J. T. (1995) Focal adhesion kinase and paxillin bind to peptides mimicking β integrin cytoplasmic domains. *J. Cell. Biol.* **130**:1181–1187.

187. Chen, H.-C., Appedu, P. A., Parsons, J. T., Hildebrand, J. D., Schaller, M. D., and Guan, J. L. (1995) Interaction of the focal adhesion kinase with cytoskeletal protein talin. *J. Biol. Chem.* **270**:16995–16999.

188. Hildebrand, J. D., Schaller, M. D., and Parsons, J. T. (1995) Paxillin, a tyrosine phosphorylated focal adhesion-associated protein binds to the carboxyl terminal domain of focal adhesion kinase. *Mol. Cell Biol.* **6**:637–647.

189. Ilic, D., Furuta, Y., Kanazawa, S., Takeda, N., Sobue, K., Nakatsuji, N., et al. (1995) Reduced cell motility and enhanced focal adhesion contact formation in cells from FAK-deficient mice. *Nature* **377**:539–544.

190. Owens, L. V., Xu, L., Craven, R .J., Dent, G. A., Weiner, T. M., Kornberg, L., et al. (1995) Overexpression of focal adhesion kinase (p125FAK) in invasive human tumors. *Cancer Res.* **55**:2752–2755.

191. Bishop, J. M. (1991) Molecular themes in oncogenesis. *Cell* **64**:235–248.

192. Hanks, S. K., Quinn, A. M., and Hunter, T. (1988) The protein kinase family: conserved features and deduced phylogeny of the catalytic domains. *Science* **241**:42–52.

193. Pawson, T. and Gish, G. D. (1992) SH2 and SH3 domains: from structure to function. *Cell* **71**:359–362.

194. Resh, M. D. (1993) Interaction of tyrosine kinase neoproteins with cellular membranes *Biochim. Biophys. Acta* **1155**:307–322.

195. Cartwright, C. A., Mamajiwalla, S., Skolnick, S. A., Eckhart, W., and Burgess, D. R. (1993) Intestinal crypt cells contain higher lev-els of cytoskeletal-associated pp60^{c-src} protein tyrosine kinase activity than do differentiated enterocytes. *Oncogene* **8**:1033–1039.

196. Burgess, D. R., Jiang, W., Mamajiwalla, S., and Kinsey, W. (1989) Intestinal crypt stem cells possess high levels of cytoskeletal-associated phosphotyrosine-containing proteins and tyrosine kinase activity relative to differentiated enterocytes. *J. Cell. Biol.* **109**:2139–2144.

197. Foss, F. M., Veillette, A., Sartor, O., Rosen, N., and Bolen, J. B. (1989) Alterations in the expression of pp60^{c-src} and p56^{lck} associated with butyrate-induced differentiation of human colon carcinoma cells. *Oncogene Res.* **5**:13–23.

198. Brickell, P. M. (1992) The pp60c-src family of protein-tyrosine kinases: structure, regulation, and function. *Crit. Rev. Oncogenesis* **3**:401–446.

199. Park, J. and Cartwright, C. A. (1995) Src activity increases and Yes activity decreases during mitosis of human colon carcinoma cells. *Mol. Cell. Biol.* **15**:2374–2382.

200. Cartwright, C. A., Meisler, A. I., and Eckhart, W. (1990) Activation of the pp60^{c-src} protein kinase is an early event in colonic carcinogenesis. *Proc. Natl. Acad. Sci. USA* **87**:558–562.

201. Talamonti, M. S., Roh, M. S., Curley, S. A., and Gallick, G. E. (1991) The c-src oncogene participates in the development of human colorectal liver metastases. *Surg. Forum* **42**:422–424.

202. Talamonti, M. S., Roh, M. S., Curley, S. A., and Gallick, G. E. (1993) Increase in activity and expression of pp60c-src during progressive stages of human colorectal carcinoma. *J. Clin. Invest.* **91**:53–60.

203. Cartwright, C. A., Coad, C. A., and Egbert, B. M. (1994) Elevated c-SRC tyrosine kinase activity in premalignant epithelia of ulcerative colitis. *J. Clin. Invest.* **93**:509–515.

204. Cartwright, C. A., Kamps, M. P., Meisler, A. I., Pipas, J. M., and Eckhart (1989) pp60^{c-src} activation in human colon carcinoma. *J. Clin. Invest.* **83**:2025–2033.

205. Sakai, T., Kawakatsu, H., Fujita, M., Yano, J., and Owada, M. K. (1998) An epitope localized c-Src negative regulatory domain is a potential marker in early stage of colonic neoplasms. *Lab. Invest.* **78**:219–225.

206. Park, J., Meisler, A. I., and Cartwright, C. A. (1993) c-yes tyrosine kinase activity in human colon carcinoma. *Oncogene* **8**:2627–2635.

207. Han, N. M., Curley, S. A., and Gallick, G. E. (1996) Differential activation of pp60c-src and pp62c-yes in human colorectal liver metastases. *Clin. Cancer Res.* **2**:1397–1404.

208. Termuhlen, P. M., Curley, S. A., Talamonti, M. A., Saboorian, M. H., and Gallick, G. E. (1993) Site-specific differences in pp60c-src activity in human colorectal metastases. *J. Surg. Res.* **54**:293–298.

209. Irby, R., Mao, W., Coppola, D., Jove, R., Gamero, A., Cuthbertson, D., et al. (1997) Overexpression of normal c-Src in poorly metastatic human colon cancer cells enhances primary tumor growth but not metastatic potential. *Cell Growth Diff.* **8**:1287–1295.

210. Staley, C. A., Parikh, N. U., and Gallick, G.E. (1997) Decreased tumorigenicity of a human colon adenocarcinoma cell line by an antisense expression vector specific for c-src. *Cell Growth Diff.* **8**:269–274.

211. Fleming, R. Y., Ellis, L. M., Parikh, N. U., Liu, W., Staley, C. A., and Gallick, G. E. (1997) Regulation of vascular endothelial growth factor expression in human colon carcinoma cells by activation of *src* kinase. *Surgery* **122**:501–507.

212. Ellis, L. M., Staley, C. A., Liu, W., Fleming, R. Y., Porikh, N. U., Bucana, C. D., et al. (1998) Down-regulation of vascular endothelial growth factor in a human colon carcinoma cell line transfected with an antisense expression vector specific for c-src. *J. Biol. Chem.* **273**:1052–1057.

213. Crouch, D. H., Fincham, V. J., and Frame, M. C. (1996) Targeted proteolysis of the focal adhesion kinase p125FAK during c-Myc-induced apoptosis is suppressed by integrin signaling. *Oncogene* **12**:2689–2696.

214. Wen, L.-P., Fahrni, J. A., Troie, S., Guan, J. L., Orth, K., and Rosen, G. D. (1997) Cleavage of focal adhesion kinase by caspases during apoptosis. *J. Biol. Chem.* **272**:26056–26061.

215. Frisch, S. M., Vuori, K., Ruoslahti, E., and Chan-Hui, P. Y. (1996) Control of adhesion-dependent cell survival by focal adhesion kinase. *J. Cell. Biol.* **134**:793–799.

216. Xu, L. H., Owens, L. V., Sturge, G. C., Yang, X., Liu, E. T., Craven, R. J., et al. (1996) Attenuation of the expression of the focal adhesion kinase induces apoptosis in tumor cells. *Cell Growth Diff.* **7**:413–418.

217. Hungerford, J. E., Compton, M. T., Matter, M. L., Hoffstrom, B. G., and Otey, C. A. (1996) Inhibition of pp125FAK in cultured fibroblasts results in apoptosis. *J. Cell. Biol.* **135**:1383–1390.

218. Khwaja, A., Rodriguez-Viviana, R., Wennstrom, S., Warne, P. H., and Downward, J. (1997) Matrix adhesion and Ras transformation both activate a phosphoinositide 3-OH kinase and oriteun kinase B/Akt cellular survival pathway. *EMBO J.* **16**:2783–2793.

219. Mazure, N. M., Chen, E. Y., Laderoute, K. R., and Giaccia, A. J. (1997) Induction of vascular endothelial growth factor by hypoxia is modulated by a phosphoinositol 3-kinase/Akt signaling pathway in Ha-*ras*-transformed cells through a hypoxia inducible factor-1 trancriptional element. *Blood* **90**:3222–3231.

14 Molecular Genetic Alterations in Primary Hepatocellular Neoplasms

Hepatocellular Adenoma, Hepatocellular Carcinoma, and Hepatoblastoma

JOE W. GRISHAM, MD

THE PRIMARY HEPATOCELLULAR NEOPLASMS

The primary hepatocellular neoplasms—hepatocellular adenoma (HCA), hepatocellular carcinoma (HCC), and hepatoblastoma (HBL)—compose a clinically important group of human neoplasms. Together they constitute one of the most numerous organ-specific tumor groups. These tumors occur at all ages and are diagnostically and therapeutically challenging. Early diagnosis of hepatocellular neoplasms is inefficient, and treatment of HCC is currently ineffective, although treatment of hepatoblastoma is more successful. On the other hand, identification of the major etiologic agents of primary hepatocellular neoplasms appears to be more comprehensive and complete than for any other group of organ-specific neoplasms, and the mechanisms by which etiologic agents perturb hepatocellular survival and function are being elucidated.

HEPATOCELLULAR CARCINOMA A cancer composed of neoplastic hepatocytes, HCC one of the most common human malignant neoplasms, with 437,000 estimated new cases enumerated worldwide during the most recent year surveyed *(1)*. HCC occurs in humans of all ages with an average peak incidence during the fifth to seventh decades of life. However, the incidence and age of peak incidence of HCC vary widely in human populations located in different geographic regions around the world, reflecting differences in the exposure of populations in particular environments to the factors that cause this cancer. The main causes of HCC include chronic infection with hepatitis B or C viruses (HBV/HCV), ingestion of food contaminated with aflatoxin B_1 (derived from the fungi *Aspergillus flavus* and *Aspergillus parasiticus*, which grow on improperly stored grains), affliction with any of several metabolic abnormalities, excessive consumption of beverages containing ethanol, external and internal radiation, and exposure to a few therapeutic drugs and to certain chemicals in the workplace and environment *(2)*. The etiology of HCC is clearly

multifactorial *(3)*, and numerous other agents may either augment or reduce the neoplastic potential of these main causes. Of interest, the incidence of HCC appears to have increased during the most recent decade in the United States *(4)*, the United Kingdom *(5)*, and France *(6)*, geographic areas with the lowest incidence rates worldwide.

HEPATOCELLULAR ADENOMA HCA, the benign counterpart of HCC, is composed of well-differentiated and benign, but neoplastic, hepatocytes. HCA is considered to be an uncommon liver tumor in humans, typically occurring in noncirrhotic livers in association with the use of some formulations of contraceptive and anabolic steroids, as well as with certain inherited metabolic abnormalities *(2)*. HCA occasionally progresses to malignant HCC, but only a small fraction of HCC are now recognized to develop from a previously occurring HCA in humans.

HEPATOBLASTOMA HBL is an uncommon malignant variant of HCC that usually develops during embryogenesis of the liver from fetal liver cells that are precursors of hepatocytes. Occurrence of HBL is virtually limited to children less than five yr of age, although it rarely occurs in adults. HBL is the most common primary liver tumor in children, who also may develop HCC *(7–9)* and HCA *(8,10)*. The close association between the cell of origin of HBL and HCC is suggested not only by the fact that many cells in fetal HBL express a hepatocellular phenotype, but also by the observation that surgically resected HCC may recur as HBL *(11)*.

As a fetal tumor, HBL is sometimes associated with genetically predicated developmental disorders, including Wilms tumor (nephroblastoma), Beckwith-Wiedemann syndrome, adenomatous polyposis coli, hemihypertrophy, and some congenital metabolic abnormalities *(7,12,13)*. Other than germline genetic abnormalities, only weak etiologic risk factors for HBL have been identified. In a case-control study of 75 children with HBL, parental exposures to petroleum products, paints, and metals showed a weak association, but no evidence was found to incriminate hepatitis virus infection, maternal estrogen exposure, and cigarette smoking *(14)*.

From: *The Molecular Basis of Human Cancer* (W. B. Coleman and G. J. Tsongalis, eds.), © Humana Press Inc., Totowa, NJ.

MOLECULAR PATHOGENESIS OF HEPATOCELLULAR NEOPLASMS

This review assesses current information on aberrations in the molecular genetic regulation of hepatocyte proliferation, differentiation, and death, and on the maintenance of genomic integrity, that precede and accompany the development of hepatocellular neoplasms. Although insight into the molecular pathology and pathogenesis of hepatocellular neoplasms in humans is as yet incomplete, details are rapidly being unraveled, especially for HCC and HBL. As for the neoplasms of other tissues, the molecular pathogenesis of HCC and HBL appears to involve multiple genetic aberrations in the molecular control of cell proliferation, differentiation, and death, and of the maintenance of genomic integrity sufficient to allow the emergence and growth of monoclonal populations of deviant cells that accumulate abnormally and invade.

A major question that is still unanswered is which (if any) specific molecular aberration is initially triggered by etiologic agents, and, in turn, sets off the cascade of changes that eventuate in the malignant hepatocellular phenotype. This review will attempt to identify the temporal order in which major molecular and genetic abnormalities associated with hepatocellular neoplasms may occur; documented molecular genetic alterations are correlated with the sequence of histologic and cytologic changes in liver tissues and in hepatocytes that evolve during the preneoplastic phases preceding the emergence of HCA and HCC, and the accumulation of molecular aberrations in neoplastic hepatocytes during the progression of early HCC to large, metastasizing tumors is assessed. Expanded insight into the molecular pathogenesis of HCC may well lead to improved strategies to prevent, diagnose, and treat this major neoplasm of mankind.

THE PROCESS OF HEPATOCARCINOGENESIS

NATURAL HISTORY OF HCC The descriptive natural history of HCC, including the pathological tissue patterns and clinical course, provides a map for attempting to trace the sequence of molecular genetic alterations that drive its development. Hepatocarcinogenesis is a continuous and slowly unfolding process that leads from the initial occurrence of epigenetic and/or genetic alterations in one or a few hepatocytes to the acquisition of a neoplastic genotype/phenotype by one or more affected cells, and ultimately to the gaining of the capacity to grow autonomously and to metastasize and spread to distant sites outside the liver. A population of poorly differentiated, rapidly proliferating, and invasive cells in an HCC is a direct lineal descendent of at least one of the hepatocytes that incurred genetic damage on contact with a causative agent and first expressed aberrations in its metabolic phenotype.

The ability to determine with considerable accuracy the time of infection with HBV or HCV, the major causes of HCC in humans, by detecting antibodies to viral antigens and viral nucleic acids, can accurately establish the time at which the process of hepatocarcinogenesis begins in some instances, enabling the temporal delineation of the evolving development of HCC more precisely than for perhaps any other human cancer; HCC develops slowly but irrevocably in a fraction of the patients chronically infected with HBV or HCV. The mean age at which HCC was found in Japanese patients who were HBV-positive was 56 ± 10 yr *(15)* and 52 ± 13 yr *(16)* in two studies that included 49 patients, while in HCV-positive patients the mean age at which HCC was detected was 63 ± 8 yr *(15)* and 62 ± 7 yr *(16)* among a total of 205 patients. Many years are required for HCC to become clinically evident after initial infection with either HBV or HCV. The HBV-positive Japanese patients, who were thought to have been infected as babies by contact with their infected mothers, were 20–80 yr old when HCC was diagnosed *(16)*; this temporal pattern was corroborated by a study of 19 HCC in HBV-positive Alaskan natives in which perinatal infection was identified, but who were first found to have HCC at ages ranging from 8–80 yr old *(17)*. HCV infection was acquired by transfusion with contaminated blood in many HCV-positive Japanese patients 20–60 yr before HCC was detected *(15,16)*. In all patients, development of HCC was preceded by chronic hepatitis and in most patients by cirrhosis of several years duration *(15,16)*. The temporal sequence of chronic hepatitis, cirrhosis, and HCC is well-illustrated by a study of 100 Japanese patients who were infected with HCV by transfusion with contaminated blood and became HCV-positive; 45 HCV-infected patients developed chronic hepatitis that was first discerned 10 ± 11.3 yr after transfusion, 23 developed cirrhosis first detected 21.2 ± 9.6 yr after transfusion, and 21 developed HCC first diagnosed 29.0 ± 13.2 yr after transfusion *(18)*. Of the 21 patients who developed HCC, all had chronic hepatitis, and 18/21 (86%) developed cirrhosis preceding the emergence of HCC.

Chronic Hepatitis and Cirrhosis Chronic hepatitis is a prolonged inflammation of the liver, associated with inflammatory-cell infiltration, smoldering hepatocyte death, and accelerated proliferation of residual hepatocytes to replace those that have been killed or injured. In chronic hepatitis, a mixture of B and T lymphocytes, dendritic cells, plasma cells, and macrophages infiltrates the connective tissue of portal tracts and may also infiltrate into the lobular parenchyma *(19,20)*. Where the inflammatory infiltrate touches the lobular parenchyma, cytotoxic T lymphocytes closely surround individual or small groups of hepatocytes, many of which are killed by activation of death-signaling pathways by the binding of ligands to the Fas receptor (Fas) and the tumor necrosis factor type 1 receptor (TNFR-1) *(21)*. Lymphocytes and macrophages accumulate in chronically inflamed liver because of the increased expression of chemotactic cytokines by endothelial cells of portal vessels and interlobular sinusoids, and because lymphocytes express the relevant receptors for these adhesion molecules *(20)*. Sinusoidal and portal-vascular endothelial cells constitutively express a variety of adhesion molecules and receptors for inflammatory-cell ligands, which are upregulated in chronic inflammation, together with the induced expression of other attraction molecules *(22–25)*.

Inflammatory cells that infiltrate the liver in chronic hepatitis express numerous cytokines, including chemotactic cytokines of the CC and CXC types, and immunomodulatory cytokines, including tumor necrosis factor-α (TNF-α), various interleukins (IL), and several interferons (IFN) *(20)*. The chemotactic cytokines attract additional chronic inflammatory cells and induce higher levels of expression of adhesion molecules and receptors for inflammatory-cell ligands by endothelial cells. The immunomodulatory cytokines stimulate both inflammatory cells and resident liver cells, including hepatocytes, to secrete a variety of cytokines, growth factors, and proteases. The complex mixture of cytokines, growth factors, and proteases that is triggered by chronic hepatitis stimulates both destruction and repair of liver cells and tissue (20). Many hepatocytes are damaged or killed as a result both of the cytotoxicity of activated T lymphocytes and of inflammatory cytokines such as TNF-α and Fas ligand (FasL); oxidative damage to hepatocytes is reflected by the increased formation of 8-hydroxyguanosine in DNA of livers that are the site of chronic hepatitis (26). Residual hepatocytes are stimulated to proliferate by cell loss, as well as by some of the cytokines and growth factors generated by inflammatory cells. The liver matrix and vasculature are also greatly modified during chronic inflammation associated with both destruction and synthesis of connective tissue elements and with the formation of new blood vessels, which sometimes causes the delicate connective-issue stroma of the healthy liver to be replaced by dense fibrosis.

Cirrhosis is a diffuse form of hepatic fibrosis, which results from severe, long-standing chronic hepatitis with extensive necrosis (27). Cirrhosis is characterized by the subdivision of the normally continuous liver parenchyma into nodular aggregates of a few million hepatocytes, each of which is segregated by encircling bands (septa) of collagenous connective tissue (27). Collagenous connective tissue is deposited in the areas of hepatocellular necrosis and tissue destruction, in association with the deposition of other matrix proteins and the formation of new vessels. Cirrhosis is one of the strongest risk factors for HCC in humans (28), and it is a precursor of about 60% of HCC world-wide. Although cirrhosis frequently precedes HCC, it is not necessary for the development of this neoplasm, because about 40% of HCC world-wide develop in the absence of cirrhosis in patients who have only chronic hepatitis and less severe fibrosis that results from exposure to the same etiologic agents that cause cirrhosis. Whether cirrhosis develops prior to HCC may reflect the intensity of exposure to etiologic agents and/or to the extent of chronic inflammatory-cell infiltration and the amount of hepatocellular necrosis.

Phenotypic Alterations and Dysplasia In the setting of simultaneous hepatocellular necrosis and proliferation, nodular aggregates of hepatocytes may develop in either cirrhotic or noncirrhotic livers that are the site of chronic hepatitis. Many hepatocytes proliferate repeatedly in either setting, often forming nodules up to 3–5 mm in diameter, and the cell populations of these hyperplastic nodules are often monoclonal. A nodule of an average size of 3–5 mm may contain more than a million hepatocytes and require 20–30 cell doublings of one parental cell, involving repeated proliferative cycles. Hyperplastic hepatocytes may express a variety of aberrant metabolic phenotypes before evident genomic abnormalities occur. Alterations in the metabolic phenotype of a few hepatocytes, evidenced by the occurrence of foci of phenotypically altered hepatocytes (FAH) is one of the earliest morphologic changes that has been detected in hepatocytes during the process of hepatocarcinogenesis. Hepatocytes in FAH aberrantly express and store

various metabolic products, such as glycogen, lipid, and iron, often forming glycogen-storing (clear-cell) foci, some of which ultimately overexpress RNA to become basophilic foci. FAH were first found more or less fortuitously in the nonneoplastic liver tissues adjacent to HCC (29–36).

Karhunen and Pentillä (37) prospectively identified FAH on the basis of aberrant storage of glycogen or iron in the livers of 11/95 persons (12%) who were subjected to consecutive unselected medicolegal autopsies. Foci of phenotypically altered hepatocytes were clustered in livers of patients who consumed more than 90 gm/d of ethanol or who had cirrhosis, and they were accompanied by non-neoplastic hepatocellular nodules or HCA in five livers (37). Bannasch et al. (38) and Su et al. (39) systematically examined 163 explanted and resected livers from transplant patients for the presence of FAH, and characterized their phenotypic properties and size distributions. Three major types of FAH—glycogen-storing, mixed-cell type, and basophilic—were found in 84/111 cirrhotic livers (76%), more frequently in livers containing HCC (29/32, 91%) than in those without HCC (55/79, 70%), and more foci were found in cirrhosis in the absence of HCC but associated with chronic infection with HBV or HCV, or with chronic ethanol abuse (37/47, 79%), than with cirrhosis due to other causes (12/21, 57%) (39). Glycogen-storing foci were smaller than mixed-cell foci, which were more often associated with the formation of larger nodules and the development of small-cell (dysplastic) change (39). Glycogen-storing foci appear to contain hepatocytes with the earliest preneoplastic changes, and mixed-cell foci, containing both glycogen-storing and basophilic cells, represent more advanced lesions. Hyperplastic (hypercellular) foci composed of cells with small-cell change appear to be the direct precursors of dysplastic nodules (40), which have a high probability of undergoing malignant transformation (41).

Emergence and Progression of HCC The first cytologically identifiable HCC develop in or near (and presumably from) dysplastic hepatocytes that form small foci or larger nodules (40,41). Cirrhotic nodules in which dysplasia and HCC develop are typically those that enlarge (up to 8–10 mm in diameter) due to relatively high rates of cell proliferation, and are variously called adenomatous hyperplasias or macroregenerative nodules (42) or multilobular nodules (43). Nodules that contain dysplastic changes are called atypical adenomatous hyperplasias, type II macroregenerative nodules (42), or dysplastic nodules (43), indicating a propensity to transform into HCC. Similar nodules with or without dysplasia may also develop in noncirrhotic livers that are the site of chronic hepatitis (44,45), and dysplasia may also develop focally in a few hepatocytes that do not form nodules (40).

Hirohashi's group has categorized HCC as "early" and "advanced" (40,46). Early HCC can contain such a small number of malignant cells that they may not form nodular lesions, but more nearly resemble foci, and the newly emerging malignant cells may proliferate slowly (40). Malignant hepatocytes proliferate rapidly in advanced HCC and the tumors grow expansively to form enlarging nodules that compress adjacent nontumor tissue (40). The cytological differentiation of neoplastic hepatocytes deteriorates in coordination with the growth of HCC from small to large size (47): malignant cells in small,

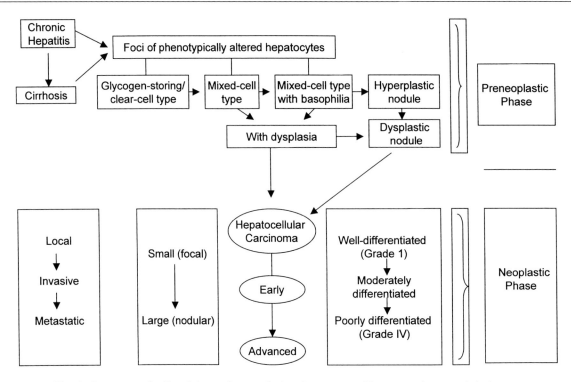

Fig. 1. Sequence of cell and tissue changes during the process of hepatocarcinogenesis in humans.

early HCC are usually well-differentiated (Grade I or II) and become poorly differentiated (Grade IV) in large tumors, associated with local invasion and distant metastasis. After becoming clinically apparent, HCC is rapidly progressive and uniformly fatal. Survival of patients varies with the sizes of tumors at diagnosis and with the growth rates of HCC *(48)*, which have doubling times that vary from 1–35 mo. The doubling time of 64 untreated HCC accumulated from three studies was 129.1 ± 98.1 d, and the median was 100 d *(49–51)*. Among 61 patients with HCC that were less than 3–5 cm in diameter, 56% survived for 2 yr *(48,52)*. In the absence of cirrhosis, HCC may reach a large size as a single lesion before it becomes clinically evident, whereas patients with cirrhosis usually seek medical care before a large HCC develops. The sequence of cell and tissue changes during the development of HCC is depicted schematically in Fig. 1.

IMPORTANT TISSUE CHANGES DURING HEPATO-CARCINOGENESIS The following cellular changes that typify livers in which HCC is likely to develop appear to represent particularly important preneoplastic events that facilitate or permit the ultimate evolution of HCC.

Increased Hepatocytic Proliferation In nondiseased livers hepatocytes are long-lived with little turnover, but both cell formation and cell death are increased in chronic hepatitis, cirrhosis, and HCC. In combination, these changes often allow affected hepatocytes to accumulate, and permit the development and accumulation of molecular genetic aberrations. Tarao et al. *(53)* determined the fraction of hepatocytes located in the S phase of the cell cycle by incubating freshly biopsied tissues with bromodeoxyuridine (BrdU) in vitro and detecting the nuclei that incorporated the BrdU into DNA by immunohistochemistry with an antibody to BrdU–DNA. In 6 livers with-

out cirrhosis or HCC, the labeling index was 0.25 ± 0.09%, as compared to 2.1 ± 1.7% in 19 cirrhotic livers (alcoholic and posthepatitic) without HCC, 3.3 ± 1.5% in the nontumorous areas of 17 cirrhotic livers that contained HCC, and 7.2 ± 2.9% in 19 HCC *(53)*. The BrdU labeling index of HCC cells increased with decreasing HCC differentiation; in 3 well-differentiated HCC the labeling index was 4.7 ± 2.3%, in 7 moderately differentiated HCC the labeling index was 6.3 ± 1.5%, and in 4 poorly differentiated HCC the labeling index was 10.7 ± 2.1 *(53)*. In another study of 30 cirrhotic livers containing HCC, the BrdU labeling index was 2.4 ± 1.4% in the nontumorous cirrhotic areas and 5.2 ± 3.2% in the HCC *(54)*; the BrdU labeling index in 4 well-differentiated HCC was 3.3 ± 2.3%, in 19 moderately differentiated HCC it was 4.3 ± 2.2%, and in 6 poorly differentiated HCC it was 9.2 ± 3.8% *(54)*. Among 25 HCC of grades I and II, the labeling index was 4.5 ± 2.0%, as compared to 11.1 ± 2.1% among 5 HCC of grades III and IV *(55)*.

These results on hepatocyte proliferation have been corroborated and extended by other studies which have applied more indirect methods to detect the fraction of hepatocytes that are cycling, including the use of antibodies to assess (by immunohistochemistry) the fraction of cells that express proliferating cell nuclear antigen (PCNA) and a nuclear antigen known as Ki-67. In all instances hepatocyte proliferation steadily increased in association with the morphological changes from nondiseased liver, to cirrhotic liver, to HCC, and, where examined, from well-differentiated to poorly differentiated HCC *(38–40,56–60)*. For example, Tiniakos and Brunt *(60)* found PCNA labeling indices (which are relatively higher than are indices for BrdU incorporation or Ki-67 labeling) of 4.2 ± 0.4% for 13 cirrhotic nodules, 2.1 ± 0.65% for 3 macroregenerative nodules, 10.6 ± 1.87% for 3 noncirrhotic regenerative nodules, 15.3 ± 3.22% for 11 dysplastic nodules (macroregenerative nodules, type II), and 23.3 ± 6.1% for 8 HCC. Matsuno et al. *(61)* demonstrated that the PCNA labeling index of the cirrhotic areas of 8 livers containing HCC was 3.0 ± 2.0%, while the labeling index in 8 atypical macroregenerative (dysplastic) nodules or low-grade HCC was 7.6 ± 5.0%, and that of 8 high-grade (poorly differentiated) HCC was 26.5 ± 18.3%.

Increased rates of proliferation also characterize the cells in the earliest FAH. Bannasch et al. *(38)* found that 3.7 ± 2.6% of the hepatocytes were PCNA-positive in 49 foci of various types from 7 livers, as compared to 0.84 ± 0.53% of the hepatocytes in areas of the same livers outside the altered foci. These observations were extended in a larger study of 111 cirrhotic livers by Su et al. *(39)* in which the PCNA labeling index was less than 0.25% in 35 nondiseased livers and in extrafocal hepatocytes of diseased livers. PCNA labeling was also low in 72 amphophilic foci and in 176 glycogen-storing foci that lacked areas of small-cell dysplastic change, while PCNA indices were 1.8 ± 0.53% in 294 amphophilic mixed-cell foci, and 2.9 ± 1.5% in 29 basophilic mixed-cell foci. In all instances the PCNA index was increased further in each of these types of altered foci that also contained small-cell change (dysplasia) as indicated by elevated cell density (in 44 glycogen-storing foci with dysplasia it was 2.6 ± 1.3%, in 99 amphophilic mixed-cell dysplastic foci it was 4.5 ± 1.3%, and in 31 basophilic mixed-cell dysplastic foci it was 7.1 ± 2.1%) *(39)*. These investigators found a PCNA index of 11.0 ± 3.7% in 66 well-differentiated HCC and of 41.6 ± 13.9% in 50 poorly differentiated HCC *(39)*, indicating that a continuum of increasing cell proliferation extends from dysplastic basophilic foci to HCC. Sugitani et al. *(40)* also found that cell proliferation increased dramatically from early to advanced HCC; the PCNA indices in early and advanced HCC were 3.5 ± 3.6% and 31.9 ± 26.8%, respectively.

LeBail et al. *(62)* examined the PCNA index and the density of hepatocytes (which increases with small-cell dysplastic change as a function of cell size) in cirrhotic nodules, in ordinary adenomatous hyperplasia (without dysplasia), and in atypical adenomatous hyperplasia (dysplastic nodules). In cirrhotic nodules the hepatocyte density was 1760 ± 160 cells/mm² and the PCNA index was 4.7 ± 3.9%, in 17 ordinary adenomatous hyperplasias cell density was 2170 ± 150 cells/mm² and PCNA index was 3.1 ± 3.0%, while in 18 dysplastic nodules (atypical adenomatous hyperplasia) cell density was 2700 ± 150 cells/mm² and PCNA index was 6.1 ± 3.7% *(62)*. Comparable values for 11 HCC included cell density of 3120 ± 200 cells/mm² and PCNA index of 18.7 ± 4.9% *(62)*. Hino et al. *(56)* and Kubo et al. *(58)* also demonstrated increasing cell proliferation in HCC of higher grades, and Kubo et al. *(58)* and Tiniakos and Brunt *(60)* showed that larger HCC are accompanied by higher rates of cell proliferation.

A high rate of hepatocyte proliferation in cirrhotic livers is a strong predictor of the risk of developing HCC *(63)*. Tarao et al. *(53,54,64)*, Ng et al. *(65)*, and Borzio et al. *(63)* found that high rates of HCC cell proliferation are associated with shortened patient survival. In a small case-control study of 18 patients with chronic HCV infection who subsequently developed HCC, matched by age and severity of chronic liver disease with

18 chronically infected patients who did not develop HCC, the former group had higher indices of PCNA expression in hepatocytes *(66)*.

In nondiseased livers the rates of proliferation and cell death, including necrosis and apoptosis (measured by nick end-labeling techniques) are in near balance. Studies of apoptosis by Hino et al. *(56)*, Grasl-Kraupp *(57)*, Kubo et al. *(58)*, Tannapfel et al. *(59)* and Wu et al. *(67)* have all demonstrated that increased rates of apoptosis accompany increased rates of hepatocyte proliferation as HCC develops in chronically inflamed and cirrhotic livers, and that high rates of apoptosis are correlated with shortened disease-free survival in patients with HCC *(68)*. However, the rates of cell formation always exceed the rates of apoptotic cell death and many populations of aberrant hepatocytes expand.

Formation of Monoclonal Hepatocyte Populations A monoclonal population is one that arises from a single progenitor cell through multiple cycles of proliferation. The importance of monoclonality is that it allows genetic changes that develop in a parental cell to accumulate in and permeate the subsequent population composed of its descendents, which may give rise to subsequent clonal populations containing new genetic aberrations. Clonality of hepatocellular nodules (cirrhotic nodules, dysplastic nodules, and adenomatous hyperplasias), HCA and HCC have been assessed by several methods, including the pattern of integration of HBV DNA into hepatocyte genomes, the random suppression of X-linked polymorphic gene loci in females, and DNA fingerprinting using polymerase chain reaction (PCR) of minisatellite repeated sequences or of arbitrary primers. Of these methods, the pattern of integration of HBV DNA provides the most sensitive and specific distinction between monoclonal and polyclonal populations of cells in instances in which the integration of HBV DNA into the hepatocyte genome has occurred. The sites of HBV DNA integration into the cellular genome are random and unique to each affected cell. Identical patterns of loss of allelic heterozygosity and chromosome structural alterations also provide evidence suggesting monoclonal expansion.

Almost every small HCC examined and reported (105/109, 95%) has been found to be monoclonal based on the pattern of integration of HBV DNA, the random silencing of a polymorphic X-linked gene in females, and/or DNA fingerprinting with minisatellite probes *(69–82)*. Sirivatnauksorn et al. *(83)* demonstrated that enlarging HCC undergo clonal divergence, correlated with increased tumor size. Using fingerprint analysis of HCC DNA performed by generating PCR fragments with arbitrary primers, they found that each of 18 HCC smaller than 6 mm in diameter (mean diameter = 4.7 mm) was monoclonal, whereas each of 13 HCC larger than 6 mm (mean diameter = 15.4 mm) contained multiple, divergent clones *(83)*.

Integration of HBV DNA in a clonal pattern has also been detected in apparently nonneoplastic hepatocytes of chronically infected livers *(69,84–86)*, and Shafritz et al. *(69)* identified identical integration patterns in an HCC and adjacent nontumorous tissue, suggesting that the HCC developed as a clonal outgrowth from the non-neoplastic cells. Aoki and Robinson *(73)* first examined the clonality of individual cirrhotic nodules in livers of patients with chronic HBV infection

and discovered that at least 6% contained monoclonal populations of hepatocytes. Subsequently, Yasui et al. *(87)* studied 83
cirrhotic nodules from 11 cases of HBV-related cirrhosis and
found that 26 (31%) of the nodules were monoclonal, and
Aihara et al. *(78)* found that 33/76 cirrhotic nodules (43%) from
HCV-related cirrhosis were monoclonal on the basis of restriction fragment-length polymorphisms (RFLP) of the X-linked
phosphoglycerokinase gene in females. Tsuda et al. *(72)* demonstrated that two atypical adenomatous hyperplasias (dysplastic nodules) were monoclonal as indicated by HBV-DNA
integration pattern, and that a small HCC arising in one of the
dysplastic nodules contained cells with the same pattern of
HBV-DNA integration and represented a clonal outgrowth
from the dysplastic cells. Aihara et al. *(80)* also found that each
of 5 dysplastic nodules was monoclonal by the expression pattern of the X-linked polymorphic phosphoglycerokinase gene
in females, and that 6/10 dysplastic nodules were monoclonal
by DNA fingerprinting with a minisatellite probe; one of these
dysplastic nodules also had loss of heterozygosity (LOH) of a
locus on chromosome 7pter-p22 *(80)*.

Taken together these observations show that monoclonal
populations of hepatocytes, often phenotypically altered and/
or dysplastic, develop at an early stage of hepatocarcinogenesis,
long before the involved hepatocytes are recognized to be either neoplastic or malignant and possibly coincident with the
development of some FAH. Repetitive clonal proliferation from
one parental cell to produce a large population of descendents
provides the opportunity to accumulate in a relatively large
population of cells genetic aberrations that have developed in
one precursor cell.

Remodeling of the Liver Matrix The liver matrix is radically modified in concert with chronic hepatitis and cirrhosis
(88), prior to the development of HCC. The matrix of the
nondiseased hepatic lobular parenchyma is located predominantly in the space of Disse between hepatocytes and the endothelial cells that line sinusoids; liver sinusoids are unique
capillary-sized vessels that lack a basal lamina and contain
fenestrated endothelium. The perisinusoidal space in healthy
livers contains discontinuous collagen IV fibers, abundant
fibronectin, thrombospondin, and scanty and focally displayed
tenascin, but lacks laminin *(89–93)*. Perlecan is also abundantly
expressed in the perisinusoidal spaces of nondiseased livers,
and syndecan-1 is strongly expressed by hepatocytes and biliary epithelial cells *(94)*. Heparan sulfate chains are expressed
in the membranes of hepatocytes and in the space of Disse *(94)*.
In the cirrhotic liver, collagen IV, fibronectin, and tenascin are
increased in amount, beginning at the peripheral ends of sinusoids and extending into nodules; laminin is also newly expressed at these locations *(89–91,93)*. Coupled with these
stromal changes, sinusoids in cirrhotic livers acquire the ultrastructural appearance of conventional capillaries, with a continuous layer of endothelium and a prominent, electron dense
basal lamina *(95)*. Most of these matrix components of basal
lamina are increased further in macroregenerative nodules
(adenomatous hyperplasias) *(93)* and in well-differentiated
HCC, but the expression of most matrix components is decreased in poorly differentiated HCC *(89–93,95–97)*, suggesting that matrix proteins modulate the differentiated phenotypes

of neoplastic hepatocytes *(89)*. Expression of syndecan-1 and
perlecan were increased in 14 HCC (which were not graded);
perlecan was heavily expressed in the pericapillary spaces of
HCC, and the pattern of expression of syndecan-1 in hepatocytes was changed from a basilateral membrane location to a
honeycomb pattern with cytoplasmic and nuclear staining in
some neoplastic cells *(94)*; syndecan-4 was also highly expressed by neoplastic hepatocytes, while the expression of
sydecan-2 and sydecan-3 were increased in vessel walls, endothelial cells, mesenchymal cells, and nerves *(94)*. The concentration of the enzyme N-acetylglucosaminyltransferase-V,
which initiates the β1-6 branching of cell-related branched oli-
gosaccharides, was increased in HCC as compared to
nondiseased liver *(98)*; in 5 nondiseased livers the activity of
this enzyme was 7.0 ± 6.2 pmol product/h/mg protein, as compared to 324 ± 270 pmol product/h/mg protein in 33 HCC and
85 ± 21 pmol product/h/mg protein in 6 nontumorous liver
tissues adjacent to HCC. The average enzyme activity also
increased significantly with increasing tumor grade, suggesting that enzyme activity correlated with tumor progression *(98)*.

Hepatocytes normally express α integrins 1 and 5, while
sinusoidal endothelial cells express 1, 2, and 5, and biliary
epithelial cells express 2, 3, 5, and 6. The β1 integrin is the
common β subunit for the various α/β dimers *(99)*. Integrin
expression on hepatocytes is normally confined to the cell-
matrix interface *(100–102)*. A global increase in the expression
of integrins α_1/β_1 and α_5/β_1 characterized macroregenerative
nodules *(93)* and well-differentiated HCC *(89,91,93,100,101,
103)*, but the pattern of expression changed from cell-membrane polarization to diffusely cytoplasmic, suggesting a redis-
tribution of these matrix receptors in HCC *(103)*. The
expression of α_5 integrin was downregulated in poorly differentiated HCC *(97)*, which coincidentally acquired the ability to
express integrins α_2, α_3, and α_6, in addition to α_1 and α_5
(91,93,101,103,104). The B isoforms of α_6 and β_1 integrins
were preferentially expressed in HCC as compared to
nondiseased liver tissue *(103,104)*. Overexpression of α_6
integrin and of laminin in HCC was highly correlated with
increased tumor-cell proliferation *(93,100)*.

Hepatocyte-hepatocyte adhesion, which is mediated by several molecules (including N-cam, Ep-Cam, E-cadherin,
annexin-I, CD24, and CD44), has been examined in many HCC
(91,101,105–114). Expression of annexin-I, a Ca++-dependent
membrane-binding protein, was increased by more than 20-
fold in HCC as compared to nondiseased liver *(109)*, with the
highest expression occurring in poorly differentiated HCC associated with elevated cell proliferation. Annexin-I, which is a
substrate for tyrosine phosphorylation by tyrosine kinases on
growth-factor receptors such as endothelial growth factor receptor (EGFR), was heavily phosphorylated on tyrosine residues in HCC *(109)*. E-cadherin was highly expressed on 197/
220 well-differentiated HCC (90%), but on only 39/70 poorly
differentiated HCC (56%) summed from six studies
(91,105,108,110,113,115). The expression of the gap-junction
protein, connexin 32, was also decreased in HCC *(115)*. Reduced expression of E-cadherin correlated with increased methylation of CpG residues in the promoter region of the
E-cadherin gene *(113)*, and LOH of loci near the E-cadherin

gene was also found in 18/28 HCC (64%) *(116)*. In contrast, the N-cam adhesion molecule (CAM), which is not expressed in nondiseased liver *(91,101)*, was rarely upregulated in poorly differentiated HCC *(91)*, but not in any well-differentiated tumors *(91,101)*.

The mean serum level of the intracellular adhesion molecule, I-CAM-1, was higher in patients with HCC as compared to patients with mild liver disease or with cirrhosis without HCC. However, the serum level of I-CAM-1 did not discriminate between individual patients with or without HCC because of overlapping values *(117)*. Ep-Cam, a Ca^{++}-independent cell adhesion molecule, which was expressed on fetal liver but not on hepatocytes of adults, was upregulated in only 2/10 HCC, as compared to 10/11 cholangiocarcinomas *(114)*.

Using differential display reverse transcription (RT)-PCR, Huang and Hsu identified the neoexpression by HCC of CD24, a glycoprotein involved in signal activation and cell adhesion. CD24 mRNA was expressed in 73/110 HCC (66%), and expression strongly correlated with p53 mutation and poor differentiation *(107)*. Expression of the CD44 antigen, also a transmembrane glycoprotein involved in cell-cell and cell-matrix interactions, has been examined in 147 HCC *(106,111,112)*. Haramaki et al. *(106)* found that metastatic HCC tumor cells located in tissues were uniformly negative, while those in peritoneal ascitic fluid were positive. However, both Mathew et al. *(111)* and Terris et al. *(112)* found that the hematopoietic isoform of CD44 (CD44H or CD44v6) was expressed by HCC that invaded intrahepatic vessels (43/123, 35%), but only rarely by HCC that did not show vascular invasion. CD44 expression did not correlate with tumor grade, tumor size, or patient survival *(111,112)*.

Matrix metalloproteinases, enzymes which dissolve matrix proteins, are strongly expressed by inflammatory cells in chronic hepatitis, and play an important role in the modification of the liver matrix in chronic hepatitis and cirrhosis; they continue to be expressed at high levels by neoplastic HCC cells. The matrix metalloproteinase-1 (MMP-1) gene was expressed by many cells in well-differentiated HCC but not by cells in poorly differentiated HCC *(89,118)*. MMP-9 gene transcripts were detected in 16/23 HCC (70%), and in 15/16 MMP-9-positive HCC (94%) the expression was more intense than in the adjacent nontumorous liver tissue *(119)*. MMP-2 was identified in 18/23 HCC (78%), and 8/18 positive HCC (44%) showed higher expression than did the surrounding nontumorous liver tissue *(119)*. Furthermore, expression of both MMP-9 and MMP-2 transcripts was significantly higher in HCC with capsular invasion *(119)*. The mean plasma level of MMP-9 was 62 ng/mL (range 13–600 ng/mL) in 100 patients with HCC, as compared to a mean of 28 ng/mL (range 13–66 ng/mL) in 21 HCC-free patients with chronic hepatitis and 35 ng/mL (16–86 ng/mL) in 24 HCC-free patients with cirrhosis *(120)*. HCC patients with tumors that invaded portal veins had higher plasma levels of MMP-9 (mean, 79 ng/mL; range 36–660 ng/mL) than did those without portal venous invasion (mean, 44 ng/mL; range 13–210 ng/mL). Although plasma levels correlated with vascular invasion, they did not correlate with tumor size *(120)*. HCC also expressed tissue inhibitor of metalloproteinase-1 (TIMP-1) and metalloproteinase-2 (TIMP-2) at levels higher

than in the surrounding nontumorous liver *(119,121)*. In general, TIMP-1 was expressed at a higher level than TIMP-2, and the level of expression tended to parallel the expression of MMP; expression did not correlate with either HCC grade or size *(119,121)*.

De Petro et al. *(122)* examined the expression of mRNA for urokinase-type plasminogen activator (uPA), uPA receptor (uPAR), and tissue-type PA (tPA) in 25 HCC and adjacent nontumorous liver tissue by RT-PCR (relative to fibronectin mRNA). Transcription of all three molecules was more highly expressed in HCC and in adjacent cirrhotic liver than in livers the site of chronic hepatitis or cirrhosis without HCC, or in nondiseased livers. The relative levels of uPA and uPAR mRNAs were always higher in HCC than in adjacent nontumorous liver tissue, and the relative level of uPA (but not tPA) was correlated with the length of survival after surgical resection. Morita et al. *(123)* examined the cellular location of uPAR mRNA (*in situ* hybridization) in 31 HCC and in adjacent liver. Tumor cells in most HCC expressed uPAR mRNA at variable intensities greater than the adjacent liver; no uPAR mRNA was detected in nondiseased livers. uPAR mRNA was expressed in 14/16 HCC with vascular invasion (88%) as compared to 8/15 HCC without vascular invasion (53%), but there was no association between uPAR mRNA expression and HCC grade or size although the period of disease-free survival after tumor resection was significantly longer for patients whose tumors were uPAR-negative *(123)*.

Morita et al. *(123)* detected uPAR protein by immunohistochemistry in HCC cells, especially those cells located at the interfaces between tumor and matrix, and by Western-blot analysis of protein extracts of HCC. However, Akahane et al. *(124)* found that uPAR protein was expressed (immunohistochemistry) by CD68-positive macrophages in 25 HCC, and not by tumor cells except in one poorly differentiated HCC. Invasive HCC contained more prominent uPAR-positive macrophages than did noninvasive tumors. In agreement, Dubuisson et al. *(125)* found that both uPA and uPAR mRNAs (*in situ* RT-PCR) and proteins (immunohistochemistry) were predominantly expressed by CD68-positive macrophages and occasionally by αSMA (smooth muscle antigen) -positive myofibroblasts in 26 HCC. However, in 6/26 HCC (23%) occasional cytokeratin 7-positive tumor cells expressed both uPA and uPAR *(125)*. Levels of uPA in the plasma were increased in patients with HCC *(126,127)*, suggesting the use of this analyte as a tumor marker for HCC *(126)*. However, plasma levels of uPA are also elevated in chronic hepatitis and cirrhosis *(128,129)*, reflecting the extensive remodeling of the tissue matrix.

Taken together these observations indicate that the plasmin system and the complex of tissue proteinases/proteinase-inhibitors, which regulate the remodeling of the liver matrix, are also involved in vascular invasion and spread of HCC.

Neoangiogenesis Formation of new blood vessels, which occurs in parallel with matrix remodeling, is an essential step in the development and progression of HCC. Radiographic perfusion studies have shown that even small HCC (<2 cm) are usually more vascular than is the surrounding non-neoplastic liver tissue *(130)*. In addition, the proportion of arterial blood received by HCC is increased over that supplied to the adjacent nontumorous tissue *(130)*. Grigioni et al. *(95)* and Haratake et al. *(131,132)* demonstrated that the liver sinusoids undergo major modifications to become structurally similar to conventional capillaries in cirrhosis and HCC. Unlike the sinusoids of the normal liver, tumor capillaries contain an unfenestrated, continuous layer of endothelial cells that are surrounded by a thick basal lamina, subtended by prominent pericapillary cells, a change that is first seen in cirrhotic livers. The extensive alterations in the tumor capillaries are also reflected in the antigenic modifications of their lumenal membranes. Tumor capillaries express ABH blood groups, *Ulex europaeus* lectin, von Willebrand-related antigen, and CD34 antigen, whereas the endothelial cells of adjacent sinusoids in the nontumorous liver tissue do not express these antigens or express them only weakly in the immediately periportal areas *(133–139)*.

CD34 is a major antigenic marker of tumor vessels in HCC; the mean density of microvessels marked by CD34 in 43 HCC and adjacent tissue was 23 ± 5 per 0.74 mm^2 tissue in chronic hepatitis and 297 ± 88 per 0.74 mm^2 tissue in HCC *(137)*. HCC were categorized as either more or less hypervascular by a relative vascularity of $290/0.74$ mm^2, and the higher vascular density was significantly associated with HCC size, differentiation, and disease-free interval following surgical resection *(137)*. Toyoda et al. *(130)* found that the expression of CD34 correlated with tumor differentiation and reflected relative arterial-blood flow estimated by CT-arterial tomography. El-Assal et al. *(139)* also found that the density of vessels correlated with disease-free survival. In contrast, Kimura et al. *(138)* found no correlation between intratumoral microvessel density (MVD) and HCC differentiation or invasiveness. Ueda et al. *(135)* found that 73 HCC contained more aberrant arterial-type vessels than did either 43 ordinary or 30 atypical adenomatous hyperplastic nodules. The relative number and relative luminal area of vessels in HCC were 93.6 and 92.0%, respectively, as compared to 46.8 and 52.5% for atypical adenomatous nodules and to 20.7 and 17.5% for ordinary adenomatous nodules, suggesting a step-wise increase *(135)*. This conclusion was supported by Park et al. *(140)*, who detected arterial vessels immunohistochemically using an antibody to smooth-muscle actin. Arterial vessels that were not paired with veins increased progressively in 20 low-grade and 27 high-grade dysplastic nodules and in 20 HCC.

Dhillon et al. *(134)* demonstrated that vessels in HCA expressed CD34 as did those in HCC and Scott et al. *(141)* identified higher expression of CD34 in a focus of HCC developing in an HCA than in the surrounding HCA.

Plasma levels of endothelin-1 (ET-1), a vasoactive peptide produced by endothelium, were markedly higher in patients with HCC than in control patients without HCC *(142)*. Both ET-1 peptide (immunohistochemistry) and ET-1 mRNA (*in situ* hybridization) were expressed by 14/20 HCC (70%); both neoplastic hepatocytes and intratumoral endothelial cells stained for ET-1 *(142)*. Neither ET-1 mRNA or protein were detected in non-neoplastic liver tissue adjacent to HCC or in liver tissue lacking HCC *(142)*.

NATURAL HISTORIES OF HCA AND HBL The natural histories of HCA and HBL are more obscure in their early phases of development than is that for HCC. HCA is an uncommonly recognized liver tumor in humans, and the early hepatocellular changes that precede its development are uncertain. HCA is typically diagnosed in a liver that is otherwise relatively normal structurally, usually lacking both chronic hepatitis and cirrhosis. It seems possible, however, that HCA are underdiagnosed in humans, and that some cirrhotic nodules may be equivalent to HCA. In keeping with this idea, benign tumors of most tissues are precursors of the malignant tumors that are composed of the same type of cell, and this relationship characterizes HCA and HCC in rodent livers *(2)*. Although the cellular development of HCA is not clear it may be identical to the changes that lead to HCC, because FAH have been detected in non-neoplastic liver tissue adjacent to HCA *(37,143)*. Furthermore, hepatocytes in 10 HCA from two studies showed increased rates of proliferation by PCNA labeling, but always less than 5% *(10,144)*, and 9/10 HCA examined were composed of monoclonal populations of hepatocytes, as indicated by the patterns of inactivation of the X-linked polymorphic androgen-receptor gene in females *(81,145)*. Monoclonality is generally considered to be a defining characteristic of neoplastic cell populations *(80)*, suggesting that 30–40% of the cirrhotic nodules, which are monoclonal *(78,87)* may actually be benign neoplasms analogous to the HCA in noncirrhotic livers. Phenotypically, the hepatocytes in HCA also resemble those in FAH, they are well-differentiated and frequently store an excess of certain metabolic products, such as lipid or glycogen. It seems possible that the HCA, which may reach 15 cm or more in diameter in noncirrhotic livers, may represent FAH that have grown to large size without developing dysplasia, because occasional HCA develop dysplastic foci and evolve into HCC. HCA often appear to be poorly supported by a collagenous matrix, and as a consequence, large HCA may rupture, causing rapid bleeding. A possible sequence of cellular changes during the development of HCA is shown in Fig. 2.

Most HBL in humans originate during the embryogenesis of the liver from hepatocyte-precursor cells *(146,147)*, and some are present at birth *(7,8)*. The early preneoplastic stages of HBL are not known. Although HBL may be massive in size when first discovered clinically, the adjacent non-neoplastic liver tissue is usually normal by routine histological examination *(7)*. Appropriate studies to detect FAH in livers containing HBL have not appeared in the literature. HBL contain epithelial cells that resemble hepatocytes more (fetal HBL) or less (embryonal HBL), and they often contain elements with aberrant epithelial differentiations (squamous), as well as mesenchymal-like differentiations, including cartilaginous and osteoid-like *(7,8)*, neuroendocrine *(148)*, melanocytic *(149)*, and other differentiations *(150)*. The cellular elements of HBL that express mesenchymal differentiations appear also to arise from epithelial precursors *(151)*. In common with HBL, HCC may also rarely express various mesenchymal differentiations *(152,153)*, and HBL can arise from HCC in adults *(11)*. Most HBL include a mixture of different epithelial differentiations, and the better-differentiated fetal components of HBL may resemble HCA morphologically *(154)*, although fetal HBL do not have an entirely benign course *(9)*. The outcome of HBL depends on the size and differentiation of the tumor. Fetal HBL have a better

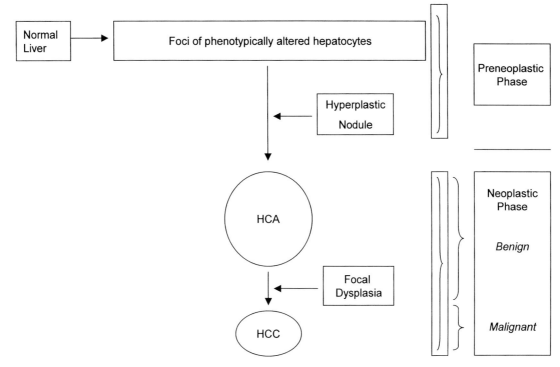

Fig. 2. Possible sequence of cellular changes during development of hepatocellular adenoma and conversion to hepatocellular carcinoma.

outcome than do embryonal, and the embryonal component may determine the success of therapy *(9,155)*.

As with HCC, extensive changes in matrix and blood vessels characterize HBL, less marked in fetal HBL and more marked in embryonal HBL *(156,157)*. In general, the matrix alterations in HBL resemble those found in HCC *(156)*. HBL show elevated rates of cell proliferation. The PCNA labeling index was $30.1 \pm 10.0\%$ in 4 HBL in one study *(10)*. Cell proliferation was highest in cells with embryonal differentiation *(158)*, and high rates of cell proliferation correlated with poor prognosis *(155)*.

ABERRANT REGULATION OF CELL PROLIFERATION IN HEPATOCARCINOGENESIS

As described earlier, HCC develops in a tissue setting in which hepatocytes proliferate continuously at levels much greater than in the nondiseased liver. The proliferative hepatic microenvironment in which HCC develops is characterized by the elevated expression (or re-expression) of several mitogenic and comitogenic growth factors/receptors, and of inflammatory cytokines and hormones/receptors, which may also function as mitogens or comitogens for hepatocytes.

MITOGENIC GROWTH FACTORS AND GROWTH FACTOR RECEPTORS

Transforming Growth Factor-α Transforming growth factor-α (TGF-α) was expressed by hepatocytes in chronic hepatitis (12/20, 60%) and cirrhosis (22/22, 100%), but not in hepatocytes in nondiseased liver (0/12) *(159)*. In nondiseased liver, TGF-α was expressed mainly by epithelial cells of bile ducts, but weakly or not at all by hepatocytes (160–164). Proliferated bile ducts and oval and transitional cells also expressed

TGF-α *(165)*. As compared to normal liver, the relative expression of *TGF-α* mRNA in chronic hepatitis (n = 6) was 4.5 ± 3.0-fold higher, and in cirrhosis (n = 3) it was 6.0 ± 3.5-fold higher *(166)*. The level of TGF-α expression was highly correlated with the fraction of PCNA-labeled hepatocytes in both of the studies of Masuhara et al. *(166)* and Harada et al. *(167)*, although Yamaguchi et al. *(168)* failed to detect such a correlation. TGF-α was most intensely expressed by dysplastic hepatocytes infected with HBV *(160,162,163,165,169)* or HCV *(170)*. Supporting this impression, transfection of cultured liver cells with HBV genomic DNA upregulated *TGF-α* expression *(171)*, and the pre-S1 gene of HBV transactivated the *TGF-α* gene in cultured human cells *(172)*. IFN treatment of patients with chronic HBV hepatitis was associated with reduced expression of TGF-α *(173)*.

TGF-α was detected by immunohistochemistry in tissue sections of 238/354 HCC (67%) accumulated from several individual studies that used various anti-TGF-α antibodies *(160–164, 169,174–176)*. As compared to adjacent nontumorous (but chronically inflamed) tissues, TGF-α was overexpressed in 53/86 HCC (62%), expressed at about the same intensity in 18/86 (21%), and expressed at a lower intensity in 15/86 (17%) *(175)*. About the same fraction of well-differentiated (48/63, 76%), moderately differentiated (34/46, 74%), and poorly differentiated (7/11, 64%) HCC expressed TGF-α *(160,162,163,169)*, but the intensity of expression *(160,169)* and the fraction of tumor cells that strongly expressed TGF-α *(163,164)* were highest in the better-differentiated tumors. In HCC composed of juxtaposed well-differentiated and poorly differentiated components, the former expressed TGF-α more strongly *(169)*. The molecular mechanism(s) by which TGF-α expression is upregulated in inflamed liver and HCC is not known, but may in part reflect the transactivating properties of HBV and HCV proteins.

Serum levels of TGF-α were elevated in 80 patients with HCC and cirrhosis (45 ± 40 pg/mL), as compared to 182 healthy patients with presumably normal livers (21 ± 15 pg/mL) or to 44 patients with cirrhosis alone (25 ± 19 pg/mL) (177). In another study, the TGF-a serum level was 5.6 ± 2.1 pg/mL in 53 control subjects without liver disease, 33 ± 8 pg/mL in 35 patients with chronic hepatitis, 404 ± 173 pg/mL in 33 patients with cirrhosis (without HCC), and 100 ± 39 pg/mL in 55 patients with HCC (167). In cirrhotic patients, serum TGF-α was positively correlated with the severity of disease as indicated by Child's classification (167). Increased amounts of TGF-α were excreted in the urine of patients with HCC (33 patients with normal liver, 4.9 ± 2.8 μg/g creatinine; 31 patients with HCC, 21.5 ± 20.3 μg/g creatinine) (178).

Epidermal Growth Factor Epidermal growth factor (EGF) was also identified in HCC (14/56, 25%) in one study (179), but expression did not correlate with any of the diagnostic or prognostic characteristics of the tumors. Furthermore, urinary excretion of EGF was not elevated in patients with HCC (178). However, gel filtration and radioreceptor assay in the urine of HCC patients detected several EGF-related growth factors of low molecular weight (180). These low molecular weight EGF-related growth factors were not identified, and they may represent breakdown products of TGF-α/EGF (180).

Epidermal Growth Factor Receptor The epidermal growth-factor receptor (EGFR), the cognate receptor for TGF-a and EGF was detected by immunohistochemistry at approximately similar intensities in both HCC and adjacent nontumorous liver tissue (175,176). EGFR mRNA expression was increased in chronic hepatitis, cirrhosis, and HCC, in correlation with increased cell proliferation as indicated by expression of PCNA (167). Quantification of EGFR confirmed that it was highly expressed both in normal liver (11.4 ± 9.2 fmol/mg protein, n = 18) and in HCC (8.9 ± 14.6 fmol/mg protein, n = 25) (181), and the EGFR gene was hypomethylated in some HCC (182). TGF-α and EGFR were co-expressed in individual cells of HCC (174), providing an autocrine pathway for self-sustaining cellular-growth stimulation.

ErbB2/HER2 The EGFR-related receptor, ErbB2/HER2, which has no recognized ligand and forms heterodimers with EGFR, HER3, and HER4, was variably detected by immunohistochemistry in HCC. In three studies, 4/35 HCC (11%) expressed ErbB2 focally on membranes of tumor cells (183–185), and it was also detected focally on hepatocytes in 2/15 cirrhotic livers (13%) (184). However, Tang et al. (176) detected ErbB2 protein in 60/75 (80%) of HCC. Furthermore, Heinze et al. (186) found elevated levels of ErbB2 protein in the cytosolic fractions of many HCC by monoclonal enzyme-linked immunosorbent assay (ELISA) assay. Levels of ErbB2 protein in 31 HCC ranged from 0.02–4.5 U/mg protein, with a median level of 0.43 U/mg protein; significantly fewer patients (10%) with ErbB2 tumor levels greater than 0.43 U/mg protein survived for 2 yr than did those with lower ErbB2 tumor levels (22%) (186). In keeping with these latter observations, the serum concentration of ErbB2 peptide was elevated significantly

in 22 patients with HCC (1244 ± 578 U/mL), as compared to 23 normal control subjects (911 ± 389 U/mL); 12/22 HCC patients (52%) had serum levels greater than one standard deviation (SD) above the mean level found in control subjects (187). ErbB2 peptide was also elevated in the sera of 12 patients with cirrhosis, but without HCC (1498 ± 701 U/mL) (187).

ErbB2 protein was not found by immunohistochemistry on tumor cells in any of 10 HBL (184,185).

Insulin-like Growth Factor-2 Normal liver tissue contained insulin-like growth factor-2 (IGF-2) at the concentration of 41.3 ± 18.7 ng/g (n = 6), cirrhotic liver not the site of HCC contained 133.2 ± 52 ng/g (n = 10), and HCC contained 369.2 ± 373.5 μg/gm (n = 10) (188). Less sensitive immunohistochemical detection of IGF-2 protein in liver tissues by several investigators generally reflected these observations. Positive immunohistochemical reaction for IGF-2 was found in none of 29 normal livers (189), in none of 10 livers the site of acute hepatitis (189), in 58/109 livers (53%) the site of chronic hepatitis (169,189), in 172/237 (73%) cirrhotic livers (169,189,190), and in 182/231 HCC (79%) (169,189–192). Immunohistochemical staining of IGF-2 in hepatocytes was usually spotty and weak in cirrhotic livers and more intense in HCC, supporting the quantitative data that this growth factor was more highly overexpressed in the latter. In situ and Northern-blot hybridization and RNase protection assay of IGF-2 mRNA generally corroborated the immunohistochemical analyses (170,188,190, 193–198). IGF-2 protein and the proliferation marker Ki-67 were co-localized predominantly in the same cells in 10 HCC, suggesting that IGF-2 expression correlated closely with tumor-cell proliferation (199).

Despite production of IGF-2 by HCC, the serum levels of this growth factor were not elevated in patients with this tumor; the serum concentration of IGF-2 was 738 ± 189 μg/L in 23 patients without HCC and 475 ± 205 μg/L in 32 patients with HCC (200). In another study, the normal range for serum IGF-2 was described as 1073–1216 ng/mL, whereas the serum concentration of IGF-2 among 7 patients with HCC was 532 ± 373 ng/mL (188).

During embryonic and fetal development, the IGF-2 gene is expressed monoallelically (201) from the P2, P3, and P4 promoters of the paternal allele only (202), with about 70% of the transcripts in hepatocytes resulting from P3 activity (203). The H19 gene, which is imprinted to the maternal allele, is coordinately expressed with IGF-2 (204). The IGF-2 gene P1 promoter is activated postnatally in the liver and gradually becomes dominant in association with loss of imprinting and acquisition of biallelic transcription from both paternal and maternal alleles (202), in coordination with downregulation of the H19 gene (204). The P1 promoter is responsible for over 50% of the IGF-2 transcripts in the nondiseased adult liver, and for biallelic transcription (203). Activity of the P1 promoter was silenced in many HCC, being weakly expressed or undetectable in 49/53 HCC (93%) in three studies (191,198,205), while the P3 promoter was upregulated in many (19/37) of these tumors (51%). The H19 gene was re-expressed from the maternal allele in parallel with monoallelic re-expression of IGF-2 from the P3 promoter (206,207), and H19 expression has been suggested to be a tumor marker for HCC (206).

Allelic heterozygosity was retained at the *IGF-2* locus in 38/39 informative HCC (97%), but 24/39 demonstrated marked allelic imbalance or monoallelic transcription, and in all 31 the activity of the P1 promoter was lost *(198,208)*. Although *IGF-2* expression was determined to be biallelic in 3/3 informative HCC in another study, promoter usage in these tumors was not ascertained *(209)*. Many HCC showed variable allelic imbalance in *IGF-2* gene transcription, with unequal transcription from each allele *(208,210)*. Among 34 informative HCC allelic imbalance was extreme, approaching monoallelic transcription in all tumors *(208,210)*, but in another study only 7/18 informative HCC (39%) demonstrated marked allelic imbalance *(211)*. Takeda et al. *(210)* found that the paternal allele was active in monoallelic transcription in 4/4 HCC, and Uchida et al. *(211)* found that *IGF-2* transcription was imprinted to the paternal allele in 3/3 HCC even in the face of retention of P1 promoter activity.

Allelic imbalance of the *IGF-2* locus was also found in livers that were the sites of chronic hepatitis and cirrhosis; 13/19 cases of chronic hepatitis (68%) and 4/5 cases of cirrhosis (80%) showed mild to marked allelic imbalance at the *IGF-2* gene in the absence of HCC *(210)*. Furthermore, Aihara et al. *(208)* demonstrated *IGF-2* allelic imbalance in 3/7 dysplastic nodules (43%). The fetal status of monoallelic transcription was clearly re-established during the formation of HCC, because HCC typically developed in adult livers in which *IGF-2* mRNA is expressed from both alleles. Because increased expression was associated with monoallelic transcription, loss of imprinting (LOI) of the *IGF-2* locus is not involved in the increased expression if *IGF-2* in HCC in contrast to some other tumors *(212)*. Complex alterations in promoter usage and the correlated allelic transcriptional imbalance appear to be associated with the increased expression of *IGF-2* that characterizes HCC and the hyperplastic hepatocellular lesions that precede HCC.

Infantile HBL also overexpressed *IGF-2 (213,214)*. The P1 promoter was downregulated in each of three informative HBL, and the P2 and P3 promoters were upregulated *(214)*, as in HCC. Upregulation of the P3 promoter was associated with its demethylation in 6/7 HBL, but the methylation of the downregulated P1 promoter was not altered *(215)*. Inactivation of the *H19* gene has been associated with aberrant promoter usage and expression of the *IGF-2* gene in HBL *(214–216)*. Fukuzawa et al. *(216)* found that the *H19* gene was inactivated by loss of the maternal allele or by hypermethylation in 7/8 (88%) sporadic HBL. This observation suggests that the *H19* gene may function as a regulator of the *IGF-2* gene. However, among 16 informative HBL, monoallelic transcription of the *IGF-2* gene (imprinting) was retained in 12 (75%) *(214,216–218)*. Thus, increased *IGF-2* expression in HBL, as in HCC, does not appear to be a result from acquired biallelic expression (i.e., LOI).

Insulin-Like Growth Factor-1 Receptor and Insulin Receptor IGF-2 sends metabolic and mitogenic signals through the insulin-like growth factor-1 receptor (IGF-1R) and the insulin receptor (IR). These receptors are expressed ubiquitously on normal cells, but no studies have been found that document their levels of expression in HCC or HBL. Likewise, little is known about IGF binding proteins (IGFBP), which can

modulate the activity of IGF-2, although Kondoh et al. *(219)* found that the IGFBP-1 gene was upregulated in 4/5 HCC. In agreement with this observation, Donaghy et al. *(220)* detected significant upregulation of IGFBP-1 expression in 35 patients with chronic hepatitis and cirrhosis, while expression of IGFBP-3 was significantly downregulated.

Mannose 6-Phosphate/IGFII Receptor The mannose 6-phosphate/IGF-2 receptor (M6P/IGF-2R), sometimes called IGF-2R, contains a binding site for IGF-2. However, binding of IGF-2 to M6P/IGF-2R does not elicit signal transduction, but instead shuttles the growth factor to lysosomes, where it is destroyed. Thus, M6P/IGF-2R competes with IGF-1R and IR for available IGF-2. Expression of mRNA for *M6P/IGF-2R* was markedly reduced in 7/11 HCC (64%), and reduced expression correlated with diminished immunohistochemical staining of receptor protein on neoplastic hepatocytes *(221)*. LOH of the *M6P/IGF-2R* locus on chromosome 6q26-q27 was found in 57/100 HCC (57%) *(222–226)*, in 2/3 benign HCA (66%) *(221)*, and in 5/8 hepatocellular dysplasias (63%) *(224)*. The remaining allele was mutated in 11/57 HCC with LOH (19%) *(224–227)*. Cirrhotic nodules adjacent to HCC that showed LOH of the *M6P/IGF-2R* gene had lost the same allele as the HCC in 9/10 instances studied (90%) *(224)*, suggesting that these HCC developed as clonal outgrowths of cirrhotic nodules in which LOH of *M6P/IGF-2R* had initially occurred. Cirrhotic nodules adjacent to HCC lacking LOH of *M6P/IGF-2R* also retained both alleles in three instances examined *(224)*. Homozygous deletion of the *M6P/IGF-2R* was reported in 5/34 (15%) HCC *(223)*. It is not clear why the studies by DeSouza et al. *(222,223)*, Yamada et al. *(224)*, and Oka et al. *(226)* found LOH in 56/78 (72%) HCC and mutations in 11/35 (31%) HCC, while Wada et al. *(225)* detected only one LOH of the *M6P/IGF-2R* gene in 22 informative HCC (5%), and no mutations of exons 27, 28, and 31 of the gene in 27 HCC.

Insulin-Like Growth Factor-1 The liver is the major source of insulin-like growth factor-1 (IGF-1) in adults, but this growth factor appears to play no role in HCC. Transcription of the *IGF-1* gene was downregulated in 7/7 HCC *(195)*, and the serum level was sharply reduced in 32 HCC patients (26.9 ± 32.6 µg/L) as compared to 23 control subjects (277.1 ± 101.7 µg/L) (200). Serum *IGF-I* was also reduced in 35 patients with chronic hepatitis and cirrhosis (mean level 81 ng/mL, range 38–155 ng/mL) as compared to 10 healthy controls (mean level 193 ng/mL, range 151–235 ng/mL). IGF-1 synthesis may be inhibited in HCC patients by the relatively high serum levels of IGF-2, which may inhibit growth-hormone (GH) secretion from the pituitary *(200)*. An alternate reason for sharply decreased IGF-2 production in HCC and cirrhosis may be the paucity of growth-hormone receptors (GHR) on hepatocytes of HCC and cirrhotic liver *(195)*. Chang et al. (228) failed to detect GHR on HCC, although the number of cases studied was small. Absence of GHR would block the ability of GH to stimulate transcription of the *IGF-1* gene by affected liver cells.

Hepatocyte Growth Factor Hepatocyte growth factor (HGF) is expressed in normal livers by sinusoidal and mesenchymal cells and biliary epithelial cells, but not by hepatocytes *(229,230)*. In contrast, HGF protein was found by immunohistochemistry in neoplastic hepatocytes of 136/214 HCC (64%)

accumulated from several individual studies *(175,229–233)*, as well as in neoplastic hepatocytes of 2/2 benign HCA, and in non-neoplastic hepatocytes of 88/109 adjacent nontumorous tissues *(174,228)*. Okano et al. *(230)* found that hepatocytes in 4/7 cases of acute hepatitis (57%), 12/20 cases of chronic hepatitis (60%), and 6/9 cases of cirrhosis (67%) stained intensively for HGF, in contrast to none of 26 HCC. Neoplastic cells in HCC stained more intensely for HGF than did adjacent nontumorous hepatocytes in 20% of cases, about the same in 48%, and less in 32% *(175)*. However, immunohistochemical localization of HGF in normal and neoplastic hepatocytes was thought to reflect receptor-mediated uptake and not synthesis *(175)*. Furthermore, localization of HGF in neoplastic hepatocytes did not correlate with the rates of cell proliferation *(232)* or with patient survival *(233)*. Additionally, some investigators have either not detected *HGF* mRNA in HCC *(234)* or have found it to be present at about one-third the level in nonneoplastic liver *(235)*. However, *HGF* mRNA was detected in hepatocytes in acute and chronic hepatitis and cirrhosis *(166,234)*, and in HCC *(236)*, and Ho et al. *(236)* found that *HGF* and *IL-6* mRNAs were expressed simultaneously in 11/13 (85%) HCC and in the adjacent cirrhotic livers. Serum levels of HGF were elevated in 39 patients with HCC (1.06 ± 1.05 ng/mL) and in 27 patients with cirrhosis (1.05 ± 0.64 ng/mL), as compared to 200 subjects with normal livers (0.27 ± 0.08 ng/mL), 9 patients with acute hepatitis (0.45 ± 0.23 ng/ml), and 40 patients with chronic hepatitis (0.40 ± 0.16 ng/mL); however, the highest serum levels were found in 6 patients with fulminant hepatic failure (16.4 ± 14.7 ng/mL) *(237)*. In contrast, Okano et al. *(230)* did not detect any differences in the mean levels of serum HGF among patients with acute or chronic hepatitis, cirrhosis, and HCC. Elevated levels of HGF in the sera of patients with cirrhosis and HCC may reflect release from the remodeling hepatic matrix.

Von Schweinitz et al. *(238)* detected HGF in mesenchymal components of HBL, but not in epithelial cells of the tumors. Serum levels of HGF were greater than 1000 pg/mL in 10/23 HBL patients as compared to less than 610 pg/mL in 3 healthy children; serum HGF values in untreated children with HBL ranged from 169–10,183 pg/mL (mean 889 pg/mL), and increased from 608–15,000 pg/mL (mean 4,556 pg/mL) within 72 h after hepatic resection. Because HBL tumor cells expressed the HGF receptor, c-met, Von Schweinitz et al. *(238,239)* suggested that the elevated level of serum HGF present in many patients both before and after treatment could stimulate the growth of the tumor and of any residual tumor cells remaining after treatment. The level of serum HGF increased after HBL resection by partial hepatectomy and sometimes following chemotherapy alone, and increased serum HGF was associated with rapid recurrence and growth of the tumor *(239)*.

HGF Receptor (c-met) Both c-met and a related receptor c-ron (a receptor for HGF-like protein) are expressed by normal hepatocytes and these receptors continue to be expressed by neoplastic cells in HCC *(240)*. Expression of both HGF and c-met on neoplastic hepatocytes could allow increased mitogenic stimulation of c-met to occur if availability of HGF is sufficient. Using immunohistochemistry, c-met expression was detected on neoplastic hepatocytes in 235/281 HCC (84%) summated from several individual studies *(175,229,230,232,*

233,240–245), and *c-met* mRNA was considered to be overexpressed in 137/244 HCC (56%) *(175,230,232,240,243–245)*. Quantification of *c-met* mRNA confirmed overexpression in 11 HCC (0.41 ± 0.20 pg/mg total mRNA) as compared to 4 normal livers (0.20 ± 0.15 pg/mg total mRNA) *(234)*. Elevated c-met expression correlated with increased cell proliferation *(232,245)* and poor survival of patients with HCC *(233)*. Expression of c-met also correlated with poor differentiation of HCC in two studies *(244,243)*, but not in three others *(232,233,243)*. Using cultured HCC tumor cells, Chen et al. *(240)* showed that expression of c-met was upregulated by HGF, EGF, and the inflammatory cytokines TNF-α, IL-1, and IL-6.

Somatic mutations in the kinase domain (exons 15–19) of the *c-met* gene were found in 3/10 (30%) HCC occurring in children younger than 15 yr, but the *c-met* gene was not mutated in any of 26 HBL in children or in any of 16 HCC occurring in adults *(246)*. Tumor epithelial cells in HBL expressed c-met by immunohistochemistry *(238)*.

CO-MITOGENIC GROWTH FACTORS AND GROWTH-FACTOR RECEPTORS

Adrenergic Receptors The density of α1 adrenergic receptors (α1AdR) was decreased in 22 HCC (39.9 fmol/mg protein) and increased in the 22 adjacent nontumor liver tissues (139.9 ± 66.3 fmol/mg protein), as compared to 24 normal liver tissues (61.9 ± 19.7 fmol/mg protein); dissociation constants for binding of prazosin to α1AdR did not differ significantly among these tissues (269.3 ± 178.6 pM in HCC; 336.4 ± 168.3 pM in adjacent nontumorous tissues; 210.1 ± 31.4 pM in normal liver tissues) *(247)*. The density of α1AdR on tumor cells was reduced in 19/22 HCC (86%) and unchanged in three. The density of β2 adrenergic receptors (β2AdR) was significantly increased in 22 HCC (197.1 ± 122.5 fmol/mg protein), as compared to either 22 nontumorous adjacent liver tissues (98.4 ± 39.2 fmol/mg protein) or to 24 normal livers (89.7 ± 17.9 fmol/mg protein); receptor dissociation constants for binding of pindolol did not differ significantly among these groups (168.5 ± 81.9 pM in HCC; 153.6 ± 58.2 pM in adjacent nontumorous liver tissue; 112.5 ± 32.1 pM in normal liver) *(247)*. The density of β2AdR was increased on 19/22 HCC (86%) and unchanged on three. In keeping with the greater receptor density, adenyl cyclase activity (measured by cAMP production) was stimulated by isoproterenol to a significantly greater extent in HCC tissues (66.6 ± 34.7 pmol/min/mg protein) than in either normal liver (29.6 ± 7.0 pmol/min/mg protein) or nontumorous adjacent tissue (32.4 ± 13.6 pmol/min/mg protein *(247)*.

Fibroblast Growth Factors Acidic fibroblast growth factor (aFGF) was detected in 18/56 HCC (32%), basic fibroblast growth factor (bFGF) in 15/56 HCC (27%), and both aFGF and bFGF were detected concurrently by immunohistochemistry in 11/56 HCC (20%) *(179,248)*. In nondiseased and cirrhotic livers, FGF was present only in vascular endothelial cells and macrophages *(179)*. In HCC, FGF was expressed focally by neoplastic hepatocytes and increased expression correlated with the extent of tumor vascularity *(179)*. Transcripts of the *bFGF* gene were detected in 20/46 HCC (42%) in three studies *(249–251)*. FGF receptors have not received detailed study in HCC. However, in a parallel hybridization analysis of multiple protein kinase genes, Tsou et al. *(252)* detected overexpression of *FGFR-4* in HCC and in cultured HCC cell lines as compared to undiseased liver.

VASCULAR GROWTH FACTORS AND GROWTH FACTOR RECEPTORS Each of the growth factors and most of the hormones that are mitogenic and antimitogenic for hepatocytes also stimulate angiogenesis, as do a number of other growth factors and hormones that affect the liver (for list see *253*). Vascular endothelial growth factor (VEGF) is also mitogenic for hepatocytes.

Vascular Endothelial Growth Factor Overexpression of vascular endothelial growth factor (VEGF) transcripts (12/20 HCC, 60%) concurred with overexpression of bFGF transcripts (9/20 HCC, 45%) and correlated with tumor hypervascularity *(254)*. VEGF was detected immunohistochemically in neoplastic hepatocytes of 131/183 HCC (72%) accumulated from several individual studies, the extent of staining ranging from weak to strong *(139,254–257)*, and by Northern-blot analysis in protein extracted from 21/28 HCC (75%) *(258)*. Strong expression of VEGF was detected immunohistochemically in neoplastic hepatocytes in 49/101 HCC (49%) *(255,256)*; in contrast, VEGF was detected immunohistochemically in both hepatocytes and mesenchymal cells of cirrhotic livers *(139)*, but only in the mesenchymal tissue of portal tracts in 6 normal livers, and not in hepatocytes *(254)*. VEGF mRNA transcripts were detected by RT-PCR in 102/139 HCC (73%) *(139,251,259–261)*, and in 20/74 adjacent nontumorous liver tissues (27%) *(259,261)*. Three *VEGF* isoforms found in normal tissues, $VEGF_{121}$, $VEGF_{165}$, and $VEGF_{189}$, were also produced in HCC *(255,259)*, but $VEGF_{206}$ was not *(255)*, although all four isoforms were expressed in HCC cell lines *(256)*.

The relationship of *VEGF* expression to HCC size and differentiation, and tumor vascularity is uncertain. In fact, Shimoda et al. *(261)* failed to detect a significant difference in the expression of transcripts (by RT-PCR) for $VEGF_{165}$ and $VEGF_{189}$ among 8 control livers, 18 instances of chronic hepatitis (HCV-related), and 10 HCC (as well as adjacent nontumorous tissue). VEGF expression was strongest in areas of HCC that contained Bcl2-positive tumor cells *(257)*. In relation to HCC differentiation, strong expression of VEGF was detected immunohistochemically in tumor cells in none of 12 well-differentiated HCC less than 1 cm diameter, while 3/14 well-differentiated HCC larger than 1 cm (21%), 11/12 moderately differentiated HCC (92%), and 11/13 poorly differentiated HCC (85%) expressed this growth factor *(255)*. However, in another study *(256)*, strong expression of VEGF was reported in 7/10 well-differentiated HCC (70%), compared to 13/26 moderately differentiated HCC (50%) and 4/14 poorly differentiated HCC (29%). In this same study, 6/9 tumors less than 1.5 cm in diameter (67%) strongly expressed VEGF, as compared to 12/22 HCC (55%) between 1.5 and 3 cm, and 6/19 HCC (32%) larger than 3 cm *(256)*. In yet another study in which *VEGF* gene transcripts were detected by RT-PCR in 16/23 HCC (70%) and in 9/23 adjacent nontumorous liver tissues (39%), no correlation was found between VEGF expression and either tumor vascularity *(259)*, or size *(259,260)*. All of the HCC in the study of Suzuki et al. *(259)* were greater than 1.5 cm in size and all but one was already hypervascular. However, El-

Assal et al. *(139)* also found that neither *VEGF* mRNA nor protein expression were correlated with microvascular density or histopathologic features of 71 HCC. Li et al. *(260)* and Zhou et al. *(258)* detected higher expression of *VEGF* in HCC associated with tumor thrombi in portal veins than in HCC without portal-vein invasion. One must conclude that despite numerous studies, the exact role of VEGF in hepatocarcinogenesis is not clear.

Platelet-Derived Endothelial-Cell Growth Factors Jinno et al. *(262)* found that the plasma level of platelet-derived endothelial-cell growth factors (PDECGF) (measured by ELISA) was significantly elevated in 34 patients with HCC (6.0 ± 2.5 U/mL) as compared to 40 patients with cirrhosis (4.6 ± 1.1 U/mL), 26 patients with chronic hepatitis (4.3 ± 0.6 U/mL), and 17 healthy individuals (4.2 ± 0.5 U/mL). The cytoplasm of the majority of tumor cells was diffusely stained for PDECGF by immunohistochemistry, whereas only a few hepatocytes in nondiseased livers stained weakly. Zhou et al. *(258)* detected PDECGF by Northern-blot analysis and 19/28 HCC (68%), as compared to 10/28 adjacent nontumorous tissues (36%). Expression of PDECGF was positively correlated with expression of VEGF, and expression was higher in HCC with portal-vein tumor thrombi than in those without.

INFLAMMATORY CYTOKINES The inflammatory cells that infiltrate the liver in chronic hepatitis and cirrhosis are a rich source of cytokines, and the expression of certain inflammatory cytokines/receptors is also induced in hepatocytes, endothelial cells, and macrophages (Kupffer cells) of the liver *(20)*. In addition to their activities in mediating inflammation, immune responses, and apoptotic cell death, some inflammatory cytokines are also essential participants in the regulation of hepatocyte proliferation (especially TNF-α and IL-6) *(263)*. It seems likely that these highly active cell-modulating molecules, which are so plentiful in livers in which HCC develop, are directly involved in the development of HCC, but this possibility has not yet been examined.

ANTIMITOGENIC GROWTH FACTORS AND GROWTH-FACTOR RECEPTORS

Transforming Growth Factor-β1 Transforming growth factor-β1 (TGFβ1) is expressed predominantly by mesenchymal cells in portal tracts and along sinusoids in normal livers, but only weakly or not at all by hepatocytes *(264–266)*. Likewise, in chronic hepatitis and cirrhosis TGFβ1 was immunolocalized predominantly to mesenchymal cells in areas of inflammation and fibrosis and not to hepatocytes *(264,265,267)*. *TGFβ1* mRNA was increased in livers with chronic hepatitis and cirrhosis by 2-fold to 14-fold *(159,165,268)*, and the level of expression correlated with the level of *proα1(1)-collagen* mRNA *(268)* or with serum procollagen peptide III *(159)*. Using a highly sensitive competitive RT-PCR technique, Roulot et al. *(269)* found that *TGFβ1* mRNA was increased over 200-fold in 35 livers the site of chronic hepatitis, as compared to 6 livers that lacked inflammation or fibrosis. However, they found no association between the elevated expression of *TGFβ1* transcripts and either the serum concentration of the amino-terminal peptide of collagen III or the histological indices of liver fibrosis. Elevated expression of TGFβ1 was associated with expression of apoptotic markers in cirrhotic livers *(270)*.

TGFβ1 mRNA was highly overexpressed in 34 HCC *(271–273)*, and the growth factor was localized to neoplastic hepatocytes in many HCC by immunohistochemistry *(266,272)*. TGFβ1 protein expression in HCC was inversely correlated with the PCNA index *(174)*, suggesting that the growth factor maintained a degree of negative control over tumor-cell proliferation. *TGFβ2* and *TGFβ3* mRNAs were also increased to an extent similar to that for *TGFβ1* mRNA *(273)*. The level of *TGFβ1* mRNA and protein were correlated in 6 HCC *(272)*. The plasma level of TGFβ1 was greatly elevated in 26 patients with HCC (19.3 ± 19.5 ng/mL), as compared to 20 subjects with normal livers (1.4 ± 0.8 ng/mL) *(274,275)*, to 12 patients with chronic hepatitis (3.0 ± 3.1 ng/mL), and to 11 patients with cirrhosis (3.7 ± 2.1 ng/mL) *(275)*. Among 17 patients with HCC, the plasma concentration of TGFβ1 correlated positively with tumor vascularity as assessed by angiography *(276)*. Resection or embolization of HCC was followed by a decrease in the serum level of TGFβ1 *(274,275)*. Urinary excretion of TGFβ1 was also increased in 140 patients with HCC (64.1 ± 47.3 µg/g creatinine), as compared to 50 patients with cirrhosis (28.9 ± 10.0 µg/g creatinine), 30 patients with chronic hepatitis (15.5 ± 3.64 mg/g creatinine), and 50 subjects with normal livers (14.9 ± 10.5 mg/g creatinine) *(277)*. Urinary excretion of TGFβ1 decreased after resection or embolization of HCC *(277)*.

TGFβ Receptors TGFβ inhibits the proliferation of hepatocytes and affects other cellular processes by binding to heterodimeric complexes of TGFβ1 receptors I and II (TGFβRI and TGFβRII), which are expressed by normal hepatocytes *(175,221,265)*. TGFβRII was not expressed by neoplastic hepatocytes in 18/25 HCC (72%), and expression was reduced in the other 7, as indicated by detection of both mRNA and protein *(265)*. Likewise, the level of *TGFβRI* mRNA was reduced by an average of 40% in 10/11 HCC, and receptor protein was reduced by 33%; in these same tumors *TGFβRII* mRNA was reduced by an average of 51% in 8/11 HCC and receptor protein was reduced by 30% *(220)*. However, Kiss et al. *(175)* and Abou-Shady et al. *(273)* detected TGFβRII by immunohistochemistry in each of 104 HCC, and the receptor was decreased as compared to adjacent nontumorous liver in only 25/104 HCC (24%). The mechanisms by which TGFβ1 receptors are downregulated or inactivated in some HCC are not known. Searches for mutations in microsatellite sequences of the TGFβ1RII gene A$_{10}$ tract located in exon 3 and the poly-GT tract located in exon 7 found none in 10 HCC examined by Vincent et al. *(278)*, none in 30 HCC evaluated by Kawate et al. *(279)*, and none in 46 HCC studied by Salvucci et al. *(280)*. However, Furuta et al. *(281)* reported that 32/73 HCC (44%) contained microdeletions in the A$_{10}$ tract (loss of one adenine), converting the microsatellite tract to A$_9$ and producing a frameshift that resulted in a downstream stop codon; no alterations were found in the poly-GT tract. The frequency of microdeletions in the TGFβ1RII gene was correlated with HCC differentiation, occurring in 4/14 (29%) well-differentiated, 10/25 (40%) moderately differentiated, and 18/34 (53%) poorly differentiated HCC *(281)*. An identical microdeletion was found in 3/20 (15%) cirrhotic nodules, suggesting that this mutation may precede the emergence of HCC *(281)*.

The M6P/IGFIIR is involved in the activation of latent TGF-β (as well as in the catabolism of IGF-2). Expression of the M6P/IGF-2R was markedly reduced on 7/11 HCC *(221)*. Inactivation of the M6P/IGF-2R occurred by a combination of LOH (found in 57/100 HCC) *(222–226)* and mutation of the remaining allele (found in 11/57 HCC with LOH, or 19%) *(224–227)*.

HORMONES AND HORMONE RECEPTORS Insulin, GH, thyroid hormone, parathyroid hormone, and the sex-steroids are conventionally considered to be comitogenic for hepatocytes *(263)*. However, all are mitogenic for hepatocytes in vivo under some circumstances, and all may be involved in the development of some HCC through this or other mechanisms.

Insulin and Insulin Receptor In Type II diabetes mellitus, which is characterized by insulin resistance with compensatory hyperinsulinemia, the liver is chronically exposed to elevated levels of insulin, pro-insulin, and to split products of pro-insulin *(282)*. These products can stimulate the proliferation of hepatocytes by binding to and activating IR and IGF-1R. The overexpression of insulin receptor substrate-1 by HCC supports the involvement of insulin and IGF in development of HCC *(283–285)*. Type II diabetes mellitus is associated epidemiologically with increased risk to primary liver cancers, predominantly HCC *(282)*, and with early recurrence of HCC after resection *(286)*. Increased risk to primary liver cancer persists in diabetic patients even when corrected for the strong HCC risk factors of alcoholism, cirrhosis, and hemochromatosis; in fact, patients who were both diabetic and also had one of the other risk factors had a greatly amplified risk as compared to patients without diabetes but who had the other risk factors *(282)*.

Growth Hormone and Growth Hormone Receptor The role of GH and GHR in HCC has not been appropriately examined. No data on GH levels in HCC have been found, but the serum level of GH is significantly increased in patients with chronic hepatitis and cirrhosis, as compared to healthy patients *(220)*. The serum level of IGF-1 through which GH produces many of its metabolic effects was decreased in patients with chronic hepatitis and cirrhosis *(220)*. It was also very low in 32 patients with HCC (26.9 ± 32.6 ug/L) as compared to 23 control subjects (277.1 ± 101.7 ug/L) *(200)*, and the transcription of the *IGF-1* gene was downregulated in 7/7 HCC *(200)*. Repression of IGF-1 production in HCC may result from the lack of expression of GHR by HCC *(195)*, because Chang et al. *(228)* failed to detect the expression of GHR in any of 6 HCC by radioreceptor assay using radiolabeled recombinant GH. In 7 nondiseased livers, the capacity of high-affinity GHR was 20.7 ± 11.5 fmol/mg protein and the affinity constant was 0.66 ± 0.20 nM, and the capacity of low-affinity GHR was 64.7 ± 32.1 fmol/mg with an affinity constant of 8.9 ± 3.3 nM. GHR was not detected on any of the 6 HCC nor on the cells of 5 adjacent cirrhotic livers, although it was expressed by one adjacent liver that was the site of chronic hepatitis *(228)*.

Thyroid Hormone and Thyroid Hormone Receptors Lin et al. *(287)* found that the genes for thyroid hormone nuclear receptors α and β (TRα1 and TRβ1) were truncated in 9/16 HCC (56%). In addition, point mutations were detected in TRα1 in 10/16 HCC (63%) and in TRβ1 in 12/16 HCC (76%), with hot-spots of mutation in amino acid codons 209–228 and 245–

256 in the TRα1 gene *(287)*. The TRβ1 protein was overexpressed in 10 HCC, while the expression of TRα1 varied. Truncation and mutation of the receptors did not alter thyroid-hormone binding, but diminished or abolished binding of the receptors to DNA. Lin et al. *(287,288)* suggested that the mutant thyroid-hormone receptors may have lost the ability to repress hepatocyte proliferation. Overexpression of TRβ1 was associated with increased invasiveness of HCC, and correlated with low expression of the *nm23* gene *(289)*.

Hyperthyroxinemia occurs in many patients with HCC correlated with elevated plasma levels of thyroxine-binding protein, which is produced by the liver *(290–292)*. The thyroxine-binding globulin produced in association with HCC had impaired binding properties for thyroxine, but the elevated plasma levels of thyroxine were not associated with evidence of hyperthyroidism *(293,294)*. When patients with cirrhosis were evaluated repeatedly for HCC and elevated levels of thyroxine-binding globulin, the expression of the aberrant binding protein was strongly correlated with ultimate emergence of HCC *(292)*. Although this relationship suggests a pathogenic role for thyroxine-binding protein in hepatocarcinogenesis, a mechanism is not known.

Arbuthnot et al. *(295)* demonstrated that expression of the c-*erbA* oncogene, which is homologous to TR, was markedly enhanced in 6 HCC and adjacent nontumorous tissue as detected by RNA blot hybridization. The gene was not rearranged.

Sex Steroids The most intense study of the role of hormones in HCC has centered on androgens, estrogens, and their receptors, which appear to be of considerable importance in the development of HCA and HCC in humans. The incidence of HCC is two- to fourfold higher in males, irrespective of the etiologic agents involved, indicating an important male sex-determined developmental susceptibility. Furthermore, abnormal metabolism of sex steroids is a feature of cirrhosis, a liver disease in which most HCC arise, and the benign counterpart of HCC, HCA, occurs most frequently in association with chronic use of exogenous estrogenic or anabolic steroids. Guéchot et al. *(296)* measured the plasma levels of testosterone, dihydrotestosterone, androstenedione, dehydroepiandrosterone, estrone, and estradiol in 15 cirrhotic patients with HCC, 15 cirrhotic patients without HCC, and 10 healthy control patients. As compared to the healthy controls, both groups of male cirrhotic patients had hypogonadism with hyperestrogenemia, associated with decreased plasma levels of testosterone and increased levels of estrone and estradiol. Plasma levels of testosterone, dihydrotestosterone, and dehydroepiandrosterone were diminished further in those cirrhotic patients, who also had HCC, while the levels of androstenedione, estrone, and estradiol did not differ from the levels found in cirrhotic patients without HCC. These results show that the androgen/estrogen ratio is markedly altered at the time HCC develops in cirrhotic patients, and raise the possibility that these alterations may play a determinative role in HCC development.

Yu and Chen *(297)* showed that the risk to the eventual development of HCC in a population of Taiwanese men was correlated with the serum level of testosterone prior to the clinical appearance of HCC. In this study, serum samples were collected from 9691 Taiwanese men, and the initial testoster-

one levels in the 35 individuals who developed HCC during an average follow-up of 4.6 yr were compared with 140 patients who had not developed HCC, matched by age and known HCC risk factors (evidence of HBV and HCV infection, alcohol usage, diet, and previous liver disease). Testosterone levels greater than 5.69 ug/mL were found in the serum gathered 4.6 yr previously from 18/35 patients (51%) who developed HCC during that interval, whereas 48/140 (34%) of the matched controls who did not develop HCC had comparable serum testosterone levels. The relative risk for the development of HCC for men who had testosterone levels in the upper tertile was 4.1 (95% confidence limits 1.3–13.2), and the association of the testosterone level with HCC risk was independent of the other risk factors for HCC (viral infections, ethanol abuse, etc.). The results are compatible with the hypothesis that testosterone has an etiological role in HCC development, perhaps as one of multiple risk factors, and suggests that testosterone may be involved in hepatocarcinogenesis even at physiological levels. These results also suggest that the low serum levels of testosterone that occur generally in male patients with long-standing cirrhosis may mask the importance of testosterone in the early development of HCC in some individuals. Guéchot et al. *(298)* treated 17 patients with HCC with D-tryptophan-6-luetinizing hormone-releasing hormone for up to 6 mo; although serum testosterone levels were sharply reduced, there was no effect on HCC growth in this small number of patients.

The association between the therapeutic use of certain formulations of contraceptive steroids and the risk to development of both HCA and HCC further highlights an important role for steroid hormones in development of HCC *(299)*. Anabolic androgenic steroids also appear to be associated with increased risk to the development of HCA and HCC, although the epidemiologic evidence is less well-substantiated *(300,301)*.

Androgen Receptors The sex steroids act by binding to cognate cytosolic receptors, after which the bound receptors migrate to the nucleus where dimerized receptor/ligand complexes function as transcription factors for genes with the appropriate promoter sequences. Although not found in the first studies by Iqbal et al. *(302)*, androgen receptors (AR) were later detected in protein extracts from the majority of nondiseased livers using binding/displacement assays, with levels of approx 6–35 fmol/mg protein and binding affinities in the vicinity of 2–30 nM *(303–305)*. Eagon et al. *(305)* also detected AR in nuclei isolated from hepatocytes of nondiseased livers. Nakagama et al. *(306)* detected *AR* mRNA by RT-PCR from nondiseased livers, although at a level that was undetectable by Northern-blot hybridization of unfractionated cellular RNA. AR have also been detected in protein extracts from 28/41 cirrhotic livers (68%) *(303,307–309)* and in 4/4 adenomatous hyperplastic nodules *(305)* at similar concentrations and with similar binding affinities as was found in nondiseased livers.

Detection of AR has been reported in 197/306 HCC (64%) at concentrations of 2–400 fmol/mg protein with binding affinities of 0.2–50 nM *(302–304,307–315)*. *AR* mRNA was also detected by RT-PCR in 7/8 HCC *(306)*. The frequency with which HCC expressed AR was reported to be lower in women (7/19, 37%), as compared to men (about 65%) *(310)*. These results showed that in AR-expressing HCC the concentration of AR was higher than in the adjacent nontumorous liver tissues *(303,304),* and Nagasue et al. *(307)* demonstrated that radiolabeled testosterone was actively concentrated by HCC tumor nodules at levels greatly exceeding the surrounding nontumorous liver tissue. A larger fraction of smaller HCC (<3 cm in diameter) (22/29, 77%) expressed AR than did the larger tumors (>3 cm) (6/14, 43%) *(314).* There was no correlation between the levels of AR expressed by HCC and by adjacent nontumorous liver tissue *(307,314).* Expression of AR by HCC was correlated with the probability of recurrence of resected neoplasms. Nagasue et al. *(307)* found the five yr recurrence rate of AR-positive HCC was 68% (21/31) with only 17% surviving for five yr, as compared to a five-yr recurrence rate of 35% (5/14) of AR-negative HCC, with 62% surviving for five yr. These results were supported by Boix et al. *(314)* who found that the probability of recurrence within two yr of resection was 50% for the AR-positive HCC as compared to 20% for the AR-negative tumors.

Estrogen Receptors The nondiseased liver expresses estrogen receptors (ER) at concentrations usually found to range from 2–6 fmol/mg protein with binding affinities of about 2 nM measured by binding/displacement assays *(302,304,316,317),* whereas cirrhotic-liver tissue expressed ER at similar to slightly higher concentrations than nondiseased liver *(303,318).* ER was detected in 98/255 HCC (38%) at levels that generally ranged from 1–15 fmol/mg protein with binding affinities in the range of 1–3 nM. In most instances, ER levels in HCC were not higher than in adjacent nontumorous liver, and there was no correlation between the levels in tumorous and nontumorous livers. ER were also detected immunohistochemically in 5–68% of the nuclei in 6/8 HCC (75%) using a monoclonal antibody (MAb) *(319),* as well as in 5–45% of the nuclei in cirrhotic livers and in 35–53% of the nuclei in 4/4 nondiseased livers. Nagasue et al. *(318)* found that ER-negative HCC were slightly larger than ER-positive tumors, but the ER status was not significantly correlated with long-term survival. A study in which 68 patients with ER-positive or ER-negative HCC were followed for up to five yr after the tumors were surgically resected, showed only a modest difference in survival. The five-yr survival rate for 21 patients with ER-positive HCC was 10% (2/21), whereas that for 47 patients with ER-negative HCC was 23% (11/47) *(320).*

Villa et al. *(321)* used RT-PCR to identify variant *ER* transcripts of 296 base pairs that lacked exon 5 of the hormone-binding domain in 7/7 HCC from male patients, but not in any of 7 HCC from female patients. The HCC in males that contained variant ER lacked wild-type ER and did not bind estradiol, unlike HCC in females, which contained a level of 37 ± 9 fmol/mg of wild-type ER protein, and in adjacent nontumorous liver tissue which contained 15 ± 5 fmol/mg of wild-type ER protein *(321).* Villa et al. *(321)* speculated that the variant *ER* transcripts may have retained constitutive transcriptional activity without requiring occupancy by estrogenic steroids. In a larger series of 40 male and female patients with HCC, Villa et al. *(322)* found that the wild-type *ER* transcript was the only form expressed in HCC in 5/25 men (20%) and in 5/15 women (33%), whereas 9/25 HCC in men (36%) and 3/15 HCC in

women (20%) expressed only the variant *ER* transcript; a mixture of wild-type and variant *ER* transcripts was expressed in all of the remaining HCC, 11/25 men (44%) and 7/15 women (47%). Examination of *ER* transcripts in liver tissue at the site of chronic hepatitis and cirrhosis (the latter with and without dysplasia) by Villa et al. *(322)* disclosed that wild-type transcripts predominated in chronic hepatitis and cirrhosis without dysplasia, although variant *ER* transcripts formed a minor component in 27/39 men (69%) and 9/22 women (41%). Variant transcripts were more strongly expressed in cirrhotic tissues with dysplasia, suggesting that the variant transcripts arose in a few preneoplastic cells, which were amplified by cell proliferation prior to the emergence of HCC *(322).*

Villa et al. *(323)* suggested that the failure of tamoxifen to slow growth of HCC *(324)* might result from the expression of variant ER to which this drug could not bind. They found that the tumor-doubling time of 4 HCC that expressed only variant ER was 42 ± 11 d, as compared to 175 ± 94 d for 4 HCC that expressed only wild-type ER *(323).* Tamoxifen-treatment increased the doubling-time of HCC with wild-type ER to 401 ± 144 d. Negestrol, an antiestrogenic drug whose action is independent of receptor binding, was used to treat the 4 patients with HCC expressing variant ER, and treatment was associated with a prolongation of tumor-doubling time to 344 ± 334 d *(323).* While suggestive, these results require a larger blinded study to be convincing.

A weak interaction between the co-expression of AR and ER in HCC was suggested by the analysis of recurrence rates in 57 patients whose HCC were resected *(312).* The five yr survival of 15 patients whose HCC expressed neither AR nor ER (AR⁻/ER⁻) was 67% (10/15), compared to 50% (2/4) for patients whose HCC were AR⁻/ER⁺; in contrast the five-yr survival was nil both for 25 patients whose HCC were AR⁺/ER⁻ and 13 patients whose HCC were AR⁺/ER⁺. AR positivity appeared to be the major determinant of survivability.

ER were detected in 4/5 HCA at levels somewhat higher than in the surrounding nontumorous liver (10–16 fmol/mg protein) *(317,325,326).* Progesterone receptors (PR) were detected in 2/2 HCA at levels (11–16 fmol/mg protein) slightly higher than that in nontumorous liver *(326).* Only two HBL have been evaluated for expression of ER *(302,327),* and one for expression of PR *(325).* In this study, ER levels were within the range expected in nontumorous liver, whereas the PR level was high at 6.2 fmol/mg protein *(325).* PR have also been detected in 17/22 HCC at low levels (0.8–0.9 fmol/mg protein) *(328).* In contrast, another study found no PR-positive tumors among 26 HCC *(313).* PR were detected immunohistochemically with a MAb in neither 4 nondiseased livers nor in 8 HCC, whereas 9–18% of the nuclei in 4/14 cirrhotic livers (29%) stained positively for PR *(319).*

Taken together, these results suggest that steroid hormones and their receptors, especially androgens and to a lesser extent estrogens, play a positive (stimulating) role in the development of HCC in humans. Although a considerable amount of work has been performed, the overall insight into the role of the sex steroids is still incomplete and more definitive studies are needed.

Retinoic Acid Receptors Three retinoic acid receptor (RAR) genes, α, β, and δ, which belong to the thyroid- and steroid-hormone family of nuclear receptors, have been identified and shown to have tissue-specific patterns of expression; *RARα* and *RARβ* genes are expressed at low levels in the liver *(329,330)*. The *RARβ* gene was initially identified in an HCC near an HBV genomic insertion site (331–334). *RARδ* does not appear to be expressed in the liver *(335)*. Retinoic acid appears to be a general modulator of cell growth and differentiation, and RARβ may have a special role in HCC; De Thé et al. *(332)* found that 6/7 HCC overexpressed the *RARβ* gene, which was not expressed in nondiseased livers. However, Sever and Locker *(336)* failed to confirm the elevated expression of *RARβ* in 4 HCC. Instead, they concluded that the expression of the *RARα* gene was markedly upregulated in HCC (and also in one HCA) but the *RARβ* gene was expressed at the low level found for both genes in nondiseased liver *(336)*. Sever and Locker *(336)* also found that unless modified, the probes frequently used did not distinguish between the two genes, and they speculated that De Thé et al. *(332)* were actually detecting the elevated expression of the *RARα* gene.

Receptors for Intestinal Regulatory Peptides Reubi et al. *(337)* used autoradiography to detect receptor-mediated binding of radiolabeled somatostatin, vasoactive intestinal peptide (VIP), substance P, and cholecystokinin (gastrin) in 59 HCC. Using this evidence, they concluded that somatostatin receptors were expressed in 24/59 HCC (41%), VIP receptors in 28/59 HCC (47%), and substance P receptors in 3/59 HCC (5%), but gastrin receptors were not detected *(337)*. In contrast, Caplin et al. *(338)* detected gastrin receptors by immunohistochemistry on 21/23 HCC (91%), as well as the expression of progastrin and glycine-extended gastrin in tumor cells. The meaning of these observations is not clear, but may reflect partial neuroendocrine differentiation of some HCC.

MITOGENIC AND ANTIMITOGENIC SIGNALING PATHWAYS Binding of mitogenic and comitogenic growth factors to their cognate receptors located on a cell's surface membrane or in its cytosol energizes the passage of mitogenic signals to the cell nucleus. The mitogen-activated protein kinase (MAPK) cascade has been most studied in HCC, but other transduction pathways are also involved. Several molecular species participate in the transfer of a signal from the tyrosine phosphorylated receptors to the nucleus through the MAP kinase pathway, not all of which have been examined in HCC. Studies on the GRB2, SOS, and c-raf molecules have not appeared in the literature. Mitogenic signal pathways other than MAPK cascade, including the JAK/STAT pathway, also have apparently not been examined in HCC. Antimitogenic signaling from TGFβ1 receptors involves the Smad pathway.

Insulin Receptor Substrate-1 Insulin receptor substrate-1 (IRS-1), which transfers phosphorylation signals from the activated IR to GRB2 and SOS, was overexpressed in 5/5 HCC as compared to adjacent nontumorous liver tissue *(283,284)*. *IRS-1* gene expression was increased over two-fold in 9/22 HCC (40%) as compared to adjacent nontumorous liver tissue, and the extent of *IRS-1* expression was significantly related to tumor size *(285)*. In animal models, *IRS-1* overexpression ac-

tivated downstream signaling molecules, including GRB2, SHP2, and the MAPK cascade *(285)*.

Ras Expression of p21 ras protein has been assessed by immunohistochemistry using various antibodies raised to purified or synthetic protein. At high dilutions of antibody, decoration of hepatocytes in most normal livers was found, but with more dilute antibody staining of neoplastic cells was achieved in some HCC and cirrhotic livers while cells in normal livers were not stained, suggesting that the level of p21 ras was higher in these proliferative lesions. Under such conditions, absence of staining of p21 ras was found in 44 normal livers *(339–344)*, while neoplastic cells in 130/265 HCC (49%), accumulated from several individual studies, were stained intensely *(176,339, 341–344)*. Hepatocytes in cirrhotic nodules also reacted positively in 111/167 cirrhotic livers (66%) *(339,341–344)*; hepatocytes were more strongly stained in cirrhotic livers adjacent to HCC (80/92, 87%) than in cirrhotic livers not accompanied by HCC (10/32, 31%), and intense staining of foci of dysplastic hepatocytes (16/16, 100%) and of hepatocytes in adenomatous hyperplastic nodules (17/18, 94%) was noted *(339)*. Additionally, intense staining of hepatocytes in cirrhotic livers (5/5, 100%) and hepatocellular adenomas (4/4, 100%) was observed *(344)*, and hepatocytes infected with HBV were most strongly stained *(339,342)*. However, Lee et al. *(340)* did not find a correlation between HBV infection and p21 ras expression by immunohistochemistry, but they detected p21 ras protein expression in only one of 14 HCC suggesting that they used an insensitive antibody. Staining was most uniform in well-differentiated tumors, whereas it was heterogeneous in moderately differentiated tumors and undetectable in poorly differentiated tumors *(339)*. These observations suggest that p21 ras expression is upregulated in HCC and in the non-neoplastic tissue lesions that precede the development of HCC (chronic hepatitis and cirrhosis), especially in dysplastic and HBV-infected cells.

Studies on the expression of mRNA specifically by c-H-*ras*, c-K-*ras*, and c-N-*ras* genes in HCC and surrounding liver tissue have produced variable results, reflecting the relatively insensitive detection methods that were usually used (Northern hybridization of whole mRNA without the use of polyA selection or PCR amplification). For example, c-K-*ras* mRNA expression was detected in all of 50 livers that were the sites of acute hepatitis, chronic hepatitis, and cirrhosis, but c-H-*ras* mRNA was not detected *(345)*. Zhang et al. *(346)* and Tang et al. *(176)* found that c-H-*ras* mRNA was increased in 13/13 HCC as compared to adjacent nontumorous liver tissue, but expression of c-K-*ras* mRNA was not increased *(346)*. Himeno et al. *(347)* did not detect either c-H-*ras* or c-N-*ras* mRNAs in 26 HCC or in surrounding nontumorous tissue, whereas, Gu et al. *(348)* found that c-N-*ras* mRNA was overexpressed in 6/9 HCC, although c-H-*ras* and c-K-*ras* transcripts were unaffected. Zhang et al. *(349)* found that c-N-*ras* mRNA was overexpressed by up to four-fold in 12 HCC as compared to adjacent nontumorous tissue. The contradictory nature of these results suggests that additional studies are needed to reconcile the potential role of the c-*ras* genes in HCC.

The c-N-*ras* gene was amplified and rearranged in 2/9 HCC *(348)*, and it was also amplified two-fold to five-fold in the nontumorous tissue adjacent to 5/12 HCC *(349)*. Loss of one c-H-*ras* allele was detected in 1/19 HCC and in the surrounding nontumorous tissue *(350)*. Likewise, the c-H-*ras* gene locus was hypermethylated in 1/19 HCC and in the tissue surrounding this tumor *(350)*, but no alteration of the methylation status of the c-K-*ras* gene was noted in any of 3 HCC *(182)*.

In HCC accumulated from several individual studies, only three activating mutations of the c-H-*ras* gene were found in codon 12 in 3/141 HCC (2.1%), none at codon 13 in 24 HCC, and none at codon 61 in 56 HCC *(350–355)*. Activating mutations of the c-K-*ras* gene were detected at codon 12 in only 2/86 HCC (2.3%), at codon 13 in none of 24 HCC, and at codon 61 in 1/50 HCC (2.0%) *(352,353,355–358)*. Activating mutations of the c-N-*ras* gene were not identified at codon 12 in any of 43 HCC, and none were found in any of 24 HCC at codon 13, but this gene was mutated at codon 61 in 4/73 HCC (5.5%) *(352,353,355,356)*. An activating mutation in the c-N-*ras* gene was also found in 1 HCC by transfection of HCC DNA combined with molecular cloning *(359)*.

The low level of mutation detected in these studies suggests that mutational activation of c-*ras* genes does not play a prominent role in the development of HCC in humans. However, as noted earlier, p21 ras protein appears to be increased in most HCC, suggesting that the ras-MAPK pathway is hyperactive in HCC in the absence of c-*ras* gene mutation. Nevertheless, in a small fraction of HCC c-*ras* gene mutation may be an important and early molecular event in the genesis of HCC. In 6 HCC in which a c-*ras* gene mutation was found in HCC, an identical mutation was found in hepatocytes of the surrounding nontumorous liver tissue *(350,353)*, suggesting that in these instances the ras gene mutation occurred early in a clone of preneoplastic hepatocytes from which the HCC ultimately developed.

MEK1, MEK2 and ERK1, ERK2 The mitogen-activated protein-kinase kinases (MEK1 and MEK2) and the extracellular signal-regulated kinases (ERK1 and ERK2) were significantly elevated in 5 HCC as compared to the adjacent nonneoplastic liver tissue *(360)*. Expression of MEK1 and MEK2, and ERK1 and ERK2 was evaluated by Western blotting of protein extracts using antibodies to these molecules. MEK1 expression in particulate fractions of HCC was increased by 4.2 ± 1.6-fold and MEK2 by 3.6 ± 1.1-fold as compared to adjacent nontumorous liver. Using parallel hybridization analysis of protein kinase genes, Tsou et al. *(252)* found that a MEK kinase (MEKK-3) was strongly upregulated in HCC and HCC cell lines as compared to normal liver.

ERK1 was increased in the particulate fractions of 5 HCC by 5.4 ± 2.1-fold and ERK2 by 6.6 ± 1.3-fold, while soluble ERK1 was increased by 2.9 ± 0.2-fold and soluble ERK2 by 3.1 ± 1.1-fold the level of that in adjacent non-neoplastic liver *(360)*. The functional ability of ERK2 to phosphorylate myelin basic protein was also significantly increased (particulate fraction, 3.2 ± 0.50-fold; cytosolic fraction, 6.0 ± 2.3-fold), as compared to that of ERK2 from adjacent nontumorous liver tissue. These observations on ERK1 and ERK2 were confirmed and extended in a larger study of 26 HCC *(361)*. Activities of ERK1 and ERK2 (measured by phosphorylation of myelin basic protein) were increased up to three-fold in 15/26 HCC (58%), as com-

pared to activities in adjacent nontumorous liver, and by an even greater extent in 17/26 HCC (65%), as compared to the lower activities found in two nondiseased livers. ERK1 and ERK2 were localized (by immunohistochemistry) most intensely in the nuclei of neoplastic cells in HCC and to a lesser extent in cytoplasm. The activities of ERK1 and ERK2 correlated significantly with the extent of expression of c-*fos* *(361)*. Furthermore, expression of cyclin D1 protein (immunoblot) also correlated significantly with expression of c-fos protein (361). These observations strongly support a direct connection between increased activation of the MAP kinase signal pathway, activation of nuclear transcription factors (c-myc, c-fos, c-jun), and increased cell cycling, as indicated by increased levels of cyclin D1 protein.

Increased overall activity of the mitogen-activated signal transduction pathways is indicated by heightened tyrosine kinase activity, reflected by the tyrosine kinase activity of p60 src protein. The tyrosine kinase activity of p60 src protein was two-fold to five-fold higher in 20 HCC than in the adjacent cirrhotic or nondiseased tissues, as measured by enolase phosphorylation or by autophosphorylation *(362)*. Activation of tyrosine kinase rather than increased enzyme protein was responsible for the augmented activity because the amounts of p60 src protein in these tissues, as judged by Western-blot analysis, did not vary *(362)*. Activity of p60 src protein tyrosine kinase increased further during progression of HCC, as shown by the significantly higher activity in 5 poorly differentiated HCC as compared to 15 moderately differentiated and 5 well-differentiated tumors *(362)*.

G Proteins The seven membrane-spanning receptors are activated when occupied by appropriate adrenergic compounds, transmitting a signal through the heterotrimeric G-proteins to the downstream effectors adenyl cyclase/cyclic adenosine monophosphate. The $G_{i\alpha}$ regulatory proteins were generally upregulated in 6 HCC as compared to adjacent nontumorous tissue *(363)*. $G_{i\alpha1}$ was increased in 5/6 HCC by 2.8 ± 0.77-fold, and showed no change in 1/6 HCC *(363)*. $G_{i\alpha1-2}$ was increased by 2.2 ± 0.21-fold in 4/6 HCC and unchanged in 2/6 (363). $G_{i\alpha3}$ was increased in 4/6 HCC by 1.5 ± 0.06-fold and decreased in 2/6 by approx 40% *(363)*. The functional activity of G_{ia} proteins demonstrated a four-fold increase in 4/6 HCC as indicated by pertussis toxin-catalyzed ADP-dependent phosphorylation, and showed no change in 2/6 HCC *(363)*. In contrast, $G_{s\alpha}$ proteins were significantly decreased in all HCC (6/6) by 70 ± 8%, and the functional activity was similarly decreased as indicated by stimulation of adenyl cyclase activity by agonist and forskolin (HCC, 3.8 ± 1.1 pmol/mg/min; adjacent liver, 11.8 ± 1.6 pmol/mg/min).

c-myc and c-fos Nuclear transcription factors including c-myc, c-fos, and c-jun are regulated through the MAP kinase pathway. Increased expression of p62 c-myc protein was found in 61/109 HCC (56%) summated from several individual studies *(340,342,343,364–366)*, in some instances being expressed at 15-fold the level in adjacent nontumorous liver *(364)*. Expression of p62 c-myc protein was also increased in livers the site of chronic hepatitis *(343)* and cirrhosis *(342,365)* as compared to normal liver. Gan et al. *(365)* found that the expression level of p62 c-myc protein was increased in both well-differentiated (relative expression = 224) and poorly differentiated (relative expression = 264) HCC, as compared to normal liver (RE 110) and cirrhotic liver (relative expression = 153). In general agreement, Saegusa et al. *(366)* found that p62 c-myc protein expression was not increased in either of two well-differentiated HCC, as contrasted to increased expression detected in 15/29 (52%) moderately differentiated HCC and in 4/9 (44%) poorly differentiated HCC.

Increased expression of c-*myc* mRNA was also detected in 68/74 HCC (92%) accumulated from several individual studies *(346–349,367)*. Expression of c-*myc* gene transcripts was also higher in 23/23 HCC than in adjacent nontumorous livers *(346,349,364)*. Gan et al. *(365)* found a steady increase in the expression of c-*myc* transcripts in cirrhotic liver (relative expression = 240) and HCC (relative expression = 297–438) as compared to normal liver (relative expression = 111). Haritani et al. *(345)* detected no c-myc transcripts in liver tissues in nonneoplastic diseases using relatively insensitive Northern blotting of whole RNA. Alterations in the expression of N-*myc* gene appeared to reflect those of c-*myc* in some instances *(348)*, but not all *(347)*.

In addition to upregulation by the activated MAPK pathway, increased expression of the c-*myc* gene in HCC involves both its hypomethylation and amplification. The c-*myc* gene was substantially hypomethylated in 15/27 HCC (55%) *(182,368)*, which particularly involved the third exon *(368)*. Kaneko et al. *(182)* and Nambu et al. *(368)* also found that the c-*myc* gene was hypomethylated in 5/15 (33%) of the adjacent cirrhotic livers, suggesting that hypomethylation is an early event underlying increased c-myc expression during the development of HCC. The c-*myc* gene was amplified in 50/163 HCC (31%) studied by four investigators *(340,351,369–372)*, but gene amplification was not found in any of 8 non-neoplastic liver tissues adjacent to the HCC in which it was amplified *(340)*. Amplification of the c-*myc* gene was associated with poor HCC differentiation, occurring in 12/40 well-differentiated HCC (30%) and in 12/22 moderately and poorly differentiated tumors (55%), as well as with poor prognosis *(371,372)* and large tumor size, high tumor-cell proliferation, and p53 overexpression *(372)*. Amplification and rearrangement of the N-*myc* gene was also described in 2/10 HCC (20%) *(348)*, and a polymorphism in the L-*myc* gene, leading to a lack of the SS L-*myc* genotype, was associated with an 8.7-fold increase in susceptibility to HCC *(373)*.

The c-*myc* (but not the N-*myc*) gene was overexpressed in 2/2 HBL *(374)*, but neither gene was amplified in 10 HBL *(375)*.

Although fewer studies have examined the c-*fos* gene in HCC, its patterns of expression *(361,364)* and methylation *(376)* in cirrhotic liver and HCC appear to reflect that of c-*myc*; expression of c-fos protein (immunoblot) was increased in 12/46 HCC (26%) *(361)*. Other signal pathway-activated transcription factors remain to be intensely studied in HCC, although Ito et al. *(361)* found that expression of c-*jun* was increased in 13/26 HCC (50%).

Smad Pathway The passage of growth-inhibiting signals from the binding of TGF-β to TGFβ1R/2R heterodimers activates the Smad pathway. One allele of the *Smad4* (*DPC4*) gene was deleted in 8/54 HCC (15%) *(377,378)*, but no gene muta-

tions were found by direct sequencing in the HCC that contained LOH *(377)*, and none were identified in either the *Smad2* or the *Smad4* gene by PCR-single-strand conformation polymorphism among 30 HCC *(279)*. Among 35 HCC, one mutation was detected in exon 10 of *Smad2* (2.9%) and two mutations were found in *Smad4* (exons 8 and 9) (5.7%) by direct sequencing *(379)*.

CYCLINS

Cyclin D1 The cyclins and cyclin-regulatory molecules, which control the passage of hepatocytes through the cell cycle, are regulated by c-myc in concert with other transcription factors. Cyclin D1 protein was overexpressed in 50/129 HCC (39%) *(361,380)* and increased expression was significantly associated with a shortened disease-free interval after resection of HCC *(380)*. Amplification of the *cyclin D1* gene by 3-fold to 20-fold was detected in 12/100 HCC (12%) *(361,381,382)*. In HCC containing an amplified *cyclin D1* gene, the cyclin D1 protein was overexpressed in 20/29 HCC (70%) *(361,381)*, and D1 mRNA was overexpressed in 5/5 *(382)*. The *int-2* gene, also located at chromosome 11q13, was co-amplified along with the *cyclin D1* (*Bcl1*) gene in 7/91 HCC (8%) *(382,383)*. The *cyclin D1* gene was neither amplified nor overexpressed in adjacent nontumorous liver tissue *(381)*. In contrast to these results, Peng et al. *(384)* found that expression of *cyclin D1* mRNA (determined by RT-PCR with internal control and by Northern blotting) was increased in 4/71 HCC (6%), but decreased expression was more common, occurring in 29/71 HCC (41%). The basis for these differences in expression of *cyclin D1* in HCC is not apparent.

Kim et al. *(385)* reported the overexpression of cyclin D1 protein in 13/17 HBL (76%) and of cyclin-dependent kinase 4 (CDK4) in 15/17 HBL (88%) based on the subjective assessment of immunohistochemical staining of histological sections. Both cyclin D1 and CDK4 were overexpressed concurrently in 11/17 HBL *(385)*. Risk of HBL recurrence was positively correlated with the highest subjective level of cyclin D1 staining *(385)*.

Iolascon et al. *(386)* found a shift in the type of *cyclin D* gene expressed among 7 HBL. Using analyses of expressed RNA (RT-PCR) and protein (immunoblot), the level of cyclin D1 was decreased, and the levels of cyclin D2 and cyclin D3 were increased in HBL *(386)*.

Cyclin E Overexpression of the *cyclin E* gene occurred in 77/175 HCC (44%) *(380,384)* and in 5/71 adjacent nontumorous liver tissues (7%) *(384)*. Concordance of RT-PCR with Northern blotting was over 90% for both genes; staining of cyclin E protein by immunohistochemistry was detected in 42/52 HCC (81%), and the correlation of RT-PCR and immunohistochemical staining in HCC was 92% *(384)*. Peng et al. *(384)* found that simultaneous upregulation of *cyclin E* and downregulation of *cyclin D1* were significantly associated with *p53* mutation (occurring in 25/71 HCC, 35%), tumors greater than 5 cm, advanced tumor grade (III-IV), poor four-year survival, and local tumor invasion *(384)*. Peng et al. *(384)* and Ito et al. *(380)* examined the expression of both cyclin D1 and cyclin E proteins in the same groups of HCC. Peng et al. *(384)* found that cyclin D1 was downregulated when cyclin E was overexpressed. However, it is not clear whether cyclin D1 and cyclin E overexpression occurred simultaneously or in different HCC in the study of Ito et al. *(380)*. However, it seems possible that overexpression of either of *cyclin D* or *cyclin E* genes can activate cell- cycle transit.

Antibodies to cyclin D1 and cyclin E were not found in sera from any of 100 patients with HCC *(387)*.

Cyclin A Overexpression of cyclin A protein was detected by Western blotting in 12/31 HCC (39%) *(388)* and *cyclin A* mRNA (measured by Northern blot) was overexpressed in 18/43 HCC (42%) *(389)*. Cyclin A protein overexpression was associated with gene amplification (Southern blotting) in 6/12 HCC (50%) *(388)*. The cyclin A-associated protein, Skp2, was also overexpressed in 17/31 HCC (55%), and cyclin A and Skp2 were overexpressed concurrently in 11 of these 17 tumors *(388)*. Cyclin A expression level was positively and highly correlated with the fraction of tumor cells in S/G_2 phases of the cell cycle (388,389), and negatively correlated with length of survival *(388)*. In one HCC, HBV genomic DNA was integrated into the *cyclin A* gene *(390)*, leading to its truncation and to the production of a cyclin A-HBV fusion protein. In this case, the N-terminus of the cyclin A protein (the signal for protein degradation) was deleted and replaced by HBV pre-S2/S sequences (including the pre-S2/S promoter), and the resulting fusion protein was highly expressed and resisted degradation *(391)*. However, HBV infection was not correlated generally with the expression status of the *cyclin A* gene *(388)*, and the observation of *cyclin A* gene alteration by HBV integration *(390,391)* appears to have been a random and rare event. Allelic loss (LOH) at the *cyclin A* gene locus on chromosome 4q27 was found in only 1/20 informative HCC (5%) *(392)*. Autoantibodies to cyclin A were detected in the sera in 8% of patients with autoimmune primary biliary cirrhosis *(393)*, but in only 1% of patients (1/100) with HCC *(387)*.

Cyclin B1 The precise role of cyclin B in the unregulated proliferation of HCC is not clear. Although unscheduled expression of cyclin B1 (in other than in the G_2/M phases of the cell cycle) of has been detected by flow cytometry in 18/28 primary malignancies *(394)*, only one HCC was included in the study and cyclin B1 was not overexpressed that tumor. However, autoantibodies to cyclin B1 have been detected in the sera of 15/100 patients (15%) with HCC *(387)*, suggesting that aberrant expression of *cyclin B1* may be a more prominent feature of HCC than has been yet discerned.

CYCLIN-DEPENDENT KINASE INHIBITORS

p16INK4A Total absence of the cyclin-dependent kinase inhibitor (CKI) p16[INK4A] (also called CDKN2A) protein was found in 16/41 HCC (39%) by Western blotting *(395,396)* and in 29/60 HCC (48%) by immunohistochemistry *(397)*, and it was reduced or absent in 37/60 HCC (62%) *(397)*. Transcripts of the *p16[INK4A]* gene were expressed in 22/22 HCC examined by RT-PCR, even when the protein was not detected *(395)*. The *p16[INK4A]* gene was hypermethylated in 95/185 HCC (51%) summated from several studies *(397–401)*. Methylation of greater than 65% of the available sites in the gene correlated with complete suppression of protein expression, whereas lesser extents of methylation were associated with reduced

protein expression *(397)*. Lack of p16[INK4A] protein expression was more frequent in poorly differentiated HCC in one study *(397)*. The p16[INK4A] protein was absent from 1/5 well-differentiated HCC (20%), 13/26 moderately differentiated HCC (50%), and 15/29 poorly differentiated HCC (52%) *(397)*. However, Hui et al. *(395)* found that p16[INK4A] protein was absent from an approximately equal portion of early HCC (2/9, 22%) and advanced HCC (8/40, 20%).

Other genetic aberrations may also lead to reduced or absent expression of the *p16[INK4A]* gene in some HCC. Intragenic somatic mutations of the *p16[INK4A]* gene were detected in 15/312 HCC (5%) *(395–400,402–405)*. Homozygous deletion of the *p16[INK4A]* gene was found in 32/300 HCC (10%) *(395–397,399,400,402–404)*, and LOH of loci on chromosome 9p near the *p16[INK4A]* locus were identified in 67/183 HCC (37%) *(396,398,400,402,404,405)*. LOH on 9p were found with a similar frequency of about 20–35% in all of the individual studies except that of Liew et al. *(400)*, in which 29/48 HCC (60%) showed LOH at a locus in the 9p21 region. Somatic intragenic mutations of the *p16[INK4A]* gene were quite variable in different studies, ranging from 33% (8/24 HCC) in one study *(395)*, 4–6% in two others *(402,404)*, to none in several studies that included over 200 HCC *(396–399,405)*. All of the homozygous deletions were found in three studies which showed frequencies of 25/41 HCC (61%) *(396)*, 5/48 HCC (10%) *(400)* and 2/24 (8%) *(403)*, whereas four studies that included 177 HCC found none *(395,397,402,404)*. Bonilla et al. *(405)* detected microsatellite aberrations suggesting small rearrangements or instabilities in 4/17 HCC (24%). Therefore, it appears that the major mechanism that suppresses p16[INK4A] protein expression in sporadic HCC is gene hypermethylation. Among 16 HCC in which the *p16[INK4A]* gene was hypermethylated, methylated *p16[INK4A]* DNA was also detected in the serum/plasma of 13 (81%) *(401)*. Interestingly, Chaubert et al. *(398)* identified germline mutations of the *p16[INK4A]* gene in 4/26 HCC-bearing patients (15%), with the somatic loss of the wild-type allele in 2/4 HCC that carried the germ-line mutation. The four patients with germ-line mutations of the *p16[INK4A]* gene developed HCC at a relatively early age and in the absence of cirrhosis *(398)*. Furthermore, the mutation occurred in a mother and her son with HCC, suggesting its involvement in familial susceptibility to HCC *(398)*.

Contrasting with these results from several studies, Ito et al. *(380)* detected low levels of p16[INK4A] protein by immunoblot analysis in both HCC and adjacent nontumorous liver tissue in a study that included 104 HCC and 90 nontumorous tissues; they detected higher concentrations of p16[INK4A] by immunoblot in protein from isolated nuclei than in total cellular proteins, and suggested that p16[INK4A] protein was actually increased in HCC. They also reported that a larger fraction of HCC nuclei were immunohistochemically positive for p16[INK4A] protein ($45.5 \pm 28.5\%$) than were nuclei in adjacent nontumorous liver tissue ($18.2 \pm 21.0\%$) *(380)*. The basis for these conflicting observations remains to be discovered.

Iolascon et al. *(386)* examined the expression of the *p16[INK4A]*, *p15[INK4B]*, and *p18[INK4C]* genes in 14 HBL; they found that the *p16[INK4A]* gene (α-transcript) and the *p15[INK4B]* gene were transcriptionally silenced in both 9 HBL and in matched normal livers, while the $p16^{INK4A}$ gene (β-transcript) and $p18^{INK4C}$ gene were expressed in both HBL and normal liver. Also, they found that all of these genes were structurally unmodified in HBL, as compared to normal livers; specifically no LOH were found in 6 loci around chromosome 9p21 (the location of $p16^{INK4A}$ and $p15^{INK4B}$ genes) or in 5 loci around chromosome 1p32 (the location of the $p18^{INK4C}$ gene).

p21WAF1/CIP1 The CKI p21$^{WAF1/CIP}$ protein was expressed at a higher level in 151/201 HCC (75%) than in surrounding nontumorous liver tissue, as indicated by immunohistochemical staining of tissue sections *(380,406)*. The staining of p21$^{WAF1/CIP1 \, protein}$ was confined to a small fraction of nuclei of both HCC ($5.5 \pm 9.8\%$) and nontumorous liver ($2.7 \pm 5.3\%$), and the protein was only weakly detected by immunohistochemistry *(380)*. Expression of $p21^{WAF1/CIP1}$ is controlled at least partly by *p53*. Both p21$^{WAF1/CIP1}$ and p53 proteins were expressed in parallel in 28/97 HCC (30%), but in 35/97 HCC (36%) p21$^{WAF1/CIP1}$ staining occurred in the absence of *p53* expression, and in 20/97 HCC (21%) *p53* expression occurred in the absence of p21$^{WAF1/CIP1}$ staining *(406)*. Expression of p21$^{WAF1/CIP1}$ did not occur in 4/6 HCC with *p53* mutations in exons 5–9 (67%), while the protein was expressed in the remaining two HCC with *p53* mutations *(401)*. Expression of $p21^{WAF1/CIP1}$ and *p53* mRNA in HCC were weakly correlated, and expression of p21$^{WAF1/CIP1}$ above the median level was associated with HCC that had fewer multiple nodules, but not with tumor grade or size *(406)*. However, a higher fraction of nuclei were stained immunohistochemically for p21$^{WAF1/CIP1}$ in HCC with intrahepatic metastasis than in those tumors without intrahepatic spread *(380)*.

Decreased expression of $p21^{WAF1/CIP1}$ mRNA (Northern blot and RT-PCR) was demonstrated in 23/40 HCC (58%) accumulated from two studies *(407,408)*, and in both of these studies the level of expression of $p21^{WAF1/CIP1}$ transcripts was significantly lower in HCC than in the surrounding nontumorous liver *(407,408)*. Mutations in the *p53* gene occurred in 5/21 HCC examined by Hui et al. *(408)*, all of which expressed very low levels of $p21^{WAF1/CIP1}$ transcripts. However, correspondence between reduced expression of $p21^{WAF1/CIP1}$ mRNA and mutated *p53* was not perfect, because 3/21 HCC, which expressed very low levels of $p21^{WAF1/CIP1}$ transcripts, contained an intact *p53* gene *(403)*. Nevertheless, the relative expression of $p21^{WAF1/CIP1}$ mRNA in HCC was significantly lower in those tumors with mutated *p53* (0.73 ± 0.13 U, n = 6), than in those with wild-type *p53* (1.00 ± 0.21 U, n = 14) *(407)*. Similarly, the level of $p21^{WAF1/CIP1}$ mRNA expressed in 6 HCC with mutations in the *p53* gene (0.73 ± 0.13 U) was significantly lower than in the adjacent nontumorous liver tissue (0.97 ± 0.13 U), whereas there was no significant difference in the level of $p21^{WAF1/CIP1}$ mRNA expression in the 14 HCC with wild-type *p53* (1.00 ± 0.21 U) and in the adjacent nontumorous liver tissue *(407)*. Although $p21^{WAF1/CIP1}$ expression was significantly reduced in 12/19 HCC, a mutated *p53* gene was found in only one *(407)*. Furutani et al. *(407)* also found that the $p21^{WAF1/CIP1}$ gene was mutated in 1/19 HCC, (codon 49, CGTÆCAT) and Watanabe et al. *(409)* detected various aberrations in the $p21^{WAF1/CIP1}$ gene in 2/3 HCC, including a mutation in codon 43 (CAG→CTG) in one tumor and a gene rearrangement and ampli-

fication in the other. In these studies the overall mutation frequency of the $p21^{WAF1/CIP1}$ gene was 2/22 HCC (9%) *(408,409)*.

p27Kip1 Transcripts for the CKI $p27^{Kip1}$ (RT-PCR) were significantly reduced (ratio of $p27^{Kip1}$ mRNA/β-*actin* mRNA) in 21 HCC (0.49 ± 0.24), as compared to the adjacent nontumorous liver tissue (0.57 ± 0.22) *(410)*. Expression of $p27^{Kip1}$ transcripts was significantly reduced in 11/21 HCC (52%) *(410)*. However, the expression level of $p27^{Kip1}$ was not correlated with either HCC differentiation or tumor size. In contrast, Ito et al. *(380)* reported that p27^{Kip1} protein (analyzed by immunoblot) was upregulated in HCC and that a higher fraction of HCC nuclei than of nuclei in adjacent nontumorous tissue were immunohistochemically positive. However, they found that high expression of p27^{Kip1} (more than 50% of nuclei staining immunohistochemically) was associated with longer disease-free survival after tumor resection *(380)*. Relatively decreased expression of p27^{Kip1} was also associated with HCC showing portal invasion, poor differentiation, and larger size *(380)*. These results suggest that even relatively small changes in $p27^{KIP1}$ expression are correlated with the growth and metastasis of HCC. Although the expression of $p27^{KIP1}$ is partly regulated by TGF-β, direct correlation of the expression of both molecules in HCC have not been found.

Expression of $p27^{Kip1}$, $p21^{WAF/CIP1}$, and the status of the $p16^{INK4A}$ gene were assessed in the same set of 17 HCC *(395,408,410)*. Abnormal expression of one or more of these CKIs occurred in 15/17 HCC (88%); in 9/17 HCC (53%) only one CKI was abnormal, 5/17 HCC (29%) contained abnormalities in two CKIs, and in 1/17 (6%) all three were abnormal *(410)*. These observations suggest that aberrant expression of the CKIs are important molecular elements in the development of HCC.

p57Kip 2 Neither LOH nor mutations of the $p57^{Kip2}$ gene were found in 17 HCC *(405)*.

Rb1 AND E2F-1 Rb1 Lack of expression of pRb (detected by immunohistochemistry) characterized 125/231 HCC (54%) *(380,411–413)*, while overexpression was detected in 15/81 HCC (19%) *(413)*. Most studies have focused on the reduced expression or lack of expression of pRb in tumor tissues. Loss of expression correlated closely with allelic deletion of the *Rb1* gene *(412)*. LOH of the *RB1* gene occurred in 10/21 HCC (48%), all but one of which also lacked expression of pRb, and in 2/9 HCC (22%) the remaining allele contained tumor-specific mutations (small deletions) *(412)*. One HCC that did not express pRb contained a rare polymorphism or germ-line mutation in the *RB1* gene (which was not found in tissues of 65 other persons). Zhang et al. *(412)* speculated that the promoter sequences of the remaining alleles might be hypermethylated in the other instances in which LOH alone was associated with lack of expression of the pRb. However, the promoter region of the *Rb1* gene was not hypermethylated among 19 HCC examined by Hada et al. *(414)* although pRb was not expressed.

LOH of the *Rb1* gene was reported in an additional 45/140 HCC (32%) accumulated from studies by several investigators *(378,415–421)*. In individual studies, the frequency of LOH ranged from 3/31 HCC (10%) *(416)* to 11/15 HCC (73%) *(421)*. In addition to these studies using *Rb1*-specific probes, Zhang et al. *(412)* and Kuroki et al. *(420)* allelotyped chromosome 13q with multiple probes that spanned both sides of the *Rb1* locus on chromosome 13q14.3. Kuroki et al. *(420)* found LOH of 80% (8/10 HCC) and 94% (16/17 HCC) with probes located on either side of the *Rb1* locus, while Zhang et al. *(412)* found LOH in the immediate vicinity of the *Rb1* locus in each of 8 HCC (100%). LOH of the *Rb1* locus was sometimes coupled with retention of some *Rb1* gene sequences, leading to the opinion that a breakpoint in chromosome 13q was located within the *Rb1* locus *(417)*. Additionally, an interstitial deletion in the *Rb1* gene was detected in 1/25 HCC (4%) *(418)*, and homozygous deletion and replication error were found in 2/7 HCC (29%) *(358)*.

LOH of the *Rb1* gene also occurred in 20/31 nonneoplastic cirrhotic nodules (65%) adjacent to 11 HCC in which the *Rb1* gene showed LOH, and the same alleles were lost in both HCC and adjacent cirrhotic nodules in most instances, while both *Rb1* alleles were retained in cirrhotic nodules adjacent to 4 HCC that also retained both *Rb1* alleles *(421)*. These observations suggest that the HCC with *Rb1* LOH were clonal outgrowths from cirrhotic nodules in which *Rb1* LOH had developed as a preneoplastic change. However, in another study the cirrhotic nodules surrounding HCC that contained *Rb1* gene LOH all retained both *Rb1* genes *(420)*. These results and those of two other studies suggest that *Rb1* gene LOH is a late change associated with HCC progression. In one study, all 100% (21/21 tumors) of early, well-differentiated HCC contained two *Rb1* genes (biallelic), while in 27% (6/22) of more advanced and less well-differentiated HCC only one *Rb1* gene was detected *(415)*. In agreement with these results, LOH of the *Rb1* gene occurred in only 1/4 well-differentiated HCC (25%) and in 8/17 moderately and poorly differentiated HCC (47%) *(412)*.

LOH of the *Rb1* gene or lack of pRb expression and mutation of the *p53* gene were often identified in the same HCC; of 7 HCC with a mutated *p53* gene, 6 also contained a monoallelic *Rb1* gene *(415)*, and p53 protein characteristic of a mutated gene was detected by immunohistochemistry in 4 of 5 HCC that lacked expression of pRb *(411)*.

E2F-1 No mutations or deletions were identified in the pRb-binding domain of *E2F-1* in 24 liver tumors studied along with 382 other cancers *(422)*.

p53, mdm2, AND p73

p53 Zhao et al. *(423)* examined the expression of p53 protein by immunohistochemistry of paraffin sections of HCC and of cirrhotic and normal livers using five different anti-p53 antibodies (CM-1, 1801, 240, 420, and DO-7). Nuclear staining varied from 62% of HCC for CM-1 and 27% for 1801, to nearly zero for the other antibodies, which occasionally stained cytoplasm or cell membranes in HCC *(423)*. Normal hepatocytes in cirrhotic livers never stained with any antibody, nor did hepatocytes showing large cell dysplasia, but staining was found in small dysplastic cells in 8/37 cirrhotic livers that were the sites of HCC (22%) and in 22/66 cirrhotic livers without HCC (33%) *(423)*.

Expression of p53 protein in HCC and in adjacent nontumorous liver tissues was examined in several other studies using either immunohistochemistry of tissue sections or immunoblotting of extracted protein. Antibody 1801 was used in 10 studies (44%), CM-1 in 8 studies (35%), and various other

antibodies in 6 studies (22%) employing immunohistochemistry, and antibody 421 was used in both studies using immunoblotting. Weak cytoplasmic expression of p53 protein was found in 11/253 noncancerous livers (4%) *(424–430)*. Ojanguren et al. *(429)* found that none of 6 HCA stained positively by immunohistochemistry for p53.

Expression (overexpression) of p53 protein was detected in the nuclei of a variable fraction of neoplastic hepatocytes among 1109 HCC accumulated from several independent studies, some nuclei stained in 343 (31%) *(424–447)*. Overexpression of p53 mRNA was found in 15/18 HCC (83%), and correlated closely with overexpression of protein *(425,437)*. Feitelson et al. *(448)* and Hosono et al. *(449)* detected increased expression of p53 protein by immunoblotting of protein extracted from HCC. The frequency with which HCC showed nuclear staining for p53 by immunohistochemistry was positively correlated with tumor grade and size; nuclei stained in 8/42 well-differentiated HCC (19%), in 8/25 moderately differentiated HCC (32%), and in 6/9 poorly differentiated HCC (67%) *(434,450)*. In studies in which HCC were categorized only as better-differentiated (or low grade) and less-differentiated (or high grade), 20–42% of the former and 39–43% of the latter showed nuclear staining for p53 *(436,443,447)*. Hsu et al. *(436)* found that nuclei stained for p53 in 26% of HCC less than 2 cm in diameter and in 39% of HCC greater than 5 cm in diameter; similarly, Qin et al. *(450)* found that nuclei were stained for p53 in one of 4 HCC less than 5 cm in diameter (25%), as compared to 7/19 HCC between 5.1 cm and 10 cm in diameter (37%), and 5/7 HCC greater than 10 cm in diameter (71%). Nakopoulou et al. *(443)* found that p53 protein staining in HCC was positively correlated with tumor cell proliferation, as indicated by the PCNA index.

Livni et al. *(428)* and Nakopoulou et al. *(443)* detected p53-staining in 28/74 nontumorous tissues (38%) adjacent to p53-positive HCC. Livni et al. *(428)* also detected immunohistochemically positive hepatocytes in 3/21 cirrhotic livers (14%) that lacked HCC, but they did not find p53-staining in any of 12 livers with chronic hepatitis or in 13 livers without disease. Both Livni et al. *(428)* and Nakopoulou et al. *(443)* posited that the changes in the p53 molecule that enabled it to be detected immunohistochemically occurred early in the process of hepatocarcinogenesis. However, Kang et al. *(430)* detected p53 immunostaining in 4/8 HCC (50%), in 4/9 high-grade dysplastic nodules (type II macroregenerative nodule) (44%) but in none of 17 low-grade dysplastic nodules and 25 cirrhotic nodules, suggesting that p53 overexpression occurred at a later stage of HCC development.

Among several independent studies, 359/871 informative HCC (41%) showed LOH of the *p53* gene *(354,378,415,417–419,424,431,444,449,451–470,475,478,484,486)*. Except for two studies, LOH was not found in nontumorous liver tissue; Kishimoto et al. *(466)* described *p53* gene LOH in 8/14 HCC, and in 5/8 cirrhotic nodules adjacent to HCC that contained LOH, but in none of 6 cirrhotic nodules adjacent to HCC that lacked *p53* gene LOH, and Tsopanomichalou et al. *(471)* detected *p53* gene LOH in 5/25 livers (20%) that were the site of chronic hepatitis or cirrhosis and in 1/8 livers (13%) that contained various nontumorous lesions. Kishimoto et al. *(466)* also found that the affected alleles were identical in individual HCC and adjacent cirrhotic nodules, and suggested that *p53* LOH developed in preneoplastic hepatocytes from which HCC were derived as a clonal outgrowth *(466)*. The frequency of LOH in individual studies ranged from none of 9 HCC (0%) in Alaskan natives *(464)* to 8/10 HCC (80%) in Japanese natives *(460)*. The frequency of *p53* gene LOH was related to the size of HCC, suggesting that *p53* LOH were associated with progression of HCC; LOH were found in 5/13 HCC (39%) less than 2.0 cm in diameter as compared to 19/35 HCC (54%) between 2.1 and 8.0 cm, and 13/17 HCC (76%) larger than 8.1 cm *(461)*. Tanaka et al. *(460)* found that in 10 HCC containing focal areas of two different histological grades, LOH were more frequent in the higher grade; no LOH were found in two grade I areas, while 4/7 grade II areas contained p53 LOH as did all of 11 grade III and IV areas.

Oda et al. *(462)* identified a complex pattern of *p53* LOH and mutation in a single HCC that formed three overlapping nodules: a larger nodule composed of grade I HCC, and two smaller inner nodules composed of grade II and grades II–III HCC, respectively. The smaller, higher-grade nodules were speculated to have arisen from the larger, lower-grade nodule because they were entirely contained within it. The larger, low-grade nodule lacked both LOH and mutation of the *p53* gene; the *p53* gene of one of the smaller nodules contained a mutation in codon 163, but no LOH, whereas the other contained a codon 249 mutation and loss of the wild-type allele. This pattern suggests that both clonal divergence and *p53* mutation/LOH occurred during tumor progression.

Mutation of the *p53* gene appears to occur in conjunction with LOH; some authors suggest that mutation precedes LOH and others that it follows. Rare mutations of the *p53* gene were identified in nontumorous livers from patients without HCC who lived in areas where the general populations were exposed to high dietary levels of aflatoxin B$_1$ *(472)*, and a mutation was found in intron 6 of the *p53* gene in the nondiseased liver of a patient exposed chronically to irradiation from thoratrast, and who had four extrahepatic neoplasms that also had mutations of the *p53* gene *(473)*. In surgically resected livers, Kang et al. *(430)* detected no *p53* gene mutations in exons 5–8 among 25 cirrhotic nodules or among either 17 low-grade dysplastic nodules or 9 high-grade dysplastic nodules, but identified such mutations in 2/9 HCC (22%). Iwamoto et al. *(474)* found mutations in the *p53* gene in the nontumorous liver tissue of 30/76 (39%) atom-bomb survivors who had HCC; there was no relationship between mutation frequency and irradiation dose in the nontumorous liver tissue, although the mutation frequency in HCC increased with dose from the high background frequency found in the nontumorous liver.

In data summated from numerous individual studies mutations in the *p53* gene were detected in exons 5–9 in 547/2029 (27%) *(354,358,384,406,408,415,425–427,430–432, 438–438–442,444,446,449,453,454,457,458,460,463,464,470, 475–483,485,487–495,500)*. In individual studies the fraction of HCC that contained a mutated *p53* gene ranged from 0/9 HCC *(431)*, 0/7 HCC *(480)*, 0/9 *(439)*, 0/14 *(464)*, 0/15 *(488)*, and 0/70 *(497)*, to 17/26 (65%) *(477,478)*. The fraction of HCC that contain mutations in the *p53* gene appears to be related to

the grade and size of HCC, among other variables. In five studies, the fraction of HCC that contained mutations of the *p53* gene was highest in the more poorly differentiated HCC *(441,460,478,486,490)*. A mutated *p53* gene was found in 10/68 well-differentiated HCC (15%), in 34/95 moderately differentiated HCC (36%), and in 38/79 poorly differentiated HCC (48%) *(441,460,478,486)*. Shi et al. *(490)* also found that 17% of HCC less than 5 cm in diameter contained *p53* mutations, compared to 33% of HCC larger than 5 cm in diameter. The length of survival of patients with HCC containing *p53* gene mutations was shorter than was that of patients whose HCC did not have mutations in the *p53* gene *(494)*, and the disease-free interval following resection was shorter in patients whose HCC contained *p53* mutations than in those whose tumors lacked *p53* gene mutations *(441)*.

Mutation of the third base of codon 249 of the *p53* gene was detected in 189/2272 HCC (8%) accumulated from several individual studies *(345,358,384,406,408,415,424–427,430,432, 437–442,444–446,449,453,454,456–458,460,463,464,470,475–482,485,487–490,492–506)*. In individual studies, the fraction of HCC that contained codon 249 mutation ranged from 0/10 HCC *(501)*, 0/59 HCC *(504)*, 0/47 HCC *(437)*, 0/13 HCC *(505)*, 0/22 HCC *(463)*, and 0/44 HCC *(490)*, to 8/16 HCC, (50%) *(454)*, 21/36 HCC (58%) *(456)*, and 10/15 (67%) *(503)*. The fraction of HCC that contain codon 249 mutations appears to reflect exposure to aflatoxin B$_1$ in the diet, but it is impossible to be certain about the role of this agent in individual patients. It seems clear that HCC that occur in patients in which the population is exposed to high levels of dietary aflatoxin B$_1$ have *p53* mutations that contain a high fraction involving a G to T transversion at the third base of codon 249 *(498)*. However, full confidence in the possible causal relationship between aflatoxin B$_1$ exposure and this specific mutation is prevented because of the existence of potentially confounding situations, including the difficulty of accurately quantifying the chronic exposure of individuals to aflatoxin and the possible interactive effects of chronic infection with HBV, which is highly prevalent in geographic areas in which the population is at risk from aflatoxin exposure *(507,508)*. Exposure of cultured human HepB2 liver cells to metabolically activated aflatoxin B$_1$ was found to produce adducts at codon 249 of the *p53* gene in studies that used RFLP-based PCR assays to focus on this particular codon *(509)*. However, a more recent study that exposed similar cells to metabolically activated aflatoxin B$_1$ under circumstances similar to those used by the earlier study *(509)*, but which applied ligation-mediated PCR to detect adducts, identified multiple adducts at codons 226, 243, 244, 245, 248, and 249 of exon of the *p53* gene, and also found that the codon 249 adduct was removed most rapidly *(510)*. Further studies are required to settle this important issue. Splice-site mutations (at intronic-exonic junctions) in the *p53* gene have been detected in 4/45 HCC (9%) *(483)*. Intronic mutations have also been identified in a study in which the *p53* gene was completely sequenced *(492)*.

Immunohistochemical detection of p53 protein in hepatocyte nuclei suggests that the protein is overexpressed and/or stabilized. Mutation of the *p53* gene could be responsible either for stabilization or lack of expression of the protein, depending on the nature of the mutation. On the other hand, stabilization of the p53 protein could be effected by means other than mutation, such as by complexing with the HBV X-antigen *(448,511–515)*. Several studies have assessed the relationship between mutation of the *p53* gene and overexpression of p53 protein as detected by immunohistochemistry. Using only the *p53* mutations at codon 249, the concordance between immunohistochemical staining of nuclei and gene mutation were relatively poor; in three studies in which immunohistochemistry demonstrated nuclear staining of p53 protein in 46/122 HCC (38%), codon 249 was mutated in only 5/122 (4%) *(424,437,493)*, and among the five HCC that contained a *p53* gene mutated at codon 249, four (80%) stained and one (20%) did not *(424,493)*. The association between *p53* gene mutation and nuclear staining with p53 protein is somewhat better when the mutational analysis is not limited to codon 249, but includes other coding sequences, which in most studies has been limited to exons 5–8 or 5–9, because few studies have sequenced the entire gene. Nuclear staining by immunohistochemistry was found in 131/412 HCC (32%) accumulated from several studies, and *p53* mutations were detected in 114/347 (33%) of the HCC *(424–427,430–432,436,439,440,442,445,446)*. Among 84 HCC that contained mutations at some codon in exons 5–8 or 5–9 of the *p53* gene, 64 showed nuclear staining by immunohistochemistry (76%) and 20 did not stain (24%), whereas among 52 HCC containing wild-type (unmutated) *p53* genes, the nuclei of 14 stained (27%) and nuclei of 38 did not stain (73%) *(436,440,446,493)*. Among 122 HCC in which nuclei stained for p53 by immunohistochemistry, 72 (59%) contained mutated *p53* genes, whereas among 77 HCC that were unstained, the *p53* gene was mutated in 12 (16%) *(427,436,440,445,493)*. Thus, the concordance between mutation at some site and nuclear staining appears to vary between 65 and 85%, suggesting that *p53* gene mutation is a major, but not the sole, factor responsible for nuclear staining of HCC by p53 immunohistochemistry.

Serum antibodies to p53 protein were detected in 73/502 patients with HCC (15%) accumulated from several studies *(445,493,516–519)*, but in none of 107 patients with various non-neoplastic liver diseases including acute hepatitis, chronic hepatitis, and cirrhosis *(516,519)*. Antibodies to p53 were moderately specific indicators of mutation and overexpression of the p53 gene in HCC *(492)*; 10/19 patients (52%) whose HCC overexpressed mutated p53 protein also had serum antibodies to the protein, whereas only 4/19 patients (21%) with HCC that did not overexpress p53 had circulating antibodies *(493)*. Although serum anti-p53 antibody was specific for HCC, it was not a sensitive indicator, and seemed to reflect the extent to which p53 protein accumulated within HCC tumor cells *(519)*. Survival of HCC patients with circulating anti-p53 antibodies was shorter than for patients lacking antibodies in one study *(518)*, but another study found the opposite relationship *(514)*.

Overexpression of p53 protein was detected immunohistochemically in 17/25 HBL (68%) *(439,520,521)*, predominantly in embryonal areas, as compared to fetal or mesenchymal areas *(520)*. LOH of the *p53* gene was detected in only one of 7 HBL (14%) *(480)*, and mutations of the *p53* gene were found

in only 10/173 HBL (6%) *(437,480,521,522)*. Kar et al. *(437)* found a codon 249 mutation (the only codon investigated) in one of 3 HBL, and all of the remaining mutations were detected in the study of Oda et al. *(521)*; in this study exons 5–8 were investigated in 10 HBL and mutations were found in 9 of them. Remarkably, eight sporadic HBL were reported to contain the same point mutation involving the first base of codon 156, whereas other mutations were located in codons 244, 273, and 279; three HBL had double mutations in the *p53* gene *(521)*. Seven of nine of the HBL that contained mutated *p53* genes showed nuclear p53 by immunohistochemistry *(521)*. This result contrasts with the observations of Kennedy et al. *(439)* who detected nuclear p53 by immunohistochemistry in 10/15 HBL, all of which lacked mutations in exons 5–8. Furthermore, Ohnishi et al. *(522)* and Kusafuka et al. *(523)* failed to detect a mutation in exons 5–9 in any of 49 HBL, but they did not investigate the presence in HBL of p53 protein by immunohistochemistry. The reasons for these striking disparities are not apparent from the published data.

mdm2 In a study that included two HCC among several types of cancers, low levels of both mdm2 protein (Western blot) and *mdm2* mRNA (RT-PCR) were detected in HCC, as well as weak staining of p53 protein *(524)*. The *mdm2* gene was not amplified in either of these HCC, but contained a mutation in both tumors that produced a premature stop codon and yielded a truncated protein that reacted weakly with antibody *(524)*. Qiu et al. *(496)* found that the level of *mdm2* transcripts (compared to the level of β-actin transcripts) was significantly higher in 42 HCC (52 ± 5.5% of β-actin) than in adjacent nontumorous liver tissue (26.2 ± 5.1%). Expression of *mdm2* was not significantly correlated with tumor size, but it was significantly correlated with tumor invasiveness. In 23 invasive HCC, *mdm2* mRNA expression was 62.6 ± 8.5% of β-actin expression as compared to 39.1 ± 5.1% in 19 noninvasive HCC *(496)*. Of most interest, Qiu et al. *(496)* found that *mdm2* mRNA expression was significantly higher in 23 HCC lacking p53 gene mutations (62.1 ± 8.4%) than in 18 HCC that contained mutated *p53* genes (38.5 ± 4.8%); among 10 HCC that expressed *mdm2* transcripts at greater than the median level (62% of β-actin), only one HCC (10%) contained a mutated *p53* gene, whereas in 32 HCC that expressed *mdm2* transcripts below the median level, the p53 gene was mutated in 17 (55%). Furthermore, *mdm2* gene expression was significantly higher in 13 HCC that recurred or metastasized within 1 yr following excision of the primary tumor (61.0 ± 8.5%) than in 19 HCC which did not recur or metastasize during one year after excision (40.6 ± 4.4%) *(496)*. Further studies on the relationship of *mdm2* expression to p53 sequestration in HCC are needed.

Among 38 HBL examined primarily for *p53* mutations, the *mdm2* gene was not amplified in any (Southern blot) *(522)*.

p73 The *p73* gene encodes a protein that is homologous to *p53* and the p73 protein activates some p53-responsive genes, suggesting that it may have similar regulatory functions *(525)*. Furthermore, the *p73* gene is imprinted, and it is located at chromosome 1p36.33 in an area that is frequently deleted in HCC, suggesting that it may be functionally inactivated in HCC. In a study of 48 HCC, LOH of the *p73* locus was identified in 5/25 informative HCC (20%), but mutations were not found, although polymorphisms were frequent *(525)*. In fact, overexpression of *p73* in HCC appears to be more frequent than lack of expression; *p73* mRNA (detected by *in situ* hybridization) was overexpressed in 25/74 HCC (34%) and p73 protein (detected by immunohistochemistry) was overexpressed in 61/193 HCC (32%) *(526)*. Heightened expression of *p73* was associated with poorly differentiated HCC and significantly reduced patient survival. No correlation was found between the expression of *p73* and *p53* in HCC in this study *(526)*.

The Wingless Signal Pathway The Wingless (Wnt) signal transduction cascade integrates the adenomatous polyposis coli (APC) protein, axin, β-catenin, and E-cadherin to transmit signals from the cell surface, through the frizzled receptor, to the nucleus; APC and E-cadherin modulate the availability of β-catenin to activate nuclear transcription factors.

APC Aberrations in the *APC* gene appear to be uncommon in HCC in adults. Only 9/118 HCC (8%) showed LOH of the *APC* locus and mutations were found in none of 69 HCC accumulated from several individual studies *(419,468,527–530)*. Furthermore, Legoix et al. *(531)* detected no *APC* mutations among 30 HCC specifically selected because they lacked a mutation in the β-*catenin* gene. However, children in families carrying a germ-line mutation in the *APC* gene are at heightened risk for development of tumors of the liver (especially HBL), as well as of carcinoma of the colon *(532–535)*. Bala et al. *(536)* reported that a 10-cm hepatocellular tumor occurring in a two-yr-old child contained a CGA to TGA mutation in codon 1451 of the *APC* gene, which was combined with the loss of the wild-type allele. The child and its mother, who died at 26 yr of age of colon cancer, carried the *APC* mutation in their germ-lines (536). In addition to inactivation of the *APC* gene by mutation and allelic deletion, the child's liver tumor also contained a mutation in codon 175 of the *p53* gene, without loss of the wild-type allele, but the c-H-*ras*, c-K-*ras*, and N-*ras* genes were not mutated *(536)*. A small fraction of the HBL that occur sporadically in children who lack apparent germ-line gene defects in the *APC* gene also contain somatic *APC* gene aberrations; among four studies the *APC* gene was mutated in 9/80 HBL (11%), and LOH occurred in 5/21 informative HBL (24%) *(528,537–539)*.

β-Catenin Expression of β-catenin by immunohistochemistry was increased in 55/66 HCC (83%), as compared to normal liver, chronic hepatitis, and cirrhosis *(108,540)*, with staining of tumor cell membranes, cytoplasm, and nuclei *(540)*. Overexpression of β-catenin occurred in all grade I HCC (3/3), in 43/55 grade II HCC (78%), and in 5/8 grade III HCC (62%), suggesting that overexpression correlated inversely with differentiation *(108)*. In four studies, the β-*catenin* gene contained mutations or deletions in 50/242 HCC (21%) *(530,531,540–542)*. Mutations clustered in exon 3, frequently involving the β-catenin degradation targeting box at the phosphorylation site for glycogen synthase kinase-3β (GSK-3β) *(530,531,540,541)*, and were associated with accumulation of β-catenin protein *(530,540–542)*, which was concentrated in tumor cell nuclei *(530)*. Mutations in the β-*catenin* gene were correlated with increased tumor-cell proliferation *(540)*, but not with HCC differentiation or size. Mutations showed no correlation with either HCV or HBV infection *(531)*, although Huang et al.

(530) found a high rate of mutation of the β-*catenin* gene in a group of HCC (9/22, 41%) that were derived from patients chronically infected with HCV. Legoix et al. *(531)* found that β-*catenin* mutations were negatively associated with the fractional allelic loss and with allelic deletions on chromosomes 1p, 4q, and 16q, suggesting alternate molecular genetic pathways in different HCC.

In 3 sporadic HBL, β-catenin protein was overexpressed in association with mutations in exon 3 of the GSK-3β binding site *(538)*. Larger studies of 70 sporadic HBL, also detected mutations and deletions in the β-*catenin* degradation targeting box (codons 32, 34, and 41) in 37 (53%) *(539,543)*. β-catenin accumulated in nuclei and cytoplasm in tumors with a mutated gene, and was detected in both mesenchymal and epithelial cellular components of the HBL *(540)*.

E-Cadherin Expression of E-cadherin was detected in 113/142 HCC (80%) in three studies, and in all normal and cirrhotic livers *(105,110,113,115,544)*. Reduced or extinguished expression of E-cadherin was related to poor differentiation of HCC, being found in six studies in 0/106 grade I lesions, in 23/114 grade II lesions (20%), in 24/60 grade III lesions (40%), and in 7/10 grade IV lesions (70%) *(91,105,108,110,113,115)*, and with tumor invasion and early recurrence *(544)*. Among 3 HCC that lacked E-cadherin (by Western blot and immunohistochemistry), mRNA was also reduced in two *(544)*. Reduced expression of E-cadherin protein correlated significantly with increased methylation of CpG residues in the promoter region of the *E-cadherin* gene, as compared to adjacent nontumorous liver tissue *(113,545)*, and frequent LOH in the region of the *E-cadherin* gene on chromosome 16q were found in 18/28 HCC (64%), although neither the expression of E-cadherin protein nor the status of the remaining allele (mutation, deletion, hypermethylation) were determined *(116)*. LOH of the *haptoglobin* locus on chromosome 16q correlated with LOH of *E-cadherin* in over 90% of instances examined *(116)*, suggesting that LOH of this site can be used as a surrogate for *E-cadherin* gene LOH. In an independent study, the *haptoglobin* locus showed LOH in 8/14 (58%) informative HCC *(546)*. These results suggest that aberrations in the Wnt-β-catenin-E-cadherin pathway have an important role in the pathogenesis of HCC occurring in adults and of HBL in children.

MISCELLANEOUS TUMOR-RELATED GENES

Various Tumor-Suppressor Genes Using microsatellite markers, Piao et al. *(378)* detected allelic losses (LOH) of the tumor-suppressor genes *BRCA1* (3/26 HCC, 12%), *EXT1* (5/25 HCC, 20%), *VHL* (2/24 HCC, 8%), and *WT1* (1/22 HCC, 5%). In addition, Piao et al. *(378)* and MacDonald et al. *(468)* found LOH of the *DCC* locus in 5/66 HCC (8%).

BRCA2 Katagiri et al. *(547)* sequenced the entire coding region of the *BRCA2* gene in 60 HCC, identifying mutations in 3 (5%). Two of the mutations were missense mutations carried in the germ line, suggesting the possibility that the mutation might predispose patients to the development of HCC.

FHIT Panagopoulos et al. *(548)* detected aberrant gene transcripts containing exonic deletions in nondiseased liver tissue, as well as in other supposedly normal tissues, and concluded that abnormal *FHIT* gene (the *fragile histidine triad* gene located on chromosome 3p14.2) transcripts were not a reliable genetic marker of neoplasia. Several studies on HCC and adjacent nontumorous liver tissue confirmed that altered *FHIT* transcripts were often found in nonneoplastic liver, but also that the gene was more frequently abnormal in HCC. Chen et al. *(549)* found one normal transcript of the *FHIT* gene together with aberrant transcripts that lacked 3 or more exons in 12/18 HCC (67%), as well as in 8/18 adjacent nontumorous liver tissues (44%). Schlott et al. *(550)* found aberrant *FHIT* gene transcripts, variably lacking exons 4–5, exons 4–6, exons 5–6, and exon 8 in all 10 HCC examined, but these aberrations were also found in all non-neoplastic liver samples. However, other aberrant transcripts lacking exons 5–7 and exons 5–8 were not found in non-neoplastic liver specimens, but were present in HCC and in samples of focal nodular hyperplasia *(550)*. Gramantieri et al. *(551)* detected aberrant *FHIT* transcripts in 13/18 HCC (72%) and in 3/24 nontumorous cirrhotic liver tissues (13%), but in none of 4 noncirrhotic, nontumorous livers. Aberrant transcripts arose by exonic deletions, with fusion of exons 3 or 4 with exons 8 or 9 to produce truncated transcripts. LOH of the *FHIT* gene was detected in 3/28 HCC (11%). The presence of truncated *FHIT* transcripts in HCC was associated with a higher rate of relapse and a shorter time to recurrence *(551)*. Yuan et al. *(552)* found that FHIT protein (detected by immunohistochemistry) was lacking in 5/10 HCC (50%) from Qidong China, but not in any of 10 nontumorous livers. Furthermore, they detected microsatellite instability (MSI) and/or allelic loss of the *FHIT* gene in 10/34 informative HCC (29%). These observations on HCC tissues were supported by studies on cultured HCC cell lines *(552)*. Downregulation of the *FHIT* gene was detected (Northern blot) in 9/14 cell lines (64%), and absence of FHIT protein (Western blot) in 4 of the 9 cell lines in which expression of the *FHIT* gene was reduced (44%). Additionally, structural alterations of chromosome 3p were found in 8/13 HCC cell lines (62%), with deletions or translocations involving chromosome 3p14.2, identified by fluorescence *in situ* hybridization (FISH) with a probe spanning the *FHIT* locus *(552)*.

The *FHIT* gene is the most fragile chromosome locus in the human genome, uniquely sensitive to various types of chromosome-damaging agents, and it is a translocation breakpoint in several neoplasms. Because the *FHIT* gene appears to be extremely sensitive to DNA damage, aberrations in nontumorous livers may reflect the effects of agents that increase risk of HCC. Although HCC appear to show more extensive alterations than does nontumorous liver, further studies of this interesting gene are needed.

KAI1 The *KAI1* gene, which codes for an integral membrane glycoprotein of the TM4 family was highly expressed (by Northern blot and *in situ* hybridization) in 10 nondiseased livers, but it was downregulated by 2.6-fold in 39 HCC (553). Among HCC, *KAI1* mRNA expression was significantly reduced in those with metastasis, as compared to nonmetastatic HCC; expression was not detected in 8/22 HCC metastases, and it was greatly reduced in the remaining 14 *(553)*.

nm23 Expression of nucleoside diphosphate kinase, a protein homologous to the *nm23* gene product, was studied by immunohistochemistry in 42 HCC, which had either distant or intrahepatic metastases *(554,555)*; the intensity of immunohis-

tochemical staining was described as less strong in tumors associated with metastases than in those without *(554,555)*. Staining intensity of nucleoside diphosphate kinase did not correlate with either grade of differentiation or tumor size *(554)*. Boix et al. *(556)* found that expression of *nm23-H1* mRNA (Northern blot) was related to recurrence of HCC in 17 cirrhotic patients with solitary HCC nodules during 30 mo after surgically resecting the tumors; 8/10 patients (80%) free of recurrent HCC after 30 mo expressed *nm23-H1* mRNA at levels 3–45-fold greater than did the adjacent nontumorous liver tissue, whereas only one of 7 patients (14%) whose HCC recurred during 30 mo expressed *nm23-H2* mRNA at the level of the surrounding nontumorous liver tissue *(556)*. Yamaguchi et al. *(557)* detected nm23-H1 and nm23-H2 protein by immunohistochemistry in 25 HCC; depending on the antibody used the cytoplasm of neoplastic hepatocytes was stained in 60–68% of the HCC. There was no relationship between staining for nm23-H1 protein and HCC grade, size, or vascular invasiveness, but 7/10 (70%) of the intrahepatic metastases did not stain and patients whose tumors expressed both nm23-H1 and nm23-H2 proteins survived considerably longer than did those patients whose tumors expressed neither protein *(557)*. Similarly, Iizuka et al. *(558)* found that the expression of *nm23-H1* mRNA and protein (but not the expression of *nm23-H2* mRNA) correlated inversely with the frequency of intrahepatic metastases, but not with tumor grade. However, Shimada et al. *(559)* found no differences in the expression of nm23-H1 protein among 13 patients with single intrahepatic HCC nodules, 7 patients with intrahepatic HCC satellite nodules, and 7 patients with metastases of HCC outside the liver; both the main HCC and the intrahepatic satellite nodules frequently overexpressed nm23-H1 protein. Among metastatic HCC, only one of 7 showed low expression of nm23-H1 protein, and in this instance the primary intrahepatic tumor also expressed nm23-H1 protein weakly *(559)*. These investigators concluded that nm23-H1 expression was not a reliable indicator of either intrahepatic or distant metastasis of HCC. Loss of one allele of the *nm23* gene was detected in 4/22 HCC (18%) *(378)*. Further definitive studies are needed to determine the role of *nm23* gene expression in HCC.

PTEN/MMAC1 Kawamura et al. *(560)* detected LOH of the *PTEN/MMAC1* gene located on chromosome 10q23 in 25/89 informative HCC (28%), and that somatic mutations involved 5/25 remaining alleles (20%). Mutations included three frame-shift mutations, a 1-bp deletion at codon 83–84 in exon 4, two 4-bp deletions located at codon 318–319 in exon 8, and two C to G transversion mutations at –9 bp from the initiation codon in the 5′-noncoding region of exon 1. The results indicate that combined LOH and intragenic mutation in different alleles in a fraction of HCC inactivate the *PTEN/MMAC1* gene. Yao et al. *(561)* sequenced the entire *PTEN/MMAC1* gene in 96 unselected HCC and identified mutations in three of them (3%): missense mutations in exon 5 (codon 144) and exon 7 (codon 255), and a putative splice site mutation in intron 3. They did not examine allelic loss of this locus in HCC.

Tg737 Isfort et al. *(562)* found tumor-specific deletions of exon 3, 5, 14, or 22 of the *Tg737* gene by PCR in 4/11 HCC

(36%), but not in adjacent nontumorous liver. The *Tg737* gene, which was first identified by positional cloning from a transgenic mouse line with autosomal recessive polycystic kidney disease, codes for a protein that can regulate proliferation and sporulation in fission yeast and is defective in HCC in rats *(562)*. However, Bonura et al. *(563)* failed to identify any alterations, including deletion or rearrangement, in the *Tg737* gene in 23 HCC or in normal liver tissue in humans using both PCR and Southern-blot analysis.

MAG Ljubimova et al. *(564)* identified a gene, which they termed *MAG* (for malignancy associated gene), that was expressed in 8/10 HCC (80%), in 2/2 macroregenerative nodules, and 16/16 cirrhotic livers, but in none of 4 normal livers. The *MAG* sequence contained a short stretch of homology with the c-*met* gene and a larger stretch homologous with the *ERCC2* gene cluster. MAG expression was also found in the liver during embryogenesis, as well as in several other neoplasms and their preneoplastic counterparts *(564)*.

MAGE/GAGE Family Members of the *MAGE* (melanoma antigen) and *GAGE* (T-cell antigen) gene family have been examined in HCC by several investigators. The *MAGE-1* gene was expressed in 43/65 HCC (66%), but in only 5/65 adjacent nontumorous liver tissues that were the sites of chronic hepatitis or cirrhosis (8%) *(565,566)*. Neither of two HCC smaller than 2 cm in diameter expressed *MAGE-1*, contrasted to 16/18 HCC larger than 2 cm (89%). However, correlation of *MAGE-1* expression with HCC differentiation was not found *(565)*. Kariyama et al. *(567)* found that *MAGE-1* mRNA (RT-PCR) was expressed in 25/33 HCC (77%) and *MAGE-3* mRNA was expressed in 14/33 HCC (42%); in agreement MAGE-1 protein was detected (immunoblot) in 12/15 HCC (80%) and MAGE-3 protein in 8/15 HCC (53%). Expression of MAGE-1 or MAGE-3 did not correlate with HCC differentiation or clinical stage. Similarly, expression of MAGE-1 or MAGE-4 was not correlated with any HCC growth characteristic other than portal-vein invasion *(568)*. Tahara et al. *(568)* studied the expression of all 12 members of the *MAGE-1* gene family in 22 HCC by PCR. *MAGE-1* and *MAGE-3* genes were expressed in approx 68% of HCC, *MAGE-8* in 46%, and *MAGE-2*, *MAGE-6*, *MAGE-10*, *MAGE-11*, and *MAGE-12* in about 30% each; 19/22 HCC (86%) expressed at least one *MAGE* gene. MAGE-3 protein was detected by immunoblot and immunohistochemistry in 11/22 HCC (50%).

Tsuzurahara et al. *(569)* found that levels of MAGE-4 protein were significantly elevated in sera of patients with HCV-related HCC and cirrhosis, as compared to controls; sera of patients with HCV-related HCC (n = 45) contained 2.2 ± 2.7 ng/mL (21/45 patients had serum levels > 1.04 ng/mL), sera of patients with HCV-related cirrhosis (n = 55) contained 1.1 ± 1.1 ng/mL (18/55 patients had serum levels > 1.04 ng/mL), and two groups of control patients each had 0.33 ± 0.24 ng/mL (n = 49) and 0.39 ± 0.33 ng/mL (n = 92). In contrast, serum levels of MAGE-4 protein did not differ from the controls in patients with cirrhosis or HCC related to HBV *(569)*. It is of interest that Tahara et al. *(568)* found that the majority of the patients whose HCC expressed either MAGE-1 or MAGE-4 proteins were HCV-positive and HBsAg-negative. *GAGE-1* and *GAGE-2*

mRNA were detected in 6/10 HCC by RT-PCR, but not in any of 10 nondiseased livers *(550)*.

HIP/PAP By differentially screening an HCC cDNA library, Lasserre et al. *(570)* found that transcription of the *HIP/PAP* gene was elevated in 7/29 HCC (24%), and they showed the gene to have significant homology with the human PSP/PTP/reg proteins, which are members of the C-type lectin family. In addition to HCC, the HIP/PAP protein was expressed by intestinal neuroendocrine and Paneth cells and by both islet and acinar cells of the pancreas, but not by non-neoplastic hepatocytes or other liver cells *(571)*. The gene was expressed by 10–50% of the neoplastic cells in 5 HCC and it was especially prominent in tumor cells that formed pseudoglands *(571)*. Recombinant HIP/PAP protein promoted the interaction of laminin and fibronectin but did not bind efficiently to collagens I or IV or to heparan sulfate proteoglycan *(571)*. Lasserre et al. *(572,573)* speculated that the HIP/PAP gene product may function as a growth promoter in HCC, because it appears to promote regeneration of pancreatic-islet cells.

DNA Transforming Activity Ochiya et al. *(574)* detected transforming activity in high molecular-weight DNA isolated from 4/11 HCC after transfecting the DNA into NIH 3T3 cells by calcium phosphate precipitation. The transforming activity was amplified in secondary assays of DNA isolated from the primarily transfected NIH 3T3 cells. DNA containing human *Alu* sequences was isolated from two of the secondary transfectants in rodent cells, and the restriction patterns of the two isolates appeared to be identical. The DNA cloned from one transfectant showed no analogy to known oncogenes by restriction analysis. Preliminary studies suggested that the human sequence came from a gene located on human chromosome 2, but a sequence analysis was not published, and no further studies of this presumptive HCC-related gene, called *lca*, have been found.

ABERRANT REGULATION OF APOPTOSIS

APOPTOTIC SIGNALING Cell death (apoptotic) signals are generated in multiple ways, including through the transcriptional actions of wild-type p53 (responding mainly to DNA damage) and c-myc, as well as through the binding of ligands to certain receptors on the cell surface. The major hepatocyte receptors that entrain cell-death signals include TNFR-1 and Fas, also known as CD95 and APO-1, in response to receptor occupancy by TNF-α and FasL, respectively. Apoptotic signaling involves complex intracellular molecular pathways, which include the Bcl2 class of molecules that either promote or inhibit this event. There have been comparatively few studies of cell-death signaling pathways in HCC and precursor lesions, but some of the results are provocative.

Fas AND FasL *Fas* is weakly expressed in nondiseased liver as detected by RT-PCR *(575–578)*, although detection of Fas on normal hepatocytes by immunohistochemistry has not been uniform. Hiramatsu et al. *(579)* and Mochizuki et al. *(580)* failed to detect Fas on hepatocytes in any of 18 HCC, but Strand et al. *(581)* found strong expression on 76–100% of the hepatocytes in 5 normal livers by *in situ* hybridization; the differences possibly reflect the different methods used. In any event, it is clear that Fas is strongly upregulated in patients with severe chronic hepatitis due to infection with either HCV (54/61 patients, 89%) *(579,582)* or HBV (26/28 patients, 92%) *(580),* and it was strongly and uniformly expressed on hepatocytes of 25 cirrhotic livers associated with HBV and HCV infections, and with ethanol abuse *(581).* Kubo et al. *(58)* also found strong expression of Fas on 23.2 ± 17.2% of the hepatocytes in 35 cirrhotic livers by immunohistochemistry. Fas expression was strongly downregulated in HCC as compared to the adjacent nontumorous livers, and was restricted to small, focal groups of neoplastic hepatocytes (42/66 HCC, 64%), or was lacking entirely (23/66 HCC, 35%) *(581,582).* Similarly, Fas was expressed on only 6.3 ± 8.8% of neoplastic cells in the study of Kubo et al. *(58)* as compared to 23.2 ± 17.2% of hepatocytes in adjacent liver tissue, and Shin et al. *(583)* also found that the expression of Fas transcripts was reduced in 6 HCC as compared to the surrounding liver using RNase protection assay.

In addition to loss of Fas, Strand et al. *(581)* and Nagao et al. *(582)* found that neoplastic hepatocytes in 26/66 HCC (39%) analyzed by *in situ* hybridization or immunohistochemistry had acquired the ability to express strongly the FasL; mature FasL proteins of 42 kDa and 40 kDa expressed by two *FasL* mRNA-positive HCC, but not by two *FasL* mRNA-negative HCC *(581).* Corroborating the expression of functional FasL by HCC cells, Strand et al. *(581)* also found that FasL-expressing HCC cells killed cytotoxic T lymphocytes on contact with the latter. They proposed that loss of expression of Fas and gain of expression of FasL by neoplastic hepatocytes rendered HCC less sensitive to damage by cytotoxic T lymphocytes *(581).* This hypothesis was supported by the studies of Nagao et al. *(582)* who found that patients with Fas-negative HCC had more frequent intrahepatic metastases and significantly shorter disease-free intervals after resection than did patients with Fas-positive HCC; in addition they demonstrated that patients with FasL-negative HCC also had shorter disease-free intervals after resection *(582).* Nagao et al. *(582)* also found that all of the Fas-negative cases of HCC were immunohistochemically positive for p53, whereas none of the Fas-negative HCC stained for p53; they proposed that p53 may have a role in regulating Fas expression.

Higher serum levels of soluble Fas (sFas) were detected in patients with cirrhosis or HCC than in control patients without these liver lesions *(582,584).* Jodo et al. *(584)* found that the mean serum level of sFas (measured by sandwich ELISA) among 59 healthy control patients was 0.29 ng/mL (range 0–4.9 ng/mL), as compared to 2.2 ng/mL (range 0.24–8.4 ng/mL) for 27 cirrhotic patients and 4.1 ng/mL (0.14–29.2 ng/mL) for 61 patients with HCC. Serum sFas levels were significantly higher in HCC patients with multiple rather than single tumor nodules, and resection of single tumor nodules was followed by a rapid decline in serum sFas. Nagao et al. *(582)* corroborated these relative differences in serum levels of sFas in cirrhosis and HCC, and showed that the sFas was produced by HCC cells that contained a truncated *sFas* gene (RF-PCR), and not by circulating lymphocytes. Both Jodo et al. *(584)* and Nagao et al. *(582)* suggested that sFas might block the Fas/FasL system by neutralizing FasL, and thereby facilitate the escape of HCC cells from immune surveillance.

Taken together, the results of these studies suggest that loss of expression of Fas, increased expression of sFas, and gain of expression of FasL by neoplastic hepatocytes, in combination, allow many HCC to escape from surveillance by cytotoxic T lymphocytes. Escape from immune surveillance may play a major role in the progression of HCC. However, less decisive results were found by Kubo et al. *(58)* who detected both Fas and FasL by immunohistochemistry in 35 HCC and adjacent nontumorous tissues, and by Shin et al. *(583)* who found transcripts for *Fas, FasL, TNFR1,* and several downstream death signal-transduction molecules in 6 HCC and adjacent nontumorous tissue using RNase-protection assays. Both of these studies found that *Fas* expression was reduced in HCC, in agreement with Strand et al. *(581)* and Nagao et al. *(582),* but unlike several other investigators both Kubo et al. *(58)* and Shin et al. *(583)* detected FasL in adjacent nontumorous livers, as well as in HCC. Kubo et al. *(58)* claimed that FasL was expressed by 8.5 ± 8.3% of cirrhotic hepatocytes, whereas the studies of Shin et al. *(583)* were not capable of localizing FasL to specific cells. It is possible that in both of these studies, the cytotoxic T lymphocytes infiltrating cirrhotic livers that were infected by HBV or HCV were the sources of FasL in the nontumorous livers. Shin et al. *(583)* found that the several molecules in the signal-transduction pathways from Fas and TNFR1 were also expressed in HCC and in adjacent nontumorous liver tissue, although the level of expression of these molecules was not quantified.

Sugimoto et al. *(585)* detected CD40, a transmembrane glycoprotein of the TNFR family that lacks death domains, by immunohistochemistry in 27/45 HCC (60%) but not in any of 25 livers the site of chronic hepatitis or cirrhosis, and in none of 5 nondiseased livers. Studies in HCC cell lines in vitro showed that CD40 expression protected cells from apoptosis induced by TNF-α or antibody to Fas. Sugimoto et al. *(585)* suggested that expression of CD40 protected HCC cells from immune attack by increasing their resistance to apoptosis mediated by TNFR and Fas pathways.

Lee et al. *(586)* detected both Fas and FasL in each of 23 HBL by immunohistochemistry. Simultaneously, 20/23 HBL expressed *sFas* (detected by RT-PCR), which might help protect HBL cells from self-inflicted killing by occupying FasL sites *(586).* Expression of Fas-associated phosphatase, which interacts with the suppressive domain of Fas, by 19/23 HBL was interpreted as supporting their hypothesis *(586).*

Bcl2 The antiapoptotic molecule, Bcl2, was not expressed (immunohistochemistry) by hepatocytes in either normal livers *(587–589),* or in chronic hepatitis *(589,590).* Bcl2 was focally expressed in hepatocytes of 10/22 cirrhotic livers (45%) *(589,590),* but in only 8/107 HCC (7%) *(251,582,587,588,590);* it was more strongly expressed in 7/12 HCC (58%), which were treated by transcatheter chemoembolization and which were presumably under oxidative stress *(257).* The antiapoptotic molecule Bcl-X$_L$ was also expressed weakly in cirrhotic livers *(589).* Metallothionein was detected in 11/13 HCC (85%) *(591),* suggesting that HCC tumor cells are relatively more protected against free-radical injury than are hepatocytes in the adjacent nontumorous liver tissue. Bcl2 was not expressed in any of 23 HBL *(586).* These incomplete results suggest that the Bcl2 class of molecules may not play a major role in the development of HCC, but further studies are needed.

ABERRANT REGULATION OF CELLULAR DIFFERENTIATION

The hepatocyte-enriched nuclear factors (HNF) are transcription factors that in combination are responsible for determining the differentiated phenotypes expressed by hepatocytes. Only two studies have examined the expression of HNF1α and HNF1β in HCC. In addition to HNF-1, hepatocytes express several other hepatocyte-enriched transcription factors, including HNF-3, HNF-4, HNF-6, and C/EBP isoforms. The expression of these other hepatocyte differentiation factors has not yet been investigated in HCC.

The ratio of expressed HNF1α and HNF1β correlated with the differentiation of HCC: among 37 HCC the ratios of $HNF1\alpha$ to $HNF1\beta$ mRNA (as measured by RT-PCR) varied from 100 to 0.01; two grade I HCC expressed a ratio of $HNF1\alpha$ to $HNF1\beta$ of 100; 4 HCC, one grade I, two grade I–II, and one grade II expressed $HNF1\alpha$ to $HNF1\beta$ ratios of 10; 16 HCC, all grade II, expressed $HNF1\alpha$ to $HNF1\beta$ ratios of 1.0; 12 HCC, one grade II, one grade II-III, 9 grade III, and one grade III–IV, expressed $HNF1\alpha$ to $HNF1\beta$ ratios of 0.1; and 3 HCC, one grade III, and two grade IV, expressed $HNF1\alpha$ to $HNF1\beta$ ratios of 0.01 (592). These results, indicating that ratios of HNF1α to HNF1β expressed by HCC are highly correlated with tumor differentiation, were supported by a study of 28 HCC, which showed that the level of HNF1α (detected by Western blot) in tumors, relative to the level expressed in adjacent nontumorous tissue, reflected the HCC differentiation grade; in 12 grade I HCC, the ratio of HNF1α in tumors to that in adjacent nontumor tissue was 1.9 ± 0.43; in 8 grade II HCC, it was 0.66 ± 0.29; in 6 grade III HCC, it was 0.41 ± 0.20; and in two grade IV HCC, it was 0.18 ± 0.12 (585). Among well-differentiated HCC, 8/12 (66%) stained strongly for HNF1α by immunohistochemistry, whereas only 1 of 12 (8%) stained for HNF1β; among moderately differentiated HCC, 1 of 8 (12%) stained for HNF1α, whereas 2 of 8 (25%) stained for HNF1β; and among 8 poorly differentiated HCC none stained for HNF1a, whereas 2 of 8 (25%) stained for HNF1β (593).

Kishimoto et al. (594) identified a new b-Zip transcription factor, which they termed HTF, in normal liver and found it to be upregulated by 1.8–3.4-fold in HCC. They speculated that HTF has a specific role in predicating the phenotypic properties of normal hepatocytes, and that aberrant expression may play a role in hepatocarcinogenesis.

ABERRANT REGULATION OF TELOMERES

TELOMERE DYNAMICS Chromosome ends, telomeres, are capped by $(TTAGGG)_n$ sequences repeated up to several hundred times. Telomeric DNA is not replicated completely by a cell's DNA synthesis machinery during S phase, but requires a special molecular complex, which consists of template RNA, telomerase reverse transcriptase (which includes the hTERT catalytic subunit that regulates overall activity of the complex), and telomerase-associated protein (595,596). The overall synthetic activity of this molecular complex is termed telomerase. Functional telomerase is not expressed by somatic cells in normal human tissues, including normal liver (597–601), and as a consequence telomeres shorten by a few hundred kilobases each time a normal human somatic-cell cycles. Complete erosion of telomeres causes chromosome ends to be sticky (analogous to a double strand break; dsb), and may provide the basis for structural rearrangements of affected chromosomes. Telomere erosion, which facilitates the development of aneuploidy, coupled with re-expression of telomerase, which enables affected cells to become immortal, may have critical roles in the development of cancer in many tissues, including the liver.

Telomerase Telomerase activity (measured by the terminal repeat assay protocol (TRAP) assay with or without an internal standard) was expressed weakly in 30/128 (23%) nontumorous livers that were the sites of chronic hepatitis or cirrhosis and located adjacent to HCC (595,597,599–602), but it was expressed strongly in 143/159 HCC (90%) accumulated from several individual studies (595,597,598–601,603). Hisatomi et al. (602) measured hTERT mRNA by PCR and showed that it correlated closely with telomerase activity. The fraction of HCC that expressed high levels of either telomerase or hTERT included 26/37 well-differentiated tumors (70%), 53/58 moderately differentiated tumors (91%), and 22/22 poorly differentiated tumors (100%) (596–598,601,602).

Several studies have attempted to quantitate the telomerase assay. Nakashio et al. (601) used a semiquantitative TRAP assay with an internal standard to quantify amounts of protein extracted from frozen liver tissues, normalizing the relative level of telomerase expressed by liver tissue to the number of cell equivalents of cultured gastric cells (MKN-1 cells, which express high levels of telomerase). They found that none of 25 adjacent liver tissues that included normal livers and chronic liver diseases expressed telomerase activity at greater than the equivalent activity expressed by 10 MKN-1 cell-equivalents/ 0.6 mg of liver tissue protein, whereas 32/37 HCC (86%) expressed telomerase at levels greater than this value, some HCC expressing telomerase as high as >200 MKN-1 cell-equivalents/0.6 mg protein (601).

Kojima et al. (604) applied a semiquantitative telomerase assay normalized to expression in cultured HeLa cells, with the activity in 1000 HeLa cells equivalent to 100 arbitrary telomerase units (ATU); telomerase activities in HeLa cells were proportional between 20 and 2000 cells. Eleven cirrhotic livers without HCC expressed 0.41 ± 0.50 ATU/6 µg of liver tissue protein, 27 nontumorous liver tissues adjacent to HCC expressed 4.5 ± 7.4 ATU/6 µg protein, and 24 HCC less than 3 cm in diameter expressed 140.6 ± 195.9 ATU/6 µg protein; 4 adenomatous hyperplasias expressed 5.5 ± 4.5 ATU/6 µg protein (604).

Nakashio et al. (601) found that the relative level of telomerase activity was correlated inversely with differentiation: 15 well-differentiated tumors expressed the equivalent of 31.3 ± 30.4 MKN-1 cell equivalents/0.6 mg of liver-tissue protein, whereas 17 moderately differentiated tumors expressed 92.2 ± 78.3 MKN-1 cell equivalents/0.6 mg protein, and 5 poorly differentiated tumors expressed 125.8 ± 45.7 MKN-1 cell equivalents/0.6 mg protein. Kojima et al. (599) found that 10 well-differentiated HCC (grades 1 and II) expressed 139.8 ± 209.6 ATU/6 µg protein, while 4 moderately differentiated

HCC expressed 119.2 ± 174.6 ATU/6 μg protein and 2 poorly differentiated HCC expressed 144 ± 80.ATU/6 μg protein. These observations suggest that telomerase is re-expressed at an early step in the process of hepatocarcinogenesis and that it is involved in tumor progression. Supporting the opinion that telomerase reactivation occurs as an early step in hepatocarcinogenesis, 9/12 (75%) high-grade dysplastic nodules dissected from cirrhotic livers adjacent to HCC also expressed telomerase *(600,603)*.

Ogami et al. *(605)* evaluated the relative amount of *telomerase* mRNA (by RT-PCR with internal control and normalized to *β-actin* mRNA) in 5 nondiseased livers, 41 livers the site of chronic hepatitis or cirrhosis, and 23 HCC; in addition they localized the cellular sites of *telomerase* mRNA in tissue sections by *in situ* RT-PCR. The mean relative telomerase mRNA level was about 10-fold greater in HCC than in chronic hepatitis and cirrhosis, and about 100-fold greater in HCC than in nondiseased liver; *telomerase* mRNA increased progressively in moderately and poorly differentiated HCC as compared to well-differentiated tumors. Intense signal for *telomerase* mRNA was localized by *in situ* PCR to many HCC tumor-cell nuclei, with the highest fraction of positive nuclei in poorly differentiated HCC; in contrast, the *telomerase* mRNA signal was localized predominantly to endothelial cells and infiltrating lymphocytes in livers without disease or that were affected by chronic hepatitis and cirrhosis, involving only occasional bile-duct epithelial cells or hepatocytes *(605)*. These results provide additional support for the opinion that telomerase is newly expressed in neoplastic hepatocytes and increases with HCC progression.

In agreement with the observation that telomerase activity increased with HCC progression, Suda et al. *(606)* found that HCC that recurred earliest after surgical resection were those that had the highest relative levels of telomerase activity. They used a fluorescence-based telomeric-repeat assay quantified by serial dilution, and incorporating an internal standard. Relative telomerase activity in the HCC of 9 patients whose tumors recurred within 15 mo following resection was 36.4 ± 27.8 arbitrary units, whereas in 11 patients whose HCC recurred later than 15 mo after resection the relative telomerase activity was 9.8 ± 7.7 arbitrary units *(606)*.

Telomere Length Data accumulated from several individual studies indicate that telomere lengths shorten progressively during the period of heightened cell proliferation that occurs in chronic liver diseases where telomerase in not expressed or is only weakly expressed, reaching a nadir in length in HCC: telomeres measured 8.3 ± 1.5 kb in 17 normal livers, 7.9 ± 1.9 kb in 45 chronic hepatitides, 6.4 ± 1.2 kb in 59 cirrhoses, and 5.3 ± 2.4 kb in 73 HCC *(597,599,600,607–610)*. Isokawa et al. *(611)* measured telomere repeat content (TRC) by blotting extracted genomic DNA with a radiolabeled $d(TTAGGG)_3$ probe, normalized to a $d(CCT)_7$ probe. The results from this methodology correlated well with telomere lengths measured through conventional means. In 7 nondiseased livers the TRC ratio was 1.07 ± 0.075, as compared to 0.89 ± 0.15 in 10 livers the site of chronic hepatitis, 0.66 ± 0.15 in 20 nontumorous liver tissues adjacent to HCC, and 0.69 ± 0.31 in 20 HCC. Although shortened in HCC, telom-

ere lengths were stable and did not change with tumor-differentiation grade of HCC *(599,600,607,608)*, perhaps reflecting the comparatively high levels of telomerase in all grades of HCC.

These results show that hepatocyte telomeres shorten significantly before HCC develops, that high levels of telomerase are re-expressed in dysplastic nodules during the pre-neoplastic phase, that high levels are maintained in HCC, and that telomeres are maintained in a shortened, but apparently stable, configuration as HCC progress.

LOSS OF GENOMIC INTEGRITY

MICROSATELLITE INSTABILITY Instability of microsatellite sequences, thought to reflect mismatch repair (MMR) deficiency, may be responsible for some of the gene mutation and LOH that occurs in HCC. Deficiency in MMR functions, associated with deletions, frameshifts, base substitutions, and small rearrangements in the microsatellite sequences of genes are reflected in alterations in their structures. Microsatellites are repetitive nucleotide sequences that are dispersed throughout both coding and noncoding regions of the human genome, occurring as dinucleotide, trinucleotide, and tetranucleotide repeats most frequently *(612)*. Evaluation of microsatellite sequence structure appears to provide a relatively sensitive and accurate method to assess the general mutability of the genome and it affords an efficient method to detect LOH. For certain neoplasms, exemplified by hereditary nonpolyposis colon cancer, elevated instability of microsatellite sequences reflects both germline and acquired defects in the MMR genes (especially *hMSH2* and *hMLH1*), conferring a mutator or replication error phenotype on the cells of affected individuals *(613)*.

Several studies have examined the status of selected MMR genes and MSI in HCC. MacDonald et al. *(468)* detected LOH of the *hMSH2* gene in 6/46 HCC (13%) and of the *hMLH1* gene in 9/46 HCC (20%), and both genes had lost one allele in 5/6 HCC that contained LOH of the *hMSH2* locus. Although the functional status of the remaining MMR gene allele was not determined in this study, examination of instability at 16 microsatellite loci showed that MSI involved at least one microsatellite locus in 16/46 HCC (36%) *(468)*. MSI was significantly greater in the cases that contained MMR gene LOH. Among 9 HCC with LOH of *hMSH2* and/or *hMLH1*, the number of unstable microsatellite loci ranged from 0.77–2.33 band shifts/microdomain, whereas among the 36 HCC that lacked LOH of *hMSH2* and/or *hMLH1* loci the number of unstable microsatellite loci averaged much less than 1.0 band shift/microdomain *(468)*. Nevertheless, LOH of the *APC* (3/45 HCC, 7%), *p53* (6/45 HCC, 13%), and *DCC* (2/45 HCC, 4%) loci did not correlate with LOH of MMR genes *(468)*, suggesting that LOH in these genes arose by a different mechanism. However, Yano et al. *(500)* found a correlation between mutation of either the *hMSH2* gene or the *p53* gene and instability involving 5 microsatellite loci among 38 HCC. As determined by direct sequencing, the *hMSH2* gene was mutated in 7/38 HCC (18%) and the *p53* gene was mutated in 6/38 HCC (16%), with no tumors containing mutations in both genes simultaneously. Among the HCC with mutations involving either the *hMSH2* or *p53* genes, 8/13 (62%) showed MSI (as indicated by a shift in at least 1/5 microsatellite loci examined), as compared to 5/25 (20%) of the HCC without these mutations. Mutations in either the *p53* or *hMSH2* genes were significantly associated with both poor survival and impaired disease-free survival after resection of HCC *(500)*.

Han et al. *(614)* examined four microsatellite loci on chromosomes 2, 3, and 17, including the *p53* locus, in 29 HCC and found that only the microsatellite locus in the *p53* gene was unstable in one tumor (3%). Kazachkov et al. *(615)* examined 9 microsatellite loci on chromosomes 2, 4, 17, and 18 in 10 HCC, and showed that in 4 HCC (40%) at least one microsatellite locus was unstable; 5 of these 10 HCC also contained multiple alterations in intronic and exonic sequences of the *p53* gene, but only one of them also showed MSI, suggesting that defective MMR could have been responsible for only 20% of the mutated *p53* genes. In a study in which 10 microsatellite loci were examined, Takagi et al. *(616)* found MSI in only 2/34 solitary HCC (6%) as compared to 4/14 HCC (29%) that formed multiple intrahepatic nodules; the *p53* gene contained an unstable microsatellite locus in neither of the two solitary HCC, but it was involved in all 4 of the multiple HCC *(616)*. In a study of MSI in patients with multiple synchronous cancers, which included four HCC, three HCC showed instability of one to four of the five microsatellite loci examined *(617)*. Kawate et al. *(279)* detected no MSI in 30 HCC by examining 5 microsatellite loci located on chromosomes 3, 13, 17, and 18, and Rashid et al. *(470)* found no MSI among 24 HCC in which 24 microsatellite loci on chromosomes 1, 4, 13, 16, and 17 were analyzed. Bonilla et al. *(405)* detected MSI in the region of the *p16INK4A* gene on chromosome 9p21-p24 in 4/14 HCC (29%). Yakushiji et al. *(618)* examined MSI in 5 cancers of a single patient who developed, either synchronously or metachronously, primary neoplasms in 6 different organs, including an HCC. All of the tumors were MSI-positive at multiple microsatellite loci; the HCC showed MSI at 7/10 loci examined, including loci on chromosomes 2, 3, 13, and 17, and in the *TGFβRII*, *M6P/IGF-2R*, and *BAX* genes *(618)*.

In their comprehensive allelotype studies of 82 HCC with 231–235 microsatellite probes, Boige et al. *(619)* and Sheu et al. *(620)* noted that most HCC exhibited MSI at a small number of loci. Boige et al. *(619)* found that the ratio of unstable microsatellite loci to the total number of loci examined averaged 0.13/HCC and ranged from none to 0.14/HCC. Sheu et al. *(620)* found that microsatellite loci detected by 12/231 markers (5%) were unstable, and that at least one microsatellite locus was unstable in 9/34 HCC (26%). Salvucci et al. *(280)* analyzed microsatellite stability in 46 HCC and adjacent nontumorous tissue, examining 8 microsatellite loci located on chromosomes 2p, 3p, 4q, 5q, 9p, 13q, 16q, and 17p, including a locus within the *hMSH2* gene. MSI was detected in at least two loci in HCC and/or adjacent nontumor liver tissue in 19/46 patients (41%), and an additional 10 patients (22%) showed instability of one microsatellite locus *(280)*. Loci on chromosome 16 were most frequently abnormal (19/46, 41%), followed by those on chromosomes 9 (9/46, 20%) and 5 (8/46, 17%) *(277)*. Kondo et al. *(621)* examined 29 microsatellite loci located on chromosomes 1, 2, 3, 4, 5, 6, 9, 10, 16, 17, 18, 19, 21, and X in 38 HCC, detecting MSI in 4 (14%).

MacDonald et al. *(468)* detected LOH of *hMSH2* and/or *hMLH1* gene loci in one benign HCA and in the nontumorous tissue adjacent to HCC or HCA in 4/9 instances (44%) in which the neoplasms also showed LOH of these loci. Salvucci et al. *(280)* also found that the adjacent nontumor tissue contained unstable microsatellite loci in 26/29 patients (90%) whose HCC were MSI-positive. The microsatellite rearrangements observed in the tumor and adjacent tissues were identical in 38% of these patients, suggesting that the HCC had developed from MSI-positive preneoplastic cells *(280)*. Progressive involvement of additional microsatellite loci during HCC development was suggested by their observation that for the 19 HCC that contained aberrations in two or more microsatellite sequences, the adjacent nontumorous tissue usually had no more than one aberrant locus *(280)*. Only rearrangement of the *D16S402* locus on chromosome 16 was associated with shortened survival *(280)*.

Salvucci et al. *(622)* also found that MSI affected hepatocytes in cirrhotic livers lacking HCC, especially in cirrhosis associated with HBV infection. Examination of microsatellite loci on chromosomes 2p, 3p, 5q, 9p, 13q, and 17p showed that in 23/38 cirrhotic livers (60%) at least one locus was unstable, including 16/18 cirrhotic livers (89%) from patients with hepatitis due to HBV, 4/10 cirrhotic livers (40%) due to HCV, and 3/10 cirrhotic livers (30%) due to chronic alcoholism *(622)*. Supporting these observations, Tsopanomichalou et al. *(471)* detected MSI in 8/22 livers the site of chronic hepatitis (36%) and 8/11 cirrhotic livers (73%) in studies examining 19 microsatellite loci on chromosomes 1, 9, and 7.

Among all of the studies reviewed, MSI was detected in at least one microsatellite locus in 90/362 HCC (25%) *(279,280,405,468,470,500,614–618,620,621)*. These results suggest that multiple HCC are more likely to develop in patients who have MSI as evidence of MMR deficiency than in those who do not. A significant fraction of HCC may develop in patients who have some extent of MMR deficiency in nontumorous liver, and who express what amounts to a mutator phenotype *(613)*. MSI appears to precede the development of HCC in some instances because it has been identified in 24/29 cirrhotic livers not the site of HCC (83%) *(471,622)*, and in 30/38 nontumorous liver tissues adjacent to HCC (79%) *(280,468)*.

MINISATELLITE ALTERATIONS In addition to the analysis of microsatellite sequences in HCC, longer repeated sequences, minisatellites, have also been examined. Minisatellites are tandemly repeated noncoding sequences of up to about 100 bp; they exhibit extreme polymorphism and high rates of mutation and recombination, and are predominantly located terminally in the genome *(612)*. Minisatellite patterns are unique to individuals and form a basis for DNA fingerprinting. Kaplanski et al. *(623)* examined 26 HCC with two multilocus minisatellite probes (designated 33.15 and 33.6), detecting rearrangements in 11/26 (42%) and 12/26 (46%) HCC, respectively. Tumor and nontumor fingerprints were identical in 12/26 instances, but in 14/26 (54%) the patterns of HCC DNA differed distinctively from that of the nonneoplastic tissue *(623)*. Somatic rearrangements observed included increased and decreased band densities and disappearance of bands, as well as the appearance of new bands;

among about 600 bands, approx 4% were rearranged in HCC *(623)*. Using single-locus probes, rearrangements were identified at 1p33-p35 in 23% of HCC, at 7q36-qter in 19%, and at 12q24.3-qter in 15%, and no association was found between any rearrangements and HBV integration or tumor size. In the 14 HCC that contained rearranged minisatellite loci, rearrangements of 1p33-p35 were identified in well to moderately differentiated HCC, whereas rearrangements at sites other than 1p33-p35 predominated in more poorly differentiated HCC *(623)*.

Aihara et al. *(80)* used the same minisatellite multilocus probes to fingerprint the DNA in 10 dysplastic nodules and 9 HCC. Six of the 10 dysplastic nodules (60%) and 6/9 HCC (67%) showed multiple band alterations with one or both probes, as compared to the non-neoplastic liver tissue *(80)*. Additionally LOH were detected with single-locus probes in one of 10 dysplastic nodules (chromosome 7p22-pter) and 2/9 HCC (chromosome 1p33-p35 and 12q24.3-qter). Divergence of the DNA fingerprints from the constitutional pattern was considered to indicate that both dysplastic nodules and HCC were monoclonal, because distinct band changes would not be detectable by Southern blotting unless the vast majority of cells in these lesions contained the same genetic alterations *(80)*. This opinion was supported by the finding that the lesions occurring in female patients were monoclonal as determined by the random inactivation of the X chromosome-linked *phosphoglycerokinase* gene *(80)*. Occurrence of extensive rearrangements in dysplastic nodules suggests that genetic instability and the accumulation of genetic aberrations began before HCC emerged.

Direct evidence of a general increase in mutation frequency in patients with chronic hepatitis, cirrhosis, and HCC, was found in a study of hemizygous and homozygous variants of the *glycophorin A* membrane component of erythrocytes from 20 patients with chronic hepatitis and cirrhosis and 30 patients with HCC, as compared to 21 healthy controls *(624)*. The hemizygous variant of *glycophorin A* was detected in $5.9 \pm 3.1 \times 10^{-6}$ control erythrocytes, compared to $7.3 \pm 4.6 \times 10^{-6}$ of the erythrocytes from patients with chronic hepatitis and cirrhosis, and $16.9 \pm 14.5 \times 10^{-6}$ of those with HCC; homozygous variants occurred in $6.3 \pm 14.5 \times 10^{-6}$ of the control erythrocytes, $8.7 \pm 6.7 \times 10^{-6}$ of the erythrocytes of patients with chronic hepatitis and cirrhosis, and $20.5 \pm 19.1 \times 10^{-6}$ of the erythrocytes of patients with HCC *(624)*. In patients who acquired HCV infection from blood transfusion, the frequency of both types of *glycophorin A* variants increased in direct proportion to the length of time following the transfusion *(624)*.

These results show that a significantly increased mutation frequency involves at least one nonhepatic indicator locus in patients with HCC, but it is not certain that this is a general phenomenon that affects multiple genes. However, in general agreement with these observations, Wu et al. *(625)* found that cultured lymphocytes collected from 28 patients with HCC were more sensitive to the induction of chromatid breaks by in vitro exposure to either bleomycin (BLEO) or benzo(a)pyrene diol epoxide (BPDE) than were lymphocytes collected from matched control patients lacking HCC. Among HCC patients, 68% showed ≥ 0.68 breaks/cell on exposure to BLEO and 80% showed ≥ 0.58 breaks/cell on exposure to BPDE, compared to

27 and 22% for healthy control patients, respectively *(625)*. Sensitivity to chromatid damage from either BLEO or BPDE was associated with increased risk to HCC, with odds ratios of 5.63 and 14.13, respectively; sensitivity to both BLEO and BPDE increased the odds ratio to 35.88. These results provide strong experimental support for host constitutional factors that affect susceptibility to gene mutation and HCC. It is also of interest that Simon et al. *(626)* found that the lymphocytes of persons chronically infected with HBV had a significantly higher incidence of chromosome aberrations than did the lymphocytes of noninfected controls.

ALLELIC LOSSES Loss of function of both alleles of a tumor-suppressor gene is a critical step in the molecular pathogenesis of cancer. Loss of gene function may result from the loss of both alleles (homozygous deletion) or from the loss of one allele coupled with the inactivation of the remaining allele by mutation, hypermethylation, and/or other possible mechanisms. Loss of gene function may occur even when one healthy allele remains through the mechanism of haploinsufficiency. Furthermore, loss of the one functional allele of imprinted genes would be sufficient to abolish the function of that gene unless the LOH was accompanied LOI of the suppressed allele.

Homozygous deletion is relatively uncommon in HCC even for tumor-suppressor genes that are frequently involved by a combination of LOH and mutation. Homozygous deletion of the *M6P/IGFIIR* gene was identified in only 5/34 HCC (18%) *(223)*, whereas about 60% of HCC examined contained LOH at this locus *(222–226)*. Similarly, the *p16^{INK4A}* gene demonstrated LOH in 67/183 HCC (37%) *(395–400,402–405)*, whereas homozygous deletion of the gene was detected in only 32/300 HCC (11%) *(395–397,399,400,402–404)*. Although LOH of the *p53* gene was identified in 258/675 HCC (38%) *(354,375,415,417–419,424,431,444,449,451–470)*, homozygous deletion was reported in only 1/37 (3%) *(431,449)*.

Detection of the loss of one allele of a gene requires that the two alleles be distinguishable by polymorphic structural differences. In this circumstance, loss of one allele can be detected by LOH. Allelic heterozygosity was initially examined by Southern hybridization with DNA probes after cutting the extracted DNA with a restriction enzyme to disclose restriction fragment length polymorphisms (RFLP) that distinguished the two alleles *(627)*. This technique is handicapped by the relatively small number of restriction fragment length polymorphisms (RFLP) probes available, by the generally low frequency of allelic heterozygosity of RFLP loci (around 20%), and by the relatively large amount of DNA required for Southern hybridization. Detection of LOH was revolutionized by the discovery of microsatellite sequences, which are multiallelic and have a frequency of allelic heterozygosity that approaches 70% *(612)*. Using primers located adjacent to particular microsatellite sequences, multiple loci can be typed allelically by PCR with small amounts of DNA from tumor samples.

Microsatellite PCR has been used to generate three comprehensive allelotypes of more than 250 HCC *(619,620,628)*, covering the 39 nonacrocentric autosomal arms with 195–275 microsatellite probes located about every 20 cM or less throughout the entire autosomal genome. Additionally, Piao et al. *(629)* examined the 39 nonacrocentric autosomal arms of 22 HCC with 68 microsatellite probes to generate a less dense allelotype.

Table 1
Fraction of Allelic Losses in HCC by Chromosome Arm

arm	Chromosome informative cases	HCC/ probes used	Number of FAL	Reference
1p	48/48	>9	0.44	(619)
	120/~85	9	0.51	(628)
	22/22	2	0.23	(629)
	19-26/6-19	13	0.63	(469)
	30/9-27	11	0.30	(633)
	6/6	7	0.70	(632)
	104/89	3	0.33	(420)
	24/9-19	3	0.46	(470)
	56/42	2	0.31	(467)
	46/22	2	0.10	(453)
	16/13	1	0.08	(452)
	63/50	1	0.30	(482)
	11/9	1	0.00	(459)
	32/18	1	0.11	(546)
1q	48/48	>7	0.23	(619)
	120/~85	7	0.44	(628)
	22/22	4	0.68	(629)
	16/4-8	2	0.32	(452)
	12/8	1	0.00	(631)
	7/0	1	0.00	(527)
	46/20	1	0.20	(453)
	14/4	1	0.00	(630)
	23/14	1	0.00	(546)
2p	48/48	>6	0.08	(619)
	120/~85	6	<0.20	(628)
	22/11	1	0.00	(629)
	46/9	2	0.00	(453)
	11/5	1	0.00	(631)
	14/4	1	0.00	(630)
2q	48/48	>8	0.08	(619)
	120/~85	8	0.35	(628)
	22/18	2	0.00	(629)
	46/18	1	0.00	(453)
	6/1	1	0.00	(546)
3p	48/48	>6	0.23	(619)
	120/~85	6	<0.20	(628)
	22/22	3	0.18	(629)
	18/18	2	0.00	(549)
	46/20	1	0.10	(453)
	29/24	1	0.08	(378)
	23/1	1	0.00	(459)
	35/14	1	0.07	(546)
3q	48/48	>7	0.17	(619)
	120/~85	7	<0.20	(628)
	22/21	2	0.14	(629)
	46/7	1	0.00	(453)
	14/6	1	0.00	(630)
4p	48/48	>3	0.08	(619)
	120/~85	3	<0.20	(628)
	22/9	1	0.22	(629)
	11/2-4	4	0.09	(631)
	46/4	1	0.00	(453)
	25/19	1	0.21	(419)
	56/9	1	0.22	(418)
	19/6	1	0.33	(417)
	14/5	1	0.20	(630)
	35/13	1	0.15	(546)
4q	48/48	>10	0.44	(619)
	120/~85	10	0.52	(628)
	22/22	4	0.73	(629)

Table 1(*cont.*)

Chromosome arm	HCC/ informative cases	Number of probes used	FAL	Reference
	41/11-34	43	0.83	(637)
	96/8-43	39	0.74	(638)
	42/14-24	13	0.77	(634)
	30/18-30	9	0.50	(636)
	11/2-5	6	0.78	(631)
	24/14-17	5	0.50	(470)
	24/18-19	3	0.46	(469)
	104/76	2	0.28	(465)
	12/7-8	2	0.14	(635)
	56/34	2	0.21	(467)
	19/5-6	2	0.17	(471)
	16/8	1	0.00	(452)
	46/20	1	0.14	(453)
	63/21	1	0.43	(482)
	35/4	1	0.00	(546)
5p	48/47	>3	0.15	(619)
	120/~85	3	<0.20	(628)
	22/15	1	0.07	(629)
	16/8	1	0.38	(452)
5q	48/48	>8	0.15	(619)
	120/~85	8	<0.20	(628)
	22/21	3	0.29	(629)
	16/8-10	3	0.50	(452)
	9/3-6	3	0.66	(527)
	46/9-10	2	0.44	(453)
	63/45	2	0.31	(482)
	29/25	2	0.20	(378)
	46/19-27	2	0.00	(529)
	25/19	1	0.05	(419)
	24/14	1	0.14	(469)
	24/2	1	0.00	(459)
6p	48/48	>6	0.06	(619)
	120/~85	6	<0.20	(628)
	22/13	1	0.08	(629)
	46/13	1	0.08	(453)
6q	48/48	>7	0.35	(619)
	120/~85	7	0.48	(628)
	22/11	1	0.27	(629)
	46/13-22	2	0.08	(453)
	11/12	1	0.00	(631)
	27/16	1	0.68	(222)
	41/3	1	0.66	(223)
	42/22	1	0.05	(225)
	27/18	1	0.61	(224)
	26/13	1	0.00	(546)
7p	48/48	>5	0.08	(619)
	120/~85	5	0.28	(628)
	22/19	1	0.11	(629)
	11/4	1	0.00	(631)
	46/10	1	0.00	(453)
	16/11	1	0.09	(452)
7q	48/48	>6	0.02	(619)
	120/~85	6	0.28	(628)
	24/12	1	0.05	(629)
	46/28	1	0.00	(452)
	16/10	1	0.11	(453)
	22/20	1	0.00	(469)
	14/11	1	0.00	(630)
	25/15	1	0.07	(546)
8p	48/48	>5	0.60	(619)

Table 1(*cont.*)

Chromosome arm	HCC/ informative cases	Number of probes used	FAL	Reference
	120/~85	5	0.40	*(628)*
	22/22	3	0.64	*(629)*
	109/22-88	40	0.60	*(641)*
	41/11-36	37	0.88	*(645)*
	142/15-87	18	0.45	*(640)*
	102/95	14	0.41	*(641)*
	102/5-89	5	0.40	*(639)*
	37/14-20	2	0.85	*(642)*
	48/?	2	0.04	*(650)*
	14/13	2	0.54	*(644)*
	63/33	1	0.42	*(482)*
	104/72	1	0.32	*(465)*
	56/40	1	0.18	*(467)*
	16/16	1	0.44	*(652)*
8q	48/48	>3	0.15	*(619)*
	120/~85	3	0.26	*(628)*
	22/22	4	0.77	*(629)*
	37/20-21	2	0.37	*(642)*
	29/24	2	0.33	*(378)*
	142/37	1	0.00	*(640)*
	46/20	1	0.20	*(453)*
	20/16	1	0.00	*(469)*
9p	48/48	>4	0.30	*(619)*
	120/~85	4	0.33	*(628)*
	22/13	1	0.23	*(629)*
	48/14-40	9	0.60	*(400)*
	23/9-21	8	0.44	*(404)*
	41/22-27	8	0.51	*(396)*
	17/14	4	0.00	*(405)*
	62/28	2	0.18	*(402)*
	26/15	1	0.20	*(398)*
9q	48/48	>5	0.21	*(619)*
	120/~85	5	0.43	*(628)*
	22/10	1	0.10	*(629)*
	16/6	1	0.17	*(452)*
	46/9	1	0.00	*(453)*
	14/8	1	0.00	*(630)*
10p	48/48	>4	0.08	*(619)*
	120/~85	4	<0.20	*(628)*
	22/21	1	0.05	*(629)*
	46/39	1	0.00	*(453)*
10q	48/48	>5	0.15	*(619)*
	120/~85	5	0.25	*(628)*
	22/21	1	0.19	*(629)*
	46/16-24	3	0.25	*(453)*
	96/89	2	0.27	*(560)*
	32/20	1	0.00	*(546)*
11p	48/48	>4	0.19	*(619)*
	120/~85	4	<0.20	*(628)*
	22/20	2	0.15	*(629)*
	14/5-11	9	0.43	*(630)*
	46/11-23	3	0.40	*(453)*
	11/4-6	2	0.00	*(631)*
	12-19/4-9	2	0.20	*(459)*
	19/6-10	2	0.17	*(417)*
	25-27/5-9	2	0.00	*(546)*
	16/5	1	0.00	*(452)*
	19/10	1	0.05	*(350)*
	56/26	1	0.15	*(418)*
	29/22	1	0.05	*(378)*

Table 1(*cont.*)

Chromosome arm	HCC/ informative cases	Number of probes used	FAL	Reference
11q	48/48	>3	0.17	*(619)*
	120/~85	3	<0.20	*(628)*
	22/19	1	0.11	*(629)*
	16/10	1	0.00	*(452)*
	46/23	1	0.13	*(453)*
	19/7	1	0.14	*(417)*
	27/2	1	0.00	*(546)*
12p	48/48	>4	0.23	*(619)*
	120/~85	4	<0.20	*(628)*
	22/8	1	0.13	*(629)*
	46/12	1	0.08	*(453)*
	14/4	1	0.00	*(630)*
12q	48/48	>5	0.23	*(619)*
	120/~85	5	<0.20	*(628)*
	22/14	1	0.07	*(629)*
	16/12	1	0.08	*(452)*
	46/14	1	0.07	*(453)*
13q	48/48	>7	0.29	*(619)*
	120/~85	7	0.53	*(628)*
	22/15	2	0.40	*(629)*
	21/4-8	15	0.43	*(412)*
	92/8-18	13	0.33	*(420)*
	56/10-27	8	0.53	*(418)*
	19/5-11	5	0.66	*(417)*
	24/9-14	5	0.38	*(470)*
	11-27/4-13	4	0.00	*(546)*
	14/2-5	3	0.75	*(630)*
	22/15	2	0.73	*(421)*
	46/13-26	2	0.20	*(453)*
	11-15/4-5	2	0.36	*(419)*
	104/87	2	0.26	*(465)*
	56/40	2	0.18	*(467)*
	11/7	1	0.14	*(631)*
	16/11	1	0.00	*(452)*
	24/17	1	0.41	*(469)*
	63/25	1	0.20	*(482)*
	29/21	1	0.33	*(378)*
14q	48/48	>6	0.27	*(619)*
	120/~85	6	0.34	(628)
	22/13	2	0.46	*(629)*
	16/10	1	0.00	*(452)*
	46/46	1	0.11	*(453)*
	23/10	1	0.10	*(459)*
	14/7	1	0.00	*(630)*
	35/17	1	0.40	*(546)*
15q	48/48	>6	0.04	*(619)*
	120/~85	6	<0.20	*(628)*
	22/18	2	0.17	*(629)*
	46/26	1	0.12	*(453)*
	20/10	1	0.30	*(469)*
	14/3	1	0.00	*(630)*
	35/10	1	0.10	*(546)*
16p	48/48	>4	0.40	*(619)*
	120/~85	4	0.22	*(628)*
	22/17	1	0.17	*(629)*
	96/53-74	10	0.48	*(648)*
	70/28-44	5	0.45	*(647)*
	35/2-16	2	0.54	*(546)*
	10-25/9-11	2	0.60	*(419)*
	38/19	2	0.74	*(455)*

Table 1(*cont.*)

Chromosome arm	HCC/ informative cases	Number of probes used	FAL	Reference
	16/10	1	0.00	*(452)*
	46/16	1	0.06	*(453)*
	43/25	1	0.28	*(415)*
16q	48/46	>4	0.39	(619)
	120/~85	4	0.31	*(628)*
	22/22	4	0.59	*(629)*
	41/35	37	0.85	*(649)*
	42/14-28	12	0.71	*(634)*
	70/26-53	10	0.57	*(647)*
	30/18-30	6	0.40	*(636)*
	24/9-16	6	0.42	*(470)*
	46/7-33	4	0.36	*(453)*
	104/87	4	0.23	*(465)*
	38/26	3	0.85	*(116)*
	56/47	3	0.26	*(467)*
	35/4-9	3	0.56	*(546)*
	33/10-19	2	0.45	*(419)*
	16/6	1	0.00	*(452)*
	20/15	1	0.00	*(469)*
	52/31	1	0.42	*(651)*
	63/50	1	0.28	*(482)*
	56/43	1	0.40	*(418)*
17p	48/46	>3	0.48	*(619)*
	120/~85	3	0.34	*(628)*
	22/13	1	0.46	*(629)*
	53/3-32	7	0.49	*(457)*
	19/6-13	6	0.53	*(455)*
	169/80	5	0.69	*(478)*
	46/7-26	4	0.50	*(453)*
	24/11-18	4	0.70	*(470)*
	19-24/13-18	3	0.38	*(469)*
	16/9-10	2	0.80	*(452)*
	63/56	2	0.57	*(482)*
	56/22-35	2	0.50	*(418)*
	29/29	2	0.66	*(378)*
	10/5	1	0.60	*(451)*
	14/9	1	0.00	*(464)*
	10/4	1	0.25	*(444)*
	33/19	1	0.58	*(419)*
	37/13	1	0.15	*(469)*
	19/17	1	0.00	*(431)*
	20/20	1	0.15	*(449)*
	16/8	1	0.63	*(454)*
	150/64	1	0.58	*(461)*
	30/30	1	0.10	*(372)*
	18/14	1	0.57	*(466)*
	13/8	1	0.38	*(354)*
	104/83	1	0.29	*(465)*
	38/30	1	0.27	*(484)*
	43/43	1	0.19	*(415)*
	20/14	1	0.36	*(458)*
	36/21	1	0.62	*(456)*
	23/21	1	0.43	*(459)*
	56/46	1	0.17	*(467)*
	34/10	1	0.80	*(460)*
	41/22	1	0.41	*(463)*
	19/14	1	0.21	*(417)*
	14/10	1	0.20	*(630)*
	14/7	1	0.14	*(546)*
17q	48/48	>5	0.04	*(619)*

Table 1(*cont.*)

Chromosome arm	HCC/ informative cases	Number of probes used	FAL	Reference
	120/~85	5	0.31	*(628)*
	22/19	3	0.21	*(629)*
	19/1-5	4	0.17	*(455)*
	53/8-13	3	0.12	*(457)*
	29/3-4	2	0.24	*(378)*
	46/21	1	0.10	*(453)*
	14/10	1	0.20	*(630)*
18p	48/48	>3	0.13	*(619)*
	120/~85	3	<0.20	*(628)*
	22/18	1	0.11	*(629)*
	29/21-29	4	0.10	*(378)*
	12/7	1	0.00	*(459)*
18q	48/48	>4	0.27	*(619)*
	120/~85	4	<0.20	*(628)*
	32/16	3	0.13	*(629)*
	25/25	3	0.24	*(377)*
	29/29	2	0.07	*(378)*
	29/21	2	0.14	*(378)*
	16/5	1	0.00	*(452)*
	46/11	1	0.09	*(453)*
	35/18	1	0.06	*(546)*
19p	48/45	>3	0.22	*(619)*
	120/~85	3	<0.20	*(628)*
	22/11	1	0.09	*(629)*
	46/28	1	0.04	*(453)*
	14/3	1	0.00	*(630)*
19q	48/44	>4	0.07	*(619)*
	120/~85	4	<0.20	*(628)*
	22/10	1	0.10	*(629)*
20p	48/47	>2	0.02	*(619)*
	120/~85	2	<0.20	*(628)*
	22/16	1	0.06	*(629)*
	46/39	1	0.00	*(453)*
20q	48/48	>4	0.06	*(619)*
	120/~85	4	<0.20	*(628)*
	22/17	1	0.00	*(629)*
	16/5	1	0.20	*(452)*
	35/15	1	0.00	*(546)*
21q	48/47	>3	0.23	*(619)*
	120/~85	3	<0.20	*(628)*
	22/17	1	0.18	*(629)*
	14/4	1	0.00	*(630)*
	10/4	1	0.25	*(546)*
22q	48/47	>4	0.09	*(619)*
	120/~85	4	<0.20	*(628)*
	22/14	1	0.07	*(629)*
	22-23/0-15	5	0.35	*(459)*
	63/28	1	0.32	*(482)*
	14/7	1	0.00	*(630)*

Several earlier studies used RFLP and/or microsatellite probes to perform less complete allelotypes of HCC, applying from 22–44 probes for loci located on 13–33 nonacrocentric autosomal arms of a total of 123 HCC *(452,453,546,630,631)*. Even more limited allelotypes have resulted from the application of 9–15 RFLP and/or microsatellite probes for loci located on 5–9 nonacrocentric autosomal arms of a total of 356 HCC *(417–419,459,465,467,482)*. In many studies only a single,

anonymous probe often represented an entire chromosome arm, and the results were often uninformative. However, several studies have applied multiple probes to map loci on particular chromosome arms: specific chromosome arms that have been more densely allelotyped with multiple RFLP or microsatellite probes include 1p *(469,470,632,633)*, 4q *(470,634–638)*, 5q *(527)*, 8p *(639–646)*, 9p *(396,400,404)*, 13q *(412,420,470)*, 16p *(647–649)*, 16q *(470,634,636,647–649)*, 17p *(455,457,*

Table 2
Chromosome Arms with Frequent Allelic Losses in HCC Correlated with "Hotspots" for
Breakage/LOH and with Known or Putative Tumor-Suppressor Genes[a]

Chromosome Arm	Fractional Allelic Loss[b]	Number of Studies With ≥2 Probes/Arm	Breakage/ LOH Hotspots	Known or Putative Tumor Suppressor Genes Tested in HCC (Location) [%LOH]
1p	0.36 ± 0.17	8	p36.1-p36.3 p13-p21	p73 (1p36) [5/25; 20%]
1q	0.42 ± 0.20	4	q31-q32	
4q	0.52 ± 0.24	11	q11-q12 q21 q24-q26 q26-q27 q28 q28-qter q31 q33	
5q	0.33 ± 0.19	7	q21-q22 q35-qter	APC (5q21) [9/11; 8%] MCC (5q21) [0/5; 0%]
6q	0.30 ± 0.20	3	q26-q27	M6P/IGFIIR (6q26-q27) [57/100; 57%]
8p	0.58 ± 0.18	8	p21-p23.1 p21 p21.3-p22	EXT1 (8p24.1) [8/24; 33%] PRLTS [5/14; 36%] DLC-1 [7/16; 43%]
			p22 p23	
8q	0.38 ± 0.23	5	q22-q24	
9p	0.39 ± 0.15	6	p21-p22	p16INK/ARF (9p21-p22) [67/183; 37%]
13q	0.42 ± 0.22	13	q12-q13 q14-q14.3 q22 q32	BRCA2 (13q12-q13) [no studies] Rb1 (13q14) [45/140; 32%]
14q	0.36 ± 0.10	3		
16p	0.49 ± 0.18	16	p13-pter	
16q	0.47 ± 0.19	12	q22-q23.2	E-cadherin (16q22.1) [18/28; 64%]
17p	0.53 ± 0.14	10	p13 p11.2-p13.3	p53 (17p13.1) [259/678; 38%]

[a]Data taken from Table 1 and references therein.
[b]Fractional allelic loss is expressed as mean ± SD.

470,478), and 22p (459). Some of these single chromosome arm allelic maps have applied probes as densely as every 2 cM on average (646).

Two of the most complete and dense allelotype analyses (619,628) generally agree in the assessments of the fraction of allelic losses per HCC, as well as in the identification of the specific chromosome arms that undergo significant allelic losses during the development and progression of HCC. The mean fraction of allelic loss per HCC (FAL or FAL index) averaged 12.8% (628) and 20% (619), and ranged from 0–42% for both studies. The less dense allelotype study of Piao et al. (629) found a mean allelic loss per HCC of 24% and a range of 0–43%. In each of these studies only one or two HCC lacked any allelic losses. Allelic losses were not distributed equally among the nonacrocentric chromosome arms in HCC and HBL,

indicating that they are not random. Chromosome arms showing significant allelic losses in each of the two comprehensive allelotypes of Boige et al. (619) and Nagai et al. (628) included 1p, 1q, 4q, 6q, 8p, 9p, 13q, 14q, 16p, 16q, and 17p. The allelotype study of Piao et al. (629) identified significant allelic losses at 1q, 4q, 5q, 8p, 8q, 13q, 14q, 16q, and 17p. Thus, there is general agreement among these three allelotype studies on the occurrence of significant allelic losses on chromosome 1p (2/3 studies), 1q (3/3), 4q (3/3), 6q (2/3), 8p (3/3), 8q (2/3), 9p (2/3), 13q (3/3), 14q (3/3), 16p (2/3), 16q (3/3), and 17p (3/3). One study out of the three also found allelic losses that reached a level of significance on 2q, 5q, 7p and 7q, 9q, 17q, and 18q.

The results of the comprehensive allelotype study of Sheu et al. (620) differed somewhat from those of Boige et al. (619), Nagai et al. (628), and Piao et al. (629) possibly because the

Table 3
Testing of Known Tumor Suppressor Gene Loci on Chromosome Arms that Show Infrequent Allelic Losses in HCC[a]

Chromosome arm	Fractional allelic loss	Number of studies with ≥3 probes	Known or putative tumor suppressor genes tested in HCC (location) [%LOH]
3p	<0.20 ± 0.03	3	*FHIT* (3p14) [3/18; 11%]
			VHL (3p25) [2/24; 8%]
10q	0.22 ± 0.05	5	*PTEN/MMAC* (10q23) [25/89; 28%]
11p	<0.30 ± 0.13	4	*WT1* (11p13) [1/22; 5%]
			IGFII (11p15.1) [1/39; 3%]
17q	<0.17 ± 0.10	5	*BRCA1* (17q21.3) [3/26; 12%]
			nm23 (17q21.7) [4/22; 18%]
18q	<0.20 ± 0.07	3	*Smad4/DPC4* (18q12.1) [8/54; 11%]
			DCC (18q21) [3/21; 14%]

[a]Data taken from Table 1 and references therein.

HCC analyzed by Sheu et al. *(620)* were smaller in size and may have represented less highly progressed tumors. In contrast to the other studies, 11/34 HCC (32%) analyzed by Sheu et al. *(620)* contained no LOH, and the FAL index of only two HCC exceeded 25%; the remaining 23 HCC had FAL indices of less than 10%. Six chromosomes (5, 9, 11, 13, 16, and 17) had LOH frequencies of 24–47% *(620)*, but the other chromosome arms were infrequently affected.

Table 1 presents the results of allelotype studies in HCC, including the less comprehensive studies. Including studies that have applied 2–43 probes/chromosome arm, 13 arms of 10 chromosomes (1p, 1q, 4q, 5q, 6q, 8p, 8q, 9p, 13q, 14q, 16p, 16q, and 17p), consistently show LOH in HCC with FAL of greater than 0.3/arm (Table 2), indicating that these deletions are not random and suggesting that they likely have recurring mechanistic roles in HCC. The other chromosome arms show LOH in HCC usually of considerably less than 0.3/arm, and the occasional deletions at these sites may reflect random LOH resulting from the general genomic instability of progressing HCC, although they may still be important elements in the pathogenesis of a few HCC. High-frequency sites (hotspots) of LOH and chromosome breakage have been identified on many of the chromosome arms that show significant, nonrandom allelic losses in HCC and candidate tumor-suppressor genes have been mapped to some of these sites in HCC (Table 2).

Actual or putative tumor suppressor genes that show the highest frequency of LOH in HCC include *M6P/IGFIIR* at 6q26-q27, *p16^INK4A* at 9p21-p22, *Rb1* at 13q14, *E-cadherin* at 16q22.1, and *p53* at 17p13.1, each of which has shown LOH from 38–64% of all informative HCC reported. However, possible tumor suppressor genes that are located in or near hotspots for LOH on 1p36 (*p73*), 5q21 (*APC*), and 13q12-q13 (*BRCA1*) all show LOH frequencies of 20% or less when locus-specific probes are used and potential candidate HCC-related genes for 1q, 4q, 8q, 14q, and 16p have not been nominated, suggesting that several tumor-suppressor genes involved in HCC are still unidentified.

Two potential tumor-suppressor genes (designated *PRLTS* and *DLC-1*) have been cloned from the chromosome 8p21.3-

p22 region that is frequently deleted in HCC. Using yeast artificial chromosome (YAC) and cosmid cloning techniques to develop probes, Fujiwara et al. *(650)* isolated a cDNA clone from this region that contained 1502 bp, including 616 bp of 5'-untranslated sequence, a 1125 bp open reading frame, and 316 bp of 3'-untranslated sequence. Northern blot analysis showed that the cDNA covered most of the transcript, detected as a 1.6 kb band. The deduced 375-amino-acid sequence was significantly similar to the extracellular domain of the PDGF receptor β, and the gene was designated *PRLTS*, for PDGF *r*eceptor β-*l*ike *t*umor *s*uppressor. The *PRLTS* gene contained somatic point mutations in 2/48 HCC (4%), which also showed LOH of the opposite allele, suggesting that it expressed major characteristics of a tumor suppressor gene. Subsequently, Chinen et al. *(651)* isolated 45 exon-like fragments from the chromosome 8p21.3-p22 region that included a fragment homologous to the PDGF receptor β.

Using a PCR-based subtractive hybridization technique to produce probes, Yuan et al. *(652)* cloned a cDNA of 600 bp from a human library. The cloned cDNA hybridized to a major 7.5 kb mRNA transcript and a minor 4.5 kb mRNA transcript, which were expressed by several normal human tissues, but not by many HCC. The full-length cDNA of 3850 bp, which was cloned by 5' and 3' RACE from a cDNA library, encoded a protein of 1091 amino acids, thought to be a human counterpart of the rat RhoGAP protein, a member of the ras-related family of signal-transduction molecules. The gene was named *DLC-1* (for Deleted in Liver Cancer), and was shown by FISH to be located on chromosome 8p21.3-p22. LOH of the *DLC-1* gene was detected in 7/16 HCC (43%) and the gene was not expressed in 4/14 HCC (29%), as expected for a tumor-suppressor gene *(652)*. Whether transcription was suppressed by a combination of deletion and mutation of the two alleles or the some other mechanism has not been determined.

The chromosome arms that lack identified hotspots as determined by LOH studies, may still contain genes that are important elements in the combinatorial molecular pathogenesis of HCC. Several tumor-suppressor genes known or suspected to be involved in other neoplasms are located on these arms, but

Table 4
Fraction of Allelic Losses in HBL by Chromosome Arm[a]

Chromosome arm	HBL/ informative cases	Number of probes used	FAL	Reference
1p	32/5-10	8	0.22	(656)
1q	32/8-9	7	0.22	(656)
11p	6/2-5	10	0.67	(654)
	18/2-6	8	0.33	(655)
	3/3	3	0.66	(653)
11q	6/1-5	3	0.20	(654)
	18/5	1	0.40	(655)
17p	7/5	1	0.20	(480)

[a]Chromosomal arms have not been comprehensively allelotyped in HBL.

most have shown low LOH frequencies in HCC when analyzed by locus-specific probes (Table 3).

Chromosome arms in HBL have not been allelotyped comprehensively. Loci on 1p, 1q, 11p, 11q, and 17p have shown allelic losses in greater than 20% of HBL *(480,653–656)*. Little et al. *(657)* reported LOH of the *INS* and *CALC* loci and Kiechle-Schwarz *(658)* detected LOH of the *INS, PTH, CALC,* and c-H-*ras* loci on chromosome 11p13-p15.1 in two HBL. Simms et al. *(659)* found that the non-neoplastic hepatocytes in 2 of 3 patients with HBL were mosaic for the 11p15.5 LOH (*INS* locus); one HBL arose from a precursor cell containing a pre-existing allelic loss, whereas the other did not. Allelotype studies on HBL are summarized in Table 4.

LOH on chromosome arms 1p and 1q were not correlated with differentiation of HBL *(656)*, but correlation between allelic losses on individual chromosome arms with tumor size and differentiation has generally been found for HCC. Allelic losses on 4q *(637)*, 8p *(640)*, 13q *(412,415)*, 16q *(643)*, and 17p *(415,458,461,477)* all increased in association with deteriorating differentiation of HCC.

Although more than 20% of the nonacrocentric chromosome arms contain allelic deletions in advanced, highly progressed HCC *(619,628,629)*, the relationship between the fraction of allelic losses in individual HCC and their differentiation, size, and/or clinical stage was not examined in detail in these studies; Piao et al. *(629)* presented evidence that HCC with high FAL indices were more likely to be poorly differentiated than were HCC with low FAL indices. This relationship was examined further by Piao et al. *(378)* in a study of the allelic status of 10 well-known tumor-suppressor genes (*APC, BRCA1, DCC, Smad4, EXT1, nm23, p53, Rb1, VHL,* and *WT1*) involving 8 chromosome arms (3p, 5q, 8q, 11p, 13q, 17p, 17q, and 18q) in 29 HCC. The FAL index for 17 well-differentiated HCC was 0.16 ± 0.12 and for 12 poorly differentiated HCC it was 0.31 ± 0.15, indicating that allelic losses at the loci for these 10 tumor-suppressor genes accumulated during the progression of HCC as reflected by poor differentiation. Although these data reflected all 10 tumor-suppressor genes, several of which are not known to be involved specifically in HCC, it was corroborated by the allelic status of the *p53* gene, which showed LOH in all 12 poorly differentiated HCC, but in only 7/17 (41%) well-differentiated HCC *(378)*. Furthermore, the HCC

in the well-differentiated group averaged 1.4 ± 1.1 LOH per tumor, whereas those in the poorly differentiated group contained 2.6 ± 1.1 LOH per tumor *(378)*.

Accumulation of multiple LOH on nine chromosome arms during the progression of HCC from small, well-differentiated tumors to large, poorly differentiated tumors (Table 5) has been specifically examined *(418,465,467,482)*. Nishida et al. *(418)* studied loci on 4p, 11p, 13q, 16q, and 17p in 56 HCC, whereas Kuroki et al. *(465)*, Tamura et al. *(467)*, and Konishi et al. *(482)* examined loci on 1p, 4q, 8p, 13q, 16q, and 17p in 104, 56, and 63 HCC, respectively. Kuroki et al. *(465)* also studied loci on 5q and 22q. Kuroki et al. *(465)* found that small, well-differentiated HCC, which they termed early and which included 11 tumors, lacked any allelic losses except on chromosome arm 1p in 2/11 HCC (18%). In contrast, among the advanced HCC in their study, moderately and poorly differentiated tumors contained LOH on all of the chromosome arms studied, and well-differentiated tumors lacked allelic losses on only chromosome arm 16q *(465)*. Well-differentiated HCC contained allelic losses on 0.18 ± 0.13 of the chromosome arms examined, whereas in moderately differentiated HCC 0.33 ± 0.08 of the chromosome arms contained deletions, and in poorly differentiated HCC 0.38 ± 0.66 of the chromosome arms were affected *(465)*; the observations of Nishida et al. *(418)* showed a similar correlation of increased allelic loss with poor differentiation, and they found that poorly differentiated HCC contained 2.4 ± 0.97 LOH per tumor. Similar observations were made by Konishi et al. *(482)* and Tamura et al. *(467)*, who found that well-differentiated HCC contained an average of 0.5–0.7 LOH per tumor (range 0–3), moderately differentiated HCC an average of 1.0–2.0 LOH per tumor (range 0–4), and poorly differentiated HCC an average of 2–3 LOH tumor (range 1–8). In addition to accumulation of LOH, the fraction of tumors showing loss of expression of *p16^INK4A* increased in poorly differentiated HCC *(395,397)*, as did the incidence of mutation of the *p53* gene *(441,460,478,486)*. Accumulation of β-catenin *(108)* and reduced expression of E-cadherin *(105,108,110,113,115)* were also related to HCC differentiation.

Using a novel technique for DNA fingerprinting, Sirivatnauksorn et al. *(83)* provided further evidence that progression of HCC is associated with the acquisition of additional genetic abnormalities and the emergence of new clones con-

Table 5
Accumulation of Genetic Changes with Increasing Tumor Grade

Deletions on chromosome arm	Early	Well-differentiated	Moderately differentiated	Poorly differentiated	References
1p	18%	10%	30%	35%	(465,467,482)
4q	0%	18%	33%	54%	(465,467,482)
5q	ND[a]	20%	30%	35%	(482)
8p	ND	20%	46%	56%	(465,467,482)
13q	0%	7%	25%	41%	(418,465,467,482)
16q	0%	4%	24%	48%	(418,465,467,482)
17p	0%	20%	48%	59%	(418,465,467,482)
LOH/HCC	ND	1.4 ± 1.1		2.6 ± 1.1	
		0.7 (0–3 range)	2.0 (0–4 range)	3.0 (1–8 range)	(378,418,467,482)
FAL Index	ND	0.18 ± 0.13		0.38 ± 0.66	
		0.16 ± 0.12	0.33 ± 0.08	0.31 ± 0.15	(465,378)
p53 Mutation	ND	15%	36%	48%	(441,460,478,486)
Rb1 LOH	0%	25%	47%[b]	47%[b]	(412,415)

[a]Not determined.
[b]LOH at the Rb1 locus was determined in a group of neoplasms containing both moderately differentiated and poorly differentiated tumors.

taining these new aberrations. They examined 31 HCC nodules of various sizes from 8 patients. Each nodule was dissected from the tissue site and divided into two or more segments for DNA fingerprint analysis by electrophoresis of PCR fragments generated with arbitrary primers. All HCC less than 6 mm in diameter (n = 18, mean diameter 4.7 mm, range 3–6 mm) consisted of monoclonal populations, showing identical DNA fingerprint patterns in each segment. In HCC larger than 6 mm in diameter (n = 13, mean diameter 15.4 mm, range 7–30 mm) all segments showed different fingerprint patterns, indicating polyclonal divergence. Furthermore, when multiple HCC were synchronously present, each showed a unique DNA fingerprint pattern (660). Expansion of genetic aberrations as reflected in the DNA fingerprints was associated with deterioration of the differentiation of tumors. In aggregate, these results on accumulation of genomic aberrations suggest that many allelic deletions occur relatively late in the process of hepatocarcinogenesis, with the majority developing during the progression phase that accompanies the emergence of less differentiated, larger, and more aggressive HCC.

Several attempts have been made to identify LOH that occur early in the process of hepatocarcinogenesis before the emergence of HCC. Investigators have searched non-neoplastic cirrhotic nodules located adjacent to HCC for LOH on chromosome arms that may have developed as a preneoplastic change; identification of the same genetic aberration in cirrhotic nodules and adjacent HCC could imply that the HCC emerged as a neoplastic clonal outgrowth from the adjacent nonneoplastic nodular hepatocytes. Nishida et al. (418) detected no LOH involving 13 loci on 5 chromosome arms (4p, 11p, 13q, 16p, 17p) in 42 cirrhotic nodules adjacent to HCC, even when the HCC located in the same livers contained LOH on one or more of these same chromosome arms. They speculated that their failure to identify LOH in cirrhotic nodules, as contrasted to HCC, may have reflected that the former did not contain monoclonal populations (418). However, recent stud-

ies have shown that many cirrhotic nodules are composed of monoclonal populations of hepatocytes (78,87). Subsequently, several investigators have identified LOH of the same chromosomal site in HCA and HCC, and in cirrhotic nodules located adjacent to an HCC.

Yamada et al. (224) identified identical LOH in 90% of the cirrhotic nodules juxtaposed to 11 HCC that contained LOH on 6q26-q27 (M6P/IGFIIR locus); in contrast, cirrhotic nodules adjacent to 7 HCC that lacked the 6q LOH also lacked this deletion. Boige et al. (619) suggested that development of LOH on 8p was an early change because this specific arm deletion did not correlate with the tumor FAL index, possibly implying that 8p LOH were generated before the bulk of the LOH that form the basis for the FAL index. Furthermore, Boige et al. (619) found an 8p deletion as the only deleted arm in an HCC, and they also identified this chromosomal aberration in a benign HCA. Supporting the opinion that LOH on 8p was an early change in HCC development, Kishimoto et al. (644) detected allelic deletion on 8p in 7/13 HCC and in 16/23 cirrhotic nodules adjacent to these HCC; the pattern of 8p LOH was identical in HCC and many cirrhotic nodules, and no 8p LOH were found in cirrhotic nodules adjacent to HCC that also lacked 8p LOH. Similar observations have also been made for LOH on 13q14 at the Rb1 locus (421), and on 17p at the p53 locus (466). In all instances, the same allele was deleted in the non-neoplastic hepatocytes of cirrhotic nodules and in the neoplastic hepatocytes of HCC, providing evidence that in these instances the LOH may have occurred initially in the former and that the neoplastic cells developed as a secondary clonal population.

Tsopanomichalou et al. (471) detected allelic losses on chromosomes 1, 9, and 17 (at 5–8 microsatellite loci) in liver tissue from patients with chronic hepatitis (n = 20) and cirrhosis (n = 11) but without HCC. In chronic hepatitis, allelic losses were detected in 5.5 ± 4.9% on chromosome 1, in 5.0 ± 3.5% on chromosome 9, and in 14.4 ± 8.9% on chromosome 17; comparable figures for cirrhotic livers were 17.5 ± 12.8% on chro-

Table 6
Karyotypes of Hepatocellular Carcinomas[a]

Case	Karyotype	Reference
1	46, XY, +del(1)(p22), der(1)t(1;?)(p32;?), +der(5)t(5;?)(q34;?), del(6)(q13), inv(9)(p12q12), -13, -16, der(22)t(22;?)(q12;?)	(667)
2	46, X, -Y	(668)
3	71-79, XX, -Y(3n+1-), der(1)t(1;?)(p36;?)del(1)(p11), +der(1)t(1;?)(q21;?), +del(1)(q32), +3, +der(6)t(6;8)(q12;q13), +der(6), -8, 9p+, +del(9)(q13), del(10)(q24), der(12)t(12;?)(p13;?), invdup12)(q11q24), der(13)t(!10;13)(q11;p13), -16, -17, -21, +1-9mar/45, +X, -Y	(668)
4	76-79, XXY, +der(1)t(1q;?), +del(1)(q25), der(1)del(1)(p34)del(1)(q42), +del(1)(p13), +7, +11, +12, +18, +2mar	(669)
5	106-113, XXXYY, del(1)(p22), -4, -5, -8, i(8)(q10), i(9), add(9)(p24), -10, -13, -13, -15, add(16)(q24), -16, -17, -17, -18, -18, add(21)(q10)x2, -22, +7, -13mar	(670)
6	72-76, XY, -X, del(1)(p32), +add(1)(q10), +del(6)(q15), +7, -8, -9, -10, -11, -12, +13, +15, -16, -17, +18, +20, -21, -22, +4-8mar	(670)
7	45, X, -Y, del(1)(p34), del(1)(p22), -4, -5, -13, der(16)add(16)(q24)+2mar	(670)
8	66-72, XY, -X, +del(1)(p32), +add(1)(q10), -4, -6, +7, -8, +11, der(13;15)(q10;p10), i(14)(q10), -16, -17, -21, -22, +1-3mar(	670
9	62-92, XX, -Y, +3, +6, +6, +7, +7, +8, +10, +13, +15, +16, +20, -21-22, +3mar/78, XX, -Y, der(1)t(p36;q21), +4, +6, +6, +7, +7, i(8)(q10), +10, +15, +20, -21, -22, +3mar	(671)
10	64-72, XY, t(1;?)(q21;?), +der(1)t(1;?)(q21;?), -3, -5, -18, tder(?)(?;12)(?;q13), +4mar/a second abnormal clone appeared to represent a doubling of this one	(672)
11	45, X-Y/43-46 X-Y, +2	(673)
12	Massive nonclonal rearrangements	(673)
13	61-66, XXY, del(1)(p11), +del(1)(q12), add(2)(q36), del(3)(p12), del(4)(q22), -5, -6, ins(6;8)(p21;q22-q24), add(8)(p11), -9, +11, +12, -13, -14, -15, +1-7mar	(673)
14	47, XX, +mar	(674)
15	46, XY, der(1)add(1)(p36)t(1;2;7)(q42;q22;q22), der(2)t(1;2;7), i(6)(p10), der(7)t(1;2;7), -12, der(17)del(17)(p11)add(17)(q25)[i3]/45, XY, -13/47, XY, +der(7)t(1;2;7)	(674)
16	45, XY, der(2)t(2;8)(q33;q13), t(7;22)(q22;q11), -8, add(10)(q22), +17, der(17)t(17;21)(p11;q11)x2, -21/45, XY, der(1)t(1;1)(p36;q25)[6]/90, XXYYx2/45, X, -Y	(674)
17	92-99, XX, -Y, -Y, +X, +X, del(1)(q12)x2, +3, ins(3)(q29q12q25), +i(3)(q10), +4, der(4;14)(q10;q10)x2, add(5)(q22)x2, der(6)t(1;6)(q25;q27)x2, add(7)(q32), -8, add(8)(q24), del(8)(p21), -11, -11, add(12)(q24), der(12)t(8;12)(q11;p11), -13, add(13)(p11)x2, -14, add(14)(p11), -15, der(16)t(12;16)(q12;q24)add(12)ins(16;?)(q24;?), -18, -18, +19, -21, -22, -22, inc	(674)
18	47, XY, +7[6]/46, XY, -Y[9]/46, XY[46]	(674)
19	74-77, XX, -Y, der(1)t(1;5)(p36;q13)x2, +der(1)t(1;14)(p13;q11)x2, +2, -5, del(5)(q11q13), +6, +7, +der(7)del(7)(p15)del(7)(q32)x2, i(8)(q10)x3, -9, -14, +18, +20, -21, -22, +r, +mar	(674)
20	81-87, X, -X, -Y, -Y, del(4)(q21q25)x2, -5, -5, +8, i8(q10)x3, i(10)(p10)x2, -13, -16, del(16)(q11), add(17)(p11)x2, +19, +19, del(19)(p11)x2, der(19)t(8;19)(q13;p11)x2, -21, -21, -22, 81-87, X, -X, -Y, -Y, -12, -14, i(14)(q10), +del16/81-87, X, -X, -Y, -Y, der(X;8)(p10;q10), +6/81-87, X, -X, -Y, -Y, +del(6)(q22)/81-87, X, -X, -Y, -Y, +del(1)(p22)x2, +del(6), -i(8)(q10)x3, +r/121-126, XXX, -Y, -Y, +del(1)x2, +2, +3, -4, del(4)x2, -5, -5, +del(6)(p10), +7, i(10)(p10)x2, add(17)x2, +20, +r, inc	(674)

[a]These data were modified from Parada et al. (674).

mosome 1, 17.2 ± 16.4% on chromosome 9, and 15.4 ± 9.5% on chromosome 17, suggesting that allelic loss increased as chronic hepatitis evolved into cirrhosis. However, the interpretation of these results is complicated by detection of similar ranges of allelic loss in liver tissue from 10 patients with various liver diseases not thought to increase the risk of HCC (471); allelic loss in these control livers were detected on chromosome 1 in 10.6 ± 5.0%, on chromosome 9 in 22.4 ± 14.2%, and on chromosome 17 in 6.0 ± 6.7%. Further studies are needed on this important point.

The occurrence of LOH in benign HCA would indicate that LOH occurs prior to the development of malignancy (HCC). Boige et al. (619) detected LOH on 8p in a single HCA, but Ding et al. (661) failed to find any LOH in 6 HCA studied with 25 RFLP probes located on 21 chromosome arms (8p was not examined), including one HCA that developed synchronously

Table 7
Karyotypes of Hepatoblastoma in Children

Case	Karyotype	Reference
1	46, XY, -2, der(19)t(4;19)(q12;q13), +mar	(675)
2	47, XX, +18	(676)
3	47, XX, +18	(677)
4	47, XY, +20, dmin	(678)
5	47, XY, +20, dmin	(678)
6	93, XXXX, +i(8)(q10)/93, XXXX, del(1)(p22), +i(8q)	(679)
7	50, XY, +dic(1)(p12), +2, +8, +20	(680)
8	47, XX, del(1)(q32.1q32.2), dup(2)(q21q35), +20, dmin/50, XX, del(1), dup(2), +5, +7, i(8)(q10), +20, +22, +dmin	(680)
9	47, XX, dup(2)(q23q35), +20/47, XX, dup(2), dup(6)(p11p24), +20	(680)
10	54, Y, der(X)t(X;1)(p22;p21), +2, +6, +8, +8, inv(9)(p11q21), +12, +15, +17, +20	(680)
11	46, XY, der(4)t(2;4)(q21;q35), add(9)(q24)/47, XX, +20	(681)
12	51, XY, +2, +der(5)t(1;5)(q25;q35), +del(6)(q15), +12, +20	(682)
13	48, X, t(X;11)(q24;q25), del(2)(p21), +der(2)t(1;2)(q23;p21), inv(5)(q22q35), del(7)(q22q32), add(9)(q22)x2, del(13)(q31), +20, dmin	(682)
14	47, XX, +2q, t(3;5)(p25;q31), dup(4)(q12q26), +20	(683)
15	47, XX, +2	(684)
16	46, XY, t(10;22)(q26;q11)	(685)
17	46, XX, +18	(686)
18	46, XY, del(1)(pter-q12)	(687)
19	46, XY, del(10)(p11), del(13)(q31)	(687)
20	49-50, XX, ?dirdup(1)(pter_q42::q23_q32::q21_qter), -2, +?dirdup(2)(pter_q33::q21_qter)x2, +6, +7, +20/100-102, XXXX, -1, -1, ?dirdup(2)(pter_q33::q21_qter)x2, -4, -5, +6, -7, +9, -12, -16, -19, -19, -21, +16mar	(687)
21	47, XX, +20	(688)
22	47, XY, +2	(688)
23	46, XX, del(17)(p12)	(688)
24	46, XX, der(2)t(2;2)(p25;q21), der(22)t(1;22)(q22;p13)/47, XX, der(2)t(2;2)(p25;q21), +20, der(22)t(1;22)(q22;p13)/47, XX, der(2)t(2;2)(p25;q21), +20/48, XX, der(2)t(2;2)(p25;q21), +12, +17, -18, +20, der(22)t(1;22)(q22;p13)/50, XX, der(2)t(2;2)(p25;q21), +8, +12, +17, +20	(689)
25	49, XY, +2, der(4)t(1;4)(q12;q34), +8, +20	(689)
26	49, XY, der(4)t(1;4)(q12;q34), +8, +8, +ace/50, XY, +20/49, XY, +8, +20/46-50, XY, -8, -8, -ace, +1-5r, +mar	(690)
27	56~58, XY, +Y, +2, der(4)t(1;4)(q12;q34), +5, +6, +7, +8, +13, +19, +20, +21, 2~15dmin	(690)
28	46, XY, der(4)t(1;4)(q25;q32)/47, XY, +20/48, XY, +8, +20/49, XY, +2, +5, +20	(690)
29	47, XX, +18	(691)
30	47, XY, +2, add(4)(q35), der(9)ins(9;2)(p22;q?;q?25)+20	(692)
31	50, XY, add(1)(p32), +2, +6, add(12q), +20, add(22q)	(693)
32	53, XY, +der(2)t(1;2)(q21;q36), +7, +8, +8, +19, +20, +21	(693)
33	55, XX, t(1;4)(q21;q32), +2, -4, +i(6)(p10), +7, +8, +15, +17, +17, +19, +20	(693)
34	50, XY, +8, +16, +20, +22	(693)
35	46, XY, i(1)(q10)/47, XY, +20	(693)
36	45, XX, -12, -15, der(12)t(12;15)(q24;q13)	(693)
37	46, XY, der(2)t(1;2)(q32;q37), der(6)t(1;6)(q12;q27), der(7)t(2;7)(q23;p22), der(21)t(2;21)(q23;p12)	(694)
38	48, XX, +2, +8	(694)
39	50, XY, +2, +der(14)t(1;14)(q21;p11.1)x2, +19	(695)

in the same liver with an HCC that contained an LOH on 17p at the *p53* locus *(662)*. In contrast, DeSouza et al. *(222)* found that HCA contained a level of LOH at 6p26-p27 (the *M6P/IGFIIR* locus) that was as high as that found in HCC (HCA, 2/3, 67%; HCC, 11/16, 68%). Nevertheless, the small number of

HCA analyzed for locus deletions handicaps the interpretation of these fragmentary results.

Nagai et al. *(663–665)* investigated genomic aberrations occurring in HCC by a technique called restriction-andmark scanning, in which genomic DNA is subjected to restriction-

Table 8
Karyotype of a Hepatoblastoma in an Adult

Case	Karyotype	Reference
1	72-77, X, -X, -Y, +1, +2, +4, +7, +8, i(8)(q10)x2, -9, der(12)t(3;12)(q21;p11), der(12)t(7;12)(q31;q24),-13, +14, +?add(14)(q24), -15, +16, -17, der(17)t(Y;17)(q11;p11), +19, +20, +21, +22, +2mar/72-76, X, -X, -Y, +der(8)t(X;8)(q13;p12)/75-77, idem, del(1)(q12), +der(8)t(X;8)(q13;p12)/73-77, X, -X, -Y, del(1)(q21), del(3)(q12), inv(6)(p25q15), +der(8)t(X;8)(q13;q12)/73-77, X, -X, -Y, del(1)(q21), del(3)(q12), inv(6)(p25q15), +der(8)+cX;8)(q13;p12), +r/73-77, X, -X, -Y, i(1)(p10), del(3)(q12), inv(6)(p25q15), +der(8)t(X;8)(q13;p12)/73-77, X, -X, -Y, der(1;3)(p10;q10), -19, [10]/73-77, idem, del(1)(q12), der(1;3)(p10;q10), +der(8)t(X;8)(q13;p12)/73-77, X, -X, -Y, del(1)(q21), +der(8)t(X;8)(q13;p12), -der(12)t(3;12)(q21;p11), +der(12)t(?2;12)(p11;p11), -19/73-77, X, -X, -Y, del(1)(q12), -der(12)t(3;12)(q21;p11), +der(12)t(?2;12)(p11;p11), -19	*(696)*

enzyme digestion, the fragments end-labeled, cleaved with a second restriction enzyme, and subjected to two-dimensional electrophoresis; more than 2000 fragments (landmark sites) could be surveyed in a single gel. Nagai et al. *(664)* found that five spots were intensified by 3-fold to 100-fold in 63–88% of 16 HCC greater than 2 cm in diameter, whereas about 20 spots decreased by 12–60% in 25–88% of HCC. Subsequent studies identified similar patterns when DNA from 6 HCC less than 2 cm in diameter was analyzed *(665)*. Although this technique discloses remarkable differences in the restriction fragments generated from HCC DNA, none of the genes located in any of the DNA that form spots that either increase or decrease have been identified *(664,665)*, and assignments to specific chromosomes appear to be ambiguous *(666)*.

ABERRATIONS IN CHROMOSOME STRUCTURE AND NUMBER

Karyotypic Analysis Abnormal karyotypes have been published for 20 HCC using cells taken directly from the tumor and cultured in vitro for only short periods *(667–674)*. Most of these HCC tumor cells were aneuploid, and chromosomes contained numerous, complex, and varied structural abnormalities (Table 6). Among these 20 HCC, chromosome 1 was most frequently abnormal, with 28 structural aberrations involving both the long and short arms; chromosome 8 contained 13 structural aberrations; chromosome 6 contained 13 aberrations; and chromosomes 7, 9, 10, and 16 each contained 5–7 structural aberrations. Copies of chromosomes 5, 8, 13, 16, 17, 18, 21, 22, and Y were each lost in 5–10 HCC. Chromosomes 3, 6, 7, and 20 each showed copy number gain in 4–10 HCC. Partial imbalances involved different chromosome arms, most frequently there were losses of all or parts of 1p, 6q, 8p, 13p, 16q, and 17p; the most frequent gains involved all or parts of 1q, 8q, and 17q. Chromosome bands most often involved in structural rearrangements included chromosome 1p11, 1p22, 1p32, 1p34, 1p36, 1q10, 1q12, 1q25, 6q13-q15, 6q22-q25, 8q10, 16q24, and 17p11.

Abnormal karyotypes of 36 HBL occurring in young children *(675–695)*, and the karyotype of one HBL occurring in an adult *(696)* have been published (Table 7). All but two of the

HBL in young children were near diploid, in contrast to the majority of the HCC and the single HBL in an adult. The most common chromosomal abnormality was trisomy 20 in 23/39 HBL (59%) and trisomy 2 in 12/39 HBL (31%). In addition, 10 other HBL contained rearrangements that resulted in an increase of loci on 2q. In four HBL, only one chromosomal aberration was discerned, four with trisomy 18, two with trisomy 2, and one with trisomy 20; two other HBL with trisomy 20 as the major abnormality also contained double minute chromosomal fragments. Chromosome 8 was completely or partially duplicated in 11/39 HBL (28%). Chromosome 1 contained structural aberrations in 13/39 HBL (33%), resulting in loss of loci on 1p and gain of loci on 1q. This type of aberration of chromosome 1 was also found in 2 of 3 HBL in which only partial karyotypes were published *(697)*. Translocations involving 4q34-35 occurred in 6/39 HBL (15%).

In contrast to the HBL in young children, the HBL occurring in an adult was near-triploid (Table 8), and contained a complex variety of aberrations involving several chromosomes. Although this tumor contained extra copies of chromosomes 2 and 20, and partial duplication of chromosome 8, as in infantile HBL *(696)*, the complex karyotype resembled that of HCC. Bardi et al. *(673)* have also found excess copies of chromosome 2 in HCC in adults, and proposed that HBL and HCC contained common chromosomal abnormalities. However, there appears to be little evidence to support this suggestion, and the karyotype of an HCC that occurred in a 15-yr-old child was typical of HCC occurring in adults *(672)*.

Children with HBL and Beckwith-Wiedemann syndrome often have a constitutional aberration of chromosome 11p11-p15, which also involves the HBL *(698)*. Kiechl-Schwarz et al. *(658)* found one sporadic HBL with trisomy 11 associated with LOH at 4 loci on chromosome 11p; this HBL, as well as two others, also showed trisomy or tetrasomy for chromosome 2q, but complete karyotypes were not presented.

Fluorescence In Situ Hybridization Loss and gain of selected individual chromosomes can be examined using probes for pericentric α-satellite DNA of specific chromosomes by FISH of intact cells or nuclei. Probes for α-satellite DNA of

Table 9
Frequently Abnormal Chromosomes and Chromosomal Regions in HCC and HBL Identified by Karyotypic Analysis, FISH, and GCH[a]

Chromosome	Karyotype Breakage/ translocation	Karyotype Imbalance[b]	Karyotype Copy number	FISH Copy number	CGH Copy number
1	1p11, 1p22, 1p32 1p34, 1p36	1p- (1p-)[c]		1+	
	1q10, 1q12, 1q25	1q+ (1q+)			1q+, 1q24+
2			(2+)		2q+ (2q+)
4				4+, 4q-, 4q21-	4q-, 4q12-q22-
5					5p+, 5p11+
6	6q13-q15, 6q22-q25	6q-	6+	6+ 6q14-, 6q21-	6p+, 6p11+ 6q-
7			7+	7+	7q31(amp)[d]
8		8p-	(8+)	8+, 8p- 8p12- 8p22-	8p-
	8q10	8q+			8q+, 8q11+ 8q21-q24+ 8q21-qter+
9				9+, 9p21- 9p24-	
10				10+	
11		(11p-), (11+)			11q13(amp)
12				12+	
13		13q-			13q-
16			16+	16+	
	16q24	16q-			16q-
17	17p11	17p- 17q+		17+, 17-, 17p-	17p- 17q+
18			(18+)		
19					19p+ 19q13-q32-
20			20+, (20+)	20+	20q+, (20q+)

[a]Data were taken from the following studies: karyotypic analyses (667–695), FISH analyses (699–706), and CGH analyses (707–712).
[b]Gains are indicated by a plus (+), and losses are indicated by a minus (-).
[c]Data from hepatoblastomas are given in parentheses.
[d]Indicates amplification of the affected chromosomal region.

chromosomes 1 (699,700), 3 (701), 4 and 6 (700,701), 7 (700,702,703), 8 (699–701,703), 9 (701,703), 10 and 12 (703), 16 (702,704), 17 (700,702–705), 18 (703,704), 20 (702), and X and Y (703) have been used to assess chromosome copy numbers. Because α-satellite-specific probes detect only the centromeric regions, the results do not provide any information on losses or translocations that may involve the chromosome arms to which a centromere is attached unless locus-specific probes are also used. Intact nuclei are required to detect all centromeres accurately; in the studies reviewed here, smears or touch preparations of whole cells or nuclei were used in all studies except that of Zimmermann et al. (700), which used frozen sections of liver tissue. Because many nuclei in sectioned tissues are transected, the numbers of centromeric spots enumerated will be less than the true number of centromeres. This is demonstrated by the fact that over 85% of the normal hepatocytes examined in each of the studies that analyzed isolated cells or nuclei, detected two or four autosomic centromeres, whereas the study of Zimmermann et al. (700) detected two or more chromosomes in only 65–70% of the non-neoplastic hepatocytes. In order to control for this underdetection, careful comparison with non-neoplastic liver tissue must be made in order to enable a statistically valid assessment of the numbers of centromeres in HCC cells relative to non-neoplastic hepatocytes. Zimmermann et al. (700) appear to have adequately controlled their analysis of centromeres in sections of HCC.

A convention used in the presentation of results by all of the investigators also makes all of these studies present slightly distorted results for the assessment of chromosomal polysomy; all of the studies considered three or more centromeric spots to indicate aberrant polysomy, although a fraction of normal hepatocytes are polyploid and therefore normally polysomic, with even-numbered multiples of the diploid set, as noted by Hamon-Benais et al. (702). Because the data presented in these reports could not be uniformly corrected for the inclusion of tetraploids and octoploids, which are eusomic in the liver, we have presented the data as reported, realizing that the assessment of polysomy will be somewhat too high.

Gains and losses of chromosomes detected by FISH with centromeric probes are highlighted in Table 9. Gains of chromosome 1 appeared to be most frequent, occurring in 31/35 HCC (89%) (699,700). Gains of chromosome 8 were found in 49/81 HCC (60%) (699–701,703). Gains of chromosome 20 were identified in 4/7 HCC (57%) (702), of chromosome X in 14/26 HCC (54%) in males (703), of chromosome 6 in 25/46 HCC (54%) (700,701), of chromosome 18 in 29/58 HCC (50%) (703,704) of chromosome 3 in 8/17 HCC (47%) (701), of chromosome 16 in 21/46 HCC (46%) (701,704), of chromosome 10 in 17/38 HCC (45%) (703), of chromosome X in 5/12 HCC (42%) in females (703), of chromosome 17 in 51/121 HCC (42%) (700,702–705), of chromosome 7 in 29/74 HCC (39%) (700,702,703), of chromosome 4 in 18/43 HCC (42%) (701,703), of chromosome 9 in 22/55 HCC (40%) (701,703), and of chromosome 12 in 13/38 HCC (34%) (703).

Chromosome loss, expressed as monosomy or loss of the Y chromosome in males or of one X chromosome in females, was much more uncommon than gain, being found most frequently for chromosome 17, where it was identified in 13/47 HCC (28%) (700,702,704); and for chromosome 4, where it was found in 10/46 HCC (22%) (700,701). Chromosome loss was identified in 0–20% of HCC for chromosome 3 (701), chromosome 7 (700,702), chromosome 9 (701,703), chromosomes 10 and 12 (and Y in males) (703), chromosome 16 (700,704), and chromosome 18 (703,704).

Ohsawa et al. (703) found that the fraction of HCC containing aberrations in the numbers of chromosomes 7, 8, 9, and 17 correlated with tumor differentiation and size, and Kimura et al. (705) also found that numerical aberrations in chromosome 17 were correlated with HCC differentiation.

No abnormalities in the numbers of chromosomes 1 and 8 were found in the neoplastic hepatocytes of five benign HCA, nor in nonneoplastic hepatocytes of three cirrhotic livers; in each instance more than 85% of the hepatocytes contained 2 or 4 signals, as did hepatocytes of normal liver (699).

Huang et al. (705) examined 8 noncentromeric regions using unique sequence probes (YAC clones) for 5 chromosomes. They found that 3p14 was deleted in 2/17 HCC (12%), 4q21 in 13/17 HCC (77%), 6q14 in 8/17 HCC (47%), 6q21 in 5/17 HCC (29%), 8p12 in 6/17 HCC (35%), 8p22 in 10/17 HCC (59%), and 9p21 and 9p24 each in 4/17 HCC (24%) (see Table 9). Huang et al. (705) found that each of 17 HCC examined showed at least one deleted locus and/or was aneuploid, while one HCA examined was diploid and lacked deletions at any of the loci studied. Huang et al. (706) examined chromosome 6q14-q22 more intensely, using 8 YAC probes that span this region, in conjunction with a chromosome 6 centromeric probe. Only 1/25 HCC contained 2 copies of chromosome 6, while 16/25 HCC (64%) were polysomic and the remainder monosomic. Allelic losses in the 6q14-q22 region were detected in 12/25 HCC (48%), and 11 of the 12 affected HCC were polysomic for chromosome 6. Some of the affected HCC contained deletions that spanned the 6q14-q22 region, while all showed allelic loss at 6q14, with the minimal region of loss spanning 2 cM. Loss of 6q14 alleles correlated with longer survival (the mean survival of patients with HCC containing 6q14 loss was 60.6 mo, as compared to 16.9 mo for patients with HCC containing intact

6q14 regions), but not with other tumor or patient characteristics (706).

A single HBL was examined by FISH using centromeric probes for chromosomes 2, 3, 4, 9, and 20 (692). On the basis of G-banding of chromosomes in 11 cells, the karyotype of this HBL was 47XY, +2, add (4q35), -9, +20. FISH detected add(4q35)(wcp 4+), der(9)ins(9;2)(wcp 2+, wcp 9+), +20(wcp20+x3). Combining FISH and G-banding the HBL karyotype was interpreted as: 47XY, add (4q35), der(9;2)(p22;q?21;q?25), +20. Thus, FISH disclosed partial trisomy of 2q by insertion into chromosome 9 that was not evident in G-banded specimens (692). Further studies combining conventional karyotypic evaluation with FISH and/or comparative genomic hybridization (CGH) should improve the accuracy and precision of defining chromosome structural aberrations in HCC.

Comparative Genomic Hybridization Gains and losses of chromosome arms and bands were examined by CGH in six studies that included 247 HCC (707–712). Losses of chromatin on 4q (70% of HCC), 6q (37%), 8p (65%), 13q (37%), 16q (54%), and 17p (51%) were noted by Marchio et al. (707); whereas Kusano et al. (708) found losses on 17p (51%), 16p (46%), 13q13-14 (37%), 4q13-22 (32%), 8p (29%), and 10q (17%); Lin et al. (709) found losses on 16q (43%), 17p (20%), 13q (20%), 4q (15%), and 8p (15%); Qin et al. (710) identified losses of 4q(70%), 1p(60%), 17p(50%), 16q(40%), 19p(40%), and 8p (30%); Sakakura et al. (711) detected losses at 1p34-36 (37%), 4q12-21 (48%), 5q13-21 (35%), 6q13-16 (23%), 8p21-23 (28%), 13q (20%), 16q (33%), and 17p (37%); and Wong et al. (712) found losses on 4q (93%), 8p (37%), 13q (37%), and 16q (30%) (Table 9). Chromatin gains were found on 1q in 58% of HCC, 6p (33%), 8q (60%), and 17q (33%) by Marchio et al. (707); by Kusano et al. (708) at 1q24-25 (78%) and 8q24 (66%); by Lin et al. (709) on 8q (30%), 1q (20%), 6p (20%) and 17q (18%); by Qin et al. (710) on 1q (100%), 8q (60%), and 5q (30%); by Sakakura et al. (711) on 1q (46%), 6p (20%), 8q21-24 (31%), and 17q (43%); and by Wong et al. (712) on 1q in 72% of HCC, 8q (48%), 17q (30%), and 20q (37%). Amplified bands were found at 11q12, 12p11, 14q12, and 19q13.1 in about 20% of HCC by Marchio et al. (707), and Kusano et al. (708) also found that 11q13 was amplified in 15%; Lin et al. (709) detected amplification on 1q, 7q, and 11q11-12 in 3–5%; Sakakura et al. (711) detected amplification of 7q31 (7%), 11q13 (3%), 14q12 (6%), and 17p12 (3%). The major gains and losses of chromosome arms are summarized in Table 9.

Neither gains nor losses of chromosomal material were found in 12 cirrhotic tissues surrounding HCC, but one of three adenomatous hyperplastic nodules showed copy-number gain of the chromosome 1q32-qter and of the entire chromosome 20 (712). Among 12 HCC developing in the absence of cirrhosis copy number gains on chromosome 8q were found in all, 1q gains in 10 (83%), and 20q gains in 9 (75%); each change was significantly higher than in 55 HCC that developed in cirrhotic livers (712). Losses on 4q were also found in 9 HCC developing in a noncirrhotic liver (712). Overall, HCC developing in noncirrhotic livers contained 5.2 ± 2.9 copy number losses and 7.5 ± 2.8 copy-number gains, as compared to 3.3 ± 3.3 gains and 4.1 ± 2.7 losses in HCC developing in cirrhotic livers (712). Lin et al. *(709)* found more frequent chromosome aberrations in HCC from HBV-positive patients than in those from HBV-negative patients.

Gain of 10q was detected by Kusano et al. *(708)* only in HCV-infected cases, whereas amplification of 11q13 was found predominantly in HBV-positive tumors. Gains of 1q and 8q occurred at a high frequency (>80%) in 15 small, well-differentiated HCC, as well as in larger, more poorly differentiated tumors by Kusano et al. *(708),* who posited that these aberrations were acquired early in the process of cancer development. In contrast, the 11q13 amplification and the 13q loss were not found in any of 15 well-differentiated tumors, and the 10q loss was identified in only one, although each aberration occurred in 23% of 26 more poorly differentiated HCC, suggesting that these aberrations are closely associated with tumor progression *(708).* Losses at 1p, 4q, 8p, 16q, and 17p were all present in from 13–33% of 15 well-differentiated HCC and in 23–54% of 26 more poorly differentiated tumors, suggesting that these aberrations accumulated throughout the development of HCC; accumulation of chromosomal aberrations with increasing growth of HCC was shown clearly by the observation that 15 HCC less than 2 cm in diameter each contained an average of 4.5 chromosomal aberrations, whereas tumors that were 2–5 cm in diameter each contained an average of 7.6 aberrations, and those greater than 5 cm in diameter contained 8.8 aberrations each *(708).* Qin et al. *(710)* found that 8p loss was highly correlated with HCC metastasis.

MOLECULAR INTERACTIONS BETWEEN HBV AND HCV HEPATOCYTES

Over 65% of HCC have been attributed to chronic infection with HBV and over 20% to chronic infection with HCV *(713),* making these viruses the most important etiologic agents for HCC. This section briefly reviews evidence pertaining to the mechanisms by which genes and molecular products of HBV and HCV may interact with the hepatocellular genome and with key regulatory molecules to perturb cellular-regulatory pathways and thereby contribute to the development of the neoplastic phenotype. The general mechanisms of direct viral interference with hepatocellular molecules include integration of portions of the viral genome into the hepatocellular genome leading to distortion of DNA structure, and causing activation, extinction (deletion), or mutation of affected genes, transactivation of cellular genes by viral proteins, and inactivation of cellular regulatory proteins by binding with viral proteins.

GENOMIC INTEGRATION BY HBV DNA Multiple integrations of HBV genomic DNA into the hepatocellular genome occur during chronic viral hepatitis, cirrhosis, and HCC; clonal HBV integrants have been detected in about 80% of HCC *(714).* Although hepatocellular genomic integrants usually do not contain the entire HBV coding sequences, the HBV *X* gene and truncated *preS/S* gene sequences are frequently retained *(714).* Expression of the HBV *X* gene has been detected by immunohistochemical identification of X protein and/or *in situ* hybridization of *X* gene mRNA in a large fraction of chronic hepatitides, cirrhoses, and HCC in some studies *(515,715–718).*

The process of HBV genomic integration is associated with the production of microdeletions in the host cell genome, all of which are mutagenic and some of which provoke larger deletions and rearrangements of chromosomes *(714).* Because it is not site or sequence-specific, but random, HBV genomic integration indiscriminantly produces multiple microdeletions throughout the hepatocyte genome, some of which are amplified by the clonal growth of the cells that contain them *(714).* Amplified sites of random HBV DNA integrants into the hepatocellular genome demonstrate the monoclonality of many preneoplastic liver nodules and HCC, and highlight some of the genes in which aberrant expression may lead to clonal growth of the affected cells. The integrated HBV DNA also rearranges host genomic DNA, produces structural aberrations of chromosomes, and leads to aberrantly expressed genes *(714).* HBV genomic integration is a major factor leading to chromosome instability in HCC.

Simon and Carr *(719)* investigated a cell line which they established from an HCC by short-term culture, and demonstrated that HBV DNA integrated at chromosome 1p36 was associated with local rearrangement. Pasquenelli et al. *(720)* examined an HBV integration site located on chromosome 4 in which there was local rearrangement. Using unique cellular DNA sequences that were located adjacent to the HBV integration site, they demonstrated similar rearrangement in 3/40 HCC (8%) and 1/10 HCA (10%), but not in 40 control DNAs *(720).* Wang et al. *(390,391)* found that the *cyclin A* gene located on chromosome 4q27 was disrupted by HBV genomic integration, but LOH at this locus was identified in only 1/20 HCC (5%) *(392).* Blanquet et al. *(721)* identified an HBV DNA insertion site at chromosome 4q32.1 by *in situ* hybridization using a probe recovered from DNA at the edge of the insert. Tokino et al. *(722)* detected a HBV integration-related translocation between chromosomes 5 and 9; Rogler et al. *(723),* Fisher et al. *(724),* and Wang and Rogler *(630)* reported on deletions on chromosome 11p13-p14 in association with HBV genomic integration; and Hatada et al. *(725)* found integrated HBV DNA on chromosome 11q13.3 that was associated with amplification of the *int-2/hst-1* locus. Slagle et al. *(116)* detected LOH of the *E-cadherin* gene on 16q in conjunction with HBV integration. HBV integration sites on chromosome 17 have been identified in several studies and associated with chromosomal translocations; Hino et al. *(726)* identified a translocation between chromosomes 17 and 18, Meyer et al. *(727)* found a translocation involving both chromosomes 17, Becker et al. *(642)* identified a translocation between chromosomes 17 and 8, Tokino et al. *(722)* detected a translocation between chromosomes X and 17. Additionally, Zhou et al. *(728)* and Becker et al. *(647)* found an HBV integrant on chromosome 17p11.2-p12 near the p53 gene in different HCC, which were associated with LOH of the *p53* locus *(455,642).*

In a few instances, HBV genomic integration has occurred in specific hepatocellular-regulatory genes, perturbing gene function in ways suggesting *cis*-activation by insertional mutation. These integrations have been reported to affect the cyclin A gene, as noted earlier *(390),* the *retinoic acid β* gene *(332),* and the *EGFR* gene *(729).* Integrations of HBV DNA that perturb the function of specific genes seem to be so rare as to be virtually unique, and *cis*-activation does not appear to be a major molecular mechanism leading to HCC in humans. The majority of HBV integration sites probably occur in anonymous stretches of cellular DNA lacking identified genes.

Gene Transactivation by HBV Proteins Gene transactivation by HBV X antigen and/or truncated preS/S protein synthesized in hepatocytes in which HBV integration has occurred may be an important hepatocarcinogenic mechanism, because these integrated sequences recovered from HCC encode proteins that are transcriptionally active in hepatocytes *(730)*. Low levels of the *X* mRNA and protein have been detected in hepatocytes at all stages of hepatocarcinogenesis *(515,715–718)*. Considerable evidence now suggests that HBV X antigen is a relatively weak, but broadly active gene transactivator, and that the truncated preS/S protein may have a somewhat similar transactivating capacity. The X antigen protein interacts with several transcriptional regulatory molecules including TFIIB, ATF-2, RPB5, and CREB *(731–734)*. Among the various genes whose promoters have been reported to be transactivated or otherwise upregulated by the X antigen or preS/S protein include *IFN-β (735)*, the major histocompatibility complex (MHC) *(736)*, IL-8 *(737)*, *RNA polymerase II* and *RNA polymerase III (738)*, EGFR *(739)*, PKC *(740,741)*, c-*ras (742)*, c-*myc (743)*, c-*fos (744)*, c-*jun (728,745–747)*, TGF-α *(172)*, and *TNF-α (748–750)*. The transactivation of mitogenic growth factors and mitogenic nuclear transcription factors was correlated with increased activity of both the MAP kinase *(742,751–753)* and the JNK *(754)* signal pathways and elevated cycle transit of affected cells *(751)*.

Mutated HBV X Antigen Proteins The HBV genome is prone to undergo mutation; some viruses that contained mutated genomes have been associated with severe liver disease, including fulminant hepatitis *(755,756)*. Mutations continue to develop in the *preC/C (757)* and the *X (758)* genes after the HBV genome is integrated into the hepatocellular genome. In fact, the incidence of *X* gene mutations is more frequent than are mutations in the *preC/C* gene *(757,758)*, and the incidence of mutations and deletions in the *X* gene integrated into HCC is higher than in the *X* gene integrated in adjacent nontumorous hepatocytes. This observation suggests that *X* gene mutations occur at a higher rate in HCC cells and/or that they accumulate selectively in them *(758)*. *X* gene mutations and deletions produce a truncated C-terminal region, resulting in the continued expression of truncated protein. Using naturally occurring mutated *X* genes isolated from HCC and nontumorous liver, Sirma et al. *(759)* demonstrated that wild-type and truncated gene products have divergent effects on growth of cultured cells in vitro. When transfected into cultured cells, the wild-type *X* gene inhibited cell growth and blocked cell-cycle transit leading to apoptosis, but these inhibitory effects were abrogated by *X* gene mutations; Sirma et al. *(759)* suggested that loss of the antiproliferative and apoptotic properties of mutated X protein might render infected hepatocytes more susceptible to uncontrolled growth, and thereby contribute to the development of HCC.

MOLECULAR BINDING/INHIBITION BY HBV PROTEINS In addition to gene transactivation, the HBV X antigen may inhibit the function of key regulatory proteins in hepatocytes by protein-protein binding to form inactive complexes. Most notably, impaired function of p53 by the formation of X antigen/p53 complexes has been proposed *(448,511–515)*. The X antigen protein also has been found to impair nucleotide excision repair (NER) by interfering with the association between p53 and ERCC3, a transcription factor involved in NER *(511)*, as well as by binding to essential helicases through a p53-independent pathway *(760)*. The X antigen protein may also interfere with apoptosis at multiple control points, possibly through similar binding/inactivation mechanisms *(748,761–765)*.

Despite the many studies that have attempted to identify how the HBV *X* gene transforms hepatocytes, the mechanisms are still obscure. Indeed, it seems that the *X* gene (and possibly other HBV genes) may produce multiple molecular aberrations in infected hepatocytes that act to enhance the probability that they will undergo neoplastic transformation. Further studies are needed.

GENE TRANSACTIVATION AND PROTEIN BINDING BY HCV PROTEINS The molecular mechanisms by which HCV products alter hepatocytic function are not well-understood. HCV is an RNA virus that does not integrate into the hepatocellular genome. However, the HCV core protein, which is expressed in infected hepatocytes, may be able to transactivate some cellular genes and inactivate some hepatocellular proteins. The 5'-untranslated regions of the HCV viral gene contain putative translational control elements, which are conserved in HCV-related chronic liver diseases and HCC *(766)*. The HCV core protein has transforming potential for cultured cells *(767,768)*. Preliminary results suggest that HCV core proteins can transcriptionally regulate the c-*myc*, c-*fos*, p53, and *Rb1* genes *(768–772)*. The HCV core protein also interacts with cellular proteins as diverse as the cytoplasmic tail of the lymphotoxin-beta receptor *(773)*, the cytoplasmic components of the TNFR-1 *(774)*, and the heterogenous nuclear ribonucleoprotein *(775)*. Gene transactivations and protein-protein interactions may contribute to HCC development by modulating hepatocyte growth *(776,777)* and apoptosis *(774,776–782)*. Nevertheless, a clear picture of the mechanism of hepatocarcinogenesis in chronic HCV infection is not yet available, and further studies are needed.

ABERRANT REGULATION OF MISCELLANEOUS GENES

GLOBAL DISTORTION OF GENE EXPRESSION In addition to the proto-oncogenes and tumor suppressor genes that may be directly involved in development of HCC, the expression of many genes involved in general cellular metabolism (housekeeping genes) are also perturbed during hepatocarcinogenesis. The extent to which the expression and function of genes becomes globally distorted in HCC is currently unknown, but new techniques for analyzing the expression of multiple genes simultaneously (gene arrays) and to compare the expression of genes in matched neoplastic and normal tissues (subtractive hybridization, differential display RT-PCR (ddRT-PCR), serial analysis of gene expression, etc.) will lead to insights into the variety and number of genes that are aberrantly expressed in HCC. It seems likely that every gene is equally susceptible to genomic damage that precedes and accompanies the development of HCC, and a large fraction of them may be abnormally structured and/or regulated in highly progressed HCC.

A few studies applying some of these techniques have already appeared. Barnard et al. *(783)* generated cDNA libraries from an HCC and adjacent nontumorous tissue, and then developed two subtraction libraries (HCC minus nontumorous liver and nontumorous liver minus HCC). Screening of more than 2,000 plasmid inserts yielded 33 coding for 17 distinct sequences that were consistently expressed at higher levels in HCC or in nontumorous livers. Barnard et al. *(783)* focused their study on a single cDNA clone, which coded for acid ribosomal phosphoprotein PO (rpPO), and was overexpressed in 5/5 HCC, but not in adjacent nontumorous tissue. Huang and Hsu *(107)* used the differential display (DD) technique in paired HCC and nontumor liver tissue to reveal more than 200 candidate bands; they concentrated on three bands, one of which coded for CD24, which was overexpressed in 52/79 (HCC) (66%). Scuric et al. *(784)* used dd-PCR to identify genes that were differentially expressed in HCC and nontumorous liver tissue; among about 7,200 bands that were generated, 67 were differentially expressed in HCC and nontumorous tissue. One of these bands that was consistently expressed in HCC but not in nontumorous livers coded for a member of the aldose reductase enzyme family, which the investigators termed hepatoma-specific aldose reductase-related protein (HARP). Kondoh et al. *(219)* applied a somewhat similar technique, which they called serial analysis of gene expression, to analyze differences in expression of genes in HCC and adjacent nontumorous liver tissue. They detected more than 50,000 transcripts representing 15,000–20,000 different genes in nontumorous liver tissue and HCC. From these, 150 transcripts that showed expression differences of more than fivefold in HCC and nontumorous tissue were selected for further analysis. Twenty-eight transcripts were overexpressed in HCC and two in nontumorous tissue, but 22 of the 28 that were highly expressed in HCC were found also to be expressed more abundantly in other samples of nontumorous liver than in HCC; they focused their study on the remaining eight transcripts, which were identified as products of the *UDP-glucuronyl transferase (UGT)*, *ribosomal phosphoprotein PO (rpPO)*, *dek*, *insulin-like receptor binding protein 1 (IGFBP1)*, *galectin 4 (gal4)*, *vitronectin (vit)*, *retinoic acid-induced gene-E (Rig-E)*, and *cytochrome P450 3A4 genes*, *(CYP3A4)*; six of the genes, *UGT*, *PO*, *dek*, *IGFBP1*, *gal4*, and *vit* were more highly expressed in HCC, whereas expression of Rig-E was less highly expressed in HCC, and *CYP3A4* was upregulated in both HCC and adjacent nontumorous liver as compared to nondiseased normal liver *(219)*. As a method to detect and identify specific genes that are overexpressed or uniquely expressed in HCC, dd techniques are labor-intensive and pose major problems to distinguish between false-positives and true-positives. It appears possible that gene-array methods may ultimately enable a more global assessment of gene-expression patterns among individual HCC, preneoplastic liver lesions, and normal livers.

Several individual metabolic genes/enzymes have been studied more or less intensively in HCC. Increased activity of genes/enzymes such as DNA methyltransferase, glutamine synthase, and ornithine decarboxylase appears to be necessary for the development and growth of cancer cells. Altered functions of some metabolic enzymes may result from random genetic damage, while other enzymes may be secondarily affected by primary alterations in multifunctional regulatory pathways. Together these studies illustrate the range of functional abnormalities that characterize HCC tumor cells, and determine their phenotypic properties.

S-Adenosylmethionine Synthetase The S-adenosylmethionine synthetase (SAMS) enzyme catalyzes the formation of S-adenosylmethionine (SAM), which is the substrate for intracellular methylations, including DNA methylation. Although the normal liver and liver tissue adjacent to HCC express only liver-specific SAMS isoforms (the α and β isoforms), only the kidney-specific SAMS isoform (δ isoform) mRNA was detected by RT-PCR in 4 HCC *(785)*. Kidney-specific SAMS has a lower K_m value for methionine than does the liver-specific form, causing this isoform to be more efficient in the utilization of methionine at the low ambient level available to hepatocytes. Cai et al. *(785)* proposed that the expression of the kidney type of SAMS might give neoplastic hepatocytes a competitive growth advantage over the nonneoplastic hepatocytes.

O6-Alkylguanine-DNA-Alkyltransferase Studies by Lee et al. *(786)* on the immunohistochemical expression of O^6-alkylguanine-DNA-alkyltransferase, responsible for the repair of promutagenic DNA adduct, O^6-alkylguanine, suggest that hepatocytes in cirrhotic livers may be impaired in their capacity to repair O^6-alkylguanine adducts. This enzyme is located in the nuclei of nondiseased hepatocytes, while it was found to be segregated in the cytoplasm of hepatocytes in HBV-related cirrhosis; nevertheless, the activity of the enzyme was not altered from that found in nondiseased liver and Western blots did not indicate that the molecules were abnormal in size *(786)*.

BAT (Kan-1) Furutani et al. *(787)* examined the expression of the gene encoding bile acid CoA:amino acid N-acetyltransferase *(BAT* or *Kan-1)*, which conjugates bile acids with taurine or glycine, in 37 HCC. They showed that *BAT* mRNA expression in 37 HCC was higher than in either cholangiocarcinoma or metastatic cancers; relatively high expression of BAT, probably reflecting better differentiation, was associated with a somewhat longer disease-free interval after resection *(787)*.

Cyclooxygenase-1 and Cyclooxygenase-2 Koga et al. *(788)* examined the expression of cyclooxygenase-1 (COX-1) and cyclooxygenase-2 (COX-2) proteins in 44 HCC and adjacent nontumorous liver tissues (including 17 cases of chronic hepatitis and 27 cases of cirrhosis), and in 7 histologically normal liver tissues. COX-1 protein was weakly expressed in nondiseased liver, and upregulated by about four-fold in chronic hepatitis and cirrhosis; expression remained elevated above the normal level in 14 well-differentiated HCC, but decreased to the level of normal liver in 34 moderately differentiated HCC and to about half the normal level in poorly differentiated HCC. COX-2 was expressed at approximately the same level in normal liver and in chronic hepatitis and cirrhosis, and expression increased about 1.3-fold in 14 well-differentiated HCC; expression of COX-2 protein decreased significantly in 34 moderately differentiated and in 8 poorly differentiated HCC. Koga et al. *(788)* suggested that COX-2 might have a role only in early stages of hepatocarcinogenesis.

Cytochromes P450 Yu et al. *(789)* found no association between the genotypic variants of *CYP1A1* determined by PCR of DNA from leukocytes of 81 patients with HCC and 409 controls; however, the presence of the Msp or Ile-Val variant allele was significantly increased among HCC patients who smoked, suggesting that polycyclic aromatic hydrocarbons derived from cigarette smoke may play a role in hepatocarcinogenesis.

Raunio et al. *(790)* found that CYP2A6 protein (detected by Western blot and immunohistochemistry) was heterogeneously overexpressed in 10/24 HCC (42%) and 9/16 adjacent nontumorous liver tissues (56%). CYP2A6 was also upregulated in human liver affected by chronic hepatitis and cirrhosis *(791)*. Although CYP2A6 metabolically activates several procarcinogenic chemicals, including aflatoxin B_1, increased expression in HCC was associated with better prognosis. Kondoh et al. *(219)* found that *CYP3A4* mRNA was upregulated in both HCC and adjacent nontumorous liver, as detected by a variation of dd-PCR.

DNA Methyltransferase Abnormal methylation of many genes accompanies the development of HCC *(113,477,651)*. The enzyme, DNA methyltransferase, whose transcription is upregulated at an early stage of hepatocarcinogenesis, catalyzes gene methylation. Using RT-PCR to detect *DNA methyltransferase* mRNA, Sun et al. *(792)* showed that the transcripts of this gene, as compared to β-actin mRNA, were more abundant in 28 HCC (0.34 ± 0.18) than in 6 nondiseased livers (0.14 ± 0.05); DNA methyltransferase was also elevated in 24 livers adjacent to HCC that were affected by cirrhosis or chronic hepatitis (0.30 ± 0.22) *(792)*, suggesting that the increase in the transcription of the gene for this enzyme occurs at an early stage of hepatocarcinogenesis preceding the emergence of HCC. Once HCC developed, transcription of the *DNA methyltransferase* gene did not increase further *(792)*, supporting its involvement in the earliest steps of hepatocarcinogenesis.

α-L-Fucosidase The activity of α-L-fucosidase was reduced by 25–40% in 14 HCC as compared to adjacent nontumorous tissue, although other characteristics of the enzyme, including thermostability, substrate affinity, and isoenzyme pattern were unchanged *(793)*. Despite the decreased activity in HCC, α-L-fucosidase increased in the serum of patients with HCC *(794)*; the serum activity in 32 patients with HCC was 146 ± 12 nkat/L as compared to 71 ± 6 nkat/L in 36 patients with cirrhosis and 51 ± 5 nkat/L in 30 healthy controls. Hutchinson et al. *(795)* confirmed these relative levels of α-L-fucosidase in plasma of patients with HCC (n = 6), cirrhosis (n = 6), and in normal subjects (n = 6); however, the activities in HCC and adjacent nontumorous liver did not differ significantly.

Fucosyltransferases Activities of α2-L-fucosyltransferase, α3-L-fucosyltransferase, and α6-L-fucosyltransferase

were elevated significantly in sera of 31 HCC patients as compared to 22 patients with cirrhosis and 10 healthy controls *(795)*; in contrast, the activity of α2-L-fucosyltransferase and α3-fucosyltransferase was lower in homogenates prepared from HCC (2 pmol/h/mg protein) as compared to homogenates made from adjacent nontumorous liver tissue (5 pmol/h/mg protein). Activities of galactosyltransferase and mannosyltransferase in HCC were higher than in adjacent nontumorous tissue *(795)*.

Glucose Transporters Increased (up to 20-fold) expression of mRNA (Northern blot) encoding the *facilitated glucose transporter* gene (brain type, but not of the erythrocyte type) was found in 6/10 HCC (60%) as compared to the levels in adjacent nontumorous liver tissue *(796)*.

UDP-Glucuronyltransferase *UGT1A* transcripts (Northern blot) were downregulated significantly in 12 HCC and 1 HCA, as compared to nondiseased liver tissue *(797)*. Quantification of RT-PCR products by laser densitometry (normalized to β-*actin* transcripts) confirmed the downregulation of each of the multiple transcripts of the *UGT1A* gene in HCC except for *UGT1A6*, which showed no change as compared to nondiseased liver; UGT1A protein was also reduced (immunoblot), and the benign HCA and malignant HCC showed similar changes *(797)*. Kondoh et al. *(219)* found that another member of the *UGT* gene family, *UGT2B*, was upregulated significantly in HCC as compared to adjacent nontumorous liver.

Glutamine Synthase Glutamine is an essential substrate for cell proliferation, and may be rate-limiting under normal circumstances. Matsuno and Goto *(798)* found that the activity of glutamine synthase (GS) was significantly reduced in 11 HCC (3.0 ± 0.71 nmol/min/mg protein) as compared to either 11 adjacent cirrhotic livers (7.8 ± 2.2 nmol/min/mg protein) or 15 nondiseased livers (9.8 ± 2.0 nmol/min/mg protein). In contrast, after detecting *GS* transcripts by subtractive screening of an HCC cDNA library, Christa et al. *(799)* found elevated levels of *GS* mRNA (3-fold to 46-fold increases) in 23/34 HCC (68%) as compared to the adjacent nontumorous liver tissue; increased *GS* mRNA was correlated with increased GS protein and, in 6/8 HCC selected for study, with increased GS enzyme activity (2-fold to 90-fold increases). In general agreement, Osada et al. *(800)* showed by immunohistochemical analysis that GS accumulated in 19/49 advanced HCC (39%) and by immunoblot analysis in 9/16 HCC (56%), whereas GS was not expressed in nondiseased livers except for a narrow rim of hepatocytes adjacent to terminal hepatic veins. The frequency of GS immunostaining was lowest in preneoplastic adenomatous hyperplasias (1/23, 4%), and increased progressively in early HCC (4/31, 13%) and advanced HCC (19/49, 39%), suggesting that the ability to express GS was acquired during the phase of tumor progression *(800)*. This opinion was supported by the observation that in nodule-in-nodule HCC, composed of both low-grade and high-grade HCC, the high-grade component was more often GS-positive (9/21, 43%) than was the low-grade component (1/21, 5%), and patients with single nodules of GS-positive HCC had shorter relapse-free intervals after resection than did those patients whose single nodules of HCC were GS-negative *(800)*. Osada et al. *(800)* also demonstrated that GS protein was normally ubiquinated and suggested that reduced ubiquination of GS protein was responsible for its accumulation in HCC.

Glutathione S-transferase Early studies indicated that glutathione S-transferase (GST) activity was lower in HCC than in nontumorous liver tissue *(801)*. This was confirmed in studies showing that the overall activity of GST was significantly lower in 32 HCC (163 ± 32 nmol/min/mg protein) than in 32 matched nontumorous tissues (348 ± 30 nmol/min/mg protein) *(802)* All classes of GST were lower in HCC than in nontumorous liver; the expression of GSTα and GSTπ in HCC was similar, but only 1/3 as many HCC expressed GSTμ as did the nontumorous livers *(802)*. The distribution of the *GSTM1* null genotype was also similar in HCC and nontumorous liver tissue although the total enzyme activity was less in HCC, and HBV infection was associated with lower GST activity, but had no effect on the distribution of GST types *(802)*. The results suggest that HBV infection may compromise the ability of the liver to detoxify certain chemicals by Phase II reactions, and, not surprisingly, that this detoxifying capability is further attenuated in HCC.

Glycine-N-methyltransferase Chen et al. *(803)* identified the differential expression of the *glycine-N-methyltransferase* (*GMT*) gene (which codes for an enzyme that regulates the cellular level of S-adenosylmethionine by consuming it to generate sarcosine) by differential display RT-PCR using paired cDNAs from HCC and nontumorous liver. Expression of the *GMT* gene was markedly diminished or absent from each of 7 HCC, and the GMT protein was lacking in tumor cells in contrast to normal hepatocytes.

Haptocorrin Haptocorrin, a vitamin B_{12}-binding protein, was detected by immunohistochemistry in 28/30 HCC (93%), but only rarely in adjacent nondiseased or cirrhotic livers *(804)*.

Heparanase Vlodavsky et al. *(805)* cloned the gene for heparanase, an enzyme that degrades heparan sulfate proteoglycans, from a human HCC cell line and from placenta. They demonstrated that *heparanase* mRNA (*in situ* hybridization) and protein (immunohistochemistry) were intensely expressed by HCC, but not by normal adult liver tissue.

Ornithine Decarboxylase Protein and mRNA corresponding to ornithine decarboxylase (ODC), detected by immunohistochemistry and *in situ* hybridization, respectively, were increased up to three-fold in 25 HCC as compared to nondiseased or cirrhotic livers *(365,806)*. This observation was corroborated by Tamori et al. *(807)* who also found a nearly three-fold increase in *ODC* mRNA by Northern blotting of extracted RNA in 10 HCC as compared to adjacent nontumorous liver. Furthermore, the ODC activity was increased in 32 HCC (147 ± 29 pmol/h/mg protein), as compared to 30 adjacent noncancerous tissues (23 ± 4 pmol/h/mg protein), and enzyme activities were higher in poorly differentiated than in moderately or well-differentiated HCC *(807)*. Increased ODC activity in HCC resulted in higher levels of the polyamines (putrescine, spermidine, and spermine) than in nontumorous liver tissue and the level of ODC activity was highly correlated with the level of cell proliferation as measured in 13 HCC by immunohistochemical detection of PCNA *(365)*. Point mutations were also detected in the PEST region of the ODC gene (determined by sequencing RT-PCR products

in each of 3 HCC), which increased the resistance of the ODC protein to degradation and offered a hypothetical basis for the increased ODC enzyme activity in HCC *(808)*.

Because polyamines are necessary for cell proliferation, these alterations probably give tumor cells a relative growth advantage over the adjacent non-neoplastic cells. In an expanded study, Koh et al. *(809)* examined the sequence of the ODC gene in 58 cDNA clones from 13 HCC. Mutations in the PEST region composed 38% of all mutations, and most of the remainder were located upstream of the PEST region. Mutations were not found in 11 clones from 3 well-differentiated HCC, as compared to 6 mutations in 23 clones from 5 moderately differentiated HCC (26%) and 11 mutations in 42 clones from 5 poorly differentiated HCC (42%); no mutations were found in 6 clones from 2 nondiseased livers, whereas 2 mutations were detected in 24 clones from livers that were the sites of chronic hepatitis and/or cirrhosis (7%) *(809)*. The frequency of *ODC* mutation correlated with poor differentiation and large size of HCC, suggesting that the mutant *ODC* was related to cancer progression *(809)*.

Ribosomal Phosphoprotein PO Expression of *rpPO* transcripts was increased by four-fold in two HCC as compared to matched nontumorous liver tissue *(783)*. This result was confirmed by Kondoh et al. *(219)*, who found that *rpPO* transcripts were upregulated in each of 5 HCC by 1.2-fold to 5-fold, as compared to matched adjacent nontumorous liver tissue.

Thrombomodulin Expression of thrombomodulin, which converts thrombin into an activator of protein C, was detected by immunohistochemistry in 25/141 resected HCC less than 6 cm in diameter (18%) *(810)*; thrombomodulin expression was shown to correlate with a significantly longer recurrence free interval.

Thrombopoietin Elevated serum levels of thrombopoietin (TPO) were found in each of 8 patients with HBL and shown to correlate with thrombocytosis *(811)*. The HBL were presumed to be the source of the increased TPO because RT-PCR demonstrated increased expression of *TPO* mRNA in each of the HBL *(811)*.

DISCUSSION

The sequential changes in hepatocellular phenotype that characterize the development of preneoplastic lesions and HCC serve as a map for defining the temporal order of alterations in regulatory molecules and pathways that drive the development of this neoplasm. At the cellular level, hepatocarcinogenesis is a more-or-less linear and progressive process in which successively more aberrant monoclonal populations of cells evolve. The time of infection with HBV or HCV, which are the major causes of HCC in humans and which start the process of hepatocarcinogenesis in most instances, can often be established with reasonable accuracy, and the hepatocellular alterations that follow are separable into preneoplastic and neoplastic phases by well-established histocytological criteria. During the preneoplastic phase, several emerging populations of altered cells proliferate clonally to form a series of lesions composed of abnormal cells (foci and nodules of phenotypically altered hepatocytes and foci and nodules of dysplastic hepatocytes), each new population arising from a change that occurs in a previous one. Eventually, cytologically benign HCA and/or malignant HCC evolve from this process of cellular alterations (Figs. 1 and 2). Comparison of molecular genetic changes that first appear at various points during the preneoplastic phase with those that are initially found in fully developed, benign or malignant neoplasms is the first step necessary to define a temporal order of molecular genetic changes, and ultimately, perhaps, to identify the essential early alterations in gene function that enable HCC to evolve.

Malignant progression of HCC from early, small, well-differentiated, and localized tumors to late, large, poorly differentiated, and disseminated tumors can be evaluated by using reliable tumor grading and clinical-staging schemes. The development and/or accumulation of molecular genetic changes in HCC of different histocytological grades and clinical stages may allow the identification of those changes that are associated with increasing malignancy (progression) and dissemination of HCC. Although HCA are not considered to be obligate lineal precursors of HCC in humans, these benign hepatocellular neoplasms occasionally become malignant; comparison of molecular alterations in cells of HCA and HCC may yield useful information on the molecular changes that determine the evolution of liver neoplasms from benign to malignant.

MOLECULAR GENETIC CHANGES DURING THE PRENEOPLASTIC PHASE

Infection of hepatocytes by HBV or HCV, the influx of inflammatory cells, and the death of many hepatocytes represent the earliest events that take place during the preneoplastic phase of hepatitis virus-associated HCC. Hepatocytes and other cellular and noncellular components of the liver are exposed not only to HBV and HCV (and other etiological agents), but also to complex mixtures of inflammatory cytokines, growth factors, and matrix-degrading enzymes in the chronically inflamed liver; the resulting interactions among hepatocytes, other liver cells, inflammatory cells, matrix molecules/cellular matrix receptors, growth factors, and inflammatory cytokines play major roles in the phenotypes expressed by altered hepatocytes during the early stages of hepatocarcinogenesis. The microenvironment of the liver is greatly modified by the chronic inflammatory cells and the cytokines they produce and by the inflammatory cytokine-induced stimulation of endogenous liver cells, to themselves express cytokines and growth factors; many hepatocytes are killed and the liver matrix is extensively remodeled by the actions of the inflammatory cells and cytokines. Of course, not all hepatocytes involved in chronic hepatitis and cirrhosis are affected, but a sufficient fraction are involved to make these early alterations one of the strongest risk factors for eventual development of HCC.

A major feature of the preneoplastic phase, resulting from both chronic inflammation and hepatocyte death, is a sustained increase in the proliferation of residual hepatocytes, leading to the development of multiple hepatocyte populations, many of which are monoclonal. High microenvironmental levels of several potent growth factors for receptors expressed by hepatocytes drive hepatocyte proliferation. Some of the inflammatory cytokines also promote the proliferation of hepatocytes; TNF-α and IL6 directly stimulate hepatocyte proliferation and also prime hepatocytes so that they respond more vigorously to mitogenic and comitogenic growth factors and hormones. TGF-α, IGF-2, and HGF are strongly upregulated or newly expressed by various liver cells during the preneoplastic phase. The receptor for HGF, c-met, is also upregulated, and receptors for TGF-α (EGFR) and IGF-2 (IGF1R or IR) continue to be expressed by hepatocytes at functional levels. The availability of IGF-2 to mitogenic receptors on hepatocytes appears to be increased further by the inactivation of M6P/IGF-2R, which normally shuttles IGF-2 molecules to lysosomes where they are degraded, thereby competing with authentic signaling receptors for available IGF-2 in the extracellular microenvironment. M6P/IGF-2R is inactivated by a combination of allelic deletion and mutation, and these aberrations have also been identified in a few preneoplastic hepatocytes located in dysplastic cirrhotic nodules adjacent to HCC. Simultaneously, the activity of the major antimitogenic growth factor for hepatocytes, TGF-β, is reduced even though the production of proTGF-β is increased. Functional activity of TGF-β is limited as a consequence of reduced availability of M6P/IGF-2R, the lack of which impairs the activation of proTGF-β. In addition, the receptors that transmit the TGF-β signal through the hepatocyte membrane, TGF-βRI and TGF-βRII, are downregulated in some livers during HCC development, probably by reduced gene transcription, as well as by MSI and intragenic mutations. Furthermore, the intracellular-signaling network activated by the binding of TGF-β to its receptors is defective in a subset of HCC due to mutation and/or LOH of *Smad2* and *Smad4* genes; whether these latter alterations occur during the preneoplastic phase is not yet known.

As a consequence of the intense mitogenic stimulation to which hepatocytes are subjected in livers that are the sites of chronic hepatitis and cirrhosis, the MAPK pathway is stimulated in hepatocytes, with increased levels of p21 ras protein and increased activity of MEK1, MEK2 ERK1, and ERK2, leading to the upregulation of p63 c-myc protein, a potent nuclear transcription factor. Identification of these molecular changes in a major mitogenic signaling pathway also infers that the activities of other cell cycle regulatory molecules, such as cyclins, cyclin-dependent kinases, and cyclin kinase inhibitors, are affected during the preneoplastic phase; other mitogenic signaling pathways are also probably activated, although these have not yet been investigated. Expression of both the *Rb1* and *p53* genes is altered, predominantly reflecting the mitogenic stimulation of multiple growth factors at this phase of hepatocarcinogenesis.

It is of interest that most of the molecular changes that occur during the preneoplastic phase appear to have an epigenetic basis. Increased hepatocyte proliferation seems initially to reflect paracrine stimulation from the production of mitogenic and comitogenic growth factors by infiltrating inflammatory cells and by nonparenchymal liver cells that are stimulated by inflammatory cytokines to secrete growth factors. However, reactive hepatocytes also are stimulated to express mitogenic growth factors (especially TGF-α and IGF-2 and, perhaps, HGF) for receptors they normally express, establishing the molecular basis for autocrine mitogenic cycles in hepatocytes. Transactivation of growth-promoting genes by proteins expressed by HBV and HCV may contribute to increased hepatocyte proliferation.

A major event in the hepatocarcinogenic process involves the conversion of these early epigenetic (and, therefore, potentially reversible) alterations in gene expression into irreversible structural aberrations of genes and chromosomes. Alterations in the methylation of CpG islands of gene-promoter sequences, which can either increase or decrease gene transcription, represent an important mechanism for controlling the function of many genes, and, possibly, for converting potentially reversible alterations to a virtually irreversible form. For example, hypomethylation of the c-myc gene is associated with increased gene expression in preneoplastic and neoplastic hepatocytes, while the c-myc gene is amplified in many HCC; hypomethylation precedes and may lead to gene amplification. In contrast, gene hypermethylation is associated with reduced or extinguished expression of some genes, and the hypermethylated loci appear to be sites at which allelic deletion later occurs. It is of interest that several proteins and enzymes that are responsible for the availability of methyl groups and the methylation of DNA, including S-adenosylmethionine, glycine-N-methyltransferase, and DNA methyltransferase, are coordinately upregulated in HCC, and the activation of these proteins and enzymes appears to occur at an early stage of hepatocarcinogenesis.

Increased hepatocyte proliferation during the preneoplastic phase is associated with the shortening of telomeres and, ultimately, with the upregulation of telomerase, which allows affected cells to proliferate continuously (immortal). Together with insertion of HBV DNA into cellular genomes, chromosome end-fusion as a result of telomere erosion may contribute to early chromosome structural aberrations when coupled with breakage at mitosis. In addition, impairment of DNA MMR is evident in some livers during the preneoplastic phase, with instabilities in both microsatellite and minisatellite sequences. Structural aberrations in a few genes and chromosomes have been found in hepatocytes even during the preneoplastic phase. Allelic loss in the M6P/IGF-2R gene has been identified in a few dysplastic nodules in livers lacking HCC, as well as in cirrhotic nodules adjacent to HCC. Additionally, loss of heterozygosity of the Rb1 and p53 genes have been described in the nonneoplastic hepatocytes of cirrhotic nodules adjacent to HCC in a very few instances, and, as well, loss of anonymous alleles on chromosomes 1p and 8p. Cells containing these molecular genetic changes, clonally amplified in foci and nodules are the immediate precursors of HCC.

It seems possible that most of the permanent changes in gene structure (MSI, allelic loss, and mutation) are the byproducts of the continuously accelerated hepatocyte proliferation that characterizes chronic hepatitis and cirrhosis. Integration of the HBV genome into the hepatocyte genome may accelerate this evolution by producing microdeletions randomly throughout the genome. Furthermore, heightened cell proliferation enables the amplification of hepatocytes containing genetic alterations that favor cell formation, as well as the accumulation of cells that contain multiple molecular aberrations. Accelerated hepatocyte proliferation also facilitates the development of clonal divergence leading to even more poorly regulated cells.

MOLECULAR GENETIC CHANGES IN HCA Few HCA have been studied for either their phenotypic or molecular genetic characteristics; in total, some molecular genetic features have been reported for only 30 or so HCA; more studies of these benign hepatocellular neoplasms are needed in order to determine their exact relationship to HCC and to the preneoplastic cellular lesions that precede HCC. No studies have been found that depict the phenotypic properties of HCA with the detail available for FAH or HCC. However, monoclonality has been demonstrated in 9 of the 10 HCA examined, indicating that in common with HCC and some cirrhotic nodules, HCA are often derived by the repeated proliferation of a single hepatocyte. Increased levels of HGF were found in all HCA studied, and elevations of both ER and PR were detected in over 80%, but each of these studies analyzed only 2–5 HCA. Strong immunohistochemical staining of p21 ras protein was found in most of the few HCA studied, but p53 protein was not detected. LOH of the hMSH2, hMLH2, and M6P/IGF-2R genes were also found in 1 or 2 HCA, and LOH on chromosome 8p was identified in one HCA, but no abnormalities were detected in the copy number of either chromosomes 1 or 8 by FISH analysis among 6 HCA. Furthermore, no LOH were found in multiple loci on 21 other chromosome arms by RFLP analysis among 6 HCA, or in one HCA that developed in synchrony with an HCC that showed allelic loss on chromosome 17.

Taken together, these fragmentary data suggest that HCA represent an evolutionary stage in the hepatocarcinogenesis process later in the sequence than foci or hyperplastic nodules, but earlier than HCC. However, the exact relationship of HCA to preneoplastic lesions and to HCC in humans remains to be established.

MOLECULAR GENETIC CHANGES WITH MALIGNANT CONVERSION Intense mitogenic signaling by elevated expression of mitogenic growth factors/receptors, established during the preneoplastic phase, continues in HCC. The growth factors TGF-a, IGF-2, and HGF, together with their receptors, are each expressed in a major fraction of HCC of all grades of differentiation, providing the molecular basis for constitutive autocrine mitogenic signaling. Heightened expression of c-myc is also maintained in HCC; upregulation of c-myc expression in HCC is correlated with hypomethylation or amplification in a large fraction of HCC; the frequency of amplification increases with impairment of tumor differentiation. The cyclin molecules that control the passage of hepatocytes through the G_1 phase of the cell cycle (cyclin D, cyclin E, and cyclin A) are strongly upregulated, in association with sharp reductions in the cyclin-dependent kinase inhibitors (p16^{INK4A}, p21$^{WAF1/CIP1}$, and p27^{KIP1}) that normally keep these cyclins in an inactive state. Expression of p16^{INK4A} is suppressed in many HCC in association with gene hypermethylation, occurring even in the smallest, best differentiated HCC (early HCC), with the frequency of p16^{INK4A} suppression increasing with impairment of tumor differentiation. Expression of at least one of the major cyclin-dependent kinase inhibitor molecules (p16^{INK4A}, p21$^{WAF1/CIP1}$, and p27^{KIP1}) is impaired in a major fraction of HCC in which all three molecules have been evaluated. Decreased expression of Rb1 and p53 genes, associated with allelic deletion and mutation of the remaining allele is found in many HCC, the frequency increasing with tumor progression. Overexpression and mutation of the β-*catenin* gene are also found in many HCC, associated with the nuclear accumulation of this molecule, which stimulates the transcription of additional genes associated with cell proliferation. Expression of the *E-cadherin* gene is decreased in many advanced HCC, apparently facilitating the separation and dispersal of affected tumor cells.

Neoplastic hepatocytes in many HCC develop molecular alterations that help them to avoid being killed by cytotoxic T-cells. These changes include the expression of membrane-anchored FasL, the expression of soluble FasL, and the expression of membrane-anchored CD40 (a TNFR-like molecule that lacks cytoplasmic death domains). Together these newly expressed molecules inactivate armed T-cells before they contact tumor cells, offer T-cells an inactive (decoy) receptor, and/or enable tumor cells sometimes to kill T-cells.

Progressive development of abnormalities in multiple chromosomal loci, karyotypic aberrations, allelic deletions, and mutation of specific genes correlates with the malignant conversion of preneoplastic lesions to HCC, and their subsequent growth and progression. Only rare LOH and/or mutations have been identified in hepatocytes forming either preneoplastic lesions, such as cirrhotic and dysplastic nodules, or benign HCA. Additionally, allelic deletions and gene mutations are uncommon in small, well-differentiated early HCC, but they accumulate in advanced HCC in coordination with deteriorating differentiation and with the growth of tumors to large size. LOH on chromosome 8p have been found in HCA and as the only chromosome aberration in a few HCC. Likewise, LOH on 1p, but not LOH on 4q, 13q, 16q, have been identified in small early HCCs; in contrast, these latter loci and others are sites of significant allelic losses in advanced HCC, with the frequency of LOH on the affected chromosome arms increasing as HCC grow progressively and lose differentiated properties. Among many studies that included hundreds of HCC at all stages of development, more than 30% of HCC contained allelic deletions in 14 chromosome arms (1p, 1q, 4q, 5q, 6q, 8p, 8q, 9p, 11p, 13q, 14q, 16p, 16q, and 17p). The *M6P/IGFIIR*, *E-cadherin*, *Rb1*, *p53*, *PTEN/MMAC1*, *EXT1*, and *p73* genes show allelic losses in 20–65% of HCC, and mutations of the *M6P/IGFIIR*, *Rb1*, *p53*, β-*catenin*, and *PTEN/MMAC1* genes have been detected in over 20% of the remaining alleles in HCC that show LOH at these loci. LOH on chromosome arms 1p, 4q, 5q, 8p, 13q, 16q, and 17p all occurred with increasing frequencies correlated with decreasing differentiation of HCC, indicating that the accumulation of these allelic deletions is associated with tumor progression. A similar relationship has been found with mutation of the *p53* gene and LOH of the *Rb1* gene, which increase in coordination with the progressive deterioration in the differentiation of HCC. Similarly, the expression of *p16INK4A* and *E-cadherin* is reduced, whereas expression of *telomerase* and β-*catenin* are increased as HCC differentiation is progressively impaired.

Taken together, these results suggest that malignant conversion of HCC is correlated with the occurrence of a crescendo of genetic aberrations, and that escalation of genomic instability is a major feature of progressing HCC. The functions of mul-

tiple genes, including several that are known, and many that remain unidentified, are perturbed by these changes. In addition to genes known to be involved in HCC, such as *p53* and *Rb1*, the chromosome arms that contain frequent allelic deletions include a large number of unidentified genes that may also function as tumor-suppressor genes for HCC. So-called housekeeping genes, many not directly involved in HCC development, also acquire abnormal functional properties in HCC. Together, the aberrant expression of all of these numerous genes gives cells of HCC their ultimate neoplastic phenotypic properties.

MOLECULAR GENETIC CHANGES IN HBL Molecular genetic alterations have been investigated in many HBL, but the variety of genes and gene products examined are much less than for HCC. The results of published studies suggest both similarities and differences in the molecular genetic alterations in HBL and HCC.

Although not associated with chronic inflammation, the matrix alterations described in HBL resemble those found in HCC. Only a few specific growth factor/receptor combinations have been studied in HBL; as in HCC, IGF-2 is overexpressed in the majority of HBL, and the serum levels of HGF in HBL patients are greatly elevated while the tumor cells express numerous c-met receptors. The c-*myc* gene is overexpressed in many HBL, but not amplified, and both *cyclin D1* and *CDK4* are upregulated. Unlike HCC, no abnormalities have been found in the *p16INK4A*, *p15INK4B*, and *p18INK4C* genes or products, as compared to nondiseased livers.

Overexpression of the p53 protein was detected by immunohistochemistry in over 66% of the HBL examined, but gene mutations and LOH were found in only about 15%, and the *mdm2* gene was not amplified in any. In contrast to HCC, a significant fraction of HBL contained LOH and mutation in the *APC* gene. Furthermore, germline aberrations in the *APC* gene are associated with an increased risk to development of HBL. Mutations in the degradation targeting box of the β-*catenin* gene are frequent in HBL, as is accumulation of β-catenin in HBL cells. These results suggest that aberrations in the Wnt signal-transduction pathway are particularly important in the molecular pathogenesis of HBL.

HBL have been less completely allelotyped than have HCC, but allelic losses in more than 20% of informative HBL have been detected on 1p, 1q, 11p, 11q, and 17p. Common karyotypic abnormalities include trisomy of chromosome 20, chromosome 2, and chromosome 18, duplication of portions of chromosome 8, structural aberrations of chromosome 1 with frequent losses on 1p and gain of 1q, and translocations involving chromosome 4. Trisomy of chromosomes 20, 2, and 18 are not frequently found in HCC, but structural changes in chromosomes 1, 4, and 8 occur in both neoplasms. The specific genes responsible for the effects of these chromosomal aberrations in HBL have not been identified.

TEMPORAL SEQUENCE OF MOLECULAR ABERRATIONS Knowledge of the chronology of the development of molecular genetic aberrations might be used to increase the precision with which diagnosis and prognosis of preneoplastic or early neoplastic stages of HCC can be determined, enabling early treatment to be implemented, and, as well, it might provide a basis for devising new molecular-based therapies. However, the delineation of a temporal sequence is made difficult by the complexity of molecular regulation of gene function.

In contrast to the linear sequence of cellular changes that are precursors of HCC and involve only a few types of aberrant hepatocytes, the molecular genetic aberrations associated with hepatocarcinogenesis affect several complex networks of interacting molecules that regulate the multi-faceted phenotypes of normal hepatocytes (812,813). Regulation of hepatocyte proliferation through control of the cell cycle, cell death (apoptosis), cell differentiation, and DNA repair involve multiple genes grouped into more-or-less distinct but overlapping regulatory networks. These regulatory networks involve numerous individual genes/products and contain many redundant elements, alternate pathways, and points of interaction (812,813); regulation of many cellular properties requires the action of multiple genes/molecules acting in combination. Accordingly, it seems likely that several different combinations of various aberrantly expressed genes and regulatory networks can sufficiently dysregulate hepatocyte proliferation, differentiation, and maintenance of genomic stability to enable affected cells to display aberrant phenotypes, including neoplasia. In keeping with this hypothesis, the molecular genetic aberrations found thus far in HCC are heterogeneous; the aberrations in individual genes most frequently expressed in HCC have been detected in no more than about 60% of even the most highly progressed of these cancers, implying that various combinations of aberrantly expressed genes are sufficient to drive neoplastic transformation of hepatocytes. Complexity and redundancy of cellular regulation make it difficult to identify a particular sequence of molecular genetic changes that leads repeatedly to the development of HCC, even if such a regularly involved sequence exists, or to distinguish clearly between molecular aberrations that are necessary for development of HCC and those that are not.

The initial molecular changes that have been detected during the process of hepatocarcinogenesis involve predominantly the complex regulatory networks that control the cycling of hepatocytes. These molecular changes are heralded by stimulation of mitogenic pathways by the coincident upregulation of several potent mitogenic growth factors/receptors, coupled with loss of effectiveness of the major antimitogenic regulatory pathway entrained by TGF-β; these early molecular changes are preceded and accompanied by major changes in the extracellular matrix (ECM) of the liver, and in the regulation of cell-cell and cell-matrix interactions. Associated with the elevated hepatocyte proliferation that results from the intense and ineffectively opposed mitogenic stimulation, intracellular regulatory networks that control hepatocyte cycling, chromosome telomeres, DNA MMR, apoptosis, and differentiation all develop aberrations that reduce their effectiveness in the face of chronically sustained cell proliferation. The early stimulation of hepatocyte proliferation is predominantly epigenetic and potentially reversible. The likely point-of-no-return to a normal hepatocyte phenotype is reached with the development of irreversible structural alterations in genes and chromosomes

(mutations, allelic deletions, and translocations, as well as loss and gain of entire chromosomes), which reach a crescendo in rapidly growing HCC.

Because most of the current studies have been limited to the simultaneous analysis of no more than one or two specific genes or chromosomal loci, we do not yet know how extensively molecular aberrations involve parallel and/or intersecting regulatory pathways in individual HCC. Preliminary evidence suggests both that individual regulatory pathways may be affected at multiple points, and that different regulatory pathways may be impaired simultaneously. Many of the regulatory genes/molecules that are most frequently aberrant, such as *TGF-β*, *p53*, *Rb1*, *β-catenin*, and *M6P/IGF-2R*, have roles in multiple regulatory pathways, and several constitute points at which different pathways intersect. Coincident aberrations in both *p53* and *Rb1* have been detected in a high fraction of the HCC in which both have been examined. In a study in which allelic deletions in 10 different tumor suppressor genes were assessed in 29 HCC, 3 HCC had synchronous LOH in 4/10 genes, 5 HCC had LOH in 3/10 genes, 8 HCC had LOH in 2/10 genes, and 9 HCC had LOH in 1/10 genes; only 4 HCC lacked LOH in any of the 10 genes examined. Similarly, in a study of cyclin-dependent kinase inhibitors $p16^{INK4A}$, $p21^{WAF1/CIP1}$, and $p27^{KIP1}$ in 17 HCC, expression of all three was impaired simultaneously in 1 HCC (6%), expression of two was impaired simultaneously in 5 HCC (29%), and expression of one was impaired in 9 HCC (53%). These studies indicate that synchronous aberrations in multiple genes occur in many HCC. Results of several studies have shown that the accumulation of genomic aberrations correlate with tumor progression as indicated by deteriorating differentiation and increasing size and multiplicity of tumors in individual patients. Nevertheless, small, well-differentiated HCC also may contain aberrations in several genes simultaneously, whereas the obverse condition is occasionally observed in poorly differentiated HCC. In order to gain a better understanding of the frequency with which different regulatory pathways and different combinations of aberrant genes are involved in individual HCC at different stages of development, studies applying gene arrays to the analysis of HCC are needed.

From the standpoints of prevention and therapy, efforts to prevent HBV and HCV infections appear to be most feasible, and are already being made. When prevention of viral infection or other causes of chronic hepatitis is not successful, attempts to prevent or eliminate the precursor lesions, especially chronic inflammation, at the stage of chronic hepatitis may be useful. It may be possible to reduce the inflammatory-cell infiltrates of chronic hepatitis, and reduce or shorten the period of elevated hepatocyte proliferation without compromising the generation of sufficient new hepatocytes to maintain adequate hepatic function; the outcome of current therapeutic strategies to reduce the viral load and intensity of chronic inflammation in the liver are not yet clear. Most challenging, both technically and economically, will be gene therapies designed to correct the structurally aberrant genes and chromosomes, because even newly emerged HCC may contain a bewildering variety of irreversible structural abnormalities in genes and chromosomes.

ACKNOWLEDGMENTS

The author's effort was supported in part by NIH grant CA29323 from the National Cancer Institute. The author thanks Fumi Wells, Lisa Bell, Carol Troutner, and Tammy Brewer for expert assistance in the production and editing of the manuscript. I am especially grateful to Ms. Brewer for correcting and assembling the final version.

REFERENCES

1. Parkin, D. M. (1998) The global burden of cancer. *Semin. Cancer Biol.* **8**:219–235.
2. Grisham, J. W. (1997) Interspecies comparison of liver carcinogenesis: implications for cancer risk assessment. *Carcinogenesis* **18**:59–81.
3. Harris, C. C. and Sun, T.-T. (1984) Multifactoral etiology of human liver cancer. *Carcinogenesis* **5**:697–701.
4. El-Serag, H. B. and Mason, A. C. (1999) Rising incidence of hepatocellular carcinoma in the United States. *N. Engl. J. Med.* **340**:745–750.
5. Taylor-Robinson, S. D., Foster, G. R., Arora, S., Hargreaves, S. and Thomas, H. C. (1997) Increase in primary liver cancer in the UK, 1979-1994. *Lancet* **350**:1142–1143.
6. Benhamiche, A.-M., Faivre, C., Minello, A., Clinard, F., Mitry, E., Hillon, P., et al. (1997) Time trends and age-period-cohort effects on the incidence of primary liver cancer in a well-defined French population: 1976–1995. *J. Hepatol.* **29**:802–806.
7. Ishak, K. G. and Glunz, P. R. (1967) Hepatoblastoma and hepatocarcinoma in infancy and childhood. Report of 47 cases. *Cancer* **20**:396–422.
8. Weinberg, A. G. and Finegold, M. J. (1983) Primary hepatic tumors of childhood. *Human Pathol.* **14**:512–537.
9. Haas, J. E., Muczynski, K. A., Krailo, M., Ablin, A., Land, V., Vietti, T. J., et al. (1989) Histopathology and prognosis in childhood hepatoblastoma and hepatocarcinoma. *Cancer* **64**:1082–1095.
10. Resnick, M. B., Kozakewich, H. P. W., and Perez-Atayde, A. R. (1995) Hepatic adenoma in the pediatric age group. Clinicopathological observations and assessment of cell proliferative activity. *Am. J. Surg. Pathol.* **19**:1181–1190.
11. Dumortier, J., Bizollon, T., Chevallier, M., Ducert, C., Baulieux, J., Scoazec, J.-Y., et al. (1999) Recurrence of hepatocellular carcinoma as a mixed hepatoblastoma after liver transplantation. *Gut* **45**:622–625.
12. Finegold, M. J. (1994) Tumors of the liver. *Semin. Liver Dis.* **14**:270–281.
13. Stocker, J. T. (1994) Hepatoblastoma. *Semin. Diagnostic Pathol.* **11**:136–143.
14. Buckley, J. D., Sather, H., Ruccione, K., Rogers, P. C., Haas, J. E., Henderson, B. E., et al. (1989) A case-control study of risk factors for hepatoblastoma. A report from the Children's Cancer Study Group. *Cancer* **64**:1169–1176.
15. Unoura, M., Kaneko, S., Matsushita, E., Shimoda, A., Takeuchi, M., Adachi, H., et al. (1993) High-risk groups and screening strategies for early detection of hepatocellular carcinoma in patients with chronic liver disease. *Hepato-Gastroenterology* **40**:305–310.
16. Shiratori, Y., Shiina, S., Imamura, M., Kato, N., Kanai, F., Okudaira, T., et al. (1995) Characteristic differences of hepatocellular carcinoma between hepatitis B- and C-viral infection in Japan. *Hepatology* **22**:1027–1033.
17. Lanier, A. P., McMahon, B. J., Alberts, S. R., Popper, H., and Heyward, W. L. (1987) Primary liver cancer in Alaskan natives 1980-1985. *Cancer* **60**:1915–1920.
18. Kiyosawa, K., Sodeyama, T., Tanaka, E., Gibo, Y., Yoshizawa, K., Nakano, Y., et al. (1990) Interrelationship of blood transfusion, non-A, non-B hepatitis and hepatocellular carcinoma: analysis by detection of antibody to hepatitis C virus. *Hepatology* **12**:671–675.
19. Ishak, K. G. (1994) Chronic hepatitis: morphology and nomenclature. *Modern Pathol.* **7**:690–713.
20. Simpson, K. J., Lukas, N. W., Colletti, L., Strieter, R. M., and Kunkel, S. L. (1997) Cytokines and the liver. *J. Hepatol.* **27**:1120–1132.
21. Kagi, D., Ledermann, B., Burki, K., Zinkernagel, R. M., and Hengartner, H. (1996) Molecular mechanisms of lymphocyte-mediated cytotoxicity and their role in immunological protection and protection in vivo. *Ann. Rev. Immunol.* **14**:207–232.
22. Steinhoff, G., Behrend, M., Schrader, B., Duijvestijn, A. M., and Wonigeit, K. (1993) Expression patterns of leukocyte adhesion ligand molecular on human liver endothelia: lack of ELAM-1 and CD62 inducibility on sinusoidal endothelia and distinct distribution of VCAM-1, ICAM-1, ICAM-2 and LFA-3. *Am. J. Pathol.* **142**:481–488.
23. McNab, G., Reeves, J. L., Salmi, M., Hubscher, S., Jalkanen, S., and Adams, D. H. (1996) Vascular adhesion protein-1 supports adhesion of T lymphocytes to hepatic endothelium: a mechanism for T cell circulation in the liver? *Gastroenterology* **110**:522–528.
24. Salmi, M., Adams, D., and Jalkanen, S. (1998) Cell adhesion and migration IV. Lymphocyte trafficking in the intestine and liver. *Am. J. Physiol.* **274**:G1–G6.
25. Yoong, K., McNab, G., Hübscher, S. G., and Adams, D. H. (1998) Vascular adhesion protein-1 and ICAM-1 support the adhesion of tumor-infiltrating lymphocytes to tumor endothelium in human hepatocellular carcinoma. *J. Immunol.* **160**:3978–3988.
26. Shimoda, R., Nagashima, M., Sakamoto, M., Yamaguchi, N., Hirohashi, S., Yokota, J., et al. (1994) Increased formation of oxidative DNA damage, 8-hydroxydeoxyguanosine, in human livers with chronic hepatitis. *Cancer Res.* **54**:3171–3172.
27. Anthony, P. P., Ishak, K. G., Nayak, N. C., Poulsen, H. E., Scheuer, P. J., and Sobin, L. H. (1978) The morphology of cirrhosis. Recommendations on definition, nomenclature, and classification by a working group sponsored by the World Health Organization. *J. Clin. Pathol.* **31**:395–414.
28. LaVecchia, C., Negri, E., Cavalieri d'Oro, L., and Franceschi, S. (1998) Liver cirrhosis and the risk of primary liver cancer. *Eur. J. Cancer Prevent.* **7**:315–320.
29. Bannasch, P. and Klinge, O. (1971) Hepatocelluläre glykogenose und hepatombildung beim menschen. *Virchows Arch.* **352**:157–164.
30. Cain, H. and Kraus, B. (1977) Entwicklungsstörungen der leber und leberkarzinom im säuglings-und kindesalter. *Dtsch. Med. Wochenschr.* **102**:505–509.
31. Uchida, T., Miyata, H., and Shikata, T. (1981) Human hepatocellular carcinoma and putative precancerous disorders: their enzyme histochemical study. *Arch. Pathol. Lab. Med.* **105**:180–186.
32. Hirota, N., Hamazaki, M., and Williams, G. M. (1982) Resistance to iron accumulation and presence of hepatitis B surface antigen in preneoplastic and neoplastic lesions in human hemochromatotic livers. *Hepato-Gastroenterology* **29**:49–51.
33. Terada, T. and Nakanuma, Y. (1989) Survey of iron-accumulative macroregenerative nodules in cirrhotic livers. *Hepatology* **10**:851–854.
34. Govindarajan, S., Conrad, A., Lim, B., Valinluck, B., Kim, A. M., and Schmid, P. (1990) Study of preneoplastic changes of liver cells by immunohistochemical and molecular hybridization techniques. *Arch. Pathol. Lab. Med.* **114**:1042–1045.
35. Terada, T., Kadoya, M., Nakamura, Y., and Matsui, O. (1990) Iron-accumulating adenomatous hyperplastic nodule with malignant foci in the cirrhotic liver. Histologic, quantitative iron, and magnetic resonance imaging *in vitro* studies. *Cancer* **65**:1994–2000.
36. Deugnier, Y. M., Charalambous, P., LeQuilleuc, D., Turlin, B., Searle, J., Brissot, P., et al. (1993) Preneoplastic significance of hepatic iron-free foci in genetic hemochromatosis: A study of 185 patients. *Hepatology* **18**:1363–1369.
37. Karhunen, P. J. and Pentillä, A. (1987) Preneoplastic lesions of human liver. *Hepato-Gastroenterology* **34**:10–15.
38. Bannasch, P., Jahn, U.-R., Hacker, H. J., Su, Q., Hofmann, W., Pichlmayr, R., et al. (1997) Focal hepatic glycogenosis: a putative preneoplastic lesion associated with neoplasia and cirrhosis in explanted human livers. *Int. J. Oncol.* **10**:261–268.
39. Su, Q., Benner, A., Hofmann, W. J., Otto, G., Pichlmayr, R., and Bannasch, P. (1998) Human hepatic preneoplasia: phenotypes and proliferation kinetics of foci and nodules of altered hepatocytes and

their relationship to liver cell dysplasia. *Virchows Arch.* **431**:391–406.

40. Sugitani, S., Sakamoto, M., Ichida, T., Genda, T., Asakura, H., and Hirohashi, S. (1998) Hyperplastic foci reflect the risk of multicentric development of human hepatocellular carcinoma. *J. Hepatol.* **28**:1045–1053.

41. Terasaki, S., Kaneko, S., Kobayashi, K., Nonomura, A., and Nakanuma, Y. (1998) Histological features predicting malignant transformation of nonmalignant hepatocellular nodules: a prospective study. *Gastroenterology* **115**:1216–1222.

42. Theise, N. D. (1995) Macroregenerative (dysplastic) nodules and hepatocarcinogenesis: Theoretical and clinical considerations. *Semin. Liver Dis.* **15**:360–371.

43. International Working Party (1995) Terminology of nodular hepatocellular lesions. *Hepatology* **22**:983–993.

44. Popper, H., Thung, S. N., McMahon, B. J., Lanier, A. P., Hawkins, I., and Alberts, S. R. (1988) Evolution of hepatocellular carcinoma associated with chronic hepatitis B virus infection in Alaskan Eskimos. *Arch. Pathol. Lab. Med.* **112**:498–504.

45. Theise, N. D., Lapook, J. D., and Thung, S. N. (1993) A macroregenerative nodule containing multiple foci of hepatocellular carcinoma in a noncirrhotic liver. *Hepatology* **17**:993–996.

46. Sakamoto, M., Hirohashi, S., and Shimosato, Y. (1991) Early stages of multistep hepatocarcinogenesis: adenomatous hyperplasia and early hepatocellular carcinoma. *Human Pathol.* **22**:172–178.

47. Edmundson, H. A. and Steiner, P. E. (1954) Primary carcinoma of the liver. A study of 100 cases among 48,900 necropsies. *Cancer* **7**:462–503.

48. Ebara, M., Ohto, M., Shinagawa, T., Sugiura, N., Kimura, K., Matsutani, S., et al. (1986) Natural history of minute hepatocellular carcinoma smaller than three centimeters complicating cirrhosis. A study in 22 patients. *Gastroenterology* **90**:289–298.

49. Yoshino, M. (1983) Growth kinetics of hepatocellular carcinoma. *Jpn. J. Clin. Oncol.* **13**:45-52.

50. Sheu, J.-C., Sung, J.-L., Chen, D.-S., Yang, P.-M., Lai, M.-Y., Lee, C.-S., et al. (1985) Growth rate of asymptomatic hepatocellular carcinoma and its clinical implications. *Gastroenterology* **89**:259–266.

51. Okada, S., Okazaki, N., Nose, H., Aoki, K., Kawano, N., Yamamoto, J., et al. (1993) Follow-up examination schedule of postoperative HCC patients based on tumor-volume doubling time. *Hepato-Gastroenterology* **40**:311–315.

52. Barbara, L., Benzi, G., Gaiani, S., Fusconi, F., Zironi, G., Siringo, S., et al. (1992) Natural history of small untreated hepatocellular carcinoma in cirrhosis: A multivariate analysis of prognostic factors of tumor growth rate and patient survival. *Hepatology* **16**:132–137.

53. Tarao, K., Shimizu, A., Harada, M., Kuni, Y., Ito, Y., Tamai, S., et al. (1989) Difference in the in vitro uptake of bromodeoxyuridine between liver cirrhosis with and without hepatocellular carcinoma. *Cancer* **64**:104–109.

54. Tarao, K., Ohkawa, S., Shimizu, A., Harada, M., Nakamura, Y., Okamoto, N., et al. (1993) DNA synthesis activities of hepatocytes from noncancerous cirrhotic tissue and of hepatocellular carcinoma (HCC) cells from cancerous tissue can predict the survival of hepatectomized patients. *Cancer* **71**:3859–3863.

55. Tarao, K., Shimizu, A., Harada, M., Ohkawa, S., Okamoto, N., Kuni, Y., et al. (1991) In vitro uptake of bromodeoxyuridine by human hepatocellular carcinoma and its relation to histopathologic findings and biologic behavior. *Cancer* **68**:1789–1794.

56. Hino, N., Higashi, T., Nouso, K., Nakatsukasa, H., and Tsuji, T. (1996) Apoptosis and proliferation of human hepatocellular carcinoma. *Liver* **16**:123–129.

57. Grasl-Kraupp, B., Ruttkay-Nedecky, B., Müellauer, L., Taper, H., Huber, W., Bursch, W., et al. (1997) Inherent increase of apoptosis in liver tumors: implications for carcinogenesis and tumor regression. *Hepatology* **25**:906–912.

58. Kubo, K., Matsuzaki, Y., Okazaki, M., Kato, A., Kobayashi, N., and Okita, K. (1998) The Fas system is not significantly involved in apoptosis in human hepatocellular carcinoma. *Liver* **18**:117– 123.

59. Tannapfel, A., Geissler, F., Köekerling, F., Katalinic, A., Hauss, J., and Wittekind, C. (1999) Apoptosis and proliferation in relation to histopathological variables and prognosis in hepatocellular carcinoma. *J. Pathol.* **187**:439–445.

60. Tiniakos, D. G. and Brunt, E. M. (1999) Proliferating cell nuclear antigen and Ki-67 labeling in hepatocellular nodules: a comparative study. *Liver* **19**:58–68.

61. Matsuno, Y., Hirohashi, S., Furuya, S., Sakamoto, M., Mukai, K., and Shimosato, Y. (1990) Heterogeneity of proliferative activity in nodule-in-nodule lesions of small hepatocellular carcinoma. *Jpn. J. Cancer Res.* **81**:1137–1140.

62. LeBail, B., Belleanneé, G., Bernard, P.-H., Saric, J., Balabaud, C., and Bioulac-Sage, P. (1995) Adenomatous hyperplasia in cirrhotic liver; histological evaluation, cellular density, and proliferative activity of 35 macronodular lesions in cirrhotic explants of 10 adult French patients. *Human Pathol.* **26**:897–906.

63. Borzio, M., Trerè, D., Borzio, F., Ferrari, A. R., Bruno, S., Roncalli, M., et al. (1998) Hepatocyte proliferation is a powerful parameter for predicting hepatocellular carcinoma development in liver cirrhosis. *J. Clin. Pathol. Mol. Pathol.* **51**:96–101.

64. Tarao, K., Ohkawa, S., Shimizu, A., Harada, M., Nakamura, Y., Ito, Y., et al. (1994) Significance of hepatocellular proliferation in the development of hepatocellular carcinoma from anti-hepatitis C virus-positive cirrhotic patients. *Cancer* **73**:1149–1153.

65. Ng, I. O. L., Lai, E. C. S., Fan, S. T., Ng, M., Chan, A. S. Y., and So, M. K. P. (1994) Prognostic significance of proliferating cell nuclear antigen expression in hepatocellular carcinoma. *Cancer* **73**:2268–2274.

66. Dutta, U., Kench, J., Byth, K., Kahn, M. H., Lin, R., Liddle, C., et al. (1998) Hepatocellular proliferation and development of hepatocellular carcinoma: A case-control study in chronic hepatitis C. *Human Pathol.* **29**:1279–1284.

67. Wu, P.-C., Lau, V. K.-T., Fang, J. W.-S., Lai, U. C.-H., Lai, C.-L., and Lai, J. Y.-N. (1999) Imbalance between cell proliferation and DNA fragmentation in hepatocellular carcinoma. *Liver* **19**:444–451.

68. Ito, Y., Matsuura, N., Sakon, M., Takeda, T., Nagano, H., Nakamori, S., et al. (1999) Both cell proliferation and apoptosis significantly predict shortened disease-free survival in hepatocellular carcinoma. *Br. J. Cancer* **81**:747–751.

69. Shafritz, D. A., Shouval, D., Sherman, H. I., Hadziyannis, S. J., and Kew, M. C. (1981) Integration of hepatitis B virus DNA into the genome of liver cells in chronic liver disease and hepatocellular carcinoma. Studies on percutaneous liver biopsies and post-mortem tissue specimens. *N. Engl. J. Med.* **305**:1067–1073.

70. Esumi, M., Aritaka, T., Arii, M., Suzuki, K., Tanikawa, K., Mizuo, H., et al. (1986) Clonal origin of human hepatoma determined by integration of hepatitis B virus DNA. *Cancer Res.* **46**:5767–5771.

71. Govindarajan, S., Craig, J. R., and Valinluck, B. (1988) Clonal origin of hepatitis B virus-associated hepatocellular carcinoma. *Hum Pathol* 19:403–405.

72. Tsuda, H., Hirohashi, S., Shimosato, Y., Terada, M., and Hasegawa, H. (1988) Clonal origin of atypical adenomatous hyperplasia of the liver and clonal identity with hepatocellular carcinoma. *Gastroenterology* **95**:1664–1666.

73. Aoki, N. and Robinson, W. S. (1989) State of the hepatitis B viral genomes in cirrhotic and hepatocellular carcinoma nodules. *Mol. Biol. Med.* **6**:395–408.

74. Chen, P.-J., Chen, D.-S., Lai, M.-Y., Chang, M.-H., Huang, G.-T., Yang, P.-M., et al. (1989) Clonal origin of recurrent hepatocellular carcinomas. *Gastroenterology* **96**:527–529.

75. Sakamoto, M., Hirohashi, S., Tsuda, H., Shimosato, Y., Makuuchi, M., and Hosoda, Y. (1989) Multicentric independent development of hepatocellular carcinoma revealed by analysis of hepatitis B virus integration pattern. *Am. J. Surg. Pathol.* **13**:1064–1067.

76. Hsu, H.-C., Chiou, T.-J., Chen, J.-Y., Lee, C.-S., Lee, P. H., and Peng, S.-Y. (1991) Clonality and clonal evolution of hepatocellular carcinoma with multiple nodules. *Hepatology* **13**:923–928.

77. Sheu, J.-C., Huang, G.-T., Chou, H.-C., Lee, P.-H., Wang, J.-T., Lee, H.-S., et al. (1993) Multiple hepatocellular carcinomas at an

early stage have different clonality. *Gastroenterology* **105**:1471–1476.

78. Aihara, T., Noguchi, S., Sasaki, Y., Nakano, H., and Imaoka, S. (1994) Clonal analysis of regenerative nodules in hepatitis C virus-induced liver cirrhosis. *Gastroenterology* **107**:1805–1811.

79. Kawai, S., Imazeki, F., Yokosuka, O., Ohto, M., Shiina, S., Kato, N., and Omata, M. (1995) Clonality in hepatocellular carcinoma: Analysis of methylation pattern of pleomorphic X-chromosome-linked phosphoglycerate kinase gene in females. *Hepatology* **22**:112–117.

80. Aihara, T., Noguchi, S., Sasaki, Y., Nakano, H., Monden, M., and Imaoka, S. (1996) Clonal analysis of precancerous lesion of hepatocellular carcinoma. *Gastroenterology* **111**:455–461.

81. Paradis, V., Laurent, A., Flejou, J.-F., Vidaud, M., and Bedossa, P. (1997) Evidence for the polyclonal nature of focal nodular hyperplasia of the liver by the study of X-chromosome inactivation. *Hepatology* **26**:891–895.

82. Yamamoto, T., Kajino, K., Kudo, M., Sasaki, Y., Arakawa, Y., and Hino, O. (1999) Determination of the clonal origin of multiple human hepatocellular carcinomas by cloning and polymerase chain reaction of integrated hepatitis B virus DNA. *Hepatology* **29**:1446–1452.

83. Sirivatnauksorn, Y., Sirivatnauksorn, V., Battacharaya, S., Davidson, B. R., Dhillon, A. P., Kakkar, A. K., et al. (1999) Evolution of genetic abnormalities in hepatocellular carcinomas demonstrated by DNA fingerprinting. *J. Pathol.* **189**:344–350.

84. Kam, W., Rall, L. B., Smuckler, E. A., Schmid, R., and Rutter, W. J. (1982) Hepatitis B viral DNA in liver and serum of asymptomatic carriers. *Proc. Natl. Acad. Sci. USA* **79**:7522–7526.

85. Hada, H., Arima, J., Togawa, K., Okada, Y., Morichika, S., and Nagashima, H. (1986) State of hepatitis B viral DNA in liver of patient with hepatocellular carcinoma and chronic liver disease. *Liver* **6**:189–198.

86. Tanaka, Y., Esumi, M., and Shikata, T. (1988) Frequent integration of hepatitis B virus DNA in noncancerous liver tissue from hepatocellular carcinoma patients. *J. Med. Virol.* **26**:7–14.

87. Yasui, H., Hino, O., Ohtake, K., Machinami, R., and Kitagawa, T. (1992) Clonal growth of hepatitis B virus-integrated hepatocytes in cirrhotic liver nodules. *Cancer Res.* **52**:6810–6814.

88. Martinez-Hernandez, A. and Amenta, P. S. (1995) The extracellular matrix in hepatic regeneration. *FASEB J.* **9**:1401–1410.

89. Grigioni, W. F., Garbisa, S., D'Errico, A., Baccarini, P., Stetler-Stevenson, W. G., Liotta, L. A., et al. (1991) Evaluation of hepatocellular carcinoma aggressiveness by a panel of extracellular matrix antigens. *Am. J. Pathol.* **138**:647–654.

90. Yamada, S., Ichida, T., Matsuda, Y., Miyazaki, Y., Hatano, T., Hata, K., et al. (1992) Tenascin expression in human chronic liver disease and in hepatocellular carcinoma. *Liver* **12**:10–16.

91. Scoazec, J.-Y., Flejou, J.-F., D'Errico, A., Fiorentino, M., Zamparelli, A., Bringuier, A.-F., et al. (1996) Fibrolamellar carcinoma of the liver: composition of the extracellular matrix and expression of cell-matrix and cell-cell adhesion molecules. *Hepatology* **24**:1128–1136.

92. Hayashi, K., Kurohiji, T., and Shirouzu, K. (1997) Localization of thrombospondin in hepatocellular carcinoma. *Hepatology* **25**:569–574.

93. LeBail, B., Faouzi, S., Boussaire, L., Balabaud, C., Bioulac-Sage, P., and Rosenbaum, J. (1997) Extracellular matrix composition and integrin expression in early hepatocarcinogenesis in human cirrhotic liver. *J. Pathol.* **181**:330–337.

94. Roskams, T., De Vos, R., David, G., Van Damme, B., and Desmet, V. (1998) Heparan sulphate proteoglycan expression in human primary liver tumours. *J. Pathol.* **185**:290–297.

95. Grigioni, W. F., D'Errico, A., Mancini, A. M., Biagini, G., Gozzetti, G., Mazziotti, A., et al. (1987) Hepatocellular carcinoma: expression of basement membrane glycoproteins. An immunohistochemical approach. *J. Pathol.* **152**:325–332.

96. Donato, M. F., Colombo, M., Matarazzo, M., and Paronetto, F. (1989) Distribution of basement membrane components in human hepatocellular carcinoma. *Cancer* **63**:272–279.

97. Jaskiewiez, K., Chasen, M. R., and Robson, S. C. (1993) Differential expression of extracellular matrix proteins and integrins in hepatocellular carcinoma and chronic liver disease. *Anticancer Res.* **13**:2229–2238.

98. Yao, M., Zhou, D.-P., Jiang, S.-M., Wang, O.-H., Zhou, X.-D., Tang, Z.-Y., et al. (1998) Elevated activity of N-acetylglucosaminyl-transferase V in human hepatocellular carcinoma. *J. Cancer Res. Clin. Oncol.* **124**:27–30.

99. Volpes, R., Van den Oord, J. J., and Desmet, V. J. (1991) Distribution of the VLA family of integrins in normal and pathological human liver tissue. *Gastroenterology* **101**:200–206.

100. Patriarca, C., Roncalli, M., Gambacorta, M., Cominotti, M., Coggi, G., and Viale, G. (1993) Patterns of integrin common chain β1 and collagen IV immunoreactivity in hepatocellular carcinoma. Correlations with tumor growth rate, grade and size. *J. Pathol.* **171**:5–11.

101. Volpes, R., Van den Oord, J. J., and Desmet, V. J. (1993) Integrins as differential cell lineage markers of primary liver tumors. *Am. J. Pathol.* **142**:1483–1492.

102. Couvelard, A., Bringuier, A.-F., Dauge, M.-C., Nejjari, M., Darai, E., Benifla, J.-L., et al. (1998) Expression of integrins during liver organogenesis in humans. *Hepatology* **27**:839–847.

103. Ozaki, I., Yamamoto, K., Mizuta, T., Kajihara, S., Fukushima, N., Setoguchi, Y., et al. (1998) Differential expression of laminin receptors in human hepatocellular carcinoma. *Gut* **43**:837–842.

104. Begum, N. A., Mori, M., Matsumata, T., Takenara, K., Sugimachi, K., and Bernard, G. F. (1995) Differential display and integrin alpha 6 messenger RNA overexpression in hepatocellular carcinoma. *Hepatology* **22**:1447–1455.

105. Shimoyama, Y. and Hirohashi, S. (1991) Cadherin intercellular adhesion molecule in hepatocellular carcinomas: Loss of E-cadherin expression in an undifferentiated carcinoma. *Cancer Lett.* **57**:131–135.

106. Haramaki, M., Yano, H., Fukuda, K., Momosaki, S., Ogasawara, S., and Kojiro, M. (1995) Expression of CD44 in human hepatocellular carcinoma cell lines. *Hepatology* **21**:1276–1284.

107. Huang, L.-R. and Hsu, H.-C. (1995) Cloning and expression of CD24 gene in human hepatocellular carcinoma: a potential early tumor marker gene correlates with p53 mutation and tumor differentiation. *Cancer Res.* **55**:4717–4721.

108. Ihara, A., Koizumi, H., Hashizume, R., and Uchikoshi, T. (1996) Expression of epithelial cadherin and a- and β-catenins in nontumoral livers and hepatocellular carcinomas. *Hepatology* **23**:1441–1447.

109. Masaki, T., Tokuda, M., Ohnishi, M., Watanabe, S., Fujimura, T., Miyamato, K., et al. (1996) Enhanced expression of the protein kinase substrate annexin in human hepatocellular carcinoma. *Hepatology* **24**:72–81.

110. Kozyraki, R., Scoazec, J.-Y., Flejou, J.-F., D'Errico, A., Bedossa, P., Terris, B., et al. (1996) Expression of cadherins and a-catenin in primary epithelial tumors of the liver. *Gastroenterology* **110**:1137–1149.

111. Mathew, J., Hines, J. E., Obafunwa, J. O., Burr, A. W., Toole, K., and Burt, A. D. (1996) CD44 is expressed in hepatocellular carcinoma showing vascular invasion. *J. Pathol.* **179**:74–79.

112. Terris, B., Laurent-Puig, P., Belghitti, J., Degott, C., Henin, D., and Flejou, J. F. (1997) Prognostic influence of clinicopathological feature, DNA-ploidy, CD44H and p53 expression in a large series of resected hepatocellular carcinoma in France. *Int. J. Cancer* **74**:614–619.

113. Kanai, Y., Ushijima, S., Hui, A.-M., Ochiai, A., Tsuda, M., Sakamoto, M., et al. (1997) The E-cadherin gene is silenced by CpG methylation in human hepatocellular carcinomas. *Int. J. Cancer* **71**:355–359.

114. DeBoer, C. J., VanKrieken, J. H. J. M., Janssen-VanRhijn, C., and Litvinov, S. (1999) Expression of Ep-cam in normal, regenerating, metaplastic, and neoplastic liver. *J. Pathol.* **188**:201–206.

115. Yamaoka, K., Nouchi, T., Tazawa, J., Hiranuma, S., Marumo, F., and Sato, C. (1995) Expression of gap junction protein connexin 32 and E-cadherin in human hepatocellular carcinoma. *J. Hepatology* **22**:536–539.

116. Slagle, B. L., Zhou, Y.-Z., Birchmeier, W., and Scorsone, K. A. (1993) Deletion of the E-cadherin gene in hepatitis B virus-positive Chinese hepatocellular carcinomas. *Hepatology* **18**:757–762.

117. Falletti, E., Fabris, C., Pirisi, M., Soardo, G., Vitulli, D., Toniutto, P., et al. (1996) Circulating intercellular adhesion molecule 1 predicts non-specific elevation of a1-fetoprotein. *J. Cancer Res. Clin. Oncol.* **122**:366–369.

118. Okazaki, I., Wada, N., Nakano, M., Saito, A., Takasaki, K., Doi, M., et al. (1997) Difference in gene expression for matrix metalloproteinase-1 between early and advanced hepatocellular carcinomas. *Hepatology* **25**:580–584.

119. Arii, S., Mise, M., Harada, T., Furutani, M., Ishigami, S., Niwano, M., et al. (1996) Overexpression of matrix metalloproteinase 9 gene in hepatocellular carcinoma with invasive potential. *Hepatology* **24**:316–322.

120. Hayasaka, A., Suzuki, N., Fujimoto, N., Iwama, S., Fukuyama, E., Kanda, Y., et al. (1996) Elevated plasma levels of matrix metalloproteinase-9 (92-kd type IV collagenase/gelatinase B) in hepatocellular carcinoma. *Hepatology* **24**:1058–1062.

121. Nakatsukasa, H., Ashida, K., Higashi, T., Ohguchi, S., Tsuboi, S., Hino, N., et al. (1996) Cellular distribution of transcripts for tissue inhibitor of metalloproteinases 1 and 2 in human hepatocellular carcinomas. *Hepatology* **24**:82–88.

122. DePetro, G., Tavian, D., Copeta, A., Portolani, N., Guilini, S. M., and Barlati, S. (1998) Expression of urokinase-type plasminogen activator (u-PA), u-PA receptor, and tissue-type PA messenger RNAs in human hepatocellular carcinoma. *Cancer Res.* **58**:2234–2239.

123. Morita, Y., Hayashi, Y., Wang, Y., Kanamaru, T., Suzuki, S., Kawasaki, K., et al. (1997) Expression of urokinase-type plasminogen activator receptor in hepatocellular carcinoma. *Hepatology* **25**:856–861.

124. Akahane, T., Ishii, M., Ohtani, H., Nagura, H., and Toyota, T. (1998) Stromal expression of urokinase-type plasminogen activator receptor (uPAR) is associated with invasive growth in primary liver cancer. *Liver* **18**:414–419.

125. Dubuisson, L., Monvoisin, A., Nielsen, B. S., LeBail, B., Bioulac-Sage, P., and Rosenbaum, J. (2000) Expression and cellular localization of the urokinase-type plasminogen activator and its receptor in human hepatocellular carcinoma. *J. Pathol.* **190**:190–195.

126. Huber, K., Kirchheimer, C., Ermler, D., Bell, C., and Binder, B. R. (1992) Determination of plasma urokinase-type plasminogen activator antigen in patients with primary liver cancer: Characterization as a tumor-associated antigen and comparison with a-fetoprotein. *Cancer Res.* **52**:1717–1720.

127. Hanss, M., Bonvoisin, C., Patouillard, T., Martin, D., Audigier, J. C., Descos, L., et al. (1994) Increased plasma levels of urokinase-type plasminogen activator during hepatocellular carcinoma. *Fibrinolysis* **8**:255–270.

128. Booth, N. A., Anderson, J. A., and Bennett, B. (1984) Plasminogen activators in alcoholic cirrhosis: Demonstration of increased tissue type and urokinase type activator. *J. Clin. Pathol.* **37**:772–777.

129. Sato, S., Higashi, T., Ouguchi, S., Hino, N., and Tsuji, T. (1994) Elevated plasminogen plasma levels are associated with deterioration of liver function but not with hepatocellular carcinoma. *J. Gastroenterol.* **29**:745–750.

130. Toyoda, H., Fukuda, Y., Hayakawa, T., Kumada, T., and Nakanos, S. (1997) Changes in blood supply in small hepatocellular carcinoma: correlation of angiographic images and immunohistochemical findings. *J. Hepatol.* **27**:654–660.

131. Haratake, J. and Scheuer, P. J. (1990) An immunohistochemical and ultrastructural study of the sinusoids of hepatocellular carcinoma. *Cancer* **65**:1985–1993.

132. Haratake, J., Hisaoka, M., Yamamoto, O., and Horie, A. (1992) An ultrastructural comparison of sinusoids in hepatocellular carcinoma, adenomatous hyperplasia, and fetal liver. *Arch. Pathol. Lab. Med.* **116**:67–70.

133. Terada, T. and Nakanuma, Y. (1991) Expression of ABH blood group antigens, Ulex europaeus agglutinin I, and type IV collagen in the sinusoids of hepatocellular carcinoma. *Arch. Pathol. Lab. Med.* **115**:50–55.

134. Dhillon, A. P., Colombari, R., Savage, K., and Scheuer, P. J. (1992) An immunohistochemical study of the blood vessels within primary hepatocellular tumors. *Liver* **12**:311–318.

135. Ueda, K., Terada, T., Nakanuma, Y., and Matsui, O. (1992) Vascular supply to adenomatous hyperplasia of the liver and hepatocellular carcinoma: a morphometric study. *Human Pathol.* **23**:619–626.

136. Ruck, P., Xiao, J. C., and Kaiserling, E. (1995) Immunoreactivity of sinusoids in hepatocellular carcinoma. An immunohistochemical study using lectin UEA-1 and antibodies against endothelial markers, including CD34. *Arch. Pathol. Lab. Med.* **119**:173–178.

137. Tanigawa, N., Lu, C., Mitsui, T., and Miura, S. (1997) Quantitation of sinusoid-like vessels in hepatocellular carcinoma: its clinical and prognostic significance. *Hepatology* **26**:1216–1223.

138. Kimura, H., Nakajima, T., Kagawa, K., Deguchi, T., Kakusui, M., Katagishi, T., et al. (1998) Angiogenesis in hepatocellular carcinoma as evaluated by CD34 immunohistochemistry. *Liver* **18**:14–19.

139. El-Assal, O., Yamanoi, A., Soda, Y., Yamaguchi, M., Igarashi, M., Yamamoto, A., et al. (1998) Clinical significance of microvessel density and vascular endothelial growth factor expression in hepatocellular carcinoma and surrounding liver: possible involvement of vascular endothelial growth factor in angiogenesis of cirrhotic liver. *Hepatology* **27**:1554–1562.

140. Park, Y. N., Yang, C.-P., Fernandez, G. J., Cubukcu, O., Thung, S. N., and Theise, N. D. (1998) Neoangiogenesis and sinusoidal "capillarization" in dysplastic nodules of the liver. *Am. J. Surg. Pathol.* **22**:656–662.

141. Scott, F. R., El-Refair, A., More, L., Scheuer, P. J., and Dhillon, A. P. (1996) Hepatocellular carcinoma arising in an adenoma: Value of QBend 10 immunostaining in diagnosis of liver cell carcinoma. *Histopathology* **28**:472–474.

142. Kar, S., Yousem, S. A., and Carr, B. I. (1995) Endothelin-1 expression by human hepatocellular carcinoma. *Biochem. Biophys. Res. Commun.* **216**:514–519.

143. Fischer, G., Hartmann, H., Droese, M., Schauer, A., and Bock, K. W. (1986) Histochemical and immunohistochemical detection of putative preneoplastic liver foci in women after long-term use of oral contraceptives. *Virchows Arch. B* **50**:321–337.

144. Grigioni, W. F., D'Errico, A., Bacci, F., Gaudio, M., Mazziotti, A., Gozzetti, G., et al. (1989) Primary liver neoplasms: evaluation of proliferative index using Moab Ki67. *J. Pathol.* **158**:23–30.

145. Gaffey, M. J., Iezzoni, J. C., and Weiss, L. M. (1996) Clonal analysis of focal nodular hyperplasia of the liver. *Am. J. Pathol.* **148**:1089–1096.

146. Ruck, P., Xiao, J. C., and Kaiserling, E. (1996) Small epithelial cells and the histogenesis of hepatoblastoma. Electron microscopic, immunoelectron microscopic, and immunohistochemical findings. *Am. J. Pathol.* **148**:321–329.

147. Ruck, P., Xiao, J. C., Pietsch, T., Von Schweinitz, D., and Kaiserling, E. (1997) Hepatic stem-like cells in hepatoblastoma: expression of cytokeratin 7, albumin and oval cell antigens detected by OV-1 and OV-6. *Histopathology* **31**:324–329.

148. Ruck, P., Harms, D., and Kaiserling, E. (1990) Neuroendocrine differnetiation in hepatoblastoma. An immunohistochemical investigation. *Am. J. Surg. Pathol.* **14**:847–855.

149. Ruck, P. and Kaiserling, E. (1993) Melanin-containing hepatoblastoma with endocrine differentiation. An immunohistochemical and ultrastructural study. *Cancer* **72**:361–368.

150. Manivel, C., Wick, M. R., Abenoza, P., and Dehner, L. P. (1986) Teratoid hepatoblastoma. The nosologic dilemma of solid embryologic neoplasms of childhood. *Cancer* **57**:2168–2174.

151. Abenoza, P., Manivel, J. C., Wick, M. R., Hagen, K., and Dehner, L. P. (1987) Hepatoblastoma: An immunohistochemical and ultrastructural study. *Human Pathol.* **18**:1025–1035.

152. Wang, J., Dhillon, A. P., Sankey, E. A., Wightman, A. K., Lewin, J. F., and Scheuer, P. J. (1991) 'Neuroendocrine' differentiation in primary neoplasms of the liver. *J. Pathol.* **163**:61–67.

153. Akasofu, M., Kawahara, E., Kaji, K., and Nakanishi, I. (1999) Sarcomatoid hepatocellular carcinoma showing rhabdomyoblastic differentiation in the adult cirrhotic liver. *Virchows Arch.* **434**:511–515.

154. Ferrell, L. (1995) Malignant liver tumors that mimic benign lesions: analysis of five distinct lesions. *Semin. Diag. Pathol.* **12**:64–76.

155. Von Schweinitz, D., Hecker, H., Schmidt-von-Arndt, G., and Harms, D. (1997) Prognostic factors and staging systems in childhood hepatoblastoma. *Int. J. Cancer* **74**:593–599.

156. Ruck, P., Xiao, J. C., and Kaiserling, E. (1995) Immunoreactivity of sinusoids in hepatoblastoma. An immunohistochemical study of lectin UEA-1 and antibodies against endothelium-associated antigens, including CD-34. *Histopathology* **26**:451–455.

157. Ruck, P. and Kaiserling, E. (1992) Extracellular matrix in hepatoblastoma: an immunohistochemical investigation. *Histopathology* **21**:115–126.

158. Rugge, M., Sonego, F., Pollice, L., Perilongo, G., Guido, M., Basso, G., et al. (1998) Hepatoblastoma: DNA nuclear content, proliferative indices, and pathology. *Liver* **18**:128–133.

159. Castilla, A., Prieto, J., and Fausto, N. (1991) Transforming growth factors β1 and a in chronic liver disease: effects of interferon alpha therapy. *N. Engl. J. Med.* **324**:933–940.

160. Hsia, C. C., Axiotis, C. A., Di Bisceglie, A. M., and Tabor, E. (1992) Transforming growth factor-alpha in human hepatocellular carcinoma and coexpression with heptitis B surface antigen in adjacent liver. *Cancer* **70**:1049–1056.

161. Collier, J. D., Guo, K., Gullick, W. J., Bassendine, M. F., and Burt, A. D. (1993) Expression of transforming growth factor alpha in human hepatocellular carcinoma. *Liver* **13**:151–155.

162. Schaff, Z., Hsia, C. C., Sarosi, I., and Tabor, E. (1994) Overexpression of transforming growth factor-a in hepatocellular carcinoma and focal nodular hyperplasia from European patients. *Human Pathol.* **25**:644–651.

163. Morimitsu, Y., Hsia, C. C., Kojiro, M., and Tabor, E. (1995) Nodules of less-differentiated tumor within or adjacent to hepatocellular carcinoma: relative expression of transforming growth factor-a and its receptor in the different areas of tumor. *Human Pathol.* **26**:1126–1132.

164. Nalesnik, M.A., Lee, R.G., and Carr, B.I. (1998) Transforming growth factor alpha (TGFα) in hepatocellular carcinomas and adjacent parenchyma. *Human Pathol.* **29**:228-234.

165. Hsia, C. C., Thorgeirsson, S. S., and Tabor, E. (1994) Expression of hepatitis B surface and core antigens and transforming factor-a in "oval cells" of the liver in patients with hepatocellular carcinoma. *J. Med. Virol.* **43**:216-221.

166. Masuhara, M., Yasunaga, M., Tanigawa, K., Tamura, F., Yamashita, S., Sakaida, I., et al. (1996) Expression of hepatocyte growth factor, transforming growth factor a, and transforming factor β1 messenger RNA in various human liver diseases and correlation with hepatocyte proliferation. *Hepatology* **24**:323–329.

167. Harada, K., Shiota, G., and Kawasaki, H. (1999) Transforming growth factor-a and epidermal growth factor receptor in chronic liver disease and hepatocellular carcinoma. *Liver* **19**:318–325.

168. Yamaguchi, M., Yu, L., Hishikawa, Y., Yamanoi, A., Kubota, H., and Nagasue, N. (1997) Growth kinetic study of human hepatocellular carcinoma using proliferating cell nuclear antigen and Lewis Y antigen: their correlation with transforming growth factor-a and β1. *Oncology* **54**:245–251.

169. Park, B. C., Huh, M. H., and Seo, J. H. (1995) Differential expression of transforming growth factor a and insulin-like growth factor II in chronic active hepatitis B, cirrhosis and hepatocellular carcinoma. *J. Hepatol.* **22**:286–294.

170. Tanaka, S., Takenaka, K., Matsumata, T., Mori, R., and Sugimachi, K. (1996) Hepatitis-C-virus replication is associated with expression of transforming growth factor-a and insulin-like growth factor-II in cirrhotic livers. *Digest. Dis. Sci.* **41**:208–215.

171. Tabor, E., Farshid, K., Di Bisceglie, A., and Hsia, C. C. (1992) Increased expression of transforming growth factor a after transfection of a human hepatoblastoma cell line with the hepatitis B virus. *J. Med. Virol.* **37**:271–273.

172. Ono, M., Morisawa, K., Nie, J., Ota, K., Taniguchi, T., Saibara, T., et al. (1998) Transactivation of transforming growth factor a gene by hepatitis B virus preS1. *Cancer Res.* **58**:1813–1816.

173. Morimitsu, Y., Kleiner, D. E., Jr., Conjeevaram, H. S., Hsia, C. C., DiBisceglie, A. M., and Tabor, E. (1995) Expression of transforming growth factor alpha in the liver before and after interferon alfa therapy for chronic hepatitis B. *Hepatology* **22**:1021–1026.

174. Yamaguchi, K., Carr, B. I., and Nalesnik, M. A. (1995) Concomitant and isolated expression of TGF-alpha and EGF-R in human hepatoma cells supports the hypothesis of autocrine, paracrine, and endocrine growth of human hepatoma. *J. Surg. Oncol.* **58**:240–245.

175. Kiss, A., Wang, N.-J., Xie, J.-P., and Thorgeirsson, S. S. (1997) Analysis of transforming growth factor (TGF)-α/epidermal growth factor receptor, hepatocyte growth factor/c-met, TGF-β receptor type II, and p53 expression in human hepatocellular carcinomas. *Clin. Cancer Res.* **3**:1059–1066.

176. Tang, Z., Qin, L., Wang, X., Zhou, G., Liao, Y., Weng, Y., et al. (1998) Alterations of oncogenes, tumor suppressor genes and growth factors in hepatocellular carcinoma: with relation to tumor size and invasiveness. *Chinese Med. J.* **111**:313–318.

177. Tomiya, T. and Fujiwara, K. (1996) Serum transforming growth factor a as a marker of hepatocellular carcinoma complicating cirrhosis. *Cancer* **77**:1056–1060.

178. Yeh, Y.-C., Tsai, J.-F., Chuang, L.-Y., Yeh, H.-W., Tsai, J.-H., Florine L., et al. (1987) Elevation of transforming growth factor a and its relationship to the epidermal growth factor and a-fetoprotein levels in patients with hepatocellular carcinoma. *Cancer Res.* **47**:896–901.

179. Motoo, Y., Sawabu, N., and Nakanuma, Y. (1991) Expression of epidermal growth factor and fibroblast growth factor in human hepatocellar carcinoma: an immunohistochemical study. *Liver* **11**:272–277.

180. Chuang, L.-Y., Tsai, J.-H., Yeh, Y.-C., Chang, C.-C., Yeh, H.-W., Guh, J.-Y., et al. (1991) Epidermal growth factor-related transforming growth factors in the urine of patients with hepatocellular carcinoma. *Hepatology* **13**:1112–1116.

181. Hamazaki, K., Yunoki, Y., Tagashira, H., Mimura, T., Mori, M., and Orita, K. (1997) Epidermal growth factor receptor in human hepatocellular carcinoma. *Cancer Detect. Prev.* **21**:355–360.

182. Kaneko, Y., Shibuya, M., Nakayama, T., Hayashida, N., Toda, G., Endo, Y., et al. (1985) Hypomethylation of c-*myc* and epidermal growth factor receptor genes in human hepatocellular carcinoma and fetal liver. *Jpn. J. Cancer Res.* **76**:1136–1140.

183. Mori, S., Akiyama, T., Morishita, Y., Shimizu, S.-I., Sakai, K., Sudoh, K., et al. (1987) Light and electron microscopical demonstration of c-*erb*B-2 gene product-like immunoreactivity in human malignant tumors. *Virchows Arch. B* **54**:8–15.

184. Brunt, E. M. and Swanson, P. E. (1992) Immunoreactivity for c-erbB-2 oncopeptide in benign and malignant diseases of the liver. *Am. J. Clin. Pathol.* **97**:s53–s61.

185. Collier, J. D., Guo, K., Mathew, J., May, F., Bennett, M. K., Corbett, I. P., et al. (1992) c-*erb*B-2 oncogene expression in hepatocellular carcinoma and cholangiocarcinoma. *J. Hepatol.* **14**:377–380.

186. Heinze, T., Jonas, S., Kärsten, A., and Neuhaus, P. (1999) Determination of the oncogenes p53 and c-erbB2 in the tumor cytosols of advanced hepatocellular carcinoma (HCC) and correlation with survival time. *Anticancer Res.* **19**:2501–2504.

187. Luo, J.-C., Yu, M.-W., Chen, C.-J., Santella, R. M., Carney, W. P., and Brandt-Rauf, P. W. (1993) Serum c-*erb*B-2 oncopeptide in hepatocellular carcinogenesis. *Med. Sci. Res.* **21**:305–307.

188. Cariani, E., Seurin, D., Lasserre, C., Franco, D., Binoux, M., and Brechot, C. (1990) Expression of insulin-like growth factor II (IGF-2) in human primary liver cancer: mRNA and protein analysis. *J. Hepatol.* **11**:226–231.

189. Su, Q., Liu, Y.-F., Zhang J.-F., Zhang, S.-X., Li, D.-F., et al. (1994) Expression of insulin-like growth factor II in hepatitis B, cirrhosis and hepatocellular carcinoma: its relationship with hepatitis B virus antigen expression. *Hepatology* **20**:788–799.

190. Fiorentino, M. Grigioni, W. F., Baccarini, P., D'Errico, A., De Mitri, M. S., Pisi, E., et al. (1994) Different in situ expression of insulin-like growth factor type II in hepatocellular carcinoma: An in situ hybridization and immunohistochemical study. *Diag. Mol. Pathol.* **3**:59–65.

191. Sohda, T., Yun, K., Iwata, K., Soejima, H., and Okumura, M. (1996) Increased expression of insulin-like growth factor 2 in hepatocellular carcinoma is primarily regulated at the transcriptional level. *Lab. Invest.* **75**:307–311.

192. Sohda, T., Kamimura, S., Iwata, K., Shijo, H., and Okumura, M. (1997) Immunohistochemical evidence of insulin-like growth factor II in human small hepatocellular carcinoma with hepatitis C virus infection: relationship to fatty change in carcinoma cells. *J. Gastroenterol. Hepatol.* **12**:224–228.

193. Cariani, E., Lasserre, C., Seurin, D., Hamelin, B., Kemeny, F., Franco, D., et al. (1988) Differential expression of insulin-like growth factor II mRNA in human primary liver cancers, benign liver tumors, and liver cirrhosis. *Cancer Res.* **48**:6844–6849.

194. Cariani, E., Lasserre, C., Kemeny, F., Franco, D., and Brechot, C. (1991) Expression of insulin-like growth factor II, a-fetoprotein and hepatitis B virus transcripts in human primary liver cancer. *Hepatology* **13**:644–649.

195. Su, T. S., Liu, W.-Y., Han, S.-H., Jansen, M., Yang-Fen, T.L., P'eng, F.-K., et al. (1989) Transcripts of insulin-like growth factors I and II in human hepatoma. *Cancer Res.* **49**:1773–1777.

196. D'Arville, C. N., Nouri-Aria, K. T., Johnson, P., and Williams, R. (1991) Regulation of insulin-like growth factor II gene expression by hepatitis B virus in hepatocellular carcinoma. *Hepatology* **13**:310–315.

197. Lamas, E., LeBail, B., Housset, C., Boucher, O., and Brechot, C. (1991) Localization of insulin-like growth factor-II and hepatitis B virus mRNAs and proteins in human hepatocellular carcinomas. *Lab. Invest.* **64**:98–104.

198. Li, X., Nong, Z., Ekström, C., Larsson, E., Nordlinder, H., Hofmann, W. J., et al. (1997) Disrupted *IGF2* promoter control by silencing of promoter P1 in human hepatocellular carcinoma. *Cancer Res.* **57**:2048–2054.

199. Sohda, T., Oka, Y., Iwata, K., Gunn, J., Kamimura, S., Shijo, H., et al. (1997) Co-localization of insulin-like growth factor II and the proliferation marker MIB1 in hepatocellular carcinoma cells. *J. Clin. Pathol.* **50**:135–137.

200. Daughaday, W. H., Wu, J.-C., Lee, S.-D., and Kapadia, M. (1990) Abnormal processing of pro-IGF-2 in patients with hepatoma and in some hepatitis B virus antibody-positive asymptomatic individuals. *J. Lab. Clin. Med.* **116**:555–562.

201. Davies, S. M. (1994) Developmental regulation of genomic imprinting of the IGF2 gene in human liver. *Cancer Res.* **54**:2560–2562.

202. Ekström, T. J., Cui, H., Li, X., and Ohlsson, R. (1995) Promoter-specific *IGF2* imprinting status and its plasticity during human liver development. *Development* **121**:309–316.

203. Li, X., Cui, H., Sandstedt, B., Nordlinder, H., Larsson, E., and Ekström, T. J. (1996) Expression levels of the insulin-like growth factor-II gene (IGF-2) in the human liver: developmental relationships of the four promoters. *J. Endocrinol.* **149**:117–124.

204. Lustig, O., Ariel, I., Ilan, J., Lev-Lehman, E., DeGroot, N., and Hochberg, A. (1994) Expression of the imprinted H19 gene in the human fetus. *Mol. Reprod. Dev.* **38**:239–246.

205. Nardone, G., Romano, M., Calabro, A., Pedone, P. V., DeSio, I., Persico, M., et al. (1996) Activation of fetal promoters of insulin-like growth factor II gene in hepatitis C virus-related chronic hepatitis, cirrhosis, and hepatocellular carcinoma. *Hepatology* **23**:1304–1312.

206. Ariel, I., Miao, H. Q., Ji, X. R., Schneider, T., Roll, D., deGroot, N., et al. (1998) Imprinted H19 oncofetal RNA is a candidate tumour marker for hepatocellular carcinoma. *Mol. Pathol.* **51**:21–25.

207. Sohda, T., Iwate, K., Soejima, H., Kamimura, S., Shijo, H., and Yun, K. (1998) In situ detection of insulin-like growth factor II (IGF2) and H19 gene expression in hepatocellular carcinoma. *J. Human Genetics* **43**:49–53.

208. Aihara, T., Noguchi, S., Miyoshi, Y., Nakano, H., Sasaki, Y., Nakamura, Y., et al. (1998) Allelic imbalance of insulin-like growth factor II gene expression in cancerous and precancerous lesions of the liver. *Hepatology* **28**:86–89.

209. Kim, K.-S. and Lee, Y.-I. (1997) Biallelic expression of *H19* and *IGF2* genes in hepatocellular carcinoma. *Cancer Lett.* **119**:143–148.

210. Takeda, S., Kondo, M., Kumada, T., Koshikawa, T., Ueda, R., Nishio, M., et al. (1996) Allelic-expression imbalance of the insulin-like growth factor 2 gene in hepatocellular carcinoma and underlying disease. *Oncogene* **12**:1589–1592.

211. Uchida, K., Kondo, M., Takeda, S., Osada, H., Takahashi, T., Nakao. A., et al. (1997) Altered transcriptional regulation of the insulin-like growth factor 2 gene in human hepatocellular carcinoma. *Mol. Carcinogenesis* **18**:193–198.

212. Feinberg, A. P., Kalikin, L. M., Johnson, L. A., and Thompson, J. S. (1994) Loss of imprinting in human cancer. *Cold Spring Harbor Symp. Quant. Biol.* **59**:357–364.

213. Akmal, S. N., Yun, K., MacLay, J., Higami, Y., and Ikeda, T. (1995) Insulin-like growth factor 2 and insulin-like growth factor binding protein 2 expression in hepatoblastoma. *Human Pathol.* **26**:846–851.

214. Li, X., Adam, G., Cui, H., Sandstedt, B., Ohlsson, R., and Ekström, T. J. (1995) Expression, promoter, usage and parental imprinting status of insulin-like growth factor II (IGF2) in human hepatoblastomas: Uncoupling of IGF2 and H19 imprinting. *Oncogene* **11**:221–229.

215. Li, X., Kogner, P., Sandstedt, B., Haas, O. A., and Ekström, T. J. (1998) Promoter-specific methylation and expression alterations of *igf2* and *h19* are involved in human hepatoblastoma. *Int. J. Cancer* **75**:176–180.

216. Fukuzawa, R., Umizawa, A., Ochi, K., Urano, F., Ikeda, H., and Hata, J.-I. (1999) High frequency of inactivation of the imprinted H19 gene in "sporadic" hepatoblastoma. *Int. J. Cancer* **82**:490–497.

217. Davies, S. M. (1993) Maintenance of genomic imprinting at the IGF2 locus in hepatoblastoma. *Cancer Res.* **53**:4781–4783.

218. Rainier, S., Dobry, C. J., and Feinberg, A. P. (1995) Loss of imprinting in hepatoblastoma. *Cancer Res.* **55**:1836–1838.

219. Kondoh, N., Wakatsuki, T., Ryo, A., Hada, A., Aihara, T., Horiuchi, S., et al. (1999) Identification and characterization of genes associated with hepatocellular carcinogenesis. *Cancer Res.* **59**:4990–4996.

220. Donaghy, A., Ross, R., Gimson, A., Hughes, S. C., Holly, J., and Williams, R. (1995) Growth hormone, insulin-like growth factor-1, and insulinlike growth factor binding proteins 1 and 3 in chronic liver disease. *Hepatology* **21**:680–688.

221. Sue, S. R., Chari, R. S., Kong, F.-M., Mills, J. J., Fine, R. L., Jirtle, R. L., et al. (1995) Transforming growth factor-beta receptors and mannose 6-phosphate/insulin-like growth factor-II receptor expression in human hepatocellular carcinoma. *Ann. Surg.* **222**:171–178.

222. DeSouza, A. T., Hankins, G. R., Washington, M. K., Fine, R. L., Orton, T. C., and Jirtle, R. L. (1995) Frequent loss of heterozygosity on 6q at the mannose 6-phosphate/insulin-like growth factor II receptor locus in human hepatocellular tumors. *Oncogene* **10**:1725–1729.

223. Piao, Z., Choi, Y., Park, C., Lee, W. J., Park, J.-H., and Kim, H. (1997) Deletion of the M6P/IGF2r gene in primary hepatocellular carcinoma. *Cancer Lett.* **120**:39–43.

224. Yamada, T., DeSouza, A. T., Finkelstein, S., and Jirtle, R. L. (1997) Loss of the gene encoding mannose 6-phosphate/insulin-like growth factor II receptor is an early event in liver carcinogenesis. *Proc. Natl. Acad. Sci. USA* **94**:10351–10355.

225. Wada, I., Kanda, H., Nomura, K., Kato, Y., Machinami, R., and Kitagawa, T. (1999) Failure to detect genetic alteration of the mannose-6-phosphate/insulin-like growth factor 2 receptor (M6P/IGF2R) gene in hepatocellular carcinomas in Japan. *Hepatology* **29**:1718–1721.

226. Oka, Y., Killian, J. K., Jang, H.-S., Tohara, K., Sakaguchi, S., Takahara, T., et al. (2001) *M6P/IGF2R* is mutated in hepato *Proc. Am. Assoc. Cancer Res.* **42**:61,62.

227. DeSouza, A. T., Hankins, G. R., Washington, M. K., Orton, T. C., and Jirtle, R. L. (1995) M6P/IGF2R gene is mutated in human hepatocellular carcinomas with loss of heterozygosity. *Nature Gen.* **11**:447–449.

228. Chang, T. C., Lin, J. J., Yu, S. C., and Chang, T. J. (1990) Absence of growth-hormone receptor in hepatocellular carcinoma and cirrhotic liver. *Hepatology* **11**:123–126.

229. Ljubimova, J. Y., Petrovic, L. M., Wilson, S. E., Geller, S.A., and Demetriou, A. A. (1997) Expression of HGF, its receptor *c-met, c-myc,* and albumin in cirrhotic and neoplastic human liver tissue. *J. Histochem. Cytochem.* **45**:79–87.

230. Okano, J.-I., Shiota, G., and Kawasaki, H. (1999) Expression of hepatocyte growth factor (HGF) and HGF receptor (c-met) proteins in liver diseases: an immunohistochemical study. *Liver* **19**:151–159.

231. Yoshinaga, Y., Matsuno, Y., Fujita, S., Nakamura, T., Kikuchi, M., Shimosato, Y., and Hirohashi, S. (1993) Immunohistochemical detection of hepatocyte growth factor/scatter factor in human cancerous and inflammatory lesions of various organs. *Jpn. J. Cancer Res.* **84**:1150–1158.

232. D'Errico, A., Fiorentino, M., Ponzetto, A., Daikuhara, Y., Tsubouchi, H., Brechot, C., et al. (1996) Liver hepatocyte growth factor does not always correlate with hepatocellular proliferation in human liver lesions: its specific receptor *c-met* does. *Hepatology* **24**:60–64.

233. Ueki, T., Fujimoto, J., Suzuki, T., Yamamoto, H., and Okamoto, E. (1997) Expression of hepatocyte growth factor and its receptor *c-met* proto-oncogene in hepatocellular carcinoma. *Hepatology* **25**:862–866.

234. Noguchi, O., Enomoto, N., Ikeda, T., Kobayashi, F., Marumo, F., and Sato, C. (1996) Gene expressions of *c-met* and hepatocyte growth factor in chronic liver disease and hepatocellular carcinoma. *J. Hepatol.* **24**:286–292.

235. Selden, C., Farnaud, S., Ding, S. F., Habib, N., Foster, C., and Hodgson, H. J. F. (1994) Expression of hepatocyte growth factor mRNA, and a c-met mRNA (hepatocyte growth factor receptor) in human liver tumours. *J. Hepatol.* **21**:227–234.

236. Ho, R. T. H., Liew, C. T., and Lai, K. N. (1999) The expression of hepatocyte growth factor (HGF) and interleukin 6 (IL-6) in damaged human liver and kidney tissues. *Hepato-Gastroenterology* **46**:1904–1909.

237. Shiota, G., Okano, J.-I., Kawasaki, H., Kawamoto, T., and Nakamura, T. (1995) Serum hepatocyte growth factor levels in liver diseases: clinical implications. *Hepatology* **21**:106–112.

238. Von Schweinitz, D., Fuchs, J., Glüer, S., and Pietsch, T. (1998) The occurrence of liver growth factor in hepatoblastoma. *Eur. J. Pediatric Surg.* **8**:133–136.

239. Von Schweinitz, D., Faundez, A., Trichmann, B., Birnbaum, T., Koch, A., Hecker, H., et al. (2000) Hepatocyte growth factor-scatter factor can stimulate post-operative tumor cell proliferation in childhood hepatoblastoma. *Int. J. Cancer* **85**:151–159.

240. Chen, Q., Seol, D.-W., Carr, B., and Zarnegar, R. (1997) Expression and regulation of *Met* and *Ron* proto-oncogenes in human hepatocellular carinoma tissues and cell lines. *Hepatology* **26**:59–66.

241. Di Renzo, M. F., Narsimhan, R. P., Olivero, M., Bretti, S., Giordano, S., Medico, E., et al. (1991) Expression of the Met/HGF receptor in normal and neoplastic human tissues. *Oncogene* **6**:1997–2004.

242. Prat, M., Narismhan, R. P., Crepaldi, T., Nicotra, M. R., Natali, P. G., and Comoglio, P. M. (1991) The receptor encoded by the human *c-met* oncogene is expressed in hepatocytes, epithelial cells and solid tumors. *Int. J. Cancer* **49**:323–328.

243. Boix, L., Rosa, J. L., Ventura, F., Castells, A., Bruix, J., Rodés, J., et al. (1994) c-*met* mRNA overexpression in human hepatocellular carcinoma. *Hepatology* **19**:88–91.

244. Suzuki, K., Hayashi, N., Yamada, Y., Yoshihara, H., Miyamoto, Y., Ito, Y., et al. (1994) Expression of the c-*met* protooncogene in human hepatocellular carcinoma. *Hepatology* **20**:1231–1236.

245. Grigioni, W. F., Fiorentino, M., D'Errico, A., Ponzetto, A., Crepaldi, T., Prat, M., et al. (1995) Overexpression of c-*met*

protooncogene product and raised Ki67 index in hepatocellular carcinomas with respect to benign liver conditions. *Hepatology* **21**:1543–1546.

246. Park, W. S., Dong, S. M., Kim, S. Y., Na, E. Y., Shin, M. S., Pi, J. H., et al. (1999) Somatic mutations in the kinase domain of the *Met*/hepatocyte growth factor receptor gene in childhood hepatocellular carcinomas. *Cancer Res.* **59**:307–310.

247. Bevilacqua, M., Norbiato, G., Chebat, E., Baldi, G., Bertora, P., Regalia, E., et al. (1991) Changes in alpha-1 and beta-2 adrenoceptor density in human hepatocellular carcinoma. *Cancer* **67**:2543–2551.

248. Motoo, Y., Sawabu, N., Yamaguchi, Y., Terada, T., and Nakanuma, Y. (1993) Sinusoidal capillarization of human hepatocellular carcinoma: possible promotion by fibroblast growth factor. *Oncology* **50**:270–274.

249. Shimoyama, Y., Gotoh, M., Ino, Y., Sakamoto, M., Kato, K., and Hirohashi, S. (1991) Characterization of high-molecular-mass forms of basic fibroblast growth factor produced by hepatocellular carcinoma cells: possible involvement of basic fibroblast growth factor in hepatocarcinogenesis. *Jpn. J. Cancer Res.* **82**:1263–1270.

250. Li, D., Bell, J., Brown, A., and Berry, C. L. (1994) The observation of angiogenic and basic fibroblast growth factor gene espression in human colonic adenocarcinomas, gastric adenocarcinomas, and hepatocellular carcinomas. *J. Pathol.* **172**:171–175.

251. Mise, M., Arii, S., Higashituji, H., Furutani, M., Niwano, M., Harada, T., et al. (1996) Clinical significance of vascular endothelial growth factor and basic fibroblast growth factor gene expression in liver tumor. *Hepatology* **23**:455–464.

252. Tsou, A. P., Wu, K. M., Tsen, T. Y., Chi, C. W., Chiu, J. H., Lui, W. Y., et al. (1998) Parallel hybridization analysis of multiple protein kinase genes: identification of gene expression patterns characteristic of human hepatocellular carcinoma. *Genomics* **50**:331-340.

253. Nelson, N. J. (1999) Angiogenesis research is on fast forward. *J. Natl. Cancer Inst.* **91**:820–822.

254. Chow, N.-H., Hsu, P.-I., Lin, X.-Z., Yang, H.-B., Chan, S.-H., Cheng, K.-S., et al. (1997) Expression of vascular endothelial growth factor in normal liver and hepatocellular carcinoma: An histochemical study. *Human Pathol.* **28**:698–703.

255. Torimura, T., Sata, M., Ueno, T., Kin, M., Tsuji, R., Suzaku, K., et al. (1998) Increased expression of vascular endothelial growth factor is associated with tumor progression in hepatocellular carcinoma. *Human Pathol.* **29**:986–991.

256. Yamaguchi, R., Yano, H., Iemura, A., Ogasawara, S., Haramaki, M., and Kojiro, M. (1998) Expression of vascular endothelial growth factor in human hepatocellular carcinoma. *Hepatology* **28**:68–77.

257. Kobayashi, N., Ishii, M., Ueno, Y., Kisara, N., Chida, N., Iwasaki, T., et al. (1999) Co-expression of Bcl-2 protein and vascular endothelial growth factor in hepatocellular carcinomas treated by chemoembolization. *Liver* **19**:25–31.

258. Zhou, J., Tang, Z.-Y., Fan, J., Wu, Z.-Q., Li, X.-M., Liu, Y.-K., et al. (2000) Expression of platelet-derived endothelial cell growth factor and vascular endothelial growth factor in hepatocellular carcinoma and portal vein tumor thrombus. *J. Cancer Res. Clin. Oncol.* **126**:57–61.

259. Suzuki, K., Hayashi, N., Miyamoto, Y., Yamamoto, M., Ohkawa, K., Ito, Y., et al. (1996) Expression of vascular permeability factor/vascular endothelial growth factor in human hepatocellular carcinoma. *Cancer Res.* **56**:3004–3009.

260. Li, X. M., Tang, Z. Y., Zhou, G., Lui, Y. K., and Ye, S. L. (1998) Significance of vascular endothelial growth factor mRNA expression in invasion and metastasis of hepatocellular carcinoma. *J. Exp. Clin. Cancer Res.* **17**:13–17.

261. Shimoda, K., Mori, M., Shibuta, K., Banner, B. F., and Bernard, G. F. (1999) Vascular endothelial growth factor/vascular permeability factor mRNA expression in patients with chronic hepatitis C and hepatocellular carcinoma. *Int. J. Oncol.* **14**:353–359.

262. Jin-no, K., Tanimizu, M., Hyodo, I., Nishikawa, Y., Hosokawa, Y., Endo, H., et al. (1998) Circulating platelet-derived endothelial cell

growth factor increases in hepatocellular carcinoma patients. *Cancer* **82**:1260–1267.

263. Michalopoulos, G. K. and DeFrances, M. C. (1997) Liver regeneration. *Science* **276**:60–66.

264. Milani, S., Herbst, H., Schuppan, D., Stein, H., and Surrenti, C. (1991) Transforming growth factors β1 and β2 are differentially expressed in fibrotic liver disease. *Am. J. Pathol.* **139**:1221–1229.

265. Bedossa, P., Peltier, E., Terris, B., Franco, D., and Poynard, T. (1995) Transforming growth factor-beta 1 (TGF-β1) and TGF-β1 receptors in normal, cirrhotic and neoplastic human livers. *Hepatology* **21**:760–766.

266. Orsatti, G., Hytiroglou, P., Thung, S. N., Ishak, K. G., and Paronetto, F. (1997) Lamellar fibrosis in the fibrolamellar variant of hepatocellular carcinoma: a role for transforming growth factor beta. *Liver* **17**:152–156.

267. Nagy, P., Schaff, Z., and Lapis, K. (1991) Immunohistochemical detection of transforming growth factor-β1 in fibrotic liver diseases. *Hepatology* **14**:269–273.

268. Annoni, G., Weiner, F. R., and Zern, M. A. (1992) Increased transforming growth factor-β1 gene expression in human liver disease. *J. Hepatol.* **14**:259–264.

269. Roulot, D., Durand, H., Coste, T., Rautureau, J., Strosberg, A. D., Benarous, R., et al. (1995) Quantitative analysis of transforming growth factor β1 messenger RNA in the liver of patients with chronic hepatitis C: absence of correlation between high levels and severity of disease. *Hepatology* **21**:298–304.

270. Takiya, S., Tagaya, T., Takahashi, K., Kawashima, H., Kamiya, M., Fukuzawa, Y., et al. (1995) Role of transforming growth factor β1 on hepatic regeneration and apoptosis in liver diseases. *J. Clin. Pathol.* **48**:1093–1097.

271. Ito, N., Kawata, S., Tamura, S., Takaishi, K., Yabuuchi, I., Matsuda, Y., et al. (1990) Expression of transforming growth factor-β1 mRNA in human hepatocellular carcinoma. *Jpn. J. Cancer Res.* **81**:1202–1205.

272. Ito, N., Kawata, S., Tamura, S., Takaishi, K., Shirai, Y., Kiso, S., et al. (1991) Elevated levels of transforming growth factor β messenger RNA and its polypeptide in human hepatocellular carcinoma. *Cancer Res.* **51**:4080–4083.

273. Abou-Shady, M., Baer, H. U., Friess, H., Berberat, P., Zimmermann, A., Graber, H., et al. (1999) Transforming growth factor betas and their signaling receptors in human hepatocellular carcinoma. *Am. J. Surg.* **177**:209–215.

274. Shirai, Y., Kawata, S., Ito, N., Tamura, S., Takaishi, K., Kiso, S., et al. (1992) Elevated levels of transforming growth factor-β in patients with hepatocellular carcinoma. *Jpn. J. Cancer Res.* **83**:676–679.

275. Shirai, Y., Kawata, S., Tamura, S., Ito, N., Tsushima, H., Takaishi, K., et al. (1994) Plasma transforming growth factor-β1 in patients with hepatocellular carcinoma. Comparison with chronic liver diseases. *Cancer* **73**:2275–2279.

276. Ito, N., Kawata, S., Tamura, S., Shirai, Y., Kiso, S., Tsushima, H., et al. (1995) Positive correlation of plasma transforming growth factor-β1 levels with tumor vascularity in hepatocellular carcinoma. *Cancer Lett.* **89**:45-48.

277. Tsai, J.-F., Chuang, L.-Y., Jeng, J.-E., Yang, M.-L., Chang, W.-Y., Hsieh, M.-Y., et al. (1997) Clinical relevance of transforming growth factor-β1 in the urine of patients with hepatocellular carcinoma. *Medicine* **76**:213–226.

278. Vincent, F., Hagiwara, K., Ke, Y., Stoner, G. D., Demetrick, D. J., and Bennett, W. P. (1996) Mutation analysis of the transforming growth factor β type II receptor in sporadic human cancers of the pancreas, liver, and breast. *Biochem. Biophys. Res. Commun.* **223**:561–564.

279. Kawate, S., Takenoshita, S., Ohwada, S., Mogi, A., Fukusato, T., Makita, F., et al. (1999) Mutation analysis of transforming growth factor beta type II receptor, Smad2, and Smad4 in hepatocellular carcinoma. *Int. J. Oncol.* **14**:127–131.

280. Salvucci, M., Lemoine, A., Saffroy, R., Azoulay, D., Lepere, B., Gaillard, S., et al. (1999) Microsatellite instability in European hepatocellular carcinoma. *Oncogene* **18**:181–187.

281. Furuta, K., Misao, S., Takahashi, K., Tagaya, T., Fukuzawa, Y., Ishikawa, T., et al. (1999) Gene mutation of transforming growth factor β1 type II receptor in hepatocellular carcinoma. *Int. J. Cancer* **81**:851–899.

282. Adami, H.-O., Chow, W.-H., Nyren, O., Berne, C., Linet, M. S., Ekbom, A., et al. (1996) Excess risk of primary liver cancer in patients with diabetes mellitus. *J. Natl. Cancer Inst.* **88**:1472–1477.

283. Nishiyama, M. and Wands, J. R. (1992) Cloning and increased expression of an insulin receptor substrate-1-like gene in human hepatocellular carcinoma. *Biochem. Biophys. Res. Commun.* **183**:280–285.

284. Furusaka, A., Nishiyama, M., Ohkawa, K., Yamori, T., Tsuruo, T., Yonezawa, K., et al. (1994) Expression of insulin receptor substrate-1 in hepatocytes: an investigation using monoclonal antibodies. *Cancer Lett.* **84**:85–92.

285. Tanaka, S., Mohr, L., Schmidt, E. V., Sugimachi, K., and Wands, J. R. (1997) Biological effects of insulin receptor substrate-1 overexpression in hepatocytes. *Hepatology* **26**:598–604.

286. Ikeda, Y., Shimada, M., Hasegawa, H., Gion, T., Kajiyama, K., Shirabe, K., et al. (1998) Prognosis of hepatocellular carcinoma with diabetes mellitus after hepatic resection. *Hepatology* **27**:1567–1571.

287. Lin, K.-H., Shieh, H.-Y., Chen, S.-L., and Hsu, H.-C. (1999) Expression of mutant thyroid hormone nuclear receptors in human hepatocellular carcinoma cells. *Mol. Carcinogenesis* **26**:53–61.

288. Lin, K.-H., Zhu, X.-G., Hsu, H.-C., Chen, S.-L., Shieh, H.-Y., Chen, S.-T., et al. (1997) Dominant negative activity of mutant thyroid hormone alpha 1 receptors from patients with hepatocellular carcinoma. *Endocrinology* **138**:5308–5315.

289. Lin, K.-H., Lin, Y.-W., Lee, H.-F., Liu, W.-L., Chen, S.-T., Chang, K. S., et al. (1995) Increased invasive activity of human hepatocellular carcinoma cells is associated with an overexpression of thyroid hormone β1 nuclear receptor and low expression of the anti-metastatic nm23 gene. *Cancer Lett.* **98**:89–95.

290. Nelson, R. B. (1979) Thyroid-binding globulin in hepatoma. *Arch. Intern. Med.* **139**:1063.

291. Kalk, W. J., Kew, M. C., Danielwitz, M. D., Jacks, F., Van Der Walt, L. A., and Levin, J. (1982) Thyroxine-binding globulin and thyroid function tests in patients with hepatocellular carcinoma. *Hepatology* **2**:72–76.

292. Alexopoulos, A., Hutchinson, W., Bari, A., Keating, J. J., Johnson, P. J., and Williams, R. (1988) Hyperthyroxinemia in hepatocellular carcinoma: relation to thyroid binding globulin in the clinical and preclinical stages of the disease. *Br. J. Cancer* **57**:313–316.

293. Hutchinson, W. L., Johnson, P. J., White, Y. S., and Williams, R. (1989) Differential hormone-binding characteristics of thyroxine-binding globulin in hepatocellular carcinoma and cirrhosis. *J. Hepatology* **9**:265–271.

294. Hutchinson, W. L., White, Y. S., Fagan, E. A., Johnson, P. J., and Williams, R. (1991) Impaired binding properties of thyroxine-binding globulin in hepatocellular carcinoma and chronic liver disease. *Hepatology* **14**:116–120.

295. Arbuthnot, P., Kew, M., Parker, I., and Fitschen, W. (1989) Expression of c-*erbA* in human hepatocellular carcinoma. *Anticancer Res.* **9**:885–888.

296. Guéchot, J., Piegny, N., Ballet, F., Vanbourdolle, M., Giboudeau, J., and Poupon, R. (1988) Sex hormone imbalance in male alcoholic patients with and without hepatocellular carcinoma. *Cancer* **62**:760–762.

297. Yu, M.-W. and Chen, C.-J. (1993) Elevated serum testosterone levels and risk of hepatocellular carcinoma. *Cancer Res.* **53**:790–794.

298. Guéchot, J., Peigney, N., Ballet, F., Vaubourdolle, M., Giboudeau, J., and Poupon, R. (1989) Effect of D-tryptophan-6-luetinizing hormone-releasing hormone on the tumoral growth and plasma sex steroid levels in cirrhotic patients with hepatocellular carcinoma. *Hepatology* **10**:346–348.

299. Hsing, A. W., Hoover, R. N., McLaughlin, J. K., Co-Chien, H. T., Wacholder, S., Blot, W. J., et al. (1992) Oral contraceptives and primary liver cancer among young women. *Cancer Causes Control* **3**:43–48.

300. Sweeney, E. C. and Evans, D. J. (1976) Hepatic lesions in patients treated with synthetic anabolic steroids. *J. Clin. Pathol.* **29**:626–633.

301. Boyd, P. R. and Mark, G. J. (1977) Multiple hepatic adenomas and a hepatocellular carcinoma in a man on oral methyl testosterone for eleven years. *Cancer* **40**:1765–1770.

302. Iqbal, M. J., Wilkinson, M. L., Johnson, P. J., and Williams, R. (1983) Sex steroid receptor proteins in foetal, adult and malignant human liver tissue. *Br. J. Cancer* **48**:791–796.

303. Nagasue, N., Ito, A., Yukaya, H., and Ogawa, Y. (1985) Androgen receptors in hepatocellular carcinoma and surrounding parenchyma. *Gastroenterology* **89**:643–647.

304. Eagon, P. K., Francavilla, A., DiLeo, A., Elm, M. S., Gennari, L., Mazzaferro, V., et al. (1991) Quantitation of estrogen and androgen receptors in hepatocellular carcinoma and adjacent normal human liver. *Digest. Dis. Sci.* **36**:1303–1308.

305. Eagon, P. K., Elm, M. S., Stafford, E.A., and Porter, L. E. (1994) Androgen receptor in human liver: Characterization and quantitation in normal and diseased liver. *Hepatology* **19**:92–100.

306. Nakagama, H., Gunji, T., Onishi, S., Kaneko, T., Ishikawa, T., Makino, R., et al. (1991) Expression of androgen receptor mRNA in human hepatocellular carcinomas and hepatoma cell lines. *Hepatology* **14**:99–102.

307. Nagasue, N., Yukaya, H., Chang, Y.-C., Ogawa, Y., Kohno, H., and Ito, A. (1986) Active uptake of testosterone by androgen receptors of hepatocellular carcinomas in humans. *Cancer* **57**:2162–2167.

308. Nagasue, N., Yamanoi, A., Kohno, H., Kimoto, T., Chang, Y., Taniura, H., et al. (1992) Androgen receptor in cirrhotic liver, adenomatous hyperplastic nodule and hepatocellular carcinoma in the human. *Hepato-Gastroenterology* **39**:455–460.

309. Onishi, S., Murakami, T., Moriyama, T., Mitamura, K., and Imawari, M. (1989) Androgen and estrogen receptors in hepatocellular carcinomas and the surrounding noncancerous liver tissue. *Hepatology* **6**:440–443.

310. Nagasue, N., Chang, Y.-C., Hayashi, T., Galizia, G., Kohno, H., Nakamura, T., et al. (1989) Androgen receptor in hepatocellular carcinoma as a prognostic factor after hepatic resection. *Ann. Surg.* **209**:424–427.

311. Nagasue, N., Kohno, H., Chang, Y.-C., Hayashi, T., Utsumi, Y., Nakamura, T., et al. (1989) Androgen and estrogen receptors in hepatocellular carcinoma and the surrounding liver in women. *Cancer* **63**:112–116.

312. Nagasue, N., Yu, L., Yukaya, H., Kohno, H., and Nakamura, T. (1995) Androgen and estrogen receptors in hepatocellular carcinoma and surrounding liver parenchyma: impact on intrahepatic recurrence after hepatic resection. *Br. J. Surg.* **82**:542–547.

313. Boix, L., Bruix, J., Castells, A., Fuster, J., Bru, C., Visa, J., et al. (1993) Sex hormone receptors in hepatocellular carcinoma. Is there a rationale for hormonal treatment? *J. Hepatol.* **17**:187–191.

314. Boix, L., Castells, A., Bruix, J., Sole, M., Bru, C., Fuster, J., et al. (1995) Androgen receptors in hepatocellular carcinoma and surrounding liver: relationship with tumor size and recurrence rate after surgical resection. *J. Hepatol.* **22**:616–622.

315. Zhang, X., He, L., Lu, Y., Liu, M., and Huang, X. (1998) Androgen receptor in primary hepatocellular carcinoma and its clinical significance. *Chin. Med. J.* **111**:1083–1086.

316. Porter, L. E., Elm, M. S., Van Thiel, D. H., Dugas, M. C., and Eagon, P. K. (1983) Characterization and quantitation of human hepatic estrogen receptor. *Gastroenterology* **84**:704–712.

317. Porter, L. E., Elm, M. S., Van Thiel, D. H., and Eagon, P. K. (1987) Hepatic estrogen receptor in human liver disease. *Gastroenterology* **92**:735–745.

318. Nagasue, N., Ito, A., Yukaya, H., and Ogawa, Y. (1986) Estrogen receptors in hepatocellular carcinoma. *Cancer* **57**:87–91.

319. Ciocca, D. R., Jorge, A. D., Jorge, O., Milutin, C., Hosokawa, R., Lestren, M. D., et al. (1991) Estrogen receptors, progesterone receptors and heat-shock 27-kD protein in liver biopsy specimens from patients with hepatitis B virus infection. *Hepatology* **13**:838–844.

320. Nagasue, N., Kohno, H., Chang, Y.-C., Yamanoi, A., Nakamura, T., Yukaya, H., et al. (1990) Clinicopathologic comparisons between estrogen receptor-positive and -negative hepatocellular carcinomas. *Ann. Surg.* **212**:150–154.

321. Villa, E., Camellini, L., Dugani, A., Zucchi, F., Grottola, A., Merighi, A., et al. (1995) Variant estrogen receptor messenger RNA species detected in human primary hepatocellular carcinoma. *Cancer Res.* **55**:498–500.

322. Villa, E., Dugani, A., Moles, A., Camellini, L., Grottola, A., Buttafuco, P., et al. (1998) Variant liver estrogen receptor transcripts already occur at an early stage of chronic liver disease. *Hepatology* **27**:983–988.

323. Villa, E., Dugani, A., Fantoni, E., Camellini, L., Buttafuco, P., Grottola, A., et al. (1996) Type of estrogen receptor determines response to antiestrogen therapy. *Cancer Res.* **56**:3883–3885.

324. Castells, A., Bruix, J., Bru, C., Ayuso, C., Roca, M., Boix, L., et al. (1995) Treatment of hepatocellular carcinoma with tamoxifen: a double-blind placebo-controlled trial in 120 patients. *Gastroenterology* **109**:917–922.

325. Friedman, M. A., Demanes, D. J., and Hoffman, P. G. Jr. (1982) Hepatomas: hormone receptors and therapy. *Am. J. Med.* **73**:362–366.

326. Carbone, A. and Vecchio, F. M. (1986) Presence of cytoplasmic progesterone receptors in hepatic adenomas. A report of two cases. *Am. J. Clin. Pathol.* **85**:325–329.

327. Demanes, D. J., Friedman, M. A., McKerrow, J. H., and Hoffman, P. G. (1982) Hormone receptors in hepatoblastoma: a demonstration of both estrogen and progesterone receptors. *Cancer* **50**: 1828–1832.

328. Nagasue, N., Kohno, H., Yamanoi, A., Kimoto, T., Chang, Y.-C., and Nakamura, T. (1991) Progesterone receptor in hepatocellular carcinoma. Correlation with androgen and estrogen receptors. *Cancer* **67**:2501–2505.

329. Petkovich, M., Brand, N. J., Krust, A., and Chambon, P. (1987) A human retinoic acid receptor which belongs to the family of nuclear receptors. *Nature* **330**:444–450.

330. De Thé, H., Marchio, A., Tiollais, P., and Dejean, A. (1989) Differential expression and ligand regulation of the retinoic acid receptor alpha and beta genes. *EMBO J.* **8**:429–433.

331. Dejean, A., Bougueleret, L., Grzeschik, K.-H., and Tiollais, P. (1986) Hepatitis B virus DNA integration in a sequence homologous to v-*erb*-A and steroid receptor genes in hepatocellular carcinoma. *Nature* **322**:70–72.

332. De Thé, H., Marchio, A., Tiollais, P., and Dejean, A. (1987) A novel steroid thyroid hormone receptor-related gene inappropriately expressed in human hepatocellular carcinoma. *Nature* **330**:667–670.

333. Brand, N., Petkovich, M., Krust, A., Chambon, P., De The, H., Marchio, A., et al. (1988) Identification of a second human retinoic acid receptor. *Nature* **332**:850–853.

334. Benbrook, D., Lernhardt, E., and Pfahl, M. (1988) A new retinoic acid receptor identified from a hepatocellular carcinoma. *Nature* **333**:669–672.

335. Krust, A., Kastner, P., Petkovich, M., Zelent, A., and Chambon, P. (1989) A third human retinoic acid receptor, hRAR-g. *Proc. Natl. Acad. Sci. USA* **86**:5310–5314.

336. Sever, C. E. and Locker, J. (1991) Expression of retinoic acid α and β receptor genes in liver and hepatocellular carcinoma. *Mol. Carcinogenesis* **4**:138–144.

337. Reubi, J. C., Zimmermann, A., Jonas, S., Waser, B., Neuhaus, P., Läderach, U., et al. (1999) Regulatory peptide receptors in human hepatocellular carcinomas. *Gut* **45**:766–774.

338. Caplin, M., Khan, K., Savage, K., Rode, J., Varro, A., Michaeli, D., et al. (1999) Expression of gastrin in hepatocellular carcinoma, fibrolamellar carcinoma, and cholangiocarcinoma. *J. Hepatol.* **30**:519–526.

339. Nonomura, A., Ohta, G., Hayashi, M., Izumi, R., Watanabe, K., Takayanagi, N., et al. (1987) Immunohistochemical detection of *ras* oncogene p21 product in liver cirrhosis and hepatocellular carcinoma. *Am. J. Gastroenterol.* **82**:512–518.

340. Lee, H.-S., Rajagopalan, M. S., and Vyas, G. N. (1988) A lack of direct role of hepatitis B virus in the activation of *ras* and c-*myc*

oncogenes in human hepatocellular carcinogenesis. *Hepatology* **8**:1116–1120.

341. Jagirdar, J., Nonomura, A., Patil, J., Thor, A., and Paronetto, F. (1989) ras oncogene p21 expression in hepatocellular carcinoma. *J. Exp. Pathol.* **4**:37–46.

342. Tiniakos, D., Spandidos, D. A., Kakkanas, A., Pintzas, A., Pollice, L., and Tiniakos, G. (1989) Expression of *ras* and *myc* oncogenes in human hepatocellular carcinoma and non-neoplastic liver tissues. *Anticancer Res.* **9**:715–722.

343. Tiniakos, D., Spandidos, D. A., Yiagnisis, M., and Tiniakos, G. (1993) Expression of ras and c-myc proteins and hepatitis B surface antigen in human liver disease. *Hepato-Gastroenterology* **40**:37–40.

344. Radosevich, J. A., Gould, K. A., Koukoulis, G. K., Haines, G. K., Rosen, S. T., Lee, I., et al. (1993) Immunolocalization of *ras* oncogene p21 in human liver diseases. *Ultrastruct. Pathol.* **17**:1–8.

345. Haritani, H., Esumi, M., Uchida, T., and Shikata, T. (1991) Oncogene expression in the liver tissue of patients with nonneoplastic liver disease. *Cancer* **67**:2594–2598.

346. Zhang, X. K., Huang, D.P., Chiu, D. K., and Chiu, J. F. (1987) The expression of oncogenes in human developing liver and hepatomas. *Biochem. Biophys. Res. Commun.* **142**:932–938.

347. Himeno, Y., Fukuda, Y., Hatanaka, M., and Imura, H. (1988) Expression of oncogenes in human liver disease. *Liver* **8**:208–212.

348. Gu, J.-R., Hu, L.-F., Cheng, Y.-C., and Wan, D.-F. (1986) Oncogenes in human primary hepatic cancer. *J. Cell. Physiol.* **4**:13–20.

349. Zhang, X.-K., Huang, D., Qiu, D.-K., and Chiu, J. (1990) The expression of c-*myc* and c-N-*ras* in human cirrhotic livers, hepatocellular carcinomas and liver tissue surrounding the tumors. *Oncogene* **5**:909–914.

350. Ogata, N., Kamimura, T., and Asakura, H. (1991) Point mutation, allelic loss and increased methylation of c-Ha-*ras* gene in human hepatocellular carcinoma. *Hepatology* **13**:31–37.

351. Fukuda, K., Ogasawara, S., Maruiwa, M., Yano, H., Murakami, T., and Kojiro, M. (1988) Structural alterations in c-*myc* and c-Ha-*ras* proto-oncogenes in human hepatocellular carcinoma. *Kurume Med. J.* **35**:77–87.

352. Tada, M., Omata, M., and Ohto, M. (1990) Analysis of *ras* gene mutations in human hepatic malignant tumors by polymerase chain reaction and direct sequencing. *Cancer Res.* **50**:1121–1124.

353. Challen, C., Guo, K., Collier, J. D., Cavanagh, D., and Bassendine, M. F. (1992) Infrequent point mutations in codons 12 and 61 of *ras* oncogenes in human hepatocellular carcinomas. *J. Hepatol.* **14**:342–346.

354. Kress, S., Jahn, U.-R., Buchmann, A., Bannasch, P., and Schwarz, M. (1992) p53 mutations in human hepatocellular carcinomas from Germany. *Cancer Res.* **52**:3220–3223.

355. Leon, M. and Kew, M. C. (1995) Analysis of *ras* gene mutations in hepatocellular carcinoma in Southern African blacks. *Anticancer Res.* **15**:859–862.

356. Tsuda, H., Hirohashi, S., Shimosato, Y., Ino, Y., Yoshida, T., and Terada, M. (1989) Low incidence of point mutation of c-Ki-*ras* and N-*ras* oncogenes in human hepatocellular carcinoma. *Jpn. J. Cancer Res.* **80**:196–199.

357. Stork, P., Loda, M., Bosari, S., Wiley, B., Poppenhusen, K., and Wolfe, H. (1991) Detection of K-*ras* mutations in pancreatic and hepatic neoplasms by non-isotopic mismatched polymerase chain reaction. *Oncogene* **6**:857–862.

358. Imai, Y., Oda, H., Arai, M., Shimizu, S., Nakatsuru, Y., Inoue, T., et al. (1996) Mutational analysis of the *p53* and K-*ras* genes and allelotype study of the *Rb-1* gene for investigating the pathogenesis of combined hepatocellular-cholangiocellular carcinomas. *Jpn. J. Cancer Res.* **87**:1056–1062.

359. Takada, S. and Koike, K. (1989) Activated N-*ras* gene was found in human hepatoma tissue but only in a small fraction of the tumor cells. *Oncogene* **4**:189–193.

360. Schmidt, C. M., McKillop, I. H., Cahill, P. A., and Sitzmann, J. V. (1997) Increased MAPK expression and activity in primary human hepatocellular carcinoma. *Biochem. Biophys. Res. Commun.* **236**:54–58.

361. Ito, Y., Sasaki, Y., Horimoto, M., Wada, S., Tanaka, Y., Kasahara, A., et al. (1998) Activation of mitogen-activated protein kinases/extracellular signal-related kinases in human hepatocellular carcinoma. *Hepatology* **27**:951–958.

362. Masaki, T., Okada, M., Shiratori, Y., Rengifo, W., Matsumoto, K., Maeda, S., et al. (1998) pp60^{c-src} activation in hepatocellular carcinoma of humans and LEC rats. *Hepatology* **27**:1257–1264.

363. Schmidt, C. M., McKillop, I. H., Cahill, P. A., and Sitzman, J. V. (1997) Alterations in guanine nucleotide regulatory protein expression and activity in human hepatocellular carcinoma. *Hepatology* **26**:1189–1194.

364. Arbuthnot, P., Kew, M., and Fitschen, W. (1991) c-*fos* and c-*myc* oncoprotein expression in human hepatocellular carcinomas. *Anticancer Res.* **11**:921–924.

365. Gan, F.-Y., Gesell, M. S., Alousi, M., and Luk, G. D. (1993) Analysis of ODC and c-*myc* gene expression in hepatocellular carcinoma by *in situ* hybridization and immunohistochemistry. *J. Histochem. Cytochem.* **41**:1185–1196.

366. Saegusa, M., Takano, Y., Kishimoto, H., Wakabayashi, G., Nohga, K., and Okudaira, M. (1993) Comparative analysis of *p53* and c-*myc* expression and cell proliferation in human hepatocellular carcinomas: An enhanced immunohistochemical approach. *J. Cancer Res. Clin. Oncol.* **119**:737–744.

367. Su, T. S., Lin, L. H., Lui, W. Y., Chang, C. M., Chou, C. K., Ting, L.P., et al. (1985) Expression of c-*myc* gene in human hepatomas. *Biochem. Biophys. Res. Commun.* **132**:264–268.

368. Nambu, S., Inoue, K., and Saski, H. (1987) Site-specific hypomethylation of the c-*myc* oncogene in human hepatocellular carcinoma. *Jpn. J. Cancer Res.* **78**:695–704.

369. Fujiwara, Y., Monden, M., Mori, T., Nakamura, Y., and Emi, M. (1993) Frequent multiplication of the long arm of chromosome 8 in hepatocellular carcinoma. *Cancer Res.* **53**:857–860.

370. Peng, S. Y., Lai, P. L., and Hsu, H. C. (1993) Amplification of the c-*myc* gene in human hepatocellular carcinoma: biologic significance. *J. Formosan. Med. Assoc.* **92**:866–870.

371. Abou-Elella, A., Gramlich, T., Fritsch, C., and Gansler, T. (1996) c-*myc* amplification in hepatocellular carcinoma predicts unfavorable prognosis. *Mod. Pathol.* **9**:95–98. 219.

372. Kawate, S., Fukusato, T., Ohwada, S., Watanuki, A., and Morishita, Y. (1999) Amplification of c-*myc* in hepatocellular carcinoma: correlation with clincopathologic features, proliferative activity and p53 overexpression. *Oncology* **57**:157–163.

373. Taylor, J. A., Bell, A., and Nagorney, D. (1993) L-*myc* proto-oncogene alleles and susceptibility to hepatocellular carcinoma. *Int. J. Cancer* **54**:927–930.

374. Nisen, P. D., Zimmerman, K. A., Cotter, S. V., Gilbert, F., and Alt, F. W. (1986) Enhanced expression of the N-*myc* gene in Wilms' tumors. *Cancer Res.* **46**:6217–6222.

375. Tsuda, H., Shimosato, Y., Upton, M. P., Yukota, J., Terada, M., Ohira, M., et al. (1988) Retrospective study on amplification of N-*myc* and c-*myc* genes in pediatric solid tumors and its association with prognosis and tumor differentiation. *Lab. Invest.* **59**:321–327.

376. Choi, E. K., Uyeno, S., Nishida, N., Okumoto, T., Fujimura, S., Aoki, Y., et al. (1996) Alterations of c-*fos* methylation in the processes of aging and tumorigenesis in human liver. *Mutat. Res.* **354**:123–128.

377. Schutte, M., Hruban, R. H., Hedrick, L., Cho, K. R., Nasady, G. M., Weinstein, C. L., et al. (1996) *DPC4* gene in various tumor types. *Cancer Res.* **56**:2527–2530.

378. Piao, Z., Kim, H., Jeon, B.K., Le, W. J., and Park, C. (1997) Relationship between loss of heterozygosity of tumor suppressor genes and histologic differentiation in hepatocellular carcinoma. *Cancer* **80**:865–872.

379. Yakicier, M. C., Irmak, M. B., Romano, A., Kew, M., and Ozturk, M. (1999) Smad2 and Smad4 mutations in hepatocellular carcinoma. *Oncogene* **18**:4879–4883.

380. Ito, Y., Matsuura, N., Sakon, M., Miyoshi, E., Noda, K., Takeda, T., et al. (1999) Expression and prognostic roles of the G1-S modula-

tors in hepatocellular carcinoma: p27 independently predicts the recurrence. *Hepatology* **30**:90–99.

381. Nishida, N., Fukuda, Y., Komeda, T., Kita, R., Sando, T., Furukawa, M., et al. (1994) Amplification and overexpression of cyclin D1 gene in aggressive human hepatocellular carcinoma. *Cancer Res.* **54**:3107–3110.

382. Zhang, Y. J., Jiang, W., Chen, C. J., Lee, C. S., Kahn, S. M., Santella, R. M., et al. (1993) Amplification and overexpression of cyclin D1 in human hepatocellular carcinoma. *Biochem. Biophys. Res. Commun.* **196**:1010–1016.

383. Tanigami, A., Tokino, T., Takita, K.-I., Ueda, M., Kasumi, F., and Nakamura, Y. (1992) Detailed analysis of an amplified region at chromosome 11q13 in malignant tumors. *Genomics* **13**:21–24.

384. Peng, S.-Y., Chou, S.-P., and Hsu, H.-C. (1998) Association of downregulation of cyclin D1 and of overexpression of cyclin E with p53 mutation, high tumor grade and poor prognosis in hepatocellular carcinoma. *J. Hepatol.* **29**:281–289.

385. Kim, H., Ham, E. K., Kim, Y. I., Chi, J. G., Lee, H. S., Park, S. H., et al. (1998) Overexpression of cyclin D1 and cdk4 in tumorigenesis of sporadic hepatoblastomas. *Cancer Lett.* **131**:1776–1783.

386. Iolascon, A., Giordani, L., Moretti, A., Basso, G., Borriello, A., and Della Ragione, F. (1998) Analysis of CDKN2A, CDKN2B, CDKN2C, and cyclin Ds gene status in hepatoblastoma. *Hepatology* **27**:989–995.

387. Covini, G., Chan, E. K. L., Nishioka, M., Morshed, S. A., Reed, S. I., and Tan, E. M. (1997) Immune response to cyclin B1 in hepatocellular carcinoma. *Hepatology* **25**:75–80.

388. Chao, Y., Shih, Y.-L., Chiu, J.-H., Chan, G.-Y., Lui, W.-Y., Yang, W. K., et al. (1998) Overexpression of cyclin A but not Skp2 correlates with the tumor relapse of human hepatocellular carcinoma. *Cancer Res.* **58**:985–990.

389. Paterlini, P., Flejou, J.-F., DeMitri, M. S., Pisi, E., Franco, D., and Bréchot, C. (1995) Structure and expression of the cyclin A gene in human primary liver cancer. Correlation with flow cytometric parameters. *J. Hepatol.* **23**:47–52.

390. Wang, J., Chenivesse, X., Henglein, B., and Bréchot, C. (1990) Hepatitis B virus integration in a cyclin A gene in a hepatocellular carcinoma. *Nature* **343**:555–557.

391. Wang, J., Zindy, F., Chenivesse, X., Lamas, E., Henglein, B., and Bréchot, C. (1992) Modification of cyclin A expression by hepatitis B virus DNA integration in a hepatocellular carcinoma. *Oncogene* **7**:1653–1656.

392. DeMitri, M. S., Pisi, E., Bréchot, C., and Paterlini, P. (1993) Low frequency of allelic loss in the cyclin A gene in human hepatocellular carcinomas: A study based on PCR. *Liver* **13**:259–261.

393. Strassburg, C. P., Alex, B., Zindy, F., Gerken, G., Lüttig, B., zum Büschenfelde, K.-H. M., et al. (1996) Identification of cyclin A as a molecular target of antinuclear antibodies (ANA) in hepatic and non-hepatic autoimmune diseases. *J. Hepatol.* **25**:859–866.

394. Gorczyca, W., Sarode, V., Juan, G., Melamed, M. R., and Darzynkiewicz, Z. (1997) Laser scanning cytometric analysis of cyclin B1 in primary human malignancies. *Mod. Pathol.* **10**:457–462.

395. Hui, A.-M., Sakamoto, M., Kanai, Y., Ino, Y., Gotoh, M., Yokota, J., et al. (1996) Inactivation of *p16^{INK4}* in hepatocellular carcinoma. *Hepatology* **24**:575–579.

396. Piao, Z., Park, C., Lee, J.-S., Yang, C. H., Choi, K. Y., and Kim, H. (1998) Homozygous deletions of the CDKN2 gene and loss of heterozygosity of 9p in primary hepatocellular carcinoma. *Cancer Lett.* **122**:201–207.

397. Matsuda, Y., Ichida, T., Matsuzawa, J., Sugimura, K., and Asakura, H. (1999) *p16^{INK4}* is inactivated by extensive CpG methylation in human hepatocellular carcinoma. *Gastroenterology* **116**:394–400.

398. Chaubert, P., Gayer, R., Zimmermann, A., Fontolliet, C., Stamm, B., Bosman, F., et al. (1997) Germ-line mutations of the *p16^{INK4} (MTS1)* gene occur in a subset of patients with hepatocellular carcinoma. *Hepatology* **25**:1376–1381.

399. Lin, Y.-W., Chen, C.-H., Huang, G.-T., Lee, P.-H., Wang, J.-T., Chen, D.-S., et al. (1998) Infrequent mutations and no methylation of CDKN2A (p16/MTS1) and CDKN2B (p15/MTS2) in hepatocellular carcinoma in Taiwan. *Eur. J. Cancer* **34**:1789–1795.

400. Liew, C. T., Li, H.-M., Lo, K.-W., Leow, C. K., Chan, J. Y. H., Hin, L. Y., et al. (1999) High frequency of p16^{INK4A} gene alterations in hepatocellular carcinoma. *Oncogene* **18**:789–795.

401. Wong, I. H. N., Dennis Lo, Y. M., Zhang, J., Liew, C.-T., Ng, M. H. L., Wong, N., et al. (1999) Detection of aberrant *p16* methylation in the plasma and serum of liver cancer patients. *Cancer Res.* **59**:71–73.

402. Kita, R., Nishida, N., Fukuda, Y., Azechi, H., Matsuoka, Y., Komeda, T., et al. (1996) Infrequent alterations in the *p16^{INK4A}* gene in liver cancer. *Int. J. Cancer* **67**:176–180.

403. Qin, L.-X., Tang, Z.-Y., Liu, K.-D., Ye, S.-L., He, B., Zhang, Y., et al. (1996) Alterations of CDKN2(p16/MTS1) exon 2 in human hepatocellular carcinoma. *Oncology Rep.* **3**:405–408.

404. Biden, K., Young, J., Buttenshaw, R., Searle, J., Cooksley, G., Xu, D.-B., et al. (1997) Frequency of mutation and deletion of the tumor suppressor gene CDKN2A (MTS1/p16) in hepatocellular carcinoma from an Australian population. *Hepatology* **25**:593–597.

405. Bonilla, F., Orlow, I., and Cordon-Cardo, C. (1998) Mutational study of p16CDKN2/MTS1/INK4A and p57KIP2 genes in hepatocellular carcinoma. *Int. J. Oncol.* **12**:583–588.

406. Qin, L. F., Ng, I. O., Fan, S. T., and Ng, M. (1998) p21/WAF1, p53 and PCNA expression and *p53* mutation status in hepatocellular carcinoma. *Int. J. Cancer* **79**:424–428.

407. Furutani, M., Arii, S., Tanaka, H., Mise, M., Niwano, M., Harada, T., et al. (1997) Decreased expression and rare somatic mutation of the CIP1/WAF1 gene in human hepatocellular carcinoma. *Cancer Lett.* **111**:191–197.

408. Hui, A.-M., Kanai, Y., Sakamoto, M., Tsuda, H., and Hirohashi, S. (1997) Reduced p21^{WAF1/CIP1} expression and p53 mutation in hepatocellular carcinomas. *Hepatology* **25**:575–579.

409. Watanabe, H., Fukuchi, K., Takagi, Y., Tomoyasu, S., Tsuruoka, N., and Gomi, K. (1995) Molecular analysis of Cip1/Waf1 (p21) gene in diverse types of human tumors. *Biochim. Biophys. Acta* **1263**:275–280.

410. Hui, A.-M., Sun, L., Kanai, Y., Sakamoto, M., and Hirohashi, S. (1998) Reduced p27^{Kip1} expression in hepatocellular carcinomas. *Cancer Lett.* **132**:67–73.

411. Hsia, C. C., DiBisceglie, A. M., Kleiner, D. E., Farshid, M., and Tabor, E. (1994) *RB* tumor suppressor gene expression in hepatocellular carcinomas from patients infected with the hepatitis B virus. *J. Med. Virol.* **44**:67–73.

412. Zhang, X., Xu, H.-J., Murakami, Y., Sachse, R., Yashima, K., Hirohashi, S., et al. (1994) Deletions of chromosome 13q, mutations in *Retinoblastoma 1*, and retinoblastoma protein state in human hepatocellular carcinoma. *Cancer Res.* **54**:4177–4182.

413. Hui, A.-M., Li, X., Makuuchi, M., Takayama, T., and Kubota, K. (1999) Over-expression and lack of retinoblastoma protein are associated with tumor progression and metastasis in hepatocellular carcinoma. *Int. J. Cancer* **84**:604–608.

414. Hada, H., Koide, N., Morita, T., Shiraha, H., Shinji, T., Nakamura, M., et al. (1996) Promoter-independent loss of mRNA and protein of the Rb gene in a human hepatocellular carcinoma. *Hepato-Gastroenterology* **43**:1185–1189.

415. Murakami, Y., Hayashi, K., Hirohashi, S., and Sekiya, T. (1991) Aberrations of the tumor suppressor p53 and retinoblastoma genes in human hepatocellular carcinomas. *Cancer Res.* **51**:5520–5525.

416. Nakamura, T., Iwamura, Y., Kaneko, M., Nakagawa, K., Kawai, K., Mitamura, K., et al. (1991) Deletions and rearrangements of the retinoblastoma gene in hepatocellular carcinoma, insulinoma and some neurogenic tumors as found in a study of 121 tumors. *Jpn. J. Clin. Oncol.* **21**:325–329.

417. Walker, G. J., Hayward, N. K., Falvey, S., and Cooksley, W. G. E. (1991) Loss of somatic heterozygosity in hepatocellular carcinoma. *Cancer Res.* **51**:4367–4370.

418. Nishida, N., Fukada, Y., Kokuryu, H., Sadamoto, T., Isowa, G., Honda, K., et al. (1992) Accumulation of allelic loss on arms of chromosomes 13q, 16q and 17p in advanced stages of human hepatocellular carcinoma. *Int. J. Cancer* **51**:862–868.

419. Fujimoto, Y., Hampton, L. L., Wirth, P. J., Wang, N. J., Xie, J. P., and Thorgeirsson, S. S. (1994) Alterations of tumor suppressor

genes and allelic losses in human hepatocellular carcinoma in China. *Cancer Res.* **54**:281–285.

420. Kuroki, T., Fujiwara, Y., Nakamori, S., Imaoka, S., Kanematsu, T., and Nakamuri, Y. (1995) Evidence for the presence of two tumor-suppressor genes for hepatocellular carcinoma on chromosome 13q. *Br. J. Cancer* **72**:383–385.

421. Ashida, K., Kishimoto, Y., Nakamoto, K., Wada, K., Shiota, G., Hirooka, Y., et al. (1997) Loss of heterozygosity of the retinoblastoma gene in liver cirrhosis accompanying hepatocellular carcinoma. *J. Cancer Res. Clin. Oncol.* **123**:489–495.

422. Nakamura, T., Monden, Y., Kawashima, K., Naruke, T., and Nishimura, S. (1996) Failure to detect mutations in the retinoblastoma protein-binding domain of the transcription factor E2F-1 in human cancers. *Jpn. J. Cancer Res.* **87**:1204–1209.

423. Zhao, M., Zhang, N.-X., Laissue, J. A., and Zimmermann, A. (1994) Immunohistochemical analysis of p53 protein overexpression in liver cell dysplasia and hepatocellular carcinoma. *Virchows Arch.* **424**:613–621.

424. Goldblum, J. R., Bartos, R. E., Carr, K. A., and Frank, T. S. (1993) Hepatitis B and alterations of the p53 tumor suppressor gene in hepatocellular carcinoma. *Am. J. Surg. Pathol.* **17**:1244–1251.

425. Ng, I. O. L., Chung, L. P., Tsang, S. W. Y., Lam, C. L., Lai, E. C. S., Fan, S. T., et al. (1994) p53 gene mutation spectrum in hepatocellular carcinomas in Hong Kong Chinese. *Oncogene* **9**:985–990.

426. Ng, I. O., Srivastava, G., Chung, L. P., Tsang, S. W., and Ng, M. M. (1994) Overexpression and point mutations of p53 tumor suppressor gene in hepatocellular carcinomas in Hong Kong Chinese people. *Cancer* **74**:30–37.

427. Volkmann, M., Hofmann, W .J., Müller, M., Räth, U., Otto, G., Zentgraf, H., et al. (1994) p53 overexpression is frequent in European hepatocellular carcinoma and largely independent of codon 249 hot spot mutations. *Oncogene* **9**:195–204.

428. Livni, N., Eid, A., Ilan, Y., Rivkind, A., Rosenmann, E., Blendis, L. M., et al. (1995) p53 expression in patients with cirrhosis with and without hepatocellular carcinoma. *Cancer* **75**:2420–2426.

429. Ojanguren, I., Ariza, A., Castellà, E. M., Fernández-Vasalo, A., Mate, J. L., and Navas-Palacios, J. J. (1995) p53 immunoreactivity in hepatocellular adenoma, focal nodular hyperplasia, cirrhosis and hepatocellular carcinoma. *Histopathology* **26**:63–68.

430. Kang, Y. K., Kim, C. J., Kim, W. H., Kim, H. O., Kang, G. H., and Kim, Y. I. (1998) p53 mutation and overexpression in hepatocellular carcinoma and dysplastic nodules in the liver. *Virchows Arch.* **432**:27–32.

431. Hosono, S., Lee, C.-S., Chou, M.-J., Yang, C.-S., and Shih, C. (1991) Molecular analysis of the p53 alleles in primary hepatocellular carcinomas and cell lines. *Oncogene* **6**:237–243.

432. Challen, C., Lunec, J., Warren, W., Collier, J., and Bassendine, M. F. (1992) Analysis of the p53 tumor-suppressor gene in hepatocellular carcinomas from Britain. *Hepatology* **16**:1362–1366.

433. Hsia, C. C., Kleiner, D. E., Axiotis, C. A., De Bisceglie, A., Nomura, A. M., Stemmermann, G. N., et al. (1992) Mutations of *p53* gene in hepatocellular carcinoma: roles of hepatitis B virus and aflatoxin contamination in the diet. *J. Natl. Cancer Inst.* **84**:1638–1641.

434. Laurent-Puig, P., Flejou, J.-F., Fabre, M., Bedossa, P., Belghitti, J., Grayal, F., et al. (1992) Overexpression of p53: a rare event in a large series of white patients with hepatocellular carcinoma. *Hepatology* **16**:1171–1175.

435. Choi, S. W., Hytiroglu, P., Geller, S. A., Kim, S. M., Chung, K. W., Park, D.H., et al. (1993) The expression of p53 antigen in primary malignant epithelial tumors of the liver: An immunohistochemical study. *Liver* **13**:172–176.

436. Hsu, H.-C., Tseng, H.-J., Lai, P.-L., Lee, P.-H., and Peng, S.-Y. (1993) Expression of *p53* gene in 184 unifocal hepatocellular carcinomas: association with tumor growth and invasiveness. *Cancer Res.* **53**:4691–4694.

437. Kar, S., Jaffe, R., and Carr, B. I. (1993) Mutation at codon 249 of *p53* gene in a human hepatoblastoma. *Hepatology* **18**:566–569.

438. Shieh, Y. S. C., Nguyen, C., Vocal, M. V., and Chu, H.-W. (1993) Tumor-suppressor *p53* gene in hepatitis C and B virus-associated hepatocellular carcinoma. *Int. J. Cancer* **54**:558–562.

439. Kennedy, S. M., MacGeogh, C., Jaffe, R., and Spurr, N. K. (1994) Overexpression of the oncoprotein p53 in primary hepatic tumors of childhood does not correlate with gene mutations. *Human Pathol.* **25**:438–442.

440. Bourdon, J. C., D'Errico, A., Paterlini, P., Grigioni, W., May, E., and Debuire, B. (1995) p53 protein accumulation in European hepatocellular carcinoma is not always dependent on *p53* gene mutation. *Gastroenterology* **108**:1176–1182.

441. Hayashi, H., Sugio, K., Matsumata, T., Adachi, E., Takenaka, K., and Sugimachi, K. (1995) The clinical significance of *p53* gene mutation in hepatocellular carcinomas from Japan. *Hepatology* **22**:1702–1707.

442. Kubicka, S., Trautwein, C., Schrem, H., Tillmann, H., and Manns, M. (1995) Low incidence of p53 mutations in European hepatocellular carcinomas with heterogeneous mutation as a rare event. *J. Hepatol.* **23**:412–419.

443. Nakopoulou, L., Janinis, J., Giannopoulou, I., Lazaris, A. C., Koureas, A., and Zacharoulis, D. (1995) Immunohistochemical expression of p53 protein and proliferating cell nuclear antigen in hepatocellular carcinoma. *Pathol. Res. Pract.* **191**:1208–1213.

444. DeBenedetti, V. M. G., Welsh, J. A., Yu, M. C., and Bennett, W. P. (1996) p53 mutations in hepatocellular carcinoma related to oral contraceptive use. *Carcinogenesis* **17**:145–149.

445. Soini, Y., Chia, S. C., Bennett, W. P., Groopman, J. D., Wang, J. S., DeBenedetti, V. M., et al. (1996) An aflatoxin-associated mutational hotspot at codon 249 in the p53 tumor suppressor gene occurs in hepatocellular carcinomas from Mexico. *Carcinogenesis* **17**:1007–1012.

446. Lunn, R. M., Zhang, Y.-J., Wang, L.-Y., Chen, C.-J., Lee, P.-H., Lee, C.-S., et al. (1997) *p53* mutations, chronic hepatitis B virus infection and aflatoxin exposure in hepatocellular carcinoma in Taiwan. *Cancer Res.* **57**:3471–3477.

447. Nakashima, Y., Hsia, C. C., Yuwen, H., Minemura, M., Nakshima, O., Kojiro, M., et al. (1998) p53 overexpression in small hepatocellular carcinomas containing two different histologic grades. *Int. J. Oncology* **12**:455–459.

448. Feitelson, M. A., Zhu, M., Duan, L.-X., and London, W. T. (1993) Hepatitis B x antigen and p53 are associated *in vitro* and in liver tissues from patients with primary hepatocellular carcinoma. *Oncogene* **8**:1109–1117.

449. Hosono, S., Chou, M.-J., Lee, C.-S., and Shih, C. (1993) Infrequent mutation of p53 gene in hepatitis B virus positive primary hepatocellular carcinomas. *Oncogene* **8**:491–496.

450. Qin, G., Su, J., Ning, Y., Duan, X., Luo, D., and Lotlikar, P. D. (1997) p53 protein expression in patients with hepatocellular carcinoma from the high incidence area of Guangxi, Southern China. *Cancer Lett.* **121**:203–210.

451. Bressac, B., Galvin, K. M., Liang, T. J., Isselbacher, K. J., Wands, J. R., and Ozturk, M. (1990) Abnormal structure and expression of *p53* gene in human hepatocellular carcinoma. *Proc. Natl. Acad. Sci. USA* **87**:1973–1977.

452. Ding, S.-F., Habib, N. A., Dooley, J., Wood, C., Bowles, L., Delhanty, J. D. (1991) Loss of constitutional heterozygosity on chromosome 5q in hepatocellular carcinoma without cirrhosis. *Br. J. Cancer* **64**:1083–1087.

453. Fujimori, M., Tokino, T., Hino, O., Kitagawa, T., Imamura, T., Okamoto, E., et al. (1991) Allelotype study of primary hepatocellular carcinoma. *Cancer Res.* **51**:89–93.

454. Hsu, I. C., Metcalf, R. A., Sun, T., Welsh, J. A., Wang, N. J., and Harris, C. C. (1991) Mutational hotspot in the *p53* gene in human hepatocellular carcinoma. *Nature* **350**:427–428.

455. Slagle, B. L., Zhou, Y.-Z., and Butel, J. S. (1991) Hepatitis B virus integration event in human chromosome 17p near the p53 gene identifies the region of the chromosome commonly deleted in virus-positive hepatocellular carcinomas. *Cancer Res.* **51**:49–54.

456. Scorsone, K. A., Zhou, Y.-Z., Butel, J. S., and Slagel, B. L. (1992) p53 mutations cluster at codon 249 in hepatitis B virus-positive hepatocellular carcinomas from China. *Cancer Res.* **52**:1635–1638.

457. Nishida, N., Fukuda, Y., Kokuryu, H., Toguchida, J., Yandell, D. W., Ikenaga, M., et al. (1993) Role and mutational heterogeneity of

the *p53* gene in hepatocellular carcinoma. *Cancer Res.* **53**:368–372.

458. Nose, H., Imazeki, F., Ohto, M., and Omata, M. (1993) *p53* gene mutations and 17p allelic deletions in hepatocellular carcinoma from Japan. *Cancer* **72**:355–360.

459. Takahashi, K., Kudo, J., Ishibashi, H., Hirata, Y., and Niho, Y. (1993) Frequent loss of heterozygosity on chromosome 22 in hepatocellular carcinoma. *Hepatology* **17**:794–799.

460. Tanaka, S., Toh, Y., Adachi, E., Matsumata, T., Mori, R., and Sugimachi, K. (1993) Tumor progression in hepatocellular carcinoma may be mediated by *p53* mutation. *Cancer Res.* **53**:2884–2887.

461. Hsu, H.-C., Peng, S.-Y., Lai, P.-L., Sheu, J.-C., Chen, D.-S., Lin, L.-I., et al. (1994) Allelotype and loss of heterozygosity of p53 in primary and recurrent hepatocellular carcinomas. A study of 150 patients. *Cancer* **73**:42-47.

462. Oda, T., Tsuda, H., Sakamoto, M., and Hirohashi, S. (1994) Different mutations of the p53 gene in nodule-in-nodule hepatocellular carcinoma as evidence for multistage progression. *Cancer Lett.* **83**:197–200.

463. Teramoto, T., Satonaka, K., Kitazawa, S., Fujimori, T., Hayashi, K., and Maeda, S. (1994) *p53* gene abnormalities are closely related to hepatoviral infections and occur in a late stage of hepatocarcinogenesis. *Cancer Res.* **54**:231–235.

464. DeBenedetti, V. M. G., Welsh, J. A., Trivers, G. E., Harpster, A., Parkinson, A. J., Lanier, A. P., et al. (1995) *p53* is not mutated in hepatocellular carcinomas from Alaska natives. *Cancer Epidemiol. Biomarkers Prev.* **4**:79–82.

465. Kuroki, T., Fujiwara, Y., Tsuchiya, E., Nakamori, S., Imaoka, S., Kanematsu, T., et al. (1995) Accumulation of genetic changes during development and progression of hepatocellular carcinoma: loss of heterozygosity of chromosome arm 1p occurs at an early stage of hepatocarcinogenesis. *Genes Chromosomes Cancer* **13**:163–167.

466. Kishimoto, Y., Shiota, G., Kamisaki, Y., Wada, K., Nakamoto, K., Yamawaki, M., et al. (1997) Loss of the tumor suppressor p53 gene at the liver cirrhosis stage in Japanese patients with hepatocellular carcinoma. *Oncology* **54**:304-310.

467. Tamura, S., Nakamori, S., Kuroki, T., Sasaki, Y., Furukawa, H., Ishikawa, O., et al. (1997) Association of cumulative allelic losses with tumor aggressiveness in hepatocellular carcinoma. *J. Hepatol.* **27**:669–676.

468. MacDonald, G. A., Greenson, J. K., Saito, K., Cherian, S. P., Appelman, H. D., and Boland, C. R. (1998) Microsatellite instability and loss of heterozygosity at DNA mismatch repair gene loci occurs during hepatic carcinogenesis. *Hepatology* **28**:90–97.

469. Hammond, C., Jeffers, L., Carr, B. I., and Simon, D. (1999) Multiple genetic alterations, 4q28, a new suppressor region, and potential gender differences in hepatocellular carcinoma. *Hepatology* **29**:1479–1485.

470. Rashid, A., Wang, J.-S., Qian, G.-S., Lu, B.-X., Hamilton, S. R., and Groopman, J.R. (1999) Genetic alterations in hepatocellular carcinomas: association between loss of chromosome 4q and *p53* gene mutations. *Br. J. Cancer* **80**:59–66.

471. Tsopanomichalou, M., Kouroumanlis, E., Ergazaki, M., and Spandidos, D. A. (1999) Loss of heterozygosity and microsatellite instability in human non-neoplastic hepatic lesions. *Liver* **19**:305–311.

472. Aguilar, F., Harris, C. C., Sun, T., Hollstein, M., and Cerutti, P. (1994) Geographic variation of p53 mutational profile in nonmalignant human liver. *Science* **264**:1317–1319.

473. Iwamoto, K. S., Mizuno, T., Kurata, A., Masuzawa, M., Mori, T., and Seyama, T. (1998) Multiple, unique, and common p53 mutations in a thoratrast recipient with four primary cancers. *Human Pathol.* **29**:412–416.

474. Iwamoto, K. S., Mizuno, T., Tokuoka, S., Mabuchi, K., and Seyama, T. (1998) Frequency of p53 mutations in hepatocellular carcinomas from atom bomb survivors. *J. Natl. Cancer Inst.* **90**:1167–1168.

475. Bressac, B., Kew, M., Wands, J., and Ozturk, M. (1991) Selective G to T mutations of p53 gene in hepatocellular carcinoma from southern Africa. *Nature* **350**:429–431.

476. Buetow, K. H., Sheffield, V. C., Zhu, M., Zhou, T., Shen, F.-M., Hino, O., et al. (1992) Low frequency of p53 mutations observed in a diverse collection of primary hepatocellular carcinomas. *Proc. Natl. Acad. Sci. USA* **89**:9622–9626.

477. Oda, T., Tsuda, H., Scarpa, A., Sakamoto, M., and Hirohashi, S. (1992) Mutation pattern of the *p53* gene as a diagnostic marker for multiple hepatocellular carcinoma. *Cancer Res.* **52**:3674–3678.

478. Oda, T., Tsuda, H., Scarpa, A., Sakamoto, M., and Hirohashi, S. (1992) *p53* gene mutation spectrum in hepatocellular carcinoma. *Cancer Res.* **52**:6358–6364.

479. Sheu, J.-C., Huang, G.-T., Lee, P.-H., Huang, J.-C., Chou, H.-C., Lai, M.-Y., et al. (1992) Mutation of *p53* gene in hepatocellular carcinoma in Taiwan. *Cancer Res.* **52**:6098–6100.

480. Debuire, B., Paterlini, P., Pontisso, P., Basso, G., and May, E. (1993) Analysis of the *p53* gene in European hepatocellular carcinomas and hepatoblastomas. *Oncogene* **8**:2303–2306.

481. Hollstein, M. C., Wild, C. P., Bleicher, F., Chutimataewin, S., Harris, C. C., Srivatanakul, P., et al. (1993) p53 mutations and aflatoxin B$_1$ exposure in hepatocellular carcinoma patients from Thailand. *Int. J. Cancer* **53**:51–55. 264.

482. Konishi, M., Kikuchi-Yanoshita, R., Tanaka, K., Sato, C., Tsuruta, K., Maeda, Y., et al. (1993) Genetic changes and histopathological grades in human hepatocellular carcinomas. *Jpn. J. Cancer Res.* **84**:893–899.

483. Lai, M.-Y., Chang, H.-C., Li, H.-P., Ku, C.-K., Chen, P.-J., Sheu, J.-C., et al. (1993) Splicing mutations of the *p53* gene in human hepatocellular carcinoma. *Cancer Res.* **53**:1653–1656.

484. Li, D., Cao, Y., He, L., Wang, N. J., and Gu, J.-R. (1993) Aberrations in the p53 gene in human hepatocellular carcinoma from China. *Carcinogenesis* **14**:169–173.

485. Diamantis, I. D., McGandy, C., Chen, T.-C., Liaw, Y.-F., Gudat, F., and Bianchi, L. (1994) A new mutational hotspot in the p53 gene in human hepatocellular carcinoma. *J. Hepatology* **20**:553–556.

486. Hsu, H.-C., Peng, S.-Y., Lai, P.-L., Chu, J.-S., and Lee, P.-H. (1994) Mutations of p53 gene in hepatocellular carcinoma (HCC) correlate with tumor progression and patient prognosis: a study of 138 patients with unifocal HCC. *Int. J. Oncol.* **4**:1341–1347.

487. Unsal, H., Yakicier, C., Marcais, C., Kew, M., Volkmann, M., Zentgraf, H., et al. (1994) Genetic heterogeniety of hepatocellular carcinoma. *Proc. Natl. Acad. Sci. USA* **91**:822–826.

488. Vesey, D. A., Hayward, N. K., and Cooksley, W. G. E. (1994) p53 gene in hepatocellular carcinomas from Australia. *Cancer Detect. Prevent.* **18**:123–130.

489. Andersson, M., Jönsson, M., Nielsen, L. L., Vyberg, M., Visfeldt, J., Storm, H. H., et al. (1995) Mutations in the tumor suppressor gene *p53* in human liver cancer induced by a-particles. *Cancer Epidemiol. Biomarkers Prev.* **4**:765–770.

490. Shi, C. Y., Phang, T. W., Lin, Y., Wee, A., Li, B., Lee, H. P., et al. (1995) Codon 249 mutation of the p53 gene is a rare event in hepatocellular carcinomas from ethnic Chinese in Singapore. *Br. J. Cancer* **72**:146–149.

491. He, B., Tang, Z. Y., Liu, K. D., and Zhou, G. (1996) Analysis of the cellular origin of hepatocellular carcinoma by p53 genotype. *J. Cancer Res. Clin. Oncol.* **122**:763–766.

492. Kazachkov, T., Khaoustov, V., Yoffe, B., Solomon, H., Klintmalm, G. B. G., and Tabor, E. (1996) p53 abnormalities in hepatocellular carcinoma from United States patients: Analysis of all 11 exons. *Carcinogenesis* **17**:2207–2212.

493. Ryder, S. D., Rizzi, P. M., Volkmann, M., Metivier, E., Pereira, L. M. M. B., Galle, P. R., et al. (1996) Use of specific ELISA for detection of antibodies directed against p53 protein in patients with hepatocellular carcinoma. *J. Clin. Pathol.* **49**:295–299.

494. Honda, K., Sabisa, E., Tullo, A., Papeo, P. A., Saccone, C., Poole, S., et al. (1998) *p53* mutation is a poor prognostic indicator for survival of patients with hepatocellular carcinoma undergoing surgical tumor ablation. *Br. J. Cancer* **77**:776–782.

495. Pontisso, P., Belluco, C., Bertorelle, R., De Moliner, L., Chieco-Bianchi, L., Nitti, D., et al. (1998) Hepatitis C virus infection associated with hepatocellular carcinoma: lack of correlation with p53 abnormalities in Caucasian patients. *Cancer* **83**:1489–1494.

496. Qiu, S.-J., Ye, S.-L., Wu, Z.-Q., Tang, Z.-Y., and Liu, Y.-K. (1998) The expression of the *mdm2* gene may be related to the aberration of the *p53* gene in human hepatocellular carcinoma. *J. Cancer Res. Clin. Oncol.* **124**:253–258.

497. Boix-Ferrero, J., Pellin, A., Blesa, R., Adrados, M., and Llombart-Bosch, A. (1999) Absence of *p53* gene mutations in hepatocarcinomas from a Mediterranian area of Spain. A study of 129 archival tumor samples. *Virchows Arch.* **434**:497–501.

498. Shimizu, Y., Zhu, J.-J., Han, F., Ishikawa, T., and Oda, H. (1999) Different frequencies of *p53* codon-249 hot-spot mutations in hepatocellular carcinomas in Jiang-su province of China. *Int. J. Cancer* **82**:187–190.

499. Vautier, G., Bomford, A. B., Portmann, B. C., Metivier, E., Williams, R., and Ryder, S. D. (1999) *p53* mutations in British patients with hepatocellular carcinoma: clustering in genetic hemochromatosis. *Gastroenterology* **117**:154–160.

500. Yano, M., Asahara, T., Dohi, K., Mizuno, T., Iwamoto, K. S., and Seyama, T. (1999) Close correlation between p53 or hMSH2 gene mutation in the tumor and survival of hepatocellular carcinoma patients. *Int. J. Cancer* **14**:447–451.

501. Hayward, N. K., Walker, G. J., Graham, W., and Cooksley, E. (1991) Hepatocellular carcinoma mutation. *Nature* **352**:764.

502. Ozturk, M. (1991) p53 mutation in hepatocellular carcinoma after aflatoxin exposure. *Lancet* **338**:1356–1359.

503. Coursaget, P., Depril, N., Chabaud, M., Nandi, R., Mayelo, V., LeCann, P., et al. (1993) High prevalence of mutations at codon 249 of the p53 gene in hepatocellular carcinomas from Senegal. *Br. J. Cancer* **67**:1395–1397.

504. Hayashi, H., Sugio, K., Matsumata, T., Adachi, E., Urata, K., Tanaka, S., et al. (1993) The mutation of codon 249 in the *p53* gene is not specific in Japanese hepatocellular carcinoma. *Liver* **13**:279–281.

505. Terris, B., Marcio, A., Tiollais, P., and Dejean, A. (1993) The p53 gene in human hepatocellular carcinomas. *J. Hepatology* **17**:422.

506. Yang, M., Zhou, H., Kong, R. Y., Fong, W. F., Ren, L. Q., Liao, X. H., et al. (1997) Mutations at codon 249 of p53 gene in human hepatocellular carconoma from Tongan, China. *Mutat Res.* **381**:25–29.

507. Lasky, T. and Magder, L. (1997) Hepatocellular carcinoma *p53* G→T transversions at codon 249: the fingerprint of aflatoxin exposure? *Environ. Health Perspect.* **105**:392–397.

508. Montesano, R., Hainaut, P., and Wild, C. P. (1997) Hepatocellular carcinoma: from gene to public health. *J. Natl. Cancer Inst.* **89**:1844–1851.

509. Aguilar, F., Hussain, S. P., and Cerutti, P. (1993) Aflatoxin B1 induces the transversion of G→T in codon 249 of the p53 gene in human hepatocytes. *Proc. Natl. Acad. Sci. USA* **90**:8586–8590.

510. Denissenko, M. F., Koudriakova, T. B., Smith, L., O'Connor, T. R., Riggs, A. D., and Pfeifer, G. P. (1998) The *p53* codon 249 mutational hotspot in hepatocellular carcinoma is not related to selective formation or persistence of aflatoxin B1 adducts. *Oncogene* **17**:3007–3014.

511. Wang, X. W., Forrester, K., Yeh, H., Feitelson, M. A., Gu, J. R., and Harris, C. C. (1994) Hepatitis B virus X protein inhibits p53 sequence-specific DNA binding, transcriptional activity, and association with transcription factor ERCC3. *Proc. Natl. Acad. Sci. USA* **91**:2230–2234.

512. Henkler, F., Waseam, N., Golding, M. H., Alison, M. R., and Koshy, R. (1995) Mutant p53 but not hepatitis B virus X protein is present in hepatitis B virus-related human hepatocellular carcinoma. *Cancer Res.* **55**:6084–6091.

513. Puisieux, A., Ji, J., Guillot, C., Legros, Y., Soussi, Y., Isselbacher, K., et al. (1995) p53-mediated cellular response to DNA damage in cells with replicative hepatitis B virus. *Proc. Natl. Acad. Sci. USA* **92**:1342–1342.

514. Truant, R., Antunovic, J., Greenblatt, J., Prives, C., and Cromlish, J. A. (1995) Direct interaction of the hepatitis B virus HBx protein with p53 leads to inhibition by HBx of p53 response element-directed transactivation. *J. Virol.* **69**:1851–1859.

515. Greenblatt, M. S., Feitelson, M. A., Zhu, M., Bennett, W. P., Welsh, J. A., Jones, R., et al. (1997) Integrity of p53 in hepatitis B X anti-gen-positive and negative hepatocellular carcinoma. *Cancer Res.* **57**:426–432.

516. Volkmann, M., Müller, M., Hofmann, W. J., Meyer, M., Hagelstein, J., Räth, U., et al. (1993) The humoral immune response to p53 in patients with hepatocellular carcinoma is specific for malignancy and independent of the a-fetoprotein status. *Hepatology* **18**:559–565.

517. Angelopoulou, K., Diamantis, E. P., Sutherland, D. J. A., Kellen, J. A., and Bunting, P. S. (1994) Prevalence of serum antibodies against the p53 tumor suppressor gene protein in various cancers. *Int. J. Cancer* **58**:480–487.

518. Shiota, G., Kishimoto, Y., Suyama, A., Okubo, M., Katayama, S., Harada, K.-I., Ishida, M., et al. (1997) Prognostic significance of serum anti-p53 antibody in patients with hepatocellular carcinoma. *J. Hepatol.* **27**:661–668.

519. Saffroy, R., Lelong, J.-C., Azoulay, D., Salvucci, M., Reynes, M., Bismuth, H., et al. (1999) Clinical significance of circulating anti-p53 antibodies in European patients with hepatocellular carcinoma. *Br. J. Cancer* **79**:604–610.

520. Ruck, P., Xiao, J.-C., and Kaiserling, E. (1994) p53 protein expression in hepatoblastoma: an immunohistochemical investigation. *Pediatric Pathol.* **14**:79–85.

521. Oda, H., Nakatsuru, Y., Imai, Y., Sugimura, H., and Ishikawa, T. (1995) A mutational hot spot in the p53 gene is associated with hepatoblastomas. *Int. J. Cancer* **60**:786–790.

522. Ohnishi, H., Kawamura, M., Hanada, R., Kaneko, Y., Tsunoda, Y., Hongo, T., et al. (1996) Infrequent mutations of the *TP53* gene and no amplification of the *MDM2* gene in hepatoblastomas. *Genes Chromosomes Cancer* **15**:187–190.

523. Kusafuka, T., Fukuzawa, M., Oue, T., Komoto, Y., Yoneda, A., and Okada, A. (1997) Mutation analysis of p53 gene in childhood malignant solid tumors. *J. Pediatric Surg.* **32**:1175–1180.

524. Schlott, T., Reimer, S., Jahns, A., Ohlenbusch, A., Ruschenberg, I., Nagel, H., et al. (1997) Point mutations and nucleotide insertions in the MDM2 zinc finger structure of human tumors. *J. Pathol.* **182**:54–61.

525. Mihara, M., Nimura, Y., Ichimiya, S., Sakiyama, S., Kajikawa, S., Adachi, W., et al. (1999) Absence of mutation of the p73 gene localized at chromosome 1p36.3 in hepatocellular carcinoma. *Br. J. Cancer* **79**:164–167.

526. Tannapfel, A., Wasner, M., Krause, K., Geissler, F., Katalinic, A., Hauss, J., et al. (1999) Expression of p73 and its relation to histopathology and prognosis of hepatocellular carcinoma. *J. Natl. Cancer Inst.* **99**:1154–1158.

527. Ding, S. F., Delhanty, J. D., Dooley, J. S., Bowles, L., Wood, C. B., and Habib, N. A. (1993) The putative tumor suppressor gene on chromosome 5q for hepatocellular carcinoma is distinct from the MCC and APC genes. *Cancer Detect. Prev.* **17**:405–409.

528. Kurahashi, H., Takami, K., Oue, T., Kusafuka, T., Okada, A., Tawa, A., et al. (1995) Biallelic inactivation of the *APC* gene in hepatoblastoma. *Cancer Res.* **55**:5007-5011.

529. Chen, T.-C., Hsieh, L.-L., Ng, K.-F., Jeng, L.-B., and Chen, M.-F. (1998) Absence of APC gene mutation in the mutation cluster region in hepatocellular carcinoma. *Cancer Lett.* **134**:23–28.

530. Huang, H., Fujii, H., Sankila, A., Mahler-Araujo, B. M., Matsuda, M., Calhomas, G., et al. (1999) β-catenin mutations are frequent in human hepatocellular carcinomas associated with hepatitis C virus infection. *Am. J. Pathol.* **155**:1795–1801.

531. Legoix, P., Bluteau, O., Bayer, J., Perret, C., Balabaud, C., Belghiti, J., et al. (1999) Beta-catenin mutations in hepatocellular carcinoma correlate with a low rate of loss of heterozygosity. *Oncogene* **18**:4044–4046.

532. Garber, J. E., Li, F. P., Kingston, J. E., Krush, A. J., Strong, J. C., Finegold, M. J., et al. (1988) Hepatoblastoma and familial adenomatous polyposis. *J. Natl. Cancer Inst.* **80**:1626–1628.

533. Giardiello, F. M., Petersen, G. M., Brensinger, J. D., Luce, M. C., Cayouette, M. C., Bacon, J., et al. (1996) Hepatoblastoma and APC gene mutation in familial adenomatous polyposis. *Gut* **39**:867–869.

534. Hughes, L. J. and Michels, V. V. (1992) Risk of hepatoblastoma in familial adenomatous polyposis. *Am. J. Med. Genet.* **43**:1023–1025.

535. Iwama, T. and Mishima, Y. (1994) Mortality in young first-degree relatives of patients with familial adenomatous polyposis. *Cancer* **73**:2065–2068.

536. Bala, S., Wúnsch, P. H., and Ballhausen, W. G. (1997) Childhood hepatocellular adenoma in familial adenomatous polyposis: mutations in adenomatous polyposis coli gene and *p53*. *Gastroenterology* **112**:919–922.

537. Oda, H., Imai, Y., Nakatsuru, Y., Hata, J., and Ishikawa, T. (1996) Somatic mutations of the *APC* gene in sporadic hepatoblastomas. *Cancer Res.* **56**:3320–3323.

538. Bläker, H., Hoffman, W. J., Rieker, R. J., Penzel, R., Graf, M., and Oho, H. F. (1999) β-catenin accumulation and mutation of the CTNNB1 gene in hepatoblastoma. *Genes Chromosomes Cancer* **25**:399–402.

539. Koch, A., Denkhaus, D., Albrecht, S., Leuschner, I., von Schweinitz, D., and Pietsch, T. (1999) Childhood hepatoblastomas frequently carry a mutated degradation targeting box of the β-catenin gene. *Cancer Res.* **59**:269–273.

540. Van Nhieu, J. T., Renard, C. A., Wei, Y., Cherqui, D., Zafrani, E. S., and Buendia, M.-A. (1999) Nuclear accumulation of mutated β-catenin in hepatocellular carcinoma is associated with increased cell proliferation. *Am. J. Pathol.* **155**:703–710.

541. De La Coste, A., Romagnolo, B., Billuart, P., Renard, C.-A., Buendia, M.-A., Sourbane, O., et al. (1998) Somatic mutations of the β-catenin gene are frequent in mouse and human hepatocellular carcinomas. *Proc. Natl. Acad. Sci. USA* **95**:8847–8851.

542. Miyoshi, Y., Iwao, K., Nagasawa, Y., Aihara, T., Sasaki, Y., Imaoka, S., et al. (1998) Activation of the β-catenin gene in primary hepatocellular carcinomas by somatic alterations involving exon 3. *Cancer Res.* **58**:2524–2527.

543. Wei, Y., Fabre, M., Branchereau, S., Gauthier, F., Perilongo, G., and Buendia, M.-A. (2000) Activation of β-catenin in epithelial and mesenchymal hepatoblastomas. *Oncogene* **19**:498–504.

544. Huang, G.-T., Lee, H.-S., Chen, C.-H., Sheu, J.-C., Chiou, L.-L., and Chen, J.-S. (1999) Correlation of E-cadherin expression and recurrence of hepatocellular carcinoma. *Hepato-Gastroenterology* **46**:1923–1927.

545. Yoshiura, K., Kanai, Y., Ochiai, A., Shimoyama, Y., Sugimura, T., and Hirohashi, S. (1995) Silencing of the E-cadherin invasion-suppressor gene by CpG methylation in human carcinomas. *Proc. Natl. Acad. Sci. USA* **92**:7416–7419.

546. Zhang, W. D., Hirohashi, S., Tsuda, H., Shimosato, Y., Yokota, J., Terada, M., et al. (1990) Frequent loss of heterozygosity on chromosomes 16 and 4 in human hepatocellular carcinoma. *Jpn. J. Cancer Res.* **81**:108–111.

547. Katagiri, T., Nakamura, Y., and Miki, Y. (1996) Mutations in the *BRCA2* gene in hepatocellular carcinoma. *Cancer Res.* **56**:4575–4577.

548. Panagopoulos, I., Thelin, S., Mertens, F., Mitelman, F., and Aman, P. (1997) Variable *FHIT* transcripts in non-neoplastic tissues. *Genes Chromosomes Cancer* **19**:215–219.

549. Chen, Y.-J., Chen, P.-H., and Chang, J.-G. (1998) Aberrant *FHIT* transcripts in hepatocellular carcinomas. *Br. J. Cancer* **77**:417–420.

550. Schlott, T., Ahrens, K., Ruschenberg, I., Reimer, S., Hartmann, H., and Droese, M. (1999) Different gene expression of MDM2, GAGE-1,-2 and FHIT in hepatocellular carcinoma and focal nodular hyperplasia. *Br. J. Cancer* **80**:73–78.

551. Gramantieri, L., Chieco, P., DiTomaso, M., Masi, L., Piscaglia, F., Brillanti, S., et al. (1999) Aberrant fragile histidine triad gene transcripts in primary hepatocellular carcinoma and liver cirrhosis. *Clin. Cancer Res.* **5**:3468–3475.

552. Yuan, B.-Z., Keck-Waggoner, C., Zimonjic, D. B., Thorgeirsson, S. S., and Popescu, N. C. (2000) Alterations of FHIT gene in human hepatocellular carcinoma. *Cancer Res.* **60**(4):1049–1053. In press.

553. Guo, X.-Z., Friess, H., DiMola, F. F., Heinicke, J.-M., Abou-Shady, M., Graber, H. U., et al. (1998) KAI1, a new metastasis suppressor gene, is reduced in metastatic hepatocellular carcinoma. *Hepatology* **28**:1481–1488.

554. Nakayama, T., Ohtsuru, A., Nakao, K., Shima, M., Nakata, K., Watanabe, K., et al. (1992) Expression in human hepatocellular carcinoma of nucleoside diphosphate kinase, a homologue of the nm23 gene product. *J. Natl. Cancer Inst.* **84**:1349–1354.

555. Fujimoto, Y., Ohtake, T., Nishimori, H., Ikuta, K., Ohhira, M., Ono, M., et al. (1998) Reduced expression and rare genomic alteration of nm23-H1 in human hepatocellular carcinoma and hepatoma cell lines. *J. Gastroenterol.* **33**:368–375.

556. Boix, L., Bruix, J., Campo, E., Sole, M., Castells, A., Fuster, J., et al. (1994) *nm23-H1* expression and disease recurrence after surgical resection of small hepatocellular carcinoma. *Gastroenterology* **107**:486–491.

557. Yamaguchi, A., Urano, T., Goi, T., Takeuchi, K., Niimoto, S., Nakagawara, G., et al. (1994) Expression of human nm23H1-1 and nm23H-2 proteins in hepatocellular carcinoma. *Cancer* **73**:2280–2284.

558. Iizuka, N., Oka, M., Noma, T., Nakazawa, A., Hirose, K., and Suzuki, T. (1995) *NM23-H1* and *NM23-H2* messenger RNA abundance in human hepatocellular carcinoma. *Cancer Res.* **55**:652–657.

559. Shimada, M., Taguchi, K., Hasegawa, H., Gion, T., Shirabe, K., Tsuneyoshi, M., et al. (1998) Nm23-H1 expression in intrahepatic or extrahepatic metastases of hepatocellular carcinoma. *Liver* **18**:337–342.

560. Kawamura, N., Nagai, H., Bando, K., Koyama, M., Matsamoto, S., Tajiri, T., et al. (1999) *PTEN/MMAC1* mutations in hepatocellular carcinomas: somatic inactivation of both alleles in tumors. *Jpn. J. Cancer Res.* **90**:413–418.

561. Yao, Y. J., Ping, X. L., Zhang, H., Chen, F. F., Lee, P. K., Ahsan, H., et al. (1999) *PTEN/MMAC1* mutations in hepatocellular carcinomas. *Oncogene* **18**:3181–3185.

562. Isfort, R., Cody, D., Doersen, C.-J., Richards, W., Yodar, B., Wilkinson, J., et al. (1997) The tricopeptide repeat containing Tg737 gene is a liver neoplasia tumor suppressor gene. *Oncogene* **15**:1797–1803.

563. Bonura, C., Paterlini-Bréchot, P., and Bréchot, C. (1999) Structure and expression of Tg737, a putative tumor suppressor gene, in human hepatocellular carcinomas. *Hepatology* **30**:677–681.

564. Ljubimova, J. Y., Wilson, S. E., Petrovic, L. M., Ehrenman, K., Ljubimov, A. V., Demetriou, A. A., et al. (1998) Novel human malignancy-associated gene (*MAG*) expressed in various tumors and in some tumor preexisting conditions. *Cancer Res.* **58**:4475–4479.

565. Yamashita, N., Ishibashi, H., Hayashida, K., Kudo, J., Takenaka, K., Itoh, K., et al. (1996) High frequency of the *MAGE-1* gene expression in hepatocellular carcinoma. *Hepatology* **24**:1437–1440.

566. Liu, B.-B., Ye, S.-L., He, P., Liu, Y.-K., and Tang, Z.-Y. (1999) *MAGE-1* and *MAGE* gene expression may be associated with hepatocellular carcinoma. *J. Cancer Res. Clin. Oncol.* **125**:685–689.

567. Kariyama, K., Higashi, T., Kobayashi, Y., Nouso, K., Nakatsukasa, H., Yamano, T., et al. (1999) Expression of MAGE-1 and -3 genes and gene products in human hepatocellular carcinoma. *Br. J. Cancer* **81**:1080–1087.

568. Tahara, T., Mori, M., Sadanaga, N., Sakamoto, Y., Kitano, S., and Makuuchi, M. (1999) Expression of the MAGE gene family in hepatocellular carcinoma. *Cancer* **85**:1234–1240.

569. Tsuzurahara, S., Sata, M., Iwamoto, O., Shichijo, S., Kojiro, M., Tanikawa, K., et al. (1997) Detection of MAGE-4 protein in the sera of patients with hepatitis-C virus-associated hepatocellular carcinoma and liver cirrhosis. *Jpn. J. Cancer Res.* **88**:915–918.

570. Lasserre, C., Christa, L., Simon, M.-T., Vernier, P., and Bréchot, C. (1992) A novel gene (HIP) activated in primary human liver cancer. *Cancer Res.* **52**:5089–5095.

571. Christa, L., Carnot, F., Simon, M.-T., Levavasseur, F., Stinnakre, M.-G., Lasserre, C., et al. (1996) HIP/PAD is an adhesive protein expressed in hepatocarcinoma, normal paneth, and pancreatic cells. *Am. J. Physiol.* **271**:G993–G1002.

572. Lasserre, C., Simon, M.-T., Ishikawa, H., Diriong, S., Nguyen, V. C., Christa, L., et al. (1994) Structural organization and chromo-

somal localization of a human gene (*HIP*/PAP) encoding a C-type lectin overexpressed in primary liver cancer. *Eur. J. Biochem.* **224**:29–38.

573. Lasserre, C., Colnot, C., Bréchot, C., and Poirier, F. (1999) HIP/PAP gene, encoding a c-type lectin overexpressed in primary liver cancer, is expressed in nervous system as well as in intestine and pancreas of the postimplantation mouse embryo. *Am. J. Pathol.* **154**:1601–1610.

574. Ochiya, T., Fujiyama, A., Fukushige, S., Hatada, I., and Matsubara, K. (1986) Molecular cloning of an oncogene from a human hepatocellular carcinoma. *Proc. Natl. Acad. Sci. USA* **83**:4993–4997.

575. Leithauser, F., Ohein, J., Mechtersheimer, G., Koretz, K., Brüderlein, S., Henne, C., et al. (1993) Constitutive and induced expression of APO-1, a member of the NGFITNF receptor super family, in normal and neoplastic cells. *Lab. Invest.* **69**:415–429.

576. Galle, P. R., Hofmann, W. J., Walczak, H., Schaller, H., Otto, G., Stremmel, W., et al. (1995) Involvement of the CD95 (APO-1/Fas) receptor and ligand in liver damage. *J. Exp. Med.* **182**:1223–1230.

577. Xerri, L., Devilard, E., Hassoun, J., Mawas, C., and Birg, F. (1997) Fas ligand is not only expressed in immune privileged organs but also coexpressed with Fas in various epithelial tissues. *J. Clin. Pathol. Mol. Pathol.* **50**:87–91.

578. Afford, S. C., Randhwa, S., Eliopoulos, A. G., Hubscher, S. G., Young, L. S., and Adams, D. H. (1999) CD40 activation induces apoptosis in cultured human hepatocytes via induction of cell surface Fas ligand expression and amplifies Fas-mediated hepatocyte death during allograft rejection. *J. Exp. Med.* **189**:441–446.

579. Hiramatsu, N., Hayashi, N., Katayama, K., Mochizuki, K., Kawanishi, Y., Kasahara, A., et al. (1994) Immunohistochemical detection of Fas antigen in liver tissue of patients with chronic hepatitis C. *Hepatology* **19**:1354–1359.

580. Mochizuki, K., Hayashi, N., Hiramatsu, N., Katayama, K., Kawanishi, Y., Kasahara, A., et al. (1996) Fas antigen expression in liver tissues of patients with chronic hepatitis B. *J Hepatology* **24**:1–7.

581. Strand, S., Hofmann, W. J., Hug, H., Müller, M., Otto, G., Strand, D., et al. (1996) Lymphocyte apoptosis induced by CD95 (APO-1/Fas) ligand-expressing tumor cells: a mechanism of immune invasion? *Nature Med.* **2**:1361–1366.

582. Nagao, M., Nakajima, Y., Hisanaga, M., Kayagaki, N., Kanehiro, H., Aomatsu, Y., et al. (1999) The alteration of Fas receptor and ligand system in hepatocellular carcinomas: How do hepatoma cells escape from the host immune surveillance *in vivo*? *Hepatology* **30**:413–421.

583. Shin, E.-C., Shin, J.-S., Park, J. H., Kim, J.-J., Kim, H., and Kim, S. J. (1998) Expression of Fas-related genes in human hepatocellular carcinomas. *Cancer Lett.* **134**:155–162.

584. Jodo, S., Kobayashi, S., Nakajima, Y., Matsunaga, T., Nakayama, N., Ogura, N., et al. (1998) Elevated serum levels of soluble Fas/APO-1 (CD95) in patients with hepatocellular carcinoma. *Clin. Exp. Immunol.* **112**:166–171.

585. Sugimoto, K., Shiraki, K., Ito, T., Fujikawa, K., Takase, K., Tameda, Y., et al. (1999) Expression of functional CD40 in human hepatocellular carcinoma. *Hepatology* **30**:920–926.

586. Lee, S. H., Shin, M. S., Lee, J. Y., Park, W. S., Kim, S. Y., Jang, J. J., et al. (1999) *In vivo* expression of soluble Fas and FAP-1: possible mechanisms of Fas resistance in human hepatoblastomas. *J. Pathol.* **188**:207–212.

587. Charlotte, F., L'Hermine, A., Martin, N., Gelyn, Y., Nollet, M., Gaulard, P., et al. (1994) Immunohistochemical detection of *bcl-2* normal and pathological human liver. *Am. J. Pathol.* **144**:460–465.

588. Zhao, M., Zhang, N.-X., Economou, M., Blaha, I., Laissue, J. A., and Zimmermann, A. (1994) Immunohistochemical detection of bcl-2 protein in liver lesions; bcl-2 protein is expressed in hepatocellular carcinomas but not in liver cell dysplasia. *Histopathology* **25**:237–245.

589. Frommel, T. O., Yong, S., and Zarling, E. J. (1999) Immunohistochemical evaluation of Bcl-2 gene family expression in liver of hepatitis C and cirrhotic patients: a novel mechanism to explain the high incidence of hepatocarcinoma in cirrhotics. *Am. J. Gastroenterol.* **94**:172–178.

590. Nakopoulou, L., Stefanaki, K., Vourlakou, C., Manolaki, H., Gakiopoulou, H., and Michalopoulos, G. (1999) Bcl-2 protein expression in acute and chronic hepatitis cirrhosis and hepatocellular carcinoma. *Pathol. Res. Pract.* **195**:19–24.

591. Deng, D. X., Chakrabati, S., Waalkes, M. P., and Cherian, M. G. (1998) Metallothionein and apoptosis in primary human hepatocellular carcinoma and metastatic adenocarcinoma. *Histopathology* **32**:340–347.

592. Ninomiya, T., Hayashi, Y., Saijon, K., Ohta, K., Yoon, S., Nakabayashi, H., et al. (1996) Expression ratio of hepatocyte nuclear factor-1 to variant hepatocyte nuclear factor-1 in differentiation of hepatocellular carcinoma and hepatoblastoma. *J. Hepatology* **25**:445–453.

593. Wang, W., Hayashi, Y., Ninomiya, T., Ohta, K., Nakabayashi, H., Tamaoki, T., et al. (1998) Expression of HNF-1a and HNF-1β in various histological differentiations of hepatocellular carcinoma. *J. Pathol.* **184**:272–278.

594. Kishimoto, T., Kokura, K., Ohkawa, N., Makino, Y., Yoshida, M., Hirohashi, S., et al. (1998) Enhanced expression of a new class of liver-enriched b-Zip transcription factors, hepatocarcinogenesis-related transcription factor, in hepatocellular carcinomas of rats and humans. *Cell Growth Differ.* **9**:337–344.

595. Nakayama, J., Tahara, H., Tahara, E., Saito, M., Ito, K., Nakamura, H., et al. (1998) Telomerase activation by hTRT in human normal fibroblasts and hepatocellular carcinomas. *Nature Genetics* **18**:65–68.

596. Wada, E., Hisatomi, H., Moritoyo, T., Kanamaru, T., and Hikiji, K. (1998) Genetic diagnostic test of hepatocellular carcinoma by telomerase catalytic subunit mRNA. *Oncology Rep.* **5**:1407–1412.

597. Tahara, H., Nakanishi, T., Kitamoto, M., Nakashio, R., Shay, J. W., Tahara, E., et al. (1995) Telomerase activity in human liver tissue: comparison between chronic liver disease and hepatocellular carcinomas. *Cancer Res.* **55**:2734–2736.

598. Ohta, K., Kanamaru, T., Yamamoto, M., and Saitoh, Y. (1996) Clinical significance of telomerase activity in hepatocellular carcinoma. *Kobe J. Med. Sci.* **42**:207–217.

599. Kojima, H., Yokosuka, O., Imazeki, F., Saisho, H., and Omata, M. (1997) Telomerase activity and telomere length in hepatocellular carcinoma and chronic liver disease. *Gastroenterology* **112**:493–500.

600. Miura, N., Horikawa, I., Nishimoto, A., Ohmura, H., Ito, H., Hirohashi, S., et al. (1997) Progressive telomere shortening and telomerase reactivation during hepatocellular carcinogenesis. *Cancer Genet. Cytogenet.* **93**:56–62.

601. Nakashio, R., Kitamoto, M., Tahara, H., Nakanishi, T., Ide, T., and Kajiyama, G. (1997) Significance of telomerase activity in the diagnosis of small differentiated hepatocellular carcinoma. *Int. J. Cancer* **74**:141–147.

602. Hisatomi, H., Nagao, K., Kanamura, T., Endo, H., Tomimatsu, M., and Hikiji, K. (1999) Levels of telomerase catalytic subunit mRNA as a predictor of potential malignancy. *Int. J. Oncol.* **14**:727–732.

603. Hytiroglou, P., Kotoula, V., Thung, S.N., Tsokos, M., Fiel, M. I., and Papadimitriou, C.S. (1998) Telomerase activity in precancerous hepatic nodules. *Cancer* **82**:1831–1838

604. Kojima, H., Yokosuka, O., Kato, N., Shiina, S., Imazeki, F., Saisho, H., et al. (1999) Quantitative evaluation of telomerase activity in small liver tumors: analysis of ultrasonography-guided liver biopsy specimens. *J. Hepatol.* **31**:514–520.

605. Ogami, M., Ikura, Y., Nishiguchi, S., Kuroki, T., Ueda, M., and Sakurai, M. (1999) Quantitative analysis and in situ localization of human telomerase RNA in chronic liver disease and hepatocellular carcinoma. *Lab. Invest.* **79**:15–26.

606. Suda, T., Isokawa, O., Aoyagi, Y., Nomoto, M., Tsukada, K., Shimizu, T., et al. (1998) Quantitation of telomerase activity in hepatocellular carcinoma: a possible aid for a prediction of recurrent disease in the remnant liver. *Hepatology* **27**:402–406.

607. Kitada, T., Seki, S., Kawakita, N., Kuroki, T., and Monna, T. (1995) Telomere shortening in chronic liver diseases. *Biochem. Biophys. Res. Commun.* **211**:33–39.

608. Ohashi, K., Tsutsumi, M., Kobitsu, K., Fukada, T., Tsujiuchi, T., Okajima, E., et al. (1996) Shortened telomere length in hepatocellular carcinomas and corresponding background liver tissues of patients infected with hepatitis virus. *Jpn. J. Cancer Res.* **87**:419–422.

609. Ohashi, K., Tsutsumi, M., Nakajima, Y., Kobitsu, K., Nakano, H., and Konishi, Y. (1996) Telomere changes in human hepatocellular carcinomas and hepatitis virus infected noncancerous livers. *Cancer* **77**:1747–1751.

610. Urabe, Y., Nouso, K., Higashi, T., Nakatsukasa, H., Hino, N., Ashida, K., et al. (1996) Telomere length in human liver diseases. *Liver* **16**:293–297.

611. Isokawa, O., Suda, T., Aoyagi, Y., Kawai, H., Yokota, T., Takahashi, T., et al. (1999) Reduction of telomeric repeats as a possible predictor for development of hepatocellular carcinoma: convenient evaluation by slot-blot analysis. *Hepatology* **30**:408–412.

612. Ramel, C. (1997) Mini- and Microsatellites. *Environ. Health Perspect.* **105**:781–789.

613. Loeb, L. A. (1998) Cancer cells exhibit a mutator phenotype. *Adv. Cancer Res.* **72**:25–56.

614. Han, H.-J., Yanagisawa, A., Kato, Y., Park, J.-G., and Nakamura, Y. (1993) Genetic instability in pancreatic cancer and poorly differentiated type of gastric cancer. *Cancer Res.* **53**:5087–5089.

615. Kazachkov, Y., Yoffe, B., Khaoustov, V. I., Solomon, H., Klintmalm, G. B., and Tabor, E. (1998) Microsatellite instability in human hepatocellular carcinoma: relationship to p53 abnormalities. *Liver* **18**:156–161.

616. Takagi, K., Esumi, M., Takano, S., and Iwai, S. (1998) Replication error frequencies in primary hepatocellular carcinoma: a comparison of solitary primary versus multiple primary cancers. *Liver* **18**:272–276.

617. Horii, A., Han, H.-J., Shimada, M., Yanigasawa, A., Kato, Y., Ohta, H., et al. (1994) Frequent replication errors at microsatellite loci in tumors of patients with multiple primary cancers. *Cancer Res.* **54**:3373–3375

618. Yakushiji, H., Sinsuke, M., Matsukura, S., Sato, S., Ogawa, A., Sasatomi, E., et al. (1999) DNA mismatch repair in curatively resected sextuple primary cancers in different organs: a molecular case report. *Cancer Lett.* **142**:17–22.

619. Boige, V., Laurent-Puig, L., Fouchet, P., Flejou, J. F., Monges, G., Bedossa, P., et al. (1997) Concerted nonsyntenic allelic losses in hyperploid hepatocellular carcinoma is determined by a high-resolution allelotype. *Cancer Res.* **57**:1986–1990.

620. Sheu, J.-C., Lin, Y.-W., Chou, H.-C., Huang, G.-T., Lee, H.-S., Lin, Y.-H., et al. (1999) Loss of heterozygosity and microsatellite instability in hepatocellular carcinoma in Taiwan. *Br. J. Cancer* **80**:468–476.

621. Kondo, Y., Kanai, Y., Sakamoto, M., Mizokami, M., Ueda, R., and Hirohashi, S. (1999) Microsatellite instability associated with hepatocarcinogenesis. *J. Hepatol.* **31**:529–536.

622. Salvucci, M., Lemoine, A., Azoulay, D., Sebagh, M., Bismuth, H., Reyns, M., et al. (1996) Frequent microsatellite instability in post hepatitis B viral cirrhosis. *Oncogene* **13**:2681–2685.

623. Kaplanski, C., Srivatanakul, P., and Wild, C. (1997) Frequent rearrangements at minisatellite loci D1S7 (1p33-35), D7S22 (7q36-ter) and D12S11 (12q24.3-ter) in hepatitis B virus-positive hepatocellular carcinomas from Thai patients. *Int. J. Cancer* **72**:248–254.

624. Okada, S., Ishii, H., Nose, H., Okusaka, T., Kyogoku, A., Yoshimori, M., et al. (1997) Evidence for increased somatic cell mutations in patients with hepatocellular carcinoma. *Carcinogenesis* **18**:445–449.

625. Wu, X., Gu, J., Patt, Y., Hassan, M., Spitz, M. R., Beasley, R. P., et al. (1998) Mutagen sensitivity as a susceptibility marker for human hepatocellular carcinoma. *Cancer Epidemiol. Biomarkers Prev.* **7**:567–570.

626. Simon, D., London, T., Hann, H.-W., and Knowles, B. B. (1991) Chromosome abnormalities in peripheral blood cells of hepatitis B virus chronic carriers. *Cancer Res.* **51**:6176–6179.

627. Gusella, J. F. (1986) DNA polymorphism and human disease. *Ann. Rev. Biochem.* **55**:831–854.

628. Nagai, H., Pineau, P., Tiollais, P., Buendia, M. A., and Dejean, A. (1997) Comprehensive allelotyping of human hepatocellular carcinoma. *Oncogene* **14**:2927–2933.

629. Piao, Z., Park, C., Park, J.-H., and Kim, H. (1998) Allelotype analysis of hepatocellular carcinoma. *Int. J. Cancer* **75**:29–33.

630. Wang, H. P. and Rogler, C. E. (1988) Deletion in human chromosome arms 11p and 13q in primary hepatocellular carcinomas. *Cytogenet. Cell Genet.* **48**:72–78.

631. Buetow, K. H., Murray, J. C., Israel, J. L., London, W. T., Smith, M., Kew, M., et al. (1989) Loss of heterozygosity suggests tumor suppressor gene responsible for primary hepatocellular carcinoma. *Proc. Natl. Acad. Sci. USA* **86**:8852–8856.

632. Simon, D., Knowles, B. B., and Weith, A. (1991) Abnormalities of chromosome 1 and loss of heterozygosity on 1p in primary hepatomas. *Oncogene* **6**:765–770.

633. Yeh, S.-H., Chen, P.-J., Chen, H.-L., Lai, M.-Y., Wang, C.-C., and Chen, D.-S. (1994) Frequent genetic alterations at the distal region of chromosome 1p in human hepatocellular carcinomas. *Cancer Res.* **54**:4188–4192.

634. Yeh, S.-H., Chen, P.-J., Lai, M.-Y., and Chen, D.-S. (1996) Allelic loss on chromosomes 4q and 16q in hepatocellular carcinoma: association with elevated a-fetoprotein production. *Gastroenterology* **110**:184–192.

635. Leon, M. and Kew, M. C. (1996) Loss of heterozygosity in chromosome 4q12-q13 in hepatocellular carcinoma in southern African blacks. *Anticancer Res.* **16**:349–351.

636. Chou, Y.-H., Chung, K.-C., Jeng, L.-B., Chen, T.-C., and Liaw, Y.-F. (1998) Frequent allelic loss on chromosomes 4q and 16q associated with human hepatocellular carcinoma in Taiwan. *Cancer Lett.* **123**:1–6.

637. Piao, Z., Park, C., Park, J.-H., and Kim, H. (1998) Deletion mapping of chromosome 4q in hepatocellular carcinoma. *Int. J. Cancer* **79**:356–360.

638. Bando, K., Nagai, H., Matsumoto, S., Koyama, M., Kawamura, N., Onda, M., et al. (1999) Identification of a 1-cM region of common deletion on 4q35 associated with progression of hepatocellular carcinoma. *Genes Chromosomes Cancer* **25**:284–289.

639. Emi, M., Fujiwara, Y., Nakajima, T., Tsuchiya, E., Tsuda, H., Hirohashi, S., et al. (1992) Frequent loss of heterozygosity for loci on chromosome 8p in hepatocellular carcinoma, colorectal cancer, and lung cancer. *Cancer Res.* **52**:5368–5372.

640. Emi, M., Fujiwara, Y., Ohata, H., Tsuda, H., Hirohashi, S., Koike, M., et al. (1993) Allelic loss at chromosome band 8p21.3-p22 is associated with progression of hepatocellular carcinoma. *Genes Chromosomes Cancer* **7**:152–157.

641. Fujiwara, Y., Ohata, H., Emi, M., Okui, K., Koyama, K., Tsuchiya, E., et al. (1994) A 3-Mb physical map of the chromosome region 8p21.3-p22, including a 600-kb region commonly deleted in human hepatocellular carcinoma, colorectal cancer, and non-small cell lung cancer. *Genes Chromosomes Cancer* **10**:7–14.

642. Becker, S. A., Zhou, Y.-Z., and Slagle, B. L. (1996) Frequent loss of chromosome 8p in hepatitis B virus-positive hepatocellular carcinomas from China. *Cancer Res.* **56**:5092–5097.

643. Kanai, Y., Ushijima, S., Tsuda, H., Sakamoto, M., Sugimura, T., and Hirohashi, S. (1996) Aberrant DNA methylation on chromosome 16 is an early event in hepatocarcinogenesis. *Jpn. J. Cancer Res.* **87**:1210–1217.

644. Kishimoto, Y., Shiota, G., Wada, K., Kitano, M., Nakamoto, K., Kamisaki, Y., et al. (1996) Frequent loss in chromosome 8p loci in liver cirrhosis accompanying hepatocellular carcinoma. *J. Cancer Res. Clin. Oncol.* **122**:585–589.

645. Piao, Z., Kim, N.-G., Kim, H., and Park, C. (1999) Deletion mapping of the short arm of chromosome 8 in hepatocellular carcinoma. *Cancer Lett.* **138**:227–232.

646. Pineau, P., Nagai, H., Prigent, S., Wei, Y., Gyapay, G., Weissenbach, J., et al. (1999) Identification of three distinct regions on the short arm of chromosome 8 in hepatocellular carcinoma. *Oncogene* **18**:3127–3134.

647. Tsuda, H., Zhang, W., Shimosato, Y., Yokota, J., Terada, M., Sugimura, T., Miyamura, T., and Hirohashi, S. (1990) Allele loss on chromosome 16 associated with progression of human hepatocellular carcinoma. *Proc. Natl. Acad. Sci. USA* **87**:6791–6794.

648. Koyama, M., Nagai, H., Bando, K., Ito, M., Moriyama, Y., and Emi, M. (1999) Localization of a target region of allelic loss to a 1-cM interval on chromosome 16p13.13 in hepatocellular carcinoma. *Jpn. J. Cancer Res.* **90**:951–956.

649. Piao, Z., Park, C., Kim, J. J., and Kim, H. (1999) Deletion mapping of chromosome 16q in hepatocellular carcinoma. *Br. J. Cancer* **80**:850–854.

650. Fujiwara, Y., Ohata, H., Kuroki, T., Koyama, K., Tsuchiya, E., Monden, M., et al. (1995) Isolation of a candidate tumor suppressor gene on chromosome 8p21.3-p22 that is homologous to an extracellular domain of the PDGF receptor beta gene. *Oncogene* **10**:891–895.

651. Chinen, K., Isomura, M., Izawa, K., Fujiwara, Y., Ohata, H., Iwamasa, T., et al. (1996) Isolation of 45 exon-like fragments from 8p22-p21.3, a region that is commonly deleted in hepatocellular, colorectal, and non-small cell lung cancers. *Cytogenet. Cell. Genet.* **75**:190–196.

652. Yuan, B.-Z., Miller, M. J., Keck, C. L., Zimonjic, D. B., Thorgeirsson, S. S., and Popescu, N. C. (1998) Cloning, characterization, and chromosomal localization of a gene frequently deleted in human liver cancer (*DLC-1*) homologous to rat *RhoGAP*. *Cancer Res.* **58**:2196–2199.

653. Koufos, A., Hansen, M. F., Copeland, N. G., Jenkins, N. A., Lampkin, B. C., and Cavanee, W. K. (1985) Loss of heterozygosity in three embryonal tumours suggests a common pathogenic mechanism. *Nature* **316**:330–334.

654. Byrne, J. A., Simms, L. A., Little, M. H., Algar, E. M., and Smith, P .J. (1993) Three non-overlapping regions of chromosome arm 11p allele loss identified in infantile tumors of adrenal and liver. *Genes Chromosomes Cancer* **8**:104–111.

655. Albrecht, S., von Schweinitz, D., Waha, A., Kraus, J. A., von Deimling, A., and Pietsch, T. (1994) Loss of maternal alleles on chromosome arm 11p in hepatoblastoma. *Cancer Res.* **54**:5041–5044.

656. Kraus, J. A., Albrecht, S., Wiestler, O. D., von Schweinitz, D., and Pietsch, T. (1996) Loss of heterozygosity on chromosome 1 in human hepatoblastoma. *Int. J. Cancer* **67**:467–471.

657. Little, M. H., Thomson, D. B., Hayward, N. K., and Smith, P. J. (1988) Loss of alleles on the short arm of chromosome 11 in a hepatoblastoma from a child with Beckwith-Wiedemann syndrome. *Human Genet.* **79**:186–189.

658. Kiechle-Schwarz, M., Scherer, G., and Kovacs, G. (1989) Cytogenetic and molecular studies on six sporadic hepatoblastomas. *Cancer Genet. Cytogenet.* **41**:286a.

659. Simms, L. A., Reeve, A. E., and Smith, P. J. (1995) Genetic mosaicism at the insulin locus in liver associated with childhood hepatoblastoma. *Genes Chromosomes Cancer* **13**:72–73.

660. Sirivatnauksorn, Y., Sirivatnauksorn, V., Battacharaya, S., Davidson, B. R., Dhillon, A. P., Kakkar, A. K., et al. (1999) Genomic heterogeneity in synchronous hepatocellular carcinomas. *Gut* **45**:761–766.

661. Ding, S.-F., Delhanty, J. D. A., Carillo, A., Dalla Serra, G., Bowles, L., and Dooley, J. S. (1993) Lack of demonstrable chromosome allele loss in hepatocellular adenoma. *Int. J. Oncol.* **2**:977–979.

662. Ding, S.-F., Jalleh, R. P., Dooley, J., Wood, C. B., and Habib, N. A. (1993) Chromosome 17 allele loss in hepatocellular carcinoma but not in synchronous liver adenoma. *Eur. J. Surg. Oncol.* **19**:195–197.

663. Nagai, H., Hirotsune, S., Komatsubara, H., Hatada, I., Mukai, T., Hayashizaki, Y., et al. (1993) Genomic analysis of human hepatocellular carcinomas using Restriction Landmark Genomic Scanning. *Cancer Detect. Prev.* **17**:399–404.

664. Nagai, H., Ponglikitmongkol, M., Mita, E., Omachi, Y., Yoshikawa, H., Saeki, R., et al. (1994) Aberration of genomic DNA in association with human hepatocellular carcinomas detected by 2-dimensional gel analysis. *Cancer Res.* **54**:1545–1550.

665. Nagai, H., Ponglikitmongkol, M., Fujimoto, J., Yamamoto, H., Kim, Y. S., Konishi, N., et al. (1998) Genomic aberrations in early stage hepatocellular carcinomas. *Cancer* **82**:454–461.

666. Yoshikawa, H., Nagai, H., Oh, K. S., Tamai, S., Fujiyama, A., Nakanishi, T., et al. (1997) Chromosome assignment of aberrant NotI restriction DNA fragments in primary hepatocellular carcinoma. *Gene* **197**:129–135.

667. Simon, D., Munoz, S. J., Maddrey, W. C., and Knowles, B. B. (1990) Chromosomal rearrangements in a primary hepatocellular carcinoma. *Cancer Genet. Cytogenet.* **45**:255–260.

668. Bardi, G., Johansson, B., Pandis, N., Heim, S., Mandahl, N., Andren-Sandberg, A., et al. (1992) Cytogenetic findings in three primary hepatocellular carcinomas. *Cancer Genet. Cytogenet.* **58**:191–195.

669. Werner, M., Nolte, M., Georgii, A., and Klempnauer, J. (1993) Chromosome 1 abnormalities in hepatocellular carcinoma. *Cancer Genet. Cytogenet.* **66**:130a.

670. Chen, H.-L., Chen, Y.-C., and Chen, D.-S. (1996) Chromosome 1p aberrations are frequent in human primary hepatocellular carcinoma. *Cancer Genet. Cytogenet.* **86**:102–106.

671. Lowichik, A., Schneider, N. R., Tonk, V., Ansari, M. Q., and Timmons, C. F. (1996) Report of a complex karyotype in recurrent metastatic fibrolamellar hepatocellular carcinoma and a review of hepatocellular carcinoma cytogenetics. *Cancer Genet. Cytogenet.* **88**:170–174.

672. Hany, M. A., Betts, D. R., Schmugge, M., Schonle, E., Niggli, F. K., Zachmann, M., et al. (1997) A childhood fibrolamellar hepatocellular carcinoma with increased aromatase activity and near triploid karyotype. *Med. Pediatric Oncol.* **28**:136–138.

673. Bardi, G., Rizou, H., Michailakis, E., Dietrich, C., Pandis, N., and Heim, S. (1998) Cytogenetic findings in three primary hepatocellular carcinomas. *Cancer Genet. Cytogenet.* **104**:165–166.

674. Parada, L. A., Hallén, M., Tranberg, K.-G., Hägerstrand, I., Bondeson, L., Mitelman, F., et al. (1998) Frequent rearrangements of chromosomes 1, 7, and 8 in primary liver cancer. *Genes Chromsomes Cancer* **23**:26–35.

675. Petkovic´, I., Nakic´, M., and Cepulic´, M. (1985) Cytogenetic analysis of hepatoblastoma. *Cancer Genet.Cytogenet.* **15**:369–371.

676. Dasouki, M. and Barr, M. Jr. (1987) Brief clinical report trisomy 18 and hepatic neoplasia. *Am. J. Med. Genet.* **27**:203–205.

677. Mamlok, V., Nichols, M., Lockhart, L., and Mamlok, R. (1989) Trisomy 18 and hepatoblastoma. *Am. J. Med. Genet.* **33**:125–128.

678. Mascarello, J. T., Jones, M. C., Kadota, R. P., and Krous, H. F. (1990) Hepatoblastoma characterized by trisomy 20 and double minutes. *Cancer Genet. Cytogenet.* **47**:243–247.

679. Bardi, G., Johansson, B., Pandis, N., Békássy, A. N., Kullendorff, C.-M., Hägerstrand, I., et al. (1991) *i(8q)* as the primary structural chromosome abnormality in a hepatoblastoma. *Cancer Genetics Cytogenet.* **51**:281–283.

680. Fletcher, J.A., Kozakewich, H.P., Pavelka, K., Grier, H.E., Shamberger, R.C., Korf, B., et al. (1991) Consistent cytogenetic aberrations in hepatoblastoma: a common pathway of genetic alterations in embryonal liver and skeletal muscle malignancies? *Genes Chromosomes Cancer* **3**:37-43.

681. Rodriguez, E., Reuter, V.E., Mies, C., Bosl, G.J., and Chiganti, R.S.K. (1991) Abnormalities of 2q: a common genetic link between rhabdomyosarcoma and hepatoblastoma? *Genes Chromosomes Cancer* **3**:122-127.

682. Soukup, S. W. and Lampkin, B. L. (1991) Trisomy 2 and 20 in two hepatoblastomas. *Genes Chromosomes Cancer* **3**:231–234.

683. Annerén, G., Nordlinder, H., and Hedborg, F. (1992) Chromosome alterations in an alpha-fetoprotein-producing hepatoblastoma. *Genes Chromosomes Cancer* **4**:99–100.

684. Bardi, G., Johansson, B., Pandis, N., Heim, S., Mandahl, N., Bekassy, A., et al. (1992) Trisomy 2 is the sole chromosomal abnormality in a hepatoblastoma. *Genes Chromosomes Cancer* **4**:78–80.

685. Hansen, K., Bagtas, J., Mark, H. F., Homans, A., and Singer, D. B. (1992) Undifferentiated small cell hepatoblastoma with a unique chromosomal translocation: a case report. *Pediatric Pathol.* **12**:457–462.

686. Tanaka, K., Uemoto, S., Asonuma, K., Katayama, T., Utsunomiya, H., Akiyama, Y., et al. (1992) Hepatoblastoma in a 2-year-old girl with trisomy 18. *Eur. J. Pediatric Surg.* **2**:298–300.

687. Dressler, L. G., Duncan, M. H., Varsa, E. E., and McConnell, T. S. (1993) DNA content measurement can be obtained using archival material for DNA flow cytometry. A comparison with cytogenetic analysis in 56 pediatric solid tumors. *Cancer* **72**:2033–2041.

688. Tonk, V. S., Wilson, K. S., Timmons, C. F., and Schneider, N. R. (1994) Trisomy 2, trisomy 20, and del(17p) as sole chromosomal abnormalities in three cases of hepatoblastoma. *Genes Chromosomes Cancer* **11**:199–202.

689. Swarts, S., Wisecarver, J., and Bridge, J. A. (1996) Significance of extra copies of chromosome 20 and the long arm of chromosome 2 in hepatoblastoma. *Cancer Genet. Cytogenet.* **91**:65–67.

690. Schneider, N. R., Cooley, L. D., Finegold, M. J., Douglass, E. C., and Tomlinson, G. E. (1997) The first recurring chromosome translocation in hepatoblastoma: der(4)t(1;4)(q12;q34). *Genes Chromosomes Cancer* **19**:291–294.

691. Teraguchi, M., Nogi, S., Ikemoto, Y., Ogino, H., Kohdera, U., Sakaida, N., et al. (1997) Multiple hepatoblastomas associated with trisomy 18 in a 3-year-old girl. *Pediatric Hematol. Oncol.* **14**:463–467.

692. Balogh, E., Swanton, S., Kiss, C., Jakab, Z. S., Secker-Walker, L. M., and Oláh, E. (1998) Fluorescence in situ hybridization reveals trisomy 2q by insertion into 9p in hepatoblastoma. *Cancer Genet. Cytogenet.* **102**:148–150.

693. Sainati L., Leszl, A., Stella, M., Montaldi, A., Perilongo, G., Rugge, M., et al. (1998) Cytogenetic analysis of hepatoblastoma: hypothesis of cytogenetic evolution in such tumors and results of a multicentric study. *Cancer Genet. Cytogenet.* **104**:39–44.

694. Nagata, T., Mugishima, H., Shichino, H., Suzuki, T., Chin, M., Koshinaga, S., et al. (1999) Karyotypic analysis of hepatoblastoma. Report of two cases and review of the literature suggesting chromosomal loci responsible for pathogenesis of this disease. *Cancer Genet. Cytogenet.* **114**:42–50.

695. Park, J. P., Ornvold, K. T., Brown, A. M., and Mohandas, T. K. (1999) Trisomy 2 and 19, and tetrasomy 1q and 14 in hepatoblastoma. *Cancer Genet. Cytogenet.* **115**:86–87.

696. Parada, L. A., Bardi, G., Hallen, M., Hagerstrand, I., Tranberg, K.-G., Mitelman, F., et al. (1997) Cytogenetic abnormalities and clonal evolution in an adult hepatoblastoma. *Am. J. Surg. Pathol.* **21**:1381–1386.

697. Douglass, E. C., Green, A. A., Hayes, F. A., Etcubanas, E., Horowitz, M., and Williams, J. A. (1985) Chromosome 1 abnormalities: a common feature of pediatric solid tumors. *J. Natl. Cancer Inst.* **75**:51–54.

698. Haas, O. A., Zoubek, A., Grümayer, E. R., and Gadner, H. (1986) Constituional interstitial deletion of 11p11 and pericentric inversion of chromosome 9 in a patient with Wiedemann-Beckwith syndrome and hepatoblastoma. *Cancer Genet. Cytogenet.* **23**:95–104.

699. Nasarek, A., Werner, M., Nolte, M., Klempnauer, J., and Georgii, A. (1995) Trisomy 1 and 8 occur frequently in hepatocellular carcinoma but not in liver cell adenoma and focal nodular hyperplasia. A fluorescence in situ hybridization study. *Virchows Arch.* **427**:373–378.

700. Zimmermann, U., Feneux, D., Mathey, G., Gayral, F., Franco, D., and Bedossa, P. (1997) Chromosomal aberrations in hepatocellular carcinomas: relationship with pathological features. *Hepatology* **26**:1492–1498.

701. Huang, S.-F., Hsu, H.-C., and Fletcher, J. A. (1999) Investigation of chromosomal aberrations in hepatocellular carcinomas by fluorescence in situ hybridization. *Cancer Genet. Cytogenet.* **111**:21–27.

702. Hamon-Benais, C., Ingster, O., Terris, B., Couturier-Turpin, M.-H., Bernheim, A., and Feldmann, G. (1996) Interphase cytogenetic studies of human hepatocellular carcinomas by fluorescent *in situ* hybridization. *Hepatology* **23**:429–435.

703. Ohsawa, N., Sakamoto, M., Saito, T., Kobayashi, M., and Hirohashi, S. (1996) Numerical chromosome aberrations in hepatocellular carcinoma detected by fluorescence *in situ* hybridization. *J. Hepatol.* **25**:655–662.

704. Kato, A., Kubo, K., Kurokawa, F., Okita, K., Oga, A., and Murakami, T. (1998) Nurmerical aberrations of chromosomes 16, 17, and 18 in hepatocellular carcinoma: a FISH and FCM analysis of 20 cases. *Digest. Dis. Sci.* **43**:1–7.

705. Kimura, H., Kagawa, K., Deguchi, T., Nakajima, T., Kakusui, M., Ohkawara, T., et al. (1996) Cytogenetic analyses of hepatocellular carcinoma by in situ hybridization with a chromosome-specific DNA probe. *Cancer* **77**:271–277.

706. Huang, S.-F., Hsu, H.-C., Cheng, Y.-M., and Chang, T.-C. (2000) Allelic loss at chromosome band 6q14 correlates with favorable prognosis in hepatocellular carcinoma. *Cancer Genet. Cytogenet.* **116**:23–27.

707. Marchio, A., Meddeb, M., Pineau, P., Danglot, G., Tiollais, P., Bernheim, A., et al. (1997) Recurrent chromosomal abnormalities in hepatocellular carcinoma detected by comparative genomic hybridization. *Genes Chromosomes Cancer* **18**:59–65.

708. Kusano, N., Shiraishi, K., Kubo, K., Oga, A., Okita, K., and Sasaki, K. (1999) Genetic aberrations detected by comparative genomic hybridization in hepatocellular carcinomas: their relationship to clincopathological features. *Hepatology* **29**:1858–1862.

709. Lin, Y.-W., Sheu, J.-C., Huang, G.-T., Lee, H.-S., Chen, C.-H., Wang, J.-T., et al. (1999) Chromosomal abnormality in hepatocellular carcinoma by comparative genomic hybridization in Taiwan. *Eur. J. Cancer* **35**:652–658.

710. Qin, L.-X., Tang, Z.-Y., Sham, J.S.T., Ma, Z.-C., Ye, S.-L., Zhou, X.-D., et al. (1999) The association of chromosome 8p deletion and tumor metastasis in human hepatocellular carcinoma. *Cancer Res.* **59**:5662–5665.

711. Sakakura, C., Hagiwara, A., Taniguchi, H., Yamaguchi, T., Yamaguchi, H., Takahashi, T., et al. (1999) Chromosomal aberrations associated with hepatitis C virus infection detected by comparative genomic hybridization. *Br. J. Cancer* **80**:2034–2039.

712. Wong, N., Lai, P., Lee, S.-W., Fan, S., Pang, E., Liew, C.-T., et al. (1999) Assessment of genetic changes in hepatocellular carcinoma by comparative genomic hybridization analysis. Relationship to disease stage, tumor size, and cirrhosis. *Am. J. Pathol.* **154**:37–43.

713. Stuver, S. O. (1998) Towards global control of liver cancer? *Semin. Cancer Biol.* **8**:299–306.

714. Tokino, T. and Matsubara, K. (1991) Chromosomal sites for hepatitis B virus integration in human hepatocellular carcinoma. *J. Virol.* **65**:6761–6764.

715. Haruna, Y., Hayashi, N., Katayama, K., Yuki, N., Kasahara, A., Sasaki, Y., et al. (1991) Expression of x protein and hepatitis B virus replication in chronic hepatitis. *Hepatology* **13**:417–421.

716. Wang, W. L., London, W. I., and Feitelson, M. A. (1991) Hepatitis B virus X antigen in hepatitis B virus carrier patients with liver cancer. *Cancer Res.* **51**:4971–4977.

717. Paterlini, P., Poussin, K., Kew, M., Franco, D., and Bréchot, C. (1995) Selective accumulation of the x transcript of the hepatitis in patients negative for hepatitis B surface antigen with hepatocellular carcinoma. *Hepatology* **21**:313–321.

718. Su, Q., Schröder, C. H., Hoffmann, W. J., Otto, G., Pichlmayr, R., and Bannasch, P. (1998) Expression of hepatitis B virus X protein in HBV-infected livers and hepatocellular carcinoma. *Hepatology* **27**:1109–1120.

719. Simon, D. and Carr, B. I. (1995) Integration of hepatitis B virus and alteration of the 1p36 region found in cancerous tissue of primary hepatocellular carcinoma with viral replication evidenced only in noncancerous, cirrhotic tissue. *Hepatology* **22**:1393–1398.

720. Pasquinelli, C., Garreau, F., Bougueleret, L., Cariani, E., Grzeschik, K. H., Thiers, V., et al. (1988) Rearrangement of a common cellular DNA domain on chromosome 4 in human primary liver tumors. *J. Virol.* **62**:629–632.

721. Blanquet, V., Garreau, F., Chenivesse, X., Bréchot, C., and Turleau, C. (1988) Regional mapping to 4q32.1 by in situ hybridization of a DNA domain rearranged in human liver cancer. *Human Genet.* **80**:274–276.

722. Tokino, T., Fukushige, S., Nakamura, T., Nagaya, T., Murotsu, T., Shiga, K., et al. (1987) Chromosome translocation and inverted duplication associated with integrated hepatitis B virus in hepatocellular carcinomas. *J. Virol.* **61**:3848–3854.

723. Rogler, C. E., Sherman, M., Su, C. Y., Shafritz, D. A., Summers, J., Shows, T. B., et al. (1985) Deletion in chromosome 11p associated

with a hepatitis B integration site in hepatocellular carcinoma. *Science* **230**:319–322.

724. Fisher, J. H., Scoggin, C. H., and Rogler, C. E. (1987) Sequences which flank an 11p deletion bserved in an hepatocellular carcinoma map to 11p13. *Human Genet.* **75**:66–69.

725. Hatada, I., Tokino, T., Ochiya, T., and Matsubara, K. (1988) Co-amplification of integrated hepatitis B virus DNA and transforming gene *hst-1* in a hepatocellular carcinoma. *Oncogene* **3**:537–540.

726. Hino, O., Shows, T. B., and Rogler, C. E. (1986) Hepatitis B virus integration site in hepatocellular carcinoma at chromosome 17;18 translocation. *Proc. Natl. Acad. Sci. USA* **83**:8338–8342.

727. Meyer, M., Wiedorn, K. H., Hofschneider, P. H., Koshy, R., and Caselmann, W. H. (1992) A chromosome 17:7 translocation is associated with a hepatitis B virus DNA integration in human hepatocellular carcinoma DNA. *Hepatology* **15**:665–671.

728. Zhou, Y.-Z., Slagle, B. L., Donehower, L. A., vanTuinen, P., Ledbetter, D. H., and Butel, J. S. (1988) Structural analysis of a hepatitis B virus genome integrated into chromosome 17p of a human hepatocellular carcinoma. *J Virol* **62**:4224–4231.

729. Zhang, X. K., Egan, J. O., Huang, D., Sun, Z.-L., Chien, V. K., and Chiu, J. F. (1992) Hepatitis B virus DNA integration and expression of an *erb* B-like gene in human hepatocellular carcinoma. *Biochem. Biophys. Res. Commun.* **188**:344–351.

730. Schlueter, V., Meyer, M., Hofschneider, P. H., Koshy, R., and Caselmann, W. H. (1994) Integrated hepatitis B virus X and 3′ truncated preS/S sequences derived from human hepatomas encode functionally active transactivators. *Oncogene* **9**:3335–3344.

731. Maguire, H. F., Hoeffler, J. P., and Siddiqui, A. (1991) HBVx protein alters the DNA binding specificity of CREB and ATF-2 by protein-protein interactions. *Science* **252**:842–844.

732. Cheong, J. H., Yi, M., Lin, Y., and Murakami, S. (1995) Human RPB5, a subunit shared by eukaryotic nuclear RNA polymerases, binds human hepatitis B virus X protein and may play a role in X transactivation. *EMBO J.* **14**:143–150.

733. Williams, J. S. and Andrisani, O. M. (1995) The hepatitis B virus X protein targets the basic region-leucine zipper domain of CREB. *Proc. Natl. Acad. Sci. USA* **92**:3819–3823.

734. Lin, Y., Nomura, T., Cheong, J., Dorjsuren, D., Iida, K., and Murakami, S. (1997) Hepatitis B virus X protein is a transcriptional modulator that communicates with transcription factor II B and the RNA polymerase II subunit 5. *J. Biol. Chem.* **272**:7132–7139.

735. Twu, J. S. and Schloemer, R. H. (1987) Transcriptional trans-activation function of hepatitis B virus. *J. Virol.* **61**:3448–3453.

736. Zhou, D. X., Tarablous, A., Ou, J. H., and Yen, T. S. (1990) Activation of class 1 major histocompatibility complex gene expression by hepatitis B virus. *J. Virol.* **64**:4025–4028.

737. Mahe, Y., Mukaida, N., Kuno, K., Akiyama, N., Ikeda, N., Matsushima, K., et al. (1991) Hepatitis B virus X protein transactivates human interleukin-8 gene through acting on nuclear factor kB and CCAAT/enhancer-binding protein-like *cis*-elements. *J. Biol. Chem.* **266**:13759–13763.

738. Aufiero, B. and Schneider, R .J. (1990) The hepatitis B virus X-gene product transactivates both RNA polymerase II and III promoters. *EMBO J.* **9**:497–504.

739. Menzo, S., Clementi, M., Alfani, E., Bagnarelli, P., Iacovacci, S., Manzin, A., et al. (1993) Transactivation of epidermal growth factor receptor gene by the hepatitis B virus x-gene product. *Virology* **196**:878–882.

740. Cross, J. C., Wen, P., and Rutter, W. J. (1993) Transactivation by hepatitis B virus X protein is promiscuous and dependent on mitogen-activated cellular serine/threonine kinases. *Proc. Natl. Acad. Sci. USA* **90**:8078–8082.

741. Kekulé, A. S., Lauer, U., Weiss, L., Luber, B., and Hofschneider, P. H. (1993) Hepatitis B virus transactivator HBx uses a tumour promoter signalling pathway. *Nature* **361**:742–745.

742. Benn, J. and Schneider, R. J. (1994) Hepatitis B virus HBx protein activates Ras-GTP complex formation and establishes a Ras, Raf, MAP kinase signalling cascade. *Proc. Natl. Acad. Sci.USA* **91**:10350–10354.

743. Balsano, C., Avantaggiati, M. L., Natoli, G., DeMarzio, E., Will, H., Perricaudet, M., et al. (1991) Full-length and truncated versions of the hepatitis B virus (HBV) X protein (pX) transactivate the c-*myc* protoncogene at the transcriptional level. *Biochem. Biophys. Res. Commun.* **176**:985–992.

744. Avantaggiati, M. L., Natoli, G., Balsano, C., Chirillo, P., Artini, M., De Marzio, E., et al. (1993) The hepatitis B virus (HBV) pX transactivates the c-*fos* through multiple *cis*-acting elements. *Oncogene* **8**:1567–1574.

745. Twu, J. S., Lai, M. Y., Chen, D. S., and Robinson, W. S. (1993) Activation of protooncogene c-*jun* by the x-protein of the hepatitis B virus. *Virology* **192**:346–350.

746. Natoli, G., Avantaggiati, M. L., Chirillo, P., Costanzo, A., Artini, M., Balsano, C., et al. (1994) Induction of the DNA-binding activity of c-*jun*/c-*fos* heterodimers by the hepatitis B virus transactivator pX. *Mol. Cell. Biol.* **14**:989–998.

747. Zhou, M. X., Watabe, M., and Watabe, K. (1994) The X gene of human hepatitis B virus transactivates the c-*jun* and alpha-fetoprotein genes. *Arch. Virol.* **134**:369–378.

748. Su, F. and Schneider, R. J. (1997) Hepatitis B virus HBx protein sensitizes cells to apoptortic killing by tumor necrosis factor a. *Proc. Natl. Acad. Sci. USA* **94**:8744–8749.

749. Kim, H., Lee, H., and Yun, Y. (1998) X-gene product of hepatitis B virus up-regulates tumor necrosis factor alpha gene expression in hepatocytes. *Hepatology* **28**:1012–1013.

750. Lara-Pezzi, E., Majano, P. L., Gomez-Gonzalo, M., Garcia-Monzon, C., Moreno-Otero, R., Levrero, M., et al. (1998) The hepatitis B virus x protein up-regulates tumor necrosis factor alpha gene expression in hepatocytes. *Hepatology* **28**:1013–1021.

751. Benn, J. and Schneider, R. J. (1995) Hepatitis B virus HBx protein deregulates cell cycle checkpoint controls. *Proc. Natl. Acad. Sci. USA* **92**:11215–11219.

752. Doria, M., Klein, N., Lucito, R., and Schneider, R. J. (1995) The hepatitis B virus HBx protein is a dual specificity cytoplasmic activator of Ras and nuclear activator transcription factors. *EMBO J.* **14**:4747–4757.

753. Klein, N. P. and Schneider, R. J. (1997) Activation of Src family kinases by hepatitis B virus HBx protein and coupled signalling to Ras. *Mol. Cell. Biol.* **17**:6427–6436.

754. Benn, J., Su, F., Doria, M., and Schneider, R. J. (1996) Hepatitis B virus HBx protein induces transcription factor AP-1 by activation of extracellular signal-regulated and c-*jun* N-terminal itogen-activated protein kinases. *J. Virol.* **70**:4978–4985.

755. Liang, T. J., Hasegawa, K., Rimon, N., Wands, J. R., and Ben-Porath, E. (1991) A hepatitis virus mutant associated with an epidemic of fulminant hepatitis. *N. Engl. J. Med.* **324**:1707–1709.

756. Laskus, T., Radkowski, M., Nowicki, M., Wang, L.-F., Vargus, H., and Rakela, J. (1998) Association between hepatitis B virus core promoter rearrangements and hepatocellular carcinoma. *Biochem. Biophys. Res. Commun.* **244**:812–814.

757. Minami, M., Poussin, K., Kew, M., Okanoue, T., Bréchot, C., and Paterlini, P. (1996) Precore/core mutations of hepatitis B virus in hepatocellular carcinomas developed in noncirrhotic livers. *Gastroenterology* **111**:691–700.

758. Poussin, K., Dienes, H., Sirma, H., Urban, S., Beaugrand, M., Franco, D., Schirmacher, P., Bréchot, C., and Paterlini Bréchot, C. (1999) Expression of mutated hepatitis B virus X genes in human hepatocellular carcinomas. *Int. J. Cancer* **80**:497–505.

759. Sirma, H., Giannini, C., Poussin, K., Paterlini, P., Kremsdorf, D., and Bréchot, C. (1999) Hepatitis B virus X mutants, present in hepatocellular carcinoma tissue, abrogate both the antiproliferative and transactivation effects of HBx. *Oncogene* **18**:4848–4859.

760. Jia, W., Wang, X.-W., and Harris, C. C. (1999) Hepatitis B virus x protein inhibits nucleotide excision repair. *Int. J. Cancer* **80**:875–879.

761. Wang, X. W., Gibson, M. K., Vermeulen, W., Yeh, H., Forrester, K., Stürzbecher, H.-W., et al. (1995) Abrogation of p53-induced apoptosis by the hepatitis B virus X gene. *Cancer Res.* **55**:6012–6016.

762. Chirillo, P., Pagano, S., Natoli, G., Puri, P. L., Burgio, V. L., Balsano, V. L., et al. (1997) The hepatitis B virus X gene induces p53-mediated programmed cell death. *Proc. Natl. Acad. Sci. USA* **94**:8162–8167.

763. Elmore, L. W., Hancock, A. R., Chang, S. F., Wang, X. W., Chang, S., Callahan, C. P., et al. (1997) Hepatitis B virus X protein and p53 tumor suppressor interactions in the modulation of apoptosis. *Proc. Natl. Acad. Sci. USA* **94**:14707–14712.

764. Gottlob, K., Fulco, M., Levrero, M., and Graessmann, A. (1998) The hepatitis B virus HBx protein inhibits caspase 3 activity. *J. Biol. Chem.* **273**:33347–33353.

765. Terradillos, O., Pollicino, T., Lacoeur, H., Tripodi, M., Gougeon, M. L., Tiollais, P., et al. (1998) p53-independent apoptotic effects of the hepatitis B virus HBx protein in vivo and in vitro. *Oncogene* **17**:2115–2123.

766. Sullivan, D. and Gerber, M. A. (1994) Conservation of hepatitis C virus 5′ untranslated sequences in hepatocellular carcinoma and the surrounding liver. *Hepatology* **19**:551–553.

767. Sakamuro, D., Furukawa, T., and Takegami, T. (1995) Hepatitis C virus nonstructural protein NS3 transforms NIH 3T3 cells. *J. Virol.* **69**:3893–3896.

768. Ray, R. B., Lagging, L. M., Meyer, K., and Ray, R. (1996) Hepatitis C virus core protein cooperates with ras and transforms primary rat embryo fibroblasts to tumorigenic phenotype. *J. Virol.* **70**:4438–4443.

769. Kim, D. W., Suzuki, R., Harada, T., Saito, I., and Miyama, T. (1994) Transsuppression of gene expression by hepatitis C viral core protein. *Jpn. J. Med. Sci. Biol.* **47**:211–220.

770. Shih, C., Chen, C., Chen, S., Wu, C., and Lee, Y. (1995) Modulation of the *trans*-activity of hepatitis C virus core protein by phosphorylation. *J. Virol.* **69**:1160–1171.

771. Ray, R. B., Steele, R., Meyer, K., and Ray, R. (1997) Transcriptional repression of p53 promoter by hepatitis C virus core protein. *J. Biol. Chem.* **272**:10983–10986.

772. Ray, R. B., Steele, R., Meyer, K., and Ray, R. (1998) Hepatitis C virus core protein represses p21WAF1/Cip1/Sid1 promoter activity. *Gene* **208**:331–336.

773. Matsumoto, M., Hseih, T. Y., Zhu, N., Van Arsdale, T., Huang, S. B., Jeng, K. S., et al. (1997) Hepatitis C virus core protein interacts with the cytoplasmic tail of lymphotoxin-beta receptor. *J. Virol.* **71**:1301–1309.

774. Zhu, N., Khoshnan, A., Schneider, R., Matsumoto, M., Dennert, G., Ware, C., et al. (1998) Hepatitis C virus core protein binds to the cytoplasmic domain of tumor necrosis factor (TNF) receptor 1 and enhances TNF-induced apoptosis. *J. Virol.* **72**:3691–3697.

775. Hsieh, T. Y., Matsumoto, M., Chou, H. C., Schneider, R., Hwang, S. B., Lee, A. S., et al. (1998) Hepatitis C virus core protein interacts with heterogenous nuclear ribonucleoprotein K. *J. Biol. Chem.* **273**:17651–17659.

776. Ghosh, A. K., Steale, R., Meyer, K., Ray, R., and Ray, R. B. (1999) Hepatitis C virus NS5A protein modulates cell cycle regulatory genes and promotes cell growth. *J. General Virol.* **80**:1179–1183.

777. Tsuchihara, K., Hijikata, M., Fukuda, K., Kuroki, T., Yamamoto, N., and Shimotohno, K. (1999) Hepatitis C virus core protein regulates cell growth and signal transduction pathway transmitting growth stimuli. *Virology* **258**:100–107.

778. Fujita, T., Ishido, S., Muramatsu, S., Itoh, M., and Hotta, H. (1996) Suppression of actinomycin D-induced apoptosis by the NS3 protein of hepatitis C virus. *Biochem. Biophys. Res. Commun.* **229**:825–831.

779. Ray, R. B., Meyer, K., and Ray, R. (1996) Suppression of apoptotic cell death by hepatitis C virus core protein. *Virology* **226**:176–182.

780. Ray, R. B., Meyer, K., Steele, R., Shrivastava, A., Aggarwal, B. B., and Ray, R. (1998) Inhibition of tumor necrosis factor (TNF-alpha)-mediated apoptosis by hepatitis C virus core protein. *J. Biol. Chem.* **273**:2256–2259.

781. Ruggieri, A., Harada, T., Matsuura, Y., and Miyamura, T. (1997) Sensitization to Fas-mediated apoptosis by hepatitis C virus core protein. *Virology* **229**:68–76.

782. Marusawa, H., Hijikata, M., Chiba, T., and Shimotohno, K. (1999) Hepatitis C virus core protein inhibits Fas- and tumor necrosis factor alpha-mediated apoptosis via NF-kappa B activation. *J. Virol.* **73**:4713–4720.

783. Barnard, G. F., Staniunas, R. J., Bao, S., Mafune, K.-I., Steele, G.-D. Jr., Gollan, J. L., et al. (1992) Increased expression of human ribosomal phosphoprotein PO messenger RNA in hepatocellular carcinoma and colon carcinoma. *Cancer Res.* **52**:3067–3072.

784. Scuric, Z., Stain, S. C., Anderson, W. F., and Hwang, J.-J. (1998) New member of aldose reductase family proteins overexpressed in human hepatocellular carcinoma. *Hepatology* **27**:943–950.

785. Cai, J., Sun, W.-M., Hwang, J.-J., Stain, S. C., and Lu, S. C. (1996) Changes in S-adenosylmethionine synthetase in human liver cancer: molecular characterization and significance. *Hepatology* **24**:1090–1097.

786. Lee, S. M., Portmann, B. C., and Margison, G. P. (1996) Abnormal intracellular distribution of O^6-alkylguanine-DNA-alkyltransferase in hepatitis B cirrhotic liver: a potential cofactor in the development of hepatocellular carcinoma. *Hepatology* **24**:987–990.

787. Furutani, M., Arii, S., Higashitsuji, H., Mise, M., Niwano, M., Harada, T., et al. (1996) *Kan-1* (Bile acid CoA:amino acid N-acyltransferase) messenger RNA as a novel predictive indicator for prognosis of hepatocellular carcinoma after partial hepatectomy. *Hepatology* **24**:1441–1445.

788. Koga, H., Sakisaka, S., Ohishi, M., Kawaguchi, T., Taniguchi, E., Sasatomi, K., et al. (1999) Expression of cyclooxygenase-2 in human hepatocellular carcinoma: relevance to tumor differentiation. *Hepatology* **29**:688–696.

789. Yu, M.-W., Chiu, Y.-H., Yang, S.-Y., Santella, R. M., Chern, H.-D., Liaw, Y.-F., et al. (1999) Cytochrome P450 1A1 genetic polymorphisms and risk of hepatocellular carcinoma among chronic hepatitis B carriers. *Br. J. Cancer* **80**:598–603.

790. Raunio, H., Juvonen, R., Pasanen, M., Pelkonen, O., Pääkkö, P., and Soini, Y. (1998) Cytochrome P4502A6 (Cyp2A6) expression in human hepatocellular carcinoma. *Hepatology* **27**:427–432.

791. Kirby, G. M., Batist, G., Alpert, L., Lamoureux, E., and Cameron, R. G. (1996) Overexpression of cytochrome P-450 isoforms involved in aflatoxin B1 bioactivation in human liver with cirrhosis and hepatitis. *Toxicol. Pathol.* **24**:458–467.

792. Sun, L., Hui, A.-M., Kanai, Y., Sakamoto, M., and Hirohashi, S. (1997) Increased DNA methyltransferase expression is associated with an early stage of human hepatocarcinogenesis. *Jpn. J. Cancer Res.* **88**:1165–1170.

793. Leray, G., Deugnier, Y., Jouanolle, A.-M., Lehry, D., Bretagne, J.-F., Campion, J.-P., et al. (1989) Biochemical aspects of a-L-fucosidase in hepatocellular carcinoma. *Hepatology* **9**:249–252.

794. Deugnier, Y., David, V., Brissot, P., Mabo, P., Delamaire, D., Messner, M., et al. (1984) Serum a-L-fucosidase: a new marker for the diagnosis of primary hepatic cancer? *Hepatology* **4**:889–892.

795. Hutchinson, W. L., Du, M.-Q., Johnson, P. J., and Williams, R. (1991) Fucosyltransferases: differential plasma and tissue alterations in hepatocellular carcinoma and cirrhosis. *Hepatology* **13**:683–688.

796. Su, T.-S., Tsai, T.-F., Chi, C.-W., Han, S.-H., and Chou, C.-K. (1990) Elevation of facilitated glucose-transporter messenger RNA in human hepatocellular carcinoma. *Hepatology* **11**:118–122.

797. Strassburg, C. P., Manns, M. P., and Tukey, R. H. (1997) Differential down-regulation of the *UDP-glucuronosyltransferase 1A* locus is an early event in human liver and biliary cancer. *Cancer Res.* **57**:2979–2985.

798. Matsuno, T. and Goto, I. (1992) Glutaminase and glutamine synthase activities in human cirrhotic liver and hepatocellular carcinoma. *Cancer Res.* **52**:1192–1194.

799. Christa, L., Simon, M.-T., Flinois, J.-P., Gebhardt, R., Bréchot, C., and Lasserre, C. (1994) Overexpression of glutamine synthetase in human primary liver cancer. *Gastroenterology* **106**:1312–1320.

800. Osada, T., Sakamoto, M., Nagawa, H., Yamamoto, J., Matsuno, Y., Iwamatsu, A., et al. (1999) Acquisition of glutamine synthetase expression in human hepatocarcinogenesis. Relation to disease re-

currence and possible regulation by ubiquitin-dependent proteolysis. *Cancer* **85**:819–831.

801. Sherman, M., Campbell, J. A. H., Titmuss, S. A., Kew, M. C., and Kirsch, R. E. (1983) Glutathione *S*-transferase in human hepatocellular carcinoma. *Hepatology* **3**:170–176.

802. Zhou, T., Evans, A. A., London, W. T., Xia, X., Zou, H., Shen, F.-M., et al. (1997) Glutathione *S*-transferase expression in hepatitis B virus-associated human hepatocellular carcinogenesis. *Cancer Res.* **57**:2749–2753.

803. Chen, Y. M., Shiu, J. Y., Tzeng, S. J., Shih, L. S., Chen, Y. J., Lui, W. Y., et al. (1998) Characterization of glycine-N-methyltransferase-gene expression in human hepatocellular carcinoma. *Int. J. Cancer* **75**:787–793.

804. Boisson, F., Fremont, S., Migeon, C., Nodari, F., Droesch, S., Gerard, P., et al. (1999) Human haptocorrin in hepatocellular carcinoma. *Cancer Detect. Prevent.* **23**:86–89.

805. Vlodavsky, I., Friedmann, Y., Elkin, M., Aingorn, H., Atzmon, R., Ishai-Michaeli, R., et al. (1999) Mammalian heparanase: gene cloning, expression and function in tumor progression and metastasis. *Nature Med.* **5**:793–802.

806. Gan, F. Y., Gesell, M. S., Moshier, J. A., Alousi, M., and Luk, G. D. (1992) Detection of ornithine decarboxylase messenger RNA in human hepatocellular carcinoma by in situ hybridization. *Epithelial Cell Biol.* **1**:13–17.

807. Tamori, A., Nishiguchi, S., Kuroki, T., Koh, N., Kobayashi, K., Yano, Y., et al. (1995) Point mutation of ornithine decarboxylase gene in human hepatocellular carcinoma. *Cancer Res.* **55**:3500–3503.

808. Tamori, A., Nishiguchi, S., Kuroki, T., Seki, S., Kobayashi, K., Kinoshita, H., et al. (1994) Relationship of ornithine decarboxylase activity and histological findings in human hepatocellular carcinoma. *Hepatology* **20**:1179–1186.

809. Koh, N., Tamori, A., Nishiguchi, S., Kuroki, T., Seki, S., Kobayashi, K., et al. (1999) Relationship between ornithine decarboxylase gene abnormalities and human hepatocarcinogenesis. *Hepato-Gastroenterology* **46**:1100–1105.

810. Suehiro, T., Shimada, M., Matsumata, T., Taketomi, A., Yamamoto, K., and Sugimachi, K. (1995) Thrombomodulin inhibits hepatic spread in human hepatocellular carcinoma. *Hepatology* **21**:1285–1290.

811. Komura, E., Matsumura, T., Kato, T., Tahara, T., Tsunoda, Y., and Sauada, T. (1998) Thrombopoietin in patients with hepatoblastoma. *Stem Cells* **16**:329–333.

812. Kohn, K. W. (1999) Molecular interaction map of the mammalian cell cycle control and DNA repair systems. *Mol. Cell. Biol.* **10**:2703–2734.

813. McCormick, F. (1999) Signalling networks that cause cancer. *Trends Cell Biol.* **9**:M53–M56.

15 The Molecular Basis of Breast Carcinogenesis

APRIL CHARPENTIER, PhD AND C. MARCELO ALDAZ, MD, PhD

INTRODUCTION

Breast cancer is the most common malignancy affecting women today. This disease has reached epidemic proportions in the industrialized world, afflicting as many as one in eight women *(1)*, and causing approx 45,000 deaths per year *(2,3)*. In response to this major public health problem, research funding is being used to identify key steps in breast carcinogenesis with the goal of developing effective means for preventing, diagnosing, and treating this devastating disease.

Overwhelming evidence has accumulated indicating that breast cancer is a genetically based disease in which spontaneous mutation and/or genetic predisposition play primary roles. Environmental and epigenetic influences are also important, however, their contribution to breast carcinogenesis is, at present, not well understood. The major determinants for development of breast cancer consist of: 1) the specific genetic makeup of an individual woman, and 2) exposure to endogenous or exogenous actors (Fig. 1). For example, an important endogenous risk factor would include the extent of exposure to a woman's own ovarian hormones *(4)*. Early age at menarche and nulliparity have been linked to an increased risk for developing breast cancer. It is likely that the extent of endogenous hormone exposure is genetically pre-determined or at least influenced by genetic factors. Examples of exogenous factors would include lifestyle choices such as diet, alcohol intake, and cigarette smoking (Fig. 1). Physical-environmental causes, such as ionizing radiation, have been shown to increase the likelihood of breast-cancer development *(5,6)*. Also, although the topic is controversial and less understood, we should mention the potential role of environmental pollutants and hormone disrupters *(7,8)*. Taken together, it is then the combination of the genetic constitution, plus the influence of multiple endogenous and exogenous factors that, ultimately, will determine

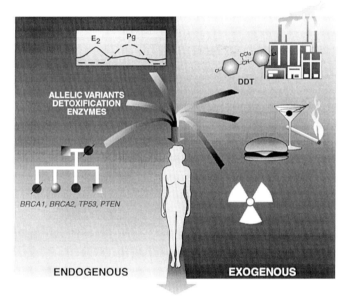

Fig. 1. Diagrammatic depiction of the multiple endogenous and exogenous factors that contribute to breast cancer risk. Ultimately, it is the combination of multiple factors along with the unique genetic composition of each individual woman that plays a decisive role in defining the risk for tumor development. This etiologic complexity is also responsible for the characteristic heterogeneity of breast cancer.

the overall risk of any particular woman for developing breast cancer.

Numerous mutated genes have been shown to be linked to breast-cancer development. However, most experts agree that there are probably many more important breast-cancer genes to be discovered. This overview focuses on the currently identified genes as well as genetic aberrations, which may lead to the identification of as-yet-unknown genes key to breast carcinogenesis. In addition, epigenetic factors that significantly con-

From: *The Molecular Basis of Human Cancer* (W. B. Coleman and G. J. Tsongalis, eds.), © Humana Press Inc., Totowa, NJ.

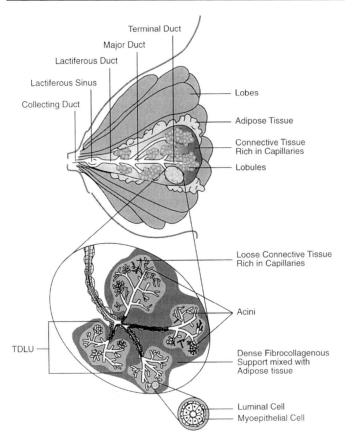

Fig. 2. Normal breast structure and histology. Adapted from Tavassoli 1992 *(12)*.

tribute to breast carcinogenesis, such as the hormonal regulation of cell proliferation, are discussed.

HISTOPATHOLOGY OF NORMAL AND NEOPLASTIC BREAST

NORMAL BREAST TISSUE In order to correlate the genetics of breast cancer to the clinical manifestations, an overview of the histology of both normal and cancerous breast tissue is required. The mammary glands are derived from modified sweat glands and basically represent downgrowths of the epidermis. In the adult woman, the mammary gland is composed of approx 15–20 lobes of branched tubuloalveolar glands. Dense fibrous-connective tissue separates the lobes. Each lobe in turn is subdivided into multiple lobules. Mammary lobules are located at the deepest end of the duct system. These lobules form clusters identified as blind-ending terminal ductules, or acini. These structures are embedded in a loose connective tissue rich in capillaries. Dense fibrocollagenous support mixed with abundant adipose tissue fills the interlobular spaces. The main collecting ducts (i.e., the lactiferous ducts) are lined by stratified squamous epithelium near the opening to the nipple. A short distance from the surface, each lactiferous duct presents a dilated portion known as the lactiferous sinus, where the epithelial lining shows a transition to a two-layer cuboidal epithelium. Throughout the rest of the duct system and acini the epithelium consists of one layer of luminal cuboidal cells and a basal layer of myoepithelial cells (Fig. 2).

The development and differentiation of the mammary gland is hormonally regulated. The ovarian hormones estrogen and progesterone control breast development, especially during puberty. Full or complete differentiation of the mammary gland takes place during pregnancy and lactation, a time when the hormone prolactin plays a fundamental role. The explosive growth that the mammary epithelium undergoes during pregnancy causes the mammary tree to branch dramatically, increasing the number of acini. This level of differentiation constitutes what Russo and colleagues have described as lobule type 3 *(9)*. Wellings has suggested that the majority of breast carcinomas originate in what is known as the terminal ductal-lobular unit (TDLU) *(10)* also known as lobule type 1 *(9)*. The TDLU has only 6–10 terminal ductules/lobules and is equivalent to the less differentiated state of mammary gland development found predominantly in the breast of the nulliparous women *(9)*.

INVASIVE CARCINOMA The most frequently observed invasive breast carcinoma is the infiltrating (invasive) ductal carcinoma (IDCA). IDCA represents approx 75–80% of the total invasive breast cancer cases *(11)*. Most invasive ductal carcinomas display the typical phenotype of well to poorly differentiated adenocarcinomas. Another type of invasive breast carcinoma, which accounts for approx 10–15% of the total invasive breast-cancer cases, is the infiltrating lobular carcinoma (ILCA) *(11)*. ILCA has a very distinctive infiltrating growth pattern, characterized by the pathognomonic presence of isolated cells or cord of cells (i.e., Indian-files pattern) *(11)*. This tumor type also presents a different clinical and metastatic pattern than the invasive ductal type *(13)*. For example, patients with ILCA have been reported to have a higher risk of developing multifocal and contralateral breast cancer than patients with IDCA *(14)*. It is important to remember, that the designation of ductal and lobular carcinomas does not imply that ductal carcinomas originate exclusively in ducts and lobular carcinomas in lobules. In fact, it has been suggested that both ductal and lobular tumor types originate in the TDLU *(10)*.

PREINVASIVE AND HYPERPLASTIC LESIONS In an attempt to clearly identify stages of breast-cancer development, standardized terminology is used to refer to important changes in the morphology of the breast epithelium that have been noted by pathologists. This is shown schematically in Fig. 3.

The identification and nomenclature of potentially premalignant lesions of the human breast have been a matter of controversy for many years. Among the noninvasive breast lesions, ductal carcinoma *in situ* (DCIS) is the most common and best-characterized precursor to invasive carcinoma. Some researchers have also proposed models where there is a direct transition from normal to malignant epithelium, without any visible evidence of a preneoplastic stage *(15)*. Nevertheless, evidence placing DCIS as a major precursor lesion of invasive carcinomas is substantial. For instance, the majority of IDCAs have an *in situ* component *(16)*. Women displaying biopsy-proven DCIS have an increased risk for development of subsequent invasive breast cancer *(17)*, and a high rate of recurrence of invasive carcinoma is observed in women who have had breast-conserving treatment of DCIS *(18)*. Taken together, these findings strongly suggest *in situ* carcinomas are precursors to

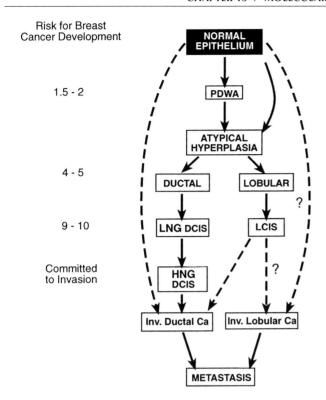

Risk for Breast
Cancer Development

1.5 - 2

4 - 5

9 - 10

Committed
to Invasion

Fig. 3. Putative model of breast cancer histopathological progression and corresponding estimated breast-cancer risk. This schematic is based on the results form studies by Page and Dupont *(20)*. A woman with proliferative disease without atypia has a 1.5–2 times greater risk for developing breast cancer than the general population, whereas a women with atypical hyperplasia exhibit a four- to fivefold greater risk. Women with DCIS and LCIS are at a much higher risk of progressing to invasive cancer. LNG, low nuclear grade; HNG, high nuclear grade

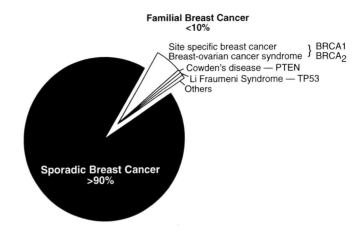

Fig. 4. Sporadic breast-cancer incidence and hereditary breast-cancer incidence.

invasive carcinomas. A more insidious lesion is lobular carcinoma *in situ* (LCIS). LCIS is characterized by a uniform population of generally small and loosely cohesive cells growing in a solid occlusive fashion. On the other hand the more common DCIS represents a highly heterogeneous group of lesions ranging from microscopic to grossly detectable intraductal carcinomas and *in situ* carcinomas with areas of stromal microinvasion.

When breast neoplastic cells begin proliferating outside their site of origin (beyond the containment of the basement membrane), and the microinvasion spreads further, the neoplasia is then termed invasive carcinoma. IDCAs are not necessarily the result of DCIS nor are ILCAs the obligated direct result of LCIS. In fact, there is some evidence that LCIS may play an important role as a precursor of IDCAs as well (Fig. 3) *(19)*. It should be mentioned, however, that the relationship of LCIS as a precursor lesion of invasive breast cancer is a matter of controversy *(19)*. It has been suggested that due to its morphologically diffuse and generalized nature, the presence of LCIS indicates that the whole breast epithelium is at risk of malignant transformation. It is possible that the distinction between DCIS or LCIS may be indicative of important differences in their genetic pathways during breast carcinogenesis.

Mammary epithelial hyperplastic lesions, which demonstrate only some of the characteristics of *in situ* carcinoma, are frequently identified in the clinic. These lesions are called atypi-

cal hyperplasias (AH) *(20)*. Atypical hyperplasias can either be ductal (ADH) or lobular (ALH) in type. Finally, other less-advanced hyperplastic lesions, which are only associated with a slightly increased risk for breast-cancer development, are known as proliferative disease without atypia. These lesions lack the qualitative and quantitative histologic features of AH *(20)*, meaning that they comprise a variety of epithelial hyperplastic lesions from mild to florid, but do not show signs of atypia.

FAMILIAL AND SPORADIC BREAST CANCER FORMS

Family history constitutes the strongest known risk factor for development of breast cancer. Women who have a family tree in which several blood relatives were afflicted with breast cancer exhibit a greater chance of developing breast cancer than the general population. Because of this fact, in the last few years intense research has focused on identifying the breast-cancer susceptibility genes that are passed from generation to generation in cancer-prone families. However, the inherited forms of breast cancer account for only 5–10% of total breast-cancer incidence (Fig. 4). The remaining 90–95% of women who develop breast cancer do not appear to segregate for an inherited susceptibility allele. Nonfamilial cases of breast cancer are termed sporadic *(21)*, a label that does not indicate the frequency of this disease. In fact, sporadic breast cancers represent the most frequently occurring form of disease.

Analysis of family pedigrees suggests the existence of various types of inherited breast cancers, consistent with models of autosomal dominant transmission of a highly penetrant susceptibility allele *(21)*. The major familial breast-cancer forms include *(23)*: 1) site-specific breast cancer, which is the most frequent and occurs in families in the absence of any other familial occurring neoplasm; 2) breast and ovarian cancer syndrome, which is characterized by early-onset and high rate of bilaterality; 3) Li-Fraumeni cancer syndrome, which is characterized by early onset of breast cancer, bilaterality, and association with other familial cancers, such as leukemia, sarcomas, brain tumors, and adrenocortical carcinoma; and 4) Cowden's disease, which is a rare condition also known as multiple hamartoma syndrome and is characterized by multiple mucocutaneous hamartomatous lesions, both benign and malignant.

In addition to the above forms the Muir Torre Syndrome, which is a variant of Lynch II syndrome, also includes breast cancer. This rare syndrome is caused by mutations in DNA mismatch repair (MMR) genes and is associated with microsatellite instability (MSI) *(24,25)*.

BREAST-CANCER SUSCEPTIBILITY GENES

BRCA1 We have witnessed tremendous progress within recent years in the identification of genes responsible for several of the inherited breast cancer types. In 1990, genetic-linkage analysis of affected families identified a gene predisposing individuals for early-onset breast cancer. This locus (termed *BRCA1* for Breast Cancer 1), was mapped to chromosome region 17q21 *(26,27)*. Furthermore it was estimated that this tumor-susceptibility allele, would account for 45% of families with high incidence of site-specific breast cancer and approx 80% of families identified as carriers of the early-onset breast- and ovarian-cancer syndrome *(28)*. After intense effort, the gene itself was cloned in 1994 by Miki and coworkers *(29)*. Mutations in *BRCA1* were found to co-segregate with the predisposing haplotype in affected kindred *(29)*. Thus, a woman who has a mutation in the *BRCA1* gene has a high risk of developing breast cancer and this risk increases over her lifetime reaching a peak by the age of 70 with a risk of 87% *(28)*.

BRCA1 is a large gene with 22 exons encoding 1,863 amino acids, that shows very little homology to other known genes, and has several alternative spliced forms. Based on the fact that the predicted amino acid sequence of the BRCA1 protein has a ring-finger motif close to its amino-terminus and a leucine heptad repeat within its sequence, speculation was made that BRCA1 may function as a transcription factor *(30)*. *BRCA1* mutations are scattered throughout the entire coding region. Interestingly, a frequently found mutation (185delAG) is also found to be present in 1% of women from Ashkenazi Jewish descent *(31)*. Most commonly the germline mutations affecting *BRCA1* are small insertions and deletions causing frameshifts, which produce stop codons, and result in truncation of the protein product.

The *BRCA1* gene product appears to play a much smaller role in nonfamilial breast cancer. As with other tumor-suppressor genes, it was expected that mutations of *BRCA1* would be frequent in sporadic breast-cancer forms, particularly due to the common finding of 17q loss of heterozygosity in most breast tumors *(32–35)*. However, no mutations in *BRCA1* have been found in nonfamilial breast- cancer cases. It has been suggested that subcellular mislocation of the BRCA1 protein may play a role in sporadic breast cancer. In normal breast epithelial cells, BRCA1 is localized in the nucleus, whereas in the majority of breast-cancer cell lines and in malignant pleural effusions from breast-cancer patients and in some primary tumors it is localized mainly to the cytoplasm *(36)*. Some groups have suggested that BRCA1 is a secreted protein because it contains certain homology regions to granins, a protein found in secretory granules *(37)*. Conflicting with this suggestion, the nuclear localization originally reported in normal cells was later confirmed by other groups *(38)*. Some evidence has also accumulated

indicating that normal *BRCA1* may act as a tumor-suppressor gene inhibiting tumor growth *(26,39)*. At present the function of BRCA1 is controversial and therefore requires additional investigation. However, both BRCA1 and BRCA2 have been shown to bind and co-localize in the nucleus with the DNA repair protein RAD51, but further analysis is needed to define the role of these proteins in this pathway *(38,40,41)*. Furthermore, it was recently suggested that BRCA1 is required for transcription coupled repair of oxidative damage *(42)*. These investigators showed that cells deficient in BRCA1 are impaired in their ability to carry out transcription-coupled repair of oxidative damage *(42)*. This would imply that BRCA1 may be playing an important role as guardian of genomic integrity.

BRCA2 A second breast cancer susceptibility gene termed *BRCA2* was isolated in 1995 *(43)*. *BRCA2* was originally mapped by linkage analysis to chromosome arm 13q12-q13 *(44)*. Similar to *BRCA1*, *BRCA2* is a large gene encoding for 3,418 amino acids and has several splice variants. Germline mutations of this gene predispose a person to early-onset, site-specific breast cancer, and moderately predispose affected women to ovarian cancer. Families that carry a mutated *BRCA2* gene exhibit a higher incidence of male breast cancer, and a higher predisposition to prostate, pancreatic, colon, and other cancers *(43)*. As with *BRCA1*, the germline mutations identified are spread throughout the coding sequence of *BRCA2*, and most frameshift mutations that result in a truncated gene product. A particular *BRCA2* germline mutation (6174delT) is frequently found (1%) in Ashkenazi Jewish women *(45)*. Like *BRCA1*, *BRCA2* appears to play no major role in sporadic breast cancer, because only very few somatic mutations were observed in these tumors. The function of the BRCA2 protein is uncertain as well.

Very recently the contribution of *BRCA1* and *BRCA2* to inherited breast cancer was assessed by linkage and mutation analysis in a series of 237 families with a history of breast cancer chosen at random without regard to the existence of other cancers *(46)*. Linkage to *BRCA1* was observed in 52% of the families, to *BRCA2* in 32%, and to neither of these genes in 16% of the families, indicating the existence of other predisposing genes. The vast majority (81%) of the breast/ovarian-cancer families were associated with *BRCA1* mutation, 14% due to *BRCA2*, whereas 76% of families with both female and male cancer cases were due to *BRCA2*. *BRCA2* carriers appear to have a similar lifetime cancer risk as *BRCA1* carriers but a lower risk before age 50 *(46)*.

p53 Germline *p53* mutations have been found in affected families and shown to be causative of the Li-Fraumeni cancer-predisposition syndrome *(47,48)*. Breast cancer is one of the neoplasms affecting patients with this syndrome. In these patients, breast tumors are characterized by early-onset, bilaterality, and association with other familial neoplasias, such as leukemia, soft-tissue sarcomas, osteosarcoma, brain tumors, and adrenocortical carcinoma. In tumors from patients with Li-Fraumeni syndrome, loss of the wild-type *p53* allele occurs frequently, with retention of the mutant allele. This observation suggests that inactivation of p53 function is essential to tumorigenesis in tumors characteristic of this syndrome.

Contrary to the previously described tumor-susceptibility genes, *p53*, a known tumor-suppressor gene, has been shown to play an important role in sporadic breast-cancer progression as well. However, germline mutations of this gene in the general population are rare. *p53*, located on chromosome arm 17p13, is somatically mutated in 25–45% of primary breast carcinomas *(49)*. All evidence indicates that *p53* is one of the most frequently affected genes in breast cancer.

PTEN Recently, a new putative tumor-suppressor gene, *PTEN*, has been identified on chromosome 10q23.3. *PTEN* is responsible for the familial predisposition of Cowden's disease *(50–52)*. Breast cancer is a component of this rare syndrome. The majority of the women who have a mutated *PTEN* gene develop breast neoplasia and approximately half of these cases progress to carcinoma. The amino acid sequence of PTEN resembles two different types of proteins: tyrosine phosphatases (enzymes that remove phosphate groups from the amino acid tyrosine in other proteins), and tensin (a protein that helps connect the cell's internal skeleton of protein filaments to its external environment) *(53)*. Homozygous deletions and mutations affecting *PTEN* have been found in both prostate and glioblastoma cancer cell lines. Somatic inactivating mutations of *PTEN* were associated with numerous primary prostate and endometrial carcinomas *(54,55)*. However, practically no somatic mutations affecting *PTEN* have been described in sporadic forms of breast cancer *(56,57)*.

PUTATIVE BREAST-CANCER SUSCEPTIBILITY GENES: ATM AND C-H-RAS Several years ago, it was suggested that heterozygous carriers of a defective Ataxia telangiectasia (*ATM*) gene are at increased risk (three- to fivefold) of developing breast cancer *(58)*. However, later studies concluded that there was no clear association between the *ATM* mutants and the risk of early-onset or familial breast cancer in general *(59,60)*. Nevertheless, it is an issue of importance because *ATM* heterozygotes represent a high percentage of the population (0.5–5%). At this point, the role of *ATM* as a factor for increasing breast-cancer risk in the general population is unclear.

Other potential breast-cancer susceptibility alleles are the polymorphic variants of the c-H-*ras* gene minisatellite sequence *(61,62)*. These studies reported a positive association between rare c-H-*ras* alleles and breast cancer *(61,62)*. However, controversial results have been reported by other research groups *(63)* and further confirmation of the positive association between these rare alleles with breast cancer is required.

COMMON ENZYMES ALLELIC VARIANTS THAT MAY CONTRIBUTE TO BREAST-CANCER RISK Through molecular epidemiology studies, it is becoming apparent that the combination of a specific genetic makeup plus exposure to specific exogenous factors (environmental, chemical, and/or physical carcinogens) play decisive roles in defining individual risk for tumor development. The heterogeneity of the genetic background found in the general population would explain why certain individuals develop cancer, whereas others do not even when exposed to a similar dose of a particular carcinogenic agent (as with cigarette-smoke exposure and lung-cancer risk). Therefore, as previously suggested, breast-cancer etiology may be explained by: 1) inherited predisposition to develop cancer, 2) inherited predisposition to accumulate new mutations, and

3) exogenous exposures *(64)* (Fig. 1). This would be the basis for the expected etiologic heterogeneity found in the general population. Thus, although breast cancers are classified as a single disease, not all are caused by the same set of etiologic agents. Most likely, different population subgroups will respond differently to similar carcinogenic insults.

Numerous studies have focused on a series of allelic variants that would confer increased tumor susceptibility. Several of these genes encode enzymes involved in detoxification pathways that the organism utilizes to eliminate xenobiotics. In most cases, a phenotypic polymorphism in the metabolic rate of specific chemicals correlated with the finding of genotypic polymorphisms (allelic variants), that could be detected as restriction fragment-length polymorphism (RFLP) variants. A good example of such polymorphism affecting breast cancer is seen with the cytochrome P450 (*CYP*) superfamily of enzymes. These phase I enzymes are responsible for the oxidative metabolism of diverse endogenous and exogenous substrates, such as steroids, prostaglandins, fatty acids, foreign chemicals, and drugs. Cytochrome P450 enzymes are responsible for the biotransformation of xenobiotics to toxic intermediate metabolites (phase I). The level of expression for a specific *CYP* gene and the catalytic activity of its gene product can vary dramatically among individuals of the general population due to the highly polymorphic nature of these enzymes. The phase II detoxification enzymes are responsible for the conjugation reaction necessary for the efficient excretion of toxic compounds. These enzymes transform toxic compounds into more hydrophilic forms for excretion. The phase II enzymes are also polymorphic in nature. Ambrosone and Shields *(65)* have suggested that women who have genetic polymorphisms that could result in greater activation, or impaired detoxification of aromatic and heterocyclic amines (NAT1, NAT2, CYP1A2 enzymes), polycyclic aromatic hydrocarbons (GSTM1, CYP1A1 enzymes), and nitroso compounds (CYP2E1 enzyme) may be at greater risk for developing breast cancer. Recently it was reported that the GSTM1 homozygous null phenotype was associated with increased risk of developing breast cancer, and similar associations were observed with polymorphic variants of the enzymes GSTT1 and GSTP1 *(66)*. On the other hand, it has been shown that cigarette smokers who are carriers of *BRCA1* or *BRCA2* mutations have a lower breast-cancer risk than subjects with mutations who never smoked, indicating that somehow smoking appears to reduce breast-cancer risk in these patients *(67)*. This confuses the significance of published observations in the field and indicates the amount of work that lies ahead in order to clarify our understanding of the interaction of environmental carcinogens and breast-cancer genetic predisposition.

SOMATIC CHROMOSOMAL AND GENETIC ABNORMALITIES IN BREAST CANCER

CYTOGENETICS OF BREAST CANCER Numerous studies have been performed in order to characterize the role of chromosomal abnormalities in breast cancer. However, as is the case with other solid tumors of epithelial origin, it has been difficult to identify the significant cytogenetic changes among the large number of apparently random alterations. This is due

Table 1
Summary of Genetic Aberrations in Sporadic Breast Cancer[a]

Chromosomal region	Cytogenetic finding	CGH finding	Invasive % LOH	DCIS % LOH	Possible target(s)	Possible consequence(s)
1p	-1p		32	8		
1q	+1q	+1q	30	16		
3p		-3p	22	0		
3q			25	0		
5p			18	0		
5q			13	0		
6p	-6	+6p	30	0		
6q	-6, -6q	-6q, +6q	26	8		
7p	+7	+7p	32	32	EGFR	Overexpression
7q	+7		25	24		
8p	-8, -8p	-8p	18	10		
8q	-8, +8q	+8q	20	22	c-myc	Overexpression
9p	-9p		58	30	$p16^{INK4A}$	Dysregulation
9q			24	0		
10p			11	0		
10q			15	0	PTEN	↓ Expression
11p	-11, -11p	-11p	28	0		
11q	-11, -11q	+11q	30	12	cyclin D1	Overexpression
13q	-13	-13q	30	18	Rb1, BRCA2, Brush-1	↓ Expression
16p	-16		40	0		
16q	-16, -16q		48	27	CDH1	↓ Expression
17p	-17, -17p	-17p	57	33	p53	Inactivation
17q	-17		36	31	BRCA1, NME1	↓ Expression
17q		+17q			c-erbB2	Overexpression
18p			25	0		
18q			48	12	bcl2	Dysregulation
19p			18	0		
19q		+19q	14	0	cyclin E	Overexpression
20q		+20q13	17	6	AIB1	Lverexpression
21q			17	5		
22q	-22		36	0		
Xp	-X		22			
Xq	-X		8			

[a]Data are adopted from refs. *(68,69,74,81,116).*

to the clonal heterogeneity characteristic of breast cancer as well as to the inherent difficulties in obtaining high-quality metaphase chromosome preparations from solid tumors. Nevertheless, the prevalence of several specific chromosomal aberrations have been noted. The most frequent tend to be numerical alterations of whole chromosome copy number, including trisomies of chromosomes 7 and 18, and monosomies of chromosomes 6, 8, 11, 13, 16, 17, 22, and X *(68).* The most common aberrations in nonmetastatic, near-diploid tumors consist of loss of chromosomes 17 and 19, trisomy of chromosome 7, and over-representation of chromosome arms 1q, 3q, and 6p *(69).* Structural alterations include terminal deletions and unbalanced nonreciprocal translocations, most frequently involving chromosomes 1, 6, and 16q. Breakpoints for structural abnormalities cluster to several chromosomal segments, including 1p22-q11, 3p11, 6p11-p13, 7p11-q11, 8p11-q11, 16q, and 19q13 *(69).* In particular, 16q was shown to participate systematically in translocations with chromosome 1q and to display frequent deletions. In fact, some investigators have suggested that specific abnormalities affecting chromosome

16q may represent early cytogenetic aberrations because they were observed in the absence of other anomalies *(70,71).*

A recently developed molecular cytogenetic technique called comparative genomic hybridization (CGH), allows for the analysis of chromosome copy-number abnormalities involving segments of at least 10 Mb *(72).* Because CGH involves hybridizing differentially labeled genomic DNA from a tumor and a normal-cell population to the same normal metaphase, it circumvents some of the difficulties encountered in conventional karyotyping. Through such analyses, nearly every tumor analyzed revealed increased or decreased DNA sequence copy number *(73).* The most common regions of increased copy number in breast cancer as determined by CGH include 1q, 8q, 17q22-q24, and 20q13. Regions of decreased DNA copy number were also observed, including 3p, 6q, 8p, 11p, 12q, 13q, 16q, and 17p *(74).* For some of these regional losses, candidate genes exist that may be the target of deletion in the progression to a malignant phenotype (Table 1). When both loss and gain of DNA copy number as determined by CGH were compared with survival data in a series of node-negative breast tumors, only copy-number losses were significant for recurrence and overall survival *(75)*. However, as is the case with conventional cytogenetics, CGH studies failed to reveal any characteristic abnormalities that occur in the majority of breast tumors or to identify any abnormalities that could be considered essential for breast-tumor development or progression.

PROTO-ONCOGENES AND GENE AMPLIFICATION

In human breast cancer as in other solid tumors, the most common aberration affecting proto-oncogenes appears to be gene amplification. Abundant evidence demonstrates that large regions of DNA, possibly as large as an entire chromosome arm, can be amplified as a contiguous unit. The importance of this to breast-cancer development is still unclear, although it suggests that genes within these regions are overexpressed, due to their increased copy number. Chromosomal regions that are overrepresented in tumor cells are frequently associated with the presence of activated proto-oncogenes. Proto-oncogenes encode proteins involved in cascade of events leading to growth in response to mitogenic factors. Alteration in the normal function of proto-oncogenes, through mutation or increased expression, can result in a constant growth stimulus and a constitutive mitogenic response. Aberration of a single allele of an oncogene can be sufficient to lead to dysregulation of growth control. Current data suggest that of the numerous proto-oncogenes described to date, only a few may have a role in breast tumorigenesis.

CHROMOSOMAL REGIONS AFFECTED BY GENE AMPLIFICATION

THE c-erbB2 LOCUS AT CHROMOSOME 17q12 In 1987, c-*erbB2* was demonstrated to be amplified in 20–40% of breast cancers, and this amplification was shown to be consistently accompanied by overexpression of c-*erbB2* mRNA and protein levels *(76,77)*. In later studies, increased copy number of the long arm of chromosome 17 (17q), which contains the c-*erbB2* gene, demonstrated a 50–100 fold amplification in some cases as determined by *in situ* hybridization analysis *(72)*.

The fact that c-*erbB2* is overexpressed in a high percentage of breast cancers suggests its involvement in breast tumorigenesis *(78,79)*. Therefore, in recent years, the diagnostic and possible treatment value of c-*erbB2* overexpression has been extensively studied. Early studies suggested a prognostic value of c-*erbB2* overexpression in node-negative breast cancer. However, more recent studies using larger data sets did not support these early observations and question the prognostic value for c-*erbB2* expression breast tumors. Nonetheless, expression of c-*erbB2* may have value in predicting response to specific therapies *(80)*. C-*erbB2* overexpression has been associated with increased resistance to chemotherapy *(82)*, and tumors that are positive for the estrogen receptor (ER) and overexpress c-*erbB2* are less likely to respond to hormone therapy *(83)*. Studies have also shown that activation or overexpression of c-*erbB2* in transgenic mice results in the genesis of mammary tumors *(84)*, whereas neutralizing antibodies against c-erbB2 protein lead to tumor regression *(85)*. In fact, Herceptin, the antibody against c-erbB2, is presently be-

ing tested in the clinic to treat breast cancer patients *(86, 87,87a)*.

The c-*erbB2* proto-oncogene is a member of the epidermal growth factor receptor (EGFR) family. All of the family members, which include *EGFR*, c-*erbB2*, c-*erbB3*, and c-*erbB4*, have been shown to be overexpressed in breast cancer. In addition, overexpression of ligands for these receptors, such as transforming growth factor-α (TGF-α), have been associated with neoplastic transformation in transgenic mouse models *(88)*. This family of receptors encodes transmembrane glycoproteins with tyrosine kinase activity. However, although the family members demonstrate significant sequence homology, their ligand specificities and related biochemical and biological responses of the individual receptors are distinct *(89)*. Thus, although these receptors show similarity in their ability to regulate cell proliferation, the mechanisms of action associated with each member of the receptor superfamily are diverse.

THE c-myc LOCUS AT CHROMOSOME 8q Amplification of chromosome 8q results in increased copy number of the c-*myc* proto-oncogene. This proto-oncogene is known to be overexpressed, through amplification or dysregulation in many breast cancers *(90)*. The c-*myc* proto-oncogene is a member of a small family of genes that encode related proteins that function as sequence-specific transcription factors *(91)*. Activation of the c-*myc*, N-*myc,* and L-*myc* genes has been described in many human cancers *(92)*. In normal cells, c-*myc* expression is rapidly induced following mitogenic stimulation, and its activity is absolutely dependent on the presence of growth factors *(93)*. The c-myc protein is commonly implicated in mediating the transition of cells from quiescence to proliferation *(94)*. Therefore, c-myc is considered to be a positive regulator of cell growth and its activation is thought to confer a growth advantage upon a tumor cell. Conversely, c-myc has also been demonstrated to induce apoptosis under some physiological conditions, a function more consistent with a negative regulator of cell growth *(95,96)*. A possible explanation for this bifunctional activity lies in the fact that in order for c-myc to act as a promoter of cell proliferation-appropriate serum growth factors (stimulating growth via a separate pathway), must be present *(92)*. Therefore, it has been suggested that in the absence of growth regulators, overexpression of c-*myc* results in the transmission of conflicting signals to the nucleus, which in turn initiates programmed cell death (apoptosis).

The c-*myc* gene is amplified in approx 25% of breast carcinomas *(90)*. Overexpression of c-*myc* in transgenic mice results in mammary tumors *(97)*, and amplification of c-*myc* has been associated with high-grade tumors in humans *(98)*. Of additional interest, c-*myc* expression is modulated by the presence of estrogen in estrogen-responsive cell lines, and constitutively high c-*myc* expression is observed in hormone-dependent lines, probably because of increased stability of the transcript *(99)*.

THE CYCLIN D1 LOCUS AT CHROMOSOME 11q13 Chromosome 11q13 is amplified in 15–20% of breast cancers, and is associated with poor patient prognosis *(100)*. The *cyclin D1* gene, located in this region, is thought to be the target of such amplification. *Cyclin D1* is overexpressed in 45% of breast carcinomas, most of which are both estrogen- and progester-

one-receptor positive *(101,102)*. Studies show that transgenic mice that are homozygous null for *cyclin D1* fail to undergo proliferative changes of the mammary epithelium associated with pregnancy, thereby indicating a significant role for *cyclin D1* in normal steroid-induced proliferation of the mammary epithelium *(103)*. Transgenic mice that overexpress *cyclin D1* develop mammary carcinomas *(104)*. Analysis of *cyclin D1* expression by mRNA *in situ* hybridization shows a high level of *cyclin D1* expression in 76% of low-grade carcinoma *in situ*, further suggesting a role for cyclin D1 in the tumorigenesis of the breast *(105)*.

Mapped within the same region of 11q13 is the *int2* gene. Transgenic mice that express an *int2* transgene develop multifocal preneoplastic hyperplasia of the mammary gland, which can give rise to focal mammary tumors *(106)*. The possibility that an additional gene responsible for breast tumorigenesis within this amplified region is *int2* is controversial because corresponding increases in mRNA and protein levels for *int2* rarely correspond to amplification status. Thus, the possibility remains that a yet-unknown gene located close to *int2* might have a biological effect, whether *int2* itself is merely co-amplified remains to be seen.

THE AIB1 LOCUS AT CHROMOSOME 20q13 The *AIB1* gene (for amplified in breast cancer) was recently identified as a leading candidate for the amplification of chromosome 20q13. Amplification of this chromosomal region occurs in 15–30% of cases of breast-cancer cases *(107)*. *AIB1* was found amplified in all ER-positive cell lines and has been suggested to function as a nuclear steroid-receptor coactivator *(107)*. Thus, *AIB1* amplification may contribute to the development of steroid-dependent breast cancers by interacting with the ER to enhance the effects of estrogen on tumor cells.

TUMOR SUPPRESSORS AND LOSS OF HETEROZYGOSITY

Based on statistical analysis of clinical observations, Knudson was the first to suggest that retinoblastoma was a cancer caused by two mutational events *(108)*. In the hereditary form of retinoblastoma, the first mutation is present in the germline and the second mutation is acquired somatically. This type of genetic predisposition results in early onset and a tendency toward bilateral tumorigenesis. In the sporadic form, both mutations are somatic, resulting in a tendency toward unilaterally and late onset. It was later suggested that these two mutational events could occur within separate alleles of a regulatory gene *(109)*. Supporting this, cytogenetic analysis of retinoblastoma revealed characteristic deletions of the long arm of chromosome 13. Subsequent analysis of the same chromosome region led to the cloning of *Rb1* and identification of aberrant transcripts encoded from the remaining allele *(110)*. As a consequence of these studies, a precedent emerged where inactivation of one allele of a tumor suppressor is accomplished by mutation, leading to the eventual deletion of the remaining normal allele through chromosomal aberrations and thus loss of heterozygosity (LOH) is thereby observed at the suppressor locus. This precedent is now considered the convention for tumor-suppressor gene inactivation and similar observations have been made for several other putative tumor-suppressor

genes, including *APC, DCC, VHL,* and *p53 (111)*. Therefore, LOH is considered indirect evidence for the existence of a suppressor gene within the affected chromosomal region.

BREAST CANCER ALLELOTYPE

The mechanisms giving rise to LOH usually involve large segments of chromosomal DNA, making it possible to utilize adjacent genes or noncoding sequences as molecular markers to identify and map regions of chromosome deletion where tumor-suppressor genes may reside. A useful group of molecular markers for mapping LOH are the naturally occurring simple sequence length polymorphisms, termed microsatellite sequences. The majority of microsatellite sequences are dinucleotide repeats (primarily $(CA)_n$) that are repeated in tandem at variable number interspersed throughout the genome *(112)*. These sequences demonstrate a mean heterozygosity of 70% and recent mapping efforts reported an average spacing of 199 kb in the human genome *(113)*. Through known linkage maps and comparison to physical maps, it is possible to select highly polymorphic microsatellites at any position within the genome. Further, through polymerase chain reaction (PCR) amplification of these microsatellites and comparison with normal DNA from the same patient, it is possible to generate a comprehensive map of allelic imbalances and losses (allelotype) occurring in a neoplasm.

Numerous studies have analyzed the breast-cancer allelotype, and numerous regions of allelic imbalance have been described using microsatellite PCR and/or RFLP analysis. Devilee and Cornelisse *(68)*, reviewed data from more than 30 studies of breast cancer, revealing a consensus of imbalances affecting 12 chromosome arms at a frequency of more than 25% (Table 1). Chromosome arms 1p, 1q, 3p, 6q, 8p, 11p, 13q, 17q, 18q, and 22q were affected at a frequency of 25–40%, whereas chromosome arms 16q and 17p were affected in more than 50% of tumors *(68)*. In addition, chromosome arm 9p, has recently been reported to be affected by allelic imbalances and losses in numerous breast carcinomas *(114)*. In general, the loss of genetic material in many of these regions has been corroborated by either CGH or classic cytogenetic data *(68,115)*. Some of these regions are known to harbor tumor-suppressor genes whose loss has been demonstrated through a variety of techniques, including Southern-blot analysis and fluorescence *in situ* hybridization (FISH) using gene-specific single-copy probes *(111)*.

Although there is overwhelming evidence that these genetic losses occur, inherent difficulties exist in determining the relevance of such losses to breast carcinogenesis. In most cases, the tumors analyzed were of the invasive type and/or advanced stages of progression, leading to the question of whether these losses are causative factors of tumorigenesis or consequences of the general genomic instability inherent to tumors. It is possible that certain losses may be selected for in the progression or clonal evolution of a tumor to a more advanced type but not strictly necessary for the genesis of the tumor. Some of these questions could be addressed in part through comparative allelotyping of both noninvasive and invasive tumors.

The relative timing and frequency of allelic losses of commonly affected regions in breast cancer was estimated by comparing the allelotype of preinvasive ductal carcinomas (DCIS) and invasive carcinomas *(81)*. The allelotypic analysis of DCIS samples revealed that chromosomal regions 3p, 3q, 6p, 11p, 16p, 18p, 18q, and 22q were not affected by a high frequency of loss; on the other hand, analyses of these same regions of invasive tumors showed them to be affected in 10–40% of cases *(81)* (Table 1). These findings are in agreement with those of Radford et al., who examined 61 DCIS samples *(116)*. Because allelic losses affecting these regions were not frequently observed at the noninvasive DCIS stage, it can be concluded that alterations of these chromosomal regions are late events in breast-cancer progression. More importantly, allelic imbalances observed on chromosome arms 7p, 7q, 16q, 17p, and 17q *(81)*, as well as 9p as reported by others *(117)*, appear to represent early changes because they occur frequently in DCIS (Table 1).

MOLECULAR TARGETS OF ALLELIC LOSS

CHROMOSOME REGION 17p13 The short arm of chromosome 17, is subject to allelic loss in more than 50% of IDCAs, and approx 30% of noninvasive ductal carcinomas *(81,116,118)*. This high frequency of allelic loss suggested that a tumor suppressor of relevance to breast tumorigenesis resides in this region. Indeed, tumor-suppressor *p53* maps to chromosome band 17p13 and is known to harbor somatic mutation in 25–45% of primary breast carcinomas *(49)*. Recently *p53* mutations were identified in mammary DCIS but not in epithelial hyperplasia *(119)*. It has been suggested that *p53* mutation analysis may serve as a marker for identifying preinvasive lesions at increased risk of developing invasive carcinoma.

We have already discussed the relevance of germline *p53* mutations as the cancer-predisposing alteration in the Li-Fraumeni syndrome *(47,48)*. In tumors from patients with Li-Fraumeni syndrome, loss of the wild-type allele is observed in conjunction with retention of the mutant *p53* allele.

Functional studies of cells with mutant *p53* indicate a change of phenotypes, including cellular immortalization, loss of growth suppression, and fourfold increase in protein half-life, which leads to p53 protein accumulation. Such an accumulation of p53 protein is observed by immunohistochemical analysis in roughly 30–50% of sporadic breast carcinomas, and has been proposed to be an indicator of higher risk of recurrence in patients with tumors positive for *p53* expression *(120)*. It appears that *p53* inactivation through mutation and LOH is intrinsically linked to the development of subsequent further genomic instability as suggested by *in vitro* findings, and as demonstrated in experimental models of mammary cancer *(121)*.

Although *p53* is most likely the driving force for allelic loss on 17p, some reports indicate that there may exist another distinct locus on this chromosomal arm that may be a target of allelic loss in breast carcinogenesis. In an analysis of 141 breast tumors, Cornelis et al. observed a strong association between *p53* mutation and allelic loss of the *p53* locus *(122)*. However, in cases where *p53* mutation was not observed, allelic loss of the distal region of 17p13.3 was always observed, sometimes without *p53* allele loss. Similar findings of distal deletion of 17p were also observed in DCIS (116). Although these findings support the existence of a second gene as target of allelic loss,

additional studies will be required to verify its existence and to determine its role in breast tumorigenesis.

CHROMOSOME REGION 17q21-q22 The long arm of chromosome 17 has recently been subjected to extensive analysis aimed at identification of the locus responsible for a subset of familial breast cancers linked to 17q *(123)*. As a result, the *BRCA1* gene was isolated by positional cloning as discussed in preceding sections *(29)*. However, when sporadic breast tumors with allelic loss of 17q were examined for *BRCA1* coding sequence alterations, only about 10% of those with LOH revealed any change of sequence, and those mutations were found to be present in the germline of affected individuals *(124)*.

Another known putative suppressor gene localized to this chromosomal region, termed *nm23* or *NME1*, has been shown to undergo allelic loss in as much as 60% of breast carcinomas *(125)*. However, analysis of *NME1* has not revealed evidence of mutations *(126)*. An additional possible explanation for allelic loss at 17q is the existence of a yet-unidentified gene within this region as the target for LOH *(122)*.

CHROMOSOME REGION 13q14 Loss of the *Rb1* region 13q14 has been reported for numerous neoplasms including small-cell lung carcinoma (SCLC), bladder carcinoma, osteosarcoma, and breast carcinoma *(111)*. Loss of 13q14 is suggested to represent an early alteration in a subset of breast tumors because 15–20% of these tumors at the DCIS stage exhibit this allelic loss *(81,116)*. However, when allelic loss and *Rb1* gene expression are examined in the same breast tumors, no correlation between the two is observed. This suggests that *Rb1* inactivation is not accomplished by allelic deletion and that another gene may be the target of such 13q14 loss *(127)*. A second breast-cancer susceptibility gene, *BRCA2*, has been mapped to chromosome 13q12-q13 *(43)*. This observation suggested that the *BRCA2* gene may be involved in sporadic breast cancer as well. However, similar to the findings with *BRCA1* on 17q, when sporadic breast tumors were analyzed for mutation of *BRCA2*, mutations were infrequent, suggesting that *BRCA2* is not the gene being targeted by allelic deletion *(128–130)*. *Brush-1* is another gene that has been mapped to 13q12-q13, proximal to *Rb1*. Analysis of *Brush-1* expression showed it to be low to absent in 6 of 13 breast-cancer lines and decreased in 100% (4/4) of tumors showing LOH of 13q12-q13 *(131)*. However, no sequence analysis has yet been reported, and the question of whether decreased expression of *Brush-1* results from allelic loss involving large regions of another gene has yet to be addressed.

CHROMOSOME REGION 16q Chromosome 16q has been suggested as a site for the occurrence of primary cytogenetic structural abnormalities in the development of breast cancer *(70,71)*. In particular, the long arm of chromosome 16 was shown to systematically participate in nonrandom translocations with chromosome 1. Breast-cancer allelotype studies have also shown the common occurrence of allelic losses affecting the long arm of chromosome 16 *(132–134)*. In addition, frequent allelic losses affecting chromosome 16q have also been reported for DCIS *(81,116,133)*.

It has been suggested that more than one putative tumor-suppressor resides in the chromosome region 16q. At least two regions of chromosome 16q have consistently been reported to show LOH: 16q21 and 16q24.2-qter *(132–134)*. In most recent studies, high-resolution allelotyping of chromosome 16 in DCIS lesions have identified three distinct regions with a very high incidence (about 70% or more) of allelic losses *(41)*. Two of the three regions agree with previously described areas: 16q21 at locus *D16S400* and 16q24.2 at locus *D16S402 (41)*. However, the region with the highest incidence of LOH observed lies within 16q23.3-q24.1 close to marker *D16S518 (41)*.

The *CDH1* gene, which encodes the E-cadherin cell-adhesion protein that is implicated as an invasion suppressor protein, is one possible candidate target of the LOH at chromosome 16q21. This gene has been demonstrated to be mutated at a high frequency in ILCAs of the breast. The lack of E-cadherin expression is suggested to account for the infiltrative growth pattern characteristic of lobular carcinomas *(135)*. However, the more common, invasive ductal carcinomas do not show high incidence of *CDH1* gene mutations. In addition to mutation, another mechanism for inhibition of *CDH1* expression involves CpG methylation within the promoter region of the gene *(136,137)*. Expression of a second cadherin gene, which encodes H-cadherin protein, maps to region 16q24 *(138)* was reported to be absent or reduced in several breast-cancer cell lines. Recently, a putative tumor suppressor gene, *WWOX*, was identified in 16a 23–24, the area known as a common fragile site, FRA16D, which is frequently affected in breast cancer *(138a)*. Further studies are necessary to identify additional possible targets for the common allelic losses observed to affect this autosome in breast cancer.

CHROMOSOMAL REGION 9p Chromosomal region 9p21 has been shown to be affected by allelic loss or imbalance in more than 58% of IDCAs and 30% of DCIS, suggesting it may be involved in breast tumorigenesis *(114,117)*. Previously, the *p16^INK4A* tumor-suppressor gene was identified within this region by positional cloning and shown to be affected by homozygous deletions in 60% of breast-carcinoma lines *(139)*. However, when primary breast tumors were analyzed for mutation of the *p16^INK4A* coding region, few mutations were found *(114)*. More recent analysis, including FISH determination of gene copy number, methylation of the 5' region, and analysis of expression, indicate that *p16^INK4A* appears to be a target of abnormalities in approx 40% of breast tumors *(140)*. These observations substantiate a role for *p16^INK4A* inactivation in the tumorigenesis of the breast and as a target of 9p allelic loss. However, some breast tumors show overexpression of *p16^INK4A*, indicating that involvement of this gene as well as that of *p14^ARF* (homolog of mouse *p19^ARF*), encoded at the same locus in an alternative reading frame is more complex than previously thought.

CELL-CYCLE DYSREGULATION IN BREAST CANCER

Cell replication in eukaryotes proceeds through an orderly cascade of events as cells progress through the cell cycle, under the regulation of numerous positive and negative protein effectors. At the top of the cell-cycle control hierarchy are the cyclins, whose expression and stability oscillate in a cell-cycle phase-dependent manner. The expression of certain cyclin genes can be upregulated by different mitogenic stimuli, for example, the

upregulation of *cyclin D1* by estrogen *(141)*. Each of these cyclins can associate in a specific manner with corresponding cyclin-dependent kinases (cdks). Cyclins compete with cdk inhibitors, which have the ability to displace the cyclin subunit and form an inactive complex with the cdks. Active cdks phosphorylate and inactivate target proteins with transcription-repressing activity *(143)* (Fig. 5).

Of the cell cycle restriction points, the G_1-S transition is best-characterized in breast cancer. Key players in early G_1 and after the passage of cells from G_0 to G_1 include: cyclins D1-D3, cdk4, and cdk6; the specific inhibitors of these cdks (p15^INK4B, p16^INK4A, p18^INK4C, and p19^INK4D); and the CDK substrates (pRb and pRb-like proteins). Later in G_1 and fueled by E2F-1 transcriptional activation, cyclin E and its partner cdk2, become important players in the G_1-S transition. Collectively, these proteins are known elements responsible for regulating progression through G_1 and as a consequence loss of function or abnormalities in the expression of an individual protein can lead to cell-cycle dysregulation and altered cell proliferation.

An additional family of CDK inhibitory proteins also exists which includes, p21^cip1, p27^kip1, and p57^KIP2. Of the proteins mentioned, pRb, cyclin D1, cyclin E, p16^INK4A, and p27^KIP1 have all been implicated in breast carcinogenesis. As previously mentioned, *cyclin D1* has been shown to be both amplified in 10–20% of breast tumors and overexpressed in the majority of breast tumors *(101,102,105)*. Cyclin D1 competes with p16^INK4A for heterodimerization with the cdks. When cyclin D1 is more abundant than p16^INK4A, it binds to and activates cdk4 and cdk6 (Fig. 5). Recently *cyclin D1* mRNA and *ER* expression were found to be positively correlated in primary breast cancer (144). There is no conclusive evidence, however, demonstrating that ER directly upregulates *cyclin D1* transcription.

Recent studies have suggested that overexpression of cyclin E protein, which is often found in breast tumors, is functionally redundant to expression of cyclin D protein *(145)*. In cells overexpressing both *cyclin E* and *p16^INK4A*, the cyclin E protein can functionally replace cyclin D providing tumor cells with a growth advantage *(145)*. They do this by activating cdks, which in turn phosphorylate pRb, releasing E2F and initiating gene transcription, leading to cell-cycle progression and a self-perpetuating positive regulatory loop (Fig. 5). Interestingly, breast cancers that exhibit high cyclin E protein expression concomitant with low expression of the cdk inhibitor p27^KIP1 are associated with poor prognosis and very high patient-mortality rate *(146)*.

Inactivation of pRb itself has been described in breast cancer as a means of enhancing cell-cycle progression, although when multiple modes of inactivation are accounted for, pRb is inactivated in less then 20% of breast cancers *(127,147)*. In the vast majority of tumor lines, there is an inverse relationship between *Rb1* and *p16^INK4A* expression *(148,149)*. For instance, breast-tumor cell lines that retain *Rb1* expression have no expression of *p16^INK4A*, whereas cell lines retaining *p16^INK4A* expression often lack expression of *Rb1*. When primary breast tumors were analyzed for *p16^INK4A* expression, approx 50% showed loss of expression or reduced expression *(140)*. The loss of expression may be due to homozygous deletion, gene

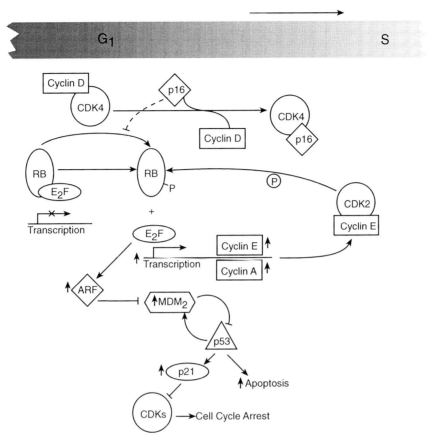

Fig. 5. The G_1-S cell-cycle restriction-point controls. Many of these critical proteins are known to be altered in breast cancer.

inactivation through methylation, or in rare instances mutation *(140)*.

The cdk inhibitor p21$^{WAF1/CIP1}$ is a universal inhibitor of cdks, inducing cell-cycle arrest at both the G_1/S and G_2/M restriction points *(150)*. Inhibition of DNA replication occurs when p21$^{WAF1/CIP1}$ complexes with the proliferating cell nuclear antigen, PCNA *(151)*. Because *p21*$^{WAF1/CIP1}$ gene transcription is regulated by p53, it has been suggested that p53-dependent cell cycle arrest is mediated by p21$^{WAF1/CIP1}$. Indeed, *p21*$^{WAF1/CIP1}$ nullizygous mice fibroblasts fail to undergo G_1 arrest when p53 is activated following DNA damage, although apoptosis is unaffected and occurs when p53 is activated in these same cells *(152)*. Accumulation of p53 protein in breast-tumor cells has been shown to be associated with *p53* mutations and a higher risk of breast-cancer recurrence *(120)*. Therefore, *p53* inactivation appears to be a critical event in the tumorigenesis of the breast. This also suggests that an additional consequence of *p53* inactivation would be abrogation of cell-cycle arrest through loss of transcriptional activation of p21$^{WAF1/CIP1}$.

Recent studies have produced evidence for an important regulatory link between the p53 and pRb pathways. At the center of this link is the recently described p14^{ARF} (previously called p19^{ARF} because of the mouse homolog). As mentioned in a preceding section, this gene is encoded at the *INK4A* locus (carried on chromosome 9p21), as an alternative reading frame of the cyclin-dependent kinase inhibitor p16^{INK4A}. It was demonstrated that the putative tumor suppressor *ARF* gene product physically interacts with mdm2 and as a consequence blocks

mdm2-induced p53 degradation and transcriptional inactivation *(153,154)*. Thus, this interaction leads to increase p53 stability and accumulation of p53 protein (Fig. 5). Further strengthening the connection between the p53 and pRb pathways, it was very recently reported that *ARF* is transcriptionally upregulated by E2F-1 *(155)*. These observations led to the speculation that perhaps abnormal cell proliferation and the associated increase in E2F-1 would result in an increase of ARF leading to cell-cycle arrest or apoptosis via p53 (Fig. 5). This would not take place if lesions in the pathway occur, such as p53 mutation or ARF inactivation *(155)*. In studies from our laboratory, we have demonstrated that both *ARF* and *p16*^{INK4A} expression levels are highly variable in breast cancer *(140)*. We observed subsets of tumors that lack expression of both genes (*p16*^{INK4A} and *ARF*) due to common inactivation events such as homozygous deletion. On the other hand, we have also observed numerous tumors that dramatically overexpressed *ARF*.

APOPTOSIS AND BREAST CANCER

Closely linked to the deregulation of the cell cycle are the molecular pathways leading to programmed cell death (apoptosis). When DNA is altered during replication, cell-cycle control checkpoints interrupt DNA replication and/or mitosis in order to allow DNA repair to occur. If the DNA damage cannot be adequately repaired, apoptosis is induced. At first much of cancer research focused on uncontrolled cell proliferation, now researchers are aware of the important role cell death has in maintaining homeostasis. Nonetheless, much remains to be done in terms of understanding the sequence of events that occur during apoptosis, which of them are essential to the normal process, and what is role of these processes in breast carcinogenesis. As already mentioned, p53 plays an important role in directing cells into apoptosis when DNA damage occurs. Other key players include the family of bcl2 proteins and ICE (interleukin 1ß-converting enzyme).

The bcl2 protein is a potent repressor of apoptosis, conferring survival advantage to cells expressing it. On the other hand, bax, another bcl2 family member, is capable of countering the death repressor activity of bcl2. Bax has been found to exist as a homodimer and is also capable of forming heterodimers with bcl2 *in vivo (156)*. Therefore the ratio of bax to bcl2 in a given cell may dictate whether the cell survives upon receiving apoptotic stimuli. This type of homeostatic control by the ratio of homodimers and heterodimers can be expanded to include several members of the bcl2 family. Some bcl2 family members act as promoters of apoptosis (like bax), while other members inhibit apoptosis (like bcl2). Although not a member of the bcl2 family, c-*myc* has been shown to cooperate with *bcl2* to achieve immortalization of tumor cells *(92)*. Bcl2 protein expression is highly variable in breast cancer and it has been suggested that high expression is associated with favorable clinicopathological features *(157,158)*. Recently a study analyzed the expression of *bcl2, bax, bcl-X*, and *bak* in small, nonmetastatic breast carcinomas, correlated levels of expression with apoptosis *(159)*. *Bcl2* expression but not *bcl-X* expression was associated with loss of apoptosis. Expression of *bax* and *bak* were significantly associated with increased apoptosis in the breast carcinomas. These large gene families form complex sets of interactions that may balance the scale either towards or away from apoptosis. To date, insufficient evidence is available to suggest whether alterations in pathways of apoptosis play a relevant role in breast carcinogenesis.

ESTROGEN AND BREAST CANCER

The role of estrogen as an important factor in the etiology and progression of human breast cancer has been well-documented. It was already observed 100 years ago that ovariectomy could lead to breast-cancer regression in premenopausal patients *(160)*. The extent of exposure to ovulatory cycles is one of the most important endogenous causes associated with a higher risk for development of sporadic breast cancer *(4)*. However, although the association of estrogen in the development of breast cancer is well-established, the fundamental mechanism(s) by which this hormone modulates cell growth and tumor development are not yet clear.

It is known from in vitro and in vivo studies that the mechanism of estrogen action is mediated through its binding to the ER, which in turn binds specific enhancer regions on the DNA and regulates gene transcription *(161)*. The interaction of estrogen with its receptors and the recruitment of accessory cofactor proteins to bind DNA and activate gene transcription has been the focus of intense recent research *(162)*. Nonetheless, important questions still remain. What are the main gene targets upon which estrogen acts to exert a growth response? What is the chronology of such events?

Estrogen has been shown to increase the pool of cells synthesizing DNA by recruiting noncycling cells into the cell cycle and by reducing the length of the G_1 phase *(163)*. The ability of estrogen to regulate the transcription of c-*myc* and c-*fos* is believed to be partly responsible for the stimulatory effects of estrogen on the cell cycle *(164)*. Entry into S phase was found to be preceded by increased activity of both cdk4 and cyclin E-cdk2 and hyperphosphorylation of pRb, all within the first 3–6 h of estradiol treatment *(165)*. The increase in cdk4 activity was accompanied by increases in *cyclin D1* mRNA and protein, indicating that an initiating event in the activation of cdk4 was increased *cyclin D1* gene expression. In addition, cyclin D1 has been shown to directly enhance transcription of *ER*-related genes *(166)*. Cyclin D1 does this without binding cdk4 and in the absence of estrogen, thereby identifying an additional role for cyclin D1 in promoting cell growth. However, the effects of estrogen on *cyclin D1* expression may not be a direct effect of the ER on the *cyclin D1* gene promoter. The ability of protein-synthesis inhibitors to abolish *cyclin D1* mRNA induction by estrogen, suggests intermediary proteins could be involved *(165)*. Clearly our understanding of how estrogen exerts its effects on breast tissue requires further analysis.

NEW TECHNOLOGIES AND FUTURE DIRECTIONS

It is estimated that within the next few years we will have compiled gene sequence information for the entire human genome. However, if we are to use this tremendous amount of information gained to improve the treatment of breast-cancer patients, it is imperative that we bridge the gap between genes and their relationship to a particular pathophysiological outcome. To date the majority of molecular biology research has focused on abnormalities of the genome such as mutation, gene amplification, and LOH. Identifying defects in the genome associated with breast cancer is the first level of genomic complexity. The next level of complexity is characterizing the changes in gene expression as a cell progresses from normal to malignant.

Present-day advances in gene expression technology are allowing researchers to study this next level of genomic complexity by defining global changes in gene expression. Technologies such as SAGE (Serial Analysis of Gene Expression) and microarray technologies are at the cutting edge of cancer research. Ultimately, the ability to understand the detailed mechanisms of tumor progression, from the very early stages of carcinogenesis through metastasis will allow researchers to identify key components and interactions of the malignant pathway.

The knowledge found by defining global and specific alterations in the transcription of premalignant and malignant cells, will allow researchers to concentrate on gene targets that better serve as diagnostic and prognostic tools. Ultimately, it will be ideal to achieve a very precise matching of specific treatment modalities to individual tumors exhibiting a characteristic growth profile, culminating with design of more rationale (molecularly based) therapeutic approaches.

ACKNOWLEDGMENT

The authors wish to thank contributing colleagues Andrzej Bednarek, Feng Jiang, Kathleen Hawkins, and Kendra Laflin, as well as Michelle Gardiner for her secretarial assistance and Chris Yone for art work. This work was supported by Grants DAMD 17-94-J-4078 and DAMD 17-96-1-6252 from the U.S. Army Breast Cancer Program; NIH Grant R01 CA59967; and Susan G. Komen Breast Cancer Foundation.

REFERENCES

1. Feuer, E., Wun L., Boring C., Flanders W., Timmel M., and Tong T. (1993) The lifetime risk of developing breast cancer. *J. Natl. Cancer Inst.* **85**:892–897.
2. Kelsey, J. and Horn-Ross, P. (1993) Breast cancer: magnitude of the problem and descriptive epidemiology. *Epidemiol. Rev.* **15**:7–16.
3. Wingo, P. A., Tong R., and Bolden, S. (1995) Cancer Statistics, 1995. *Ca: Cancer J. Clin.* **45**:8–30.
4. Pike, M., Spicer, D., Dahmoush, L., and Press, M. (1993) Estrogens, progesterones, normal breast cell proliferation, and breast cancer risk. *Epidemiol. Rev.* **15**:17.
5. McGregor, H., Land, C., Choi, K., Tokuoka, S., Liu, P., Wakabayashi, T., and Beebe, C. (1977) Breast cancer incidence among atomic bomb survivors, Hiroshima and Nagasaki, 1960–1969. *J. Natl. Cancer Inst.* **59**:799–811.
6. Bhatia, S., Robison, L., Oberlin, O., Greenberg, M., Bunin, G., Fossati-Bellani, F., et al. (1996) Breast cancer and other second neoplasms after childhood Hodgkin's disease. *N. Engl. J. Med.* **334**:745–751.
7. el-Bayoumy, K. (1992) Environmental carcinogens that may be involved in human breast cancer etiology. *Chem. Res. Toxicol.* **5**:585–590.
8. Wolff, M. and Weston, A. (1997) Breast cancer risk and environmental exposures. *Environ. Health Perspect.* **4**:891–896.
9. Russo, J., Rivera, R., and Russo, I. (1992) Influence of age and parity on the development of the human breast. *Breast Cancer Res. Treat.* **23**:211–218.
10. Wellings, S., Jensen, H., and Marcum, R. (1975) An atlas of subgross pathology of 16 human breasts with special reference to possible precancerous lesions. *J. Natl. Cancer Inst.* **55**:231–275.
11. Rosen, P. P. (1979) The pathological classification of human mammary carcinoma: past, present and future. *Ann. Clin. Lab. Sci.* **9**:144–156.
12. Tavassoli, F. (1992) *Pathology of the Breast.* Appleton & Lange, Norwalk, CT.
13. Silverstein, M., Lewinsky, B., Waisman, J., Gierson, E., Colburn, W., Senofsky, G., et al. (1994) Infiltrating lobular carcinoma. Is it different from infiltrating duct carcinoma? *Cancer* **73**:1673–1677.
14. Dixon, J. M., Anderson, T. J., Page, D. L., Lee, D., Duffy, S. W., and Stewart, H. J. (1983) Infiltrating lobular carcinoma of the breast: an evaluation of the incidence and consequence of bilateral disease. *Br. J. Surg.* **70**:513–516.
15. Ponten, J., Holmberg, L., Trichopoulos, D., Kallioniemi, O., Kvale, G., Wallgren, A., et al. (1990) Biology and natural history of breast cancer. *Int. J. Cancer* **5**:5–21.
16. Alpers, C. and Wellings, S. (1985) The prevalence of carcinoma in situ in normal and cancer-associated breasts. *Human Pathol.* **16**:796–807.
17. Dupont, W. and Page, D. (1985) Risk factors for breast cancer in women with proliferative breast disease. *N. Engl. J. Med.* **312**:146–151.
18. Solin, L., Recht, A., Kurtz, J., Kuske, R., McNeese, M., McCormick, B., et al. (1991) Ten-year results of breast-conserving surgery and definitive irradiation for intraductal carcinoma (ductal carcinoma in situ) of the breast. *Cancer* **68**:2337–2344.
19. Lakhani, S. R., Collins, N., Sloane, J. P., and Stratton, M. R. (1995) Loss of heterozygosity in lobular carcinoma in situ of the breast. *J. Clin. Pathol.* **48**:M74–M78.
20. Page, D. and Dupont, W. (1992) Benign breast disease: indicators of increased breast cancer risk. *Cancer Detect. Prevent.* **16**:93–97.
21. Newman, B., Austin, M., Lee, M., and King, M.-C. (1988) Inheritance of human breast cancer: evidence for autosomal dominant transmission in high-risk families. *Proc. Natl. Acad. Sci. USA* **85**:3044–3048.
22. Claus, E. B., Risch, N., and Thompson, W. D. (1991) Genetic analysis of breast cancer in the cancer and steroid hormone study. *Am. J. Human. Genet.* **48**:232–242.
23. Anderson, D. (1991) Familial versus sporadic breast cancer. *Cancer* **70**:1740–1746.
24. Liu, B., Parsons, R., Papadopoulos, N., Nicolaides, N. C., Lynch, H. T., Watson, P., et al. (1996) Analysis of mismatch repair genes in hereditary non-polyposis colorectal cancer patients. *Nature Med.* **2**:169–174.
25. Kolodner, R., Hall ,N., Lipford, J., Kane, M., Rao, M., Morrison, P., et al. (1994) Structure of the human MSH2 locus and analysis of two Muir-Torre kindreds for MSH2 mutations. *Genomics* **24**:516–526.
26. Bowcock, A. M., Anderson, L. A., Friedman, L. S., Black, D. M., Osborne-Lawrence, S., Rowell, S. E., et al. (1993) THRA1 and D17S183 flank an interval of <4cM for the breast-ovarian cancer gene (BRCA1) on chromosome 17q21. *Am. J. Human Genet.* **52**:718–722.
27. Chamberlain, J., Boehnke, M., Frank, T., Kiousis, S., Xu, J., Guo, S., et al. (1993) BRCA1 maps proximal to D17S579 on chromosome 17q21 by genetic analysis. *Am. J. Human Genet.* **52**:792–798.
28. Easton, D., Bishop, D., Ford, D., and Crockford, G. (1993) Genetic linkage analysis in familial breast and ovarian cancer: results from 214 families. The Breast Cancer Linkage Consortium. *Am. J. Human Genet.* **52**:678–701.
29. Miki, Y., Swensen, J., Shattuck-Eidens, D., Futreal, P., Harshman, K., Tavtigian, S., et al. (1994) A strong candidate for the breast and ovarian cancer susceptibility gene BRCA1. *Science* **266**:66–71.
30. Chapman, M. and Verma, I. (1996) Transcriptional activation by BRCA1. *Nature* **382**:678–679.
31. Cornelisse, C., Cornelis, R., and Devilee, P. (1996) Genes responsible for familial breast cancer. *Pathol. Res. Practice* **192**:684–693.
32. Futreal, P., Söderkvist, P., Marks, J., Iglehart, J., Cochran, C., Barrett, J., et al. (1992) Detection of frequent allelic loss on proximal chromosome 17q in sporadic breast carcinoma using microsatellite lenght polymorphisms. *Cancer Res.* **52**:2624–2627.
33. Cropp, C., Champeme, M.-H., Lidereau, R., and Callahan, R. (1993) Identification of three regions on chromosome 17q in primary human breast carcinomas which are frequently deleted. *Cancer Res.* **53**:5617–5619.
34. Saito, H., Inazawa, J., Saito, S., Kasumi, F., Koi, S., Sagae, S., et al. (1993) Detailed deletion mapping of chromosome 17q in ovarian and breast cancers: 2-cM region on 17q21.3 often and commonly deleted in tumors. *Cancer Res.* **53**:3382–3385.
35. Devilee, P. and Cornelisse, C. (1990) Genetics of human breast cancer. *Cancer Surv.* **9**:605–630.
36. Chen, Y., Chen, C., Riley, D., Allred, D., Chen, P., Von Hoff, D., et al. (1995) Aberrant subcellular localization of BRCA1 in breast cancer. *Science* **270**:789–791.
37. Jensen, R., Thompson, M., Jetton, T., Szabo, C., van der Meer, R., Helou, B., et al. (1996) BRCA1 is secreted and exhibits properties of a granin. *Nature Genet.* **12**:303–308.
38. Scully, R., Ganesan, S., Brown, M., DeCaprio, J., Cannistra, S., Feunteun, J., et al. (1996) Localization of BRCA1 in human breast and ovarian cancer cells. *Science* **272**:122.
39. Smith, S., Easton, D., Evans, D., and Ponder, B. (1992) Allele losses in the region 17q12-q21 in familial breast and ovarian cancer involve the wild-type chromosome. *Nature Genet.* **2**:128.
40. Scully, R., Chen, J., Plug, A., Xiao, Y., Weaver, D., Feunteun, J., Ashely, T., et al. (1997) Association of BRCA1 with Rad51 in mitotic and meiotic cells. *Cell* **88**:265–275.
41. Chen, T., Sahin, A., and Aldaz, C. (1996) Deletion map of chromosome 16q in ductal carcinoma *in situ* of the breast: refining a putative tumor suppressor gene region. *Cancer Res.* **56**:5605–5609.

42. Gowen, L., Avrutskaya, A., Latour, A., Koller, B., and Leadon, S. (1998) BRCA1 required for transcription-coupled repair of oxidative DNA damage. *Science* **281**:1009–1012.

43. Wooster, R., Neuhausen, S., Mangion, J., Quirk, Y., Ford, D., Collins, N., et al. (1994) Localization of a breast cancer susceptibility gene, BRCA2, to chromosome 13q12-13. *Science* **265**:2088–2090.

44. Wooster, R., Bignell, G., Lancaster, J., Swift, S., Seal, S., Mangion, J., et al. (1995) Identification of the breast cancer susceptibility gene BRCA2. *Nature* **378**:789–792.

45. Struewing, J., Abeliovich, D., Peretz, T., Avishai, N., Kaback, M., Collins, F., et al. (1995) The carrier frequency of the BRCA1 185delAG mutation is approximately 1 percent in Ashkenazi Jewish individuals. *Nature Genet.* **11**:198–200.

46. Ford, D., Easton, D. F., Stratton, M., Narod, S., Goldgar, D., Devilee, P., et al. (1998) Genetic heterogeneity and penetrance analysis of the BRCA1 and BRCA2 genes in breast cancer families. *Am. J. Human Genet.* **62**:676–689.

47. Malkin, D., Li, F., Strong, L., Fraumeni, J. J., Nelson, C., Kim, D., et al. (1990) Germline p53 mutations in a familial syndrome of breast cancer, sarcomas, and other neoplasms. *Science* **250**:1233–1238.

48. Srivastava, S., Zou, Z., Pirollo, K., Blattner, W., and Chang, E. (1990) Germ-line transmission of a mutated p53 gene in a cancer-prone family with Li-Fraumeni syndrome. *Nature* **348**:747–749.

49. Osborne, R., Merlo, G., Mitsudomi, T., Venesio, T., Liscia, D., Cappa, A., et al. (1991) Mutations in the p53 gene in primary human breast cancers. *Cancer Res.* **51**:6194–6198.

50. Nelen, M., Padberg, G., Peeters, E., Lin, A., van den Helm, B., Frants, R., et al. (1996) Localization of the gene for Cowden disease to chromosome 10q22-23. *Nature Genet.* **13**:114–116.

51. Liaw, D., Marsh, D., Li, J., Dahia, P., Wang S., Zheng, Z., et al. (1997) Germline mutations of the PTEN gene in Cowden disease, an inherited breast and thyroid cancer syndrome. *Nature Genet.* **16**:64–67.

52. Steck, P., Pershouse, M., Jasser, S., Yung, W., Lin, H., Ligon, A., et al. (1997) Identification of a candidate tumour suppressor gene, MMAC1, at chromosome 10q23.3 that is mutated in multiple advanced cancers. *Nature Genet.* **15**:356–362.

53. Li, J., Yen, C., Liaw, D., Podsypania, K., Bose, S., Wang, S., et al. (1997) PTEN, a putative protein tyrosine phosphatase gene mutated in human brain, breast, and prostate cancer. *Science* **275**:1876–1878.

54. Cairns, P., Okami, K., Halachmi, S., Halachmi, N., Esteller, M., Herman, J., et al. (1997) Frequent inactivation of PTEN/MMAC1 in primary prostate cancer. *Cancer Res.* **57**:4997–5000.

55. Risinger, J., Hayes, A., Berchuck, A., and Barrett, J. (1997) PTEN/MMAC1 mutations in endometrial cancers. *Cancer Res.* **57**:4736–4738.

56. Rhei, E., Kang, L., Bogomolniy, F., Federici, M., Borgen, P., and Boyd, J. (1997) Mutation analysis of the putative tumor suppressor gene PTEN/MMAC1 in primary breast carcinoma. *Cancer Res.* **57**:3657–3659.

57. Ueda, K., Nishijima, M., Inui, H., Watatani, M., Yayoi, E., Okamura, J., et al. (1998) Infrequent mutations in the PTEN/MMAC1 gene among primary breast cancers. *Jpn. J. Cancer Res.* **89**:17–21.

58. Gatti, R., Berkel, I., Boder, E., Braedt, G., Charmley, P., Concannon, P., et al. (1988) Localization of an ataxia-telangiectasia gene to chromosome 11q22-23. *Nature* **336**:577–580.

59. FitzGerald, M., Bean, J., Hegde, S., Unsal, H., MacDonald, D., Harkin, D., et al. (1997) Heterozygous ATM mutations do not contribute to early onset of breast cancer. *Nature Genet.* **15**:307–310.

60. Chen, J., Birkholtz, G., Lindblom, P., Rubio, C., and Lindblom, A. (1998) The role of ataxia-telangiectasia heterozygotes in familial breast cancer. *Cancer Res.* **58**:1376–1379.

61. Krontiris, T., Devlin, B., Karp, D., Robert, N., and Risch, N. (1993) An association between the risk of cancer and mutations in the HRAS1 minisatellite locus. *N. Engl. J. Med.* **329**:517–523.

62. Garrett, P., Hulka, B., Kim, Y., and Farber, R. (1993) HRAS protooncogene polymorphism and breast cancer. *Cancer Epidemiol. Biomarkers Prevent.* **2**:131–138.

63. Hall, J., Huey, B., Morrow, J., Newman, B., Lee, M., Jones, E., et al. (1990) Rare HRAS alleles and susceptibility to human breast cancer. *Genomics* **6**:188–191.

64. Rebbeck, T., Couch, F., Kant, J., Calzone, K., Deshano, M., Peng, Y., et al. (1996) Genetic heterogeneity in hereditary breast cancerz: role of BRCA1 and BRCA2. *Am. J. Human Genet.* **59**:547–553.

65. Ambrosone, C. B. and Shields, P. G. (1997) Molecular epidemiology of breast cancer. *In: Etiology of Breast and Gynecological Cancers,* vol. 396 (Aldaz, C.M., Gould, M.N., McLachlan, J. and Slaga, T. J., rds), Wiley-Liss, New York, pp. 83–99.

66. Helzlsouer, K., Selmin, O., Huang, H., Strickland, P., Hoffman, S., Alberg, A., et al. (1998) Associate between glutathione S-transferase M1, P1, and T1 genetic polymorphisms and development of breast cancer. *J. Natl. Cancer Inst.* **90**:512–518.

67. Brunet, J., Ghadirian, P., Rebbeck, T., Lerman, C., Garber, J., Tonin, P., et al. (1998) Effect of smoking on breast cancer in carriers of mutant BRCA1 or BRCA2 genes. *J. Natl. Cancer Inst.* **90**:761–766.

68. Devilee, P. and Cornelisse C. (1994) Somatic genetic changes in human breast cancer. *Biochim. Biophys. Acta* **1198**:113–130.

69. Thompson, F., Emerson, J., Dalton, W., Yang, J.-M., McGee, D., Villar, H., et al. (1993) Clonal chromosome abnormalities in human breast carcinomas I. Twenty-eight cases with primary disease. *Genes Chromosomes Cancer* **7**:185–193.

70. Dutrillaux, B., Gerbault-Seureau, M. and Zafrani, B. (1990) Characterization of chromosomal anomalies in human breast cancer. A comparison of 30 paradiploid cases with few chromosome changes. *Cancer Genet. Cytogenet.* **49**:203–217.

71. Pandis, N., Heim, S., Bardi, G., Idvall, I., Mandahl, N., and Mitelman, F. (1992) Whole-arm t(1;16) and i(1q) as sole anomalies identify gain of 1q as a primary chromosomal abnormality in breast cancer. *Genes Chromosomes Cancer* **5**:235–238.

72. Kallioniemi, A., Kallioniemi, O.-P., Sudar, D., Rutovitz, D., Gray, J., Waldman, F., et al. (1992) Comparative genomic hybridization for molecular cytogenetic analysis of solid tumors. *Science* **258**:818–820.

73. Kallioniemi, A., Kallioniemi, O.-P., Piper, J., Tanner, M., Stokke, T., Chen, L., et al. (1994) Detection and mapping of amplified DNA sequences in breast cancer by comparative genomic hybridization. *Proc. Natl. Acad. Sci. USA* **91**:2156–2160.

74. Gray, J., Collins, C., Henderson, I., Isola, J., Kallioniemi, A., Kallioniemi, O.-P., et al. (1994) Molecular cytogenetics of human breast cancer. *Cold Spring Harbor Symp. Quant. Biol.* **59**:645–652.

75. Isola, J., Kallioniemi, O., Chu, L., Fuqua, S., Hilsenbeck, S., Osborne, C., et al. (1995) Genetic aberrations detected by comparative genomic hybridization predict outcome in node-negative breast cancer. *Am. J. Pathol.* **147**:905–911.

76. Venter, D. J., Tuzi, N. L., Kumar, S., and Gullick, W. J. (1987) Overexpression of the c-erbB-2 oncoprotein in human breast carcinomas: Immunohistological assessment correlates with gene amplification. *Lancet* **2**:69–72.

77. Slamon, D. J., Godolphin, W., Jones, L. A., Holt, J. A., Wong, S. G., Keith, D. E., et al. (1989) Studies of the HER-2/neu proto-oncogene in human breast and ovarian cancer. *Science* **244**:707–712.

78. Berger, M., Locher, G., Saurer, S., Gullick, W., Waterfield, M., Groner, B. et al. (1988) Correlation of C-ERBB-2 gene amplification and protein expression in human breast carcinoma with nodal status and nuclear grading. *Cancer Res.* **48**:1238–1243.

79. Zhou, D., Battifora, H., Yokota, J., Yamamoto, T., and Cline, M. (1987) Association of multiple copies of the c-erbb-2 oncogene with spread of breast cancer. *Cancer Res.* **47**:6123–6125.

80. Ravdin, P. and Chamness, G. (1995) The c-erbB-2 proto-oncogene as a prognostic and predictive marker in breast cancer: a paradigm for the development of other macromolecular markers : a review. *Gene* **159**:19–27.

81. Aldaz, C., Chen, T., Sahin, A., Cunningham, J., and Bondy, M. (1995) Comparative allelotype of in situ and invasive human breast cancer: high frequency of microsatellite instability in lobular breast carcinomas. *Cancer Res.* **55**:3976–3981.

82. Muss, H. B., Thor, A. D., Berry, D. A., Kute, T., Liu, E. T., Koerner, F., et al. (1994) c-erbB-2 expression and response to adjuvant

therapy in women with node- positive early breast cancer. *N. Engl. J. Med.* **330**:1260–1266.

83. Leitzel, K., Teramoto, Y., Konrad, K., Chinchilli, V. M., Volas, G., Grossberg, H., et al. (1995) Elevated serum c-erbB-2 antigen levels and decreased response to hormone therapy of breast cancer. *J. Clin. Oncol.* **13**:1129–1135.

84. Muller, W., Sinn, E., Pattengale, P., Wallace, R., and Leder, P. (1988) Single-step induction of mammary adenocarcinoma in transgenic mice bearing the activated c-neu oncogene. *Cell* **54**:105–115.

85. Petit, A., Rak, J., Hung, M., Rockwell, P., Goldstein, N., Fendly, B., et al. (1997) Neutralizing antibodies against epidermal growth factor and ErbB-2/neu receptor tyrosine kinases down-regulate vascular endothelial growth factor production by tumor cells in vitro and in vivo: angiogenic implications for signal transduction therapy of solid tumors. *Am. J. Pathol.* **151**:1523–1530.

86. Wright, M., Grim, J., Deshane, J., Kim, M., Strong, T., Siegal, G., et al. (1997) An intracellular anti-erbB-2 single-chain antibody is specifically cytotoxic to human breast carcinoma cells overexpressing erbB-2. *Gene Ther.* **4**:317–322.

87. Eccles, S., Court, W., Box, G., Dean, C., Melton, R., and Springer, C. (1994) Regression of established breast carcinoma xenografts with antibody- directed enzyme prodrug therapy against c-erbB2 p185. *Cancer Res.* **54**:5171–5177.

87a. Baselga, J., (2001) Clinical trials of Herceptin (trastuzumab). *Eur. J. Canc.* **37**: 518–524.

88. Sandgren, E. P., Luetteke, N. C., Palmiter, R. D., Brinster, R. L., and Lee, D. C. (1990) Overexpression of TGF alpha in transgenic mice: induction of epithelial hyperplasia, pancreatic metaplasia, and carcinoma of the breast. *Cell* **61**:1121–1135.

89. Cohen, B. D., Siegall, C. B., Bacus, S., Foy, L., Green, J. M., Hellstrom, I., et al. (1998) Role of epidermal growth factor receptor family members in growth and differentiation of breast carcinoma. *Biochem. Soc. Symp.* **63**:199–210.

90. Visscher, D., Wallis, T., Awussah, S., Mohamed, A., and Crissman, J. (1997) Evaluation of MYC and chromosome 8 copy number in breast carcinoma by interphase cytogenetics. *Genes Chromosomes Cancer* **18**:1–7.

91. Chin, L., Liegeois, N., DePinho, R., and Schreiber-Agus, N. (1996) Functional interactions among members of the Myc superfamily and potential relevance to cutaneous growth and development. *J. Invest. Dermatol. Symp. Proc.* **1**:128–135.

92. White, E. (1996) Life, death and the pursuit of apoptosis. *Genes Dev.* **10**:1–15.

93. Alexandrow, M. G., Kawabata, M., Aakre, M., and Moses, H. L. (1995) Overexpression of the c-Myc oncoprotein blocks the growth-inhibitory response but is required for the mitogenic effects of transforming growth factor beta 1. *Proc. Natl. Acad. Sci. USA* **92**:3239–3243.

94. Evan, G. and Littlewood, T. (1993) The role of c-myc in cell growth. *Curr. Opin. Genet. Dev.* **3**:44–49.

95. Shi, Y., Glynn, J., Guilbert, L., Cotter, T., Bissonnette, R., and Green, D. (1992) Role for c-myc in activation-induced apoptotic cell death in T cell hybridomas. *Science* **257**:212–214.

96. Steiner, P., Rudolph, B., Muller, D., and Eilers, M. (1996) The functions of Myc in cell cycle progression and apoptosis. *Prog. Cell Cycle Res.* **2**:73–82.

97. Leder, A., Pattengale, P., Kuo, A., Stewart, T., and Leder, P. (1986) Consequences of widespread deregulation of the c-myc gene in transgenic mice: multiple neoplasms and normal development. *Cell* **45**:485–495.

98. Varley, J., Swallow, J., Brammar, W., Whittaker, J., and Walker, R. (1987) Alterations to either C-ERBB-2 (NEU) or C-MYC proto-oncogenes in breast carcinomas correlate with poor short-term prognosis. *Oncogene* **1**:423–430.

99. Shiu, R., Watson, P., and Dubik (1993) c-myc oncogene expression in estrogen-dependent and independent breast cancer. *Clin. Chem.* **39**:353–355.

100. Lammie, G. and Peters, G. (1991) Chromosome 11q13 abnormalities in human cancer. *Cancer Cells* **3**:413–420.

101. Gillett, C., Fantl, V., Smith, R., Fisher, C., Bartek, J., Dickson, C., et al. (1994) Amplification and overexpression of cyclin D1 in breast cancer detected by immunohistochemical staining. *Cancer Res.* **54**:1812–1817.

102. Bartkova, J., Lukas, J., Muller, H., Lutzhft, D., Strauss, M., and Bartek, J. (1994) Cyclin D1 protein expression and function in human breast cancer. *Int. J. Cancer* **57**:353–361.

103. Sicinski, P., Donaher, J. L., Parker, S., Li, T., Fazeli, A., Gardner, H., et al. (1995) Cyclin D1 provides a link between development and oncogenes in the retina and breast. *Cell* **82**:621–630.

104. Wang, T., Cardiff, R., Zukerberg, L., Lees, E., Arnold, A., and Schmidt, E. (1994) Mammary hyperplasia and carcinoma in MMTV-cyclin D1 transgenic mice. *Nature* **369**:669–671.

105. Weinstat-Saslow, D., Merino, M., Manrow, R., Lawrence, J., Bluth, R., Wittenbel, K., et al. (1995) Overexpression of cyclin D mRNA distinguishes invasive and in situ breast carcinomas from nonmalignant lesions. *Nature Med.* **1**:1257–1260.

106. Muller, W., Lee, F., Dickson, C., Peters, G., Pattengale, P., and Leder, P. (1990) The int-2 gene product acts as an epithelial growth factor in transgenic mice. *EMBO J.* **9**:907–913.

107. Anzick, S. L., Kononen, J., Walker, R. L., Azorsa, D. O., Tanner, M. M., Guan, X. Y., et al. (1997) AIB1, a steroid receptor coactivator amplified in breast and ovarian cancer. *Science* **277**:965–968.

108. Knudson, A. (1971) Mutation and cancer: statistical study of retinoblastoma. *Proc. Natl. Acad. Sci. USA* **68**:820–823.

109. Comings, D. (1973) A general theory of carcinogenesis. *Proc. Natl. Acad. Sci. USA* **70**:3324–3328.

110. Goodrich, D. and Lee, W.-H. (1993) Molecular characterization of the retinoblastoma susceptibility gene. *Biochim. Biophys. Acta* **1155**:43–61.

111. Cox, L., Chen, G., and Lee, E. Y.-H. P. (1994) Tumor suppressor genes and their roles in breast cancer. *Breast Cancer Res. Treat.* **32**:19–38.

112. Weber, J. and May, P. (1989) Abundant class of human DNA polymorphisms which can be typed using the polymerase chain reaction. *Am. J. Human Genet.* **44**:388–396.

113. Hudson, T. J., Stein, L. D., Gerety, S. S., Ma, J., Castle, A. B., Silva, J., et al. (1995) An STS-based map of the human genome. *Science* **270**:1945–1954.

114. Brenner, A. and Aldaz, C. (1995) Chromosome 9p allelic loss and p16/CDKN2 in breast cancer and evidence of p16 inactivation in immortal breast epithelial cells. *Cancer Res.* **55**:2892–2895.

115. Trent, J., Yang, J.-M., Emerson, J., Dalton, W., McGee, D., Massey, K., et al. (1993) Clonal chromosome abnormalities in human breast carcinomas II. Thirty-four cases with metastatic disease. *Genes Chromosomes Cancer* **7**:194–203.

116. Radford, D., Fair, K., Phillips, N., Ritter, J., Steinbrueck, T., Holt, M., et al. (1995) Allelotyping of ductal carcinoma in situ of the breast: deletion of loci on 8p, 13q, 16q, 17p and 17q. *Cancer Res.* **55**:3399–3405.

117. Fujii, H., Marsh, C., Cairns, P., Sidransky, D., and Gabrielson, E. (1996) Genetic divergence in the clonal evolution of breast cancer. *Cancer Res.* **56**:1493–1497.

118. Radford, D., Fair, K., Thompson, A., Ritter, J., Holt, M., Steinbrueck, T., et al. (1993) Allelic loss on a chromosome 17 in ductal carcinoma in situ of the breast. *Cancer Res.* **53**:2947–2949.

119. Done, S., Arneson, N., Ozcelik, H., Redston, M., and Andrulis, I. (1998) p53 mutations in mammary ductal carcinoma in situ but not in epithelial hyperplasias. *Cancer Res.* **58**:785–789.

120. Ozbun, M. and Butel, J. (1995) Tumor suppressor p53 mutations and breast cancer: a critical analysis. *Adv. Cancer Res.* **66**:71–141.

121. Donehower, L., Godley, L., Aldaz, C., Pyle, R., Shi, Y., Pinkel, D., et al. (1995) Deficiency of p53 accelerates mammary tumorigenesis in Wnt-1 transgenic mice and promotes chromosomal instability. *Genes Dev.* **9**:882–895.

122. Cornelis, R., van Vliet, M., Vos, C., Cleton-Jansen, A.-M., van de Vijver, M., Peterse, J., et al. (1994) Evidence for a gene on 17p13.3, distal to TP53, as a target for allele loss in breast tumors without p53 mutations. *Cancer Res.* **54**:4200–4206.

123. Hall, J., Lee, M., Newman, B., Morrow, J., Anderson, L., Huey, B., et al. (1990) Linkage of early-onset familial breast cancer to chromosome 17q21. *Science* **250**:1684–1689.

124. Futreal, P., Liu, Q., Shattuck-Eidens, D., Cochran, C., Harshman, K., Tavtigian, S., et al. (1994) BRCA1 mutations in primary breast and ovarian carcinomas. *Science* **266**:120–122.

125. Leone, A., McBride, O., Weston, A., Wang, M., Anglard, P., Cropp, C., et al. (1991) Somatic allelic deletion of nm23 in human cancer. *Cancer Res.* **51**:2490–2493.

126. Cropp, C., Lidereau, R., Leone, A., Liscia, D., Cappa, A., Campbell, G., et al. (1994) NME1 protein expression and loss of heterozygosity mutations in primary human breast tumors. *J. Natl. Cancer Inst.* **86**:1167–1169.

127. Borg, A., Zhang, Q.-X., Alm, P., Olsson H., and Sellberg, G. (1992) The retinoblastoma gene in breast cancer: allele loss is not correlated with loss of gene protein expression. *Cancer Res.* **52**:2991–2994.

128. Miki, Y., Katagiri, T., Kasumi, F., Yoshimoto, T., and Nakamura, Y. (1996) Mutation analysis in the BRCA2 gene in primary breast cancers. *Nature Genet.* **13**:245–247.

129. Teng, D., Bogden, R., Mitchell, J., Baumgard, M., Bell, R., Berry, S., et al. (1996) Low incidence of BRCA2 mutations in breast carcinoma and other cancers. *Nature Genet.* **13**:241–244.

130. Lancaster, J. M., Wooster, R., Mangion, J., Phelan, C. M., Cochran, C., Gumbs, C., et al. (1996) BRCA2 mutations in primary breast and ovarian cancers. *Nature Genet.* **13**:238–240.

131. Schott, D., Chang, J., Deng, G., Kurisu, W., Kuo, W., Gray, J., et al. (1994) A candidate tumor suppressor gene in human breast cancers. *Cancer Res.* **54**:1393–1396.

132. Sato, T., Tanigami, A., Yamakawa, K., Akiyama, F., Kasumi, F., Sakamoto, G., et al. (1990) Allelotype of breast cancer: cumulative allele losses promote tumor progression in primary breast cancer. *Cancer Res.* **50**:7184–7189.

133. Tsuda, H., Callen, D., Fukutomi, T., Nakamura, Y., and Hirohashi, S. (1994) Allele loss on chromosome 16q24..2-qter occurs frequently in breast cancer irrespectively of differences in phenotype and extent of spread. *Cancer Res.* **54**:513–517.

134. Cleton-Jansen, A., Moerland, E., Kuipers-Dijkshoorn, N., Callen, D., Sutherland, G., Hansen, B., et al. (1994) At least two different regions are involved in allelic imbalance on chromosome arm 16q in breast cancer. *Genes Chromosomes Cancer* **9**:101–107.

135. Berx, G., Cleton-Jansen, A., Nollet, F., de Leeuw, W., van de Vijver, M., Cornelisse, C., et al. (1995) E-cadherin is a tumour/invasion suppressor gene mutated in human lobular breast cancers. *EMBO J.* **14**:6107–6115.

136. Yoshiura, K., Kanai, Y., Ochiai, A., Shimoyama, Y., Sugimura, T., and Hirohashi, S. (1995) Silencing of the E-cadherin invasion-suppressor gene by CpG methylation in human carcinomas. *Proc. Natl. Acad. Sci. USA* **92**:7416–7419.

137. Rimm, D., Sinard, J., and Morrow, J. (1995) Reduced α-catenin and E-cadherin expression in breast cancer. *Lab. Invest.* **72**:506–512.

138. Lee, S. (1996) H-cadherin, a novel cadherin with growth inhibitory functions and diminished expression in human breast cancer. *Nature Med.* **2**:776–782.

138a. Bedmarck, A. K., Laflin, K. J., Daniel, K. J., Lino, Q., Hawkins, K. A., Aldez, C. M. (2000) WWOX, a novel WWdomain, containing protein mapping to human chomosome 16a 23.3–24.1 a region frequently affected in breast cancer. *Cancer Res.* **60**: 2140–2145.

139. Kamb, A., Gruis, N., Weaver-Feldhaus, J., Qingyun, L., Harshman, K., Tavtigian, S., et al. (1994) A cell cycle regulator potentially involved in genesis of many tumor types. *Science* **264**:436–440.

140. Brenner, A., Paladugu, A., Wang, H., Olopade, O., Dreyling, M., and Aldaz, C. (1996) Preferential loss of expression of p16^{INK4a} rather than p19^{ARF} in breast cancer. *Clin. Cancer Res.* **2**:1993–1998.

141. Altucci, L., Addeo, R., and Cicatiello, L. (1996) 17β-estradiol induces cyclin D1 gene transcription, p36D1-p34cdk4 complex activation and p105Rb phosphorylation during mitogenic stimulation of G1-arrested human breast cancer cells. *Oncogene* **12**:2315–2324.

142. Sherr, C. (1994) G1 phase progression: cycling on cue. *Cell* **79**:551–555.

143. Sherr, C. (1996) Cancer cell cycles. *Science* **274**:1672–1677.

144. Hui, R., Cornish, A., Mcclelland, R., Robertson, J., Blamey, R., Musgrove, E., et al. (1996) Cyclin D1 and estrogen receptor messenger RNA levels are positively correlated in primary breast cancer. *Clin. Cancer Res.* **2**:923–928.

145. Graybablin, J., Zalvide, J., Fox, M., Kinckerbocker, C., Decaprio, J., and Keyomarsi, K. (1996) Cyclin E, a redundant cyclin in breast cancer. *Proc. Natl. Acad. Sci. USA* **93**:15215–15220.

146. Porter, P., Malone, K., Heagerty, P., Alexander, G., Gatti, L., Firpo, E., et al. (1997) Expression of cell-cycle regulators p27^{Kip1} and cyclin E, alone and in combination, correlate with survival in young breast cancer patients. *Nature Med.* **3**:222–225.

147. Varley, J., Armour, J., Swallow, J., Jeffreys, A., Ponder, B., T'Ang, A., et al. (1989) The retinoblastoma gene is frequently altered leading to loss of expression in primary breast tumours. *Oncogene* **4**:725–729.

148. Okamoto, A., Demetrick, D., Spillare, E., Hagiwara, K., Hussain, S., Bennett, W., et al. (1994) Mutations and altered expression of p16INK4 in human cancer. *Proc. Natl. Acad. Sci. USA* **91**:11045–11049.

149. Parry, D., Bates, S., Mann, D., and Peters, G. (1995) Lack of cyclin D-Cdk complexes in Rb-negative cells correlates with high levels of p16$^{INK4/MTS1}$ tumour suppressor product. *EMBO J.* **14**:503–511.

150. Xiong, Y., Hannon, G., Zhang, H., Casso, D., Kobayashi, R., and Beach, D. (1993) p21 is a universal inhibitor of cyclin kinases. *Nature* **366**:701–704.

151. Waga, S., Hannon, G., Beach, D., and Stillman, B. (1994) The p21 inhibitor of cyclin-dependent kinases controls DNA replication by interaction with PCNA. *Nature* **369**:574–578.

152. Brugarolas, J., Chandrasekaran, C., Gordon, J., Beach, D., Jacks, T., and Hannon, G. (1995) Radiation-induced cell cycle arrest compromised by p21 deficiency. *Nature* **377**:552–557.

153. Pomerantz, J., Schreiber-Agus, N., Liegeois, N., Silverman, A., Alland, L., Chin, L., et al. (1998) The Ink4a tumor suppressor gene product, p19^{Arf}, interacts with MDM2 and neutralizes MDM2's inhibition of p53. *Cell* **92**:713–723.

154. Zhang, Y., Xiong, Y., and Yarbrough, W. G. (1998) ARF promotes MDM2 degradation and stablizes p53: ARF-INK4a locus deletion impairs both the Rb and p53 tumor suppression pathways. *Cell* **92**:725–734.

155. Bates, S., Phillips, A. C., Clark, P. A., Stott, F., Peters, G., Ludwig, R. L., et al. (1998) p14ARF links the tumour suppressors RB and p53. *Nature* **395**:124–125.

156. Oltvai, Z., Milliman, C., and Korsmeyer, S. (1993) Bcl-2 heterodimerizes in vivo with a conserved homolog, Bax, accelerates programmed cell death. *Cell* **74**:609–619.

157. Joensuu, H., Pylkkanen, L., and Toikkanen, S. (1994) Bcl-2 protein expression and long-term survival in breast cancer. *Am. J. Pathol.* **145**:1191–1198.

158. Barbareschi, M., Caffo, O., Veronese, S., Leek, R., Fina, P., Fox, S., et al. (1996) Bcl-2 and p53 expression in node-negative breast carcinoma: a study with long-term follow-up. *Human Pathol.* **27**:1149–1155.

159. Sierra, A., Castellsague, X., Coll, T., Manas, S., Escobedo, A., Moreno, A., et al. (1998) Expression of death-related genes and their relationship to loss of apoptosis in T1 ductal breast carcinomas. *Int. J. Cancer* **79**:103–110.

160. Beatson, G. (1896) On the treatment of inoperable cases of carcinoma of the mamma: suggestions for a new method of treatment, with illustrative cases. *Lancet* **ii**:104–107.

161. Fishman, J., Osborne, M., and Telang, N. (1995) The role of estrogen in mammary carcinogenesis. *Ann. NY Acad. Sci.* **768**:91–100.

162. Tsai, M. and O'Malley, B. (1994) Molecular mechanisms of action of steroid/thyroid receptor superfamily members. *Ann. Rev. Biochem.* **63**:451–486.

163. Leung, B. and Potter, A. (1987) Mode of estrogen action on cell proliferation in CAMA-1 cells: II. Sensitivity of G1 phase population. *J. Cell. Biochem.* **34**:213–225.

164. Davidson, N., Prestigiacomo, L., and Hahm, H. (1993) Induction of jun gene family members by transforming growth factor alpha but not 17 beta-estradiol in human breast cancer cells. *Cancer Res.* **53**:291–297.

165. Prall, O., Sarcevic, B., Musgrove, E., Watts, C., and Sutherland, R. (1997) Estrogen-induced activation of Cdk4 and Cdk2 during G1-Sphase progression is accompanied by increased cyclin D1 expression and decreased cyclin-dependent kinase inhibitor association with cyclin E-Cdk2. *J. Biol. Chem.* **272**:10882–10894.

166. Zwijsen, R., Wientjens, E., Klompmaker, R., van der Sman, J., Bernards, R., and Michalides, R. (1997) CDK-independent activation of estrogen receptor by cyclin D1. *Cell* **88**:405–415.

167. Zhang, L., Zhou, W., Velculescu, V., Kern, S., Hruban, R., Hamilton, S., et al. (1997) Gene expression profiles in normal and cancer cells. *Science* **276**:1268–1272.

168. Perov, C. M., Soulie, T., Eisen, M. B., van de Kijin, M., Jeffrey, S. S., Rees, C. A., et al. (2000) Molecular portraits of human breast tumors. *Nature* **406**:747–752.

16 The Molecular Basis of Prostate Carcinogenesis

ALLEN C. GAO, MD, PhD AND JOHN T. ISAACS, PhD

INTRODUCTION

Prostate cancer is a major health problem in men in the Western world. It is the most commonly diagnosed cancer in the United States, with an estimated 334,500 new cases diagnosed in 1997 (1), compared to 165,000 cases in 1993 (2). This dramatic increase in prostate cancer is due in part to an increasing elderly population and better methods for detection at an early stage in individual patients. This latter effect is related to the development of serum assays for prostate specific antigen (PSA), which has led to a substantial increase in the number of digital rectal examinations, transrectal ultrasound (US) examinations, and prostatic needle biopsies performed in the clinic. Despite the improved early detection, the death rate due to prostate cancer within the United States remains high (second only to lung cancer), with an estimated 41,800 prostate cancer deaths in 1997 (1). As the life expectancy of the male population increases over time, it is anticipated that the prevalence and mortality from the prostate cancer will also increase. Despite the high incidence of prostate cancer, the etiology and risk factors for development of this tumor remain largely unknown. However, it is recognized that factors related to heredity, environment, and lifestyle are important in prostate carcinogenesis (3).

The prostate grows from a size of about 2–3 g at puberty to reach its maximal normal size of 20 g by 20 yr of life (4). This normal growth is dependent on a physiological level of testicular androgen, which both stimulates proliferation and inhibits apoptotic death of the prostate cells (4). In the adult, the prostate is a pear-shaped glandular organ composed of a mixture of well-developed stromal tissues, predominantly smooth-muscle cells, surrounding acinar structures comprising epithelial cells with an outer fibrous capsule. The prostate gland is composed of four separated regions (5). These include: 1) the peripheral zone, constituting over 70% of the glandular prostate; 2) the central zone, constituting 25% of the glandular prostate; 3) the peri-urethral transition zone region; and 4) the anterior fibro-muscular stroma (5). The growth pattern of the prostate gland is unique in that it is one of the few organs that continues to grow throughout life, such that the size of a prostate gland from a 65-yr-old man is, on average, two- to threefold larger than that of a 20-yr-old man (6). The factors responsible for this characteristic continued growth pattern are not fully resolved but minimally require androgen (4). This continuous growth of the prostate can result in either benign prostatic hyperplasia (BPH) or prostate cancer. BPH is an overgrowth of the peri-urethral region including the transition zone and peri-urethral ducts of the prostate (5). This overgrowth involves both an increase in the number of prostate epithelial and stromal cells, predominantly smooth-muscle cells (6–9). No consistent genetic alterations have been demonstrated for stromal or epithelial cells in BPH. Due to this benign overgrowth, BPH produces clinical syndromes including urinary obstruction. BPH is a common condition in older men, with more than 50% of all men above the age of 50 having microscopic BPH and 25% eventually requiring surgery for clinical symptoms (10).

In contrast to the heterogeneous overgrowth of both stromal and epithelial cells in BPH and the lack of characteristic genetic changes, the majority of prostate cancers originate from the peripheral zone (5) as a clonal outgrowth of genetically altered epithelial cells (11,12). However, cancers can also arise in the central and transition zones (5). Owing to the genetic instability of the prostate (13–15), multiple independent malignant clones can be histologically identified within the same gland (16–18). These multiple focal lesions are clonal and display different genetic instability as measured by DNA ploidy (19), loss of heterozygosity (LOH) (17), and fluorescence in situ hybridization (FISH) analyses (20). These data demonstrate the unique genetic instability of the aging prostatic epithelium.

Studies on the etiology and molecular biology of prostate cancer have been hampered until recently by a number of factors, such as restricted access to tissues, limited availability of prostate-cancer cell lines for in vitro studies, and limited num-

From: *The Molecular Basis of Human Cancer* (W. B. Coleman and G. J. Tsongalis, eds.), © Humana Press Inc., Totowa, NJ.

ber of animal models. These limitations are rapidly being overcome and recent genetics and molecular biology studies, such as cytogenetic analysis using FISH or comparative genomic hybridization (CGH), LOH analysis, and analysis of expression and mutation in various proto-oncogenes and tumor suppressor genes, have provided a growing insight into the molecular events responsible for the initiation, promotion, and progression of prostate cancer.

HISTOPATHOLOGICAL CLASSIFICATION OF PROSTATE CANCER

The problem presented by prostate cancer is that currently it is difficult to predict the clinical course of the disease for individuals. Approximately 50% of men with prostate cancer have clinically advanced (nonorgan-confined) disease at the time of initial diagnosis (21). One-third of the remaining 50% of men with organ-confined disease (initially determined by clinical staging) actually have micrometastatic disease at the time of surgery (as determined by subsequent pathological staging) (21). In some men, prostate cancer kills the patient within a year of diagnosis. In contrast, other men survive untreated for many years with clinically undetectable localized disease. If completely localized within the prostatic capsule, prostate cancer can be cured by surgery alone through radical prostatectomy (22,23).

For most solid tumors, the histopathological indicators of biological aggressiveness have been determined through the comparison of tumor morphology with corresponding clinical outcome. The histological grade of the primary prostate cancer is evaluated using the Gleason grading system (24). In this system, grading is based upon the degree of glandular differentiation and growth pattern of the tumor as it relates to the prostatic stroma. The pattern may vary from well differentiated (grade 1) to poorly differentiated (grade 5). This system takes into account tumor heterogeneity by summing the score of both the primary and secondary tumor-growth patterns. For example, if the majority of the tumor is well-differentiated (grade 1) and the secondary growth pattern is poorly differentiated (grade 5), the combined Gleason sum would be a 6. Low Gleason sum prostate cancers (Gleason sum of 5) predictably have minimal aggressive behavior, whereas very high Gleason sum tumors (Gleason sum of 8–10) are usually highly aggressive (25). Unfortunately, the intermediate Gleason sum tumors (Gleason sum between 5 and 7) are highly unpredictable in their clinical aggressiveness (25). This limitation is of particular importance because the majority of tumors (76%) fall into this intermediate Gleason sum category (22). Thus, predicting the biological potential of the majority of prostate cancer in asymptomatic patients based on histology alone is problematic.

Prostate cancer is believed to arise from the epithelial cells that line the prostatic ducts and acini (4,11). Most carcinomas arise in the peripheral zones of the prostate gland, where prostatic intraepithelial neoplasia (PIN) are often found. PIN is characterized by the abnormal proliferation within the prostatic ducts, which appears as premalignant foci of cellular dysplasia and carcinoma in situ without stromal invasion (11,27). However, the likelihood that an individual PIN lesion evolves into clinical cancer is very low (11,26,27). The majority of the PINs

that do progress to the histologically detectable cancers never produce clinical symptoms during the lifetime of the host. Based on autopsy studies, 20% of men in the age range of 50–60 yr and 50% in the 70–80 yr range have histological deposits of cancer within their prostates that never produced clinical symptoms during their lifetime (3,12). There are approx 11 million men older than 50 yr in the United States with such cancer (21). Despite the remarkably high number of these histological cancers, the majority remain clinically silent (neither life-threatening nor life-altering), and only a portion become clinically manifest during the lifetime of the host.

The major reason that these microscopic cancers remain clinically silent is because the development of a malignant (clinically aggressive) prostate cancer from a normal prostatic glandular cell requires multiple transformation events (12). Due to the multi-step nature of prostatic carcinogenesis, cells that have undergone some but not all of the transformation steps needed to produce clinically aggressive cancers are present within the prostate tissue of aging men. It is the limited clonal outgrowth of these partially transformed cells that produces these histologically detectable, sub-clinical cancers in the prostates of aging men (12). Two fundamental questions with regard to prostatic carcinogenesis are: 1) what are the multiple molecular events associated with the initial development of histological prostate cancer, and perhaps more significantly 2) what additional molecular changes are needed for the evolution from an indolent tumor to a life-threatening cancer? The resolution of these questions hold important clinical implications related to the development of new methods for preventing and treating prostate cancer. In addition, because distant metastases are responsible for the death of the patient, defining the molecular basis of metastasis should allow the development of prognostic methods for predicting which cancers have acquired this ability and thus require aggressive systemic treatment.

GENETIC PREDISPOSITION

Germline mutations have been shown to convey genetic predisposition to several types of cancers. Like many other human cancers, prostate cancer exists in both sporadic and germ-like inheritance forms. Steinberg and Colleagues (28) reported that men with a father or brother affected with prostate cancer are twice as likely to develop prostate-cancer as men with no affected relatives. In addition, the risk of prostate cancer development increases with increasing numbers of affected family members, such that men with two or three affected first degree relatives exhibit a 5-fold to 11-fold increased risk of developing prostate cancer. Men with an inherited predisposition are not only cancer prone, but they are also likely to develop cancer at an early age. Up to 40% of prostate-cancer patients younger than 55 yr may be related to an inherited genetic defect, whereas only 5–10% of all prostate cancers are believed to involve an inherited predisposition (29). Other studies on the familial aggregation of prostate cancer have suggested the existence of germ-line inheritance of prostate cancer susceptibility genes in an autosomal dominant allele that predisposes men to develop prostate cancer independent of environmental exposures (29). Recently, a genome-wide scan performed in 66 high-risk prostate cancer families linked the

Table 1
Summary of the Genetic Alterations in Prostate Cancer Progression

Chromosomal Location	Candidate genes	Stage of occurrence	Phenotypic effect	References
1q24-q25	HPC-1 (gain)	Very early (Germline)	Increased susceptibility to prostate-cancer development	(30)
11q13	GSTπ (loss)	Very early	Increased susceptibility to prostate-cancer development	(168)
8p11-p12	? (loss)	Very early	Metastasis suppressor	93,101,104
10q24-q25	?	Early	Tumor suppressor	88,91,108,109
13q	Rb1 (loss)	Early	Tumor suppressor	(90)
2q37	Gbx2 (gain)	Middle	Proto-oncogene	(67)
8p	NKX3.1 (loss)	Middle	Tumor suppressor	107,152
11p11.2	KAI1 (loss)	Middle	Metastasis suppressor	(155)
11p13	CD44 (loss)	Middle	Metastasis suppressor	(159)
16q	E-cadherin (loss)	Middle	Tumor/metastasis suppressor	(130)
5q	α-catenin (loss)	Late	Tumor suppressor	(135)
7q31.1	? (loss)	Late	Tumor suppressor	(102)
8q (q24)	c-myc (gain)	Late	Proto-oncogene	(20)
10q23	PTEN (loss)	Late	Tumor/metastasis suppressor	115,116
17p	p53 (loss)	Late	Tumor suppressor	(138)
17pter-q23	?	Late	Metastasis suppressor	(146)
17q	BRCA1 (loss)	Late	Tumor suppressor	170,171
18q	DCC (loss)	Late	Tumor suppressor	(142)
18q	bcl2 (gain)	Late	Proto-oncogene Androgen-independence	(44–50)
19q	cCAM (loss)	Late	Tumor suppressor	(169)
X (p11-q13)	AR (gain)	Late	Androgen-independence	(79,80)

hereditary prostate-cancer susceptibility (*HPC-1*) gene(s) to the long arm of chromosome 1q24-q25 *(30)*. Thus, as with many other human cancers, numerous studies suggest that both genetic and environmental factors are involved in the etiology of prostate cancer. In contrast, some studies suggest that there is no unique clinical or pathological characteristic difference between hereditary prostate cancer and sporadic prostate cancer other than an earlier age of clinical onset *(18,31)*.

GENES AND GENETIC ALTERATIONS IN SPORADIC PROSTATE CANCER

Several types of genetic changes occur during the evolution of cancer cells. There are 1) mutations and genetic rearrangements causing activation of proto-oncogenes, resulting in a growth advantage for the altered cells; 2) mutations and genetic deletions causing inactivation or loss of tumor-suppressor genes, which normally have negative growth regulatory functions; and 3) mutations and deletions in susceptibility genes that enhance the frequency of gain of function mutations of proto-oncogenes or loss of function mutations of tumor-suppressor genes. Table 1 summarizes the candidate genes, chromosomal locations, types of alterations (loss or gain of function), phenotypic consequences, and temporal occurrence of the genetic alterations that have been reported in prostate carcinogenesis and tumor progression.

PROTO-ONCOGENES A number of proto-oncogenes including c-*ras*, c-*myc*, and c-*erbB2* have been studied in prostate cancer. The expression of these proto-oncogenes has been

detected in prostate cancer, but their expression is not been consistently correlated with initiation or progression of prostate cancer *(32)*. Some studies report c-*ras* mutations in prostate cancer. However, these mutations occur at a relatively low frequency, which is estimated to be less than 5% of prostate tumors in the United States *(33–35)*. Using the Dunning R-3327 system of rat prostate cancer cell lines as a model, Treiger and Isaacs *(36)* demonstrated that the transfection-induced overexpression of the v-H-*ras* oncogene into a tumorigenic nonmetastatic Dunning rat prostate cell line resulted in the acquisition of high metastatic ability. A quantitative overexpression in the c-H-*ras* proto-oncogenes appears to be more common in metastatic prostate cancer *(37–38)*. Overexpression of the c-H-*ras* gene product p21 does not appear to be an early event in initiation of prostate carcinogenesis, but may be involved in the subsequent progression of the cancer to a highly metastatic state via enhancement of genetic instability of the cancer cells *(39)*. Experimentally, this overexpression can greatly enhance cellular motility, which directly affects the metastatic potential of these cells *(40)*. These results suggest that enhanced expression, not mutation, of c-H-*ras* p21 protein is involved in the progression of prostate cancer.

Chromosome 8q appears to be the most frequently amplified region in prostate cancer. Gain of this region has been found in 5–16% of primary prostate cancer by CGH and FISH analyses *(41–43)*. Cher and colleagues *(41)* examined 20 patients with prostate-cancer metastases using CGH and found that 85% of the samples had 8q gain. Therefore, gain of 8q is the most common genetic alteration associated with advanced prostate cancer. The c-*myc* proto-oncogene is located on human chromosome 8q24 and encodes proteins that are members of the helix-loop-helix-leucine zipper family of transcription factors. Several studies have shown an increased c-*myc* mRNA expression in prostate cancer compared to BPH and normal tissues, and an association with tumor grade (42,43). Using FISH analysis, Jenkins et al. (20) examined human prostate tissues and demonstrated that substantial amplification of c-*myc* was strongly correlated with increasing prostate-cancer nuclear grade and immunohistochemical evidence of c-myc protein overexpression. Thus, they suggest that gain of chromosome 8 and amplification of the c-*myc* gene are potential markers of prostate-carcinoma progression.

The *bcl2* gene is a proto-oncogene located on chromosome 18q21 that encodes a membrane-bound 26 kDa protein that prolongs cell survival by inhibiting apoptosis (44–46). Expression of *bcl2* is localized to the basal epithelial cells in normal human prostate (47). The secretary epithelial cells of the normal human prostate do not express the bcl2 protein. However, some primary untreated prostate adenocarcinoma cells express this apoptosis-suppressing oncoprotein at significant levels (48). Using immunohistochemical examination for bcl2 protein expression on androgen-dependent and androgen-independent prostate carcinoma, McDonnell et al. (47) reported that bcl2 protein was undetectable in 13 of 19 cases of androgen-dependent cancers. In contrast, androgen-independent cancers displayed diffuse, high-level expression of bcl2 protein. This observation has been confirmed by Colombel and colleagues (48). These findings suggest that expression of *bcl2* is elevated following androgen ablation and is correlated with the progression of prostate cancer from androgen dependence to androgen independence. In a more recent study, Furuya and colleagues (50) evaluated the frequency of *bcl2* expression during the progression of human and rat prostate cancer from an androgen-sensitive nonmetastatic phenotype to an androgen-independent metastatic phenotype by immunocytochemical staining. They reported that there is a statistically significant association between expression of bcl2 protein and the progression of human prostate-cancer cells to a metastatic phenotype. However, *bcl2* expression is not absolutely required for androgen-independence or metastatic ability by human prostate cancer cells (50). This observation is consistent within a series of eight distinct Dunning R3327 rat prostate cancer sublines that differ widely in their progression state (50). Combining these data, the development of androgen-independence and/or metastatic ability by prostate cancer cells can be associated with the expression of bcl2 protein, but bcl2-independent mechanisms also exist for such progression (50). Experimentally, overexpression of the *bcl2* proto-oncogene in human prostate-cancer cells protects these cells from apoptotic stimuli in vitro and confers resistance to androgen depletion in vivo and such protection correlates with the ability to form hormone-refractory prostate tumors in vivo (49).

Homeobox-containing genes comprise a large family of genes whose expression regulate body plan, pattern formation, and various aspects of cell regulation and differentiation (51). The defining characteristic of this family of genes is a common DNA sequence motif termed the homeobox domain, which is a conserved structural motif of nucleotides encoding a 61 amino acid residue polypeptide sequence with DNA binding ability. On the basis of structural similarities and direct evidence that *Drosophila* homeobox domain proteins are capable of binding DNA sequences and modulating transcriptional activity, it is generally accepted that homeobox domain proteins are transcription factors (52–54). In humans, as well as in mice, there are 38 class I homeobox genes that are organized in four clusters designated as A, B, C, and D. In humans, these clusters are located on chromosomes 7, 17, 12, and 2, respectively (55). Homeobox genes are expressed during embryogenesis in a tissue-specific and often stage-related manner (56,57). A number of homeobox genes have been found to be transcriptionally active in mature tissues, including breast (58), kidney (59), and hematopoietic cell lineages (60). The evidence for the role of the homeobox gene in malignant processes was first documented in leukemia (61). It was shown that over-expression of the *HOX-7.1* gene in myoblasts inhibited terminal differentiation and induced cell transformation (62). The oncogenic potential of several *HOX* genes was demonstrated in NIH 3T3 cells (63,64). Several homeobox genes are also involved in solid tumors. Preliminary studies demonstrated that expression of homeobox genes are altered in various human carcinomas, such as breast (58), colon (65), gastric (66), lung (66), renal (59), and testicular cancers (66).

To begin to assess the possible role of homeobox genes in prostatic-cell carcinogenesis, Gao et al. (67) surveyed initially for expression of homeobox containing genes in the human TSU-PRI metastatic prostate cancer cell line. This was accomplished by reverse transcription-polymerase chain reaction (RT-PCR) using degenerate oligodeoxyribonucleotide primers to homeobox-binding sequence to generate partial cDNAs, which were cloned and sequenced. Using this method, expression of 14 members of homeobox-containing genes were detected in TSU-PRI cells. All of these expressed genes correspond to previously identified homeobox genes located within the *HOX* clusters A, B, C, and D (67). Further examination of the expression of these homeobox genes in different human prostatic cell lines by using whole cDNA slot blot and Northern-blot analyses revealed that one of the sequences corresponding to the human *GBX2* homeobox gene is overexpressed in TSU-PRI, LNCAP, PC-3, and DU145 metastatic prostate cell lines relative to the normal prostate (67). These results suggest that the homeobox gene *GBX2* may participate in the metastastic progression of prostatic cancer.

The *GBX* class of homeobox domain genes comprises six known members. These include *GBX1* (68) and *GBX2* (69) in human, *Gbx1* (70) and *Gbx2* (71) in mice, chicken *Hox7* (72), and *Xenopus laevis* homeobox gene *xgbx-2* (GenBank accession number U04867). This *GBX* family of homeobox genes shares over 97% sequence identity in the 60 amino acids of the homeobox domain (68–71). In humans, the *GBX1* and *GBX2* genes are located on chromosome 7q36 and 2q37, respectively (68). Using RNA *in situ* hybridization analysis of mouse embryos, expression of mouse *Gbx2* RNA, which is homologous to human *GBX2*, occurs during gastrulation and neurulation (73). *Gbx2* RNA is expressed in the spinal cord, hindbrain, optic vesicle, and the mandibular arch *(73),* suggesting that *Gbx2* expression is associated with the development of the nervous system.

Because the *GBX* genes consistently are overexpressed in a panel of human prostatic-cancer cell lines (including TSU-PRl, PC3, DU145, and LNCAP) compared to normal prostate, Gao et al. *(74)* designed specific primer sets for RT-PCR detection of the expression of *GBX1* and *GBX2* in human prostate cancer. These studies demonstrated that only the *GBX2* gene, but not *GBX1,* is consistently overexpressed in this panel of human prostate-cancer cell lines compared to normal human prostate *(74).* In addition, an antisense gene approach was used to examine the importance of *GBX* expression for prostate-cancer malignancy. To do this, *GBX*-overexpressing TSU-PRl and PC3 human prostatic-cancer cells were transfected with an eukaryotic expression vector containing an antisense *GBX* homeobox domain cDNA. Stable transfectant clones that expressed the antisense *GBX* homeobox domain were obtained. When tested in vitro, the clonogenic ability of all of the antisense transfectants was reduced in both cell lines. When implanted subcutaneously into nude mice, the tumorigenicity of the antisense *GBX* expression transfectants from both of the human prostatic-cancer cell lines is inhibited by more than 70% compared to the parental cells *(74).* Taken together, these results suggest that expression of *GBX* genes is required for malignant growth of human prostate cells.

Enhanced expression of thymosin beta 15 is associated with metastatic ability within the Dunning system of rat prostate cancer cells *(75).* Within this system, thymosin beta 15 expression is correlated with both motility and metastatic potential of prostate-cancer cells *(75).* Thymosin beta 15 encodes a 45-amino acid highly hydrophilic protein with no apparent transmembrane domains *(75).* Thymosin beta 15 sequesters G-actin and in doing so disturbs actin polymerization kinetics. Thymosin beta 15 is not expressed in normal or benign human prostate cells but is upregulated in human prostate cancers with increasing Gleason grades and metastatic potential *(75).* Transfection of antisense thymosin beta 15 constructs into Dunning rat prostatic-carcinoma cells demonstrates that this molecule positively regulates cell motility and metastasis *(75).*

Androgen receptor (AR) is a key mediator of androgen function within normal and malignant prostate cells. AR is nearly universally expressed in primary and metastatic sites in untreated patients and androgen-ablation recurrent patients, suggesting that AR is required for the progression of prostate cancer to metastatic stage *(76,77).* CGH analysis demonstrated that amplification of the Xq11-q13 region (where the *AR* gene is located) is common in prostate cancer recurring during androgen-ablation therapy *(78,79).* AR amplification has been detected in 30% of recurrent prostate cancers, whereas no amplification is observed in the specimens taken from the same patients prior to androgen-ablation therapy *(78).* Likewise, FISH analysis demonstrates that *AR* gene amplification occurs in 28% of the recurrent therapy-resistant tumors, but none of the untreated primary tumors *(79).* These results combine to suggest that in approx one-third of patients, failure of androgen-ablation therapy may be caused by clonal outgrowth of prostate-cancer cells with increased AR expression that are

able to continue androgen-dependent growth despite low concentrations of serum androgens *(79).* In addition to amplification, mutations in the *AR* gene can cause AR dysfunction including alterations of AR specificity, binding affinity, and expression *(80–83).* *AR* mutations occur at a low frequency in primary prostate cancer *(83,84).* In contrast, the cells in the distant metastases and androgen-ablation recurrent prostate cancer often contain *AR* mutations *(83,85).* Several mutation sites in the *AR* gene have been detected in advanced prostate cancer, which resulted in the impairment of AR function and androgen insensitivity, including alterations at codons 772 (Arg→Cys), 877 (Thr→Ala), and 907 (Gly→Arg) *(80–83).*

Trisomy of chromosome 7 has been detected in prostate cancer. Bandyk et al. *(86)* demonstrated that chromosome 7 trisomy is associated with the progression of human prostate cancer by FISH analysis of 36 specimens including 15 primary prostate carcinomas, 16 metastatic lesions, and 5 normal prostate tissues. The frequency of cells displaying trisomy of chromosome 7 is significantly increased in the advanced-stage prostate cancers but not in the early stage tumors or normal prostate tissues *(86).*

TUMOR-SUPPRESSOR GENES Loss of characteristic chromosomal regions is a hallmark of a tumor-suppressor gene and has been used to identify these genes. Because tumor-suppressor genes are negative regulators of cell growth, their inactivation is recessive at the cellular level, inactivation of both alleles being necessary if they are to contribute to the oncogenic process. This inactivation has been proposed to be involved in the "two hit" process proposed by Knudson *(87),* where the first hit may either be carried in the germline (inherited cancer) or be acquired somatically (sporadic cancer) and is commonly a point or other small mutation. The second hit usually involves gross loss of genetic material from the other allele (LOH). LOH measurements using polymorphic markers distributed along human chromosomes have often been performed in human cancers to find loci that may contain recessive tumor-suppressor genes. LOH is very common in prostate cancer, occurring in almost all chromosomes in the genome *(11,41).* Frequent LOH in primary prostate cancer has been demonstrated at the chromosomal regions 7q, 8p, 10q, 13q, 16q, 17q, and 18q *(88–101).* The chromosomal regions affected by LOH are often large and may harbor many genes.

Genetic alterations at chromosome 7q have been demonstrated in prostate cancer by cytogenetic analyses such as FISH and LOH *(98,102,103).* Oakahashi et al. *(102)* examined 54 paired prostate cancer and control DNAs by PCR analysis of 21 microsatellite loci and demonstrated that overall allelic imbalance at chromosome 7 was 30% (16/54 cases), whereas allelic imbalance at 7q was 93% (15/16 cases). The most common site of allelic loss is at 7q31.1, where LOH correlates with higher tumor grade and lymph node metastasis *(102).*

LOH at 8p appears to be the most common genetic defect in primary prostate cancer. LOH at 8p in prostate cancer has been reported in several different studies *(11,41,91,93,104).* Deletion of 8p22 has been found in approx 70% of primary prostate cancers *(93).* Vocke et al. *(104)* performed PCR-based LOH studies utilizing 25 microsatellite markers on the short arm and one locus on the long arm of chromosome 8 on 99 matched normal and tumor microdissected prostate samples. This study found 8p LOH in 86% of carcinomas, with the most frequent loss occurring in the 8p12-p21 region without correlation to tumor grade or stage. In contrast to these results, Trapman et al. *(93)* reported that loss of 8p12-p21 did correlate with advanced prostate disease. Two minimal regions of deletions, 8p11-p12 and 8p22, have been reported suggesting the presence of two different tumor-suppressor genes in this chromosomal region *(93,94,101)*. A candidate gene (designated *N33*) was recently isolated from the 8p22 region *(105,106)*. This gene encodes an 1.5 kb mRNA in most tissues including prostate and its expression is downregulated in most colon-cancer cell lines due to hypermethylation of a CpG island located at 5' end of this gene *(105)*.

Recently, He et al. *(107)* isolated *NKX3.1*, a novel human prostate-specific, androgen-regulated homeobox gene, located on human chromosome 8p21. *NKX3.1* belongs to the *Drosophila* NK homeobox gene family. This gene is expressed at high levels in adult prostate and at a much lower level in testis, but is expressed little or not at all in several other tissues. *NKX3.1* expression is upregulated by androgen in LNCAP human prostate-cancer cells, but it is not expressed by more malignant human prostate cancer cells *(107)*. These results suggest *NKX3.1* as a candidate tumor-suppressor gene for prostate cancer located on the short arm of chromosome 8.

Deletion of 10q24-q25 is another frequent event in prostate cancer that was first described by classical cytogenetic studies *(108,109)*. LOH at 10q has been reported in 30–40% of primary prostate tumors and in 25% of PIN lesions *(15,88,91)*. A recent study that examined genetic alterations using CGH and allelotyping found 10q loss in 50% of prostate cancer from untreated metastases and androgen-independent patients *(41)*. A candidate gene, *MXI1*, whose expression negatively regulates the c-*myc* proto-oncogene was mapped to this chromosomal region *(111,112)*. Mutations of the *MXI1* gene have been found in primary prostate cancers *(112)*. However, Gray et al. *(113)* reported that the majority of 10q24-q25 LOH occurs near the 10q23-q24 boundary and does not involve the *MXI1* locus, suggesting another tumor-suppressor gene resides in this chromosomal region.

The *PTEN* gene (also known as *MMAC1*), which is located at human chromosome 10q23, has been recently isolated as a candidate tumor-suppressor gene *(114,115)*. The *PTEN* gene encodes a widely-expressed 5.5 kb mRNA. The predicted protein contains sequence motifs with significant homology to the catalytic domain of protein phosphatases and to the cytoskeletal proteins tensin and auxilin *(114,115)*. Mutations in the coding region of *PTEN* were observed at a significant frequency in human cancers including glioma, prostate, kidney, and breast carcinoma *(114,115)*. The *PTEN* gene is inactivated by mutation in three prostate-cancer cell lines *(115)*. In a more recent study, Cairns and colleagues *(116)* screened 80 primary prostate tumors by microsatellite analysis and found chromosome 10q23 to be deleted in 23 cases. Further, sequence analysis of the entire coding region of the *PTEN* gene and screening for homozygous deletion with new intragenic markers in these 23 cases with 10q23 LOH identified a second mutational event in 10 (43%) tumors *(116)*. This observation established the *PTEN*

gene as a significant target for inactivation through 10q loss in sporadic prostate cancer *(116)*.

Chromosome 13q, which contains the retinoblastoma (*Rb1*) tumor suppressor gene, is frequently deleted in prostate cancer, as determined by both LOH and CGH studies *(88–90,113,114)*. *Rb1* encodes a 110 kDa phosphoprotein that functions as one of the major negative regulators of cell growth. LOH at the *Rb1* locus (13q14) has been detected in approx 25% of localized human prostate cancers *(88)*. This was confirmed by Ittmann and Brooks *(119,120)*. In a separate study, Phillips et al. *(90,117)* reported LOH at the *Rb1* locus in 24/40 (60%) informative patients with prostate cancer. Furthermore, loss of *Rb1* occurred with similar frequency in early-stage/low-grade prostate cancers and in more advanced cancers, suggesting that loss of *Rb1* is an early event in prostate tumorigenesis. In addition, decreased levels of Rb1 protein have been observed in approx 50% of surgical specimens obtained from metastatic sites of human prostate cancer *(121)*. Bookstein and colleagues found that the *Rb1* gene product is truncated in the human prostate-cancer cell line DU-145. A functional role for *Rb1* is suggested by the finding that when an intact copy of cloned *Rb1* gene was introduced into these cells, their tumorigenicity was suppressed *(122)*. Two other human prostate cell lines examined in this study apparently have normal *Rb1* gene products, indicating that *Rb1* mutation is not an universal event in prostate cancer tumorigenesis.

LOH at 16q22.1-q24 has been found in a high frequency (up to 50%) of prostate cancers *(15,88,91,100)*. CGH studies have shown loss of 16q in over 50% of untreated metastases and androgen-independent prostate cancers *(41)*, which correlated with higher Gleason score *(11)*. These studies led to an examination of putative candidate genes in this region. The *E-cadherin* gene, which maps to chromosome 16q22.1 *(123)*, is of particular interest. The product of this gene, originally termed uvomorulin by Peyrieras and colleagues *(124)*, Arc-1 by Berhrens and colleagues *(125)*, and E-cadherin by Takeichi *(126)*, was demonstrated to play a critical role in embryogenesis and organogenesis by mediating epithelial cell-cell recognition and adhesion processes. The appearance of E-cadherin protein on the surface of cells of the early mouse embryo has been shown to be required for normal development. The cadherin family of proteins is large, with expression found in numerous cell types. The role of E-cadherin in maintaining various aspects of cell differentiation led several investigators to examine E-cadherin in adenocarcinoma cells. These studies found that E-cadherin protein levels were frequently reduced or absent in cancer cell lines, and such lines were often more fibroblastic in morphology and invasive in experimental assays *(127,128)*. Vleminckx and colleagues *(129)* demonstrated that experimental inactivation of E-cadherin with either antibodies or antisense RNA resulted in the acquisition of invasive potential and that transfection of invasive adenocarcinoma cells with E-cadherin cDNA rendered the expressing cells noninvasive.

The first studies to examine E-cadherin in prostate cancer were carried out by Bussemakers and colleagues *(130)* in the Dunning rat model. These studies found a strong correlation between the lack of E-cadherin and metastatic potential, invasive potential, or both. This correlation was strengthened by the direct observation of the progression of a noninvasive, E-cadherin-positive tumor to a E-cadherin-negative, highly metastatic tumor. These observations have been extended to human prostate cancer in a series of more than 90 samples of prostate cancer examined for E-cadherin protein levels using immunohistochemistry *(131)*. Whereas all benign samples stained with uniform, strong intensity at cell-cell borders, about one half of the tumors examined showed reduced or absent E-cadherin protein staining. When compared with Gleason grade, there was a strong association between high-grade and aberrant E-cadherin staining. No tumors with Gleason grade 9 or 10 showed normal staining, whereas all tumors with a Gleason score of less than 6 had normal staining patterns. Aberrant E-cadherin staining is a powerful predictor of poor outcome, both in terms of disease progression and overall survival *(131)*.

To extend understanding of the role of E-cadherin-mediated cell-cell adhesion in prostate cancer, the synthesis and organization of this protein and its associated proteins in prostate-cancer cell lines have been examined *(132)*. Cultured normal prostatic epithelial cells make abundant E-cadherin, which forms complexes with a series of cytoplasmic proteins termed catenins (α and β). These proteins, in particular a-catenins, are thought to link E-cadherin to the microfilament cytoskeleton, and the interaction of E-cadherin with these proteins is required for induction of cell-cell adhesion *(133)*. In cultured prostate-cancer cell lines, E-cadherin levels are frequently reduced or the protein is absent. Similar observations have been made in surgical specimens of prostate cancer. Furthermore, this study provides the unexpected finding that the levels of the E-cadherin-associated protein α-catenin are also frequently reduced in prostate-cancer cells. Loss of this protein in human PC-3 prostate cancer cells is associated with their decreased ability to aggregate compared with cells expressing normal levels of E-cadherin and α-catenin. Thus, the E-cadherin-mediated pathway of cell-cell adhesion may become inactivated in a variety of ways. The lack of α-catenin expression in PC-3 cells is the result of a homozygous deletion within the α-catenin gene *(132)*. The α-catenin gene has been mapped to chromosome 5q22 *(134)*, and preliminary results indicate that LOH occurs in this chromosomal region occurs in approx 25% of prostate cancers analyzed. In a recent study, Ewing et al. *(135)* showed that a transferred portion of human chromosome 5 containing the α-catenin gene suppresses the tumorigenicity of PC-3 human prostate-cancer cells due to restoration of E-cadherin/catenin complex formation.

Elo et al. *(136)* analyzed allelic losses in 50 prostate-cancer specimens of various histological grades, and found that the most frequently deleted region is located at 16q23-24.2. Furthermore, LOH at 16q24.1-q24.2 is significantly associated with clinically aggressive behavior of the disease, metastatic disease, and higher tumor grade. This result suggests that a potentially important gene other than E-cadherin may be located at 16q24.1-q24.2 region and that this gene may be associated with prostate-cancer progression.

Loss of heterozygosity at 17p13.1, where the *p53* gene is located is one of the most common genetic changes associated with human malignancy. The wild-type p53 protein functions as a negative regulator of cell growth after DNA damage has

occurred. Although the role of *p53* mutation in prostate-cancer development is less significant than many other cancers, the association of *p53* mutation and aberrant protein expression with different stages of prostate cancer has been shown in a series of studies. Mutations in the *p53* gene are uncommon in clinically localized prostate cancer, occurring in 10–30% of tumors *(88,137,138)*. Accumulation of p53 protein has been reported in 50–60% of bone metastases and hormone-refractory primary tumors, compared with only 7–8% of primary hormone-naïve tumors and local lymph-node metastases *(139)*. Using single-strand conformational polymorphism (SSCP) analysis for *p53* mutation and immunohistochemical staining for p53 protein, Brooks et al. *(140)* examined 67 tumors derived from patients with clinically localized disease and found that *p53* gene inactivation is rare in primary prostate cancers, not essential to the development of prostate-cancer metastases, and have limited use as a prognostic marker in patients with primary or metastatic disease. Experimentally, transfection of the wild-type *p53* gene vs a mutated *p53* gene into two cell lines with *p53* mutations resulted in reduced colony formation. Revertants that overcame the growth suppressor activity of wild-type p53 protein no longer retained wild-type *p53* sequences *(141)*.

Chromosome 18q, which contains the *DCC* (for deleted in colon cancer) gene, is frequently deleted in human colorectal carcinoma *(142)*. Gao and colleagues *(143)* reported that the *DCC* gene was present and expressed in normal prostate cells. In patient samples, 12 of 14 prostate cancer cases (86%) showed reduced expression of *DCC* RNA, and 5 of 11 informative cases (45%) showed LOH at the *DCC* locus *(143)*. Carter and colleagues *(88)* reported that the frequency of LOH at the *DCC* locus was approx 17%. These results indicate that downregulation of the *DCC* gene, by either reduced expression or LOH at the *DCC* locus, can occur during the progression of prostate cancer. Although these data indicate a correlation between LOH of the *DCC* locus and prostate cancer, a functional role for *DCC* in the initiation or progression of prostate cancer has not yet been identified.

In addition to the chromosomal regions that frequently demonstrate loss in prostate cancer (including 8p, 13q, 16q, 17p, and 10q), several other chromosomal regions have been found to undergo loss in some prostate cancers, including 2cen-q31, 5cen-q31.1, 6ql4-q23, 15cen-q24, 4q13-q31.1, and 18q21.1 *(11,41)*.

In addition to tumor suppressor genes, which normally function in the regulation of cell growth, there are genes that suppress the metastatic ability of cancer cells without affecting the tumorigenicity of these cancer cells *(144)*. In order to identify the specific chromosomal regions and genes involved in metastasis suppression, somatic-cell hybrids were generated from nonmetastatic and highly metastatic rat prostate cells. The hypothesis was that if the loss or inactivation of metastasis-suppressor genes is involved in malignant progression, then somatic-cell hybrids would be nonmetastatic, because chromosomes from the nonmetastatic parental cell would supply the lost suppressor-gene functions. Ichikawa and colleagues *(144)* found that the tumorigenicity and in vivo growth rates of the somatic-cell hybrids, which contained a full complement of parental chromosomes, were not affected. However, none of the animals bearing tumors derived from somatic-cell hybrids developed distant metastases. When these nonmetastatic primary tumors were propagated in vivo, animals occasionally developed distant metastases. Cytogenetic analysis of the metastatic revertants showed a consistent loss of specific rat chromosome (144). This study demonstrated that prostatic-cancer metastasis is associated with the loss of specific chromosomes that do not affect the growth rate or tumorigenicity, only metastatic ability (144).

These results indicate that expression of genes located on certain chromosomes can suppress the metastatic ability of rat prostatic-cancer cells. One such gene, nm23, has been identified (145). The nm23 gene encodes a nucleoside diphosphate kinase whose expression is decreased in metastatic melanoma and breast-cancer cells. Preliminary studies, which quantitated the level of nm23 protein in the Dunning system, showed that the level of nm23 expression is not correlated with the metastatic ability of the cell lines (146). This suggests that decreased expression of nm23 is not involved in progression within this rodent system. The role of nm23 expression in human model systems is not fully resolved. Igawa and colleagues (147) demonstrated that the levels of nm23 mRNA and protein are more commonly increased in prostate-cancer cells from patients with clinically metastatic disease than in cells from patients with clinically localized disease. Jensen and colleagues (148) found that the level of nm23-H1 mRNA was increased twofold or more in prostate-tumor tissues compared with normal tissues in 13 of 27 (48%) patients, with a mean increase of 5.4-fold. These samples also showed an increase in the level of nm23 protein. Unlike the Igawa and colleagues study (147), the Jensen and colleagues study found no statistical correlation between the pathologic staging of the tumors and the fold increase in nm23-H1 expression. As is indicated by these reports, the potential role of nm23-H1 RNA or nm23 protein overexpression in prostate tumorigenesis has yet to be resolved.

In an attempt to identify other genes involved in the suppression of prostate-cancer metastasis, a panel of rodent prostate-cancer cells containing defined portions of human chromosomes has been constructed. The general construction scheme employs microcell-mediated chromosome transfer to specifically transfer individual human chromosomes to the recipient cells of interest (149–151). Mouse fibrosarcoma cells containing normal human chromosomes tagged with a selectable marker gene are sequentially treated with colcemid to depolymerize microtubules and cytochalasin b to depolymerize actin bundles. The treated cells are then centrifuged, and the resulting pellet contains the microcells. Microcells are, in effect, micelles that contain single or multiple chromosomes. To enrich for those containing single chromosomes, the microcells are sized by sequential filtration through ploycarbonate membranes of decreasing pore size. The purified microcells are attached to highly metastatic rat prostate-cancer cells via incubation with phytohemagglutinin and finally fused by incubation with polyethylene glycol. The recipient rat prostate cancer cells that contain the human chromosomes of interest are clonally selected in antibiotic-containing media. The clones are characterized by FISH, cytogenetics, and molecular biology methods to define the regions of the human chromosome retained in these microcell-hybrid cells. These microcell hybrids containing known regions of human chromosomes can be tested in vivo for the tumorigenicity and metastatic ability.

Using microcell-mediated chromosome-transfer methods, several chromosomal regions have been reported to suppress the metastatic potential of Dunning rat prostate-cancer cells. These include chromosome 8p21-p12 (152), chromosome 10, between the centromere and D10S215 (152), chromosome 11p11.2-p13 (154), chromosome 11q14-q21 (Gao et al., unpublished results), and chromosome 17pter-q23 (156).

With regard to the chromosome 11 microcell hybrids, spontaneous deletion of portions of human chromosome 11 in some of these clones demonstrated that the minimal portion of this chromosome capable of suppressing prostate-cancer metastasis involves a region between 11p11.2-p13 and does not include the WT1 locus (154). Although LOH or CGH analysis has not previously identified chromosome 11 as a site of common loss of genetic material in human prostate cancer, positional cloning has identified genes located on human chromosome 11p12.1-p13 that can suppress metastatic ability of prostate-cancer cells (155). KAI1, a metastasis-suppressor gene for prostate cancer located on human chromosome 11p11.2 has been isolated and demonstrated to suppress metastasis when introduced into rat prostate-cancer cells (155). Expression of KAI1 is reduced in cell lines derived from metastatic human prostate tumors (155). The KAI1 gene encodes a protein of 267 amino acids, with four hydrophobic transmembrane domains and one large extracellular hydrophilic domain with three potential N-glycosylation sites (155). KAI1 is evolutionarily conserved, expressed in many human tissues, and encodes a member of a structurally distinct family of leukocyte-surface glycoproteins (155). By immunohistochemistry, high levels of KAI1 protein are detected in the epithelial but not stromal compartment of normal prostate and benign prostatic hyperplasia tissue (156,157). In epithelial cells, KAI1 protein is expressed on the plasma membrane (156,157). KAI1 protein expression is downregulated in more than 70% of the primary prostate cancers from untreated patients (156,157). In untreated patients, downregulation of KAI1 protein occurred in all of the lymph-node metastases examined (156,157). In patients with metastatic disease who had failed androgen-ablation therapy, more than 90% of the primary prostatic cancers had downregulation of expression and 60% showed no KAI1 protein expression (156,157). In other studies, KAI1 expression was documented to be inversely correlated to both Gleason score and clinical state (157). Primers derived from the sequences flanking each exon of KAI1 were employed in an analysis of KAI1 mutation and allelic loss by the SSCP. Using this method, no point mutation or allelic loss was detected in metastases (156). No allelic loss was detected in primary and lymph-node metastases via microsatellite analysis using the marker D11S1344, which is located in the region of KAI1 (156). These results demonstrate that KAI1 protein expression is consistently downregulated during the progression of human prostate cancer to a metastatic state and that this downregulation does not commonly involve either mutation or allelic loss of the KAI1 gene (156). In a recent study, Kawana and colleagues

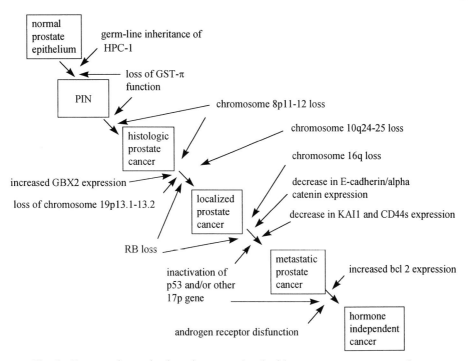

Fig. 1. Genes and genetic alterations associated with prostate cancer progression.

(158) examined LOH at polymorphic microsatellite loci on human chromosome 11 in human prostate-cancer tissues. They reported that the percentage of LOH or allelic imbalance at the *D11S1344* locus in metastatic tumors from autopsy cases was 70%, whereas *D11S1344* LOH or allelic imbalance in primary tumors from the same cases and from cases with clinically localized prostate cancer were 33 and 8%, respectively.

In addition to *KAI1*, *CD44* is another metastasis-suppressor gene located on human chromosome 11 *(159)*. The *CD44* gene is located on human chromosome 11p13 and encodes an integral transmembrane glycoprotein that participates in specific cell-cell and cell-matrix interactions *(160)*. The *CD44* gene is approx 60 kb in size and contains 20 exons, at least 10 of which are variably expressed due to alternative splicing of the mRNA *(161,162)*. *CD44* is involved in cell adhesion, serving as a receptor for the extracellular matrix (ECM) components hyaluronic acid *(163,164)* and osteopontin *(165)*. Although *CD44* appears to function in lymphocyte homing, lymphocyte activation, and ECM adhesion, the precise functions of each of the CD44 protein isoforms are not clear *(160)*. Individual isoforms differ in their ability to enhance or decrease tumorigenicity or metastatic potential when overexpressed on tumor cells *(160)*. Downregulation of the common 85 kDa form of CD44 both at the mRNA and protein level correlates with metastatic potential within the Dunning system of rat-prostate cancer sublines *(159)*. Transfection and expression of the 85 kDa form of CD44 in highly metastatic rat prostate cells results in suppression of lung metastatic potential without suppression of growth rate or tumorigenicity in vivo *(159)*. CD44 is normally expressed on the plasma membrane of human prostate glandular cells (the cells of origin for prostate cancer) *(166)*. *CD44* expression is downregulated in human prostate-cancer progression with downregulation being correlated with high tumor grade, aneuploidy, and distant metastasis *(166)*. Studies by Noordzij and

colleagues *(167)* on *CD44* expression in the radical prostatectomy specimens of 97 patients with prostate cancer and in 12 lymph-node metastases by immunohistochemical-staining methods demonstrated the prognostic value of CD44 isoforms in prostate cancer. They reported that benign prostatic glands almost always expressed the CD44 common form (or CD44s) or CD44v6; whereas in prostatic adenocarcinomas CD44s, CD44v5, and CD44v6 were expressed in 86, 23, and 69% of tumors, respectively. Gleason sum score and pT stage were correlated inversely with CD44s and CD44v6 scores *(167)*. CD44 was not found in the lymph-node metastatic tumor cells *(167)*. Loss of CD44s expression in prostate adenocarcinoma predicts a poor prognosis, independent of stage and grade *(167)*. These clinical observations are in agreement with the data that enhanced expression of the common CD44 isoform in rat prostatic-cancer cells inhibits their metastatic potential in vivo, whereas downregulation of CD44 protein expression is associated with acquisition of metastatic ability. These results suggest that CD44 is a metastasis suppressor for prostatic cancer and that immunocytochemical detection of decreased expression of the CD44s may be useful in predicting the aggressiveness of prostate cancers.

PROSTATE CANCER SUSCEPTIBILITY GENES

In addition to genetic changes, epigenetic changes (such as alterations in DNA methylation) can also affect gene expression. The methylation pattern in the promoter of the glutathione S-transferase (GST) π gene (located on chromosome 11q13) was examined to explain downregulation of this gene expression in prostate cancer *(168)*. Analysis of methylation-sensitive restriction sites within the CpG island region of the promoter revealed the virtual universality of hypermethylation of these sites in the DNA of all 30 cancers examined *(168)*. Methylation of this region was not detected in any DNA samples from either normal or hyperplastic prostate tissue *(168)*. Thus, this methylation event is the most common genomic change yet observed in prostate cancer. The GST enzyme encoded by the GSTπ gene is a key part of an important cellular pathway to prevent damage from a wide range of carcinogens; the inactivation of this enzyme could increase the susceptibility of prostate tissue to both tumor initiation and progression resulting from an increased rate of accumulated DNA damage.

SUMMARY

Molecular genetic analysis of prostate cancers indicates that the mechanisms underlying prostate carcinogenesis are complicated (Fig. 1). Both hereditary predisposition and somatic alterations are involved in the etiology of prostate cancer. Up to 5–10% of all prostate cancers have an inherited germline mutation that facilitates prostate carcinogenesis due to the inheritance of prostate-cancer susceptibility genes located at chromosome 1q24-q25. The majority of inherited or spontaneous prostate cancer may be the result of a series of somatic genetic alterations affecting many genes on several chromosomes (including 2q, 5q, 7q, 8p, 8q, 10q, 11p, 11q, 13q, 16q, 17q, 18q, 19p, and X). The earliest are those involving GSTπ gene at 11q13 and genes located on chromosome 8p11-p12. These changes predispose prostate cells to genetic alterations in many proto-oncogenes (c-*ras*, c-*myc*), tumor-suppressor genes (*Rb1*, *p53*), homeobox genes (*GBX2*), metastasis-suppressor genes (*KAI1*, *CD44s*), and survival genes (*bcl2*). Further studies are required, not only to better identify the specific changes, but to define such genetic mechanisms during specific steps in this molecular progression. In this way, better approaches to diagnosis, prognosis, therapy, and prevention for prostate cancer should be possible.

REFERENCES

1. Parker, S. L., Tong, T., Bolden, S., and Wingo, P. A. (1997) Cancer statistics, 1997. *Ca: Cancer J. Clin.* **47**:5–27.
2. Boring, C. C., Squires, T. S., and Tong, T. (1993) Cancer statistics, 1993. *Ca: Cancer J. Clin* **43**:7–26.
3. Carter, H. B. and Coffey, D. S. (1990) The prostate: an increasing medical problem. *Prostate* **16**:39–48.
4. Isaacs, J. T. (1994) Role of androgen in prostatic cancer. *Vitamins Hormones* **49**:433–502.
5. McNeal J. E. (1981) The zonal anatomy of the prostate. *Prostate* **2**:35–49,
6. Berry, S. J., Coffey, D. S., Walsh, P. C., and Ewing, L. L. (1984) The development of human benign prostatic hyperplasia with age. *J. Urol.* **132**:474–479.
7. Shapiro, E., Hartanto, V., and Lepor, H. (1992) Anti-desmin vs. anti-actin for quantifying the area density of prostate smooth muscle. *Prostate* **20**:259–267.
8. Peehl, D. M. and Sellers, R. G. (1997) Induction of smooth muscle cell phenotype in cultured human prostatic stromal cells. *Exp. Cell Res.* **232**:208–215.
9. Chung, L. W. and Davies, R. (1996) Prostate epithelial differentiation is dictated by its surrounding stroma. *Mol. Biol. Reports* **23**:13–19.
10. Isaacs, J. T. and Coffey, D. S. (1989) Etiology of BPH. *Prostate* **2**:33–58.
11. Bostwick, D. G. (1989) Prostatic intraepithelial neoplasia (PIN) *Urology* **34**:16–22.
12. Carter, H. B., Piantadosi, S., and Isaacs, J. T. (1990) Clinical evidence for and implications of the multistep development of prostate cancer. *J. Urol.* **143**:742–746.
13. Cunningham, J. M., Shan, A., Wick, M. J., McDonnell, S. K., Schaid, D. J., Tester, D. J., et al. (1996) Allelic imbalance and microsatellite instability in prostatic adenocarcinoma. *Cancer Res.* **56**:4475–4482.
14. Dahiya, R., Lee, C., McCarville, J., Hu, Q., Kaur G., and Deng, G. (1997) High frequency of genetic instability of microsatellites in human prostate adenocarcinoma. *Int. J. Cancer* **72**:762–767.
15. Watanabe., M., Imai, H., Suimazaki, J., Kotake, T., and Yatani, R. (1995) Microsatellite instability in human prostate cancer. *Br. J. Cancer.* **72**:562–564.
16. Byar, D. P., and Mostofi, F. K. (1972) Carcinoma of the prostate: prognostic evaluation of certain pathological features in 208 radical prostatectomies, examined by the step section technique. *Cancer* **30**:5–13.
17. Sakr, W. A., Macoska, J. A., Benson, P., Grignon, D. J., Wolman, S. R., Pontes J. E., and Crissman, J. D. (1994) Allelic loss in locally metastatic, multisampled prostate cancer. *Cancer Res.* **54**:3273–3277.
18. Bastacky, S. I., Wojno, K. J., Walsh, P. C., Carmichael, M. J., and Epstein, J. I. (1995) Pathological features of hereditary prostate cancer. *J. Urol.* **153**:987–992.
19. Greene, D. R., Taylor, S. R., Wheeler, T. M., and Scardino, P. T. (1991) DNA ploidy by image analysis of individual foci of prostate cancer: a preliminary report. *Cancer Res.* **51**:4084–4089.
20. Jenkins, R. B., Qian, J., Lieber, M. M., and Bostwick, D. G. (1997) Detection of c-myc oncogene amplification and chromosomal anomalies in metastatic prostatic carcinoma by fluorescence in situ hybridization. *Cancer Res.* **57**:524–53 1.
21. Scardino, P. T., Weaver, R., and Hudson, M. A. (1992) Early detection of prostate cancer. *Human Pathol.* **23**:211–222.
22. Partin, A. W., Borland, R. N., Epstein, J. I., and Brendier, C. B. (1993) Influence of wide excision of the neurovascular bundle(s) on prognosis in men with clinically localized prostate cancer with established capsular penetration. *J. Urol.* **150**:142–146.
23. Sgrignoli, A. R., Walsh, P. C., Steinberg, G. D., Steiner, M. S., and Epstein, J. I. (1994) Prognostic factors in men with stage D1 prostate cancer: identification of patients less likely to have prolonged survival after radical prostatectomy. *J. Urol.* **152**:1077–1081.
24. Gleason, D. F. (1966) Classification of prostatic carcinomas. *Cancer Chemother. Rep.* **50**:125–128.
25. Gleason, D. F. and Mellinger, G. T. (1974) Prediction of prognosis for prostatic adenocarcinoma by combined histological grading and clinical staging. *J. Urol.* **111**:58–64.
26. Epstein, J. I., Walsh, P. C., Carmichael, M., and Brendler, C. B. (1994) Pathologic and clinical findings to predict tumor extent of nonpalpable (stage T1c) prostate cancer. *JAMA* **271**:368–374.
27. Epstein, J. I. (1994) Pathology of prostatic intraepithelial neoplasia and adenocarcinoma of the prostate: Prognostic influences of stage, tumor volume, grade, and margins of resection. *Semin. Oncol.* **21**:527–541.
28. Steinberg, G. D., Carter, B. S., Beaty, T. H., Childs, B., and Walsh, P. C. (1990) Family history and the risk of prostate cancer. *Prostate* **17**:337–347.
29. Carter, B. S., Beaty, T. H., Steinberg, G. D., Childs, B., and Walsh, P. C. (1992) Mendelian inheritance of familial prostate cancer. *Proc. Natl. Acad. Sci. USA* **89**:3367–3371.
30. Smith, J. R., Freije, D., Carpten, J. D., Gronberg, H., Xu, J. X., Isaacs, S. D., Brownstein, M. J., et al. (1996) Major susceptibility locus for prostate cancer on chromosome 1 suggested by a genome-wide search. *Science* **274**:1371–1374.
31. Carter, B. S., Bova, G. S., and Beaty, T. H. (1993) Hereditary prostate cancer: epidemiologic and clinical features. *J. Urol.* **150**:797–802.
32. Strohmeyer, T. G. and Slamon, D. J. (1994) Proto-oncogenes and tumor suppressor genes in human urological malignancies. *J. Urol.* **151**:1479–1497.
33. PerRolizzi, R. G., Kreis, W., Rottach, C., Susin, M., and Broome, J. D. (1993) Mutational status of codons 12 and 13 of the N- and K-ras genes in tissue and cell lines derived from primary and metastatic prostate carcinomas. *Cancer Invest.* **11**:25–32.

34. Peehl, D. M., Wehner, N., and Stamey, T. A. (1987) Activated Ki-ras oncogene in human prostatic adenocarcinoma. *Prostate* **10**:281–289.

35. Carter, B. S., Epstein, J. I., and Isaacs, W. B. (1990). ras gene mutations in human prostate cancer. *Cancer Res.* **50**:6830–6832.

36. Treiger, B. and Isaacs, J. (1988) Expression of a transfected v-Harvey-ras oncogene in a Dunning rat prostate adenocarcinoma and the development of high metastatic ability. *J. Urol.* **140**:1580–1586.

37. Viola, M. V., Fromowitz, F., Oravez, S., Deb, S., Finkel, G., Lundy, J., et al. (1986) Expression of ras oncogene p21 in prostate cancer. *N. Engl. J. Med.* **314**:133–137.

38. Sumiya, H., Masai, M., Akimoto, S., Yatani, R., and Shimazaki, J. (1990) Histochemical examination of expression of ras p21 protein and R1881-binding protein in human prostatic cancers. *Eur. J. Cancer* **26**:786–789.

39. Ichikawa, T., Schalken, J. A., Ichikawa, Y. X., Steinberg, G. D., and Isaacs, J. T. (1991) Hras expression, genetic instability, and acquisition of metastatic ability by rat prostatic cancer cells following v-H-ras oncogene transfection. *Prostate* **18**:163–172.

40. Partin, A. W., Isaacs, J. T., Treiger, B., and Coffey, D. S. (1988) Early cell motility changes associated with an increase in metastatic ability in rat prostatic cancer cells transfected with the v-Harvey-ras oncogene. *Cancer Res.* **48**:6050–6053.

41. Cher, M. L., Bova, G. S., Moore, D. H., Small, E. J., Carroll, P. R., Pin, S. S., et al. (1996) Genetic alterations in untreated metastases and androgen-independent prostate cancer detected by comparative genomic hybridization and allelotyping. *Cancer Res.* **56**:3091–3102.

42. Fleming, W. H., Hamel, A., MacDonald, R., Ramsey, E., Pettigrew, N. M., Johnston, B., et al. (1986) Expression of the c-myc protooncogene in human prostatic carcinoma and benign prostatic hyperplasia. *Cancer Res.* **46**:1535–1538.

43. Buttyan, R., Sawczuk, I. S., Benson, M. C., Siegal, J. D., and Oisson, C. A. (1987) Enhanced expression of the c-myc protooncogene in high-grade human prostate cancers. *Prostate* **11**:327–337.

44. Tsujimoto, Y., Finger, L. R., Yunis, J., Nowell, P. C., and Croce, C. M. (1984). Cloning of the chromosome breakpoint of neoplastic B cells with the t(14,18) chromosome translocation. *Science* **226**:1097–1099.

45. Tsujimoto, Y., Yunis, J., Onorato-Showe, L., Erikson, J., Nowell, P. C., and Croce, C. M. (1984) Molecular cloning of the chromosomal breakpoint of B-cell lymphomas and leukemias with the t(11;14) chromosome translocation. *Science* **224**:1403–1406.

46. Hockenbery, D. M. (1992) The bcl-2 oncogene and apoptosis. *Semin. Immunol.* **4**:413–420.

47. McDonnell, T. J., Troncoso, P., Brisbay, S. M., Logothetis, C. X., Chung L. W., Hsieh, J. T., et al. (1992) Expression of the protooncogene bcl-2 in the prostate and its association with emergence of androgen-independent prostate cancer. *Cancer Res.* **52**:6940–6944.

48. Colombel, M., Symmans, F., Gil, S., O'Toole, K. M., Chopin, D., Benson M., et al. (1993) Detection of the apoptosis-suppressing oncoprotein bcl-2 in hormone-refractory human prostate cancers. *Am. J. Pathol.* **143**:390–400.

49. Raffo, A. J., Perlman, H., Chen, M. W., Day, M. L., Streitman, J. S., and Buttyan, R. (1995) Overexpression of bcl-2 protects prostate cancer cells from apoptosis in vitro and confers resistance to androgen depletion in vivo. *Cancer Res.* **55**:4438–4445.

50. Furuya, Y., Krajewski, S., Epstein, J. I., Reed, J. C., and Isaacs, J. T. (1996). Expression of bcl-2 and the progression of human and rodent prostatic cancers. *Clin. Cancer Res.* **2**:389–398.

51. McGinnis, W. and Krumlauf, R. (1992) Homeobox genes and axial patterning. *Cell* **68**:283–302.

52. Hoey, T., Warrior, R., Manak, J., and Levine, M. (1988) DNA-binding activities of the Drosophila melanogaster even-skipped protein are mediated by its homeo domain and influenced by protein context. *Mol. Cell. Biol.* **8**:4598–4607.

53. Hoey, T. and Levine, M. (1988) Divergent homeo box proteins recognize similar DNA sequences in Drosophila. *Nature* **332**:858–861.

54. Han, K., Levine, M. S., and Manley, J. L. (1989) Synergistic activation and repression of transcription by Drosophila homeobox proteins. *Cell* **56**:573–583.

55. Ruddle, F. H., Bartels, J. L., Bentley, K. L., Kappen, C., Murtha, M. T., and Pendleton, J. W. (1994) Evolution of Hox genes. *Ann. Rev. Genet.* **28**:423–442.

56. Simeone, A., Mavilio, F., Acampora, D., Giampaolo, A., Faielia, A, Zappavigna, V., et al. (1987) Two human homeobox genes, c1 and c8: structure analysis and expression in embryonic development. *Proc. Natl. Acad. Sci. USA* **84**:4914–4918.

57. Simeone, A., Mavilio, F., Bottero, L., Giampaolo, A., Russo, G., Faiella, A., et al. (1986) A human homeo box gene specifically expressed in spinal cord during embryonic development. *Nature* **320**:763–765.

58. Friedmann, Y., Daniel, C. A., Strickland, P., and Daniel, C. W. (1994) Hox genes in normal and neoplastic mouse mammary gland. *Cancer Res.* **54**:5981–5985.

59. Cillo, C., Barba, P., Freschi, G., Bucciarelli, G., Magli, M. C., and Boncinclli E. HOX gene expression in normal and neoplastic human kidney. *Int. J. Cancer* **51**:892–897.

60. Magli, M. C., Barba, P., Celetti, A., De Vita, G., Cillo, C., and Boncinelli, E. (1991) Coordinate regulation of HOX genes in human hematopoietic cells. *Proc. Natl. Acad. Sci. USA* **88**:6348–6352.

61. Kongsuwan, K., Webb, E., Housiaux, P., and Adams, J. M. (1988) Expression of multiple homeobox genes within diverse mammalian haemopoietic lineages. *EMBO J.* **7**:2131–2138.

62. Song, K., Wang, Y., and Sassoon, D. (1992) Expression of Hox-7.1 in myoblasts inhibits terminal differentiation and induces cell transformation. *Nature* **360**:477–481.

63. Maulbecker, C. C. and Gruss, P. (1993) The oncogenic potential of deregulated homeobox genes. *Cell Growth Diff.* **4**:431–441.

64. Aberdam, D., Negreanu, V., Sachs, L., and Blatt, C. (1991) The oncogenic potential of an activated Hox-2.4 homeobox gene in mouse fibroblasts. *Mol. Cell. Biol.* **11**:554–557.

65. De Vita, G., Barba, P., Odartchenko, N., Givel, J. C., Freschi, G., Bucciarelli, G., et al. (1993) Expression of homeobox-containing genes in primary and metastatic colorectal cancer. *Eur. J. Cancer* **29A**:887–893.

66. Redline, R. W., Hudock, P., MacFee, M., and Patterson, P. (1994) Expression of AbdB-type homeobox genes in human tumors. *Lab. Invest.* **71**:663–670.

67. Gao, A. C. and Isaacs, J. T. (1996) Expression of homeobox gene-GBX2 in human prostatic cancer cells. *Prostate* **29**:395–398.

68. Matsui, T., Hirai, M., Hirano, M., and Kurosawa, Y. (1993) The HOX complex neighbored by the EVX gene, as well as two other homeobox-containing genes, the GBX-class and the EN-class, are located on the same chromosomes 2 and 7 in humans. *FEBS Lett.* **336**:107–110.

69. Matsui, T., Hirai, M., Wakita, M., Hirano, M., and Kurosawa, Y. (1993) Expression of a novel human homeobox-containing gene that maps to chromosome 7q36.1 in hematopoietic cells. *FEBS Lett.* **322**:181–185.

70. Murtha, M. T., Leckman, J. F., and Ruddle, F. H. (1991) Detection of homeobox genes in development and evolution. *Proc. Natl. Acad. Sci. USA* **88**:10711–10715.

71. Chapman, G. and Rathjen, P. D. (1995) Sequence and evolutionary conservation of the murine Gbx-2 homeobox gene. *FEBS Lett.* **364**:289–292.

72. Fainsod, A. and Greunbaum, Y. (1989) A chicken homeo box gene with developmentally regulated expression. *FEBS Lett.* **250**:381–385.

73. Bulfone, A., Puelles, L., Porteus, M. H., Frohman, M. A., Martin, G. R., and Rubenstein, J. L. (1993) Spatially restricted expression of Dix-1, Dix-2 (Tes-1), Gbx-2, and Wnt-3 in the embryonic day 12.5 mouse forebrain defines potential transverse and longitudinal segmental boundaries. *J. Neurosci.* **13**:3155–3172.

74. Gao, A. C., Lou, W., and Isaacs, J. T. (1998) Down regulation of homeobox gene *GBX2* expression inhibits human prostate cancer clonogenic ability and tumorigenicity. *Cancer Res.* **58**:1391–1394.

75. Bao, L., Loda, M., Janmey, P. A., Anand-Apte, B., and Zetter, B. R. (1996) Thymosin beta 15: a novel regulator of tumor cell motility upregulated in metastatic prostate cancer. *Nature Med.* **2**:1322–1328.

76. Hobisch, A., Culig, Z., Radmayr, C., Bartsch, G., Klocker, H., and Hittmair, A. (1996) Androgen receptor status of lymph node metastases from prostate cancer. *Prostate* **28**:129–135.

77. Hobisch, A., Culig, Z., Radmayr, C., Bartsch, G., Klocker, H., and Hittmair, A. (1995) Distant metastases from prostate carcinoma express androgen receptor protein. *Cancer Res.* **55**:3068–3072.

78. Koivisto, P., Kononen, J., Palmberg, C., Tammela, T., Hyytinen, E., Isola, J., et al. (1997) Androgen receptor gene amplification: a possible molecular mechanism for androgen deprivation therapy failure in prostate cancer. *Cancer Res.* **57**:314–319.

79. Visakorpi, T., Hyytinen, E., Koivisto, P., Tanner, M., Keinanen, R., Palmberg, C., et al. (1995) In vivo amplification of the androgen receptor gene and progression of human prostate cancer. *Nature Genet.* **9**:401–406.

80. Choong, C. S., Sturm, M. J., Strophair, J. A. McCulloch, R. K., Tilley, W. D., Leedman, P. J., et al. (1996) Partial androgen insensitivity caused by an androgen receptor mutation at amino acid 907 (Gly/ÆArg) that results in decreased ligand binding affinity and reduced androgen receptor messenger ribonucleic acid levels. *J. Clin. Endocrinol. Metab.* **81**:236–243.

81. Marcelli, M., Tilley, W. D., Zoppi, S., Griffin, J. E., Wilson, J. D., and McPhaul, M. J. (1991) Androgen resistance associated with a mutation of the androgen receptor at amino acid 772 (Arg/ÆCys) results from a combination of decreased messenger ribonucleic acid levels and impairment of receptor function. *J. Clin. Endocrinol. Metab.* **73**:318–325.

82. McPhaul, M. J., Marcelli, M., Tilley, W. D., Griffin, J. E., Isidro-Gutierrez, R. F., Wilson, J. D. (1991) Molecular basis of androgen resistance in a family with a qualitative abnormality of the androgen receptor and responsive to high-dose androgen therapy. *J. Clin. Invest.* **87**:1413–1421.

83. Gaddipati, J. P., McLeod, D. G., Heidenberg, H. B., Sesterhenn, I. A., Finger, M. J. Moul, J. W., et al. (1994) Frequent detection of codon 877 mutation in the androgen receptor gene in advanced prostate cancers. *Cancer Res.* **54**:2861–2864.

84. Culig, Z., Hobisch, A., Cronauer, M. V., Cato, A. C., Hittmair, A., Radmayr, C., et al. (1993) Mutant androgen receptor detected in an advanced stage prostatic carcinoma is activated by adrenal androgens and progesterone. *Mol. Endocrinol.* **7**:1541–1550.

85. Tilley, W. D., Buchana, G., Hickey, T. T., and Bentel, J. M. (1996) Mutations in the androgen receptor gene are associated with progression of human prostate cancer to androgen independent. *Clin. Cancer Res.* **2**:277–285.

86. Bandyk, M. G., Zhao, L., Troncoso, P., Pisters, L. L., Palmer, J. L., von Eschenbach, A. C., et al. (1994) Trisomy 7: a potential cytogenetic marker of human prostate cancer progression. *Genes Chromosomes Cancer* **9**:19–27.

87. Knudson, A. G. (1971) Mutation and cancer: a statistical study of retinoblastoma. *Proc. Natl. Acad. Sci. USA* **68**:820–823.

88. Carter, B. S., Ewing, C. M., Ward, W. S., Treiger, B. F., Aalders, T. W., Schalken J. A., et al. (1990) Allelic loss of chromosomes 16q and 10q in human prostate cancer. *Proc. Natl. Acad. Sci. USA* **87**:8751–8755.

89. Kunimi, K., Bergerheim, U. S., Larsson, I. L., Ekman, P., and Collins, V. P. (1991) Allelotyping of human prostatic adenocarcinoma. *Genomics* **11**:530–536.

90. Phillips, S. M., Barton, C. M., Lee, S. J., Morton, D. G., Wallace, D. M., Lemoine N. R., et al. (1994) Loss of the retinoblastoma susceptibility gene (RB1) is a frequent and early event in prostatic tumorigenesis. *Br. J. Cancer* **70**:1252–1257.

91. Bergerheim, U. S., Kunimi, K., Collins, V. P., and Ekman, P. (1991) Deletion mapping of chromosomes 8, 10, and 16 in human prostatic carcinoma. *Genes Chromosomes Cancer* **3**:215–220.

92. Macoska, J. A., Trybus, T. M., Benson, P. D., Sakr, W. A., Grignon, D. J., Wojno, K. D., et al. (1995) Evidence for three tumor suppressor gene loci on chromosome 8p in human prostate cancer. *Cancer Res.* **55**:5390–5395.

93. Macoska, J. A., Trybus, T. M., Sakr, W. A., Wolf, M. C., Benson, P. D., Powell, I. J., et al. (1994) Fluorescence in situ hybridization analysis of 8p allelic loss and chromosome 8 instability in human prostate cancer. *Cancer Res.* **54**:3824–3830.

94. Bova, G. S., Carter, B. S., Bussemakers, M. J., Emi, M., Fujiwara, Y., Kyprianou, N., et al. (1993) Homozygous deletion and frequent allelic loss of chromosome 8p22 loci in human prostate cancer. *Cancer Res.* **53**:3869–3873.

95. Gao, X., Zacharek, A., Grignon, D. J., Sakr, W., Powell, I. J., Porter, A. T., et al. (1995) Localization of potential tumor suppressor loci to a <2 Mb region on chromosome 17q in human prostate cancer. *Oncogene* **11**:1241–1247.

96. Latil, A., Baron, J. C., Cussenot, O., Fournier, G., Soussi, T., Boccon-Gibod, L., et al. (1994) Genetic alterations in localized prostate cancer: identification of a common region of deletion on chromosome arm 18q. *Genes Chromosomes Cancer* **11**:119–125.

97. MacGrogan, D., Levy, A., Bostwick, D., Wagner, M., Wells, D., and Bookstein R. (1994) Loss of chromosome arm 8p loci in prostate cancer: mapping by quantitative allelic imbalance. *Genes Chromosomes Cancer* **10**:151–159.

98. Zenklusen, J. C., Thompson, J. C., Troncoso, P., Kagan, J., and Conti, C. J. (1994) Loss of heterozygosity in human primary prostate carcinomas: a possible tumor suppressor gene at 7q31.1. *Cancer Res.* **54**:6370–6373.

99. Brewster, S. F., Gingell, J. C., Browne, S., and Brown, K. W. (1994) Loss of heterozygosity on chromosome 18q is associated with muscle-invasive transitional cell carcinoma of the bladder. *Br. J. Cancer* **70**:697–700.

100. Massenkeil, G., Oberhuber, H., Hailemariam, S., Sulser, T., Diener, P. A, Bannwart, F., et al. (1994) p53 mutations and loss of heterozygosity on chromosomes 8p, 16q, 17p, and 18q are confined to advanced prostate cancer. *Anticancer Res.* **14**:2785–2790.

101. Trapman, J., Sleddens, H. F., van der Weiden, M. M., Dinjens, W. N., Konig, J. J., Schroder, F. H., et al. (1994) Loss of heterozygosity of chromosome 8 microsatellite loci implicates a candidate tumor suppressor gene between the loci D8S87 and D8S133 in human prostate cancer. *Cancer Res.* **54**:6061–6064.

102. Oakahashi, S., Shan, A. L., Ritiand, S. R., Delacey, K. A., Bostwick, D. G., Lieber, M. M., et al. (1995) Frequent loss of heterozygosity at 7q31.1 in primary prostate cancer is associated with tumor aggressiveness and progression. *Cancer Res.* **55**:4114–4119.

103. Alcaraz, A., Takahashi, S., Brown, J. A., Bergstralh, E. J., Larson-Keller, J. J., Lieber, M. M., et al. (1994) Aneuploidy and aneusomy of chromosome 7 detected by fluoresence in situ hybridization are markers of poor prognosis in prostate cancer. *Cancer Res.* **54**:3998–4002.

104. Vocke, C. D., Pozzatti, R. O., Bostwick, D. G., Florence, C. D., Jennings, S. B., Strup, S. E., et al. (1996) Analysis of 99 microdissected prostate carcinomas reveals a high frequency of allelic loss on chromosome 8p12-21. *Cancer Res.* **56**:2411–2416.

105. MacGrogan, D., Levy, A., Bova, G. S., Isaacs, W. B., and Bookstein, R. (1996) Structure and methylation-associated silencing of a gene within a homozygously deleted region of human chromosome band 8p22. *Genomics* **35**:55–65.

106. Bova, G. S., MacGrogan, D., Levy, A., Pin, S. S., and Bookstein, R., and Isaacs W. B. (1996) Physical mapping of chromosome 8p22 markers and their homozygous deletion in a metastatic prostate cancer. *Genomics* **35**:46–54.

107. He, W. W., Sciavolino, P. J., Wing, J., Augustus, M., Hudson, P., Meissner, P. S., et al. (1997) A novel human prostate-specific, androgen-regulated homeobox gene (NKX3.1) that maps to 8p21, a region frequently deleted in prostate cancer. *Genomics* **43**:69–77.

108. Atkin, N. B. and Baker, M. C. (1985) Chromosome 10 deletion in carcinoma of the prostate. *N. Engl. J. Med.* **312**:315.

109. Lundgren, R., Kristoffersson, U., Heim, S., Mandahl, N., and Mitelman F. (1988) Multiple structural chromosome rearrangements, including del(7q) and del(10q), in an adenocarcinoma of the prostate. *Cancer Genet. Cytogenet.* **35**:103–108.

110. Edelhoff, S., Ayer, D. E., Zervos, A. S., Steingrimsson, E., Jenkins, N. A., Copeland, N. G., et al. (1994) Mapping of two genes encod-

ing members of a distinct subfamily of MAX interacting proteins: MAD to human chromosome 2 and mouse chromosome 6, and MXI1 to human chromosome 10 and mouse chromosome 19. *Oncogene* **9**:665–668.

111. Shapiro, D. N., Valentine, V., Eagle, L., Yin, X., Morris, S. W., and Prochownik E. V. (1994) Assignment of the human MAD and MXI1 genes to chromosomes 2p12-p13 and 10q24-q25. *Genomics* **23**:282–285.
112. Eagle, L. R., Yin, X., Brothman, A. R., Williams, B. J., Atkin, N. B., and Prochownik E. V. (1995) Mutation of the MXI1 gene in prostate cancer. *Nature Genet.* **9**:249–255.
113. Gray, I. C., Phillips, S. M., Lee, S. J., Neoptolemos, J. P., Weissenbach J., and Spurr, N. K. (1995) Loss of the chromosomal region 10q23-25 in prostate cancer. *Cancer Res.* **55**:4800–4803.
114. Li, J., Yen, C., Liaw, D., Podsypanina, K., Bose, S., Wang, S. I., et al. (1997) PTEN, a putative protein tyrosine phosphatase gene mutated in human brain, breast, and prostate cancer. *Science* **275**:1943–1947.
115. Steck, P. A., Pershouse, M. A., Jasser, S. A., Yung, W. K., Lin, H., Ligon, A. H., et al. (1997) Identification of a candidate tumor suppressor gene, MMAC1, at chromosome 10q23.3 that is mutated in multiple advanced cancers. *Nature Genet.* **15**:356–362.
116. Cairns, P., Okami, K., Halachmi, S., Halachmi, N., Esteller, M., Herman, J. G., et al. (1997) Frequent inactivation of PTEN/MMACI in primary prostate cancer. *Cancer Res.* **57**:4997–5000.
117. Phillips, S. M., Morton, D. G., Lee, S. J., Wallace, D. M., and Neoptolemos J. P. (1994) Loss of heterozygosity of the retinoblastoma and adenomatous polyposis susceptibility gene loci and in chromosomes 10p, 10q and 16q in human prostate cancer. *Br. J. Urol.* **73**:390–395.
118. Visakorpi, T., Kallioniemi, A. H., Syvanen, A. C., Hyytinen, E. R., Karhu, R., Tammela, T., et al. (1995) Genetic changes in primary and recurrent prostate cancer by comparative genomic hybridization. *Cancer Res.* **55**:342–347.
119. Ittmann, M. M. and Wieczorek, R. (1996) Alterations of the retinoblastoma gene in clinically localized, stage B prostate adenocarcinomas. *Human Pathol.* **27**:28–34.
120. Brooks, J. D., Bova, G. S., and Isaacs, W. B. (1995) Allelic loss of the retinoblastoma gene in primary human prostatic adenocarcinomas. *Prostate* **26**:35–39.
121. Bookstein, R., Rio, P., Madreperia, S. A., Hong, F., Allred, C., Grizzle, W. E, et al. (1990) Promoter deletion and loss of retinoblastoma gene expression in human prostate carcinoma. *Proc. Natl. Acad. Sci. USA* **87**:7762–7766.
122. Bookstein, R., Shew, J. Y., Chen, P. L., Scully, P., and Lee, W. H. (1990) Suppression of tumorigenicity of human prostate carcinoma cells by replacing a mutated RB gene. *Science* **247**:712–715.
123. Natt, E., Magenis, R. E., Zimmer, J., Mansouri, A., and Scherer, G. (1989) Regional assignment of the human loci for uvomorulin (UVO) and chymotrypsinogen B (CTRB) with the help of two overlapping deletions on the long arm of chromosome 16. *Cytogenet. Cell Genet.* **50**:145–148.
124. Peyrieras, N., Hyafil, F., Louvard, D., Ploegh, H. L., and Jacob, F. (1983) Uvomorulin: a nonintegral membrane protein of early mouse embryo. *Proc. Natl. Acad. Sci. USA* **80**:6274–6277.
125. Behrens, J., Birchmeier, W., Goodman, S. L., and Imhof, B. A. (1985) Dissociation of Madin-Darby canine kidney epithelial cells by the monoclonal antibody anti-arc-1: mechanistic aspects and identification of the antigen as a component related to uvomorulin. *J. Cell Biol.* **101**:1307–1315.
126. Takeichi, M. (1991) Cadherin cell adhesion receptors as a morphogenetic regulator. *Science* **251**:1451–1455.
127. Frixen, U. H., Behrens, J., Sachs, M., Eberle, G., Voss, B., Warda, A., et al. (1991) E-cadherin-mediated cell-cell adhesion prevents invasiveness of human carcinoma cells. *J. Cell Biol.* **113**:173–185.
128. Sommers, C. L., Thompson, E. W., Torri, J. A., Kemier, R., Gelmann, E. P., and Byers, S. W. (1991) Cell adhesion molecule uvomorulin expression in human breast cancer cell lines: relationship to morphology and invasive capacities. *Cell Growth Diff.* **2**:365–372.
129. Vleminckx, K., Vakaet, L., Jr., Mareel, M., Fiers, W., and van Roy, F. (1991) Genetic manipulation of E-cadherin expression by epithelial tumor cells reveals an invasion suppressor role. *Cell* **66**:107–119.
130. Bussemakers, M. J., van Moorselaar, R. J., Giroldi, L. A., Ichikawa, T, Isaacs, J. T., Takeichi, M., et al. (1992) Decreased expression of E-cadherin in the progression of rat prostatic cancer. *Cancer Res.* **52**:2916–2922.
131. Umbas, R., Isaacs, W. B., Bringuier, P. P., Schaafsma, H. E., Karthaus, H. F., Oosterhof, G. O., et al. (1994) Decreased E-cadherin expression is associated with poor prognosis in patients with prostate cancer. *Cancer Res.* **54**:3929–3933.
132. Morton, R. A., Ewing, C. M., Nagafuchi, A., Tsukita, S., and Isaacs, W. B. (1993) Reduction of E-cadherin levels and deletion of the α-catenin gene in human prostate cancer cells. *Cancer Res.* **53**:3585–3590.
133. Ozawa, M., Baribault, H., and Kemier, R. (1989) The cytoplasmic domain of the cell adhesion molecule uvomorulin associates with three independent proteins structurally related in different species. *EMBO J.* **8**.1711–1717.
134. McPherson, J. D., Morton, R. A., Ewing, C. M., Wasmuth, J. J., Overhauser J., Nagafuchi, A., et al. (1994) Assignment of the human α-catenin gene (CTNNA1) to chromosome 5q21-q22. *Genomics* **19**:188–190.
135. Ewing, C. M., Ru, N., Morton, R. A., Robinson, J. C., Wheelock, M. J., Johnson, K.R., et al. (1995) Chromosome 5 suppresses tumorigenicity of PC3 prostate cancer cells: correlation with re-expression of α-catenin and restoration of E-cadherin function. *Cancer Res.* **55**:4813–4817.
136. Elo, J. P., Harkonen, P., Kylionen, A. P., Lukkarinen, O. L., Poutanen, M., Vihko, R., et al. (1997) Loss of heterozygosity at 16q24.1-24.2 is significantly associated with metastatic and aggressive behavior of prostate cancer. *Cancer Res.* **57**:3356–3359.
137. Mottaz, A. E., Markwalder, R., Fey, M. F., Klima, I,, Merz, V. W., Thalmann, G. N., et al. (1997) Abnormal p53 expression is rare in clinically localized human prostate cancer: comparison between immunohistochemical and molecular detection of p53 mutations. *Prostate* **31**:209–215.
138. Brewster, S. F., Browne, S., and Brown, K. W. (1994) Somatic allelic loss at the DCC, APC, nm23-HI and p53 tumor suppressor gene loci in human prostatic carcinoma. *J. Urol.* **151**:1073–1077.
139. Cohen, R. J., Cooper, K., Haffejee, Z., Robinson, E., and Becker, P. J. (1995) Immunohistochemical detection of oncogene proteins and neuroendocrine differentiation in different stages of prostate cancer. *Pathology* **27**:229–232.
140. Brooks, J. D., Bova, G. S., Ewing, C. M., Piantadosi, S., Carter, B. S., Robinson, J. C., et al. (1996) An uncertain role for p53 gene alterations in human prostate cancers. *Cancer Res.* **56**:3814–3822.
141. Isaacs, W. B., Carter, B. S., and Ewing, C. M. (1991) Wild-type p53 suppresses growth of human prostate cancer cells containing mutant p53 alleles. *Cancer Res.* **51**:4716–4720.
142. Fearon, E. R., Cho, K. R., Nigro, J. M., Kern, S. E., Simons, J. W., Ruppert, J. M., et al. (1990) Identification of a chromosome 18q gene that is altered in colorectal cancers. *Science* **247**:49–56.
143. Gao, X., Honn, K. V., Grignon, D., Sakr, W., and Chen, Y. Q. (1993) Frequent loss of expression and loss of heterozygosity of the putative tumor suppressor gene DCC in prostatic carcinomas. *Cancer Res.* **53**:2723–2727.
144. Ichikawa, T., Ichikawa, Y., and Isaacs, J. T. (1991) Genetic factors and suppression of metastatic ability of prostatic cancer. *Cancer Res.* **51**:3788–3792.
145. Steeg, P. S., Bevilacqua, G., Pozzatti, R., Liotta, L. A., and Sobel, M. E. (1988) Altered expression of NM23, a gene associated with low tumor metastatic potential, during adenovirus 2 E1a inhibition of experimental metastasis. *Cancer Res.* **48**:6550–6554.
146. Rinker-Schaeffer, C. W., Hawkins, A. L., Ru, N., Dong, J., Stoica, G., Griffin, C. A., et al. (1994) Differential suppression of mammary and prostate cancer metastasis by human chromosomes 17 and 11. *Cancer Res.* **54**:6249–6256.
147. Igawa, M., Rukstalis, D. B., Tanabe, T., and Chodak, G. W. (1994) High levels of nm23 expression are related to cell proliferation in human prostate cancer. *Cancer Res.* **54**:1313–1318.

148. Jensen, S. L., Wood, D. P., Banks, E. R., Mcroberts, W., Rangnekar, V. W. (1993) Increased levels of NM23-H mRNA associated with adenocarcinoma of the prostate. Society for Basic Urological Research Abstracts.

149. Koi, M., Shimizu, M., Morita, H., Yamada, H., and Oshimura, M. (1989) Construction of mouse A9 clones containing a single human chromosome tagged with neomycin-resistance gene via microcell fusion. *Jpn. J. Cancer Res.* **80**:413–418.

150. Koi, M., Morita, H., Shimizu, M., and Oshimura, M. (1989) Construction of mouse A9 clones containing a single human chromosome (X/autosome translocation) via micro-cell fusion. *Jpn. J. Cancer Res.* **80**:122–125.

151. Koi, M., Morita, H., Yamada, H., Satoh, H., Barrett, J. C., and Oshimura, M. (1989) Normal human chromosome 11 suppresses tumorigenicity of human cervical tumor cell line SiHa. *Mol. Carcinogenesis* **2**:12–2 1.

152. Nihei, N., Ichikawa, T., Kawana, Y., Kuramochi, H., Kugoh, H. X., Oshimura, M., et al. (1996) Mapping of metastasis suppressor gene(s) for rat prostate cancer on the short arm of human chromosome 8 by irradiated microcell-mediated chromosome transfer. *Genes Chromosomes Cancer* **17**:260–268.

153. Nihei, N., Ichikawa, T., Kawana, Y., Kuramochi, H., Kugo, H. X., Oshimura, M., et al. (1995) Localization of metastasis suppressor gene(s) for rat prostatic cancer to the long arm of human chromosome 10. *Genes Chromosomes Cancer* **14**:112–119.

154. Ichikawa, T., Ichikawa, Y., Dong, J., Hawkins, A. L., Griffin, C. A., Isaacs, W. B., et al. (1992) Localization of metastasis suppressor gene(s) for prostatic cancer to the short arm of human chromosome 11. *Cancer Res.* **52**:3486–3490.

155. Dong, J. T., Suzuki, H., Pin, S. S., Bova, G. S., Schalken, J. A., Isaacs, W. B., et al. (1996) Down-regulation of the KAI1 metastasis suppressor gene during the progression of human prostatic cancer infrequently involves gene mutation or allelic loss. *Cancer Res.* **56**:4387–4390.

156. Dong, J. T., Lamb, P. W., Rinker-Schaeffer, C. W., Vukanovic, J. X., Ichikawa T, Isaacs, J. T., et al. (1995) KAI1, a metastasis suppressor gene for prostate cancer on human chromosome 11p11.2. *Science* **268**:884–886.

157. Ueda, T., Ichikawa, T., Tamaru, J., Mikata, A., Akakura, K., Akimoto, S., et al. (1996) Expression of the KAI1 protein in benign prostatic hyperplasia and prostate cancer. *Am. J. Pathol.* **149**:1435–1440.

158. Kawana, Y., Komiya, A., Ueda, T., Kuramochi, H., Suzuki, H., Yatani, R., et al. (1997) Location of KAI1 on the short arm of human chromosome 11 and frequency of allelic loss in advanced human prostate cancer. *Prostate* **32**:205–213.

159. Gao, A. C., Lou, W., Dong, J. T., and Isaacs, J. T. (1997) CD44 is a metastasis suppressor gene for prostatic cancer located on human chromosome 11p13. *Cancer Res.* **57**:846–849.

160. Gunthert, U., Stauder, R., Mayer, B., Terpe, H. J., Finke, L. X., and Friedrichs, K. (1995) Are CD44 variant isoforms involved in human tumor progression? *Cancer Surveys* **24**:19–42.

161. Screaton, G. R., Bell, M. V., Bell, J. I., and Jackson, D. G. (1993) The identification of a new alternative exon with highly restricted tissue expression in transcripts encoding the mouse Pgp-1 (CD44) homing receptor. Comparison of all 10 variable exons between mouse, human, and rat. *J. Biol. Chem.* **268**:12235–12238.

162. Screaton, G. R., Bell, M. V., Jackson, D. G., Cornelis, F. B., Gerth, U. X., and Bell J. I. (1992) Genomic structure of DNA encoding the lymphocyte homing receptor CD44 reveals at least 12 alternatively spliced exons. *Proc. Natl. Acad. Sci. USA* **89**:12160–12164.

163. Goldstein, L. A., Zhou, D. F., Picker, L. J., Minty, C. N., Bargatze, R. F., Ding, J. F., et al. (1989) A human lymphocyte homing receptor, the hermes antigen, is related to cartilage proteoglycan core and link proteins. *Cell* **56**:1063–1072.

164. Underhill, C. (1992) CD44: the hyaluronan receptor. *J. Cell Sci.* **103**:293–298.

165. Weber, G. F., Ashkar, S., Glimcher, M. J., and Cantor, H. (1996). Receptor-ligand interaction between CD44 and osteopontin (Eta-1). *Science* **271**:509–512.

166. Kallakury, B. V., Yang, F., Figge, J., Smith, K. E., Kausik, S. J., Tacy, N. J., et al. (1996) Decreased levels of CD44 protein and mRNA in prostate carcinoma. Correlation with tumor grade and ploidy. *Cancer* **78**:1461–1469.

167. Noordzij, M. A., Steenbrugge, G.-J. V., Verkaik, N. S., Schroder, F. H., and Van der Kwast, T. H. (1997) The prognostic value of CD44 isoforms in prostate cancer patients treated by radical prostatectomy. *Clin. Cancer Res.* **3**:805–815.

168. Lee, W. H., Morton, R. A., Epstein, J. I., Brooks, J. D., Campbell, P. A., Bova, G. S., et al. (1994) Cytidine methylation of regulatory sequences near the π-class glutathione-S-transferase gene accompanies human prostate cancer carcinogenesis. *Proc. Acad. Natl. Sci. USA* **91**:11733–11737.

169. Kleinerman, D. I., Troncoso, P., Lin, S. H., Pisters, L. L., Sherwood, E. R., Brooks, T., et al. (1995) Consistent expression of an epithelial cell adhesion molecule (C-CAM) during human prostate development and loss of expression in prostate cancer: implication as a tumor suppressor. *Cancer Res.* **55**:1215–1220.

170. Gao, X., Zacharek, A., Salkowski, A., Grignon, D. J., Sakr, W., Porter, A. T., et al. (1995) Loss of heterozygosity of the BRCA1 and other loci on chromosome 17q in human prostate cancer. *Cancer Res.* **55**:1002–1005.

171. Langston, A. A., Stanford, J. L., Wicklund, K. G., Thompson, J. D., Blazej, R. G., and Ostrander, E. A. (1996) Germ-line BRCA1 mutations in selected men with prostate cancer. *Am. J. Human Genet.* **58**:881–884.

17 The Molecular Basis of Lung Carcinogenesis

Kwun M. Fong, MD, Yoshitaka Sekido, MD, PhD, and John D. Minna, MD

INTRODUCTION

Lung cancer is the leading cause of cancer deaths in the Western world. According to the World Health Organization (WHO), lung cancer kills about 1 million people worldwide each year. In the United States in 1997, lung cancer accounted for 13% of new cancer cases, and 32% of cancer deaths in males and 17% of cancer deaths in females *(1)*.

Clinically, lung cancer is usually broadly classified into two categories: nonsmall-cell lung cancer (NSCLC) and small-cell lung cancer (SCLC). This classification relies on differences in histological, clinical, and neuroendocrine (NE) differentiation characteristics, which are often expressed by SCLC cells (Table 1). NSCLC accounts for about 75% of bronchogenic carcinomas, and SCLC constitutes almost all of the remainder. However, there are a small proportion of mixed tumor types, with features of both NSCLC and SCLC.

A characteristic NE phenotype is expressed by the pulmonary NE cells of normal lung and in a subset of lung malignancies; primarily SCLC, bronchopulmonary carcinoids, and NSCLC with NE features *(2,3)*. This phenotype is characterized by: 1) specific peptide production; 2) general NE markers such as L-dopa decarboxylase, chromogranin A, synaptophysin A, neuron-specific enolase (NSE), and neural-cell adhesion molecule (NCAM); and 3) the presence of cytoplasmic dense core granules. In normal lung, pulmonary NE cells show granular cytoplasmic silver staining and may occur singly or in small clusters in the bronchi (known as neuro-epithelial bodies). They are most numerous in late fetal and early postnatal life and are relatively scant in normal adult lung, suggesting that their secretions play a major role in pulmonary development and maturation. In contrast, most NSCLC lack these properties and are comprised of three major subtypes: adenocarcinoma, squamous-cell carcinoma, and large cell carcinoma. In vitro, the NSCLC and SCLC subtypes also tend to have different biological profiles such as the adhesion of NSCLC cells to substrate, which is generally absent in SCLC cell lines. The CD44 adhesion molecule (which is involved in intercellular interactions) was found to be predominantly associated with the NSCLC phenotype, indicating that it may be a useful differentiation marker *(4)*.

Although it is still uncertain whether SCLC and NSCLC are derived from the same or different cell lineage, much progress has been made towards understanding the molecular etiology of lung cancer. Tumorigenesis is a complex process, and the current paradigm suggests that human epithelial tumours such as lung cancer arise as a result of the accumulation of multiple independent molecular lesions that affect critical genetic pathways, distinct from the random genetic damage that occurs in advanced neoplasms. Furthermore, it is believed that specific proto-oncogenes and tumor-suppressor genes are the target of somatic mutations in lung cancer, resulting from the genotoxic effects of tobacco-smoke carcinogens.

The critical cellular pathways affected directly or indirectly by the various acquired mutations are becoming apparent as the biochemical functions of the proteins encoded by the mutated genes continue to be discovered. Cancer development results from abnormal cell proliferation (with loss of the normal cellular-growth control mechanisms) and abnormalities in apoptosis (programmed cell death). Indeed, solid tumours ensue from an imbalance between cell proliferation and cell death. The regulation of these processes is extremely complex, involving positive mediators of cell proliferation (cytokines, hormones, growth factors and their specific receptors, and signaling molecules) and negative regulators of cell growth and proliferation (tumor-suppressor genes, cell-cycle regulators). Proto-oncogenes are the normal cellular counterparts of viral oncogenes. They encode proteins that are positive effectors of the transformed phenotype and may be considered positive growth regulators. Oncogenic activation of proto-oncogenes (c-*ras*, c-*myc*) typically occurs via mechanisms that target only one allele, such as gene amplification, point mutation, or transcriptional dysregulation, resulting in constitutive over-

From: *The Molecular Basis of Human Cancer* (W. B. Coleman and G. J. Tsongalis, eds.), © Humana Press Inc., Totowa, NJ.

Table 1
Characteristics of Small Cell and Nonsmall Cell Lung Cancer

	SCLC	NSCLC
Frequency	~25%	~75%
Histology	Scant cytoplasm, small hyperchromatic nuclei, fine chromatin, indistinct nucleoli, tumor in sheets	Abundant cytoplasm, pleomorphic nuclei, coarse chromatin, prominent nucleoli, squamous /glandular architecture
Neuroendocrine phenotype	~100%	Large cell neuroendocrine carcinomas and carcinoids
Peptide secretion	ACTH, AVP, calcitonin, ANF	PTH
Radiation-sensitivity	80–90% shrinkage	30–50% shrinkage
Chemo-sensitivity	High	Low
c-ras mutation	< 1%	~15–20%
c-myc amplification/overexpression	~15–30%	~5-10%
c-erbB2 over-expression	<10%	~ 30%
bcl2 expression	~75–95%	~10–35%
Aberrant CD44 expression	Generally absent	Present
Putative autocrine loops	GRP/GRP receptor, SCF/KIT	HGF/met, neuregulin/erbB
3p allele loss	>90%	~50–80%
p53 mutation	~75–100%	~50%
17p LOH	~80–90%	~70%
Abnormal p53 expression (immunohistochemistry)	~40–70%	~40–60%
Absent Rb1 expression	~90%	~15–30%
13q LOH	~75%	~40–60%
$p16^{INK4A}$ mutation	< 1 %	~10–40%
9p LOH	~20–50%	~50–75%
Absent $p16^{INK4A}$ expression (immunohistochemistry)	~0–10%	~30–70%
Other genetic deletions 5q, 8p, 11p, 18q	Present, variable	Present, variable
Telomerase expression	~100%	80–85%

expression. These activating mechanisms cause functional deregulation of the proto-oncogene, thereby leading to a gain in function or dominant effect. It is clear that some proto-oncogene products function as essential components of growth-signaling pathways. These can become abnormally activated in the course of lung-cancer development by different genetic mechanisms, and also by other yet unidentified processes not obviously involving genetic mutations. These proto-oncogene products include various growth factors, receptor tyrosine kinases, nonreceptor tyrosine kinases, membrane-associated G proteins, cytoplasmic serine/threonine kinases, and nuclear transcription factors (Fig. 1). Conversely, tumor-suppressor gene products (p53, Rb) are negative growth regulators. It is their loss of function, classically by loss of one allele and point mutation of the other allele, that contributes to malignant transformation. The requirement for the mutations to affect both alleles of the tumor-suppressor gene represents the two-hit hypothesis initially proposed by Knudson for retinoblastomas.

Another class of genes implicated in tumorigenesis encode proteins involved in DNA synthesis and repair. Notably, DNA mismatch repair (MMR) gene defects have been linked to tumors of the hereditary nonpolyposis coli syndrome. Some lung cancers also exhibit the genetic changes in certain DNA repeat sequences (termed microsatellites), which is pathognomonic of this type of defect (microsatellite instability; MSI). These observations are consistent with the possibility of a mutator phenotype in lung tumorigenesis. Cells that exhibit a mutator phenotype have sustained damage to genes that may be involved in DNA replication, repair, or chromosomal segregation, predisposing the affected cells to a cascade of additional mutations and genetic instability (5,6).

Karyotypic and molecular analyses of lung-cancer cells suggest that a number of genetic lesions accumulate in lung cells during tumorigenesis, with perhaps 10 or more lesions required for the development of an overt lung cancer. The temporal sequence and timing of these genetic lesions in the multistep process of lung carcinogenesis continues to unravel as improvements in molecular techniques increase the ability to examine DNA from tiny preneoplastic bronchial lesions that accompany overt cancers. Further, it should be noted that there may be heterogeneity in the timing and number of genetic lesions that occur during the development of lung cancers, such that alternate pathways may still result in the end product of a bronchogenic carcinoma. Although some of the molecular lesions are commonly found in both SCLC and NSCLC, others show greater specificity for one or other subtypes (Table 1). Aneuploidy, representing an abnormal total DNA content, is another frequently found characteristic of tumor cells. Like many other solid tumors that exhibit aneuploidy ranging from hypoploidy to hyperploidy, lung cancers are also often aneuploid (7,8). Several studies have assessed the value of aneuploidy as a marker of biological aggressiveness, but much of the data on the prognostic value of aneuploidy in lung cancer has been conflicting (9,10). Newer techniques have identified ex-

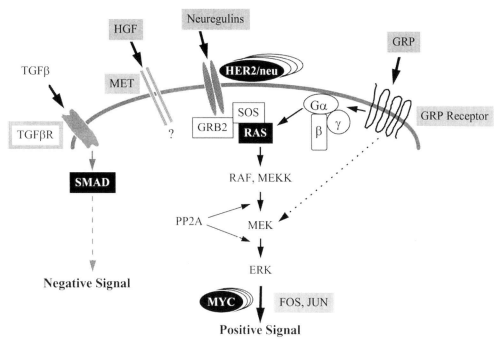

Fig. 1. Schematic representation of some of the major positive and negative signal-transduction pathways regulating cell growth in lung-cancer development. Black boxes indicate protein products whose encoding genes have frequent activating mutations (like c-*ras*) or rare inactivating mutations (*SMAD*) in lung cancer. Black ovals indicate oncogenic activation by gene amplification; either observed frequently (c-*myc*) or occasionally (c-*erbB2*) in lung cancer. Filled grey boxes indicate protein overexpression by uncertain mechanisms; (GRP, GRP receptor, neuregulins, HGF, met, fos and jun). Open gray box indicates downregulation (TGFßR).

tensive areas of aneuploidy in the respiratory epithelium of lung-cancer patients, a finding consistent with the field-cancerization theory (11).

MOLECULAR CHANGES IN OVERT LUNG CANCERS

PROTO-ONCOGENES AND GROWTH STIMULATION Proto-oncogenes may be considered genes that, when aberrantly expressed into normal cells will cause those cells, to acquire some phenotypic characteristics of cancer cells. With this working definition, perhaps about 50 or so genes may currently be classified as proto-oncogenes. Several proto-oncogenes were originally identified by virtue of their chromosomal location within DNA sequences amplified in tumor cells. In early studies, amplified chromosomal sequences were detected using cytogenetic methods. These studies identified aberrant chromosomal structures, including double-minute chromosomes (DMs) and novel staining regions called homogenously staining regions (HSRs). These DMs and HSRs may contain between twenty to several hundred copies of a specific chromosomal sequence. As the amplified sequences often involve several hundred thousand basepairs, it is possible that more than one proto-oncogene is contained within the amplified region. Comparative genomic hybridization (CGH) is a recently developed molecular cytogenetic technique that can detect genetic imbalance (both gains and losses of DNA) in a tumor genome. This powerful technique has led to the identification of several new chromosomal regions affected by either deletions or increased DNA copy number in lung-cancer genomes *(12–16)*. CGH has been applied to cell lines as well as primary or metastatic lung cancers and the chromosomal re-

gions with increased DNA copy number include 1p, 1q, 2p, 3q, 5p, 8q, 11q, 16p, 17q, 19q, and Xq. Some of these chromsomal segments, like 1p32 (L-*myc*), 2p25 (N-*myc*), and 8q24 (c-*myc*), contain known proto-oncogenes, whereas the potentially oncogenic genes in other genomic regions that demonstrate increased copy number have yet to be identified. Of the currently known proto-oncogenes, approx 20 have been shown to be mutated in human tumors and several of these are particularly prominent in the development of lung cancer. These include c-*ras* (typically activated by point mutations) as well as c-*myc* and c-*erbB* (typically activated by amplification and/or overexpression).

The ras Signal Transduction Pathway The c-*ras* gene family represent proto-oncogenes, which are important in a subset of lung cancers. The c-*ras* genes encode 21 kDa proteins, members of a large family of proteins including rho, rac, rab, that regulate cytoskeletal changes, vesicular and nuclear transport, and proliferation. The c-*ras* proto-oncogene family (c-K-*ras*, c-H-*ras*, and c-N-*ras*) is usually activated by point mutations at codons 12, 13, or 61. Mutations affect 15–20% of all NSCLC and approx 20–30% of lung adenocarcinomas, but are very uncommon in SCLC *(17)*. Mutations in c-K-*ras* account for approx 90% of the c-*ras* mutations in lung adenocarcinomas, with 85% of the c-K-*ras* changes affecting codon 12.

In unstimulated cells, c-ras protein is inactive. Following ligand binding, receptor tyrosine kinases signal the c-ras protein by interaction with downstream molecules such as Grb2 and the guanine nucleotide-exchange factor SOS. Wild-type c-ras protein is able to bind to guanosine triphosphate (GTP) but also has intrinsic GTPase activity, which can hydrolyze bound GTP to guanosine diphosphate (GDP). Active GTP-bound ras

AU:
constituitively?

protein stimulates a downstream cascade ending with MAP kinase, which migrates to the cell nucleus and subsequently activates various transcription factors. When GTP is hydrolyzed to GDP, the molecule assumes its inactive configuration and the signal-transduction pathway returns to its inactive state.

When a c-*ras* gene undergoes oncogenic missense mutations, the mutant c-ras oncoprotein loses its capability to hydrolyze GTP and the protein becomes constituitively active. The resultant inappropriate growth signal to the cell nucleus is thought to contribute to unrestrained cellular proliferation; effectively causing a gain of function. This model underscores the general concept that proto-oncogenes encode proteins with important regulatory functions and that oncogenic activation results in mutant proteins with altered function.

The majority of (70%) c-K-*ras* codon 12 mutations are G→T transversions, resulting in either glycine to cysteine (GGT→TGT) or glycine to valine (GGT→GTT) amino acid substitutions in the mutant protein. This type of mutation also affects the p53 gene in lung-cancer cells, and represent the type of DNA damage expected from bulky DNA adducts caused by the polycyclic hydrocarbons and nitrosamines in tobacco smoke *(18)*. The correlation of c-K-*ras* mutations with a smoking history further implicates a causative role of tobacco-smoke carcinogens in the acquisition of these mutations *(19)*. Mutations of c-K-*ras* are suggested to be associated with a poor prognosis in both early- and late-stage NSCLC *(20–24)*. However, other studies have challenged this suggestion. In 181 patients with lung adenocarcinoma, c-K-*ras* mutation status itself did not appear to be a good predictor of prognosis; rather, the substitution of a polar or charged amino acid may be a negative prognostic indicator *(25)*. Although it has also been suggested that c-*ras* mutations induce resistance to chemotherapy and radiation, no association between c-*ras* mutation and in vitro resistance against a range of chemotherapeutic agents was found in a panel of NSCLC cell lines *(26)*. Moreover, a recent prospective study has shown that neither chemotherapy-sensitivity nor survival correlated with c-K-*ras* mutation in patients with advanced (inoperable stage III or stage IV) lung adenocarcinoma *(27)*.

The reason for the predilection of c-*ras* mutations for the adenocarcinoma histological subtype of lung cancers is not clear. One possible explanation is that the activation of certain proto-oncogenes may result in disparate tumor-differentiation pathways. In studying this, various proto-oncogenes have been introduced into a nontumorigenic cell line BEAS-2B, derived from normal bronchial epithelial cells transfected with SV40. Overexpression of c-*myc* and c-*raf*-1, for instance, resulted in the development of large tumor cells with certain NE markers *(28)*. Indeed, the subtype specificity may be even more intriguing, because a recent study has reported that c-K-*ras* mutations were seen in parenchymal but not in bronchial adenocarcinomas, indicating genetic heterogeneity *(29)*. Furthermore, the goblet-cell subtype appears to have the highest frequency of c-K-*ras* mutations compared to the other adenocarcinoma subtypes *(30)*. Some investigators have also suggested that rare alleles of the c-H-*ras* minisatellite locus represent a major risk factor for common types of cancer, including lung cancers, but this possibility has not been firmly established *(31)*.

Another proto-oncogene, c-*raf*-1, which encodes a direct downstream effector of c-ras may also be relevant to lung carcinogenesis as one copy of c-*raf*-1 at chromosome region 3p25 is frequently deleted in human lung cancer *(32)*. On the other hand, genetic loss is not the type of abnormality expected with an oncogene according to current concepts. Nevertheless, no c-*raf*-1 mutations in lung cancer have however been detected so far *(33,34)*.

The other signal-transduction molecules downstream of c-raf-1 in this pathway include MEK (MAP kinase/ERK-activating kinase), ERK (extracellular signal-regulated kinase), and their regulatory phosphatases (such as PP2A). Constitutively active mutants of MEK have been shown to transform cells, suggesting that MEK can function as a dominant proto-oncogene. However, *MEK-1* and *MEK-2* are only rarely mutated in lung cancer *(35)*. On the other hand, the *MKK4* (for mitogen-activated protein kinase kinase 4) gene, located approx 10 cM centromeric from *p53* on 17p, has been found to be homozygously deleted in a NSCLC cell line, leading to speculation that it may be a candidate tumor suppressor *(36)*.

c-myc and Other Nuclear Proto-oncogenes Stimulation of the c-ras signal-transduction cascade ultimately activates nuclear proto-oncogene products, including c-myc, which belongs to the basic helix-loop-helix leucine-zipper (bHLHZ) class of transcription factors, and has been implicated in normal cell growth and proliferation through interaction with genes involved in DNA synthesis, RNA metabolism, and cell-cycle progression *(37)*. The c-myc proteins function by heterodimerizing with max, and resultant myc-max heterodimers have a high affinity for CACGTG consensus sequences leading to transcriptional activation of downstream genes. The max protein interacts with another bHLHZ protein, termed mad, to form a complex that is believed to antagonize myc-max function. Thus, the function of c-myc protein appears to be controlled by a complex, interactive system of positive and negative protein regulators.

The c-*myc* proto-oncogenes are the cellular homologs of a gene present in several highly oncogenic avian retroviruses. Of the well-characterized *myc* family of genes, c-*myc* is the most frequently activated in SCLC and NSCLC. On the other hand, its closely related cellular homologs, N-*myc* and L-*myc*, are usually only activated in the SCLC subtype. In fact, L-*myc* was initially isolated from the DNA of a SCLC *(38)*.

Activation of the *myc* genes occurs through gene amplification or transcriptional dysregulation, leading to protein overexpression *(39)*. These genes may be amplified from 20–115 copies per cell, and in most cases, only one member of the *myc* family is amplified. Gene amplification is generally associated with enhanced mRNA expression and increased protein production. From a review of 17 different studies, Richardson et al. calculated that 36/200 (18%) SCLC tumors and 38/122 (31%) SCLC cell lines exhibit amplification of one member of the *myc* proto-oncogene family *(17)*. In comparison, 25/320 (8%) NSCLC tumors and 3/15 (20%) NSCLC cell lines had *myc* amplification. Thus, *myc* family activation in general appears to be more frequent in SCLC than NSCLC. Furthermore, *myc* amplification occurs more frequently in cell lines derived from metastatic lesions than in primary tumors, in patients previously treated with chemotherapy, and in the variant subtype SCLC *(40)*. These observations may help explain why *myc* amplification has been reported to correlate with poor prognosis and survival.

Unlike lymphomas, *myc* translocation and point mutations have not been reported in lung cancer. On the other hand, there have been reports of L-*myc* amplification with rearrangement in which L-*myc* fuses to the *RLF* gene, thereby resulting in a chimeric protein *(41,42)*. In some cases, L-*myc* expression may be associated with neuroendocrine differentiation. For instance, all-*trans*-retinoic acid-mediated growth inhibition of a SCLC cell line was associated with increased NE differentiation and L-*myc* expression, but decreased c-*myc* expression *(43)*. Others have reported that immunohistochemically detectable myc protein overexpression correlates with a lack of histological differentiation in lung cancers *(44)*. Finally, although some studies have suggested that an *EcoRI* restriction fragment-length polymorphism (RFLP) in intron 2 of L-*myc* might be associated with lung (and other human) cancer susceptibility, metastasis, and adverse survival, other studies have shown no such correlation *(38,45)*.

Other nuclear proto-oncogenes such as c-*myb*, c-*jun*, and c-*fos* have also been implicated in lung cancer, although their precise functional importance and biological role are still being investigated. The protein products of c-*jun* and c-*fos* are heterodimeric proteins that function as immediate early transcription factors regulating cellular proliferation. However, their role in lung carcinogenesis remains unresolved. Some investigators have described higher expression of these genes in normal lung tissue adjacent to tumor than in the tumor itself. Conversely, other studies have reported higher expression in tumors with lack of expression in normal epithelium *(46–49)*.

c-erbB Receptor Tyrosine Kinases The peptide growth-factor ligands that interact with the c-erbB family of transmembrane receptor tyrosine kinases are called neuregulins, neu differentiation factors, or heregulins *(50)*. The neuregulin and c-erbB (c-erbB2, c-erbB3, and c-erbB4) families may be considered to be potential growth-stimulatory loops involved in the development of lung cancer *(51)*. On binding neuregulin, c-erbB receptors homodimerize or heterodimerize, subsequently inducing intrinsic kinase activities that initiate intracellular signal-transduction cascades such as the MAP kinase pathway. Although c-erbB2 (also known as HER2/neu) itself lacks ligand-binding ability, it plays a major coordinating role by enhancing and stabilizing dimerization. Each directly liganded receptor appears to dimerize preferentially with c-erbB2, and resulting c-erbB2-containing heterodimers have very high signaling potency.

The c-*erbB2* gene maps to chromosome 17q21, and its amplification and overexpression has been implicated in the development of several human cancers. Although amplification appears uncommon in lung cancer, c-*erbB2* is highly expressed in over a third of NSCLCs, especially in the adenocarcinoma subtype *(52–54)*. Experiments with transfected c-*erbB2* suggest that c-*erbB2* overexpression is insufficient for but contributes to tumor induction in immortalized human bronchial epithelial cells *(55)*. Additionally, an anti-c-erbB2 monoclonal

antibody MAb has been developed that can inhibit the in vitro growth of NSCLC cell lines expressing c-*erbB2* *(56)*.

Some but not all studies have suggested that c-*erbB2* overexpression correlates with a shorter survival in lung cancer *(57–59)*. In any case, other observations support the idea that c-*erbB2* overexpression may be an adverse clinical indicator in some lung-cancer patients. In one study, the transfection of a c-*erbB2* gene into a NSCLC cell line in a xenograft model led to enhanced metastatic potential *(60)*. Transfection and overexpression of the c-*erbB2* gene in a constitutively low c-*erbB2* expressing NSCLC cell line also led to the induction of a drug-resistant phenotype *(61)*. In vitro assays further suggest that c-*erbB2* overexpression may be associated with intrinsic multi-drug resistance to chemotherapy agents in NSCLCs *(62)*.

Another c-*erbB* gene family member (c-*erbB1*) encodes the epidermal growth-factor receptor (EGFR), which has a role in regulating epithelial proliferation and differentiation. Epidermal growth factor (EGF) and transforming growth factor-α (TGF-α) are prominent among the six characterized mammalian ligands that bind to the EGFR. The production of EGFR ligands (especially TGF-α) by lung-cancer cells expressing cognate receptors suggests that this system represents an important autocrine growth stimulatory loop in lung cancer *(51,63,64)*. Activation of EGFR in lung-cancer cells generally occurs by overexpression in the absence of gene amplification, and appears to be more common in NSCLC than in SCLC, possibly related to tumor stage and differentiation *(63,65)*. Knockout mice lacking EGFR have been produced that develop abnormal epithelia in several organs including the lung, in which there was impaired branching, deficient alveolization, and septation *(66,67)*.

Other Proto-oncogenes and Growth Stimulatory Loops The hepatocyte growth factor/scatter factor (HGF/SF) stimulates epithelial-cell proliferation, motogenesis, complex differentiation programs with morphogenesis, and angiogenesis. HGF appears be a potent mitogen for normal and neoplastic bronchial epithelium *(68)*. During lung development, HGF levels increase during postnatal lung maturation and its receptors are expressed on bronchial and alveolar type II cells. HGF is involved in embryonal lung budding and branching, and stimulates mitogenesis and/or motogenesis of human bronchial epithelial, alveolar type II, and SCLC cells in vitro.

HGF is expressed at very low levels in normal lung but these levels increase in response to local lung or distant injury *(69)*. The c-*met* proto-oncogene that encodes the HGF receptor is expressed in normal lung, as well as in SCLC and NSCLC. HGF is expressed in many NSCLCs (but not in SCLCs), suggesting an autocrine growth-stimulatory loop in a subset of lung cancers *(70–72)*. A study of resected lung-cancer tissue showed c-*met* expression in 34/47 (72%) adenocarcinomas and 20/52 (38%) squamous carcinomas by Western blotting and immunohistochemistry *(73)*. This study suggested a poor prognosis for patients with tumors expressing the receptor, especially adenocarcinomas. Recently, Western blotting of proteins extracted from 56 NSCLCs (predominantly adenocarcinomas) using a polyclonal anti-HGF showed that high levels of immunoreactive HGF were associated with poorer survival for patients with stage I tumors *(74)*. Although c-*met* gene mutation has been observed in a subset of sporadic papillary renal carcinomas, such investigations have not been reported in lung cancer *(75)*.

An additional autocrine growth-stimulatory loop may involve the insulin-like growth factors (IGF-1 and IGF-2) and the type 1 IGF receptor (IGF-1R), which are frequently co-expressed in both SCLC and NSCLC *(76)*. Of the IGF family, it appears that IGF-2 may be the predominant member involved with the autocrine growth stimulation of lung cancer. The c-*kit* proto-oncogene, which encodes a tyrosine kinase receptor and its ligand, stem-cell factor (SCF), are co-expressed in many SCLCs, and may thus represent another autocrine loop for lung cancers *(77,78)*. In SCLC, activation of this putative SCF/kit autocrine loop could conceivably provide a growth advantage or mediate chemo-attraction. Platelet-derived growth factor (PDGF), which is the proto-oncogene counterpart of v-*sis*, and its receptor (PDGFR) were also found to be co-expressed in lung cancer, generating another potential autocrine loop *(79)*.

In essence, many proto-oncogenes encode growth factors, regulatory peptides, or their receptors and are expressed by lung-cancer cells or adjacent normal cells, thus providing a number of autocrine or paracrine growth-stimulatory loops *(80)*. Other autocrine systems not obviously involving known proto-oncogenes also exist. In fact, the autocrine loop comprising gastrin-releasing peptide, other bombesin-like peptides (GRP/BN) and their receptors is arguably the best characterized growth-stimulatory loop in lung cancer. GRP/BN has been associated with many physiologic effects including regulation of secretion, growth, and neuromodulation. There are three human GRP/BN receptor subtypes that belong to the G-protein coupled receptor superfamily with seven predicted transmembrane domains *(81)*. The cellular responses of SCLC to GRP/BN stimulation have been extensively studied *(82)*. Preliminary data also suggests that GRP/BN may regulate the MAP kinase cascade, at least in certain tumor cells *(83)*. Immunohistochemical studies showed that approx 20–60% of SCLC cancers expressed GRP, whereas NSCLCs expressed GRP less frequently *(17)*. In comparison, expression of the three GRP/BN receptors is widespread in both SCLC and NSCLC cell lines, with most cell lines expressing at least one of the three receptors and many cell lines expressing more than one receptor *(81)*.

The effects of GRP/BN pathway inhibition also supports its role in lung carcinogenesis. The formation of soft-agar clones in vitro and the in vivo growth of nude mouse xenografts of SCLC cell lines were inhibited by a neutralizing MAb directed against the C-terminal domain of GRP/BN, as well as by antagonists of bombesin *(84,85)*. A clinical trial of the MAb has shown some anti-tumor activity among 12 patients with previously treated SCLC *(86)*.

There is good evidence that the GRP/BN and GRP receptor autocrine loop is involved in the growth of SCLC. Because none of their encoding genes appear to be genetically altered by amplifications or rearrangements, another possible mechanism is that these regulatory loops, which are required during lung embryogenesis, somehow become reactivated during lung-cancer development. In fact, GRP/BN is known to be involved in lung development and repair *(87)*. GRP/BN in embryonic pulmonary NE cells augments epithelial growth and lung branching and stimulates migration of airway epithelial cells, a process thought to be essential for healing and restoration of function after airway injury.

The bcl2 Proto-oncogene and Apoptosis Tumor cells can acquire the ability to escape apoptotic pathway by which normal cells would usually undergo programmed cell death (apoptosis) in response to appropriate conditions such as DNA damage. A large and growing number of apoptosis regulatory gene products are classified as agonists of apoptosis (including bax, bak, bcl-X$_S$, bad, bid, bik, hrk) or antagonists of apoptosis (including bcl2, bcl-X$_L$, bcl-w, bfl-1, brag-1, mcl-1, and A1) *(88)*. Two key members of the apoptotic pathway are the *bcl2* proto-oncogene product and the *p53* tumor-suppressor gene product. The bcl2 protein antagonizes the induction of programmed cell death by p53. By protecting cells from the apoptotic process, bcl2 probably plays a role in determining the chemotherapy response through repression of apoptosis in cancer cells. A *bcl2*-transfected human SCLC cell line showed higher resistance to some anti-cancer agents by inhibiting apoptosis *(89)*, and SCLC cells transfected with antisense oligodeoxynucleotides to *bcl2* mRNA showed a reduced cell viability with decreased bcl2 protein levels facilitating apoptosis *(90)*.

Expression of bcl2 protein may correlate with NE differentiation in lung cancers *(91)*, and is expressed at a relatively higher level in squamous cell carcinoma (25–35%) than in adenocarcinoma (~10%) *(91–94)*. An inverse relationship between immunohistochemical bcl2 expression and abnormal p53 expression in resected NSCLCs has been reported *(95,96)*. These results suggest the hypothesis that either *p53* mutation or upregulation of *bcl2* expression is sufficient to modify the apoptotic pathway in NSCLC, and that bcl2-positive tumors may show less aggressive behavior *(95)*. In contrast, SCLCs usually have both *p53* mutations and *bcl2* overexpression.

Immunohistochemical studies of bcl2 in lung cancer show highest expression in small-cell cancers. For instance, bcl2 protein is immunohistochemically expressed in 75–95% of SCLCs *(91,97,98)*. This observation initially seems inconsistent with the finding that SCLCs are often much more sensitive than NSCLCs to chemotherapy, a situation in which tumor death usually occurs by apoptosis. In addition, there was a paradoxical trend, albeit nonstatistically significant, towards longer survival in patients whose SCLC tumors express *bcl2* *(98)*. Furthermore, an increased survival among patients with bcl2-positive NSCLC has been observed *(92–95)*. Thus, the role of bcl2 in lung cancer is complex and likely to unfold further. Notably, the recent suggestion that bcl2 may be converted to bax-like death effectors by the caspase family of cysteine proteases may be relevant *(99)*. Alternatively, increased bcl2 immunoreactivity may possibly indicate reduced rather than enhanced function, similar to the situation of overexpression of nonfunctional mutant p53 protein.

The bcl2-related protein bax promotes apoptosis and may act as a tumor suppressor *(100)*. Furthermore, bax may be a downstream transcription target of the p53 pathway. Bax can form homodimers or complex with bcl2 to form heterodimers, and it has been suggested that the bcl2/bax ratio determines cellular apoptotic susceptibility. For instance, the immunohistochemical staining of bax and bcl2 were inversely related in 121 NE lung cancers. Most carcinoid tumors showed low bcl2 and high bax expression in contrast to the inverse situation in most SCLCs and large-cell NE cancers (101). This could potentially lead to a higher degree of apoptosis in carcinoid tumors compared to SCLCs, and correlate with their clinical behavior where carcinoid tumors are generally less metastatic than SCLC.

Tumor-Suppressor Genes and Growth Inhibition Apart from aneuploidy, lung-cancer cells are characterized by numerous cytogenetic abnormalities, including deletions and nonreciprocal translocations. Frequent deletions of chromosome region 3p14-p23 was one of the initial cytogenetic observations made in SCLC, and this finding was later found to be also applicable to NSCLC (102). Subsequently, specific deletions at several chromosomal sites have been revealed by cytogenetic methods, including karyotype analysis, and more recently, comparative genomic hybridization. Furthermore, application of molecular allelotyping has been applied to the identification of allele loss in tumor cell lines, primary tumor cells, and preneoplastic cells associated with invasive cancers. Analysis of allelic deletion by molecular allelotyping of polymorphic DNA markers can discern loss of heterozygosity (LOH). Chromosomal regions that are affected by deletion may contain tumor-suppressor genes that are important in the molecular pathogenesis of lung cancer.

Chromosomal regions 1p, 1q, 3p (several sites), 5q (APC/MCC cluster), 8p, 9p21 (p16^{INK4A}), 11p13, 11p15, 13q14 (Rb1), 17p13 (p53), and 22q, as well as several other sites have been found to be frequently involved in lung-cancer cells or cell lines derived from lung-cancer tissues (103). This leads to the notion that if most of these sites encode tumor-suppressor genes, then individual tumors must have acquired inactivation of multiple genes to become clinically evident. Some of these are common to both SCLC and NSCLC, and some are more frequent in a given histologic type. The best-characterized of these deletions appear to target genes that are now accepted as classical tumor-suppressor genes, including p53, Rb1, and p16^{INK4A}. On the other hand, there is also mounting evidence that there may be other closely situated genes that are also affected by the chromosomal deletions, particularly because these deletions may be quite large involving the whole chromosomal arm or chromosome.

p53 Mutations in the p53 gene are the most common genetic alteration found in human cancers. The p53 gene encodes a protein that functions as a transcription factor, particularly in response to DNA damage by γ-irradiation, ultraviolet (UV) irradiation, and carcinogens (104). It has been called the guardian of the genome and the guardian of the G$_1$ checkpoint. p53 is believed to play a major role in maintaining the integrity of the genome because loss of p53 function allows inappropriate survival of genetically damaged cells, leading to the evolution of a cancer cell.

DNA damage is a major upstream event in p53 activation and results in a rapid increase in the level of p53 protein, and activation of p53 as a sequence-specific transcription factor regulating expression of downstream genes. The net effect is

either a stop to cell-cycle progression to permit repair, or apoptosis in the case of irrepairable damage. p53 can itself detect and bind sites of primary DNA damage through the function of its carboxy-terminal domain. Hypoxia is also able to stimulate p53 levels and lead to apoptotic cell death (105). Oxygen delivery and blood supply becomes rate-limiting when a tumor reaches a critical size. Thus, hypoxia may act as a physiological selective agent against apoptosis-competent cells in tumors. On the other hand, such selection may allow for the expansion of clones with acquired defects in their apoptotic program genes. The genes downstream of p53 include those encoding for p21^{WAF1}, mdm2, GADD45 (growth arrest and DNA damage-inducible), bax, insulin-like growth factor binding protein (IGF-BP), and cyclin G, which participate in controlling cell cycle arrest at the G$_1$/S-phase transition and apoptosis. A link between mutant p53 and aneuploidy has been revealed by studies implicating p53 as an active component of a mitotic-spindle checkpoint and as a regulator of centrosome function. Thus, p53 appears to participate in the DNA-damage checkpoints of the cell cycle at both the G$_1$/S transition and at the G$_2$/M boundary.

The p53 gene plays a critical role in lung cancer as well as in many other types of cancers. In both SCLC and NSCLC, one copy of the chromosomal region 17p13 that contains p53 is frequently deleted, constituting the first genetic hit. Mutational inactivation of the remaining allele, the second genetic hit, occurs in 75–100% of SCLCs and ~50% of NSCLCs (18), leading to loss of p53 function. Although found throughout the entire coding region, p53 mutations in lung cancer are most common in the evolutionarily conserved exons 5–8. The types of p53 mutations include missense and nonsense mutations, splicing abnormalities, and large deletions. Evidence supporting a causative role for tobacco smoke in inducing p53 mutations comes from the observation that p53 mutations in lung tumors correlate with cigarette smoking, and that the most common p53 mutations in lung cancer are the G→T transversions, a mutation that is expected to result from the interaction of tobacco-smoke carcinogens with DNA (18). Additional evidence for a pulmonary oncogenic role for p53 dysfunction comes from the finding that transgenic mutant p53 mice develop lung cancers in addition to bone and lymphoid tumors (106). Furthermore, transfection of a wild-type p53 gene into lung-cancer cells dramatically blocked tumor cell growth due to apoptosis (not G$_1$ arrest), despite concurrent abnormalities of several other tumor-suppressor genes and oncogenes (107,108).

Many p53 mutations are missense mutations that prolong the half-life of the p53 protein to several hours, leading to increased protein levels that can be detected by immunohistochemistry as a surrogate for molecular analysis (109). Immunohistochemical studies have shown abnormal p53 expression in 40–70% of SCLCs and 40–60% of NSCLCs (101,110–113). Most studies have shown that the frequency of p53 protein overexpression is higher in squamous cell carcinomas than in adenocarcinomas.

The predictive value of p53 mutations for survival, whether assayed by immunohistochemistry or by molecular analysis, is controversial. A summary of 14 studies of the prognostic importance of p53 mutations or overexpression in NSCLC (mutational analysis (4 studies), immunostaining (8 studies), and both techniques (2 studies) yielded controversial results (114). p53 mutations predicted shortened survival in half of the four reported mutational analyses, whereas the other two found no such difference. Of the 10 immunohistochemical studies, aberrant p53 expression was associated with a shortened survival in five studies, an improved survival in three studies, and no survival effect in two studies. In one study that simultaneously analyzed both mutations and protein expression, p53 overexpression but not gene mutation predicted shortened survival. Perhaps the various p53 mutants or types of wild-type p53 protein overexpression have different effects on lung-cancer behavior. Alternatively, wild-type p53 protein expression may be immunohistochemically detectable in certain tumors due to nonmutational mechanisms of protein stabilization. Finally, different antibodies that may not be strictly comparable for detecting aberrant p53 expression have often been used.

Some 15–25% of lung cancer patients develop antibodies against the p53 protein, suggesting the possibility that mutant p53 protein overexpression can lead to a humoral immune response. Nonetheless, the p53 epitopes reacting with the patients' antibodies appear to be preferentially localized in the amino and carboxyl termini of the protein, which are often not mutated (115). Moreover, p53 antibodies also reacted well against wild-type p53 protein (116). Although p53 antibodies have been suggested as an early diagnostic marker (117), the presence of these antibodies may not be a useful prognostic marker (116,118).

In certain cancers, such as of the uterine cervix, p53 protein can be inactivated through binding by the oncogenic E6 protein of human papilloma virus (HPV). This process inactivates p53 tumor-suppressor activity by promoting degradation of the p53 protein. The epitheliotropic HPV may also be involved in some respiratory tract lesions. For example, HPV subtypes 6 and 11 are associated with most cases of tracheal and bronchial papillomatosis. Although there are reports of neoplastic transformation in these benign papillomas, it has also been suggested that HPV may also play a part in the development of de novo bronchogenic carcinomas (119–121). Morphological studies have shown occasional presence of HPV-suggestive lesions in primary squamous-cell carcinomas, and DNA hybridization studies for the presence of HPV DNA in lung cancers show conflicting results, ranging from 0–40% (122–124). Most PCR studies looking for HPV sequences suggest that any potential involvement of HPV in primary lung cancer is likely to be limited (125–128), although some investigators have found more frequent involvement using in situ hybridization and polymerase chain reaction (PCR) (129).

Because p53 is frequently mutated in lung cancers, therapeutic approaches have been initiated against mutated p53. One experimental study demonstrated inhibition of tumor growth in lung-cancer cells in an orthotopic nude mouse model by in vivo retroviral transduction of wild-type p53 (130). In human studies, direct injection of a retroviral construct containing wild-type p53 under the control of a β-actin promoter into tumors was tested in nine NSCLC patients who failed conventional treatment. Tumor regression was noted in one-third of the group and tumor growth was stabilized in three others (131).

$p21^{WAF1}$ is a p53-responsive gene, which inhibits cyclin/cyclin dependent kinase (cdk) complexes in the G_1 phase of the cell cycle, and proliferating cell nuclear antigen (PCNA). Although not somatically mutated in lung cancer (132), $p21^{WAF1}$ mRNA and protein overexpression is detected in approx 65% of NSCLC cases, especially in well-differentiated tumors. This high frequency of overexpression suggests that $p21^{WAF1}$ can be expressed independently of p53 gene/protein alterations that are so frequent in lung cancers (133). Lastly, there is a C→A polymorphism in codon 31 of the $p21^{WAF1}$ gene (ser→arg), which has been suggested to be associated with the development of lung cancer in a case control study (134).

mdm2 is an oncoprotein that can functionally inhibit p53 and pRb. By binding its transcriptional activation domain, mdm2 blocks the ability of p53 to regulate target genes. It also causes rapid reduction of p53 levels through enhanced proteasome-dependent degradation. Conversely, p53 activates the expression of the mdm2 gene in an autoregulatory feedback loop. However, phosphorylation of p53 by DNA-dependent protein kinase (DNA-PK) after DNA damage leads to reduced interaction of p53 with mdm2, most likely due to a p53 conformational change (135). In some human sarcomas and brain tumors, the chromosome 12q mdm2 gene is amplified and its protein overexpressed. In lung cancer, however, mdm2 gene amplification was only detected in 2/30 (7%) NSCLCs. Nonetheless, expression was a favorable prognostic factor (136).

A gene encoding p73, a protein that shares considerable homology with p53 was recently isolated and mapped to 1p36 (137). This is of interest as 1p36 because also a site of frequent allelic deletion in lung and other cancer cells (103). Although p73 mutations were not detected in neuroblastomas despite frequent LOH, p73 can activate the transcription of p53-responsive genes and inhibit cell growth in a p53-like manner by inducing apoptosis (138). Consequently, the possible role of p73 in lung cancers with intact p53 function needs to be tested.

THE pRb/CYCLIN D1/cdk4/p16INK4A PATHWAY

The Rb1 Gene The *Rb1* gene located in chromosomal region 13q14 encodes a nuclear phosphoprotein that was initially identified as a tumor-suppressor gene in retinoblastomas. The pRb/cyclin D1/cdk4/p16^{INK4A} pathway is central to the regulation of the G_1 to S-phase transition of the cell cycle. Hypophosphorylated pRb binds and controls other cellular proteins including the transcription factor E2F, which is essential for the G_1/S-phase transition when bound to E2F sites in cooperation with the DP family of transcription factors. Transcriptional activation is mediated by unbound E2F, whereas hypophosphorylated pRb antagonizes heterodimers formed by E2F and DP, thereby resulting in inhibition of S-phase entry. Cyclin D1/cdk4 and other cyclin/cdk complexes phosphorylate pRb with subsequent loss of its binding pocket activity that is needed to sequester the transcription factors, thereby releasing E2F and allowing entry into S phase. It is becoming more apparent that one of the four genes responsible for pRb/cyclin D1/cdk4/p16^{INK4A} pathway is mutated or functionally altered in many cancers including lung cancers (Fig. 2).

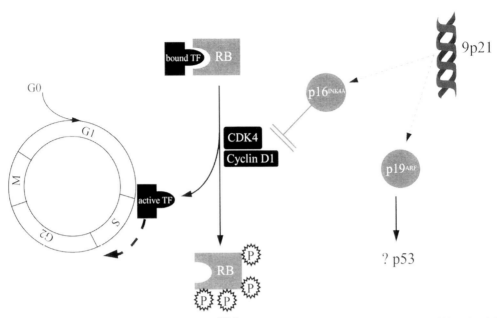

Fig. 2. Schematic diagram of the role of the RB/cyclin D1-CDK4/p16^INK4A pathway in cell-cycle regulation and a possible role of the alternative reading-frame protein p19^ARF in lung cancer. Hyperphosphorylated pRb is indicated by   TF denotes a transcription factor, e.g. E2F/DP complex. Unphosphorylated pRb binds transcription factors, which are released when pRb is phosphorylated under the stimulation of the cdk4/ cyclin D1 complex. p16^INK4A in an inhibitor of the cdk4/cyclin D1 complex.

It has also been shown that the c-ras signaling pathway may functionally link to cell-cycle regulation by pRb *(139)*. Furthermore, pRb also appears to have other functions; for instance, it can repress transcription of all three nuclear RNA polymerases classes (*Pol I*, *Pol II*, and *Pol III*) *(140)*. pRb also appears to inhibit apoptosis and may be actively involved in induction of differentiation.

In terms of interacting partners for pRb, overexpression of E2F-1 or E2F-1/DP-1 cooperates with activated c-*ras* in fibroblast-transformation assays, and these transformed cells can form tumors in nude mice. However, studies of *E2F-1*-deficient transgenic mice suggest that E2F-1 may also have a tumor-suppression function, because mice lacking *E2F-1* developed a broad spectrum of tumors including highly invasive lung adenocarcinomas *(141)*. Nonetheless, studies of E2F-1 in lung-cancer cells have not yet been reported.

Rb1 mutations together with loss of the wild-type allele have been consistently demonstrated in lung cancers *(142,143)*. The pRb protein is abnormal in over 90% of SCLCs and 15–30% of NSCLCs *(144–146)*. *Rb1* mutations in lung cancers include truncation by deletions, nonsense mutations, or splicing abnormalities. There are only a few studies of *Rb1* point mutations in lung cancer, at least partly due to its 200 kb genomic size and 27 exon structure. However, from these limited studies, most mutations result in pRb truncation *(147)*, although a rare missense mutation affecting the pRb pocket domain has been shown to cause defective pRb phosphorylation and binding to oncoproteins *(148)*.

The sensitivity for detecting *Rb1* abnormalities in SCLCs varies by detection method. Southern-blot analysis detects approx 20% of *Rb1* mutations through discernment of band loss. Northern-blot analysis can detect approx 60% of *Rb1* abnormalities based on detection of abnormal mRNA or loss of mRNA expression. Immunohistochemical methods can detect

the majority of *Rb1* mutations (approx 90%), based on loss of pRb protein expression. Thus, *Rb1* abnormalities are very frequent in SCLC, particularly in comparison to NSCLC. In NSCLC, a large study showed *Rb1* abnormalities in 2/219 (<1%) by Southern analysis, 22/219 (10%) by Northern analysis, and 53/163 (32%) by immunohistochemical analysis *(144)*. The absence of *Rb1* expression was associated with poor prognosis in NSCLCs, particularly stage I and II disease, in some but not all studies *(146,149–151)*. On the other hand, the observation of frequent LOH on chromosome 13q, but relatively less frequent *Rb1* inactivation in NSCLCs, has prompted the notion that the allelic loss on 13q targets other tumor-suppressor genes on this chromosome apart from *Rb1 (152)*.

The relatives of retinoblastoma patients who were also germline carriers of an *Rb1* mutation were about 15 times more likely to die from lung cancer than the general population *(153)*. Furthermore, functional support comes from a study showing that the re-introduction of a wild-type *Rb1* gene led to growth suppression of SCLC cells *(154)*.

There are two other members of the *Rb* gene family, *p107* and *p130*, which are structurally and functionally related genes. They have also been implicated in lung cancer to a limited extent *(155)*. One SCLC cell line was shown to have a point mutation of p130 in a splice-acceptor site, leading to loss of exon 2 and production of a truncated p130 protein *(156)*.

Cyclin D1 and cdk4 The relatively infrequent involvement of *Rb1* mutation in NSCLC compared to SCLC suggested that alternative members of this growth-suppressive pathway might be affected. Because cyclin D1 inhibits the activity of pRb by stimulating its phosphorylation by cdk4, cyclin D1 overexpression was an attractive candidate for disrupting the pRb-mediated growth-control pathway. In keeping with this, cyclin D1 was found to be overexpressed in some NSCLCs with normal pRb protein expression *(157,158)*. Cyclin D1 is

Table 2
Summary of p16^INK4A Abnormalities Reported in Nonsmall Cell Lung Cancer^a

Samples	p16^INK4A	Abnormalities ^b/ tumors studied (%)	Methods^c
Primary tumors	Mutation	60/444 (14%)	Southern, PCR-based mutation detection, FISH
	Absent expression	208/517 (40%)	Immunohistochemistry, Western
Cell lines	Mutation	76/210 (36%)	Southern, PCR-based mutation detection
	Absent expression	83/121 (69%)	Northern, RT-PCR, Western

^aAdapted from (151,168–177,179–182,184–187a), and Geradts, J, K.M. Fong, P.V. Zimmerman, R. Maynard, and J.D. Minna, unpublished data)

^bAbnormalities include homozygous deletions, point mutations, undetectable expression, and cytogenetic deletion detected by FISH.

^cFISH, fluorescent in situ hybridization.

encoded for by the CCND1 proto-oncogene, which is located on chromosome 11q13. Cyclin D1 protein was overexpressed by several-fold to 100-fold in 11/12 NSCLC cell lines compared to an immortalized nontumorigenic bronchoepithelial cell line (157). Amplification of cyclin D1 was detected in 15% of primary NSCLC tumors (158). Likewise, overexpression of cyclin D1 was observed in 47% of 53 primary NSCLC tumors (158). Cyclin D1 immunohistochemical overexpression has been reported to correlate with patient survival and Ki67 labeling (159,160). Abnormal immunostaining of cyclin D1 and pRb has been observed in epithelial cells from the resection margin of lung cancers, suggesting that these changes may be relatively early events in lung carcinogenesis (161).

In terms of cdk4, although gene amplification has been reported in 10–15% of malignant gliomas and certain other malignancies, its role in lung cancer has not yet been reported. Interestingly, the chromosome 12q13-q15 region, which harbors the cdk4 gene, also contains the mdm2 locus. Whereas cdk4 and mdm2 often show co-amplification in sarcomas and glioblastomas, some tumors show only cdk4 amplification but not mdm2 amplification, and vice versa, indicating that each gene is an independent amplification target (162).

The p16INK4A and Other cdk-Inhibitor Genes The p16^INK4A protein functions as a cell cycle modulator that appears to regulate pRb function by inhibiting cyclin D1/cdk4 activity, and represents another important genetic target for disrupting the pRb/cyclin D1/cdk4/p16^INK4A pathway. The p16^INK4A tumor-suppressor gene is located at chromosome 9p21. The short arm of chromosome 9, including 9p21, frequently undergoes allelic loss or mutation in a variety of human cancers including lung cancer (163–166). A summary of a wide variety of cancers identified several mutational hot spots (point and other mutations including deletions, insertions, and splice mutations), including some at conserved residues within the ankyrin domains of p16^INK4A (167).

p16^INK4A abnormalities have been extensively studied and reported in lung cancer (Table 2) and are found frequently in NSCLC, but rarely in SCLC. Homozygous deletion or point mutations have been observed in 10–40% of NSCLCs (168–176). Absent expression of p16^INK4A was detected by Northern

blot, Western blot, or immunohistochemical analyses in 30–70% of NSCLC. Epigenetic hypermethylation of 5′-CpG islands was suggested to cause the functional downregulation of p16^INK4A in lung cancers that lack genetic mutations of p16^INK4A (177,178). The multiple mechanisms of p16^INK4A inactivation may account for the relatively low rates of inactivating deletions and point mutations deleted in earlier genetic studies (179).

It has been suggested that p16^INK4A mutations may be associated with tumor progression and more advanced lung cancer, because higher frequencies of deletion or mutation have been observed in cultured cell lines and metastatic lesions compared to primary tumors (180). Although an immunohistochemical study of primary NSCLCs demonstrated an association of p16^INK4A-negativity with more advanced clinical stage (151), this finding was not confirmed in another study (181). Nevertheless, both studies did show that about 30–40% of early-stage primary NSCLCs lacked p16^INK4A expression. Finally, there is conflicting data as to whether the absence of p16^INK4A expression is a predictor of adverse survival in NSCLC (151,182).

It has become increasingly clear that p16^INK4A abnormalities are perhaps the most common mechanism for inactivating the pRb/cyclin D1/cdk4/p16^INK4A cell-cycle control pathway in NSCLC. Conversely, direct pRb inactivation appears to be the preferred mechanism in SCLC. Consequently, lung cancers are in general characterized by Rb1 inactivation (~90% of SCLC and 15–30% of NSCLC) or p16^INK4A inactivation (30–70% of NSCLC), either scenario leading to loss of this growth-inhibitory pathway. The apparently mutually exclusive inactivation of either Rb1 or p16^INK4A has been well-documented in NSCLC cases (151,181,183–187). Furthermore, the simultaneous inactivation of both Rb1 and p16^INK4A is uncommon, but cyclin D1 overexpression can coexist with each of these abnormalities (179). It is also noteworthy that a significant proportion of NSCLCs (10–30%) appear to be normal for both pRb and p16^INK4A, thereby implicating cyclin D1 and cdk4 alterations. The p16^INK4A locus also encodes a second protein product, p19^AKF which originates from an unrelated exon of p16^INK4A (exon 1b) spliced onto exon 2 in an alternate reading frame (188). Thus, exon 2, which is often deleted or mutated in

NSCLC, is common to both $p16^{INK4A}$ and $p19^{ARF}$. Intriguingly, mice lacking $p19^{ARF}$, but expressing functional $p16^{INK4A}$, were prone to tumor development, possibly through the p53 pathway as $p53$-negative cell lines were resistant to p19^{ARF}-induced growth arrest *(189)*. Thus the extent of $p19^{ARF}$ damage through deletions and mutations to the $p16^{INK4A}$ locus, and its possible contribution to human lung carcinogenesis requires investigation.

There are a number of other cdk-inhibitor genes including $p15^{INK4B}$, $p18^{INK4C}$, $p19^{INK4D}$, $p21^{WAF1/CIP1}$, $p27^{KIP1}$, and $p57^{KIP2}$. However, apart from $p15^{INK4B}$, mutational analyses of these genes have not detected significant genetic changes in lung cancer.

$p15^{INK4B}$ shares approx 70% amino acid similarity and is situated immediately centromeric to $p16^{INK4A}$ It also functions to restrain cell growth, probably by acting as an effector of TGF-β-mediated cell-cycle arrest *(190)*. Coordinate deletion of $p15^{INK4B}$ and $p16^{INK4A}$ frequently occur in NSCLC, but point mutations targeting $p15^{INK4B}$ itself appear to be uncommon.

The $p18^{INK4C}$ and $p19^{INK4D}$ genes have not been shown to be mutated in lung cancer *(191)*. Similarly, $p27^{KIP1}$ has not been found to be mutated in lung cancers *(192)*, but low levels of p27^{KIP1} protein were associated with a poor outcome in NSCLC patients *(193)*. The p57^{KIP2} cdk inhibitor (which maps to 11p15) is usually imprinted, with expression of the maternal allele only. Thus, $p57^{KIP2}$ expression can be downregulated by selective loss of the maternal allele, and this has been reported in 11/13 (85%) lung cancer cases with LOH of 11p15 *(194)*. Because point mutations have not been described in lung cancer, one could speculate that loss of a single allele could inactivate the imprinted $p57^{KIP2}$ gene.

Candidate 3p Tumor-Suppressor Genes It has long been known that chromosome 3p deletions occur commonly in cancers, notably lung and renal cancers. The frequent deletion of one copy of the short arm of chromosome 3 in both SCLC (>90%) and NSCLC (>80%) has provided a strong basis for the hypothesis that one or more lung-cancer tumor-suppressor genes exist on this chromosomal arm. These cytogenetic 3p deletions have been confirmed by allelotyping, which showed allelic loss not only in invasive cancers, but also in preneoplastic respiratory epithelial lesions associated with NSCLC *(102,195,196)*. Three discreet regions of 3p loss have been identified by allelotyping in lung cancers, including 3p25-p26, 3p21.3-p22 and 3p14-cen. This observation is consistent with the notion that there are probably three (or more) different tumor-suppressor genes located on 3p *(197)*. In addition, five homozygously deleted regions have been found in lung-cancer cell lines. There is one in the 3p14.2 region (*FHIT* gene location), one at 3p12-p13 (U2020 cell-line deletion) *(198,199)*, and three at the 3p21 region. These sites are considered strong candidates for the location of tumor-suppressor genes that may be important in lung tumorigenesis.

The *FHIT* gene consists of 10 exons encoding a 1.1 kb transcript, maps to 3p14.2, and encompasses approx 1 Mb of genomic DNA, which includes the human common fragile site (*FRA3B*) and the t(3;8) translocation breakpoint of familial renal-cell carcinoma. *FRA3B* is the most frequent of the common fragile sites, which are chromosomal sites prone to breakages under stress, such as aphidicolin treatment. *FHIT* is a candidate tumor-suppressor gene for lung cancers on the basis of frequent LOH in lung cancer and homozygous deletion in several lung-cancer cell lines; the latter particularly affecting NSCLC *(200–202)*. Although reverse transcription-polymerase chain reaction (RT-PCR) showed that 40–80% of lung cancers express aberrant *FHIT* transcripts, these were nearly always accompanied by wild-type *FHIT* mRNA *(200–202)*. As in other cancers, point mutations of *FHIT* are rare in lung tumors *(200,201)*, and it is possible that deletions of this allele reflect the susceptibility of the *FRA3B* fragile site to chromosomal breakage. Nevertheless, although *FHIT* abnormalities differ from the mutations and loss of wild-type transcript expression expected of classic tumor-suppressor genes, absence of FHIT protein in primary lung tumors and cell lines correlate with DNA and/or RNA abnormalities *(203)*. A recent study has shown that transfection of an exogenous wild-type *FHIT* gene results in suppression of tumorigenicity in nude mice of various human cancer cell lines, including a NSCLC cell line *(204)* Furthermore, the much more frequent *FHIT* allele loss in lung cancers from smokers (80%) compared to nonsmokers (22%) suggests that this chromosomal region is selectively targeted by the carcinogens in tobacco smoke (205).

The 3p21.3 region has been extensively examined for putative tumor-suppressor genes by several groups. The finding of several homozygously deleted lung cancer cell lines suggested a role for two 3p21.3 loci. One locus corresponds to the 370 kb minimal common deleted region identified in three cell lines with homozygous deletion *(206–208)*. Over twenty genes have been identified in this region *(208a)*. A key gene here is the RASSF1A isoform whose expression is extinguished by methylation in many long cancers *(208b, 208c)*. The other 3p21 region was identified in like manner encompasses an approx 800 kb deletion *(209)*. In addition to these loci, the *hMLH1* gene (the human homolog of the yeast *mutL* gene) resides within chromosome 3p21, but mutations of this gene have not been reported in lung cancer *(210)*.

Other candidate 3p lung cancer-suppressor genes include the von Hippel-Lindau (VHL) tumor-suppressor gene at 3p25, which is frequently mutated in renal-cell carcinoma but rarely involved in lung cancers *(211)*. Abnormalities of retinoic acid receptors (RARs) have also been implicated in lung-cancer pathogenesis. Several studies have indicated abnormalities of the expression or function of the *RARβ* gene, which maps to chromosome region 3p24, another site of frequent allele loss in lung cancer *(212–217)*. Mutational analysis, however, has failed to demonstrate lesions in *RARβ*. Additionally, the *TGFβ*-type II receptor (*TGFβRII*) gene at 3p22 is another candidate tumor suppressor.

Thus, despite intensive efforts, the identity of the putative 3p tumor-suppressor gene(s) in lung cancer remains elusive. However, because of the frequency of its involvement and apparent early, critical role in bronchogenic carcinogenesis, research efforts should continue to focus on this area.

Other Candidate Tumor-Suppressor Gene Locations Apart from the known and candidate tumor-suppressor gene locations, cytogenetic and allelotyping studies have shown allelic loss of many other chromosomal regions in lung cancer, thereby implicating involvement of other tumor-suppressor genes. These chromosomal regions include 1p, 1q, 2q, 5q, 6p, 6q, 8p, 8q, 10q, 11p, 11q, 14q, 17q, 18q and 22q *(103,218–225)*. In addition, the presence of homozygously deleted chromosomal regions 2q33, 8, and X/Y in lung cancer imply yet other unidentified tumor-suppressor genes *(234)*. The comparative genomic hybridization (CGH) technique also detected deletions at 1p, 2q, 3p, 4p, 4q, 5q, 6q, 8p, 9p, 10q, 13q, 17p, 18p, 18q, 21q, and 22q, and characterized the different deletion patterns between SCLC and NSCLC, as well as between adenocarcinoma and squamous-cell carcinoma subtypes *(12–14,16)*. Several of these chromosomal arms contain known or candidate tumor-suppressor genes (such as *WT1* at 11p13, *DCC* at 18q21, *NF2* at 22q12), but these genes have not been found to be mutated in lung cancer *(226,227)*. Regions on chromosome 5q, around the *APC* and *MCC* gene cluster are frequently deleted in lung cancer. However, *APC* mutations have not been detected in lung cancer *(227,228)*. In addition, high rates of allelic loss or homozygous deletion in the 5p13-p12 region have been reported in lung cancer *(229,230)*.

There is cytogenetic and molecular evidence of frequent allelic loss of parts of chromosome 11p in lung cancer *(222,231–233)*. Apart from allele loss in the 11p13 region, refined mapping of the telomeric 11p15.5 region has suggested the location of two distinct tumor-suppressor genes *(225)*. Loss of genetic material from 11q including the chromosomal region containing the *ATM* tumor-suppressor gene (11q23) is seen in a number of human cancers, including lung *(223)*, breast, ovary, cervix, colon, and skin. Nonetheless, *ATM* mutations have not been reported in lung cancer.

At 10q23, a candidate tumor-suppressor gene called *PTEN* was recently identified and found to be somatically mutated in various kinds of tumors including glioblastoma, and prostate, kidney, and breast cancers *(235)*. Recombinant *PTEN* appears to dephosphorylate protein and peptide substrates with a dual-specificity phosphatase activity. *PTEN* was found to be mutated in a few primary lung cancers, and several lung-cancer cell lines show homozygous deletions of this gene.

TGF-β Signaling The TGF-β family of signaling molecules regulate the proliferation of many cell types, and have been implicated in several human cancers *(236)*. The three mammalian isoforms (TGFβ1, TGFβ2, and TGFβ3) are homologous peptides that act by binding to a single common receptor complex. TGFβ1 is a potent inhibitor of proliferation of most normal cells, but responsiveness to the negative growth-regulatory effects of TGFβ1 is lost in many tumorigenic cell lines. In addition, the presence of mutant *p53* has been shown to diminish growth inhibition by TGFβ1 in human bronchial epithelial cells *(237)*. Cell-cycle regulator proteins such as cyclins, cdks, and cdk inhibitors have been implicated as the ultimate targets of TGFβ1-induced negative signals.

TGF-β ligands bind to transmembrane receptors with serine/threonine kinase activity, designated types I and II *(238)*. The TGFβRI is recruited upon binding of TGF-β to the TGFβRII, thereby forming an heterocomplex of the ligand and both receptors. Phosphorylation of the TGFβRI by the kinase of TGFβRII is essential to subsequent downstream signaling. In SCLC cell lines, resistance to growth inhibition by TGFβ1 was

shown to correlate with loss of expression of *TGFβRII* mRNA *(239)*. The *TGFβRII* gene has been mapped to chromosome 3p22 and is thus a candidate tumor-suppressor gene. Although mutations in TGFβRII have been reported in colon cancers with the MSI phenotype, this gene is rarely mutated in lung cancer *(240,241)*. It remains to be seen if another candidate tumor-suppressor gene, the *M6P/IGF2R* gene (encoding the mannose-6-phosphate/insulin-like growth-factor II receptor), which is involved in the activation of latent TGF-β, plays a significant role in lung carcinogenesis *(236)*. Notably, the *M6P/IGF2R* locus maps to chromosome 6q26-q27, a chromosomal arm that is deleted in some lung cancers *(16,242)*.

The recent identification of the SMAD family of signal-transducer proteins has unravelled the mechanisms by which TGF-β signals from the cell membrane to the nucleus. SMAD genes encode homo-oligomer proteins, which are important downstream signaling mediators of TGF-β ligand-receptor complexes when complexed in hetero-oligomeric forms. Phosphorylated SMAD proteins are translocated to the nucleus, and induce the expression of growth-regulatory genes. In one study, four SMAD genes (*SMAD1*, *SMAD3*, *SMAD5*, and *SMAD6*) were not mutated among 15 lung cancers *(243)*. However, SMAD2 and SMAD4 are suggested to function as tumor-suppressor proteins, and mutations have been identified in their corresponding genes. The *SMAD2* gene (within 18q21) was reported to be mutated in 2/57 (3.5%) lung cancers *(244)*. The *SMAD4* gene (also known as *DPC4*, for deleted in pancreatic carcinoma 4) also maps to 18q21 and has been shown to be mutated in nearly half of pancreatic cancers and approx 20% of colon cancers. In lung cancer, somatic missense and frameshift mutations of *SMAD4* occur at a low frequency (3/42 cases) *(245)*. Other components of this TGF-β pathway, such as SMAD7 protein, an inhibitor of TGF-β signaling, have yet to be studied in lung cancer *(246)*.

MOLECULAR GENETIC CHANGES IN PRENEOPLASIA Much of our knowledge of preneoplastic changes in bronchial epithelium is based on the histological appearance and alteration of bronchial epithelial cells. Before the appearance of a clinically overt lung cancer, a sequence of morphologically distinct changes (hyperplasia, metaplasia, dysplasia, and carcinoma *in situ*) can be observed in bronchial epithelium. The sequential changes for cancers that arise from the proximal airways and bronchi (predominantly squamous-cell carcinomas) have long been recognized, whereas similar changes in peripheral bronchioles and alveoli (adenocarcinomas and large-cell carcinomas) have been described more recently. A number of studies have shown that the preneoplastic cells and bronchial epithelium adjacent to cancers contain a number of genetic abnormalities that are identical to some of the abnormalities found in overt cancer cells. These include c-*myc* and c-*ras* upregulation, *cyclin D1* overexpression, p53 immunoreactivity, and DNA aneuploidy *(11,161,247–252)*. A follow-up longitudinal study of ex-chromate workers confirmed that some p53 immuno-positive dysplasias progress to subsequent squamous cell carcinoma *(251)*.

In terms of the temporal sequence of molecular changes, allelotyping analysis of precisely microdissected, preneoplastic foci suggests that 3p allelic loss is the earliest change, followed

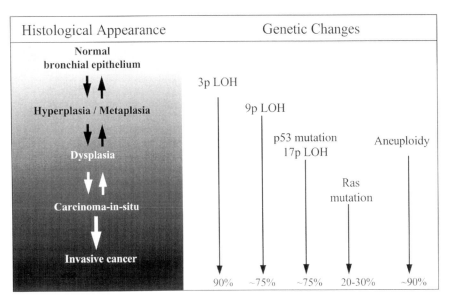

Fig. 3. Schematic representation of the approximate timing of genetic changes found in preneoplastic lesions of the respiratory epithelium accompanying primary nonsmall cell lung cancers. The data depicted in this figure are mainly derived from squamous-cell carcinomas and adenocarcinomas.

by allelic loss at 9p, 17p (and *p53* mutation), and 5q, and ultimately c-*ras* mutations *(247,253–256)*. It has been hypothesized that one or more 3p tumor-suppressor gene(s) may be critical for lung-cancer pathogenesis as abnormalities of 3p appear to be among the earliest detectable genetic lesions (Fig. 3). Based on topographical analysis, others have speculated that c-K-*ras* activation may also occur early during tumorigenesis leading to adenocarcinoma *(252)*. In this context, c-K-*ras* mutations can also be found in atypical alveolar hyperplasia, postulated by some to be the precursor lesion for adenocarcinomas *(29,257)*.

These observations are also consistent with the multi-step model of carcinogenesis and the field-cancerization theory proposed by Slaughter. This theory suggests that as the whole aerodigestive tract is repeatedly exposed to carcinogenic damage (tobacco smoke), it is at risk for developing multiple, separate foci of neoplasia *(258)*. Interestingly, the 3p, 9p, and 17p deletions showed allele specific loss, defined as deletion of the same allele in preneoplastic tissues as in the primary tumor, even when these lesions were geographically and morphologically distinct *(254)*. Possible explanations for these allele-specific changes include: 1) clonal spread of mutated cells throughout the lung; 2) inherited differences in alleles predisposing to their subsequent loss; or 3) some event occurring during lung embryogenesis affecting a particular set of alleles. In support of the clonal-spread theory, an identical *p53* point mutation was identified in multiple dysplastic lesions from both lungs of a smoker with chronic obstructive pulmonary disease, thereby indicating an unusual field-cancerization mechanism and clonal spread *(259)*.

OTHER MOLECULAR ALTERATIONS IN LUNG CANCER

MICROSATELLITE ALTERATIONS Microsatellite repeats (or short-tandem repeats, simple-sequence repeats) are highly polymorphic short-repeating sequences of DNA (such as di-

nucleotide repeats), which are widely distributed throughout the genome and have been very useful markers for genetic mapping and analyzing small amounts of tumor samples for allelic deletion. MSI, representing changes in the number of the short-tandem DNA repeats, was initially reported in hereditary nonpolyposis colon cancer (HNPCC), where it reflects mutations of DNA MMR genes (*hMSH2*, *hMLH1*, *PMS1*, and *PMS2*). Cells expressing microsatellite instability are said to exhibit the replication error phenotype (RER), which is typically detected as instability in microsatellite-repeat sequences in PCR-based assays. Changes in size of microsatellite length in tumor vs normal DNA from the same individual can involve mono-, di-, tri-, and tetra-nucleotide repeats. Although the expansion of microsatellite-repeat sequences is used as the main criteria for identification of the RER phenotype, the molecular defect responsible for the phenotype is likely to cause point mutational alterations of DNA sequences in addition to alterations in microsatellites. In contrast to this RER phenotype, a different and distinct shift of individual allelic bands occurs in lung cancer. The MSI in cancers associated with HNPCC usually affects multiple genetic loci, whereas lung cancers often show instability at only a few loci. These differences, together with the lack of reported mutations in the DNA MMR genes, have prompted suggestions that the phenomenon in lung cancers is distinct and should perhaps be called microsatellite alteration. In any case, the changes in an individual microsatellite marker appear to be clonally preserved as the tumor develops.

Of the microsatellite alteration studies in lung cancer *(260–272)*, the overall frequencies of microsatellite alteration have ranged widely. For instance, there was a 10-fold difference in the frequency of microsatellite alteration in two studies of the same NSCLC samples, 2 vs 21% *(260,261)*. Nonetheless, a summary of the reported studies suggests possible differences in frequencies of microsatellite alteration between SCLC and NSCLC as 35% (37/106) of SCLCs and 22% (160/727) of NSCLCs appeared to display microsatellite alteration at individual loci. From these studies, it can also be estimated that perhaps 1–10% of lung tumors show microsatellite alteration at multiple loci. Several possible reasons may explain the wide-range of results. The definition of MSI is variable and poorly defined. Larger tandem repeats such as tri- and tetranucleotide repeats are thought to be more susceptible than dinucleotide repeats to expansion or contraction mutations. Selection bias may result in the repeated study of those microsatellite markers known to show frequent microsatellite alteration *(266,267,271)*. Technical considerations and methodology may affect the interpretation of microsatellite alteration. Indeed, two SCLC studies yielded different frequencies of microsatellite alteration, despite having analyzed the same microsatellite markers; 6/33 (18%) for paraffin-embedded tissue *(263)* and 0/37 for fresh samples *(266)*. Furthermore, there is also the possibility of publication bias against studies with low rates of microsatellite alteration. Notwithstanding these considerations, if most tumors have at least one microsatellite alteration in a particular selection of markers, then this phenomenon could potentially be used for lung-cancer detection *(271)*

In terms of associated factors, microsatellite alterations are observed more frequently in patients with rare c-H-*ras* variable repeat (VNTR) alleles and chromosome 3p LOH *(272)* as well as in younger patients *(261,270)*. The suggestion that microsatellite alteration is more frequently observed in advanced-stage tumors is controversial *(266,269)*. The presence of microsatellite alteration has also been reported to be related to reduced survival *(269)*. In addition, one study reported that microsatellite alterations were also observed in histologically normal bronchial mucosa *(271)*.

In conclusion, it remains to be seen whether microsatellite alteration observed in lung cancer plays a causative role resulting in disruption of specific genetic targets involved in carcinogenesis, or alternatively reflects nonspecific genomic instability. Further, any potential underlying mutator phenotype defect affecting DNA synthesis and/or repair processes leading to microsatellite alteration in lung cancer remain elusive. Consequently, the role of microsatellite alterations in lung cancer should be rigorously evaluated using a standardized definition and methodology for testing a variety of markers.

ABERRANT DNA METHYLATION IN LUNG CANCER

The process of DNA methylation involves the covalent modification at the fifth carbon position of cytosine residues within CpG dinucleotides, which tend to be clustered in islands at the 5'-ends of many genes, and can be considered an epigenetic modification of DNA. In general, methylated genes are inactive, whereas unmethylated genes tend to be active. DNA methylation appears to be associated with genetic repression and necessary for proper embryonic development. The methylated CpG residues could either interfere directly with the binding of specific transcription factors to DNA, bind to specific repression factors or convert chromatin to an inactive form by altering its structure. Recent investigations have also tied in the cell-cycle factors (PCNA, p21^{WAF1}) with the regulation of methylation, leading to possible epigenetic interaction with cell-cycle regulation *(273)*.

Instead of structural deletions or point mutations, downregulation of the wild-type function of a tumor-suppres-

sor gene may occur through hypermethylation. For instance, hypermethylation in the 5'-region of the *Rb1* and *VHL* genes is associated with transcriptional silencing in retinoblastoma and renal-cancer, respectively *(274–276)*. In some NSCLCs, hypermethylation appears to be a specific mechanism for inactivating the *p16^{INK4A}* gene *(177,178)*. Conversely in SCLC, regional hypermethylation has been found at chromosome 3p, but the precise gene target is uncertain *(277)*. Given the higher frequency of absent p16^{INK4A} protein expression compared to somatic *p16^{INK4A}* mutations in primary NSCLCs, it is likely that *p16^{INK4A}* inactivation by methylation is a common event in NSCLCs. Recent in vitro work has suggested that promoter hypermethylation may also downregulate *p53* function *(278)*. Recent studies have shown that multiple genes can have their expression in activated by promotor methylation in both N5CLC and SCLC including *RARB, ECAD, HCAD, MGMT, GSTP1, DAPK, p16, FHIT, RASSF1A,* and *AVC* *(208b,208c,278a,278b)*.

Methylation plays a significant role in mediating genomic imprinting, defined as a gamete-specific modification causing differential expression of the two alleles of a gene in somatic cells. Loss of genomic imprinting could therefore lead to inappropriate expression of a gene. In fact, loss of imprinting of the *IGF2 (insulin-like growth factor 2)* gene at 11p15 has been observed in lung cancer *(279)*. In addition, located within 200 kb of the *IGF2* locus is the *H19* gene, which has been postulated to be a tumor suppressor. In some lung cancers, the *H19* gene shows loss of imprinting associated with promoter-region hypomethylation, resulting in *H19* overexpression *(280)*.

TOBACCO-SMOKE CARCINOGENS It is thought that tobacco smoke is responsible for 85–90% of all cases of lung cancer *(281)*. Tobacco smoke contains thousands of substances including carcinogens, co-carcinogens, and tumor promoters. The polycyclic hydrocarbons (such as benzo(a)pyrene), nitrosamines, and aromatic amines are the three major classes of carcinogens in tobacco smoke. There has been much study of the nitrosamines that are derived from nicotine during the burning of tobacco, especially 4-(methylnitrosamino)-1-(3-pyridyl)-1-butanone (NNK). Indeed, NNK and its metabolite, 4-(methylnitrosamino)-1-(3-pyridyl)-1-butanol (NNAL), are potent carcinogens that are specific for the lung in rodents.

The carcinogenic effects of tobacco smoke in the lung involve the induction of carcinogen-activating and inactivating enzymes, as well as covalent DNA adduct formation, which may result in DNA misreplication and mutation. DNA adducts have been identified in the bronchial tissue of lung-cancer patients and their levels correlate with the amount of tobacco-smoke exposure. Furthermore, benzo(a)pyrene, a major cigarette smoke carcinogen, was shown to form adducts selectively along the *p53* gene of bronchial epithelial cells, at the nucleotide positions known to be the major mutational hot spots in lung cancer *(282)*. Thus, targeted adduct formation rather than phenotypic selection may determine the pattern of p53 mutations in lung cancer, and the data provided a direct etiological link between a defined chemical carcinogen and lung cancer.

LUNG-CANCER SUSCEPTIBILITY Only a portion of smokers develop lung cancer, despite the fact that tobacco smoke is implicated in most cases of lung cancer. Clearly, there are other important factors operating apart from the simple inhalation of tobacco smoke. It has, for instance, been postulated that individuals may exhibit genetic polymorphisms in carcinogen-metabolizing pathways that would lead to inherited differences in lung-cancer risks associated with tobacco smoking. The relationships of human lung cancer to polymorphisms of phase I procarcinogen-activating and phase II-deactivating enzymes and intermediate biomarkers of DNA mutation, such as DNA adducts, proto-oncogene, and tumor-suppressor gene mutation, and genetic polymorphisms have recently been compiled and reviewed *(283)*. The important genetic variations in lung cancer include polymorphisms at the *cytochrome P450* gene *(CYP)* loci and the *glutathione S-transferases (GST)* M1 gene cluster.

The phase II GST enzymes are encoded by a multigene family whose proteins serve to detoxify mutagenic electrophiles *(284)*. The gene products are suggested to play a part in detoxifying epoxides of certain carcinogenic polycyclic aromatic hydrocarbons (PAH). These enzymes conjugate glutathione to a substrate generally resulting in its inactivation and excretion, although in certain cases this can lead to activation of a procarcinogen to a mutagenic product. Four gene families are known *(GSTA, GSTM, GSTP, and GSTT)* and large interindividual variations in enzyme activity are known to exist for several GSTs *(285)*. The *GSTM1* locus is homozygously null or deficient in approx 40–50% of the population. Several case-control studies have linked the null phenotype to an increased risk of lung cancer *(286,287)*, but there have also been conflicting studies *(288,289)*. A meta-analysis of 12 comparable studies suggested that the *GSTM1* null genotype is over-represented in lung cancer cases with an overall odds ratio (OR) of 1.41 (95% CI of 1.23–1.61), which did vary depending on ethnic origin, being lower in Caucasians (OR 1.17) *(290)*. Although the increased risk was modest, it potentially translates to a large number at the population level, and the authors suggested that approx 17% of new lung-cancer cases could be attributable to GSTM1 deficiency. Additionally, because GSTM1 is only weakly expressed in the lung, there has been recent interest in the protein product of *GSTP1*, which, in fact, is the major GST protein in the lung *(285,291)*. This enzyme has activity for many epoxides of PAH and could theoretically compensate for loss of GSTM1 activity. Increased expression of the *GSTP1* gene has been reported in lung tissue *(285)*. In the only study of lung cancer, the combination of *GSTM1* null and the G allele at a *GSTP1* codon 104 polymorphism (A→G substitution resulting in isoleucine→valine) was shown to be associated with more hydrophobic-DNA adducts and lung-cancer risk in Norwegian patients *(292)*. Importantly, this polymorphism is known to functionally change the enzyme kinetics of the GSTP1 protein *(293)*.

The structural gene for the phase I enzyme, cytochrome *CYP1A1* which catalyses a range of human carcinogens, has a *MspI* restriction polymorphism (designated m2) associated with an amino acid substitution in the enzymatically active site that results in a protein of high activity *(294)*. In the Japanese population, this polymorphism has been shown to be associated with an increased lung-cancer risk *(295)*. The data in

Caucasians is controversial as this association was not demonstrated in some older studies of Caucasians where the polymorphism is much rarer *(296–298)*. On the other hand, a recent study of 490 Caucasians found an estimated OR of 2.08 for the *CYP1A1* m2 allele (heterozygotes and homozygotes) and lung-cancer development *(299)*. Finally, NSCLC patients with at least one susceptible allele of the *MspI* polymorphism were associated with a shortened survival *(300)*.

Another polymorphism at residue 462 (Ile/Val) of the CYP1A1 heme-binding region, has also been associated with lung-cancer risk in Japan *(301)*. The Val-containing protein demonstrates twice as much activity as the isoleucine-containing protein *(295)*, but recent studies have shown little or no in vitro difference in their kinetic properties (302,303). In any case, the results are mixed as CYP1A1 Val/Val was twice as prevalent in Brazilian lung-cancer patients *(304)*, borderline in a German cohort *(305)*, and not increased in a Finnish cohort *(296)*.

In the complex process of multi-step carcinogenesis, it is unlikely that a single factor can completely account for an individual's susceptibility to lung cancer. For any given exposure to an environmental carcinogen, it is more likely that it is the interaction between several genetic-susceptibility factors that determines the risk of lung cancer. Consequently, the possibility that it is the combination of the bioactivating phase I (P450s) and the inactivating phase II (GSTs) carcinogen-metabolizing enzyme polymorphisms that is crucial to lung-cancer risk is biologically plausible and attractive.

The *CYP1A1 MspI* polymorphism in conjunction with the *GSTM1* null genotype has been reported to carry a ninefold increased risk of lung cancer *(287)*. This was confirmed in a second cohort of Japanese subjects where the OR of a combined *CYP1A1* m2/m2 and GSTM1 null genotype vs nonsmoker controls was 21.9 (95% CI 4.7–112.7), albeit lowered when smoking controls were compared. In the only non-Japanese cohort to be tested, a Swedish study found too few appropriate subjects for analysis *(297)*. Thus, although the data implicates a link for combination genotypes and lung-cancer risk in Japanese populations, the relatively lower prevalence of the m2 and Val allele in non-Japanese populations, estimated to be 12% and 3–16%, respectively *(283)*, suggests that this may not have been adequately studied in Caucasian populations.

CYP2D6 (debrisoquine 4-hydroxylase), another P450-metabolizing enzyme, bioactivates nicotine and NNK. The relationship between lung-cancer risk and the CYP2D6 polymorphism has been the subject of numerous studies and is still controversial *(306,307)*. Although some studies have suggested a reduction in the risk of lung cancer with the poor metabolizer phenotype and/or genotype *(308)*, others have indicated little or no role for the *CYP2D6* polymorphism in lung cancer *(307,309,310)*.

DIFFERENTIATION FACTORS Some genetic abnormalities of proto-oncogenes and tumor-suppressor genes are common to all lung cancers, but others appear more specific for certain histological subtypes. Mutation of the c-*ras* genes are specific to NSCLC, *Rb1* mutation is predominant in SCLC, and *p16^{INK4A}* mutation typically occurs in NSCLC. Aberrant expression of *CD44* is considered to be a marker for NSCLC *(4,311)*. It is possible that such specificies may represent important determinants for the phenotypical development of the histological subtypes, but the possibility that it is a secondary phenomenon remains. In support of the former suggestion, the in vitro introduction of oncogenes and tumor-suppressor genes into lung-cancer cell lines can induce phenotypic transitions among subtypes of lung cancer. For instance, the v-H-*ras* gene was shown to change the SCLC phenotype of lung-cancer cells into a NSCLC phenotype *(312)*.

A few normal bronchial epithelial cells and a substantial proportion of lung cancers, particularly exemplified by SCLC, exhibit a NE phenotype. The genetic factors responsible for NE differentiation in either normal lung or lung cancer are not understood. Candidate molecules include the achaete-scute family of bHLH transcription factors, which play a critical developmental role in neuronal commitment and differentiation of both *Drosophila* and vertebrates. The human *achaete-scute homologue-1* (*hASH1*) gene is selectively expressed in normal fetal pulmonary NE cells, as well as in lung cancers with NE features *(313)*. Additionally, pulmonary NE cells appear absent in newborn mice with *ASH1* disruptions and antisense-mediated *ASH1* depletion from lung-cancer cells results in a significant decrease in the expression of NE markers *(313)*.

TRANSGENIC ANIMAL MODELS Transgenic and knockout mice have only been minimally used to understand lung-cancer pathogenesis. Nevertheless, different transgenic animals have been generated that show dramatic developmental abnormalities including lung structure, suggesting crucial roles of the genes in normal lung development *(67)*. In terms of lung-cancer development, relatively few transgenic animals with introduced proto-oncogenes or targeted tumor-suppressor genes develop lung cancer. These include mice overexpressing mutant alleles of *p53*, lacking *E2F-1*, or that express a truncated nuclear *RARβ* *(106,141,314)*. Transgenic animal models are likely to contribute in the future to the currently limited knowledge of the functional relationship between the genes required in normal lung development and those mutated in lung cancer.

TELOMERASE ACTIVATION Vertebrates have special structures at the ends of their chromosomes (telomeres), which are composed of 5–15 kb pairs of a guanine-rich hexameric repeat (TTAGGG)n. In normal somatic cells, there is a progressive degradation of telomeres with aging. The loss of these telomeric repeats during normal cell division is thought to represent an intrinsic cellular clock by gradually shortening the telomere. The progressive telomere shortening is believed to lead to senescence and thus govern normal cellular mortality. Germ cells and some stem cells compensate for the telomere shortening by expressing a telomerase activity that replaces the hexameric repeats at the chromosomal ends. Normal somatic cells, however, do not express telomerase, presumably because they do not need to replicate or only replicate to a finite degree. Thus immortal cells may be able to proliferate indefinitely because they express telomerase activity, whereas the vast majority of normal adult cells do not.

The length of terminal telomeric restriction fragments is altered in various types of tumors, including lung cancer. Te-

lomere shortening was detected in 14/60 (23%) primary lung cancers, while 2 cases showed telomere elongation *(315)*. Telomerase is upregulated or reactivated in almost 90% of all human cancers. All SCLC and 80–85% of NSCLC were demonstrated to express high levels of telomerase activity as measured by a highly sensitive telomere-replication amplification protocol (TRAP) *(315–317)*. A high level of telomerase activity was associated with increased cell-proliferation rates and advanced pathologic stage in primary NSCLC *(317)*. In addition, telomerase activity and/or expression of the RNA component of human telomerase were frequently dysregulated in carcinoma *in situ* lesions, implicating its early involvement in the multi-stage development of lung cancer *(318)*. The catalytic subunits of human telomerase have been recently cloned and appear expressed in human cancers *(319)*. However, the regulation and expression of these catalytic subunits in lung cancer requires additional investigation. It also remains to be seen whether a novel mechanism for lengthening their telomeres, termed alternative lengthening of telomeres (or ALT) found in some immortalized cell lines with no detectable telomerase activity, is relevant to those lung cancers without high levels of telomerase expression *(320)*.

EVADING HOST IMMUNITY The major function of the immune system is to distinguish between self and nonself. The conceptual role of immune surveillance in cancer detection and elimination postulates that tumor cells express various novel tumor-specific epitopes that represent potential immune nonself targets. Thus, established cancers are thought to have effectively avoided immune recognition and elimination. Several different genetic mechanisms for escaping immune surveillance have been elucidated in lung cancer patients. It has been shown that the class I major histocompatibility complex (MHC) antigen expression is downregulated in human cancers including lung cancer *(321,322)*. These class I MHC molecules mediate presentation of endogenous antigenic peptides to cytotoxic T lymphocytes. In addition, rare mutations of the β_2-microglobulin gene, whose protein product comprises a component of the class I molecules, have also been reported in lung-cancer cells *(323)*. Indeed, transfection of a normal β_2-microglobulin gene into tumor cells restored expression of MHC class I proteins *(323)*. For the stable assembly of MHC class I complex and subsequent recognition by cytotoxic T lymphocytes, transporters associated with antigen presentation (TAP-1 and TAP-2), are necessary for conveying intracellular peptides into the endoplasmic reticulum for complex formation with class I MHC. The TAP-1 transporter has been shown to be downregulated in lung cancer *(322,324)*. Although the TAP-1 gene is not somatically mutated in lung cancer, one SCLC cell line was found to be transcriptionally silent for its wild-type allele and only expressed a genetically defective TAP allele, leading to an acquired loss of antigen-presenting ability *(325)*.

The Fas (CD95) system is an important mediator of T-cell cytotoxicity. The FasL ligand can induce activated T cells to undergo apoptosis, and this mechanism is thought to contribute to development of immunologically privileged sites. It is notable that lung-cancer cells (both lines and primary tumors) express FasL and co-culture of lung-cancer cell lines with a Fas-sensitive human T-cell line induced apoptosis in the T-

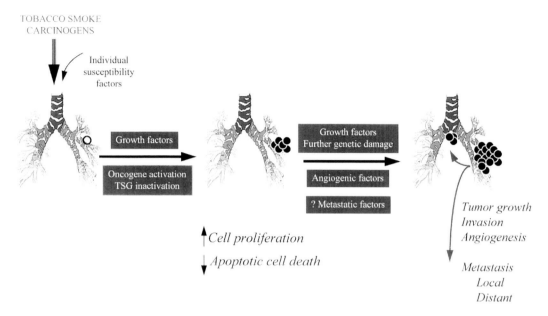

Fig. 4. Schematic overview of the interaction of genetic damage and other factors in the pathogenesis of lung cancer. TSG, tumor-suppressor gene.

cells *(326)*. Thus, the expression of FasL by neoplastic lung cells can be speculated to be a potential mechanism for evading host immunity by the peripheral deletion of tumor-reactive T-cell clones *(327,328)*.

TUMOR ANGIOGENESIS For primary and metastatic tumors to grow, it is essential that they receive an adequate blood supply, which is acquired by recruiting new blood vessels from the surrounding host vasculature. The development of new vessels leading to and within the tumor mass is required for adequate nutrient delivery and necessary at the beginning and end of metastatic dissemination. Without angiogenesis, tumors are unable to grow larger than 2–4 mm in diameter. During angiogenesis, normally quiescent endothelial cells become invasive, breaching their own basement membrane to invade the stroma during the development of new capillary buds. The number of microvessels in the tumor area, representing an index of angiogenesis, has been shown to correlate with an increased risk of metastatic disease and a worse overall survival for several types of human cancer, including lung cancer. The higher the microvessel density (MVD), the poorer the clinical outcome *(329,330)*.

The process of tumor angiogenesis is complex and controlled by a diverse family of inducers and inhibitors governing angiogenesis and regulating endothelial cell proliferation and migration *(331)*. Vascular endothelial growth factor (VEGF) and basic fibroblast growth factor (bFGF) are among the most important tumor-angiogenesis inducers. In lung cancer, VEGF expression was significantly lower in *p53*-negative and lowly vascularized NSCLCs *(332,333)*. VEGF expression was higher in lung cancers with nodal metastasis than those without *(334)*. In squamous-cell lung carcinomas, VEGF expression was inversely correlated with overall survival of patients, and the VEGF receptor flt-1 was frequently expressed *(335)*. Both the bFGF and its receptor (FGFR-1) are variably expressed in NSCLCs. Whether there is an association between bFGF ex-

pression and prognosis is currently controversial *(336,337)*. In either case, expression of another angiogenic/endothelial-cell chemotactic factor, platelet-derived endothelial cell growth factor (also called gliostatin), correlated with tumor angiogenesis and adverse prognosis in a study of node-negative NSCLC patients *(338)*.

Many inhibitors of angiogenesis are produced as propeptides. These inhibitors include angiostatin (a fragment of plasminogen), and endostatin (a fragment of collagen XVIII). Endostatin administered to Lewis lung carcinoma-bearing mice has been shown to regress tumors without inducing drug resistance during six treatment cycles *(339)*. Another inhibitor, thrombospondin-1 (TSP-1) is regulated by p53, and loss of p53 function in tumor cells is associated with reduced levels of this angiogenesis inhibitor *(340)*. Restoration of p53 function upregulates TSP-1 and impairs tumor angiogenesis. Another angiostatic factor, interferon-γ-inducible protein 10 (IP-10) was shown to inhibit human NSCLC tumorigenesis and spontaneous metastases *(341)*. Thus, it is the balance between angiogenesis inducers and inhibitors expressed from tumor cells that appears to affect the ability of the normally quiescent vasculature to form new capillaries (331). Another example comes from the finding that an imbalance in the expression of the angiogenic or angiostatic CXC chemokine family favors angiogenesis in NSCLC *(342)*.

CONCLUSIONS

Our understanding of the role of the molecular genetic changes that occur during lung-cancer pathogenesis, although in its early stages, is advancing rapidly with several specific genes and candidate chromosomal regions being identified (Fig. 4). The gene products are being classified into several important growth and cell-cycle regulatory pathways. Some of these markers appear to be important for carcinogenesis in general, whereas others show more frequent involvement in lung cancers. The challenge is to translate such understanding of the disrupted cellular physiology into clinical benefit for the patient by expanding the diagnostic and therapeutic armamentarium. Effective strategies may include: 1) early molecular diagnosis; 2) identification of high-risk individuals for developing lung cancer; 3) early treatment studies; 4) rational development of novel therapies such as tumor vaccines; 5) genetic inhibition of growth factor loops by regulation of agonists and antagonists and by other mechanisms such as MAbs; 6) epigenetic alteration of gene expression, such as by alteration of methylation; 7) manipulating intrinsic tumor chemosensitivity or radiosensitivity; 8) blocking the expression of activated proto-oncogenes; or 9) replacing defective tumor-suppressor genes.

There has been much emphasis for the molecular diagnosis of early disease or pre-invasive changes. Most cases of lung tumors that are detected by imaging have grown at least 1 cm in diameter, with a mass of a gram or more, and contain at least 10^8 to 10^9 cells, estimated to be about 30 population doublings from a single malignant cell. This only leaves a narrow window of opportunity for intervention before the tumor burden reaches the lethal range, about 10^{12} cells (approx a kilogram or another 10 population doublings) or metastatic disease develops. In other words, about three-quarters of the natural history of the cancer has occurred by the usual time of clinical detection by traditional methods. The considerable number of genetic lesions identified in overt lung cancer justifies attempts to detect corresponding lesions in preneoplastic lung tissue. If there are a few critical and consistent early lung-cancer clonal markers, one could envisage an opportunity to detect preneoplastic or early lesions by testing a panel of selected markers. An example frequently cited is the finding of *p53* mutations in a retrospective analysis of sputum samples obtained from patients undergoing screening procedures who subsequently developed lung cancer *(343)*. The hope is that intervention with chemoprevention or other means can block progression to multiple other genetic lesions in these same cells and the development of overt malignancy. In addition, other important aspects of lung-cancer development such as the genes responsible for drug resistance, tumor progression, and metastasis are being studied and need to be extended further. Already the observations on tumor angiogenesis are providing new therapeutic avenues. Thus, the paradigm proposed by Boveri and Little early this century—that cancer is essentially a genetic disease at the cellular level—and now confirmed by modern techniques, is affording us new approaches to the prevention, early detection, and treatment of lung cancer. There is now a rational hope that new therapies directed against one or more of these targets may ultimately be clinically successful in treating and curing lung cancer.

REFERENCES

1. Parker, S. L., Tong, T., Bolden, S., and Wingo, P. A. (1997) Cancer statistics, 1997. *CA: Cancer J. Clin.* **47**:5–27.
2. Williams, C. L. (1997) Basic science of small cell lung cancer. *Chest Surg. Clin. North Am.* **7**:1–19.
3. Vuitch, F., Sekido, Y., Fong, K., Mackay, B., Minna, J. D., and Gazdar, A. F. (1997) Neuroendocrine tumors of the lung. Pathology and molecular biology. *Chest Surg. Clin. North Am.* **7**:21–47.
4. Penno, M. B., August, J. T., Baylin, S. B., Mabry, M., Linnoila, R. I., Lee, V. S., et al. (1994) Expression of CD44 in human lung tumors. *Cancer Res.* **54**:1381–1387.
5. Loeb, L. A. (1991) Mutator phenotype may be required for multistage carcinogenesis. *Cancer Res.* **51**:3075–3079.
6. Loeb, L. A. (1994) Microsatellite instability: marker of a mutator phenotype in cancer. *Cancer Res.* **54**:5059–5063.
7. Barlogie, B., Drewinko, B., Schumann, J., Gohde, W., Dosik, G., Latreille, J., et al. (1980) Cellular DNA content as a marker of neoplasia in man. *Am. J. Med.* **69**:195–203.
8. Barlogie, B., Raber, M. N., Schumann, J., Johnson, T. S., Drewinko, B., Swartzendruber, D. E., et al. (1983) Flow cytometry in clinical cancer research. *Cancer Res.* **43**:3982–3997.
9. Zimmerman, P. V., Hawson, G. A., Bint, M. H., and Parsons, P. G. (1987) Ploidy as a prognostic determinant in surgically treated lung cancer. *Lancet* **2**:530–533.
10. Schmidt, R. A., Rusch, V. W., and Piantadosi, S. (1992) A flow cytometric study of non-small cell lung cancer classified as T1N0. *Cancer* **69**:78–85.
11. Smith, A. L., Hung, J., Walker, L., Rogers, T. E., Vuitch, F., Lee, E., et al. (1996) Extensive areas of aneuploidy are present in the respiratory epithelium of lung cancer patients. *Br. J. Cancer* **73**:203–209.
12. Levin, N. A., Brzoska, P., Gupta, N., Minna, J. D., Gray, J. W., and Christman, M. F. (1994) Identification of frequent novel genetic alterations in small cell lung carcinoma. *Cancer Res.* **54**:5086–5091.
13. Levin, N. A., Brzoska, P. M., Warnock, M. L., Gray, J. W., and Christman, M. F. (1995) Identification of novel regions of altered DNA copy number in small cell lung tumors. *Genes Chromosomes Cancer* **13**:175–185.
14. Schwendel, A., Langreck, H., Reichel, M., Schröck, E., Ried, T., Dietel, M., et al. (1997) Primary small-cell lung carcinomas and their metastases are characterized by a recurrent pattern of genetic alterations. *Int. J. Cancer* **74**:86–93.
15. Petersen, I., Langreck, H., Wolf, G., Schwendel, A., Psille, R., Vogt, P., et al. (1997) Small-cell lung cancer is characterized by a high incidence of deletions on chromosomes 3p, 4q, 5q, 10q, 13q and 17p. *Br. J. Cancer* **75**:79–86.
16. Petersen, I., Bujard, M., Petersen, S., Wolf, G., Goeze, A., Schwendel, A., et al. (1997) Patterns of chromosomal imbalances in adenocarcinoma and squamous cell carcinoma of the lung. *Cancer Res.* **57**:2331–2335.
17. Richardson, G. E. and Johnson, B. E. (1993) The biology of lung cancer. *Semin. Oncol.* **20**:105–127.
18. Greenblatt, M. S., Bennett, W. P., Hollstein, M., and Harris, C. C. (1994) Mutations in the p53 tumor suppressor gene: clues to cancer etiology and molecular pathogenesis. *Cancer Res.* **54**:4855–4878.
19. Slebos, R. J., Hruban, R. H., Dalesio, O., Mooi, W. J., Offerhaus, G. J., and Rodenhuis, S. (1991) Relationship between K-ras oncogene activation and smoking in adenocarcinoma of the human lung. *J. Natl. Cancer Inst.* **83**:1024–1027.
20. Slebos, R. J., Kibbelaar, R. E., Dalesio, O., Kooistra, A., Stam, J., Meijer, C. J. L. M., et al. (1990) K-ras oncogene activation as a prognostic marker in adenocarcinoma of the lung. *N. Engl. J. Med.* **323**:561–565.
21. Slebos, R. J. and Rodenhuis, S. (1992) The ras gene family in human non-small-cell lung cancer. Monographs *J. Natl. Cancer Inst. Monograph* **13**:23–29.
22. Sugio, K., Ishida, T., Yokoyama, H., Inoue, T., Sugimachi, K., and Sasazuki, T. (1992) ras gene mutations as a prognostic marker in adenocarcinoma of the human lung without lymph node metastasis. *Cancer Res.* **52**:2903–2906.
23. Mitsudomi, T., Steinberg, S. M., Oie, H. K., Mulshine, J. L., Phelps, R., Viallet, J., et al. (1991). ras gene mutations in non-small cell lung cancers are associated with shortened survival irrespective of treatment intent. *Cancer Res.* **51**:4999–5002.
24. Rosell, R., Li, S., Skacel, Z., Mate, J. L., Maestre, J., Canela, M., et al. (1993) Prognostic impact of mutated K-ras gene in surgically resected non-small cell lung cancer patients. *Oncogene* **8**:2407–2412.

25. Siegfried, J. M., Gillespie, A. T., Mera, R., Casey, T. J., Keohavong, P., Testa, J. R., et al. (1997) Prognostic value of specific KRAS mutations in lung adenocarcinomas. *Cancer Epidemiol. Biomark. Prev.* **6**:841–847.

26. Tsai, C.-M., Chang, K.-T., Perng, R.-P., Mitsudomi, T., Chen, M.-H., Kadoyama, C., et al. (1993) Correlation of intrinsic chemoresistance of non-small-cell lung cancer cell lines with HER-2/neu gene expression but not with ras gene mutations. *J. Natl. Cancer Inst.* **85**:897–901.

27. Rodenhuis, S., Boerrigter, L., Top, B., Slebos, R. J., Mooi, W. J., van't Veer, L., et al. (1997) Mutational activation of the K-ras oncogene and the effect of chemotherapy in advanced adenocarcinoma of the lung: A prospective study. *J. Clin. Oncol.* **15**:285–291.

28. Pfeifer, A. M., Mark, G. D., Malan-Shibley, L., Graziano, S., Amstad, P., and Harris, C. C. (1989) Cooperation of c-raf-1 and c-myc protooncogenes in the neoplastic transformation of simian virus 40 large tumor antigen-immortalized human bronchial epithelial cells. *Proc. Natl. Acad. Sci. USA* **86**:10,075–10,079.

29. Cooper, C. A., Carby, F. A., Bubb, V. J., Lamb, D., Kerr, K. M., and Wyllie, A. H. (1997) The pattern of K-ras mutation in pulmonary adenocarcinoma defines a new pathway of tumour development in the human lung. *J. Pathol.* **181**:401–404.

30. Tsuchiya, E., Furuta, R., Wada, N., Nakagawa, K., Ishikawa, Y., Kawabuchi, B., et al. (1995) High K-ras mutation rates in goblet-cell-type adenocarcinomas of the lungs. *J. Cancer Res. Clin. Oncol.* **121**:577–581.

31. Ryberg, D., Tefre, T., Skaug, V., Stangeland, L., Ovrebo, S., Naalsund, A., et al. (1992) Allele diversity of the H-ras-1 variable number of tandem repeats in Norwegian lung cancer patients. *Environ. Health Perspect.* **98**:187–189.

32. Graziano, S. L., Pfeifer, A. M., Testa, J. R., Mark, G. E., Johnson, B. E., Hallinan, E. J., et al. (1991) Involvement of the RAF1 locus, at band 3p25, in the 3p deletion of small-cell lung cancer. *Genes Chromosomes Cancer* **3**:283–293.

33. Miwa, W., Yasuda, J., Yashima, K., Makino, R., and Sekiya, T. (1994) Absence of activating mutations of the RAF1 protooncogene in human lung cancer. *Biol. Chem. Hoppe-Seyler* **375**:705–709.

34. Przygodzki, R. M., Finkelstein, S. D., Langer, J. C., Swalsky, P. A., Fishback, N., Bakker, A., et al. (1996) Analysis of p53, K-ras-2, and C-raf-1 in pulmonary neuroendocrine tumors. Correlation with histological subtype and clinical outcome. *Am. J. Pathol.* **148**:1531–1541.

35. Bansal, A., Ramirez, R. D., and Minna, J. D. (1997) Mutation analysis of the coding sequences of MEK-1 and MEK-2 genes in human lung cancer cell lines. *Oncogene* **14**:1231–1234.

36. Teng, D. H.-F., Perry, W. L., Hogan, J. K., Baumgard, M., Bell, R., Berry, S., et al. (1997) Human mitogen-activated protein kinase kinase 4 as a candidate tumor suppressor. *Cancer Res.* **57**:4177–4182.

37. Grandori, C. and Eisenman, R. N. (1997) Myc target genes. *Trends Biochem. Sci.* **22**:177–181.

38. Nau, M. M., Brooks, B. J., Battey, J., Sausville, E., Gazdar, A. F., Kirsch, I. R., et al. (1985) L-myc, a new myc-related gene amplified and expressed in human small cell lung cancer. *Nature* **318**:69–73.

39. Krystal, G., Birrer, M., Way, J., Nau, M., Sausville, E., Thompson, C., et al. (1988) Multiple mechanisms for transcriptional regulation of the myc gene family in small-cell lung cancer. *Mol. Cell. Biol.* **8**:3373–3381.

40. Johnson, B. E., Russell, E., Simmons, A. M., Phelps, R., Steinberg, S. M., Ihde, D. C., et al. (1996) MYC family DNA amplification in 126 tumor cell lines from patients with small cell lung cancer. *J. Cell Biochem. Suppl.* **24**:210–217.

41. Sekido, Y., Takahashi, T., Mäkelä, T. P., Obata, Y., Ueda, R., Hida, T., et al. (1992) Complex intrachromosomal rearrangement in the process of amplification of the L-myc gene in small-cell lung cancer. *Mol. Cell. Biol.* **12**:1747–1754.

42. Makela, T. P., Hellsten, E., Vesa, J., Hirvonen, H., Palotie, A., Peltonen, L., et al. (1995) The rearranged L-myc fusion gene (RLF) encodes a Zn-15 related zinc finger protein. *Oncogene* **11**:2699–2704.

43. Ou, X., Campau, S., Slusher, R., Jasti, R. K., Mabry, M., and Kalemkerian, G. P. (1996). Mechanism of all-trans-retinoic acid-mediated L-myc gene regulation in small cell lung cancer. *Oncogene* **13**:1893–1899.

44. Spandidos, D. A., Zakinthinos, S., Petraki, C., Sotsiou, F., Yiagnisis, M., Dimopoulos, A. M., et al. (1990) Expression of ras p21 and myc p62oncoproteins in small cell and non small cell carcinomas of the lung. *Anticancer Res.* **10**:1105–1114.

45. Fong, K. M., Kida, Y., Zimmerman, P. V., and Smith, P. J. (1996) MYCL genotypes and loss of heterozygosity in non-small-cell lung cancer. *Br. J. Cancer* **74**:1975–1978.

46. Volm, M., Drings, P., Wodrich, W., and van-Kaick, G. (1993) Expression of oncoproteins in primary human non-small cell lung cancer and incidence of metastases. *Clin. Exp. Metastasis* **11**:325–329.

47. Wodrich, W. and Volm, M. (1993) Overexpression of oncoproteins in non-small cell lung carcinomas of smokers. *Carcinogenesis* **14**:1121–1124.

48. Szabo, E., Riffe, M. E., Steinberg, S. M., Birrer, M. J., and Linnoila, R. I. (1996) Altered cJUN expression: an early event in human lung carcinogenesis. *Cancer Res.* **56**:305–315.

49. Levin, W. J., Press, M. F., Gaynor, R. B., Sukhatme, V. P., Boone, T. C., Reissmann, P. T., et al. (1995) Expression patterns of immediate early transcription factors in human non-small cell lung cancer. The Lung Cancer Study Group. *Oncogene* **11**:1261–1269.

50. Alroy, I. and Yarden, Y. (1997) The ErbB signaling network in embryogenesis and oncogenesis: signal diversification through combinatorial ligand-receptor interactions. *FEBS Lett.* **410**:83–86.

51. Rachwal, W. J., Bongiorno, P. F., Orringer, M. B., Whyte, R. I., Ethier, S. P., and Beer, D. G. (1995) Expression and activation of erbB-2 and epidermal growth factor receptor in lung adenocarcinomas. *Br. J. Cancer* **72**:56–64.

52. Schneider, P. M., Hung, M.-C., Chiocca, S. M., Manning, J., Zhao, X., Fang, K., et al. (1989) Differential expression of the c-erbB-2 gene in human small cell and non-small cell lung cancer. *Cancer Res.* **49**:4968–4971.

53. Shi, D., He, G., Cao, S., Pan, W., Zhang, H. Z., Yu, D., et al. (1992) Overexpression of the c-erbB-2/neu-encoded p185 protein in primary lung cancer. *Mol. Carcinogenesis* **5**:213–218.

54. Weiner, D. B., Nordberg, J., Robinson, R., Nowell, P. C., Gazdar, A., Greene, M. I., et al. (1990) Expression of the neu gene-encoded protein (P185^{neu}) in human non-small cell carcinomas of the lung. *Cancer Res.* **50**:421–425.

55. Noguchi, M., Murakami, M., Bennett, W., Lupu, R., Hui, F., Jr., Harris, C. C., et al. (1993) Biological consequences of overexpression of a transfected c-erbB-2 gene in immortalized human bronchial epithelial cells. *Cancer Res.* **53**:2035–2043.

56. Kern, J .A., Torney, L., Weiner, D., Gazdar, A., Shepard, H. M., and Fendly, B. (1993) Inhibition of human lung cancer cell line growth by an anti-p185HER2 antibody. *Am. J. Resp. Cell Mol. Biol.* **9**:448–454.

57. Tateishi, M., Ishida, T., Mitsudomi, T., Kaneko, S., and Sugimachi, K. (1991) Prognostic value of c-erbB-2 protein expression in human lung adenocarcinoma and squamous cell carcinoma. *Eur. J. Cancer* **27**:1372–1375.

58. Kern, J. A., Slebos, R. J., Top, B., Rodenhuis, S., Lager, D., Robinson, R. A., et al. (1994) C-erbB-2 expression and codon 12 K-ras mutations both predict shortened survival for patients with pulmonary adenocarcinomas. *J. Clin. Invest.* **93**:516–520.

59. Pfeiffer, P., Clausen, P. P., Andersen, K., and Rose, C. (1996) Lack of prognostic significance of epidermal growth factor receptor and the oncoprotein p185HER-2 in patients with systemically untreated non-small-cell lung cancer: an immunohistochemical study on cryosections. *Br. J. Cancer* **74**:86–91.

60. Yu, D., Wang, S. S., Dulski, K. M., Tsai, C. M., Nicolson, G. L., and Hung, M. C. (1994) c-erbB-2/neu overexpression enhances metastatic potential of human lung cancer cells by induction of metastasis-associated properties. *Cancer Res.* **54**:3260–3266.

61. Tsai, C. M., Yu, D., Chang, K. T., Wu, L. H., Perng, R. P., Ibrahim, N. K., et al. C. (1995) Enhanced chemoresistance by elevation of

p185neu levels in HER-2/neu-transfected human lung cancer cells. *J. Natl. Cancer Inst.* **87**:682–684.

62. Tsai, C.-M., Chang, K.-T., Wu, L.-H., Chen, J.-Y., Gazdar, A. F., Mitsudomi, T., et al. (1996) Correlations between intrinsic chemoresistance and HER-2/neu gene expression, p53 gene mutations, and cell proliferation characteristics in non-small cell lung cancer cell lines. *Cancer Res.* **56**:206–209.

63. Tateishi, M., Ishida, T., Mitsudomi, T., Kaneko, S., and Sugimachi, K. (1990) Immunohistochemical evidence of autocrine growth factors in adenocarcinoma of the human lung. *Cancer Res.* **50**:7077–7080.

64. Rusch, V., Baselga, J., Cordon-Cardo, C., Orazem, J., Zaman, M., Hoda, S., et al. (1993) Differential expression of the epidermal growth factor receptor and its ligands in primary non-small cell lung cancers and adjacent benign lung. *Cancer Res.* **53**:2379–2385.

65. Damstrup, L., Rygaard, K., Spang-Thomsen, M., and Poulsen, H. S. (1992) Expression of the epidermal growth factor receptor in human small cell lung cancer cell lines. *Cancer Res.* **52**:3089–3093.

66. Miettinen, P. J., Berger, J. E., Meneses, J., Phung, Y., Pedersen, R. A., Werb, Z., et al. (1995) Epithelial immaturity and multiorgan failure in mice lacking epidermal growth factor receptor. *Nature* **376**:337–341.

67. Miettinen, P. J., Warburton, D., Bu, D., Zhao, J. S., Berger, J. E., Minoo, P., et al. (1997). Impaired lung branching morphogenesis in the absence of functional EGF receptor. *Dev. Biol.* **186**:224–236.

68. Singh Kaw, P., Zarnegar, R., and Siegfried, J. M. (1995). Stimulatory effects of hepatocyte growth factor on normal and neoplastic human bronchial epithelial cells. *Am. J. Physiol.* **268**:L1012–L1020.

69. Yanagita, K., Matsumoto, K., Sekiguchi, K., Ishibashi, H., Niho, Y., and Nakamura, T. (1993) Hepatocyte growth factor may act as a pulmotrophic factor on lung regeneration after acute lung injury. *J. Biol. Chem.* **268**:21,212–21,217.

70. Rygaard, K., Nakamura, T., and Spang-Thomsen, M. (1993) Expression of the proto-oncogenes c-met and c-kit and their ligands, hepatocyte growth factor/scatter factor and stem cell factor, in SCLC cell lines and xenografts. *Br. J. Cancer* **67**:37–46.

71. Harvey, P., Warn, A., Newman, P., Perry, L. J., Ball, R. Y., and Warn, R. M. (1996) Immunoreactivity for hepatocyte growth factor/scatter factor and its receptor, met, in human lung carcinomas and malignant mesotheliomas. *J. Pathol.* **180**:389–394.

72. Olivero, M., Rizzo, M., Madeddu, R., Casadio, C., Pennacchietti, S., Nicotra, M. R., et al. (1996) Overexpression and activation of hepatocyte growth factor/scatter factor in human non-small-cell lung carcinomas. *Br. J. Cancer* **74**:1862–1868.

73. Ichimura, E., Maeshima, A., Nakajima, T., and Nakamura, T. (1996) Expression of c-met/HGF receptor in human non-small cell lung carcinomas in vitro and in vivo and its prognostic significance. *Jpn. J. Cancer Res.* **87**:1063–1069.

74. Siegfried, J. M., Weissfeld, L. A., Singh-Kaw, P., Weyant, R. J., Testa, J. R., and Landreneau, R. J. (1997) Association of immunoreactive hepatocyte growth factor with poor survival in resectable non-small cell lung cancer. *Cancer Res.* **57**:433–439.

75. Schmidt, L., Duh, F.-M., Chen, F., Kishida, T., Glenn, G., Choyke, P., et al. (1997) Germline and somatic mutations in the tyrosine kinase domain of the MET proto-oncogene in papillary renal carcinomas. *Nature Genet.* **16**:68–73.

76. Quinn, K. A., Treston, A. M., Unsworth, E. J., Miller, M. J., Vos, M., Grimley, C., et al. (1996) Insulin-like growth factor expression in human cancer cell lines. *J. Biol. Chem.* **271**:11,477–11,483.

77. Sekido, Y., Takahashi, T., Ueda, R., Takahashi, M., Suzuki, H., Nishida, K., et al. (1993) Recombinant human stem cell factor mediates chemotaxis of small-cell lung cancer cell lines aberrantly expressing the c-kit protooncogene. *Cancer Res.* **53**:1709–1714.

78. Krystal, G. W., Hines, S. J., and Organ, C. P. (1996) Autocrine growth of small cell lung cancer mediated by coexpression of c-kit and stem cell factor. *Cancer Res.* **56**:370–376.

79. Antoniades, H. N., Galanopoulos, T., Neville-Golden, J., and O'Hara, C. J. (1992) Malignant epithelial cells in primary human lung carcinomas coexpress in vivo platelet-derived growth factor

(PDGF) and PDGF receptor mRNAs and their protein products. *Proc. Natl. Acad. Sci. USA* **89**:3942–3946.

80. Viallet, J. and Sausville, E. A. (1996) Involvement of signal transduction pathways in lung cancer biology. *J. Cell. Biochem. Suppl.* **24**:228–236.

81. Fathi, Z., Way, J. W., Corjay, M. H., Viallet, J., Sausville, E. A., and Battey, J. F. (1996) Bombesin receptor structure and expression in human lung carcinoma cell lines. *J. Cell. Biochem. Suppl.* **24**:237–246.

82. Sethi, T., Langdon, S., Smyth, J., and Rozengurt, E. (1992) Growth of small cell lung cancer cells: stimulation by multiple neuropeptides and inhibition by broad spectrum antagonists in vitro and in vivo. *Cancer Res.* **52**:2737s–2742s.

83. Sharif, T. R., Luo, W., and Sharif, M. (1997) Functional expression of bombesin receptor in most adult and pediatric human glioblastoma cell lines; role in mitogenesis and in stimulating the mitogen-activated protein kinase pathway. *Mol. Cell. Endocrinol.* **130**:119–130.

84. Cuttitta, F., Carney, D. N., Mulshine, J., Moody, T. W., Fedorko, J., Fischler, A., et al. (1985) Bombesin-like peptides can function as autocrine growth factors in human small-cell lung cancer. *Nature* **316**:823–826.

85. Halmos, G. and Schally, A. V. (1997) Reduction in receptors for bombesin and epidermal growth factor in xenografts of human small-cell lung cancer after treatment with bombesin antagonist RC-3095. *Proc. Natl. Acad. Sci. USA* **94**:956–960.

86. Kelley, M. J., Linnoila, R. I., Avis, I. L., Georgiadis, M. S., Cuttitta, F., Mulshine, J. L., et al. (1997) Antitumor activity of a monoclonal antibody directed against gastrin-releasing peptide in patients with small cell lung cancer. *Chest* **112**:256–261.

87. Spurzem, J. R., Rennard, S. I., and Romberger, D. J. (1997) Bombesin-like peptides and airway repair: A recapitulation of lung development? *Am. J. Respir. Cell Mol. Biol.* **16**:209–211.

88. Yang, E. and Korsmeyer, S. J. (1996) Molecular thanatopsis: A discourse on the BCL2 family and cell death. *Blood* **88**:386–401.

89. Ohmori, T., Podack, E. R., Nishio, K., Takahashi, M., Miyahara, Y., Takeda, Y., et al. (1993) Apoptosis of lung cancer cells caused by some anti-cancer agents (MMC, CPT-11, ADM) is inhibited by bcl-2. *Biochem. Biophys. Res. Commun.* **192**:30–36.

90. Ziegler, A., Luedke, G. H., Fabbro, D., Altmann, K. H., Stahel, R. A., and Zangemeister Wittke, U. (1997) Induction of apoptosis in small-cell lung cancer cells by an antisense oligodeoxynucleotide targeting the Bcl-2 coding sequence. *J. Natl. Cancer Inst.* **89**:1027–1036.

91. Jiang, S. X., Kameya, T., Sato, Y., Yanase, N., Yoshimura, H., and Kodama, T. (1996) Bcl-2 protein expression in lung cancer and close correlation with neuroendocrine differentiation. *Am. J. Pathol.* **148**:837–846.

92. Pezzella, F., Turley, H., Kuzu, I., Tungekar, M. F., Dunnill, M. S., Pierce, C. B., et al. (1993) bcl-2 protein in non-small-cell lung carcinoma. *N. Engl. J. Med.* **329**:690–694.

93. Higashiyama, M., Doi, O., Kodama, K., Yokouchi, H., Nakamori, S., and Tateishi, R. (1997) bcl-2 oncoprotein in surgically resected non-small cell lung cancer: possibly favorable prognostic factor in association with low incidence of distant metastasis. *J. Surg. Oncol.* **64**:48–54.

94. Apolinario, R. M., van der Valk, P., de Jong, J. S., Deville, W., van Ark-Otte, J., Dingemans, A. M., et al. (1997). Prognostic value of the expression of p53, bcl-2, and bax oncoproteins, and neovascularization in patients with radically resected non-small-cell lung cancer. *J. Clin. Oncol.* **15**:2456–2466.

95. Fontanini, G., Vignati, S., Bigini, D., Mussi, A., Lucchi, M., Angeletti, C. A., et al. (1995) Bcl-2 protein: a prognostic factor inversely correlated to p53 in non-small-cell lung cancer. *Br. J. Cancer* **71**:1003–1007.

96. Kitagawa, Y., Wong, F., Lo, P., Elliott, M., Verburgt, L. M., Hogg, J. C., et al. (1996) Overexpression of Bcl-2 and mutations in p53 and K-ras in resected human non-small cell lung cancers. *Am. J. Resp. Cell Mol. Biol.* **15**:45–54.

97. Jiang, S. X., Sato, Y., Kuwao, S., and Kameya, T. (1995) Expression of bcl-2 oncogene protein is prevalent in small cell lung carcinomas. *J. Pathol.* **177**:135–138.

98. Kaiser, U., Schilli, M., Haag, U., Neumann, K., Kreipe, H., Kogan, E., et al. (1996) Expression of bcl-2—protein in small cell lung cancer. *Lung Cancer* **15**:31–40.

99. Cheng, E. H., Kirsch, D. G., Clem, R. J., Ravi, R., Kastan, M. B., Bedi, A., et al. (1997). Conversion of Bcl-2 to a Bax-like death effector by caspases. *Science* **278**:1966–1968.

100. Yin, C., Knudson, C. M., Korsmeyer, S. J., and Van Dyke, T. (1997) Bax suppresses tumorigenesis and stimulates apoptosis in vivo. *Nature* **385**:637–640.

101. Brambilla, E., Negoescu, A., Gazzeri, S., Lantuejoul, S., Moro, D., Brambilla, C., et al. (1996) Apoptosis-related factors p53, Bcl2, and Bax in neuroendocrine lung tumors. *Am. J. Pathol.* **149**:1941–1952.

102. Whang-Peng, J., Kao-Shan, C. S., Lee, E. C., Bunn, P. A., Carney, D. N., Gazdar, A. F., et al. (1982) Specific chromosome defect associated with human small-cell lung cancer; deletion 3p(14-23) *Science* **215**:181–182.

103. Virmani, A. K., Fong, K. M., Kodagoda, D., McIntire, D., Hung, J., Tonk, V., et al. (1998) Allelotyping demonstrates common and distinct patterns of chromosomal loss in human lung cancer types. *Gene Chromosomes Cancer* **21**:308–319.

104. Levine, A. J. (1997). p53, the cellular gatekeeper for growth and division. *Cell* **88**:323–331.

105. Graeber, T. G., Osmanian, C., Jacks, T., Housman, D. E., Koch, C. J., Lowe, S. W., et al. (1996) Hypoxia-mediated selection of cells with diminished apoptotic potential in solid tumours. *Nature* **379**:88–91.

106. Lavigueur, A., Maltby, V., Mock, D., Rossant, J., Pawson, T., and Bernstein, A. (1989) High incidence of lung, bone, and lymphoid tumors in transgenic mice overexpressing mutant alleles of the p53 oncogene. *Mol. Cell. Biol.* **9**:3982–3991.

107. Takahashi, T., Carbone, D., Takahashi, T., Nau, M. M., Hida, T., Linnoila, I., et al. (1992) Wild-type but not mutant p53 suppresses the growth of human lung cancer cells bearing multiple genetic lesions. *Cancer Res.* **52**:2340–2343.

108. Adachi, J., Ookawa, K., Shiseki, M., Okazaki, T., Tsuchida, S., Morishita, K., et al. (1996) Induction of apoptosis but not G1 arrest by expression of the wild-type p53 gene in small cell lung carcinoma. *Cell Growth Differ.* **7**:879–886.

109. Casey, G., Lopez, M. E., Ramos, J. C., Plummer, S. J., Arboleda, M. J., Shaughnessy, M., et al. (1996) DNA sequence analysis of exons 2 through 11 and immunohistochemical staining are required to detect all known p53 alterations in human malignancies. *Oncogene* **13**:1971–1981.

110. Eerola, A.-K., Törmänen, U., Rainio, P., Sormunen, R., Bloigu, R., Vähäkangas, K., et al. (1997) Apoptosis in operated small cell lung carcinoma is inversely related to tumour necrosis and p53 immunoreactivity. *J. Pathol.* **181**:172–177.

111. Nishio, M., Koshikawa, T., Kuroishi, T., Suyama, M., Uchida, K., Takagi, Y., et al. (1996) Prognostic significance of abnormal p53 accumulation in primary, resected non-small-cell lung cancers. *J. Clin. Oncol.* **14**:497–502.

112. Konishi, T., Lin, Z., Fujino, S., Kato, H., and Mori, A. (1997) Association of p53 protein expression in stage I lung adenocarcinoma with reference to cytological subtypes. *Human Pathol.* **28**:544–548.

113. Ishida, H., Irie, K., Itoh, T., Furukawa, T., and Tokunaga, O. (1997) The prognostic significance of p53 and bcl-2 expression in lung adenocarcinoma and its correlation with Ki-67 growth fraction. *Cancer* **80**:1034–1045.

114. Graziano, S. L. (1997) Non-small cell lung cancer: clinical value of new biological predictors. *Lung Cancer* **17**:S37–S58.

115. Schlichtholz, B., Trédaniel, J., Lubin, R., Zalcman, G., Hirsch, A., and Soussi, T. (1994) Analyses of p53 antibodies in sera of patients with lung carcinoma define immunodominant regions in the p53 protein. *Br. J. Cancer* **69**:809–816.

116. Winter, S. F., Minna, J. D., Johnson, B. E., Takahashi, T., Gazdar, A. F., and Carbone, D. P. (1992) Development of antibodies against p53 in lung cancer patients appears to be dependent on the type of p53 mutation. *Cancer Res.* **52**:4168–4174.

117. Lubin, R., Zalcman, G., Bouchet, L., Tredanel, J., Legros, Y., Cazals, D., et al. (1995) Serum p53 antibodies as early markers of lung cancer. *Nature Med.* **1**:701–702.

118. Rosenfeld, M. R., Malats, N., Schramm, L., Graus, F., Cardenal, F., Vinolas, N., et al. (1997) Serum anti-p53 antibodies and prognosis of patients with small-cell lung cancer. *J. Natl. Cancer Inst.* **89**:381–385.

119. Rahman, A. and Ziment, I. (1983) Tracheobronchial papillomatosis with malignant transformation. *Arch. Int. Med.* **143**:577–578.

120. Byrne, J. C., Tsao, M. S., Fraser, R. S., and Howley, P. M. (1987) Human papillomavirus-11 DNA in a patient with chronic laryngotracheobronchial papillomatosis and metastatic squamous-cell carcinoma of the lung. *N. Engl. J. Med.* **317**:873–878.

121. Bejui-Thivolet, F., Chardonnet, Y., and Patricot, L. M. (1990) Human papillomavirus type 11DNA in papillary squamous cell lung carcinoma. *Virch. Arch. A Pathol. Anat. Histopathol.* **417**:457–461.

122. Carey, F. A., Salter, D. M., Kerr, K. M., and Lamb, D. (1990) An investigation into the role of human papillomavirus in endobronchial papillary squamous tumours. *Resp. Med.* **84**:445–447.

123. Kulski, J. K., Demeter, T., Mutavdzic, S., Sterrett, G. F., Mitchell, K. M., and Pixley, E. C. (1990) Survey of histologic specimens of human cancer for human papillomavirus types 6/11/16/18 by filter in situ hybridization. *Am. J. Clin. Pathol.* **94**:566–570.

124. Yousem, S. A., Ohori, N. P., and Sonmez-Alpan, E. (1992) Occurrence of human papillomavirus DNA in primary lung neoplasms. *Cancer* **69**:693–697.

125. Fong, K. M., Schonrock, J., Frazer, I. M., Zimmerman, P. V., and Smith, P. J. (1995) Human papillomavirus not found in squamous and large cell lung carcinomas by polymerase chain reaction. *Cancer* **75**:2400–2401.

126. Szabo, I., Sepp, R., Nakamoto, K., Maeda, M., Sakamoto, H., and Uda, H. (1994) Human papillomavirus not found in squamous and large cell lung carcinomas by polymerase chain reaction. *Cancer* **73**:2740–2744.

127. Bohlmeyer, T., Le, T. N., Shroyer, A. L., Markham, N., and Shroyer, K. R. (1998) Detection of human papillomavirus in squamous cell carcinomas of the lung by polymerase chain reaction. *Am. J. Resp. Cell. Mol. Biol.* **18**:265–269.

128. Welt, A., Hummel, M., Niedobitek, G., and Stein, H. (1997) Human papillomavirus infection is not associated with bronchial carcinoma: evaluation by in situ hybridization and the polymerase chain reaction. *J. Pathol.* **181**:276–280.

129. Soini, Y., Nuorva, K., Kamel, D., Pollanen, R., Vahakangas, K., Lehto, V. P., et al. (1996) Presence of human papillomavirus DNA and abnormal p53 protein accumulation in lung carcinoma. *Thorax* **51**:887–893.

130. Fujiwara, T., Cai, D. W., Georges, R. N., Mukhopadhyay, T., Grimm, E. A., and Roth, J. A. (1994) Therapeutic effect of a retroviral wild-type p53 expression vector in an orthotopic lung cancer model. *J. Natl. Cancer Inst.* **86**:1458–1462.

131. Roth, J. A., Nguyen, D., Lawrence, D. D., Kemp, B. L., Carrasco, C. H., Ferson, D. Z., et al. (1996) Retrovirus-mediated wild-type p53 gene transfer to tumors of patients with lung cancer. *Nature Med.* **2**:985–991.

132. Shimizu, T., Miwa, W., Nakamori, S., Ishikawa, O., Konishi, Y., and Sekiya, T. (1996) Absence of a mutation of the p21/WAF1 gene in human lung and pancreatic cancers. *Jpn. J. Cancer Res.* **87**:275–278.

133. Marchetti, A., Doglioni, C., Barbareschi, M., Buttitta, F., Pellegrini, S., Bertacca, G., et al. (1996) p21 RNA and protein expression in non-small cell lung carcinomas: evidence of p53-independent expression and association with tumoral differentiation. *Oncogene* **12**:1319–1324.

134. Sjalander, A., Birgander, R., Rannug, A., Alexandrie, A. K., Tornling, G., and Beckman, G. (1996) Association between the p21

codon 31 A1 (arg) allele and lung cancer. *Human Heredity* **46**:221–225.

135. Shieh, S. Y., Ikeda, M., Taya, Y., and Prives, C. (1997) DNA damage-induced phosphorylation of p53 alleviates inhibition by MDM2. *Cell* **91**:325–334.

136. Higashiyama, M., Doi, O., Kodama, K., Yokouchi, H., Kasugai, T., Ishiguro, S., et al. (1997) MDM2 gene amplification and expression in non-small-cell lung cancer: immunohistochemical expression of its protein is a favourable prognostic marker in patients without p53 protein accumulation. *Br. J. Cancer* **75**:1302–1308.

137. Kaghad, M., Bonnet, H., Yang, A., Creancier, L., Biscan, J.-C., Valent, A., et al. (1997) Monoallelically expressed gene related to p53 at 1p36, a region frequently deleted in neuroblastoma and other human cancers. *Cell* **90**:809–819.

138. Jost, C. A., Marin, M. C., and Kaelin, W. G. (1997) p73 is a human p53-related protein that can induce apoptosis. *Nature* **389**:191–194.

139. Peeper, D. S., Upton, T. M., Ladha, M. H., Neuman, E., Zalvide, J., Bernards, R., et al. (1997) Ras signalling linked to the cell-cycle machinery by the retinoblastoma protein. *Nature* **386**:177–181.

140. White, R. J., Trouche, D., Martin, K., Jackson, S. P., and Kouzarides, T. (1996) Repression of RNA polymerase III transcription by the retinoblastoma protein. *Nature* **382**:88–90.

141. Yamasaki, L., Jacks, T., Bronson, R., Goillot, E., Harlow, E., and Dyson, N. J. (1996) Tumor induction and tissue atrophy in mice lacking E2F-1. *Cell* **85**:537–548.

142. Harbour, J. W., Lai, S. L., Whang-Peng, J., Gazdar, A. F., Minna, J. D., and Kaye, F. J. (1988) Abnormalities in structure and expression of the human retinoblastoma gene in SCLC. *Science* **241**:353–357.

143. Horowitz, J. M., Park, S. H., Bogenmann, E., Cheng, J. C., Yandell, D. W., Kaye, F. J., et al. (1990) Frequent inactivation of the retinoblastoma anti-oncogene is restricted to a subset of human tumor cells. *Proc. Natl. Acad. Sci.USA* **87**:2775–2779.

144. Reissmann, P. T., Koga, H., Takahashi, R., Figlin, R. A., Holmes, E. C., Piantadosi, S., et al. (1993) Inactivation of the retinoblastoma susceptibility gene in non-small-cell lung cancer. The Lung Cancer Study Group. *Oncogene* **8**:1913–1919.

145. Cagle, P. T., El-Naggar, A. K., Xu, H.-J., Hu, S.-X., and Benedict, W. F. (1997) Differential retinoblastoma protein expression in neuroendocrine tumors of the lung. Potential diagnostic implications. *Am. J. Pathol.* **150**:393–400.

146. Dosaka-Akita, H., Hu, S.-X., Fujino, M., Harada, M., Kinoshita, I., Xu, H.-J., et al. (1997) Altered retinoblastoma protein expression in nonsmall cell lung cancer: its synergistic effects with altered ras and p53 protein status on prognosis. *Cancer* **79**:1329–1337.

147. Mori, N., Yokota, J., Akiyama, T., Sameshima, Y., Okamoto, A., Mizoguchi, H., et al. (1990) Variable mutations of the RB gene in small-cell lung carcinoma. *Oncogene* **5**:1713–1717.

148. Kaye, F. J., Kratzke, R. A., Gerster, J. L., and Horowitz, J. M. (1990) A single amino acid substitution results in a retinoblastoma protein defective in phosphorylation and oncoprotein binding. *Proc. Natl. Acad. Sci. USA* **87**:6922–6926.

149. Xu, H. J., Quinlan, D. C., Davidson, A. G., Hu, S. X., Summers, C. L., Li, J., et al. (1994) Altered retinoblastoma protein expression and prognosis in early-stage non-small-cell lung carcinoma. *J. Natl. Cancer Inst.* **86**:695–699.

150. Shimizu, E., Coxon, A., Otterson, G. A., Steinberg, S. M., Kratzke, R. A., Kim, Y. W., et al. (1994) RB protein status and clinical correlation from 171 cell lines representing lung cancer, extrapulmonary small cell carcinoma, and mesothelioma. *Oncogene* **9**:2441–2448.

151. Kratzke, R. A., Greatens, T. M., Rubins, J. B., Maddaus, M. A., Niewoehner, D. E., Niehans, G. A., et al. (1996) Rb and p16INK4a expression in resected non-small cell lung tumors. *Cancer Res.* **56**:3415–3420.

152. Tamura, K., Zhang, X., Murakami, Y., Hirohashi, S., Xu, H. J., Hu, S. X., et al. (1997) Deletion of three distinct regions on chromosome 13q in human non-small-cell lung cancer. *Int. J. Cancer* **74**:45–49.

153. Sanders, B. M., Jay, M., Draper, G. J., and Roberts, E. M. (1989) Non-ocular cancer in relatives of retinoblastoma patients. *Br. J. Cancer* **60**:358–365.

154. Ookawa, K., Shiseki, M., Takahashi, R., Yoshida, Y., Terada, M., and Yokota, J. (1993) Reconstitution of the RB gene suppresses the growth of small-cell lung carcinoma cells carrying multiple genetic alterations. *Oncogene* **8**:2175–2181.

155. Baldi, A., Esposito, V., Deluca, A., Howard, C. M., Mazzarella, G., Baldi, F., et al. (1996) Differential expression of the retinoblastoma gene family members pRb/p105, p107, and pRb2/p130 in lung cancer. *Clin. Cancer Res.* **2**:1239–1245.

156. Helin, K., Holm, K., Niebuhr, A., Eiberg, H., Tommerup, N., Hougaard, S., et al. (1997) Loss of the retinoblastoma protein-related p130 protein in small cell lung carcinoma. *Proc. Natl. Acad. Sci. USA* **94**:6933–6938.

157. Schauer, I. E., Siriwardana, S., Langan, T. A., and Sclafani, R. A. (1994) Cyclin D1 overexpression vs. retinoblastoma inactivation: implications for growth control evasion in non-small cell and small cell lung cancer. *Proc. Natl. Acad. Sci. USA* **91**:7827–7831.

158. Betticher, D. C., Heighway, J., Hasleton, P. S., Altermatt, H. J., Ryder, W. D., Cerny, T., and Thatcher, N. (1996) Prognostic significance of CCND1 (cyclin D1) overexpression in primary resected non-small-cell lung cancer. *Br. J. Cancer* **73**:294–300.

159. Caputi, M., De Luca, L., Papaccio, G., D'Aponte, A., Cavallotti, I., Scala, P., et al. (1997) Prognostic role of cyclin D1 in non small cell lung cancer: an immunohistochemical analysis. *Eur. J. Histochem.* **41**:133–138.

160. Mate, J. L., Ariza, A., Aracil, C., Lopez, D., Isamat, M., Perez Piteira, J., et al. (1996) Cyclin D1 overexpression in non-small cell lung carcinoma: correlation with Ki67 labelling index and poor cytoplasmic differentiation. *J. Pathol.* **180**:395–399.

161. Betticher, D. C., Heighway, J., Thatcher, N., and Hasleton, P. S. (1997) Abnormal expression of CCND1 and RB1 in resection margin epithelia of lung cancer patients. *Br. J. Cancer* **75**:1761–1768.

162. Reifenberger, G., Ichimura, K., Reifenberger, J., Elkahloun, A. G., Meltzer, P. S., and Collins, V. P. (1996) Refined mapping of 12q13-q15 amplicons in human malignant gliomas suggests CDK4/SAS and MDM2 as independent amplification targets. *Cancer Res.* **56**:5141–5145.

163. Merlo, A., Gabrielson, E., Askin, F., and Sidransky, D. (1994) Frequent loss of chromosome 9 in human primary non-small cell lung cancer. *Cancer Res.* **54**:640–642.

164. Kishimoto, Y., Sugio, K., Mitsudomi, T., Oyama, T., Virmani, A. K., McIntire, D. D., et al. (1995) Frequent loss of the short arm of chromosome 9 in resected non-small-cell lung cancers from Japanese patients and its association with squamous cell carcinoma. *J. Cancer Res. Clin. Oncol.* **121**:291–296.

165. Neville, E. M., Stewart, M., Myskow, M., Donnelly, R. J., and Field, J. K. (1995) Loss of heterozygosity at 9p23 defines a novel locus in non-small cell lung cancer. *Oncogene* **11**:581–585.

166. Kim, S. K., Ro, J. Y., Kemp, B. L., Lee, J. S., Kwon, T. J., Fong, K. M., et al. (1997) Identification of three distinct tumor suppressor loci on the short arm of chromosome 9 in small cell lung cancer. *Cancer Res.* **57**:400–403.

167. Pollock, P. M., Pearson, J. V., and Hayward, N. K. (1996) Compilation of somatic mutations of the CDKN2 gene in human cancers: non-random distribution of base substitutions. *Genes Chromosomes Cancer* **15**:77–88.

168. Hayashi, N., Sugimoto, Y., Tsuchiya, E., Ogawa, M., and Nakamura, Y. (1994) Somatic mutations of the MTS (multiple tumor suppressor) 1/CDK4I (cyclin-dependent kinase-4 inhibitor) gene in human primary non-small cell lung carcinomas. *Biochem. Biophys. Res. Commun.* **202**:1426–1430.

169. de Vos, S., Miller, C. W., Takeuchi, S., Gombart, A. F., Cho, S. K., and Koeffler, H. P. (1995) Alterations of CDKN2 (p16) in non-small cell lung cancer. *Genes Chromosomes Cancer* **14**:164–170.

170. Xiao, S., Li, D., Corson, J. M., Vijg, J., and Fletcher, J. A. (1995) Codeletion of p15 and p16 genes in primary non-small cell lung carcinoma. *Cancer Res.* **55**:2968–2971.

171. Washimi, O., Nagatake, M., Osada, H., Ueda, R., Koshikawa, T., Seki, T., et al. (1995) In vivo occurrence of p16 (MTS1) and p15 (MTS2) alterations preferentially in non-small cell lung cancers. *Cancer Res.* **55**:514–517.

172. Shimizu, T. and Sekiya, T. (1995) Loss of heterozygosity at 9p21 loci and mutations of the MTS1 and MTS2 genes in human lung cancers. *Int. J. Cancer* **63**:616–620.

173. Rusin, M. R., Okamoto, A., Chorazy, M., Czyzewski, K., Harasim, J., Spillare, E. A., et al. (1996) Intragenic mutations of the p16(INK4), p15(INK4B) and p18 genes in primary non-small-cell lung cancers. *Int. J. Cancer* **65**:734–739.

174. Takeshima, Y., Nishisaka, T., Kawano, R., Kishizuchi, K., Fujii, S., Kitaguchi, S., et al. (1996) p16/CDKN2 gene and p53 gene alterations in Japanese non-smoking female lung adenocarcinoma. *Jpn. J. Cancer Res.* **87**:134–140.

175. Marchetti, A., Buttitta, F., Pellegrini, S., Bertacca, G., Chella, A., Carnicelli, V., et al. (1997) Alterations of P16 (MTS1) in node-positive non-small cell lung carcinomas. *J. Pathol.* **181**:178–182.

176. Wiest, J. S., Franklin, W. A., Otstot, J. T., Forbey, K., Varella-Garcia, M., Rao, K., et al. (1997) Identification of a novel region of homozygous deletion on chromosome 9p in squamous cell carcinoma of the lung: the location of a putative tumor suppressor gene. *Cancer Res.* **57**:1–6.

177. Merlo, A., Herman, J. G., Mao, L., Lee, D. J., Gabrielson, E., Burger, P. C., et al. (1995) 5'CpG island methylation is associated with transcriptional silencing of the tumour suppressor p16/CDKN2/MTS1 in human cancers. *Nature Med.* **1**:686–692.

178. Otterson, G. A., Khleif, S. N., Chen, W., Coxon, A. B., and Kaye, F. J. (1995) CDKN2 gene silencing in lung cancer by DNA hypermethylation and kinetics of p16^{INK4} protein induction by 5-aza 2'deoxycytidine. *Oncogene* **11**:1211–1216.

179. Shapiro, G. I., Edwards, C. D., Kobzik, L., Godleski, J., Richards, W., Sugarbaker, D. J., et al. (1995) Reciprocal Rb inactivation and p16INK4 expression in primary lung cancers and cell lines. *Cancer Res.* **55**:505–509.

180. Okamoto, A., Hussain, S. P., Hagiwara, K., Spillare, E. A., Rusin, M. R., Demetrick, D. J., et al. (1995) Mutations in the $^{p16INK4/MTS1/}$^{CDKN2}, p15$^{INK4B/MTS2}$, and p18 genes in primary and metastatic lung cancer. *Cancer Res.* **55**:1448–1451.

181. Kinoshita, I., Dosaka-Akita, H., Mishina, T., Akie, K., Nishi, M., Hiroumi, H., et al. (1996) Altered p16INK4 and retinoblastoma protein status in non-small cell lung cancer: Potential synergistic effect with altered p53 protein on proliferative activity. *Cancer Res.* **56**:5557–5562.

182. Taga, S., Osaki, T., Ohgami, A., Imoto, H., Yoshimatsu, T., Yoshino, I., et al. (1997) Prognostic value of the immunohistochemical detection of p16^{INK4} expression in nonsmall cell lung carcinoma. *Cancer* **80**:389–395.

183. Okamoto, A., Demetrick, D. J., Spillare, E. A., Hagiwara, K., Hussain, S. P., Bennett, W. P., et al. (1994) Mutations and altered expression of p16(ink4) in human cancer. *Proc. Natl. Acad. Sci. USA* **91**:11,045–11,049.

184. Otterson, G. A., Kratzke, R. A., Coxon, A., Kim, Y. W., and Kaye, F. J. (1994) Absence of p16INK4 protein is restricted to the subset of lung cancer lines that retains wildtype RB. *Oncogene* **9**:3375–3378.

185. Nakagawa, K., Conrad, N. K., Williams, J. P., Johnson, B. E., and Kelley, M. J. (1995) Mechanism of inactivation of CDKN2 and MTS2 in non-small cell lung cancer and association with advanced stage. *Oncogene* **11**:1843–1851.

186. Kelley, M. J., Nakagawa, K., Steinberg, S. M., Mulshine, J. L., Kamb, A., and Johnson, B. E. (1995) Differential inactivation of CDKN2 and Rb protein in non-small-cell and small-cell lung cancer cell lines. *J. Natl. Cancer Inst.* **87**:756–761.

187. Sakaguchi, M., Fujii, Y., Hirabayashi, H., Yoon, H. E., Komoto, Y., Oue, T., et al. (1996). Inversely correlated expression of p16 and Rb protein in non-small cell lung cancers: an immunohistochemical study. *Int. J. Cancer* **65**:442–445.

187a. Geradts J. Fong KM. Zimmermann PV. Maynard R. Minna JD. (1999). Correlation of abnormal RB, p16ink4a, and p53 expression

with 3p loss of heterozygosity, other genetic abnormalities, and clinical features in 103 primary non-small cell lung cancers. *Clin Cancer Res.* **5(4)**:791–800

188. Quelle, D. E., Zindy, F., Ashmun, R. A., and Sherr, C. J. (1995) Alternative reading frames of the INK4a tumor suppressor gene encode two unrelated proteins capable of inducing cell cycle arrest. *Cell* **83**:993–1000.

189. Kamijo, T., Zindy, F., Roussel, M. F., Quelle, D. E., Downing, J. R., Ashmun, R. A., et al. (1997) Tumor suppression at the mouse INK4a locus mediated by the alternative reading frame product p19^{ARF}. *Cell* **91**:649–659.

190. Hannon, G. J. and Beach, D. (1994) p15^{INK4B} is a potential effector of TGF-beta-induced cell cycle arrest. *Nature* **371**:257–261.

191. Miller, C. W., Yeon, C., Aslo, A., Mendoza, S., Aytac, U., and Koeffler, H. P. (1997) The p19(ink4d) cyclin dependent kinase inhibitor gene is altered in osteosarcoma. *Oncogene* **15**:231–235.

192. Kawamata, N., Morosetti, R., Miller, C. W., Park, D., Spirin, K. S., Nakamaki, T., et al. (1995) Molecular analysis of the cyclin-dependent kinase inhibitor gene p27/Kip1 in human malignancies. *Cancer Res.* **55**:2266 2269.

193. Esposito, V., Baldi, A., De Luca, A., Micheli, P., Mazzarella, G., Baldi, F., et al. (1997) Prognostic value of p53 in non-small cell lung cancer: relationship with proliferating cell nuclear antigen and cigarette smoking. *Human Pathol.* **28**:233–237.

194. Kondo, M., Matsuoka, S., Uchida, K., Osada, H., Nagatake, M., Takagi, K., et al. (1996) Selective maternal-allele loss in human lung cancers of the maternally expressed p57^{KIP2} gene at 11p15.5. *Oncogene* **12**:1365–1368.

195. Naylor, S. L., Johnson, B. E., Minna, J. D., and Sakaguchi, A. Y. (1987) Loss of heterozygosity of chromosome 3p markers in small-cell lung cancer. *Nature* **329**:451–454.

196. Kok, K., Osinga, J., Carritt, B., Davis, M. B., van der Hout, A. H., van der Veen, A. Y., et al. (1987) Deletion of a DNA sequence at the chromosomal region 3p21 in all major types of lung cancer. *Nature* **330**:578–581.

197. Hibi, K., Takahashi, T., Yamakawa, K., Ueda, R., Sekido, Y., Ariyoshi, Y., et al. (1992) Three distinct regions involved in 3p deletion in human lung cancer. *Oncogene* **7**:445–449.

198. Drabkin, H. A., Mendez, M. J., Rabbitts, P. H., Varkony, T., Bergh, J., Schlessinger, J., et al. (1992) Characterization of the submicroscopic deletion in the small-cell lung carcinoma (SCLC) cell line U2020. *Genes Chromosomes Cancer* **5**:67–74.

199. Latif, F., Tory, K., Modi, W. S., Graziano, S. L., Gamble, G., Douglas, J., et al. (1992) Molecular characterization of a large homozygous deletion in the small cell lung cancer cell line U2020: A strategy for cloning the putative tumor suppressor gene. *Genes Chromosomes Cancer* **5**:119–127.

200. Sozzi, G., Veronese, M. L., Negrini, M., Baffa, R., Cotticelli, M. G., Inoue, H., et al. (1996) The FHIT gene 3p14.2 is abnormal in lung cancer. *Cell* **85**:17–26.

201. Fong, K. M., Biesterveld, E. J., Virmani, A., Wistuba, I., Sekido, Y., Bader, S. A., et al. (1997) FHIT and FRA3B 3p14.2 allele loss are common in lung cancer and preneoplastic bronchial lesions and are associated with cancer-related FHIT cDNA splicing aberrations. *Cancer Res.* **57**:2256–2267.

202. Yanagisawa, K., Kondo, M., Osada, H., Uchida, K., Takagi, K., Masuda, A., et al. (1996) Molecular analysis of the FHIT gene at 3p14.2 in lung cancer cell lines. *Cancer Res.* **56**:5579–5582.

203. Sozzi, G., Tornielli, S., Tagliabue, E., Sard, L., Pezzella, F., Pastorino, U., et al. (1997) Absense of Fhit protein in primary lung tumors and cell lines with FHIT gene abnormalities. *Cancer Res.* **57**:5207–5212.

204. Siprashvili, Z., Sozzi, G., Barnes, L. D., McCune, P., Robinson, A. K., Eryomin, V., et al. (1997) Replacement of Fhit in cancer cells suppresses tumorigenicity. *Proc. Natl. Acad. Sci. USA* **94**:13,771–13,776.

205. Sozzi, G., Sard, L., De Gregorio, L., Marchetti, A., Musso, K., Buttitta, F., et al. (1997) Association between cigarette smoking and FHIT gene alterations in lung cancer. *Cancer Res.* **57**:2121–2123.

206. Daly, M. C., Xiang, R.-H., Buchhagen, D., Hensel, C. H., Garcia, D. K., Killary, A. M., et al. (1993) A homozygous deletion on chromosome 3 in a small cell lung cancer cell line correlates with a region of tumor suppressor activity. *Oncogene* **8**:1721–1729.

207. Kok, K., van den Berg, A., Veldhuis, P. M. J. F., van der Veen, A. Y., Franke, M., Schoenmakers, E. F. P. M., et al. (1994) A homozygous deletion in a small cell lung cancer cell line involving a 3p21 region with a marked instability in yeast artificial chromosomes. *Cancer Res.* **54**:4183–4187.

208. Wei, M. H., Latif, F., Bader, S., Kashuba, V., Chen, J. Y., Duh, F. M., et al. (1996) Construction of a 600-kilobase cosmid clone contig and generation of a transcriptional map surrounding the lung cancer tumor suppressor gene (TSG) locus on human chromosome 3p21.3: Progress toward the isolation of a lung cancer TSG. *Cancer Res.* **56**:1487–1492.

208a. Lerman, M. and Minna, J. (2000)The 630-kb lung cancer homozygous deletion region on human chromosome 3p21.3: identification and evaluation of the resident candidate tumor suppressor genes. The International Lung Cancer Chromosome 3p21.3 Tumor Suppressor Gene Consortium, *Cancer Res.* **60**:6116–6133.

208b. Dammann, R., Li C., Yoon, J. H., Chin, P. L., Bates, S., and Pfeifer, G. P. (200). Epigenetic in activation of a RAS association domain family protein from the lung tumour suppressor locus 2p21.3, *Nat Genet.* **25**:315–319

208c. Burbee, D., Forgacs, E., Zöchbauer-Müller, S., Shivakuma, L., Fong, K., Gao, B., et al. RASSF1A in th e 3p21.3 homozygous deletion region: epigenetic inactivation in lung and breast cancer, *Cancer Res.* **61**

209. Yamakawa, K., Takahashi, T., Horio, Y., Murata, Y., Takahashi, E., Hibi, K., et al. (1993) Frequent homozygous deletions in lung cancer cell lines detected by a DNA marker located at 3p21.3-p22. *Oncogene* **8**:327–330.

210. Papadopoulos, N., Nicolaides, N. C., Wei, Y. F., Ruben, S. M., Carter, K. C., Rosen, C. A., et al. (1994) Mutation of a mutL homolog in hereditary colon cancer. *Science* **263**:1625–1629.

211. Sekido, Y., Bader, S., Latif, F., Gnarra, J. R., Gazdar, A. F., Linehan, W. M., et al. (1994) Molecular analysis of the von Hippel-Lindau disease tumor suppressor gene in human lung cancer cell lines. *Oncogene* **9**:1599–1604.

212. Gebert, J. F., Moghal, N., Frangioni, J. V., Sugarbaker, D. J., and Neel, B. G. (1991). High frequency of retinoic acid receptor beta abnormalities in human lung cancer. *Oncogene* **6**:1859–1868.

213. Nervi, C., Vollberg, T. M., George, M. D., Zelent, A., Chambon, P., and Jetten, A. M. (1991) Expression of nuclear retinoic acid receptors in normal tracheobronchial cells and in lung carcinoma cells. *Exp. Cell Res.* **195**:163–170.

214. Geradts, J., Chen, J. Y., Russell, E. K., Yankaskas, J. R., Nieves, L., and Minna, J. D. (1993) Human lung cancer cell lines exhibit resistance to retinoic acid treatment. *Cell Growth Diff.* **4**:799–809.

215. Zhang, X. K., Liu, Y., Lee, M. O., and Pfahl, M. (1994) A specific defect in the retinoic acid response associated with human lung cancer cell lines. *Cancer Res.* **54**:5663–5669.

216. Moghal, N. and Neel, B. G. (1995) Evidence for impaired retinoic acid receptor-thyroid hormone receptor AF-2 cofactor activity in human lung cancer. *Mol. Cell. Biol.* **15**:3945–3959.

217. Houle, B., Leduc, F., and Bradley, W. E. (1991) Implication of RARβ in epidermoid (Squamous) lung cancer. *Genes Chromosomes Cancer* **3**:358–366.

218. D'Amico, D., Carbone, D. P., Johnson, B. E., Meltzer, S. J., and Minna, J. D. (1992) Polymorphic sites within the MCC and APC loci reveal very frequent loss of heterozygosity in human small cell lung cancer. *Cancer Res.* **52**:1996–1999.

219. Ohata, H., Emi, M., Fujiwara, Y., Higashino, K., Nakagawa, K., Futagami, R., et al. (1993) Deletion mapping of the short arm of chromosome 8 in non-small cell lung carcinoma. *Genes Chromosomes Cancer* **7**:85–88.

220. Sato, S., Nakamura, Y., and Tsuchiya, E. (1994) Difference of allelotype between squamous cell carcinoma and adenocarcinoma of the lung. *Cancer Res.* **54**:5652–5655.

221. Shiseki, M., Kohno, T., Nishikawa, R., Sameshima, Y., Mizoguchi, H., and Yokota, J. (1994) Frequent allelic losses on chromosomes 2q, 18q, and 22q in advanced non-small cell lung carcinoma. *Cancer Res.* **54**:5643–5648.

222. Bepler, G. and Garcia-Blanco, M. A. (1994) Three tumor-suppressor regions on chromosome 11p identified by high-resolution deletion mapping in human non-small-cell lung cancer. *Proc. Natl. Acad. Sci. USA* **91**:5513–5517.

223. Iizuka, M., Sugiyama, Y., Shiraishi, M., Jones, C., and Sekiya, T. (1995) Allelic losses in human chromosome 11 in lung cancers. *Genes Chromosomes Cancer* **13**:40–46.

224. Otsuka, T., Kohno, T., Mori, M., Noguchi, M., Hirohashi, S., and Yokota, J. (1996) Deletion mapping of chromosome 2 in human lung carcinoma. *Genes Chromosomes Cancer* **16**:113–119.

225. O'Briant, K. C. and Bepler, G. (1997) Delineation of the centromeric and telomeric chromosome segment 11p15.5 lung cancer suppressor regions LOH11A and LOH11B. *Genes Chromosomes Cancer* **18**:111–114.

226. Sekido, Y., Pass, H. I., Bader, S., Mew, D. J., Christman, M. F., Gazdar, A. F., et al. (1995) Neurofibromatosis type 2 (NF2) gene is somatically mutated in mesothelioma but not in lung cancer. *Cancer Res.* **55**:1227–1231.

227. Cooper, C. A., Bubb, V. J., Smithson, N., Carter, R. L., Gledhill, S., Lamb, D., et al. (1996) Loss of heterozygosity at 5q21 in non-small cell lung cancer: a frequent event but without evidence of apc mutation. *J. Pathol.* **180**:33–37.

228. Hosoe, S., Shigedo, Y., Ueno, K., Tachibana, I., Osaki, T., Tanio, Y., et al. (1994) Detailed deletion mapping of the short arm of chromosome 3 in small cell and non-small cell carcinoma of the lung. *Lung Cancer* **10**:297–305.

229. Wieland, I., Böhm, M., and Bogatz, S. (1992) Isolation of DNA sequences deleted in lung cancer by genomic difference cloning. *Proc. Natl. Acad. Sci. USA* **89**:9705–9709.

230. Wieland, I., Bohm, M., Arden, K. C., Ammermuller, T., Bogatz, S., Viars, C. S., et al. (1996) Allelic deletion mapping on chromosome 5 in human carcinomas. *Oncogene* **12**:97–102.

231. Bepler, G. and Koehler, A. (1995) Multiple chromosomal aberrations and 11p allelotyping in lung cancer cell lines. *Cancer Genet. Cytogenet.* **84**:39–45.

232. Ludwig, C. U., Raefle, G., Dalquen, P., Stulz, P., Stahel, R., and Obrecht, J. P. (1991) Allelic loss on the short arm of chromosome 11 in non-small-cell lung cancer. *Int. J. Cancer* **49**:661–665.

233. Fong, K. M., Zimmerman, P. V., and Smith, P. J. (1994) Correlation of loss of heterozygosity at 11p with tumour progression and survival in non-small cell lung cancer. *Genes Chromosomes Cancer* **10**:183–189.

234. Kohno, T., Morishita, K., Takano, H., Shapiro, D. N., and Yokota, J. (1994) Homozygous deletion at chromosome 2q33 in human small-cell lung carcinoma identified by arbitrarily primed PCR genomic fingerprinting. *Oncogene* **9**:103–108.

235. Li, J., Yen, C., Liaw, D., Podsypanina, K., Bose, S., Wang, S. I., et al. (1997) PTEN, a putative protein tyrosine phosphatase gene mutated in human brain, breast, and prostate cancer. *Science* **275**:1943–1947.

236. Markowitz, S. D. and Roberts, A. B. (1996) Tumor suppressor activity of the TGF-beta pathway in human cancers. *Cytokine Growth Factor Rev.* **7**:93–102.

237. Gerwin, B. I., Spillare, E., Forrester, K., Lehman, T. A., Kispert, J., Welsh, J. A., et al. (1992) Mutant p53 can induce tumorigenic conversion of human bronchial epithelial cells and reduce their responsiveness to a negative growth factor, transforming growth factor beta 1. *Proc. Natl. Acad. Sci. USA* **89**:2759–2763.

238. Heldin, C. H., Miyazono, K., and ten Dijke, P. (1997) TGF-beta signalling from cell membrane to nucleus through SMAD proteins. *Nature* **390**:465–471.

239. Nørgaard, P., Spang-Thomsen, M., and Poulsen, H. S. (1996) Expression and autoregulation of transforming growth factor beta receptor mRNA in small-cell lung cancer cell lines. *Br. J. Cancer* **73**:1037–1043.

403

240. Tani, M., Takenoshita, S., Kohno, T., Hagiwara, K., Nagamachi, Y., Harris, C. C., et al. (1997) Infrequent mutations of the transforming growth factor beta-type II receptor gene at chromosome 3p22 in human lung cancers with chromosome 3p deletions. *Carcinogenesis* **18**:1119–1121.

241. Takenoshita, S., Hagiwara, K., Gemma, A., Nagashima, M., Ryberg, D., Lindstedt, B. A., et al. (1997) Absence of mutations in the transforming growth factor-beta type II receptor in sporadic lung cancers with microsatellite instability and rare H-ras1 alleles. *Carcinogenesis* **18**:1427–1429.

242. Merlo, A., Gabrielson, E., Mabry, M., Vollmer, R., Baylin, S. B., and Sidransky, D. (1994) Homozygous deletion on chromosome 9p and loss of heterozygosity on 9q, 6p, and 6q in primary human small cell lung cancer. *Cancer Res.* **54**:232–2326.

243. Riggins, G. J., Kinzler, K. W., Vogelstein, B., and Thiagalingam, S. (1997) Frequency of Smad gene mutations in human cancers. *Cancer Res.* **57**:2578–2580.

244. Uchida, K., Nagatake, M., Osada, H., Yatabe, Y., Kondo, M., Mitsudomi, T., et al. (1996) Somatic in vivo alterations of the JV18-1 gene at 18q21 in human lung cancers. *Cancer Res.* **56**:5583–5585.

245. Nagatake, M., Takagi, Y., Osada, H., Uchida, K., Mitsudomi, T., Saji, S., et al. (1996) Somatic in vivo alterations of the DPC4 gene at 18q21 in human lung cancers. *Cancer Res.* **56**:2718–2720.

246. Hayashi, H., Abdollah, S., Qiu, Y., Cai, J., Xu, Y.-Y., Grinnell, B. W., et al. (1997) The MAD-related protein Smad7 associates with the TGFbeta receptor and functions as an antagonist of TGFbeta signaling. *Cell* **89**:1165–1173.

247. Sundaresan, V., Ganly, P., Hasleton, P., Rudd, R., Sinha, G., Bleehen, N. M., et al. (1992) p53 and chromosome 3 abnormalities, characteristic of malignant lung tumours, are detectable in preinvasive lesions of the bronchus. *Oncogene* **7**:1989–1997.

248. Nuorva, K., Soini, Y., Kamel, D., Autio-Harmainen, H., Risteli, L., Risteli, J., et al. (1993) Concurrent p53 expression in bronchial dysplasias and squamous cell lung carcinomas. *Am. J. Pathol.* **142**:725–732.

249. Bennett, W. P., Colby, T. V., Travis, W. D., Borkowski, A., Jones, R. T., Lane, D. P., et al. (1993) p53 protein accumulates frequently in early bronchial neoplasia. *Cancer Res.* **53**:4817–4822.

250. Hirano, T., Franzén, B., Kato, H., Ebihara, Y., and Auer, G. (1994) Genesis of squamous cell lung carcinoma. Sequential changes of proliferation, DNA ploidy, and p53 expression. *Am. J. Pathol.* **144**:296–302.

251. Satoh, Y., Ishikawa, Y., Nakagawa, K., Hirano, T., and Tsuchiya, E. (1997) A follow-up study of progression from dysplasia to squamous cell carcinoma with immunohistochemical examination of p53 protein overexpression in the bronchi of ex-chromate workers. *Br. J. Cancer* **75**:678–683.

252. Li, Z. H., Zheng, J., Weiss, L. M., and Shibata, D. (1994) c-k-ras and p53 mutations occur very early in adenocarcinoma of the lung. *Am. J. Pathol.* **144**:303–309.

253. Chung, G. T. Y., Sundaresan, V., Hasleton, P., Rudd, R., Taylor, R., and Rabbitts, P. H. (1995) Sequential molecular genetic changes in lung cancer development. *Oncogene* **11**:2591–2598.

254. Hung, J., Kishimoto, Y., Sugio, K., Virmani, A., McIntire, D. D., Minna, J. D., et al. (1995) Allele-specific chromosome 3p deletions occur at an early stage in the pathogenesis of lung carcinoma. *JAMA* **273**:558–563.

255. Kishimoto, Y., Sugio, K., Hung, J. Y., Virmani, A. K., McIntire, D. D., Minna, J. D., et al. (1995) Allele-specific loss in chromosome 9p loci in preneoplastic lesions accompanying non-small-cell lung cancers. *J. Natl. Cancer Inst.* **87**:1224–1229.

256. Sugio, K., Kishimoto, Y., Virmani, A. K., Hung, J. Y., and Gazdar, A. F. (1994) K-ras mutations are a relatively late event in the pathogenesis of lung carcinomas. *Cancer Res.* **54**:5811–5815.

257. Westra, W. H., Baas, I. O., Hruban, R. H., Askin, F. B., Wilson, K., Offerhaus, G. J., et al. (1996) K-ras oncogene activation in atypical alveolar hyperplasias of the human lung. *Cancer Res.* **56**:2224–2228.

258. Slaughter, D. P., Southwick, H. W., and Smejkal, W. (1953) "Field cancerization" in oral stratified squamous epithelium: clinical implications of multicentric origin. *Cancer* **6**:963–968.

259. Franklin, W. A., Gazdar, A. F., Haney, J., Wistuba, I. I., La Rosa, F. G., Kennedy, T., et al. (1997) Widely dispersed p53 mutation in respiratory epithelium. *J. Clin. Invest.* **100**:2133–2137.

260. Peltomäki, P., Lothe, R. A., Aaltonen, L. A., Pylkkänen, L., Nyström-Lahti, M., Seruca, R., et al. (1993) Microsatellite instability is associated with tumors that characterize the hereditary nonpolyposis colorectal carcinoma syndrome. *Cancer Res.* **53**:5853–5855.

261. Ryberg, D., Lindstedt, B. A., Zienolddiny, S., and Haugen, A. (1995) A hereditary genetic marker closely associated with microsatellite instability in lung cancer. *Cancer Res.* **55**:3996–3999.

262. Mao, L., Lee, D. J., Tockman, M. S., Erozan, Y. S., Askin, F., and Sidransky, D. (1994) Microsatellite alterations as clonal markers for the detection of human cancer. *Proc. Natl. Acad. Sci. USA* **91**:9871–9875.

263. Merlo, A., Mabry, M., Gabrielson, E., Vollmer, R., Baylin, S. B., and Sidransky, D. (1994) Frequent microsatellite instability in primary small cell lung cancer. *Cancer Res.* **54**:209–2101.

264. Shridhar, V., Siegfried, J., Hunt, J., del Mar Alonso, M., and Smith, D. I. (1994) Genetic instability of microsatellite sequences in many non-small cell lung carcinomas. *Cancer Res.* **54**:2084–2087.

265. Fong, K. M., Zimmerman, P. V., and Smith, P. J. (1995) Microsatellite instability and other molecular abnormalities in non-small cell lung cancer. *Cancer Res.* **55**:28–30.

266. Adachi, J., Shiseki, M., Okazaki, T., Ishimaru, G., Noguchi, M., Hirohashi, S., et al. (1995) Microsatellite instability in primary and metastatic lung carcinomas. *Genes Chromosomes Cancer* **14**:301–306.

267. Chen, X. Q., Stroun, M., Magnenat, J. L., Nicod, L. P., Kurt, A. M., Lyautey, J., et al. (1996) Microsatellite alterations in plasma DNA of small cell lung cancer patients. *Nature Med.* **2**:1033–1035.

268. Hurr, K., Kemp, B., Silver, S. A., and El-Naggar, A. K. (1996) Microsatellite alteration at chromosome 3p loci in neuroendocrine and non-neuroendocrine lung tumors. Histogenetic and clinical relevance. *Am. J. Pathol.* **149**:613–620.

269. Rosell, R., Pifarré, A., Monzó, M., Astudillo, J., López-Cabrerizo, M. P., Calvo, R., et al. (1997) Reduced survival in patients with stage-I non-small-cell lung cancer associated with DNA-replication errors. *Int. J. Cancer* **74**:330–334.

270. Sekine, I., Yokose, T., Ogura, T., Suzuki, K., Nagai, K., Kodama, T., et al. (1997) Microsatellite instability in lung cancer patients 40 years of age or younger. *Jpn. J. Cancer Res.* **88**:559–563.

271. Miozzo, M., Sozzi, G., Musso, K., Pilotti, S., Incarbone, M., Pastorino, U., et al. (1996). Microsatellite alterations in bronchial and sputum specimens of lung cancer patients. *Cancer Res.* **56**:2285–2288.

272. Lindstedt, B.-A., Ryberg, D., and Haugen, A. (1997) Rare alleles at different VNTR loci among lung-cancer patients with microsatellite instability in tumours. *Int. J. Cancer* **70**:412–415.

273. Chuang, L. S.-H., Ian, H.-I., Koh, T.-W., Ng, H.-H., Xu, G., and Li, B. F. L. (1997) Human DNA-(cytosine-5)methyltransferase PCNA complex as a target for p21(WAF1). *Science* **277**:1996–2000.

274. Herman, J. G., Latif, F., Weng, Y., Lerman, M. I., Zbar, B., Liu, S., et al. (1994) Silencing of the VHL tumor-suppressor gene by DNA methylation in renal carcinoma. *Proc. Natl. Acad. Sci. USA* **91**:9700–9704.

275. Ohtani-Fujita, N., Dryja, T. P., Rapaport, J. M., Fujita, T., Matsumura, S., Ozasa, K., et al. (1997) Hypermethylation in the retinoblastoma gene is associated with unilateral, sporadic retinoblastoma. *Cancer Genet. Cytogenet.* **98**:43–49.

276. Sakai, T., Toguchida, J., Ohtani, N., Yandell, D. W., Rapaport, J. M., and Dryja, T. P. (1991) Allele-specific hypermethylation of the retinoblastoma tumor-suppressor gene. *Am. J. Human Genet.* **48**:880–888.

277. Makos, M., Nelkin, B. D., Lerman, M. I., Latif, F., Zbar, B., and Baylin, S. B. (1992) Distinct hypermethylation patterns occur at altered chromosome loci in human lung and colon cancer. *Proc. Natl. Acad. Sci. USA* **89**:1929–1933.

278. Schroeder, M. and Mass, M. J. (1997) CpG methylation inactivates the transcriptional activity of the promoter of the human p53 tumor suppressor gene. *Biochem. Biophys. Res. Commun.* **235**:403–406.

278a. Zöchbauer-Müller, S., Fong, K. M., Maitra, A., Lam, S., Geradts, J., Ashfaq, R., et al. 5'CpG Island methylation of the FHIT gene os correlated with loss of gene expression in lung and breast cancer, *Cancer Res.* **61** in Press.

278b. Zochbauer-Muller, S., Fong, K. M., Virmani, A. K., Geradts, J., Gazdar, A. F., and Minna, J. D. Aberrant promoter methylation of multiple genes in non-small cell lung cancers, *Cancer Res.* **61**: 249-55., 2001

279. Suzuki, H., Ueda, R., Takahashi, T., and Takahashi, T. (1994) Altered imprinting in lung cancer. *Nature Genet.* **6**:332–333.

280. Kondo, M., Suzuki, H., Ueda, R., Osada, H., Takagi, K., Takahashi, T., et al. (1995). Frequent loss of imprinting of the H19 gene is often associated with its overexpression in human lung cancers. *Oncogene* **10**:1193–1198.

281. Gazdar, A. F. and Minna, J. D. (1997) Cigarettes, sex, and lung adenocarcinoma. *J. Natl. Cancer Inst.* **89**:1563–1565.

282. Denissenko, M. F., Pao, A., Tang, M., and Pfeifer, G .P. (1996) Preferential formation of benzo[a]pyrene adducts at lung cancer mutational hotspots in p53. *Science* **274**:430–432.

283. Spivack, S. D., Fasco, M. J., Walker, V. E., and Kaminsky, L. S. (1997) The molecular epidemiology of lung cancer. *Crit. Rev. Toxicol.* **27**:319–365.

284. Wolf, C. R., Smith, C. A., and Forman, D. (1994) Metabolic polymorphisms in carcinogen metabolising enzymes and cancer susceptibility. *Br. Med. Bull.* **50**:718–731.

285. Hayes, J. D. and Pulford, D. J. (1995) The glutathione S-transferase supergene family: regulation of GST and the contribution of the isoenzymes to cancer chemoprotection and drug resistance. *Crit. Rev. Biochem. Mol. Biol.* **30**:445–600.

286. Nazar-Stewart, V., Motulsky, A. G., Eaton, D. L., White, E., Hornung, S. K., Leng, Z. T., et al. (1993) The glutathione S-transferase mu polymorphism as a marker for susceptibility to lung carcinoma. *Cancer Res.* **53**:2313–2318.

287. Hayashi, S., Watanabe, J., and Kawajiri, K. (1992) High susceptibility to lung cancer analyzed in terms of combined genotypes of P450IA1 and Mu-class glutathione S-transferase genes. *Jpn. J. Cancer Res.* **83**:866–870.

288. Brockmoller, J., Kerb, R., Drakoulis, N., Nitz, M., and Roots, I. (1993) Genotype and phenotype of glutathione S-transferase class mu isoenzymes mu and psi in lung cancer patients and controls. *Cancer Res.* **53**:1004–1011.

289. Nakajima, T., Elovaara, E., Anttila, S., Hirvonen, A., Camus, A. M., Hayes, J. D., et al. (1995) Expression and polymorphism of glutathione S-transferase in human lungs: risk factors in smoking-related lung cancer. *Carcinogenesis* **16**:707–711.

290. McWilliams, J. E., Sanderson, B. J., Harris, E. L., Richert Boe, K. E., and Henner, W. D. (1995) Glutathione S-transferase M1 (GSTM1) deficiency and lung cancer risk. *Cancer Epidemiol. Biomark. Prev.* **4**:589–594.

291. Anttila, S., Hirvonen, A., Vainio, H., Husgafvel Pursiainen, K., Hayes, J. D., and Ketterer, B. (1993) Immunohistochemical localization of glutathione S-transferases in human lung. *Cancer Res.* **53**:5643–5648.

292. Ryberg, D., Skaug, V., Hewer, A., Phillips, D. H., Harries, L. W., Wolf, C. R., et al. (1997) Genotypes of glutathione transferase M1 and P1 and their significance for lung DNA adduct levels and cancer risk. *Carcinogenesis* **18**:1285–1289.

293. Zimniak, P., Nanduri, B., Pikula, S., Bandorowicz Pikula, J., Singhal, S. S., Srivastava, S. K., et al. (1994) Naturally occurring human glutathione S-transferase GSTP1-1 isoforms with isoleucine and valine in position 104 differ in enzymic properties. *Eur. J. Biochem.* **224**:893–899.

294. Kawajiri, K., Nakachi, K., Imai, K., Yoshii, A., Shinoda, N., and Watanabe, J. (1990) Identification of genetically high risk individuals to lung cancer by DNA polymorphisms of the cytochrome P450IA1 gene. *FEBS Lett.* **263**:131–133.

295. Kawajiri, K., Nakachi, K., Imai, K., Watanabe, J., and Hayashi, S. (1993) The CYP1A1 gene and cancer susceptibility. *Crit. Rev. Oncol. Hematol.* **14**:77–87.

296. Hirvonen, A., Husgafvel-Pursiainen, K., Anttila, S., Karjalainen, A., Sorsa, M., and Vainio, H. (1992) Metabolic cytochrome P450 genotypes and assessment of individual susceptibility to lung cancer. *Pharmacogenet.* **2**:259–263.

297. Alexandrie, A. K., Sundberg, M. I., Seidegard, J., Tornling, G., and Rannug, A. (1994) Genetic susceptibility to lung cancer with special emphasis on CYP1A1 and GSTM1: a study on host factors in relation to age at onset, gender and histological cancer types. *Carcinogenesis* **15**:1785–1790.

298. Tefre, T., Daly, A. K., Armstrong, M., Leathart, J. B., Idle, J. R., Brogger, A., et al. (1994) Genotyping of the CYP2D6 gene in Norwegian lung cancer patients and controls. *Pharmacogenetics* **4**:47–57.

299. Xu, X., Kelsey, K. T., Wiencke, J. K., Wain, J. C., and Christiani, D. C. (1996) Cytochrome P450 CYP1A1 MspI polymorphism and lung cancer susceptibility. *Cancer Epidemiol. Biomark. Prev.* **5**:687–692.

300. Goto, I., Yoneda, S., Yamamoto, M., and Kawajiri, K. (1996) Prognostic significance of germ line polymorphisms of the CYP1A1 and glutathione S-transferase genes in patients with non-small cell lung cancer. *Cancer Res.* **56**:3725–3730.

301. Hayashi, S., Watanabe, J., Nakachi, K., and Kawajiri, K. (1991) Genetic linkage of lung cancer-associated MspI polymorphisms with amino acid replacement in the heme binding region of the human cytochrome P450IA1 gene. *J. Biochem.* **110**:407–411.

302. Persson, I., Johansson, I., and Ingelman Sundberg, M. (1997) In vitro kinetics of two human CYP1A1 variant enzymes suggested to be associated with interindividual differences in cancer susceptibility. *Biochem. Biophys. Res. Commun.* **231**:227–230.

303. Zhang, Z.-Y., Fasco, M. J., Huang, L., Guengerich, F. P., and Kaminsky, L. S. (1996) Characterization of purified human recombinant cytochrome P4501A1-Ile462 and -Val462: assessment of a role for the rare allele in carcinogenesis. *Cancer Res.* **56**:3926–3933.

304. Hamada, G. S., Sugimura, H., Suzuki, I., Nagura, K., Kiyokawa, E., Iwase, T., et al. (1995) The heme-binding region polymorphism of cytochrome P450IA1 (CypIA1), rather than the RsaI polymorphism of IIE1 (CypIIE1), is associated with lung cancer in Rio de Janeiro. *Cancer Epidemiol. Biomark. Prevent.* **4**:63–67.

305. Drakoulis, N., Cascorbi, I., Brockmoller, J., Gross, C. R., and Roots, I. (1994). Polymorphisms in the human CYP1A1 gene as susceptibility factors for lung cancer: exon-7 mutation (4889 A to G), and a T to C mutation in the 3'-flanking region. *Clin. Invest.* **72**:240–248.

306. Caporaso, N., DeBaun, M. R., and Rothman, N. (1995) Lung cancer and CYP2D6 (the debrisoquine polymorphism): sources of heterogeneity in the proposed association. *Pharmacogenetics* **129**:129–134.

307. Christensen, P. M., Gotzsche, P. C., and Brosen, K. (1997) The sparteine/debrisoquine (CYP2D6) oxidation polymorphism and the risk of lung cancer: a meta-analysis. *Eur. J. Clin. Pharmacol.* **51**:389–393.

308. Bouchardy, C., Benhamou, S., and Dayer, P. (1996) The effect of tobacco on lung cancer risk depends on CYP2D6 activity. *Cancer Res.* **56**:251–253.

309. London, S. J., Daly, A. K., Leathart, J. B., Navidi, W. C., Carpenter, C. C., and Idle, J. R. (1997) Genetic polymorphism of CYP2D6 and lung cancer risk in African-Americans and Caucasians in Los Angeles County. *Carcinogenesis* **18**:1203–1214.

310. Legrand, M., Stucker, I., Marez, D., Sabbagh, N., Lo-Guidice, J. M., and Broly, F. (1996) Influence of a mutation reducing the catalytic activity of the cytochrome P450 CYP2D6 on lung cancer susceptibility. *Carcinogenesis* **17**:2267–2269.

311. Tran, T. A., Kallakury, B. V., Sheehan, C. E., and Ross, J. S. (1997) Expression of CD44 standard form and variant isoforms in non-small cell lung carcinomas. *Human Pathol.* **28**:809–814.

312. Falco, J. P., Baylin, S. B., Lupu, R., Borges, M., Nelkin, B. D., Jasti, R. K., et al. (1990). v-rasH induces non-small cell phenotype, with associated growth factors and receptors, in a small cell lung cancer cell line. *J. Clin. Invest.* **85**:1740–1745.

313. Borges, M., Linnoila, R. I., van de Velde, H. J., Chen, H., Nelkin, B. D., Mabry, M., et al. (1997) An achaete-scute homologue essential for neuroendocrine differentiation in the lung. *Nature* **386**:852–855.

314. Berard, J., Laboune, F., Mukuna, M., Masse, S., Kothary, R., and Bradley, W. E. (1996) Lung tumors in mice expressing an antisense RARbeta2 transgene. *FASEB J.* **10**:1091–1097.

315. Hiyama, K., Hiyama, E., Ishioka, S., Yamakido, M., Inai, K., Gazdar, A. F., et al. (1995) Telomerase activity in small-cell and non-small-cell lung cancers. *J. Natl. Cancer Inst.* **87**:895–902.

316. Kim, N.-W., Piatyszek, M. A., Prowse, K. R., Harley, C. B., West, M. D., Ho, P. L., et al. (1994) Specific association of human telomerase activity with immortal cells and cancer. *Science* **266**:2011–2015.

317. Albanell, J., Lonardo, F., Rusch, V., Engelhardt, M., Langenfeld, J., Han, W., et al. (1997) High telomerase activity in primary lung cancers: association with increased cell proliferation rates and advanced pathologic stage. *J. Natl. Cancer Inst.* **89**:1609–1615.

318. Yashima, K., Piatyszek, M. A., Saboorian, H. M., Virmani, A. K., Brown, D., Shay, J. W., et al. (1997) Telomerase activity and in situ telomerase RNA expression in malignant and non-malignant lymph nodes. *J. Clin. Pathol.* **50**:110–117.

319. Meyerson, M., Counter, C. M., Eaton, E. N., Ellisen, L. W., Steiner, P., Caddle, S. D., et al. (1997) hEST2, the putative human telomerase catalytic subunit gene, is up-regulated in tumor cells and during immortalization. *Cell* **90**:785–795.

320. Bryan, T. M., Marusic, L., Bacchetti, S., Namba, M., and Reddel, R. R. (1997) The telomere lengthening mechanism in telomerase-negative immortal human cells does not involve the telomerase RNA subunit. *Human Mol. Genet.* **6**:921–926.

321. Redondo, M., Concha, A., Oldiviela, R., Cueto, A., Gonzalez, A., Garrido, F., et al. (1991) Expression of HLA class I and II antigens in bronchogenic carcinomas: its relationship to cellular DNA content and clinical-pathological parameters. *Cancer Res.* **51**:4948–4954.

322. Korkolopoulou, P., Kaklamanis, L., Pezzella, F., Harris, A. L., and Gatter, K. C. (1996) Loss of antigen-presenting molecules (MHC class I and TAP-1) in lung cancer. *Br. J. Cancer* **73**:148–153.

323. Chen, H. L., Gabrilovich, D., Virmani, A., Ratnani, I., Girgis, K. R., Nadaf-Rahrov, S., et al. (1996) Structural and functional analysis of beta2 microglobulin abnormalities in human lung and breast cancer. *Int. J. Cancer* **67**:756–763.

324. Singal, D. P., Ye, M., and Qiu, X. (1996) Molecular basis for lack of expression of HLA class I antigens in human small-cell lung carcinoma cell lines. *Int. J. Cancer* **68**:629–636.

325. Chen, H. L., Gabrilovich, D., Tampe, R., Girgis, K. R., Nadaf, S., and Carbone, D. P. (1996) A functionally defective allele of TAP1 results in loss of MHC class I antigen presentation in a human lung cancer. *Nature Genet.* **13**:210–213.

326. Niehans, G. A., Brunner, T., Frizelle, S. P., Liston, J. C., Salerno, C. T., Knapp, D. J., et al. (1997) Human lung carcinomas express Fas ligand. *Cancer Res.* **57**:1007–1012.

327. Hahne, M., Rimoldi, D., Schroter, M., Romero, P., Schreier, M., French, L. E., et al. (1996) Melanoma cell expression of Fas(Apo-1/CD95) ligand: implications for tumor immune escape. *Science* **274**:1363–1366.

328. Strand, S., Hofmann, W. J., Hug, H., Muller, M., Otto, G., Strand, D., et al. (1996) Lymphocyte apoptosis induced by CD95 (APO-1/

Fas) ligand-expressing tumor cells: A mechanism of immune evasion? *Nature Med.* **2**:1361–1366.

329. Angeletti, C. A., Lucchi, M., Fontanini, G., Mussi, A., Chella, A., Ribechini, A., et al. (1996) Prognostic significance of tumoral angiogenesis in completely resected late stage lung carcinoma (stage IIIA-N2). Impact of adjuvant therapies in a subset of patients at high risk of recurrence. *Cancer* **78**:409–415.

330. Fontanini, G., Lucchi, M., Vignati, S., Mussi, A., Ciardiello, F., De Laurentiis, M., et al. (1997) Angiogenesis as a prognostic indicator of survival in non-small-cell lung carcinoma: a prospective study. *J. Natl. Cancer Inst.* **89**:881–886.

331. Hanahan, D. and Folkman, J. (1996) Patterns and emerging mechanisms of the angiogenic switch during tumorigenesis. *Cell* **86**:353–364.

332. Mattern, J., Koomagi, R., and Volm, M. (1996) Association of vascular endothelial growth factor expression with intratumoral microvessel density and tumour cell proliferation in human epidermoid lung carcinoma. *Br. J. Cancer* **73**:931–934.

333. Fontanini, G., Vignati, S., Lucchi, M., Mussi, A., Calcinai, A., Boldrini, L., et al. (1997) Neoangiogenesis and p53 protein in lung cancer: their prognostic role and their relation with vascular endothelial growth factor (VEGF) expression. *Br. J. Cancer* **75**:1295–1301.

334. Ohta, Y., Watanabe, Y., Murakami, S., Oda, M., Hayashi, Y., Nonomura, A., et al. (1997) Vascular endothelial growth factor and lymph node metastasis in primary lung cancer. *Br. J. Cancer* **76**:1041–1045.

335. Volm, M., Koomägi, R., and Mattern, J. (1997) Prognostic value of vascular endothelial growth factor and its receptor Flt-1 in squamous cell lung cancer. *Int. J. Cancer* **74**:64–68.

336. Volm, M., Koomägi, R., Mattern, J., and Stammler, G. (1997) Prognostic value of basic fibroblast growth factor and its receptor (FGFR-1) in patients with non-small cell lung carcinomas. *Eur. J. Cancer* **33**:691–693.

337. Takanami, I., Imamura, T., Hashizume, T., Kikuchi, K., Yamamoto, Y., Yamamoto, T., et al. (1996) Immunohistochemical detection of basic fibroblast growth factor as a prognostic indicator in pulmonary adenocarcinoma. *Jpn. J. Clin. Oncol.* **26**:293–297.

338. Koukourakis, M. I., Giatromanolaki, A., O'Byrne, K. J., Comley, M., Whitehouse, R. M., Talbot, D. C., et al. (1997) Platelet-derived endothelial cell growth factor expression correlates with tumour angiogenesis and prognosis in non-small-cell lung cancer. *Br. J. Cancer* **75**:477–481.

339. Boehm, T., Folkman, J., Browder, T., and O'Reilly, M. S. (1997) Antiangiogenic therapy of experimental cancer does not induce acquired drug resistance. *Nature* **390**:404–407.

340. Dameron, K. M., Volpert, O. V., Tainsky, M. A., and Bouck, N. (1994) Control of angiogenesis in fibroblasts by p53 regulation of thrombospondin-1. *Science* **265**:1582–1584.

341. Arenberg, D. A., Kunkel, S. L., Polverini, P. J., Morris, S. B., Burdick, M. D., Glass, M. C., et al. (1996) Interferon-gamma-inducible protein 10 (IP-10) is an angiostatic factor that inhibits human non-small cell lung cancer (NSCLC) tumorigenesis and spontaneous metastases. *J. Exp. Med.* **184**:981–992.

342. Arenberg, D. A., Polverini, P. J., Kunkel, S. L., Shanafelt, A., Hesselgesser, J., Horuk, R., et al. (1997) The role of CXC chemokines in the regulation of angiogenesis in non-small cell lung cancer. *J. Leuk. Biol.* **62**:554–562.

343. Mao, L., Hruban, R. H., Boyle, J. O., Tockman, M., and Sidransky, D. (1994) Detection of oncogene mutations in sputum precedes diagnosis of lung cancer. *Cancer Res.* **54**:1634–1637.

18 The Molecular Basis of Skin Carcinogenesis

Caterina Missero, PhD, Mariarosaria D'Errico, PhD, Gian Paolo Dotto, MD, and Eugenia Dogliotti, PhD

INTRODUCTION: SKIN STRUCTURE AND EPIDERMAL DIFFERENTIATION

The skin is constituted by two different tissues: the epidermis, which is composed mostly of squamous epithelial cells (called keratinocytes), and the underlying dermis, which is composed predominantly of dermal fibroblasts. The epidermis is organized in four distinct cell layers. The innermost basal layer consists of actively proliferating keratinocytes, which are characterized by a relatively dispersed network of keratin filaments, primarily keratin 5 (K5) and K14 *(1,2)*. As basal keratinocytes migrate toward the skin surface, proliferation ceases and terminal differentiation begins. Cells of the suprabasal spinous layer are metabolically active and express high amounts of two differentiation-specific keratins, K1 and K10 *(1,3)*. They also produce glutamine and lysine-rich envelope proteins, such as involucrin, which are crosslinked by epidermal transglutaminase and deposited at the inner surface of the cellular membrane, to form the cornified envelope *(4,5)*. In the overlying granular layer, cells contain numerous lipid-containing granules, that are released in the intercellular space. Keratinocytes at this step synthesize filaggrin and loricrin, which also contribute to the cornified envelope formation *(6,7)*. The outermost layer of the epidermis is the cornified layer. Here cells are metabolically inactive, lack a nucleus and cytoplasmic organelles, and are full of keratin filaments.

Human keratinocytes can be grown for several hundred generations in culture on a feeder layer of X-ray or mytomicin-treated fibroblasts, forming a stratified structure that resembles the epidermis, although many biochemical changes characteristic of terminal differentiation do not occur under these conditions *(8,9)*. Mouse primary keratinocytes can be grown as a proliferating monolayer when the calcium ion concentration in the medium is reduced from the standard level of 1.2–0.05 m*M* (low-calcium medium) *(9)*. Calcium addition triggers a terminal differentiation program that closely resembles that which occurs in vivo. Calcium is a prerequisite for desmosome assembly, cell stratification, and activation of the epidermal transglutaminase *(9)*. Further, calcium induces irreversible withdrawal from the cell cycle, which is an important step in this process, although cell cycle arrest is not sufficient by itself to cause terminal differentiation.

Signal-transduction events involved in the response to the extracellular increase in calcium ions have been extensively studied. Addition of calcium is associated with rapid induction of tyrosine phosphorylation, occurring as early as 2 min after treatment *(10,11)*. Phospholipase C is activated resulting in the induction of protein kinase C (PKC) activity, which may be involved in downregulating the early markers of differentiation (K1 and K10), and upregulating loricrin, filaggrin, and transglutaminase during the spinous to granular cell transition *(12–14)*.

The phorbol ester 12-O-tetradecanoylphorbol-13-acetate (TPA) is also known to induce some aspects of keratinocyte-terminal differentiation in culture, such as growth arrest, loricrin and filaggrin production, and epidermal transglutaminase activation. TPA rapidly activates PKC and induces tyrosine phosphorylation of protein substrates that are affected by calcium signaling at later times, in agreement with the notion that TPA induces only the late markers of terminal differentiation *(10,13,15)*. The phosphorylation reactions are mediated by the fyn tyrosine kinase, a member of the c-*src* gene family. Interestingly, keratinocytes lacking fyn kinase are significantly altered in their differentiation response both in vitro and in vivo, suggesting that signaling mediated by fyn plays an important role in this process *(15)*.

The nuclear factors controlling transcription of the differentiation-specific markers have been investigated for many years, and recently candidate genes involved in transcriptional regulation during terminal differentiation have been isolated. Expression of novel members of the *Ets* gene family, *Ese1* and *Jen*, and members of the POU domain protein family, Skn-1a/i and Tst-1, are induced upon terminal differentiation both in

From: *The Molecular Basis of Human Cancer:* (W. B. Coleman and G. J. Tsongalis, eds.), © Humana Press Inc., Totowa, NJ.

vitro and in vivo *(16–19)*. Interestingly, knock-out mice for the *skn-1a/i* gene display reduced loricrin expression in a normal-appearing skin, whereas mice deficient for both *Skn-1a/i* and *Tst-1* genes display an hyperplastic skin, associated with K14 expression in basal as well as suprabasal keratinocytes *(17)*. Another transcription-factor gene involved in skin differentiation is *Whn*, the winged-helix nude gene, whose mutation results in the nude phenotype in mice and rats *(20)*. The skin defect of the nude mice resides in the epithelial cells, resulting in inappropriate hair-follicle formation and thickened epidermis *(21)*. Keratinocytes isolated from nude mice exhibit a dramatically increased sensitivity to TPA-induced differentiation in vitro and exogenous expression of *Whn* in these cells suppresses expression of the TPA-responsive genes *(21)*. In addition to tissue-specific transcription factors, some ubiquitous transcription factors have been described to play a role in epithelial terminal differentiation, including SP3 *(22)*, AP-1 *(23)*, AP-2 *(24)*, and mad *(25,26)*. The mad protein is a c-myc-binding protein that is induced in keratinocyte differentiation and whose expression is lost in basal-cell carcinoma (BCC) and squamous-cell carcinoma (SCC) *(25, 26)*.

EXPERIMENTAL SKIN CARCINOGENESIS

Mouse skin provides a unique experimental system to study chemical, physical, and viral carcinogenesis. This model has been extensively used for over 20 years and has provided important insights into general mechanisms of oncogenesis in vivo (27). The external location of the skin allows monitoring of tumor formation during experimental procedures. Tumors develop relatively rapidly (2–4 mo) after carcinogen exposure, irrespective of the route of administration (topical or systemic). Of great practical relevance is that the skin model can be used to assess the carcinogenic risk of chemicals, and is highly reproducible and quantitative. Studies on the molecular mechanisms of oncogenesis have been possible because keratinocytes can be easily isolated from human and mouse skin. After establishment of primary cultures, cells can be manipulated and introduced back into the animal, in grafting-assay experiments. Recent studies have examined the contribution of individual genes in skin carcinogenesis in vivo using skin-specific transgenic and knock-out mice.

Epithelial skin cancer is the most common malignancy in humans. There are two main types of epithelial skin cancer in humans: BCC and SCC. In experimental models, rodent skin develops BCC at low-carcinogen dose and SCC at higher doses *(28)*. Susceptibility to carcinogen varies depending on the strain of mice *(29)*. Tumor formation is influenced by multiple genetic alterations, which can act at three different stages of tumor development. This process can be operationally divided into the well-characterized stages of initiation, promotion, and progression (Fig. 1).

Initiation is an irreversible step, that experimentally can be induced by a limited exposure to a carcinogen, usually as a single treatment at low dose. At the molecular level, initiation causes a genetic lesion in few normal cells of the treated area and the gene target depends on the carcinogen used. For instance, point mutations of the protoncogene c-H-*ras* are found

in high proportion in premalignant cells, indicating that this is an early event *(30,31)*.

Promotion is achieved by repeated treatments over a period of time with an agent that is thought to confer a growth advantage to the mutated cells without causing additional genetic damage. This process in the skin leads to the formation of benign tumors, called papillomas. Promoting agents can be chemicals (like TPA), or physical agents (like wounding, abrasion, and hair-follicle damage by depilation) *(32–35)*. Acute treatment with phorbol esters induces marked skin hyperplasia *(36)*. This effect may not be sufficient to explain tumor promotion because some TPA derivatives that cause hyperplasia are unable to induce papillomas. As mentioned earlier, phorbol esters are also known to promote differentiation *(37)*, and an attractive model is that initiated cells become resistant to this particular effect of the phorbol ester.

Papillomas progress to SCC following a second genetic event, which occurs spontaneously or can be induced by the same carcinogen used during initiation. Papillomas can be grouped into low-risk and high-risk for premalignant progression. Low-risk papillomas are organized structurally like the normal epidermis, with proliferation occurring primarily in the basal layers, whereas the upper layers still express the differentiation markers K1 and K10. In high-risk papillomas, proliferation occurs in each of the cellular layers of the lesion, differentiation markers K1 and K10 are undetectable, and there is aberrant expression of K13 and K19, which are not expressed in normal epidermis *(38)*. The $\alpha_6\beta_4$ integrin is detected in suprabasal and basal cells in high-risk papillomas, whereas expression is polarized to the basal surface of basal cells in normal epidermis and low-risk papillomas *(38,39)*. Benign lesions are diploid, but their hyperproliferative phenotype results in the spontaneous accumulation of nonrandom chromosomal aberrations over time, most frequently involving chromosomes 6 and 7, and involving chromosomes 4, 11, and 15 in a smaller fraction of lesions *(40–43)*. The development of aneuploidy is a consistent feature of tumor progression both in humans and in animal models *(44)*. Carcinomas can undergo a further epithelial-mesenchymal transition to give rise to highly invasive, metastatic phenotype, involving reorganization of the cytoskeleton, poor keratin organization, loss of *E-cadherin* expression and spindle-cell morphology *(45,46)*. Fusion experiments between spindle-cell carcinoma and papilloma cell lines have shown that the spindle-cell phenotype involves functional loss of genes controlling epithelial differentiation *(47)*.

Alteration of cell-cell contact is a crucial event in tumorigenesis. In addition to integrins and cadherins, gap-junctional intercellular communication (GJIC) is also altered in tumor formation. Gap-junctions are transmembrane channels that link the cytoplasm of adjacent cells, allowing passage of ions, second messengers, and small metabolites *(48)*. In vitro, GJIC is greatly reduced after TPA and neoplastic transformation by exogenous activated oncogenes. TPA acts at multiple levels, initially affecting channel permeability and then affecting the synthesis of the connexins, which are the proteins that form the channel *(49)*. Introduction of the c-H-*ras* oncogene in mouse primary keratinocytes causes a 70–80% decrease in GJIC, due

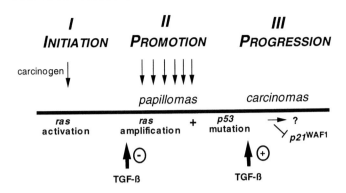

Fig. 1. Stages of chemically induced mouse skin carcinogenesis and the underlying molecular events. Initiation of mouse skin carcinogenesis is induced by a single low dose carcinogen exposure and has been causally related to activation of the c-H-*ras* proto-oncogene by single point mutation. Progression of the benign tumors (papillomas) into carcinomas is favored by several genetic events, including amplification of the activated c-*ras* oncogene, as well as loss of the *p53* tumor-suppressor gene. $p21^{WAF1/CIP1}$ is one of the best-characterized downstream targets of p53, and loss of p21$^{WAF1/CIP1}$ function promotes the neoplastic outgrowth of c-*ras*-transformed keratinocytes. TGF-β functions as an inhibitor of early stages of keratinocyte tumor development, and a promoter of later stages, at a time when tumor cells have lost sensitivity to TGF-β growth inhibition.

to changes in connexin expression and phosphorylation similar to those elicited by TPA. These two agents act together to completely suppress communication *(49,50)*. Other oncoproteins are thought to interfere with GJIC, including the human papillomavirus type 16 E5 protein *(51)*.

GJIC in mouse skin carcinoma cell lines is significantly decreased when compared to that observed in papilloma cell lines and normal mouse keratinocytes *(52)*. Connexin expression has been measured in several cell lines, representing different stages of chemically induced mouse-skin carcinogenesis. The amount of connexin proteins Cx43 and Cx26 correlates with the degree of tumor differentiation *(53)*. The overall expression of Cx43 and Cx26 appears to be elevated in papillomas and the subcellular localization of these proteins is disrupted. The expression of Cx43 and Cx26 is subsequently extinguished in SCC and communication appears to be completely lost *(53–55)*. Taken together, these data suggest that alteration in gap junctions are associated with skin neoplasia and lack of GJIC is likely to play a role in the malignant conversion of mouse epidermal cells.

THE ROLE OF PROTO-ONCOGENE C-*RAS* IN INITIATION AND PROGRESSION OF SKIN CARCINOGENESIS

As previously mentioned, c-*ras* is thought to be a main target of initiators. Dimethylbenzanthracene (DMBA), one of the most commonly used initiators, reproducibly provokes an A→T transversion at codon 61 of the c-H-*ras* gene, causing an amino acid substitution from Gln to Leu *(56)*. The methylating agent N-methyl-N'-nitro-N-nitrosoguanidine (MNNG) and methylnitrosourea (MNU) induce a G→A transition at the second base of codon 12 of the c-H-*ras* gene *(57)*. Treatment with

the initiating carcinogen can be replaced by direct application on the skin of a retrovirus encoding a mutant c-*ras* gene *(58)*.

Isolated cells harboring a mutation in the c-*ras* gene, can become transformed either by TPA treatment or by removal of surrounding normal cells. In grafting experiments, it has been shown that pure cultures of c-*ras*-transformed mouse primary keratinocytes can develop papillomas or carcinomas depending on c-*ras* expression levels and whether or not all targeted keratinocytes express the transforming oncogene *(59–62)*. Accordingly, studies on chromosomal alterations during skin-tumor progression have revealed a frequently occurring allelic imbalance involving mouse chromosome 7 (where c-H-*ras* is located) during chemical carcinogenesis, leading to an increase in the copy number of the mutant c-H-*ras* allele and/or loss of the normal allele *(40)*.

Involvement of the c-*ras* oncogene in skin tumorigenesis has also been evaluated using transgenic mice carrying an activated c-*ras* that is specifically expressed in the skin. K1 and K10 promoters have been used to drive expression of a mutant c-H-*ras* oncogene, isolated from T24 human bladder carcinoma cells *(63,64)*. Transgenic mice carrying the mutated c-H-*ras* under the control of these differentiation-specific keratin promoters develop hyperkeratosis of the skin, which become papillomas in the area subjected to biting or scratching. Promotion in these mice is achieved simply by a mild stimulus provided by wounding. These data suggest that even cells of the suprabasal compartment can be induced to form at least benign tumors. Because K1 and K10 expression is shut off during progression, the use of these promoters to study carcinogenesis might not be ideal. In subsequent studies expression of c-H-*ras* has been targeted to the basal layer of the skin using the K5 promoter *(65)*. Transgenic animals develop a high frequency of benign keratoacanthomas or papillomas, many of which subsequently progress to SCC *(65)*. Thus, targeting c-*ras* to the different skin layers results in either benign or malignant tumorigenic phenotype, depending on the differentiation stage of the target-cell population. Similarly, during chemical carcinogenesis, low-risk and high-risk papillomas may be generated by c-*ras* mutation occurring in distinct keratinocyte populations within the skin.

INACTIVATION OF TUMOR-SUPPRESSOR *P53* AND PROGRESSION TO SKIN CARCINOMA

Inactivation of tumor-suppressor genes is thought to be an important step in the transition from initiated cells to benign tumors and subsequent progression to malignancy. The tumor-suppressor gene *p53* is elevated in response to DNA damage where it mediates cell-cycle arrest and/or induction of apoptosis *(66)*. Thus, loss of p53 activity can confer a growth advantage to genetically altered cells. Loss of heterozygousity (LOH) on mouse chromosome 11, where the *p53* gene is located, occurs in a significant number of skin carcinomas and it is always accompanied by point mutation of the other *p53* allele *(67,68)*. In human skin, a high number of BCCs and SCCs show mutations in the *p53* gene, primarily as a consequence of exposure to ultraviolet (UV) radiation.

The role of *p53* in initiation, promotion, and progression has been explored using *p53*-deficient mice as a model *(69,70)*. Mice that are *p53*-deficient develop spontaneous chromosomal aberrations at a much higher rate than control animals (71). Transgenic mice with the genotype of *p53*−/− and *p53*+/− have been compared to wild-type controls in a standard skin-carcinogenesis assay, in which initiation is induced by a single treatment with DMBA, followed by promotion with TPA for 15 wks *(72)*. Loss of *p53* does not cooperate with mutant c-H-*ras* to provide a selective growth advantage in papilloma formation, but actually a decrease in papillomas formation is observed in the absence of *p53*. Papillomas isolated from *p53*-deficient mice show alterations in *E-cadherin* expression, associated with focal loss of cell-cell contacts *(73)*. Interestingly, tumor progression is dramatically accelerated in *p53*−/− mice, with some carcinomas appearing after only 10 wk of tumor promotion, in contrast to wild-type mice in which carcinomas appear only after 25 wk *(72)*. The rate of tumor progression is accelerated in *p53*+/− mice, typically due to the loss of the wild-type allele. Histologically, carcinomas isolated from the *p53*−/− and *p53*+/− mice present a more undifferentiated phenotype than those from wild-type mice. Similar results have been obtained by infecting *p53*−/− primary keratinocytes with a retrovirus carrying c-H-*ras* and grafting cells back into nude mice *(74)*. In this assay, keratinocytes lacking *p53* develop tumors that exhibit a high proliferative index and are morphologically more aggressive than tumors arising in wild-type mice. These studies suggest that loss of p53 function is a key step in the malignant progression of skin tumors.

PROTO-ONCOGENE C-*FOS* ACTIVITY IS REQUIRED FOR SKIN-TUMOR PROGRESSION

The proto-oncogene c-*fos* is one of the major targets of several signal-transduction pathways, involved in cell growth and differentiation, including signaling pathways that are mediated by c-*ras*. The c-*fos* gene belongs to a family of nuclear factors that dimerize with members of the c-*jun* family to form the active transcription complex AP-1 *(75)*. Expression of this transcription factor is constitutive in skin and does not change significantly during calcium-induced differentiation of mouse primary keratinocytes *(76–78)*. The role of c-*fos* in skin carcinogenesis has been directly tested, measuring the ability of c-*fos*-deficient mice to develop tumors *(79)*. Upon repeated treatment with the tumor promoter TPA, which is known to highly induce c-*fos* expression in vitro, c-*fos* null mice carrying a v-H-*ras* transgene, develop papillomas similarly to the c-*fos* positive controls. However, c-*fos*-deficient papillomas become very dry, hyperkeratinized, and show little vascularization over time. Whereas expression of keratin K1 and K13 are mutually exclusive in wild-type papillomas, in the *fos*-deficient ones these two keratins are co-expressed in the same cells, resulting in an altered intermediate filament network, that may contribute to the hyperkeratinized phenotype. Importantly, the affected papillomas fail to progress into malignant tumors. Furthermore resistance to tumor progression has been shown to be an intrinsic property of the c-*fos* null keratinocytes, because when these cells are grafted back into nude mice, no tumor is observed

(79). Interestingly, an activated form of c-*fos* (v-fos) expressed under the K1 promoter, can generate papillomas after long promotion treatment in the absence of an initiator *(80)*.

DYSREGULATED EXPRESSION OF TGF-β AND PROGRESSION TO MALIGNANCY IN SKIN TUMORS

Transforming growth factors β(TGF-βs) are a family of multifunctional peptides that affect cellular proliferation and differentiation and modulate extracellular matrix *(81)*. TGF-βs are involved in migration and morphogenesis during development, fibroblast proliferation, migration, and matrix deposition, and play an important role in tissue remodeling during wound healing *(82)*. TGF-β family members act as potent inhibitors of keratinocyte proliferation, TGFβ3 being 100-fold more potent that TGFβ1 and TGFβ2 *(83,84)*. TGFβ1 is produced and secreted by the keratinocytes of the basal layer, and it is thought to control their growth in an autocrine fashion, whereas TGFβ3 is secreted by the dermal fibroblasts and has been proposed to have an homeostatic role in carcinoma formation *(85–87)*. In grafting experiments, tumorigenicity of c-H-*ras*-transformed primary keratinocytes can be suppressed by the presence of normal dermal fibroblasts, and pretreatment of the transformed keratinocytes with either dermal fibroblast conditioned medium or TGFβ3 can partially inhibit tumor formation *(84)*.

Besides the effect on keratinocyte growth rate, TGF-βs are likely to have a more complex role in tumor formation, given their multiple functions in cell homeostasis. A vast amount of literature exists on the role of TGFβ1 in skin carcinogenesis. Loss of the growth response to TGF-β is a frequent event in human and mouse skin tumors, and it is considered to be one of the earliest changes of premalignant progression associated with the high-risk papilloma phenotype *(86,87)*. *TGFβ1* is highly expressed in the stroma of mouse and skin carcinomas, and in the skin after tumor-promoting stimuli, as TPA and wounding *(85,88,89)*. Acute treatment with the tumor-promoter TPA induces epidermal hyperplasia within 48–72 h, and this effect is associated with early induction of *TGFβ1* and *TGFβRII* receptor as well as *TGFβ2* and *TGFβ3* downregulation, suggesting that the different components of the TGF-β family are likely to play different roles in epidermal homeostasis *(89,90)*. Several lines of transgenic mice expressing *TGFβ1* have been generated to study its effect under basal condition and during skin carcinogenesis. In transgenic mice carrying the *TGFβ1* gene under the K10 promoter control a two- to three-fold induction in epidermal DNA labeling index is observed, in the absence of epidermal hyperplasia, suggesting that a more rapid keratinocyte turnover may occur in these animals *(90)*. However, the transgene acts as a negative regulator of cell growth, when hyperplasia is induced acutely by TPA. In a chemical carcinogenesis protocol, K10-*TGFβ1* and K6-*TGFβ1* transgenic mice develop a reduced number of papillomas, which display a more aggressive phenotype, express K13, and an altered integrin pattern *(91)*. The malignant conversion rate is increased in these transgenic mice, and there is an higher incidence of spindle cell carcinomas, suggesting that tumor cells that evade negative growth regulation, are likely to be still responsive to other aspects of TGF-β cell signaling.

In another study a human keratin K1 promoter has been used to target an activated form of *TGFβ1* to the skin *(92)*. Mice expressing the transgene exhibited a marked phenotype at birth resulting in perinatal death, their skin being very shiny and tautly stretched. Histologically, the epidermis of these mice appear thinner and hyperkeratotic, with a reduced number of hair follicles and, in contrast to the transgenic mice expressing a latent form of TGF-β protein, display a reduced number of replicating cells as judged by their labeling index. These data indicate that TGFβ1 acts in vivo as an endogenous negative regulator of basal cell proliferation. However, no carcinogenesis experiments could be performed due to the uniform perinatal lethality exhibited by this transgenic mouse strain. This dramatic phenotype is very similar to the one obtained in the skin of mice carrying a loss-of-function mutation of the *follistatin* gene, which encodes a heparan sulphate proteoglycan-binding protein that most likely functions to modulate the actions of members of the TGF-β family *(93)*.

Targeted deletion of the *TGF-β* gene has also been used to assess the role of this factor in skin carcinogenesis. *TGFβ1* null mice develop normally but die at 3–4 wk after birth due to a wasting syndrome caused by an excessive inflammatory response characterized by massive infiltration of the heart and lungs with lymphocytes and macrophages *(94)*. For this reason, a chemical carcinogenesis protocol could not be performed on the skin of these mice. Interestingly, *TGFβ1* null keratinocytes, isolated from newborn mice and transformed with c-H-*ras* in vitro, rapidly develop dysplastic papillomas or SCCs after three wk following transplantation into the skin of nude mice, whereas their wild-type counterparts produce mostly benign tumors *(95)*. No *p53* or endogenous c-*ras* mutations were detected in these early occurring carcinomas. In addition, cells isolated from the *TGFβ1* null tumors still respond to TGF-β inhibition, suggesting that the inability of keratinocytes to produce TGF-β results in malignant transformation when these cells are grafted back into nude mouse skin. These experiments are complicated by the persistent expression not only of the other two closely related members of the *TGF-β* family, but also of other more distal members of the *TGF-β* super family, like the activins and the bone morphogenetic proteins (BMPs), which are expressed in normal skin and play a role in tissue repair and remodeling *(96–98)*. The role of the other TGF-β isoforms and of BMPs and activins has not yet been addressed in skin-tumor formation. Thus, the various members of *TGF-β* family clearly play several distinct and complex roles in skin homeostasis and tumor formation, and loss of TGF-β induced growth inhibition is an important step in skin-tumor progression.

CELL-CYCLE REGULATORS AND SKIN CARCINOGENESIS

Overexpression and/or loss of function of a number of cell-cycle regulatory proteins has been implicated in skin tumorigenesis. Expression of activated proto-oncogenes (like c-*ras*) accelerate cell-cycle progression, by either inactivating nega-

tive regulators or by promoting positive mediators of cell proliferation *(99)*.

The D-type cyclins are among the G_1 cyclins that function to regulate the G_1 to S phase transition. The *cyclin D1 (cycD1)* gene is a putative proto-oncogene strongly implicated in several types of human tumors, including SCC *(99,100)*. Early-stage papillomas show only basal expression of *cycD1*, whereas overexpression is observed in most advanced papillomas and carcinomas *(101)*. The *cycD1* gene maps in the distal end of mouse chromosome 7. Because trisomy of chromosome 7 is among the genetic alterations that occur during skin-tumor progression, increased *cycD1* gene copy number has been proposed to be at least partially responsible for *cycD1* overexpression during tumorigenic progression *(102)*. Transgenic mice expressing *cycD1* under a bovine K5 promoter have been generated. Transgenic epidermis, as well as other stratified epithelia, display a dramatic increase in basal-cell proliferation, even though differentiation is unaffected. Spontaneous development of epithelial tumors is not observed in K5-*cycD1* transgenic mice, suggesting that overexpression of *cycD1* and the resulting hyperproliferation are not sufficient to induce tumors in stratified epithelia in the presence of a normal differentiation program.

Other cell-cycle regulators that have been implicated in skin carcinogenesis include the cyclin-dependent kinase (cdk) inhibitors, p16[INK4A], p15[INK4B] and p21[WAF1/CIP1] *(103)*. Association of cdk4 and cyclin D results in an active cdk4-cyclin D complex that is negatively regulated by p15[INK4B] and p16[INK4A], two related cdk inhibitors that bind and sequester cdk4 in early G_1, blocking cell cycle progression *(103)*. p15[INK4B] protein greatly accumulates in keratinocytes in response to TGF-β-induced growth arrest, suggesting that this cdk inhibitor could play an important role in cell-cycle withdrawal upon TGF-β treatment *(104)*. p16[INK4A] is suggested to be a tumor suppressor because deletion and mutation of the *p16[INK4A]* gene occurs in several types of sporadic tumors and in familial melanomas. Deletion and altered regulation of the *p16[INK4A]* and *p15[INK4B]* genes has been shown in SCC and in spindle-cell carcinomas, through examination of mouse primary tumors and derived cell lines. Mice lacking *p16[INK4A]* are viable but develop spontaneous tumors in skin and other tissues *(105)*. In contrast to wild-type mice, treatment with relatively low doses of UVB alone, or DMBA and UVB induces well-differentiated SCC in *p16[INK4A]*-deficient mice, although at low frequency *(105)*. Moreover, loss of *INK4* and activation of c-*ras* can cooperate to accelerate the development of melanoma *(106)*. In fact, mice with melanocyte-specific expression of activated c-H-*ras* on an *INK4A*-deficient background develop spontaneous cutaneous melanomas. Thus, loss of function of these two cdk inhibitors may contribute to tumor progression in a subset of skin tumors.

Another family of cdk inhibitors, comprising *p21[WAF1/CIP1]* and *p27[KIP1]* gene products, is involved in cell-cycle withdrawal in response to several regulatory pathways *(103)*. In mouse primary keratinocytes, p21[WAF1/CIP1] and p27[KIP1] protein expressions are increased shortly after induction of terminal differentiation (within hours), in association with inhibition of cdk activity and cell-cycle withdrawal *(107,108)*. p21$^{WAF1/CIP1}$ is regulated by p53 in response to DNA damage, whereas increased expression upon keratinocyte differentiation occurs independently of p53, with a mechanism that involves the transcriptional coactivator p300 *(107)*. The role of these cdk inhibitors in keratinocyte differentiation and skin-tumor formation has been analyzed, using mouse primary keratinocytes isolated from mice that are deficient for *p21$^{WAF1/CIP1}$* and *p27^{KIP1}*, respectively *(108)*. Mice lacking *p21$^{WAF1/CIP1}$* or *p27^{KIP1}* display no gross abnormality of their skin, nor spontaneous skin-tumor formation *(109–112)*. However, primary keratinocytes derived from *p21$^{WAF1/CIP1}$* knockout mice, transformed with the c-*ras* oncogene, and injected subcutaneously into nude mice exhibit a very aggressive tumorigenic behavior (Fig. 2), which is not observed in *p27^{KIP1}*-deficient keratinocytes nor in wild-type keratinocytes *(108)*. Histologically, keratinocytes from normal mice develop small numbers of benign lesions after c-*ras* transformation, whereas *p21$^{WAF1/CIP1}$*-deficient keratinocytes consistently form SCCs in all injected sites following c-*ras* transformation (Fig. 2). In this model *p21$^{WAF1/CIP1}$* acts as a tumor suppressor gene. In vitro studies have shed some light on the possible mechanisms of this effect. Keratinocytes lacking *p21$^{WAF1/CIP1}$* show a significantly increased proliferation potential under basal conditions, but undergo normal cell-cycle withdrawal upon differentiation (108). The absence of p21$^{WAF1/CIP1}$ causes profound changes in the ability of keratinocytes to undergo spontaneous or calcium-induced differentiation, because K1, involucrin, and loricrin are greatly diminished in *p21$^{WAF1/CIP1}$*-null keratinocytes (108). Thus, induction of *p21$^{WAF1/CIP1}$* is likely to play an important role at the onset of skin differentiation. Taken together, these data suggest that increased cellular-proliferation potential and partial impairment of terminal differentiation results in an imbalance that leads to tumor formation under certain circumstances. These results are in conflict with a very similar study in which c-*ras*-transformed *p21$^{WAF1/CIP1}$*-null keratinocytes have been injected into nude mice in the presence of dermal fibroblasts *(113)*. In this circumstance *p21$^{WAF1/CIP1}$*-deficient keratinocytes do not display an increased tumorigenic potential compared to c-*ras* transformed control keratinocytes. However, the role of *p21$^{WAF1/CIP1}$* in skin carcinogenesis may have been obscured by the very high number of aggressive tumors developed by the c-*ras* transformed wild-type keratinocytes, which has never been reported in similar experiments *(74)*.

c-*ras* transformed *p27^{KIP1}*-deficient keratinocytes do not display an increased tumorigenic behavior nor have an altered differentiation pattern, suggesting that the p21$^{WAF1/CIP1}$ and p27^{KIP1} provide nonredundant functions in the regulation of cell proliferation in keratinocytes. Interestingly, p27^{KIP1}-deficient keratinocytes display a partial resistance to TGF-β-mediated growth inhibition, and this level of resistance to TGF-β is greater than that exhibited by *p21$^{WAF1/CIP1}$*-deficient keratinocytes. These findings suggest that the lack of TGF-β responsiveness does not contribute to the aggressive behavior displayed by keratinocytes lacking *p21$^{WAF1/CIP1}$* (108).

p21$^{Cip1/WAF1}$ has been recently found to be a target of the human papillomavirus (HPV) oncoprotein E7 *(114,115)*. The

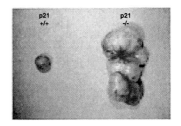

TUMORIGENICITY OF ras-TRANSFORMED KERATINOCYTES

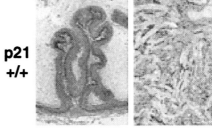

Fig. 2. The absence of p21$^{WAF1/CIP1}$ promotes aggressive tumorigenic behavior of c-ras-transformed keratinocytes. Primary keratinocytes from *p21$^{WAF1/CIP1}$* knockout mice and genetically matched wild-type controls were infected with a helper-free retrovirus encoding a v-H-*ras* gene1 d after plating, and cultivated for 6 d before subcutaneous injection into nude mice. After 3 wk, mice were euthanized and tumors were isolated for histological analysis. Top Panel, Macroscopic appearance of tumors formed by normal versus *p21$^{WAF1/CIP1}$*-deficient keratinocytes. Bottom Panel (left), Note the well-organized and papilloma-like structure of the lesions formed by v-H-*ras* transformed keratinocytes, exhibiting abundant keratinization and a high level of differentiation. Bottom Panel (right), In contrast, the tumors formed by *p21$^{WAF1/CIP1}$*-deficient keratinocytes show features typical of aggressive SCCs, with a variable degree of differentiation.

HPVs are small DNA viruses clinically associated with human cervical carcinoma. HPV E7 can override a variety of growth-regulatory mechanisms, such as TGF-β-mediated growth inhibition, p53-mediated growth arrest, and cell-cycle withdrawal during differentiation. Human keratinocyte cultures expressing *E7* show delayed onset of calcium-induced differentiation and elevated cdk2 activity, in spite of an increased *p21$^{WAF1/CIP1}$* expression. It has been shown that the oncogenic E7 protein can bind and inactivate p21$^{WAF1/CIP1}$, supporting the suggestion that p21$^{WAF1/CIP1}$ may play an important role in keratinocyte differentiation and tumor suppression.

ANIMAL MODELS FOR BCC

SSC has been extensively studied using various animal models. However, the molecular basis of BCC has not been the subject of intense investigation due to the fact that mice do not spontaneously develop BCC. Recently it has been shown that the human homolog of the *Drosophila patched* (or *ptc*) gene is mutated in human patients with the basal-cell nevus syndrome, a disease causing developmental defects and multiple BCCs. The *ptc* gene is a member of the *hedgehog* (*hh*) gene family, which encode proteins that function in the control of patterning and growth during vertebrate development *(116)*. The *ptc* gene product is a receptor for the protein product of the *sonic hedge-hog* (*shh*) gene *(117,118)*. The effects of the *shh* expression on skin formation has been investigated using transgenic mice overexpressing this extracellular factor and by grafting human keratinocytes infected with a retrovirus carrying this gene onto nude mice *(119,120)*. Both studies have shown that forced expression of *shh* induces BCC as determined both at the histological level and by measurement of molecular markers, like *bcl2* expression. Binding of the *shh* gene product to its receptor is thought to prevent normal inhibition of the *smoothened* (*smo*) signaling pathway by the *ptc* gene product, a key mediator of the signal transduction pathway that leads to the activation of the transcription factor Gli1 *(117)*. Interestingly, it has been recently shown that transgenic mice overexpressing a mutant *smo* in the skin display skin abnormalities closely resembling BBCs *(121)*. Moreover, ectopic expression of the transcription factor Gli1 in the embryonic frog epidermis results in the development of tumors *(122)*. These data provide direct evidence that the *smo*/Gli1 signal-transduction pathway is involved in BCC pathogenesis.

EXPERIMENTAL UV CARCINOGENESIS OF THE SKIN

The acute exposure of the skin to UVB-irradiation induces various biological responses which are triggered by oxidative stress and DNA damage. One of the major histologic characteristics of the UVB-exposed epidermis is the appearance of sunburn cells, which are apoptotic keratinocytes. The number of sunburn cells peaks at 24 h after exposure. Concomitant alterations induced by UVB exposure include an early suppression of keratinocyte proliferation (at 12–24 h after exposure) and delayed rebound response (at 48–96 h after exposure). This delayed hyperproliferative response results in epidermal thickening by 48 h of treatment and beyond. Expression of *p53* is strongly increased in response to UV exposure, consistent with this protein playing a key function in UV-induced growth arrest and apoptosis *(123)*. p21$^{WAF1/CIP1}$ expression is also increased after UV treatment of cells, in both a p53-dependent and p53-independent manner *(124)*. An important question that remains to be addressed is the role of p53, p21$^{WAF1/CIP1}$, and related molecules in the acute response to UV-irradiation, and in the sequence of events that lead to long term UV-induced modifications.

Chronic UVB exposure leads to dose-dependent carcinogenesis *(125–126)*. The first and most complete experimental evidence for a causal relationship between UV-irradiation and skin carcinomas comes from experiments on rodents already performed in the 1920s and 1930s. The fur is a handicap especially with UV-irradiation, and shaving could introduce a confounding stimulatory effect on tumor formation. For this reason, mice with the hairless mutation (*hr/hr*), and in particular the SKH-1 strain, have provided the best-characterized model for UV-induced skin carcinogenesis. In homozygous *hr/hr* mice, UV irradiation almost exclusively induces skin carcinomas and precursor lesions, whereas in shaved haired mice, fibrosarcomas are also found that originate from the dermis. In the hairless skin, tumor formation can be observed at a very early stage.

The tumor response of a given cohort of mice is measured in terms of prevalence (percentage of tumor-bearing animals) and yield (average number of tumors per mouse). Initial tumors are very small (~1–2 mm in size) and exhibit benign histological properties (actinic keratoses, often classified in the mouse as papillomas). Tumor progression consists in the development of larger tumors (>3 mm in size), with the histological features of SCCs. As in chemical carcinogenesis, only a fraction of benign tumors progress into their malignant counterparts, suggesting that additional stochastic events are involved.

Mutations in the *p53* gene have been implicated as an important factor in the pathogenesis of UV-induced skin cancers. To investigate the role of p53 in skin carcinogenesis, the development of skin cancers after chronic UVB exposure was examined in groups of homozygous *p53*-deficient mice and wild-type control mice (*p53$^{+/+}$*) *(127)*. At a dose of 2 J/m^2/s of UVB for 30 min three times per week, all *p53$^{-/-}$* mice developed skin tumors by wk 12, with all of these mice developing multiple tumors by wk 16. None of the p53$^{+/+}$ mice developed skin tumors after 17 wk of UV exposure. Ten *p53$^{-/-}$* tumors were examined histologically: five invasive SCCs, four SCC *in situ*, and one actinic keratosis. These are important results in that they demonstrate that loss of wild-type *p53* function significantly shortens tumor latency and predisposes the animals to the development of SCC after UV-irradiation.

Unlike human skin, UV-induced tumors with the features of BCCs are very rare in mice. The reasons for this are unclear, but may involve the fact that the experimental situation is based on relatively high doses of UV light, concentrated over a limited period of time. Higher doses of UVB (just below the erithematous dose) result in efficient tumor formation as early as 2–3 mo after the initiation of treatment. Lower doses induce tumors after a longer time interval, but with the same kinetics. It is also possible that control of epidermal self-renewal and the target cells for UV-induced carcinogenesis are substantially different in mouse vs human skin. The identity of these target cells, whether they correspond to totipotent epidermal stem cells, and how they can be influenced by the surrounding cellular environment remain key questions in experimental carcinogenesis with direct relevance to the clinical situation.

HUMAN SKIN CARCINOGENESIS

PHOTOMUTAGENESIS AND DNA REPAIR
UV Exposure Induces DNA Photoproducts In 1968 the first evidence for the involvement of DNA photoproducts in human skin carcinogenesis was published *(128)*. Cells from patients affected by the cancer-prone inherited disorder xeroderma pigmentosum (XP) were shown to be defective in excision repair of UV-induced dimers from their DNA. A large body of epidemiologic studies confirmed that sunlight (particularly UVB-irradiation) represents the predominant environmental risk factor for skin cancer *(129)*.

Solar UV induces a variety of photoproducts in DNA. The two most frequent types are the *cis-syn* cyclobutane pyrimidine dimers (CPD) and the pyrimidine pyrimidone photoproducts, or 6-4 photoproducts *(130)*. The CPDs are formed *via* a cyclobutane ring connecting the 5 and 6 positions of two adjacent pyrimidine bases like 5′-TT, 5′-TC, 5′-CT, or 5′-CC sequences. In vitro and in vivo mapping experiments have shown that the preferred target for CPD formation is 5′-TT and the least represented is 5′-CC. In mammalian genes′, CPDs have been reported at sequences containing 5-methylcytosine, that is within CpG dinucleotides. 5-methylcytosine bases are indeed the preferred target for CPD formation when cells are irradiated with natural sunlight *(131)*.

UV irradiation induces alkali-labile lesions at positions of cytosine, and less frequently thymine, 3′ to pyrimidine nucleosides. Because a strong bond between positions 6 and 4 of the two adjacent pyrimidines is established these lesions are referred to as 6-4 photoproducts. Irradiation of DNA with UV light at 313 nm or with simulated sunlight (SSL) or natural sunlight produces the Dewar valence isomer of the 6-4 photoproducts. The CPD remains the major UV-induced lesion following sunlight exposure of the skin. However, the relative yield of 6-4 photoproducts (which are formed in general at a rate of 20–30% of that of CPD) may vary as a function of the sequence context. Mapping of these lesions has shown that the preferred targets are 5′-TC and 5′-CC sequences, and 3′-bases within runs of adjacent pyrymidines *(132–134)*. In addition to CPD and 6-4 photoproducts, at low frequency UV-irradiation also produces pyrimidine and purine monoadducts. Their identification and biological significance in human cells remain unclear.

UV Photoproducts Are Repaired Efficiently by Specific Cell Enzymes Dipyrimidine photoproducts are repaired by the mechanism known as nucleotide excision repair (NER), which is highly conserved among eukaryotes. The efficiency of this repair system appears to depend on the degree of structural distortion caused by the DNA modification. Accordingly, CPDs are removed from the genome more slowly than the 6-4 photoproducts *(135)*, which cause a significantly more distorted base-pairing than the CPDs *(136)*. A total deficiency in this repair pathway is compatible with life, but affected patients (XP syndrome) exhibit a 1000-fold higher risk of skin-cancer development compared to normal subjects. The hypersensitivity of XP patients to sunlight implies that in humans NER has a major role in the removal of UV photoproducts and their persistence in the genome is a serious threat to genome stability.

To summarize briefly the reaction mechanism, the NER pathway can be subdivided into three steps: 1) lesion recognition, 2) incisions at both sides of the lesion, and 3) gap filling *(137)*. The DNA damage recognition step most likely involves the XPA protein in complex with the single-stranded binding protein RPA and possibly the XPE protein. Interestingly, these DNA damage binding proteins have a strong preference for 6-4 photoproducts over CPDs *(135)*. This differential recognition might determine the faster repair of 6-4 photoproducts as compared to CPDs.

After lesion recognition, other repair proteins like the basal transcription factor TFIIH are recruited to the lesion site *(138)*. Human TFIIH contains the XPB and XPD proteins, which possess a DNA helicase activity, which is involved in local DNA unwinding. Two incisions are made in the damaged DNA strand, one on each side of a DNA lesion. The size of the repair patch is about 25–30 nucleotides. The exact position of the incisions varies depending on the adduct. In the case of CPDs,

one incision is made 5–6 phosphodiester bonds 3′ to the lesion and another incision 22–24 bonds away from the lesion on the 5′-side *(139)*. The patch size for 6-4 photoproducts has not been determined yet. The 5′-incision is made by the ERCC1/XPF complex and the 3′-incision by the XPG protein. The NER mechanism involves the formation of an open region around a DNA lesion. Cleavage of the DNA at the borders between this region and duplex DNA is performed by structure-specific nucleases of the appropriate polarity like ERCC1/XPF and XPG *(140)*. The excised oligonucleotide is removed and finally the remaining gap is filled by a complex consisting of DNA polymerase ε, proliferating cell nuclear antigen (PCNA), and replication factor C.

UV photoproducts are not repaired with the same efficiency within all regions of the genome. In 1994, Hanawalt and co-workers discovered that CPD are in general removed several-fold faster from the transcribed genes than from the nontranscribed genes and that most of this effect is due to preferential repair of the transcribed strand *(141)*. Strand-specific repair provides an efficient mechanism to mantain transcription of essential genes, a process that is impeded by lesions like the CPD, which are able to block the progression of RNA polymerase II. This process is active on both CPD and 6-4 PP but its effect on the repair of 6-4 PP is overruled by the efficiency of the global DNA-repair system on these lesions *(142)*. In *Escherichia coli*, Selby and Sancar *(143)* isolated a transcription-repair coupling factor, which is encoded by the *mfd* gene (for mutation frequency decline), that binds to and releases the RNA polymerase blocked at the lesion site. This factor may interact with the excision-repair complex to remove the offending lesion. In human cells, the product of the *CSB* gene, ERCC6, may be the transcription-repair coupling factor *(144)* because cells that contain a defective *CSB* gene show a lack of repair of the transcribed DNA strand *(145)*.

Malfunctioning of DNA Repair Predisposes to Skin Cancer Abnormal DNA repair is associated with several human genetic diseases of which XP is the best-known. These patients, in addition to sun sensitivity, show other cutaneous abnormalities and neurological degeneration. They present a very high incidence of premalignant actinic keratosis, as well as benign and malignant skin tumors. The median age of onset of skin cancer is 8 yr, nearly 50 yrs younger than in the general population *(146)*. Complementation analysis by cell fusion has led to the identification of seven complementation groups, designated A through G, which differ in the severity of the repair deficiency. In addition to the classical XP groups, cases with typical XP clinical features but without an obvious defect in NER (almost 10% of all XP cases) are referred to as XP variants. Several XP genes have been isolated by cloning and their molecular analysis and/or protein function is fully consistent with the notion that classical XP is a disease that is due to defective NER.

Two other syndromes characterized by UV hypersensitivity are trichothiodystrophy (TTD) and Cockayne's syndrome (CS). TTD is characterized by ichthyosis, brittle hair, intelectual impairment, decreased fertility, and short stature. CS patients exhibit short stature, retinal degeneration, deafness, and various neurologic abnormalities. The relationship between these syndromes and defective DNA repair is complex. First of all, both TTD and CS patients are not especially prone to skin cancer. Although these patients are photosensitive and defective in NER at cell level, the incidence of skin cancer is not significantly different from the general population. Interestingly, the molecular characterization of these syndromes has identified in the case of TTD the involvement of the XPD and XPB genes, both subunits of the TFIIH complex, and in the case of CS a defect in the preferential repair of actively transcribed genes. These observations have led to the transcription-syndrome hypothesis, which predicts that the genes responsible for TTD and CS have dual roles in transcription and NER.

Within the XP phenotype, large variations in repair activity have been noted, ranging from 2–80% of normal levels. If XP is considered to represent the lower range of repair capabilities, those individuals expressing a reduced repair response may be at increased risk of cancer. Studies by Wei et al. *(147),* using an in vitro repair assay based on human peripheral lymphocytes *(148),* demonstrated that DNA repair capacity declines with age and is reduced in young individuals with BCC. Using the same experimental approach, Hall et al. *(149)* did not detect any significant difference in the DNA-repair capacity between patients with BCC or SCC history and control subjects. Recently, we were able to confirm the observations made by Wei et al. on Italian patients affected by BCC. These studies combine to suggest that deficiencies in DNA repair may represent a potential risk for skin- cancer development.

UV Irradiation Causes Distinct Mutations in DNA The reaction of UV with cellular DNA may cause mutations. CPD and 6-4 photoproducts are believed to be responsible for most of the cytotoxic and mutagenic effects of UV light. In bacterial as well as in mammalian cells, UVC light produces a distinct spectrum of mutations characterized by predominant C→T transitions at dipyrimidines sequences and by the occurrence of tandem-base substitutions CC→TT type (reviewed in *150).* A possible mechanism for fixation of a photolesion into a C→T transition implies that the bypass of a totally noncoding lesion occurs via insertion of an A (referred to as the A rule) across from the lesion. This would result exclusively in C→T transitions, because photolesions involving T residues would not produce mutations as a result of the insertion of the correct base (an A) opposite the T residue. Furthermore, it has been hypothesized that the high frequency of cytosine deamination in PyPy lesions may be responsible for the observed C→T transitions according to the A rule *(151).*

Most of the studies on UV mutagenesis have used germicidal lamps that emit UVC wavelengths, especially monochromatic light at 254 nm. However, the relevance of these wavelengths to sunlight-associated human skin cancer is questionable considering that UV wavelengths <280 nm (UVC) are absorbed almost completely by the earth's atmosphere. More recently the mutational specificity of UVB (290–320 nm), UVA (350–400 nm), and broad-spectrum SSL (310–1100 nm) have been analyzed in mammalian cells *(152–154).* The data revealed that although the UVB-induced mutation spectrum is very similar to UVC-induced mutation fingerprint, UVA-ex-

posed cells present a high proportion (up to 50%) of AT→TG transversions. This type of mutational event comprises a significant percentage of SSL-induced mutations (25%), whereas it was rarely detected after UVB or UVC exposure (5–9% of the total mutants). Thus, the mutagenic specificity of SSL indicates that UVA plays a significant role in solar mutagenesis. When UV-induced mutation specificity was investigated in NER-deficient cells *(154),* the mutation spectrum of both UVB and SSL showed a marked increase in tandem CC→TT transitions relative to NER-proficient cells. Moreover, the T→G transversion class disappeared from the SSL spectrum that could be entirely accounted for by the UVB-induced mutations.

The occurrence of preferential repair of the transcribed strand *(155,156)* is expected to lead to the accumulation of UV-induced mutations on the nontranscribed strand of active genes. In general this expectation has been proven experimentally using rodent-cell systems *(157–159).* In exponentially growing human cells, no strand bias in favor of the nontranscribed DNA strand was reported for UV-induced mutations *(160)* and the expected accumulation of mutations on the nontranscribed DNA strand of the target gene was only detected when G$_1$-synchronized cells were irradiated *(161).* It is important to recall that, although rodent cells present a strong difference in the repair rate of the two strands (in favor of the transcribed strand), human cells efficiently repair both strands of active genes *(156),* although the transcribed strand is repaired faster than the nontranscribed strand. By 24 hr post-irradiation, no difference between the two strands was detected by gene-specific repair assay.

UV-INDUCED PROTO-ONCOGENE MUTATIONS

Activation of Proto-oncogenes Mutational analysis of the c-*ras* genes in human melanocytic lesions *(162)* revealed that mutations are predominantly located at codon 61 of c-N-*ras* gene and are exclusively found in nodular malignant melanomas (31% mutation frequency). No c-*ras* mutations were reported in superficial spreading melanomas (SSM) nor in lentigo malignant melanomas. These findings might explain the high variability of c-*ras* mutation frequency (from 5–27%) reported in several studies *(163,164)* where the relative frequency of nodular malignant melanomas and SSM in the tumor samples was not evaluated. The absence of c-*ras* mutations in the early stage of the human melanoma strongly suggests that the modifications of this gene family may represent a late event in the development of melanoma, although no formal genetic proof exists to support this hypothesis. Whether c-*ras* mutations are a significant phenomenon in nonmelanoma skin cancers (NMSC) is also unclear *(165,166).* In a study that analyzed c-*ras* mutations in BCC and SCC from normal and XP patients *(167),* a higher frequency of c-*ras* mutations were found in XP tumors (50%) as compared to non-XP tumors (22–26%). This finding is in agreement with a key role of unrepaired UV-induced DNA lesions in c-*ras* mutations. Moreover, the majority of c-*ras* mutations were located at dipyrimidine sites, strongly suggesting that UV photodimers are involved in the molecular mechanism of proto-oncogene activation.

INACTIVATION OF TUMOR SUPPRESSOR GENES

The p53 Gene Human skin cancer is often associated with alterations of the *p53* gene. A curious exception is human melanoma, which presents a low incidence of *p53* mutations. No mutations have been reported in primary cutaneous melanomas and melanoma metastases for the conserved region of the *p53* gene (exons 5–8) *(168,169)*. The basis for the low frequency of *p53* mutations is not understood. The finding that melanomas from c-*ras* mutated/*INK4A*-deficient mice do not present p53 mutations *(170)* has led to the hypothesis that the *p16^INK4A* and *p53* genes might have overlapping tumor-suppressor functions. A direct mechanistic link between these two potent growth- and tumor-suppressor activities has yet to be established, but high levels of p19^ARF (encoded by an alternative reading frame of the *INK4A* gene) *(171)* have been observed in *p53*-deficient cells, suggesting the involvement of a regulatory feedback loop *(172)*.

The inactivation of the *p53* gene plays a major role in the etiology of NMSC. Recent studies have estimated that the incidence of UV-specific *p53* gene mutations in SCC and BCC ranges between 12% and 58% *(173–180)*. The mutation spectrum in NMSC is characterized by frequent C→T transitions (Fig. 3), and in particular a high frequency of CC→TT transitions, which represent 9% of the mutations in SCC and 12% in BCC. Both types of mutation are consistent with the mutagenic action of UV-irradiation. Although C→T transitions are common in all tumor types, tandem CC→TT transitions are exceptional in internal malignancies. Further evidence for a direct link between these mutations and UV-exposure comes from the analysis of skin tumors from DNA repair-deficient XP patients, which show a particularly high frequency of tandem CC→TT transitions *(181)*. It is interesting to recall that the same drastic increase in the relative percentage of CC→TT tandem mutations was reported in NER-deficient cells exposed to UVB or SSL *(154)*. Mutations at dipyrimidines have also been observed in normal sun-exposed skin of skin-cancer patients from Australia, suggesting that they occur at a very early stage of skin carcinogenesis *(182)*.

The distribution of *p53* mutations in skin cancers show striking differences when compared with most other types of cancers (Fig. 4). The majority of the hot-spots for skin cancer mutations suffer from slow DNA repair of UV-induced damage *(183)*. Examples of slow-repair spots are codons 196, 245, 248, 278, and 286, where more than 10% of the CPD remain 24 h after UV exposure. Other factors, like selection of forms of mutant *p53* with functional specificity for skin carcinogenesis and the rate of DNA damage at nucleotide level, might determine the mutation profile found in these tumors. When the distribution of the UV-induced *p53* mutations is analyzed, an almost even distribution of the mutations over the two strands is detected. Using human diploid-skin fibroblast as a model, Tornaletti and Pfeiffer *(183)* have shown that the average repair rate of UV-induced cyclobutane pyrimidine dimers in exons 5–9 of the *p53* gene was slower than in a control housekeeping gene and that the transcribed strand of *p53* was more rapidly repaired than the nontranscribed strand. However, as in the case of UV-treated human cells in culture, the difference in strand-specific repair might not be sufficient to leave its finger-

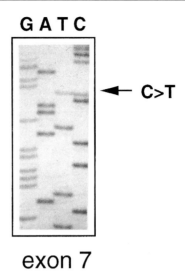

G A T C

← C>T

exon 7

Fig. 3. UV-specific mutations are present in the *p53* gene of nonmelanoma skin cancers. DNA sequencing analysis of exon 7 of the *p53* gene. DNA was extracted from a BCC biopsy, *p53* exon 7 was amplified by polymerase chain reaction (PCR), and the sequencing products were separated on a 6% urea/polyacrylamide gel and exposed to film. An arrow-head indicates the position of a C→T transition at codon 248 (nontranscribed DNA strand).

print on mutation distribution. When the analysis is confined only to tandem CC→TT transitions in NMSC, they are all located on the coding strand, suggesting that the transcription-coupled repair might act preferentially on these lesions. Also, half of the CC→TT transitions observed in NMSC are within CpG sequences, suggesting that spontaneous deamination of 5-methylcytosine may contribute to enhance the mutation rate at such sequences.

To determine whether *p53* mutations are an early or a late event in human skin-cancer development, Brash and coworkers *(184)* analyzed *p53* gene sequences in actinic keratosis biopsy samples. This condition represents an early stage in SCC development. A high p53 mutation frequency (60%) was detected in these skin lesions and the base changes found implicated sunlight as the mutagen. These results suggest that *p53* mutation is an early event in malignant conversion of the skin and contrast its role in several types of tumors where mutations in the gene occur at later stages of cancer progression. In this same study, evidence was presented that inactivating the *p53* gene (even a single allele) in mouse skin reduced the appearance of sunburn cells (apoptotic keratinocytes). The presence of a *p53* mutation (due to UV light) might therefore promote the survival of the heterozygote over the wild-type cells leading to the formation of the actinic keratosis lesion. In this model, UV light would play the dual role of both initiating and promoting carcinogen *(185)*. These combined actions of sunlight have been recently demonstrated by showing that clones of *p53*-mutated keratinocytes are present in normal human skin (initiated cells) *(186,187)* and their frequency and size increases in sun-exposed skin as compared to sun-shielded skin (during promotion) *(187)*. It is interesting to recall that, conversely, in the murine system of *p53* mutations are a late event in skin cancer development, whereas mutations are the initiating event (Fig. 1)

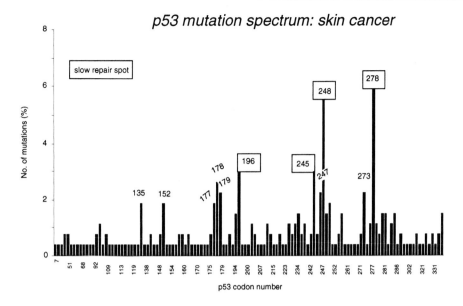

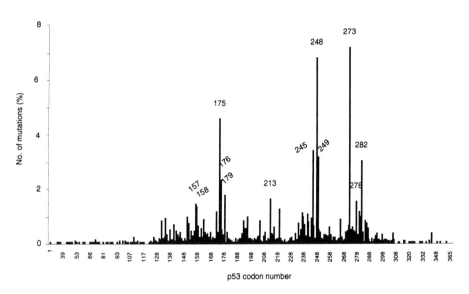

Fig. 4. The location of *p53* gene mutation in nonmelanoma skin cancers is not random. The distribution of *p53* gene mutations in nonmelanoma skin cancers (top panel) and in all human cancers (bottom panel), based on the July 1997 version of the *p53* database of the International Agency for Research on Cancer (kindly provided by P. Hainaut and T. Hernandez, IARC, Lyon, France). This database is available at URL http://www.iarc.fr/p53/homepage.htm

The p16INK4A Gene Melanoma samples present frequent loss of 9p21 *(188)*. The genomic organization of the 9p21 locus is quite complex. This region encodes for at least three potent growth inhibitor proteins, namely p16[INK4A], p15[INK4B], and p19[ARF]. Genetic alterations of the *p16[INK4A]* gene have frequently been observed in human melanoma cell lines *(189,190)*, and in some primary melanomas and metastasis (191–193). The finding of germline *p16[INK4A]* mutations in approx 50% of members of melanoma-prone families *(194)* suggested that the p16[INK4A] might be important in the etiology of inherited melanoma. Moreover, the analysis of the type of mutations detected (predominatly C→T transitions at dipyrimidine sites) might be compatible with UV mutagenesis *(195)*. More recent investigations demonstrated that the frequency of *p16[INK4A]* mutations is lower (around 10%) than initially thought. In general, the cur-

rently available data do not disprove a potential contribution of *p16[INK4A]* to melanoma susceptibility, but suggest that other critical genes responsible for melanoma susceptibility remain to be identified. Frequent LOH of 9p21 has been described in human cutaneous SCC *(196)*. Mutations in the *p16[INK4A]* have been detected in few cases of human SCC, suggesting that the inactivation of the *INK4A* locus might have some relevance to this type of skin cancer *(197)*.

The ptc Gene Patients affected by the rare nevoid basal cell carcinoma syndrome (NBCCS) have an increased frequency of BCC, medulloblastomas, and ovarian fibromas. In addition to these tumors, developmental abnormalities are a striking feature of this syndrome *(198)*. The clinical characteristics of NBCCS (early onset of multiple tumors, autosomal inheritance) suggested a heritable defect in a tumor-suppressor

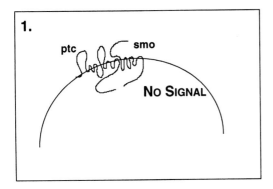

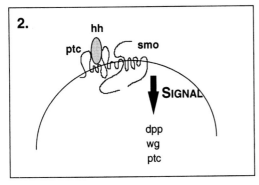

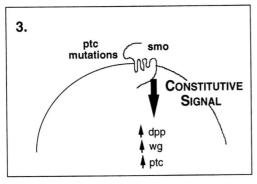

Fig. 5. Mechanism of action of the *patched* gene, a putative tumor suppressor in BCC. *Patched* (*ptch*) is a component of the *hedgehog* (*hh*) signaling pathway. Panel 1, The ptc protein represses transcription of hh target genes by inactivating the membrane protein smoothened (smo). Panel 2, The hh protein binds to ptc resulting in the activation of smo. Consequently the transcription of hh genes, like *decapentaplegic* (*dpp*), *wingless* (*wg*), and *ptc* itself, is increased. Panel 3, If ptc is functionally inactive, *smo* may be constitutively activated with subsequent unregulated overexpression of *hh* genes.

naling membrane protein smo and ptc form an inactive complex (Fig. 5, panel 1), which is reverted by hh binding to ptc (Fig. 5, panel 2). In the absence of functional ptc (Fig. 5, panel 3), the smo protein may be constitutively active with subsequent unregulated overexpression of downstream target genes, including *ptc* itself. Most of the genes in *hedgehog* pathway have been showed to be conserved in mammals and play equally critical roles in development. *Sonic hedgehog* (*shh*), the most common vertebrate homolog, is required for correct embryonic patterning. *Ptch* is expressed in all tissues that express *shh*. Because the *ptch* gene product is a suppressor of *hedgehog* function, loss of this gene might lead to abnormal expression of hedgehog proteins, including ptch itself. Northern-blot analysis of BCCs has indeed shown that ptch protein is barely detectable in normal skin, although it is expressed at variable levels in tumors *(203)*. Overexpression of *shh* has been shown to cause BCC in animal models. Recent findings *(204)* suggest that any mutation leading to the expression of the putative oncogene *Gli1* (which is also a target and mediator of *shh* signaling) in basal cells might induce BCC formation. In fact, an analysis of a large sample of human sporadic BCCs has shown that these tumors consistently express *Gli1*, but not necessarily *shh* or *ptc*. *Gli1* expression in basal cells might be an early event in BCC formation. Moreover, activating somatic missense mutations in the *smo* gene have been detected in sporadic BCCs from three patients supporting the hypothesis that *smo* can also function as an oncogene in BCCs *(121)*.

The human *ptch* gene is about 34 kb and encompasses at least 23 exons. Determination of the DNA sequence of this gene facilitated direct mutation screening in both hereditary and sporadic BCC. Although in NBCCS inactivation of both copies of *ptch* has been observed (typically loss of one allele and inactivation by point mutation of the second allele), in sporadic BCCs not all the tumors present inactivation of both copies of the gene. The type of mutations identified *(200,201,203,205–208)* are summarized in Fig. 6. Almost half are frameshift mutations or deletions/insertions of short tracts of nucleotides. The remaining *ptch* mutations are base-pair substitutions that are consistent with UV-induced mutations. C→T mutations are the predominant class of mutations and a small number of CC→TT tandem mutations have also been described. However, half of the *ptch* mutations found are not typical of UV mutagenesis (frameshift and small deletions/insertions). Furthermore, allelic loss of this locus, which is a frequent event in both hereditary and sporadic BCCs, is also unlikely to be induced by UV light. Therefore, the role of UV-irradiation in the genesis of *ptch* gene mutations remains obscure.

The mutations detected in the *ptch* gene resemble those found in most tumor-suppressor genes, frequently nonsense mutations, deletions, and insertions, leading to truncated or absent protein product *(209)*. These mutations are loss of function mutations. The pattern of mutations affecting the *p53* gene are in this sense peculiar because missense mutations are frequently detected (78% of the total mutations detected) (Fig. 6). The *ptch* gene shares characteristics with tumor suppressors genes like *APC*, which encode cytoplasmic proteins with signaling functions. Mutations in the *ptch* gene, like those of the *APC* gene, lead to development of relatively benign lesions. As

gene. Loss of heterozygosity at 9q22.3 is indeed a consistent feature of both sporadic and hereditary BCC *(199)*. Linkage analysis of NBCCS kindreds demonstrated that the gene responsible for this condition maps to the 9q22.3 region. The human homolog of the *Drosophila ptc* gene, termed *ptch*, was isolated from this chromosomal region *(200,201)*. The *ptc* gene encodes for a transmembrane glycoprotein whose function is transcriptional repression of members of the *Wnt* (*wingless*) and *TGF-β* (*decapentaplegic*) gene families, all of which encode morphogenetic proteins. The action of ptc is opposed by the product of the *hedgehog* (*hh*) gene, which encodes a secreted glycoprotein that activates transcriptionally both ptc-repressible genes and *ptc* itself *(116)*. The current model *(202)*, based on studies in *Drosophila* mutants, suggests that the sig-

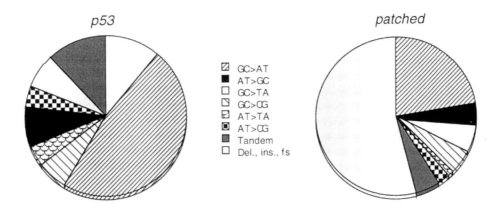

Fig. 6. The role of UV-irradiation in the occurrence of *ptch* genetic alterations is unclear. The type of mutations detected in the *p53* gene (right panel) and in the *ptch* gene (left panel) of BCCs are displayed. The *p53* mutations are derived from the IARC database (see legend to Fig. 4). *Ptch* mutations are based on data in the literature *(200,201,203,205–207)*.

speculated by Sidransky *(210)*, the effect of alterations of these so-called gatekeeper genes may be the generation of clusters of cells that do not respond properly to signals from neighboring cells, and therefore proliferate abnormally. These clusters might be the target population for a cascade of genetic events (like *p53* mutations) that will eventually lead to tumor progression.

UV-INDUCED IMMUNOSUPPRESSION AND DEVELOPMENT OF SKIN CANCER

The important role of immunosuppression in skin carcinogenesis was first demonstrated in the 1980s by Kripke *(211,212)* and Daynes et al. *(213)*, who studied UV-induced tumors in mice. Such tumors are highly antigenic and frequently immunologically rejected upon transplantation into syngeneic mice. However, in mice exposed to a short course of UV-irradiation rejection does not occur and the tumors grow rapidly *(214)*. UV irradiation alters not only rejection of UV-induced tumors but also contact hypersensitivity (CHS) and delayed-type hypersensitivity. In the CHS response, erythema, edema, and induration of the skin are induced following topical application of dinitrochlorobenzene to the skin of mice. Such effects are greatly reduced if the skin is previously irradiated by UV. The modulation of the delayed-type hypersensitivity response by UV is similar with the exception that in this case the antigen is a protein introduced by intradermal or subcutaneous route *(214,215)*. Moreover, UV-irradiation (at both chronic and acute doses) appears to decrease the CHS response even when the hapten is applied to UV-unexposed sites, demonstrating a systemic, rather than a local, impairment of immune system *(216)*.

The ability of UVB-irradiation to impair induction of CHS response is dependent on the mouse strain *(217)*. UV-irradiation impairs the CHS response induced by dinitrofluorobenzene in UVB-susceptible (UVB-S) strains but has no effect in UVB-resistant (UVB-R) strains. Similar UVB-R and UVB-S traits have been suggested for humans. The UVB-R and UVB-S phenotypes are genetically determined by polymorphic alleles at two independent genetic loci in mouse *(218)*, whereas the evidence concerning a genetic basis in humans is far from being proved *(216)*. Among subjects with histories of BCC and SCC, the frequency of the UVB-S phenotype is extremely high (>92%), significantly higher than that observed among normal

subjects of comparable age *(218)*. Moreover, 100% (10/10) of patients with a diagnosed malignant melanoma proved to be UVB-S after UV-irradiation whereas only 30–50% of healthy human volunteers presented the UVB-S phenotype *(219)*. NMSC patients with large and multiple lesions showed decreased skin-test reaction to common antigens and increased number of circulating suppressor T lymphocytes, respectively *(220)*, while patients with small NMSC lesions showed normal skin-test reactions *(221)*. Whether the relationship between immunosuppression and skin cancer is one of cause or effect remains an open question. However, the extremely high risk of developing BCC and SCC among immunosuppressed organ-transplant patients strongly suggests a causal association *(216)*.

The molecular mechanisms by which UV irradiation impairs immune response remain controversial. It is recognized that to generate a biological response, nonionizing radiation must first be absorbed by a photoreceptor molecule that converts it into a biochemical signal. A possible candidate is urocanic acid (UCA), a deamination product of histidine that is abundant in the stratum corneum of the skin. This photoreceptor undergoes photoisomerization from the *trans* to the *cis* form upon UVB-irradiation and *cis*-UCA is a potent systemic immunosuppressor *(222)*. When injected into the skin, *cis*-UCA mimics the effects of UV, causing depletion of epidermal Langherans cells (LC) and inhibition of CHS *(223)*.

Simon et al. *(224)* and Devary et al. *(225)* hypothesized that UV-irradiation activates the transcription factors AP-1 and NF-κB. These factors have been shown to increase the expression of tumor necrosis factor-α (TNF-α) and other cytokine genes *(226)*. These cytokines produce morphologic cytoskeletal changes in LC or in other antigen presenting cells, along with a decrease of class II major histocompatibility molecules. TNF-α is released from keratinocytes and is implicated in the immunosuppressive cascade of events induced by UV irradiation. It has been shown to play a role in the suppression of the CHS response in mice. This effect is completely reversed by anti-TNF-α antibodies *(227)*. UV-irradiation may also affect the capacity of keratinocytes to produce a pro-inflammatory cytokine, interferon γ (IFN-γ). A decrease of *in situ* expression of IFN-γ may be related to the direct effects of UV-irradiation on IFN-γ-producing T cells, or indirectly to a release of a mediator like interleukin-10 (IL-10) *(228)*. IL-10 is a potent inhibitor of T-helper lymphocytes and impairs LC function *(229)*. The major source of IL-10 in UV-irradiated skin seems to be the infiltrating macrophages.

UV-induced structural alterations in DNA appear to be the signal for the production of immunoregulatory cytokines *(230)*. Topical applications of an excision-repair enzyme (T4 endonuclease V) by liposomes to UV-irradiated mouse skin reduces the number of CPDs 6 h after UV-irradiation *(231)*. Remarkably, this treatment also prevented the UV-induced impairment of CHS response and the generation of local and systemic T-suppressor lymphocytes *(232)*. Control liposomes containing heat-inactivated enzyme did not produce this effect *(231)*. In other studies, lower doses of UVB induced a greater degree of immunosuppression in mice that were deficient for DNA repair than that observed in normal control mice *(233)*. Recent results *(234)* strongly suggest that the immunological response may be even more important than DNA-repair capacity in the etiology of UV-induced skin cancer. It is known that both XPD and TTD patients are characterized by a deficiency in DNA-repair capacity, due to a molecular defect at the level of the XPD gene. However, only XPD patients show an increased risk of skin cancer. Cells from XPD patients, but not from TTD patients, showed an inhibition of the intercellular adhesion molecule (*ICAM-1*) gene expression after UVB-irradiation. Furthemore, the transfection of XPD cells with the wild-type XPD cDNA completely restored normal ICAM expression.

REFERENCES

1. Fuchs, E. and Green, H. (1980) Changes in keratin gene expression during terminal differentiation of the keratinocyte. *Cell* **19**:1033–1042.
2. Fuchs, E. (1990) Epidermal differentiation: the bare essentials. *J. Cell. Biol.* **111**:2807–2814.
3. Moll, R., Franke, W. W., Volc-Platzer, B., and Krepler, R. (1982) Different keratin polypeptides in epidermis and other epithelia of human skin: a specific cytokeratin of molecular weight 46,000 in epithelia of the pilosebaceous tract and basal cell epitheliomas. *J. Cell. Biol.* **95**:285–295.
4. Rice, R. H. and Green, H. (1978) Relation of protein synthesis and transglutaminase activity to formation of the cross-linked envelope during terminal differentiation of the cultured human epidermal keratinocyte. *J. Cell. Biol.* **76**:705–711.
5. Eckert, R. L. and Green, H. (1986) Structure and evolution of the human involucrin gene. *Cell* **46**:583–589.
6. Mehrel, T., Hohl, D., Rothnagel, J. A., Longley, M. A., Bundman, D., Cheng, C., et al. (1990) Identification of a major keratinocyte cell envelope protein, loricrin. *Cell* **61**:1103–1112.
7. Markova, N. G., Marekov, L. N., Chipev, C. C., Gan, S. Q., Idler, W. W., and Steinert, P. M. (1993) Profilaggrin is a major epidermal calcium-binding protein. *Mol. Cell. Biol.* **13**:613–625.
8. Rheinwald, J. G. and Green, H. (1975) Serial cultivation of strains of human epidermal keratinocytes: the formation of keratinizing colonies from single cells. *Cell* **6**:331–343.
9. Hennings, H., Michael, D., Cheng, C., Steinert, P., Holbrook, K., and Yuspa, S. H. (1980) Calcium regulation of growth and differentiation of mouse epidermal cells in culture. *Cell* **19**:245–254.
10. Filvaroff, E., Stern, D. F., and Dotto, G. P. (1990) Tyrosine phosphorylation is an early and specific event involved in primary keratinocyte differentiation. *Mol. Cell. Biol.* **10**:1164–1173.
11. Filvaroff, E., Calautti, E., McCormick, F., and Dotto, G. P. (1992) Specific changes of *Ras* GTPase-activating protein (GAP) and a GAP-associated p62 protein during calcium-induced keratinocyte differentiation. *Mol. Cell. Biol.* **12**:5319–5328.
12. Lee, E. and Yuspa, S. H. (1991) Changes in inositol phosphate metabolism are associated with terminal differentiation and neoplasia in mouse keratinocytes. *Carcinogenesis* **12**:1651–1658.
13. Dlugosz, A. A. and Yuspa, S. H. (1993) Coordinate changes in gene expression which mark the spinous to granular cell transition in epidermis are regulated by protein kinase C. *J. Cell Biol.* **120**:217–225.
14. Punnonen, K., Denning, M., Lee, E., Li, L., Rhee, S. G., and Yuspa, S. H. (1993) Keratinocyte differentiation is associated with changes in the expression and regulation of phospholipase C isoenzymes. *J. Invest. Dermatol.* **101**:719–726.
15. Calautti, E., Missero, C., Stein, P. L., Ezzell, R. M., and Dotto, G. P. (1995) fyn tyrosine kinase is involved in keratinocyte differentiation control. *Genes Dev.* **9**:2279–2291.
16. Fischer, D. F., Gibbs, S., van De Putte, P., and Backendorf, C. (1996) Interdependent transcription control elements regulate the expression of the SPRR2A gene during keratinocyte terminal differentiation. *Mol. Cell. Biol.* **16**:5365–5374.
17. Andersen, B., Weinberg, W. C., Rennekampff, O., McEvilly, R. J., Bermingham J. R., Jr, Hooshmand, F., et al. (1997) Functions of the POU domain genes Skn-1a/i and Tst-1/Oct-6/SCIP in epidermal differentiation. *Genes Dev.* **11**:1873–1884.
18. Andreoli, J. M., Jang, S. I., Chung, E., Coticchia, C. M., Steinert, P. M., and Markova, N. G. (1997) The expression of a novel, epithelium-specific ets transcription factor is restricted to the most differentiated layers in the epidermis. *Nucleic Acids Res.* **25**:4287–4295.
19. Oettgen, P., Alani, R. M., Barcinski, M. A., Brown, L., Akbarali, Y., Boltax, J., et al. (1997) Isolation and characterization of a novel epithelium-specific transcription factor, ESE-1, a member of the ets family. *Mol. Cell. Biol.* **17**:4419–4433.
20. Nehls, M., Pfeifer, D., Schorpp, M., Hedrich, H., and Boehm, T. (1994) New member of the winged-helix protein family disrupted in mouse and rat nude mutations. *Nature* **372**:103–107.
21. Brissette, J. L., Li, J., Kamimura, J., Lee, D., and Dotto, G. P. (1996) The product of the mouse nude locus, Whn, regulates the balance between epithelial cell growth and differentiation. *Genes Dev.* **10**:2212–2221.
22. Prowse, D. M., Bolgan, L., Molnar, A., and Dotto, G .P. (1997) Involvement of the Sp3 transcription factor in induction of p21Cip1/WAF1 in keratinocyte differentiation. *J. Biol. Chem.* **272**:1308–1314.
23. Gandarillas, A. and Watt, F. M. (1995) Changes in expression of members of the fos and jun families and myc network during terminal differentiation of human keratinocytes. *Oncogene* **11**:1403–1407.
24. Leask, A., Byrne, C., and Fuchs, E. (1991) Transcription factor AP2 and its role in epidermal-specific gene expression. *Proc. Natl. Acad. Sci. USA* **88**:7948–7952.
25. Vastrik, I., Kaipainen, A., Penttila, T. L., Lymboussakis, A., Alitalo, R., Parvinen, M., et al. (1995) Expression of the mad gene during cell differentiation in vivo and its inhibition of cell growth *in vitro*. *J. Cell. Biol.* **128**:1197–1208.
26. Lymboussaki, A., Kaipainen, A., Hatva, E., Vastrik, I., Jeskanen, L., Jalkanen, M., et al. (1996) Expression of Mad, an antagonist of Myc oncoprotein function, in differentiating keratinocytes during tumorigenesis of the skin. *Br. J. Cancer* **73**:1347–1355.
27. Yuspa, S. H. (1991) Cutaneous carcinogenesis: natural and experimental, in *Physiology Biochemistry and Molecular Biology of the Skin* (L. Goldsmith, ed.), Oxford University Press, New York.
28. Rasmussen, K. S., Glenthoj, A., and Arffmann, E. (1983) Skin carcinogenesis in rats by 3-methylcholanthrene and 7,12-dimethylbenz(alpha)anthracene. Influence of dose and frequency on tumour response and its histological type. *Acta Pathol. Microbiol. Immunol. Scand. [A]* **91**:445–455.
29. Mohr, U., Emura, M., Aufderheide, M., Riebe, M., and Ernst, H. (1989) Possible role of genetic predisposition in multigeneration carcinogenesis. *IARC Sci. Publ.* **96**:93–103.
30. Nelson, M. A., Futscher, B. W., Kinsella, T., Wymer, J., and Bowden, G. T. (1992) Detection of mutant Ha-*ras* genes in chemically initiated mouse skin epidermis before the development of benign tumors. *Proc. Natl. Acad. Sci. USA* **89**:6398–6402.

31. Balmain, A., Ramsden, M., Bowden, G. T., and Smith, J. (1984) Activation of the mouse cellular Harvey-ras gene in chemically induced benign skin papillomas. *Nature* **307**:658–660.

32. Clark-Lewis, I. and Murray, A. W. (1978) Tumor promotion and the induction of epidermal ornithine decarboxylase activity in mechanically stimulated mouse skin. *Cancer Res.* **38**:494–497.

33. Argyris, T. S. (1980) Tumor promotion by abrasion induced epidermal hyperplasia in the skin of mice. *J. Invest. Dermatol.* **75**: 360–362.

34. Furstenberger, G. and Marks, F. (1983) Growth stimulation and tumor promotion in skin. *J. Invest. Dermatol.* **81**:157–162.

35. Hansen, L. A. and Tennant, R. W. (1994) Follicular origin of epidermal papillomas in v-Ha-ras transgenic TG.AC mouse skin. *Proc. Natl. Acad. Sci. USA* **91**:7822–7826.

36. Yuspa, S. H., Ben, T., Patterson, E., Michael, D., Elgjo, K., and Hennings, H. (1976) Stimulated DNA synthesis in mouse epidermal cell cultures treated with 12-O-tetradecanoyl-phorbol-13-acetate. *Cancer Res.* **36**:4062–4068.

37. Reiners, J. J., Jr. and Slaga, T. J. (1983) Effects of tumor promoters on the rate and commitment to terminal differentiation of subpopulations of murine keratinocytes. *Cell* **32**:247–255.

38. Tennenbaum, T., Weiner, A. K., Belanger, A. J., Glick, A. B., Hennings, H., and Yuspa, S. H. (1993) The suprabasal expression of alpha 6 beta 4 integrin is associated with a high risk for malignant progression in mouse skin carcinogenesis. *Cancer Res.* **53**:4803–4810.

39. Tennenbaum, T., Yuspa, S. H., Grover, A., Castronovo, V., Sobel, M. E., Yamada, Y., et al. (1992) Extracellular matrix receptors and mouse skin carcinogenesis: altered expression linked to appearance of early markers of tumor progression. *Cancer Res.* **52**:2966–2976.

40. Bremner, R. and Balmain, A. (1990) Genetic changes in skin tumor progression: correlation between presence of a mutant ras gene and loss of heterozygosity on mouse chromosome 7. *Cell* **61**:407–417.

41. Kemp, C. J., Fee, F., and Balmain, A. (1993) Allelotype analysis of mouse skin tumors using polymorphic microsatellites: sequential genetic alterations on chromosomes 6, 7, and 11. *Cancer Res.* **53**:6022–6027.

42. Boukamp, P., Peter, W., Pascheberg, U., Altmeier, S., Fasching, C., Stanbridge, E. J., et al. (1995) Step-wise progression in human skin carcinogenesis *in vitro* involves mutational inactivation of p53, rasH oncogene activation and additional chromosome loss. *Oncogene* **11**:961–969.

43. Nagase, H., Bryson, S., Cordell, H., Kemp, C. J., Fee, F., and Balmain, A. (1995) Distinct genetic loci control development of benign and malignant skin tumours in mice. *Nature Genet.* **10**:424–429.

44. Holliday, R. (1989) Chromosome error propagation and cancer. *Trends Genet.* **5**:42–45.

45. Klein-Szanto, A. J., Larcher, F., Bonfil, R. D., and Conti, C. J. (1989) Multistage chemical carcinogenesis protocols produce spindle cell carcinomas of the mouse skin. *Carcinogenesis* **10**:2169–2172.

46. Buchmann, A., Ruggeri, B., Klein-Szanto, A. J., and Balmain, A. (1991) Progression of squamous carcinoma cells to spindle carcinomas of mouse skin is associated with an imbalance of H-ras alleles on chromosome 7. *Cancer Res.* **51**:4097–4101.

47. Stoler, A. B., Stenback, F., and Balmain, A. (1993) The conversion of mouse skin squamous cell carcinomas to spindle cell carcinomas is a recessive event. *J. Cell. Biol.* **122**:1103–1117.

48. Kumar, N. M. and Gilula, N. B. (1996) The gap junction communication channel. *Cell* **84**:381–388.

49. Dotto, G. P., el-Fouly, M. H., Nelson, C., and Trosko, J. E. (1989) Similar and synergistic inhibition of gap-junctional communication by ras transformation and tumor promoter treatment of mouse primary keratinocytes. *Oncogene* **4**:637–641.

50. Brissette, J. L., Kumar, N. M., Gilula, N. B., and Dotto, G. P. (1991) The tumor promoter 12-O-tetradecanoylphorbol-13-acetate and the ras oncogene modulate expression and phosphorylation of gap junction proteins. *Mol. Cell. Biol.* **11**:5364–5371.

51. Oelze, I., Kartenbeck, J., Crusius, K., and Alonso, A. (1995) Human papillomavirus type 16 E5 protein affects cell-cell communication in an epithelial cell line. *J. Virol.* **69**:4489–4494.

52. Klann, R. C., Fitzgerald, D. J., Piccoli, C., Slaga, T. J., and Yamasaki, H. (1989) Gap-junctional intercellular communication in epidermal cell lines from selected stages of SENCAR mouse skin carcinogenesis. *Cancer Res.* **49**:699–705.

53. Budunova, I. V., Carbajal, S., Viaje, A., and Slaga, T. J. (1996) Connexin expression in epidermal cell lines from SENCAR mouse skin tumors. *Mol. Carcinogenesis* **15**:190–201.

54. Kamibayashi, Y., Oyamada, Y., Mori, M., and Oyamada, M. (1995) Aberrant expression of gap junction proteins (connexins) is associated with tumor progression during multistage mouse skin carcinogenesis in vivo. *Carcinogenesis* **16**:1287–1297.

55. Sawey, M. J., Goldschmidt, M. H., Risek, B., Gilula, N. B., and Lo, C. W. (1996) Perturbation in connexin 43 and connexin 26 gap-junction expression in mouse skin hyperplasia and neoplasia. *Mol. Carcinogenesis* **17**:49–61.

56. Quintanilla, M., Brown, K., Ramsden, M., and Balmain, A. (1986) Carcinogen-specific mutation and amplification of Ha-ras during mouse skin carcinogenesis. *Nature* **322**:78–80.

57. Brown, K., Buchmann, A., and Balmain, A. (1990) Carcinogen-induced mutations in the mouse c-Ha-ras gene provide evidence of multiple pathways for tumor progression. *Proc. Natl. Acad. Sci. USA* **87**:538–542.

58. Brown, K., Quintanilla, M., Ramsden, M., Kerr, I. B., Young, S., and Balmain, A. (1986) v-ras genes from Harvey and BALB murine sarcoma viruses can act as initiators of two-stage mouse skin carcinogenesis. *Cell* **46**:447–456.

59. Roop, D. R., Lowy, D. R., Tambourin, P. E., Strickland, J., Harper, J. R., Balaschak, M., et al. (1986) An activated Harvey ras oncogene produces benign tumours on mouse epidermal tissue. *Nature* **323**:822–824.

60. Dotto, G. P., Weinberg, R. A., and Ariza, A. (1988) Malignant transformation of mouse primary keratinocytes by Harvey sarcoma virus and its modulation by surrounding normal cells. *Proc. Natl. Acad. Sci. USA* **85**:6389–6393.

61. Greenhalgh, D. A., Welty, D. J., Player, A., and Yuspa, S. H. (1990) Two oncogenes, v-fos and v-ras, cooperate to convert normal keratinocytes to squamous cell carcinoma. *Proc. Natl. Acad. Sci. USA* **87**:643–647.

62. Brissette, J. L., Missero, C., Yuspa, S. H., and Dotto, G. P. (1993) Different levels of v-Ha-ras p21 expression in primary keratinocytes transformed with Harvey sarcoma virus correlate with benign versus malignant behavior. *Mol. Carcinogenesis* **7**:21–25.

63. Bailleul, B., Surani, M. A., White, S., Barton, S. C., Brown, K., Blessing, M., et al. (1990) Skin hyperkeratosis and papilloma formation in transgenic mice expressing a ras oncogene from a suprabasal keratin promoter. *Cell* **62**:697–708.

64. Greenhalgh, D. A., Rothnagel, J. A., Quintanilla, M. I., Orengo, C. C., Gagne, T. A., Bundman, D. S., et al. (1993) Induction of epidermal hyperplasia, hyperkeratosis, and papillomas in transgenic mice by a targeted v-Ha-ras oncogene. *Mol. Carcinogenesis* **7**:99–110.

65. Kemp, C. J., Burns, P. A., Brown, K., Nagase, H., and Balmain, A. (1994) Transgenic approaches to the analysis of ras and p53 function in multistage carcinogenesis. *Cold Spring Harbor Symp. Quant. Biol.* **59**:427–434.

66. Wang, X. W. (1997) p53 tumor-suppressor gene: clues to molecular carcinogenesis. *J. Cell. Physiol.* **173**:247–255.

67. Burns, P. A., Kemp, C. J., Gannon, J. V., Lane, D. P., Bremner, R., and Balmain, A. (1991) Loss of heterozygosity and mutational alterations of the p53 gene in skin tumours of interspecific hybrid mice. *Oncogene* **6**:2363–2369.

68. Ruggeri, B., Caamano, J., Goodrow, T., DiRado, M., Bianchi, A., Trono, D., et al. (1991) Alterations of the p53 tumor suppressor gene during mouse skin tumor progression. *Cancer Res.* **51**:6615–6621.

69. Donehower, L. A., Harvey, M., Slagle, B. L., McArthur, M. J., Montgomery C. A., Jr., Butel, J. S., et al. (1992) Mice deficient for p53 are developmentally normal but susceptible to spontaneous tumours. *Nature* **356**:215–221.

70. Jacks, T., Remington, L., Williams, B. O., Schmitt, E. M., Halachmi, S., Bronson, R. T., et al. (1994) Tumor spectrum analysis in p53-mutant mice. *Curr. Biol.* **4**:1–7.

71. Bouffler, S. D., Kemp, C. J., Balmain, A., and Cox, R. (1995) Spontaneous and ionizing radiation-induced chromosomal abnormalities in p53-deficient mice. *Cancer Res.* **55**:3883–3889.

72. Kemp, C. J., Donehower, L. A., Bradley, A., and Bailmain, A. (1993) Reduction of p53 gene dosage does not increase initiation or promotion but enhances malignant progression of chemically induced skin tumors. *Cell* **74**:813–822.

73. Cano, A., Gamallo, C., Kemp, C. J., Benito, N., Palacios, J., Quintanilla, M., et al. (1996) Expression pattern of the cell adhesion molecules. E-cadherin, P-cadherin and alpha 6 beta 4 intergrin is altered in pre-malignant skin tumors of p53-deficient mice. *Int. J. Cancer* **65**:254–262.

74. Weinberg, W. C., Azzoli, C. G., Kadiwar, N., and Yuspa, S.H. (1994) p53 gene dosage modifies growth and malignant progression of keratinocytes expressing the v-rasHa oncogene. *Cancer Res.* **54**:5584–5592.

75. Karin, M., Liu, Z. G., and Zandi, E. (1997) AP-1 function and regulation. *Curr. Opin. Cell Biol.* **9**:240–246.

76. Dotto, G. P., Gilman, M. Z., Maruyama, M., and Weinberg, R. A. (1986) c-myc and c-fos expression in differentiating mouse primary keratinocytes. *EMBO J.* **5**:2853–2857.

77. Fisher, C., Byers, M. R., Iadarola, M. J., and Powers, E. A. (1991) Patterns of epithelial expression of Fos protein suggest important role in the transition from viable to cornified cell during keratinization. *Development* **111**:253–258.

78. Smeyne, R. J., Vendrell, M., Hayward, M., Baker, S. J., Miao, G. G., Schilling, K., et al. (1993) Continuous c-fos expression precedes programmed cell death *in vivo*. *Nature* **363**:166–169.

79. Saez, E., Rutberg, S. E., Mueller, E., Oppenheim, H., Smoluk, J., Yuspa, S. H., et al. (1995) c-fos is required for malignant progression of skin tumors. *Cell* **82**:721–732.

80. Greenhalgh, D. A., Rothnagel, J. A., Wang, X. J., Quintanilla, M. I., Orengo, C. C., Gagne, T. A., et al. (1993) Hyperplasia, hyperkeratosis and benign tumor production in transgenic mice by a targeted v-fos oncogene suggest a role for fos in epidermal differentiation and neoplasia. *Oncogene* **8**:2145–2157.

81. Alevizopoulos, A. and Mermod, N. (1997) Transforming growth factor-beta: the breaking open of a black box. *Bioessays* **19**:581–591.

82. O'Kane, S. and Ferguson, M. W. (1997) Transforming growth factor betas and wound healing. *Int. J. Biochem. Cell. Biol.* **29**:63–78.

83. Bascom, C. C., Wolfshohl, J. R., Coffey R. J., Jr., Madisen, L., Webb, N. R., Purchio, A. R., et al. (1989) Complex regulation of transforming growth factor beta 1, beta 2, and beta 3 mRNA expression in mouse fibroblasts and keratinocytes by transforming growth factors beta 1 and beta 2. *Mol. Cell. Biol.* **9**:5508–5515.

84. Missero, C., Ramon Y., Cajal, S., and Dotto, G. P. (1991) Escape from transforming growth factor beta control and oncogene cooperation in skin tumor development. *Proc. Natl. Acad. Sci. USA* **88**:9613–9617.

85. Akhurst, R. J., Fee, F., and Balmain, A. (1988) Localized production of TGF-beta mRNA in tumour promoter-stimulated mouse epidermis. *Nature* **331**:363–365.

86. Pelton, R. W., Saxena, B., Jones, M., Moses, H. L., and Gold, L. I. (1991) Immunohistochemical localization of TGF beta 1, TGF beta 2, and TGF beta 3 in the mouse embryo: expression patterns suggest multiple roles during embryonic development. *J. Cell. Biol.* **115**:1091–1105.

87. Glick, A. B., Kulkarni, A. B., Tennenbaum, T., Hennings, H., Flanders, K. C., O'Reilly, M., et al. (1993) Loss of expression of transforming growth factor beta in skin and skin tumors is associated with hyperproliferation and a high risk for malignant conversion. *Proc. Natl. Acad. Sci. USA* **90**:6076–6080.

88. Kane, C. J., Hebda, P. A., Mansridge, J. N., and Hanawalt, P. C. (1991) Direct evidence for spatial and temporal regolation of transforming growth factor beta 1 expression during cutaneous wound healing. *J. Cell. Physiol.* **148**:157–173.

89. Escherick, J. S., DiCunto, F., Flanders, K. C., Missero, C., and Dotto, G. P. (1993) Transforming growth factor beta 1 induction is associated with transforming growth factors beta 2 and beta 3 downmodulation in 12-O-tetradecanoylphorbol-13-acetate-induced skin hyperplasia. *Cancer Res.* **53**:5517–5522.

90. Cui, W. (1995) Concerted action of TGF-β1 and its type II receptor in control of epidermal homeostasis in transgenic mice. *Genes Dev.* **9**:945–955.

91. Cui, W., Fowlis, J., Bryson, S., Duffie, E., Ireland, H., Balmain, A., et al. (1996) TGFβ1 inhibits the formation of benign skin tumors, but enhances progression to invasive spindle carcinomas in transgenic mice. *Cell* **86**:531–542.

92. Sellheyer, K., Bickenbach, J. R., Rothnagel, J. A., Bundman, D., Longley, M. A., Krieg, T., et al. (1993) Inhibition of skin development by overexpression of transforming growth factor beta 1 in the epidermis of transgenic mice. *Proc. Natl. Acad. Sci. USA* **90**:237–5241.

93. Matzuk, M. M., Lu, N., Vogel, H., Sellheyer, K., Roop, D. R., and Bradley, A. (1995) Multiple defects and perinatal death in mice deficient in follistatin. *Nature* **374**:360–363.

94. Kulkarni, A. B., Huh, C. G., Becker, D., Geiser, A., Lyght, M., Flanders, K. C., et al. (1993) Transforming growth factor beta 1 null mutation in mice causes excessive inflammatory response and early death. *Proc. Natl. Acad. Sci. USA* **90**:770–774.

95. Glick, A. B., Lee, M. M., Darwiche, N., Kulkarni, A. B., Karlsson, S., and Yuspa, S. H. (1994) Targeted deletion of the TGF-beta 1 gene causes rapid progression to squamous cell carcinoma. *Genes Dev.* **8**:2429–2440.

96. Hubner, G., Hu Q., Smola H., and Werner S. (1996) Strong induction of activin expression after injury suggests an important role of activin in wound repair. *Dev. Biol* **173**:490–98.

97. Blessing, M., Schirmacher P., and Kaiser S. (1996) Overexpression of bone morphogenetic protein-6 (BMP-6) in the epidermis of transgenic mice: inhibition or stimulation of proliferation depending on the pattern of transgene expression and formation of psoriatic lesions. *J. Cell. Biol.* **135**:227–239.

98. Kaplan, F. S. (1996) Skin and bones. *Arch. Dermatol.* **132**:815–818.

99. Sherr, C. J. (1996) Cancer cell cycles. *Science* **274**:1672–1677.

100. Sicinski, P., Donaher, J. L., Parker, S. B., Li, T., Fazeli, A., Gardner, H., et al. (1995) Cyclin D1 provides a link between development and oncogenesis in the retina and breast. *Cell* **82**:621–630.

101. Bianchi, A. B., Fischer, S. M., Robles, A. I., Rinchik, E. M., and Conti, C. J. (1993) Overexpression of cyclin D1 in mouse skin carcinogenesis. *Oncogene* **8**:1127–1133.

102. Robles, A. I., Larcher, F., Whalin, R. B., Murillas, R., Richie, E., Gimenez-Conti, I. B., et al. (1996) Expression of cyclin D1 in epithelial tissues of transgenic mice results in epidermal hyperproliferation and severe thymic hyperplasia. *Proc. Natl. Acad. Sci. USA* **93**:7634–7638.

103. Sherr, C. J. and Roberts, J. M. (1995) Inhibitors of mammalian G1 cyclin-dependent kinases. *Genes Dev.* **9**:1149–1163.

104. Hannon, G. J. and Beach, D. (1994) p15 INK4B is a potential effector of TGF-β-induced cell cycle arrest. *Nature* **371**:257–261.

105. Serrano, M., Lee, H., Chin, L., Cordon-Cardo, C., Beach, D., and DePinho, R. A. (1996) Role of the INK4a locus in tumor suppression and cell mortality. *Cell* **85**:27–37.

106. Chin, L., Pomerantz, J., Polsky, D., Jacobson, M., Cohen, C., Cordon-Cardo, C., et al. (1997) Cooperative effects of INK4a and ras in melanoma susceptibility *in vivo*. *Genes Dev.* **11**:2822–2834.

107. Missero, C., Calautti, E., Eckner, R., Chin, J., Tsai, L. H., Livingston, D. M., et al. (1995) Involvement of the cell-cycle inhibitor Cip1/WAF1 and the E1A-associated p300 protein in terminal differentiation. *Proc. Natl. Acad. Sci. USA* **92**:5451–5455.

108. Missero, C., Di Cunto, F., Kiyokawa, H., Koff, A., and Dotto, G. P. (1996) The absence of p21Cip1/WAF1 alters keratinocyte growth and differentiation and promotes ras-tumor progression. *Genes Dev.* **10**:3065–3075.

109. Deng, C., Zhang, P., Harper, J. W., Elledge, S. J., and Leder, P. (1995) Mice lacking p21CIP1/WAF1 undergo normal development, but are defective in G1 checkpoint control. *Cell* **82**:675–684.

110. Fero, M. L., Rivkin, M., Tasch, M., Porter, P., Carow, C. E., Firpo, E., et al. (1996) A syndrome of multiorgan hyperplasia with features of gigantism, tumorigenesis, and female sterility in p27(Kip1)-deficient mice. *Cell* **85**:733–744.

111. Kiyokawa, H., Kineman, R. D., Manova-Todorova, K. O., Soares, V. C., Hoffman, E. S., Ono, M., et al. (1996) Enhanced growth of mice lacking the cyclin-dependent kinase inhibitor function of p27(Kip1). *Cell* **85**:721–732.

112. Nakayama, K., Ishida, N., Shirane, M., Inomata, A., Inoue, T., Shishido, N., et al. (1996) Mice lacking p27(Kip1) display increased body size, multiple organ hyperplasia, retinal dysplasia, and pituitary tumors. *Cell* **85**:707–720.

113. Weinberg, W. C., Montano, N. E., and Deng, C. (1997) Loss of p21CIP1/WAF1 does not recapitulate accelerated malignant conversion caused by p53 loss in experimental skin carcinogenesis. *Oncogene* **15**:685–690.

114. Funk, J. O., Waga, S., Harry, J. B., Espling, E., Stillman, B., and Galloway, D. A. (1997) Inhibition of CDK activity and PCNA-dependent DNA replication by p21 is blocked by interaction with the HPV-16 E7 oncoprotein. *Genes Dev.* **11**:2090–2100.

115. Jones, D. L., Alani, R. M., and Munger, K. (1997) The human papillomavirus E7 oncoprotein can uncouple cellular differentiation and proliferation in human keratinocytes by abrogating p21Cip1-mediated inhibition of cdk2. *Genes Dev.* **11**:2101–2111.

116. Perrimon, H. (1995) Hedgehog and beyond. *Cell* **80**:517–520.

117. Stone, D. M., Hynes, M., Armanini, M., Swanson, T. A., Gu, Q., Johnson, R. L., et al. (1996) The tumour-suppressor gene patched encodes a candidate receptor for Sonic hedgehog. *Nature* **384**:129–134.

118. Marigo, V., Davey, R. A., Zuo, Y., Cunningham, J. M., and Tabin, C. J. (1996) Biochemical evidence that patched is the Hedgehog receptor. *Nature* **384**:176–179.

119. Fan, H., Oro, A. E., Scott, M. P., and Khavari, P. A. (1997) Induction of basal cell carcinoma features in transgenic human skin expressing Sonic Hedgehog. *Nature Med.* **3**:788–792.

120. Oro, A. E., Higgins, K. M., Hu, Z., Bonifas, J. M., Epstein E. H., Jr., and Scott, M. P. (1997) Basal cell carcinomas in mice overexpressing sonic hedgehog. *Science* **276**:817–821.

121. Xie J., Murone, M., Luoh, S. M., Ryan, A., Gu, Q., Zhang, C., et al. (1998) Activating smoothened mutation in sporadic basal-cell carcinoma. *Nature* **391**:90–92.

122. Dahmane, N., Lee, J., Robins, P., Heller, P., Ruiz, I., and Altaba, A. (1997) Activation of the transcription factor Gli1 and the sonic hedgehog signaling pathway in skin tumors. *Nature* **389**:876–881.

123. Jonason, A. S., Kunala, S., Price, G. J., Spinelli, H. M., Persing, J. A., Leffell, D. J., et al. (1996) Frequent clones of p53-mutated keratinocytes in normal human skin. *Proc. Natl. Acad. Sci. USA* **93**:14,025–14,029.

124. Loignon, M., Fetni, R., Gordon, A. J., and Drobetsky, E. A. (1997) A p53-independent pathway for induction of p21 and concomitant G1 arrest in UV-irradiated human skin fibroblasts. *Cancer Res.* **57**:3390–3394.

125. De Gruijl, F. R., Van Der Meer, J. B., and Van Der Leun, J. C. (1983) Dose-time dependency of tumor formation by chronic UV exposure. *Photochem. Photobiol.* **37**:53–62.

126. Leffel, D. J. and Brash, D. E. (1996) Sunlight and skin cancer. *Sci. Am.* **275**:52–59.

127. Li, G., Tron, V., and Ho, V. (1998) Induction of squamous cell carcinoma in p53-deficient mice after ultraviolet irradiation. *J. Invest. Dermatol.* **110**:72–75.

128. Cleaver, J. E. (1968) Defective repair replication of DNA in Xeroderma pigmentosum. *Nature* **218**:651–656.

129. International Agency for Research on Cancer. (1992) IARC Monographs on the Evaluation of Carcinogenic Risks to Humans: Solar and Ultraviolet Radiation, vol. 55. Lyon, France.

130. Pfeifer, G. P. (1997) Formation and processing of UV photoproducts: effects of DNA sequence and chromatin environment. *Photochem. Photobiol.* **65**:270–283.

131. Tommasi, S., Denissenko, M. F., and Pfeifer, G. P. (1997) Sunlight induces pyrimidine dimers preferentially at 5-methylcytosine bases. *Cancer Res.* **57**:4727–4730.

132. Lippke, J. A., Gordon, L. K., Brash, D. E., and Haseltine, W. A. (1981) Distribution of UV light-induced damage in a defined sequence of human DNA: detection of alkaline-sensitive lesions at pyrimidine nucleoside-cytidine sequences. *Proc. Natl. Acad. Sci. USA* **78**:3388–3392.

133. Brash, D. E., Seetharam, S., Kraemer, K. H., Seidman, M. M., and Bredberg, A. (1987) Photoproduct frequency is not the major determinant of UV base substitution hot spots or cold spots in human cells. *Proc. Natl. Acad. Sci. USA* **84**:3782–3786.

134. Pfeifer, G. P., Drouin, R., Riggs, A. D., and Holmquist, G. P. (1991) *In vivo* mapping of a DNA adduct at nucleotide resolution: detection of pyrimidine (6-4) pyrimidone photoproducts by ligation-mediated polymerase chain reaction. *Proc. Natl. Acad. Sci. USA* **88**:1374–1378.

135. Szymkowski, D. E., Lawrence, C. W., and Wood, R. D. (1993) Repair by human cell extracts of single (6-4) and cyclobutane thymine-thymine photoproducts in DNA. *Proc. Natl. Acad. Sci. USA* **90**:9823–9827.

136. Kim, J.-K. and Choi, B. (1995) The solution structure of DNA duplex-decamer containing the (6-4) photoproduct of thymidylyl(3'→5')thymine by NMR and relaxation matrix refinement. *Eur. J. Biochem.* **228**:849–854.

137. Wood, R. D. (1996) DNA repair in eukaryotes. *Ann. Rev. Biochem.* **65**:135–167.

138. Schaeffer, L., Roy, R., Humbert, S., Moncollin, V., Vermeulen, W., Hoeijmakers, J. H., et al. (1993) DNA repair helicase: a component of BTF2 (TFIIH) basic transcription factor. *Science* **260**:58–63.

139. Huang, J.-C., Svoboda, D. L., Reardon, J. T., and Sancar, A. (1992) Human nucleotide excision nuclease removes thymine dimers from DNA by incising the 22nd phopshodiester bond 5' and the 6th phosphodiester bond 3' to the photodimer. *Proc. Natl. Acad. Sci. USA* **89**:3664–3668.

140. O' Donovan, A., Davies, A., Moggs, J. G., West, S. C., and Wood, R. D. (1994) XPG endonuclease makes the 3' incision in human DNA nucleotide excision repair. *Nature* **371**:432–435.

141. Hanawalt, P. (1994) Transcription-coupled repair and human disease. *Science* **266**:1957–1958.

142. van Hoffen, A., Venema, J., Meschini, R., van Zeeland, A. A., and Mullenders, L. H. F. (1995) Transcription-coupled repair removes both cyclobutane pyrimidine dimers and 6-4 photoproducts with equal efficiency and in a sequential way from transcribed DNA in xeroderma pigmentosum group C fibroblasts. *EMBO J.* **14**:360–367.

143. Selby, C. P. and Sancar, A. (1991) Gene- and strand-specific repair *in vitro*: partial purification of a transcription-repair coupling factor. *Proc. Natl. Acad. Sci. USA* **88**:8232–8236.

144. Troelstra, C., Odijk, H., de Wit, J., Westerveld, A., Thompson, L. H., Bootsma, D., et al. (1990) Molecular cloning of the human DNA excision repair gene ERCC-6. *Mol. Cell. Biol.* **10**:5806–5813.

145. van Hoffen, A., Natarajan, A. T., Mayne, L. V., van Zeeland, A. A., Mullenders, L. H., and Venema, J. (1993) deficient repair of the transcribed strand of active genes in Cockayne's syndrome cells. *Nucleic Acids Res.* **21**:5890–5895.

146. Kraemer, K. H., Levy, D. D., Parris, C. N., Gozukara, E. M., Moriwaki, S., Adelberg, S., et al. (1994) Xeroderma Pigmentosum and related disorders: examining the linkage between defective DNA repair and cancer. *J. Invest. Dermatol.* **103**:96S–101S.

147. Wei, Q., Matanoski, G. M., Farmer, E. R., Hedayati, M. A., and Grossman, L. (1993) DNA repair and aging in basal cell carcinoma: a molecular epidemiology study. *Proc. Natl. Acad. Sci. USA* **90**:1614–1618.

148. Athas, W. F., Hedayati, M. A., Matanoski, G. M., Farmer, E. R., and Grossman, L. (1991) Development and field-test validation of an assay for DNA repair in circulating human lymphocytes. *Cancer Res.* **51**:5786–5793.

149. Hall, J., English, D. R., Artuso, M., Armstrong, B. K., and Winter, M. (1994) DNA repair capacity as a risk factor for non-melanocytic skin cancer: a molecular epidemiology study. *Int. J. Cancer* **58**:179–184.

150. Sage, E. (1993) Distribution and repair of photolesions in DNA: genetic consequences and the role of sequence context. *Photochem. Photobiol.* **57**:163–174.

151. Tessman, I., Liu, S.-K., and Kennedy, M. A. (1992) Mechanisms of SOS mutagenesis of UV-irradiated DNA: mostly error-free processing of deaminated cytosine. *Proc. Natl. Acad. Sci. USA* **89**:1159–1163.

152. Drobetsky, E. A., Moustacchi, E., Glickman, B. W., and Sage, E. (1994) The mutational specificity of simulated sunlight at the aprt locus in rodent cells. *Carcinogenesis* **15**:1577–1583.

153. Drobetsky, E. A., Turcotte, J., and Chateauneuf, A. (1995) A role for ultraviolet-A in solar mutagenesis. *Proc. Natl. Acad. Sci. USA* **92**:2350–2354.

154. Sage, E., Lamolet, B., Brulay, E., Moustacchi, E., Chateauneuf, A., and Drobetsky, E. A. (1996) Mutagenic specificity of solar UV light in nucleotide excision repair-deficient rodent cells. *Proc. Natl. Acad. Sci. USA* **93**:176–180.

155. Mellon, I., Bohr, V. A., Smith, C. A., and Hanawalt, P. C. (1986) Preferential DNA repair of an active gene in human cells. *Proc. Natl. Acad. Sci. USA* **83**:8878–8882.

156. Mellon, I., Spivak, G., and Hanawalt, P. C. (1987) Selective removal of transcription-blocking DNA damage from the transcribed strand of the mammalian DHFR gene. *Cell* **51**:241–249.

157. Vrieling, H., van Rooijen, M. L., Groen, N. A., Zdzienicka, M. Z., Simons, J. W. I. M., Lohman, P. H. M., et al. (1989) DNA strand specificity of the UV-induced mutations in mammalian cells. *Mol. Cell. Biol.* **9**:1277–1283.

158. Vrieling, H., Venema, J., van Rooyen, M.-L., van Hoffen, A., Menechini, P., Zdzienicka, M. Z., et al. (1991) Strand specificity for UV-induced DNA repair and mutations in the Chinese Hamster HPRT gene. *Nucleic Acids Res.* **19**:2411–2415.

159. Menichini, P., Vrieling, H., and van Zeeland, A. A. (1991) Strand specific mutation spectra in repair proficient and repair deficient hamster cells. *Mutat. Res.* **251**:143–155.

160. Palombo, F., Kohfeldt, E., Calcagnile, A., Nehls, P., and Dogliotti, E. (1992) N-methyl-N-nitrosourea-induced mutations in human cells. Effects of the transcriptional activity of the target gene. *J. Mol. Biol.* **223**:587–594.

161. McGregor, W. G., Chen, R.-H., Lukash, L., Maher, V. M., and McCormick, J. J. (1991) Cell cycle-dependent strand bias for UV-induced mutations in the transcribed strand of excision repair-proficient human fibroblasts but not in repair-deficient cells. *Mol. Cell. Biol.* **11**:1927–1934.

162. Jafari, M., Pap, T., Kirchner, S., Diener, U., Henschler, D., Burg, G., et al. (1995) Analysis of ras mutations in human melanocytic lesions: activation of the ras gene seems to be associated with the nodular type of human malignant melanoma. *J. Cancer Res. Clin. Oncol.* **121**:23–30.

163. Albino, A. P., Nanus, D. M., Mentle, I. R., Cordon-Cardo, C., McNutt, N. S., Bressler, J., et al. (1989) Analysis of ras oncogenes in malignant melanoma and precursor lesions: correlation of point mutations with differentiation phenotype. *Oncogene* **4**:1363–1374.

164. Veer, L. J. V. T., Burgering, B. M. T., Versteeg, R., Boot, A. J. M., Ruiter, D. J., Osanto, S., et al. (1989) N-ras mutations in human cutaneous melanoma from sun-exposed body-sites. *Mol. Cell. Biol.* **9**:3114–3116.

165. Pierceall, W. E., Goldberg, L. H., Tainsky, M. A., Mukhopadhyay, T., and Ananthaswamy, N. H. (1991) Ras gene mutations and amplification in human non-melanoma skin cancers. *Mol. Carcinogenesis* **4**:96–202.

166. Campbell, C., Quinn, A. G., and Rees, J. I. (1993) Codon 12 Harvey-ras mutations are rare events in non-melanoma human skin cancer. *Br. J. Dermatol.* **128**:111–114.

167. Daya-Grosjean, L., Robert, C., Drougard, C., Suarez, H., and Sarasin, A. (1993) Hight mutation frequency in ras genes of skin tumors isolated from DNA repair deficient Xeroderma Pigmentosum patients. *Cancer Res.* **53**:1625–1629.

168. Lubbe, J., Reichel, M., Burg, G., and Kleihues, P. (1994) Absence of p53 gene mutations in cutaneous melanoma. *J. Invest. Dermatol.* **102**:819–821.

169. Papp, T., Jafari, M., and Schiffmann, D. (1996) Lack of p53 mutations and loss of heterozigosity in non-cultured human melanocytic lesions. *J. Cancer Res. Clin. Oncol.* **122**:541–548.

170. Chin, L., Pomerantz, J., Polsky, D., Jacobson, M., Cohen, C., Cordon-Cardo, C., et al. (1997) Cooperative effects of INK4a and ras in melanoma susceptibility *in vivo*. *Genes Develop.* **11**:2822–2834.

171. Quelle, D. E., Zindy, F., Ashmun, R. A., and Sherr, C. J. (1995) Alternative reading frames of the INK4a tumor suppressor gene encode two unrelated proteins capable of inducing cell cycle arrest. *Cell* **83**:993–1000.

172. Quelle, D. E., Cheng, M., Ashmun, R. A., and Sherr, C. J. (1997) Cancer-associated mutations of the INK4a locus cancel cell cycle arrest by p16INK4a but not by the alternative reading frame protein p19ARF. *Proc. Natl. Acad. Sci. USA* **94**:669–673.

173. Brash, D. E., Rudolph, J. A., Simon, J. A., Lin, A., McKenna, G. J., Baden, H. P., et al. (1991) A role for sunlight in skin cancer: UV-induced p53 mutations in squamous cell carcinoma. *Proc. Natl. Acad. Sci. USA* **88**:10,124–10,128.

174. Pierceall, W. E., Mukhopadhyay, T., Goldberg, L. H., and Ananthaswamy, N. H. (1991) Mutations in the p53 tumor suppressor gene in human cutaneous squamous cell carcinomas. *Mol. Carcinogenesis* **4**:445–449.

175. Moles, J.-P., Moyret, C., Guillot, B., Jeanteur, P., Guilhou, J.-J., Theillet, C., et al. (1993) p53 gene mutations in human epithelial skin cancers. *Oncogene* **8**:583–588.

176. Ziegler, A., Leffell, D. J., Kunala, S., Sharma, H. W., Gailani, M., Simon, A. J., et al. (1993) Mutation hotspots due to sunlight in the p53 gene of nonmelanoma skin cancer. *Proc. Natl. Acad. Sci. USA* **90**:4216–4220.

177. Kubo, Y., Urano, Y., Yoshimoto, K., Iwahana, H., Fukuhara, K., Arase, S., et al. (1994) p53 gene mutations in human skin cancers and precancerous lesions: comparison with immunohistochemical analysis. *J. Invest. Dermatol.* **102**:440–444.

178. Campbell, C., Quinn, A. G., Ro, Y.-S., Angus, B., and Rees, J. L. (1993) p53 mutations are common and early events that precede tumor invasion in squamous cell neoplasia of the skin. *J. Invest. Dermatol.* **100**:746–748.

179. Rady, P., Scinicariello, F., Wagner, R. F., and Tyring, S. K. (1992) p53 mutations in basal cell carcinomas. *Cancer Res.* **52**:3804–3806.

180. D'Errico, M., Calcagnile, A. S., Corona, R., Fucci, M., Annessi, G., Baliva, G., et al. (1997) p53 mutations and chromosome instability in basal cell carcinoma developed at an early or late age. *Cancer Res.* **57**:747–752.

181. Dumaz, N., Drougard, A., Sarasin, A., and Daya-Grosjean, L. (1993) Specific UV-induced mutation spectrum in the p53 gene of skin tumors from DNA-repair-deficient xeroderma pigmentosum patients. *Proc. Natl. Acad. Sci. USA* **90**:10,529–10,533.

182. Nakazawa, H., English, D., Randell, P. L., Nagazawa, K., Martel, N., Armstrong, B. K., et al. (1994) UV and skin cancer: specific p53 gene mutations in normal skin as a biologically relevant exposure measurement. *Proc. Natl. Acad. Sci. USA* **91**:360–364.

183. Tornaletti, S. and Pfeifer, G. P. (1994) Slow repair of pyrimidine dimers at p53 mutation hotspots in skin cancer. *Science* **263**:1436–1438.

184. Ziegler, A., Jonason, A. S., Leffell, D. J., Simon, J. A., Sharma, H. W., Kimmelman, J., et al. (1994) Sunburn and p53 in the onset of skin cancer. *Nature* **372**:773–776.

185. Kamb, A. (1994) Sun protection factor p53. *Nature* **372**:730-731.

186. Ren, C.-P., Hedrum, A., Ponten, F., Nister, M., Ahmadian, A., Lundeberg, J., et al. (1996) Human epidermal cancer and accompanying precursors have identical p53 mutations different from p53 mutations in adjacent areas of clonally expanded non-neoplastic keratinocytes. *Oncogene* **12**:765–773.

187. Jonason, A. S., Kunala, S., Price, G. J., Restifo, R. J., Spinelli, H. M., Persing, J. A., et al. (1996) Frequent clones of p53-mutated keratinocytes in normal human skin. *Proc. Natl. Acad. Sci. USA* **93**:14,025–14,029.

188. Herlyn, M. (1993) *Molecular and Cellular Biology for Melanoma.* R.G. Landes, Austin, TX.

189. Kamb, A., Gruis, N. A., Weaver-Feldhaus, J., Liu, Q., Harshman, K., Tavtigian, S. V., et al. (1994) A cell cycle regulator potentially involved in genesis of many tumor types. *Science* **264**:436–439.

190. Nobori, T., Miura, K., Wu, D. J., Lois, A., Takabayashi, K., and Carson, D. A. (1994) Deletions of the cyclin-dependent kinase-4 inhibitor gene in multiple human cancers. *Nature* **368**:753–756.

191. Dracopoli, N. C. and Fountain, J. W. (1996) CDKN2 mutations in melanoma. *Cancer Surveys* **26**:115–132.

192. Gruis, N. A., Weaver-Feldhaus, J., Liu, Q., Frye, C., Eeles, R., Orlow, I., et al. (1995) Genetic evidence in melanoma and bladder cancers that p16 and p53 function in separate pathways of tumor suppression. *Am. J. Pathol.* **146**:1199–1206.

193. Platz, A., Ringborg, U., Lagerlof, B., Lundqvist, E., Sevigny, P., and Inganas, M. (1996) Mutational analysis of the CDKN2 gene in metastases from patients with cutaneous malignant melanoma. *Br. J. Cancer* **73**:344–348.

194. Goldstein, A. M. and Tucker, M. A. (1997) Screening for CDKN2A mutations in hereditary melanoma. *J. Natl. Cancer Inst.* **89**:676–678.

195. Maestro, R. and Boiocchi, M. (1995) Sunlight and melanoma: an answer from MTS1 (p16). *Science* **267**:15–16.

196. Quinn, A. G., Sikkink, S., and Rees, J. L. (1994) Basal cell carcinoma and Squamous cell carcinoma of human skin show distinct pattern of Chromosome loss. *Cancer Res.* **54**:4756–4759.

197. Kubo, Y., Urano, Y., Matsumoto, K., Ahsan, K., and Arase, S. (1997) Mutations of the INK4a locus in squamous cell carcinomas of human skin. *Biochem. Biophys. Res. Commun.* **232**:38–41.

198. Gorlin, R. J. (1987) Nevoid basel-cell carcinoma syndrome. *Medicine* **66**:98–113.

199. Quinn, A. G., Campbell, C., Healy, E., and Rees, J. L. (1994) Chromosome 9 allele loss occurs in both basal and squamous cell carcinoma of the skin. *J. Invest. Dermatol.* **102**:300–303.

200. Hahn, H., Wicking, C., Zaphiropoulos, P. G., Gailani, M. R., Shanley, S., Chidambaram, A., et al. (1996) Mutations of the human homolog of Drosophila patched in the nevoid basal cell carcinoma syndrome. *Cell* **85**:841–851.

201. Johnson, R. L., Rothman, A. L., Xie, J., Goodrich, L. V., Bare, J. W., Bonifas, J. M., et al. (1996) Human homolog of patched, a candidate gene for the basal cell nevus syndrome. *Science* **272**:1668–1671.

202. Stone, D. M., Hynes, M., Armanini, M., Swanson, T. A., Gu, Q., Johnson, R. L., et al. (1996) The tumor-suppressor gene patched encodes a candidate receptor for sonic hedgehog. *Nature* **384**:129–134.

203. Gailani, M. R., Stahle-Backdahl, M., Leffell, D. J., Glynn, M., Zaphiropoulos, P. G., Pressman, C., et al. (1996) The role of the human homologue of Drosophila patched in sporadic basal cell carcinomas. *Nature Genet.* **14**:78–81.

204. Dahmane, N., Lee, J., Robins, P., Heller, P., and Ruiz i Altaba, A. (1997) Activation of the transcription factor Gli1 and the Sonic hedgehog signalling pathway in skin tumors. *Nature* **389**:876–881.

205. Unden, A. B., Holmberg, E., Lundh-Rozell, B., Stahle-Backdahl, M., Zaphiropoulos, P. G., Toftgard, R., et al. (1996) Mutations in the human homologue of Drosophila patched (PTCH) in basal cell carcinomas and the Gorlin syndrome: different *in vivo* mechanisms of PTCH inactivation. *Cancer Res.* **56**:4562–4565.

206. Chidambaram, A., Goldstein, A. M., Gailani, M. R., Gerrard, B., Bale, S. J., DiGiovanna, J. J., et al. (1996) Mutations in the human homologue of the Drosophila patched gene in caucasian and african-american nevoid basal cell carcinoma syndrome patients, *Cancer Res.* **56**:4599–4601.

207. Wolter, M., Reifenberger, J., Sommer, C., Ruzicka, T., and Reifenberger, G. (1997) Mutations in the human homologue of the Drosophila segment polarity gene patched (PTCH) in sporadic basal cell carcinomas of the skin and primitive neuroectodermal tumors of the central nervous system, *Cancer Res.* **57**:2581–2585.

208. Wicking, C., Shanley, S., Smyth, I., Gillies, S., Negus, K., Graham, S., et al. (1997) Most germ-line mutations in the nevoid basal cell carcinoma syndrome lead to a premature termination of the PATCHED protein, and no genotype-phenotype correlations are evident, *Am. J. Human Genet.* **60**:21–26.

209. Harris, C. C. (1996) The 1995 Walter Hubert Lecture—molecular epidemiology of human cancer: insights from the mutational analysis of the p53 tumour-suppressor gene. *Br. J. Cancer* **73**:261–269.

210. Sidransky, D. (1996) Is human patched the gatekeeper of common skin cancers? *Nature Genet.* **14**:7–8.

211. Kripke, M. (1981) Immunologic mechanisms in UV radiation carcinogenesis. *Adv. Cancer Res.* **34**:69–106.

212. Kripke, M. L. (1984) Immunologic unresponsiveness induced by UV radiation. *Immunol. Rev.* **80**:87–102.

213. Daynes, R. A., Bernhard, E. J., Gurish, M. F., and Lynch, D. H. (1981) Experimental photoimmunology: immunologic ramifications of UV-induced carcinogenesis. *J. Invest. Dermatol.* **77**:77–85.

214. Kripke, M. L. (1990) Effect of UV Radiation on tumor immunity. *J. Natl. Cancer Inst.* **82**:1392–1396.

215. Elmets, C. A. and Bergstresser, P. R. (1982) Ultraviolet radiation effects on immune response. *Photochem. Photobiol.* **101**:715–719.

216. Streilein, J. W., Taylor, J. R., Vincek, V., Kurimoto, I., Shimizu, T., Tie, C., et al. (1994) Immune surveillance and sunlight-induced skin cancer. *Immunol. Today* **15**:174–179.

217. Streilein, W., Taylor, J. R., Vincek, V., Kurimoto, I., Richardson, J., Tie, C., et al. (1994) Relationship between ultraviolet radiation-induced immunosuppression and carcinogenesis. *J. Invest. Dermatol.* **103**:107S–111S.

218. Yoshikawa, T. and Streilein, J. W. (1990) Genetic basis of the effects of ultraviolet light B on cutaneous immunity. *Immunogenetics* **32**:398–405.

219. Yoshikawa, T., Rae, V., Bruins-Slot, W., Van den Berg, J. W., Taylor, J. R., and Streilein, J. W. (1990) Susceptibility to effects of UVB radiation on induction of contact hypersensitivity as a risk factor for skin cancer in humans. *J. Invest. Dermatol.* **95**:530–536.

220. Weimar, V. M., Ceilley, R. I., and Goeken, J. A. (1980) Cell-mediated immunity in patients with basal and squamous cell skin cancer. *J. Am. Acad. Dermatol.* **2**:143–147.

221. Frentz, G., da Cunha Bang, F., Munch-Petersen, B., and Wantzin, G. L. (1988) Increased number of circulating suppressor T lymphocytes in sun-induced multiple skin cancer. *Cancer* **61**:294–297.

222. Noonan, F. P. and De Fabo, E. (1992) Immunosuppression by ultraviolet B radiation: initiation by urocanic acid. *Immunol. Today* **13**:250–254.

223. Kurimoto, F. and Srteilein, J. W. (1992) Cis-urocanic acid suppression of contact hypersensitivity induction is mediated via tumor necrosis factor α. *J. Immunol.* **148**:3072–3078.

224. Simon, M., Aragane, Y., Schwarz, A., Luger, T., and Schwarz, T. (1994) UVB light induces nuclear factor kB (NF-kB) activity independently from chromosomal DNA damage in cell-free cytoplasmic extracts. *J. Invest. Dermatol.* **102**:422–427.

225. Devary, Y., Rosette, C., Di Donato, J., and Karin, M. (1993) NF-κB activation by ultraviolet light is not dependent on a nuclear signal. *Science* **261**:1442–1445.

226. Chaplin, D. and Hogquist, K. (1992) Interactions between TNF and interleukin-1, in *Tumor Necrosis Factors: The Molecules and Their Emerging Role in Medicine* (Beutler, B., ed.), Raven Press, New York, pp. 197.

227. Vermeer, M. and Streilein, J. W. (1990) Ultraviolet-B-light induced alterations in epidermal Langherans cells are mediated by tumor necrosis factor α. *Photodermatol. Photoimmunol. Photomed.* **7**:258–265.

228. Grewe, M., Gyufko, K., and Krutmann, J. (1995) Interleukin-10 production by cultured human keratinocytes: regulation by ultraviolet B and ultraviolet A1 radiation. *J. Invest. Dermatol.* **104**:3–6.

229. Enk, A. H., Angeloni, V., Udey, M. C., and Kats, S. I. (1993) Inibition of Langherans cell antigen-presenting function by IL-10: A role for IL-10 in induction of tolerance. *J. Immunol.* **151**:2390–2398.

230. Stein, B., Rahmsdorf, H., Steffen, A., Litfin, M., and Herrlich, P. (1989) UV induced DNA damage is an intermediate step in UV induced expression of human immunodeficiency virus type-1, collagenase, c-*fos* and metallothionein. *Mol. Cell. Biol.* **9**:5169–5181.

231. Kripke, M. L., Cox, P. A., Alas, L. G., and Yarosh, D. B. (1992) Pyrimidine dimers in DNA initiate systemic immunosuppression in UV-irradiated mice. *Proc. Natl. Acad. Sci. USA* **89**:7516–7520.

232. Hersey, P., Haran, G., Hasic, E., and Edwards, A. (1983) Alteration of T cell subsets and induction of suppressor T cell activity in normal subjects after exposure to sunlight. *J. Immunol.* **131**:171–174.

233. Vink, A. A., Strickland, F. M., Bucana, C., Cox, P. A., Ronza, L., Yarosh, D. B., et al. (1996) Localization of DNA damage and its role in anigen-presenting cell function in ultraviolet-irradiated mice. *J. Exp. Med.* **183**:1491–1500.

234. Ahrens, C., Grewe, M., Benreburg, M., Grether-Beck, S., Quilliet, X., Mezzina, M., et al. (1997) Photocarcinogenesis and inhibition of intercellular adhesion molecule 1 expression in cells of DNA repair defective individuals. *Proc. Natl. Acad. Sci. USA* **94**:6837–6841.

19 The Molecular Biology of Leukemias

Arnold B. Gelb, MD and L. Jeffrey Medeiros, MD

INTRODUCTION

Approximately 50% of *de novo* acute leukemias have distinctive molecular abnormalities, most frequently chromosomal translocations *(1,2)*. These translocations typically involve genes that are involved in transcription and differentiation *(3)*. As a result of the translocation, these genes are disrupted and the 5'-segment of one gene is joined to the 3'-end of a second gene to form a novel fusion gene, from which chimeric mRNA is transcribed and protein is translated. Inversions occur as well, which also create fusion genes from which novel proteins are generated *(1,3)*. In contrast, many of the known translocations that occur in chronic leukemias and malignant lymphomas affect proto-oncogenes, which are involved in cell proliferation or survival, and an antigen-receptor gene. As a result of the translocation, the proto-oncogene is brought into proximity with the involved antigen receptor gene locus, typically without disrupting the coding region of the proto-oncogene. Under the influence of the antigen-receptor gene enhancers or promoters, the proto-oncogene is constitutively expressed, resulting in increased expression (overexpression) of the normal (nonmutated) protein *(1,3)*. A common theme in such translocations are errors in the normal recombinational mechanisms involving the antigen-receptor genes.

Other molecular mechanisms have been implicated in leukemogenesis *(4)*. Point mutations cause missense or nonsense mutations that result in abnormal or truncated protein products. Gene amplification may result in overexpression of genes within the amplicon. Numerical gains or losses of chromosomes, such as trisomies or monosomies due to nondisjunction, are detected in a large subset of acute and chronic leukemias. Gene deletions, like those arising from partial chromosomal deletions or unbalanced translocations, may result in loss of one copy of a tumor-suppressor gene. Subsequent inactivation of the remaining normal copy by hypermethylation, point mutation, or deletion allows neoplastic transformation. Often more

than one mechanism is involved, leading to the accumulation of genetic lesions that culminates in leukemogenesis or subsequently contributes to disease progression.

ACUTE MYELOID LEUKEMIA

Acute myeloid leukemias (AMLs) are neoplasms composed of immature myeloid cells. AMLs are characterized by the presence of at least 30% myeloblasts in the blood or bone marrow according to the French–American–British (FAB) classification(s). These leukemias are classified on the basis of their morphological features and cytochemical reactions, as well as by immunophenotype in some cases, according to the FAB criteria *(5)*. It is also useful to determine whether AML has arisen *de novo*, is arising in the setting of a pre-existing myelodysplasia, or is secondary to chemotherapy for another disorder. A variety of cytogenetic and/or molecular abnormalities have been associated with various types of AML (Table 1).

TRANSLOCATIONS INVOLVING THE RETINOIC ACID RECEPTOR GENE

t(15;17)(q21;q21) The t(15;17)(q21;q21) occurs exclusively in acute promyelocytic leukemia (APL), classified in FAB system as M3 *(5)*. APLs represent approx 5–13% of all *de novo* AMLs in various studies *(2,6)*. There also appears to be variation in genetic predisposition to the development of APL. For example, in Los Angeles County in the United States, the incidence of APL is 24% in adult Latinos, compared with 8% in non-Latinos, and similar high incidences of APL have been reported in children from Central and South America and Italy *(6)*. The presence of the t(15;17) consistently predicts responsiveness to a specific treatment, all-*trans*-retinoic acid (ATRA). Retinoic acid is a ligand for the retinoic acid receptor α (RARα), which is involved in the t(15;17). ATRA is thought to overcome the block in cell maturation, allowing the neoplastic cells to mature and be eliminated *(7,8)*. Unlike other FAB subtypes of AML, in which a multi-step accumulation of genetic defects has been described (point mutations in genes or abnormalities of chromosome number), additional molecular abnormalities

From: *The Molecular Basis of Human Cancer* (W. B. Coleman and G. J. Tsongalis, eds.), © Humana Press Inc., Totowa, NJ.

Table 1
Cytogenetic and Molecular Abnormalities in AML

Chromosomal translocations	*Genes*	*Comments*
Involving RARα		
t(15;17)(q21;q21)	PML	DNA binding, cell proliferation
	RARα	Transcription factor
		ATRA responsive
t(11;17)(q23;q21)	PLZF	Zn-finger transcription factor
	RARα	Transcription factor
t(5;17)(q32;q21)	NPM	RNA transport/processing
	RARα	Transcription factor
Involving core-binding factor		
t(8;21)(q22;q22.3)	eto	Zn-finger transcription factor
	aml1	*runt*-like transcription factor
t(3;21)(q26;q22)	evi1, MDS1, EAP	contains Zn-finger motif
	aml1	*runt*-like transcription factor
t(12;21)(p13;q22)	TEL	*ets*-like transcription factor
	aml1	*runt*-like transcription factor
t(1;21)(p36;q22),	Unknown	Rare in AML and MDS
t(5;21)(q13;q22),	aml1	*runt*-like transcription factor
t(17;21)(q11;q22)		
inv(16)(p13;q22),	CBFβ	Stabilizes CBF binding to DNA
t(16;16)(p13;q22),	MYH11	Smooth-muscle myocingene
del(16q)		
Involving *mll*		
t(11;v)(q23;v)	mll	*Drosophila trithorax* homology
	Variable	Many partner genes, AF-9 of
		t(9;11)(p22;q23) is commonest
Involving nucleoporin genes		
t(6;9)(p23;q34)	dek	Putative transcription factor
	can	Nucleoporin
Cryptic	set	Unknown function
	can	Nucleoporin
t(7;11)(p15;p15)	HOXA9	Homeobox gene
	NUP98	Nuclear-pore complex gene
inv(11)(p15;q22)	DDX10	DEAD-box putative RNA
	NUP98	helicase
		Nuclear-pore complex gene
Involving genes of the *ets* family		
(t16;21)(p11;q22)	TLS/FUS	*EWS*-like RNA-binding protein
	erg	*ets*-like transcription factor
t(12;22)(p13;q11)	TEL	*ets*-like transcription factor
	MN1	Cloned from meningioma
Other Translocations		
t(8;16)(p11;13)	MOZ	Monocytic leukemia Zn finger
	CBP	Transcriptional activation
t(9;22)(q34;q11)	c-abl	Tyrosine kinase
	bcr	Unknown function

are rare in APL. These findings suggest that the t(15;17), by itself, is sufficient for neoplastic transformation.

Approximately 75% of patients with APL present with a bleeding diathesis, usually the result of one or more processes including disseminated intravascular coagulation, increased fibrinolysis, and thrombocytopenia, and secondary to the release of procoagulants or tissue plasminogen activator (tPA) from the granules of neoplastic promyelocytes *(8,9)*. This bleeding diathesis may be exacerbated by standard cytoreductive chemotherapy. Two morphologic variants of APL have been described, typical and microgranular (FAB

M3v); both variants carry the t(15;17) *(8–10)*. In the typical or hypergranular variant, the promyelocytes have numerous azurophilic cytoplasmic granules that often obscure the border between the cell nucleus and the cytoplasm. Cells with numerous Auer rods in bundles (so-called faggot cells) are common. In contrast, in FAB-M3v the promyelocytes contain numerous small cytoplasmic granules that are difficult to discern with the light microscope, but are easily seen by electron microscopy.

The t(15;17) is a balanced and reciprocal translocation (Fig. 1) in which the *PML* (for promyelocytic leukemia) gene on

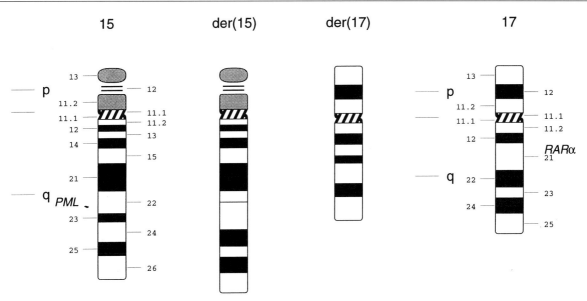

Fig. 1. Idiogram of the cytogenetic events in APL. Normal chromosomes (outer set) and derivative chromosomes (inner set) of the balanced and reciprocal translocation between the long arms of chromosomes 15 and 17, t(15;17)(q22;q12). The *PML* and *RARα* genes are normally located at 15q22 and 17q12, respectively. Adapted from Warrell et al. *(9)*.

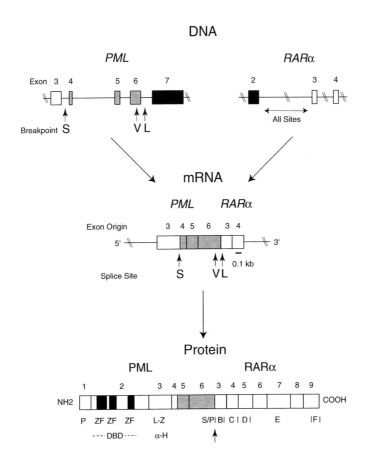

Fig. 2. Structure of the PML and RARα genes. Schematic diagrams depicting the structure of the *PML* and *RARα* genes (top), the *PML-RARα* fusion mRNA transcript (middle), and the L-form of the fusion protein (bottom). The lines represent introns, the arrows indicate three breakpoints, the open boxes represent the exons present in each type of *PML-RARα*, the shaded boxes represent exons excluded from the short (S)-form type but included in the long (L)- or variable (V)-form types, and the solid boxes indicate exons excluded from all types. Domains/motifs: P, proline-rich; S, serine-rich; ZF, zinc finger; L-Z, leucine zipper; DBD, putative DNA binding; and α-H, α-helical. B-F denotes regions of RARα (A is excluded). Adapted from Gallagher et al. *(15)*.

chromosome 15 and the *RARα* gene on chromosome 17 are disrupted and fused to form a hybrid gene (Fig. 2) *(11,12)*. The *PML-RARα* fusion gene, located on chromosome 15, encodes a chimeric mRNA and protein. On the derivative chromosome 15, both the *PML* and *RARα* genes are oriented in a head-to-tail orientation. The function of the normal *PML* gene is poorly understood. The gene is ubiquitously expressed and encodes a protein characterized by an N-terminal region with two zinc-finger-like motifs, known as a ring and a B-box, and thought to be involved in DNA binding *(8,11,12)*. A dimerization domain is also present. The normal PML protein appears to have an essential role in cell proliferation. The *RARα* gene encodes a transcription factor that binds to DNA sequences in *cis*-acting retinoic acid-responsive elements. High-affinity DNA binding also requires heterodimerization with another family of proteins, the retinoic acid X receptors. The RARα protein, from N-terminal to C-terminal, has transactivation, DNA binding, heterodimerization, and ligand-binding domains. The normal RARα protein plays an important role in myeloid differentiation.

There are three major forms of the *PML-RARα* fusion gene, corresponding to different breakpoints in the *PML* gene (Fig. 2) *(13–15)*. The breakpoint in the *RARα* gene occurs in the same general vicinity in all cases, within intron 2. Approximately 40–50% of cases have a *PML* breakpoint in exon 6 (the so-called long form, termed *bcr1*), 40–50% of cases have the *PML* breakpoint in exon 3 (the so-called short form, termed *bcr3*), and 5–10% of cases have a breakpoint in *PML* exon 6 that is variable (the so-called variable form, termed *bcr2*). In each form of the translocation, the PML-RARα fusion protein retains the 5'-DNA binding and dimerization domains of PML and the 3'-DNA binding, heterodimerization, and ligand (retinoic acid) binding domains of RARα. Recent studies indicate that the different forms of *PML-RARα* fusion mRNA correlate with clinical presentation or prognosis. In particular, the *bcr3* type of *PML-RARα* correlates with higher leukocyte counts at time of presentation and is more commonly present in the FAB-M3v variant *(14,15)*. Both higher leukocyte counts and FAB-M3v morphology are adverse prognostic findings, and the *bcr3* type of *PML-RARα* does not independently predict poorer disease-free survival *(15)*.

In addition to the PML-RARα protein, the t(15;17) results in two other abnormal proteins *(8)*. An aberrant PML protein is expressed in virtually all cells with the t(15;17), as a result of alternative mRNA splicing. This PML protein retains its DNA binding capacity and could possibly play a role in neoplastic transformation. A *RARα-PML* fusion gene is also formed, located on the derivative chromosome 17, and *RARα-PML* protein is expressed in approx 75% of cases of APL *(8,16)*. Because this protein lacks the DNA-binding regions of both normal PML and RARα, it is not thought to play a role in leukemogenesis. Furthermore, *RARα-PML* expression does not correlate with response to ATRA in vitro or with clinical outcome in vivo *(16)*.

A number of methods may be used to detect the t(15;17). Conventional cytogenetic methods detect the t(15;17) in approx 80–90% of APL cases at time of initial diagnosis. Suboptimal clinical specimens and poor-quality metaphases explain a large subset of the negative results. Fluorescence *in situ* hybridiza-

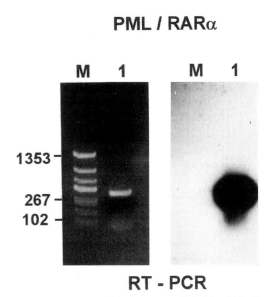

PML / RARα

RT - PCR

Fig. 3. A case of APL with the t(15;17)(q21;q21) shown by conventional cytogenetics. RT-PCR amplification demonstrated the presence of *PML-RARα* transcripts. Left panel, ethidium bromide-stained agarose gel of RT-PCR products. Lane M, φX174-pUC19/*Hae*III size markers. Lane 1, APL. Right panel, The RT-PCR products were transferred by Southern blotting to a nylon membrane and the membrane was hybridized with a ^{32}P-labeled probe specific for *PML-RARα*.

tion (FISH) is another useful method for detecting the t(15;17) in APL *(17)*. Different methods employ probes specific for either chromosome 15 or chromosome 17 (or both), and commercial kits are available. Southern-blot hybridization is another method to detect gene rearrangements that result from the t(15;17) *(18)*. The breakpoints consistently involve the second intron of the *RARa* gene and therefore probes derived from this region are the most often used. Virtually all cases of APL can be detected by Southern blot analysis using two or three genomic *RARα* probes *(18)*. RT-PCR is a very convenient method for detecting the *PML-RARα* fusion transcripts *(13)*. Primers have been designed to amplify the potential transcripts, and each type of transcript can be recognized. Results using this method are equivalent to or better than other methods at time of initial diagnosis.

Polyclonal and monoclonal antibodies (PAbs/MAbs) reactive with the PML and RARα proteins have been generated and immunohistochemical studies to assess the pattern of staining appear to be useful for diagnosis *(19,20)*. Dyck et al. *(19)* have studied a number of APLs and have shown that the pattern of PML or RARα immunostaining correlates with the presence of the t(15;17). In normal cells, PML protein is localized in 5–20 spherical structures per nucleus, known as PML oncogenic domains, that are highlighted in a punctate pattern of staining by the anti-PML antibody. RARα protein is not present in these structures. In contrast, in APL cells immunostaining for either PML or RARα reveals a microgranular pattern. Thus, the PML-RARα fusion protein is present in the microgranules. The fusion protein may prevent PML from forming normal oncogenic domains, because treatment with ATRA allows PML reorganization into these domains. Falini et al. *(20)* have used the PG-

M3 MAb to analyze a number of AMLs of non-FAB-M3 type and all showed the punctate pattern characteristic of normal PML oncogenic domains.

For the diagnosis of residual disease or early relapse after therapy, conventional cytogenetic studies, Southern-blot analysis, and immunohistochemical methods are limited by low sensitivity. In contrast, reverse transcription-polymerase chain reaction (RT-PCR) (Fig. 3) and FISH methods are very useful. The sensitivity of RT-PCR, which can detect one cell with the *PML-RARα* gene in 1×10^5 benign cells, makes this method very useful for monitoring residual disease after therapy. For the first few months after therapy, RT-PCR results may be positive with no correlation with relapse rate. However, longer than three mo after therapy, a positive RT-PCR result significantly correlates with an increased rate of relapse *(21,22)*. For example, Lo Coco et al. *(21)* studied 35 patients with APL in complete clinical remission after therapy. In this study, 11/13 (85%) patients positive by RT-PCR relapsed within 4 mo as compared with 22 RT-PCR-negative patients who did not relapse with clinical follow-up ranging from 3 mo to 5 yr. FISH methods compare favorably with RT-PCR methods, although the greater sensitivity of RT-PCR will detect disease in occasional cases that are negative by FISH *(23)*. However, FISH methods offer two advantages over RT-PCR. First, FISH studies may detect variant forms of the t(15;17) that are negative by RT-PCR. Secondly, FISH methods detect proliferating cells that presumably are more likely to correlate with active disease, in contrast with RT-PCR, that can detect both proliferating and nonproliferating cells *(23)*.

t(11;17)(q23;q21) The t(11;17)(q23;q21) has been rarely identified in AML, detected in 0.4% of all cases in one large study *(2)*. Many of the patients with t(11;17)-positive AMLs presented with a bleeding diathesis and the tumors were originally classified as APL. Licht et al. *(24)* have suggested that the neoplastic cells have cytological features intermediate between the blasts of AML FAB-M2 and the promyelocytes of APL. Unlike APLs, t(11;17)-positive AMLs respond poorly to ATRA *(24,25)*.

The t(11;17)(q23;q21) is a reciprocal and balanced translocation involving the *PLZF* (promyelocytic leukemia zinc finger) gene on chromosome 11 and the *RAR* gene on chromosome 17 *(24,25)*. Via the translocation, two fusion genes are produced, *PLZF-RARα* and *RARα-PLZF*, from which chimeric proteins are generated. It is presently uncertain which chimeric protein is leukemogenic. The structure of both chimeric proteins suggests that either can bind to DNA and influence transcription. The normal *PLZF* gene is expressed in a tissue-specific manner, particularly in cells of myeloid lineage. *PLZF* is a member of a large family of zinc-finger transcription factors and is probably involved in myeloid differentiation. The inability of ATRA to induce differentiation in t(11;17)-positive AMLs suggests that disruption of the normal *PLZF* gene, rather than the *RARα* gene (as is the case in APL), is the primary leukemogenic event. Analogous to the t(15;17), there is some variability in the breakpoints within the *PLZF* gene. The breakpoints in the *RARα* gene occur in the second intron, similar to those that occur in the t(15;17). In most reported cases, the t(11;17) was identified using conventional cytogenetic studies.

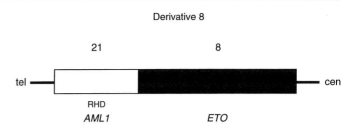

Fig. 4. The *aml1-eto* fusion gene. Schematic diagram of the structure of the *aml1-eto* fusion gene located on the derivative 8 chromosome in AML with a t(8;21)(q22;q22.3). The amino terminal *runt* homology domain (RHD) of *aml1* from 21q22 that is involved in DNA binding and interaction with *CBFβ* is conserved but the carboxy terminal transactivation domain is lost when *aml1* is joined to *eto* at 8q22.

However, in one study of six cases RT-PCR methods effectively identified *PLZF-RARα* transcripts in all cases, and both Southern-blot analysis and pulsed-field gel electrophoresis (PFGE) detected the translocation in different subsets of tumors examined *(24)*.

t(5;17)(q32;q21) Rare cases of APL carry the t(5;17)(q32;q21). In a case reported by Redner et al. *(26)*, the neoplastic cells were morphologically indistinguishable from APLs with the t(15;17) and the neoplasm responded well to ATRA. The t(5;17)(q32;q21) is a balanced and reciprocal translocation involving the *NPM* (nucleophosmin) gene on chromosome 5 and the *RARα* gene on chromosome 17. The *NPM* and *RARα* genes are fused in a 5'→3' direction, encoding a chimeric mRNA and protein. The breakpoint region in the *RARα* gene is identical to the breakpoint in the t(15;17). The *NPM* sequence involved in the case reported by Redner et al. *(26)* was identical to the *NPM* sequence identified in the *NPM-ALK* fusion gene, created by the t(2;5) that occurs in anaplastic large cell lymphomas of T/null-cell lineage. The NPM protein is a major phosphoprotein that has been mapped to the granular portion of the nucleolus. This protein is thought to play a role in ribosomal RNA transport and processing. NPM expression has been linked to cell proliferation.

TRANSLOCATIONS INVOLVING CORE BINDING FACTOR

t(8;21)(q22;q22.3) The t(8;21)(q22;q22) has been identified in approximately 8–12% of *de novo* AML *(2,27,28)*. Less commonly, the t(8;21) also has been identified in therapy-related AMLs and in myelodysplastic syndromes (MDS) *(29)*. In adults, *de novo* AMLs with the t(8;21) respond well to chemotherapy (containing AraC) with a high rate of complete remission and relatively long survival *(28)*. However, the presence of the t(8;21) in pediatric cases of AML may not predict as good a prognosis as it does in adults *(30)*. Morphologically, the majority of cases are classified as M2 using the FAB classification and approx 30–40% of all M2 cases carry the t(8;21) *(10)*. However, a subset of cases also have been classified as M4 or M1 *(10)*. The myeloblasts in AMLs associated with the t(8;21) typically have characteristic cytological features, characterized by abundant evidence of maturation, including numerous Auer rods and salmon-colored cytoplasmic granules *(10,31)*.

The t(8;21)(q22;q22) is a reciprocal chromosomal translocation involving the *eto* gene on chromosome 8 and the *aml1* gene on chromosome 21 *(29,32–34)*. As a result of this translocation, the *eto* and *aml1* genes are disrupted and fused forming a *aml1-eto* fusion gene, located on the derivative chromosome 8, that encodes chimeric mRNA (Fig. 4) and protein. The *aml1* and *eto* genes are fused in a 5'→3' orientation. The fusion protein includes the promoter and *runt*-like domains of the aml1 protein; the translocation domain of normal aml1 is replaced by sequences derived from the eto protein. A reciprocal *eto-aml1* fusion gene located on the derivative chromosome 21 has not been identified. One proposed mechanism for the role of aml1-eto in leukemogenesis is competitive inhibition of normal aml1 protein *(34)*. The breakpoints in the *aml1* gene are consistently detected in intron 5. The breakpoints in the *eto* gene are also relatively uniform, in the 5'-end of the gene. The novel protein that results from the t(8;21) has a predicted size of 83 kDa.

The *aml1* gene encodes for one of many members of a family of heterodimeric transcriptional regulatory proteins. The *aml1* gene is highly homologous with the *Drosophila runt* gene, and encodes the α subunit of core binding factor (CBF), the human counterpart of the murine nuclear polyoma enhancer binding protein (PEBP2). The binding of aml1 protein to DNA occurs via the *runt*-like central domain of the protein and also requires heterodimerization with CBF. The latter protein does not bind to DNA but improves the binding affinity of aml1. The *aml1* gene is normally expressed by myeloid and T-cells, but is not expressed in brain, lung, or gonads (unlike *eto*) *(29)*, and is thought to play an important role in hematopoietic differentiation *(35)*. Other human genes in this family include *aml2*, mapped to chromosome 1p36 and *aml3*, mapped to chromosome 6p21. The *eto* gene (also referred to in some studies as *CDR* or *MTG8*) encodes a transcription-factor protein that has two zinc-finger-motifs at its C-terminus. The *eto* gene (unlike *aml1*), is expressed in the brain, lung, and gonads, but is not normally expressed in hematopoietic cells.

A variety of methods are available to detect the t(8;21). This translocation is not difficult to recognize using conventional cytogenetics, which detects the t(8;21) in over 95% of cases *(29)*. However, rare cases have been reported in which the translocation was not detected by cytogenetics, but was detected by other molecular methods *(36)*. Genomic probes derived from the *aml1* and *eto* genes have been cloned and can be used to detect the translocation by Southern-blot analysis *(32,37)*. However, no single probe will detect all cases with the t(8;21) using this method. The large size of the genes or other mechanisms, such as DNA deletion, may explain this phenomenon. RT-PCR methods detect almost all cases with the t(8;21) and are more convenient than Southern-blot analysis (Fig. 5) *(38)*. RT-PCR methods, because of their extraordinary sensitivity, also have been used to monitor residual disease. However, initial studies with small numbers of patients have demonstrated the presence of *aml1-eto* transcripts in patients in complete clinical remission after chemotherapy or bone marrow transplantation, and who have remained in complete remission with prolonged clinical follow-up *(39,40)*. Jurlander et al. *(41)* summarized the literature: of 23 patients with *aml1-eto*-positive

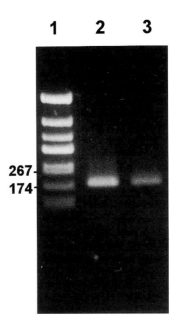

Fig. 5. RT-PCR analysis of *aml1-eto* fusion transcripts in AML. Two cases of AML with the t(8;21)(q22;q22.3) shown by conventional cytogenetics were evaluated for the presence of *aml1-eto* fusion gene transcripts using RT-PCR. Representative ethidium-stained agarose gels of the RT-PCR products are shown. Lane 1, φX174-pUC19/*Hae*III size markers. Lanes 2 and 3, RT-PCR analysis of mRNA from two different cases of AML.

AML treated with bone marrow transplantation and in clinical remission, 15 remained positive, 7 became negative, and 1 could not be evaluated. Thus, RT-PCR does not appear to effectively predict risk of relapse after therapy in patients in clinical remission *(39–41)*.

An antibody reactive with the t(8;21) chimeric protein has been developed *(42)*. Using the Kasumi cell line, which carries the t(8;21) and Western-blot analysis, this antibody detects a 64 kDa protein localized to the nucleus. This protein is smaller than the predicted size of 83 kDa, which may be the result of alternative splicing or post-translational modification. Detection of the t(8;21) protein may be diagnostically useful, although this needs to be studied further.

t(3;21)(q26;q22) The t(3;21)(q26;q22) has been reported in cases of chronic myeloid leukemia (CML) in blast crisis, in MDS, and in AMLs following treatment with topoisomerase II inhibitors, such as etoposide *(43,44)*. The breakpoint in the *aml1* gene on chromosome 21 may be identical to that in the t(8;21), but more often occurs approx 60 kb downstream. The chromosome 3q26 locus is the site of three different genes that are involved in the t(3;21): from telomere to centromere, *EAP*, *MDS1*, and *evi1*. These genes are located within approx 200 kb of each other. In each of these translocations, the 5'-end of the *aml1* gene, including sequences that encode the *runt*-like domain, is fused to the 3'-end of one of these partner genes.

In the *aml1-EAP* fusion gene, the 3'-*EAP* sequence is very small and it is not fused to *aml1* in reading frame. Thus, the aml1-EAP chimeric protein lacks transactivation activity and may exert its effect by inhibiting normal aml1 protein. In con-

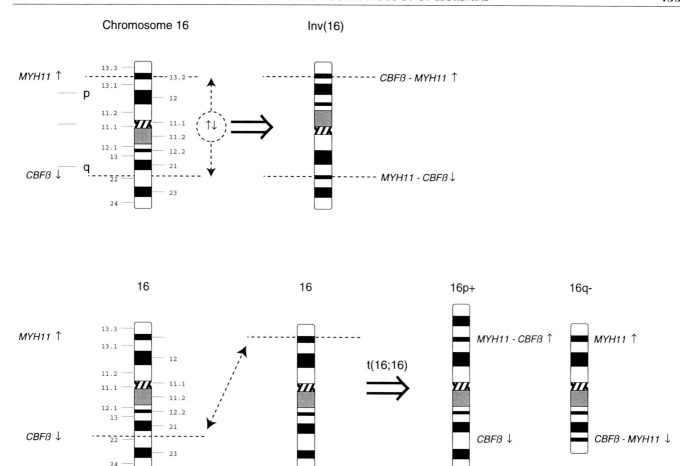

Fig. 6. Idiogram representations of inv(16) and t(16;16) chromosomal rearrangements. Top panel, In inv(16), the majority of *CBFβ* at 16q22 is joined upstream of the 3' end of *MYH11* at 16p13 forming a chimeric *CBFβ-MYH11* gene. Bottom panel, The t(16;16) results in a similar chimeric gene on 16p+. Adapted from Claxton et al. *(57).*

trast, the *aml1-MDS1* and *aml1-evi1* fusion genes contain significant 3'-sequences of the *MDS1* and *evi1* genes, suggesting that their proteins possibly have unique functions, in addition to inhibiting normal aml1 protein. For example, the 3'-end of the *evi1* gene involved in the *aml1-evi1* fusion gene encodes three zinc-finger motifs. One potential explanation for the occurrence of these different translocations, not proven, is that the entire 3q26 region is transcribed as a result of the t(3;21), and different fusion genes result from alternative splicing of mRNA *(29,45).* The normal EAP, MDS1, and evi1 proteins are not normally expressed in hematopoietic cells, but are expressed as a result of the t(3;21).

Other Translocations Inolving aml1 and eto Genes The *aml1* gene on chromosome 21q22 is also involved in other translocations *(29).* Of these, the t(12;21), resulting in a fusion between the *TEL* and *aml1* genes is most common, occurring in approx 30% of pediatric ALL. Other translocations involving *aml1* have been reported rarely in MDS and AMLs including the t(1;21)(p36;q22), t(5;21)(q13;q22), and t(17;21)(q11;q22) *(46).* One case of AML has been reported with a t(8;20)(q22;p13). In this case, the *eto* gene was overexpressed but *aml1-eto* transcripts were not identified, suggesting that the *aml1* gene was not involved. The putative gene at 20p13 is unknown *(47).*

inv(16)(p13q22) or t(16;16)(p13;q22) The inv(16) (p13q22) and, more rarely, the t(16;16)(p13;q22) have been identified in approx 5–12% of *de novo* AMLs (Fig. 6) *(2,27,48).* In most cases, the blasts have monocytic cytological features and are associated with eosinophilia. In addition, the eosinophils are usually cytologically abnormal with large and basophilic cytoplasmic granules *(10,48,49).* These neoplasms are recognized in the FAB classification as M4Eo. However, not all cases with the inv(16) are morphologically recognizable as FAB-M4Eo *(2,27).* For example, in one study by Mitelman and Heim *(2),* 85% of cases with the inv(16) were classified as M4Eo, approx 10% of cases were classified as either M2 or M5, and rare cases were classified as M1, M6, or M7. Also, the inv(16) is has been identified in rare cases of MDS and CML in blast crisis *(50–53).* The detection of the inv(16) in *de novo* AMLs is a favorable prognostic finding. Patients with AML with the inv(16) usually have a higher rate of complete response to chemotherapy, longer duration of remission, and prolonged survival as compared with patients with other forms of AML *(35,49,54).*

The inv(16)(p13q22) involves the gene that encodes the *CBF* (core binding factor or *PEBP2*) β subunit situated on chromosome 16q22 and the *MYH11* (smooth muscle myosin heavy chain) gene located at chromosome 16p13 (Fig. 6). The inversion results in a *CBFβ-MYH11* fusion gene from which chimeric mRNA and a novel protein are generated *(55,56)*. Both the *CBFβ* and *MYH11* genes are oriented 5'→3' and are transcribed in the centromeric to telomeric direction *(57)*. The t(16;16) also involves the *CBFβ* and *MYH11* genes, and results in an identical *CBFβ-MYH11* fusion gene. A reciprocal *MYH11-CBFβ* mRNA or protein has not been identified.

The CBF protein has two components, α and β, of which there are three α subunits and one βsubunit. The α subunits all share a *runt* domain sequence, which allows binding of the protein to DNA and to the β subunit. One of the α subunits is encoded by the *aml1* gene, which is disrupted in the t(8;21). The β subunit binds to the α subunit and stabilizes CBF binding to DNA. The normal *CBFβ* gene spans 50 kb with six exons. The breakpoints in the *CBFβ* gene are relatively constant. In the majority of cases, the breakpoint occurs in intron 5, at nucleotide 495 (corresponding to amino acid 165) *(57)*. However, a small subset of cases with a more proximal breakpoint at nucleotide 399 (amino acid 133) have been reported *(58)*. The normal *MYH11* gene encodes for the smooth-muscle form of the myosin heavy chain, and the gene is a member of the myosin II family *(56)*. Although the function of the CBFβ-MYH11 protein is not completely known, it is thought to bind to the enhancer or promoters of a number of genes involved in hematopoietic cell differentiation *(48)*.

The breakpoints in the *MYH11* gene are more variable than *CBFβ*; a number of different breakpoint sites have been reported, although the majority occur in a small 370 bp intron *(48,57,58)*. This common breakpoint, corresponds to nucleotide 1921 in the *MYH11* gene. At the present time, it is unclear whether different breakpoints correlate with differences in clinical findings or prognosis. Despite the variability in the different fusion genes generated by the inv(16) and t(16;16), one form of the fusion gene is created in approx 85% of cases, involving nucleotide 495 of the *CBFβ* and 1921 of *MYH11* genes. This fusion gene results in the generation of CBFβ-MYH11 protein that includes the first 165 amino acids of the normal CBFβ protein and a relatively small tail portion of the normal MYH11 protein.

Conventional cytogenetic methods, Southern-blot analysis, and RT-PCR have been used to detect the inv(16)(p13q22) and t(16;16). One major advantage of conventional cytogenetics is that this method will also identify additional chromosomal abnormalities that have been found in up to 50% of cases *(2,27,54)*. However, one potential disadvantage of karyotyping is that the inv(16) can be difficult to recognize or it may be misinterpreted as a del(16) *(50,58)*. The clustering of the breakpoints in the *CBFβ* and *MYH11* genes allows detection by Southern-blot analysis using genomic probes derived from either of the genes involved. For example, the breakpoints in the *MYH11* gene are clustered within a 14 kb *EcoRI* fragment of DNA *(56)*. RT-PCR analyses identify *CBFβ-MYH11* transcripts in most cases of AML with either the inv(16) or the t(16;16), demonstrating that the genetic consequences of both the inversion and translocation are identical *(50,57,58)*. However, the number of potential transcripts generated by the inv(16) can result in a small (<10%) subset of cases being falsely negative by RT-PCR, but detectable by conventional cytogenetics *(57,58)*.

del(16)(q22) Cases of AML also occur with deletion of chromosome 16q22. In fact, in the original report by Arthur and Bloomfield *(59)* describing involvement of chromosome 16 in AML FAB-M4Eo, the chromosome 16 abnormality was reported as a del(16)(q22). However, AMLs with del(16q22) appear to be a heterogeneous group with at least three subsets of neoplasms. In one group, the abnormality is associated with clinicopathological findings typical of inv(16)-positive AML and *CBFβ-MYH11* transcripts have been identified in cases studied by RT-PCR *(48,50)*. In a second group, re-examination of the cytogenetics has shown that the original interpretation as del(16) was incorrect; these cases were actually inv(16) *(50)*. In a third group are neoplasms with del(16q22) that have been diagnosed as chronic myelomonocytic leukemia, chronic myelomonocytic leukemia with transformation to AML, or *de novo* AML of FAB M4 or M5 types. Patients with these neoplasms have had a relatively poorer prognosis, and these neoplasms clinically behave as do AMLs without the inv(16) *(35,54,60)*.

TRANSLOCATIONS INVOLVING THE MLL GENE

11q23 Translocations Translocations involving the 11q23 locus are detected in 3–5% of all *de novo* AMLs *(61)*. In infants (age <1 yr), AMLs with 11q23 translocations typically present with hyperleukocytosis and have a poor prognosis *(62)*. In adults, AMLs with 11q23 translocations most commonly exhibit monocytic maturation and are classified as FAB M4 or M5. These AMLs do not have specific clinical features and may have a poorer prognosis than AMLs without 11q23 translocations. In addition, 80–90% of therapy-related AMLs that occur in patients previously treated with topoisomerase II inhibitors are associated with 11q23 translocations *(61,63)*. Acute lympho-blastic leukemias (ALLs) may also carry 11q23 translocations, in approx 5–10% of cases. 11q23 translocations have been detected in up to 50–60% of ALLs in infants (<1 yr) and in 5% of cases in adults *(62)*.

All 11q23 translocations disrupt the *mll* (myeloid-lymphoid leukemia or mixed lineage leukemia) gene (also known as *all1*, *hrx*, or *hrtx*) *(61,63)*. The *mll* gene is a relatively large gene that spans 100 kb with 30 exons *(61,64)*. The *mll* gene encodes a large protein, of approx 4000 amino acids with a predicted size of 431 kDa, that has three domains highly homologous to the *Drosophila trithorax* gene *(65,66)*. The *mll* gene has an amino terminus AT-hook motif and multiple zinc-finger motifs involved in protein-DNA binding and most likely encodes a transcription factor *(65,66)*. The *mll* gene is considered to be promiscuous due to the large number of partner genes on different chromosomes (up to 15 in AMLs) that may be involved in 11q23 translocations. The chromosomes most commonly involved are 4, 9, and 19. Other chromosomes less commonly involved in 11q23 translocations include chromosomes 1, 2, 5, 6, 10, 14, 15, 17, 22, and X *(67)*.

Despite the large size of the *mll* gene, the breakpoints are clustered in an area between exons 5 and 11, within 8.3 kb of each other *(61,63)*. There is a correlation between the location of the breakpoints in *de novo* vs therapy-related AML. Using the *XbaI* restriction enzyme, the 8.3 kb fragment of DNA can be divided into a 5' 4.6 kb region I and a 3'-3.9 kb region II according to Broeker et al. *(68)*. *De novo* AMLs more commonly have breakpoints in the 5'-region I. In contrast, most cases of therapy-related AML have 3'-region II breakpoints *(68)*. The presence of scaffold-attachment regions and possible topoisomerase II consensus binding sites in the 3'-region II may explain the increased likelihood of region II breakpoints in therapy-related AMLs *(68)*.

Conventional cytogenetics may be the most complete method to assess for the presence of 11q23 abnormalities *(67)*. This technique allows the detection of translocations involving 11q23 and also identifies all possible partner chromosomes. However, a subset of AMLs with 11q23 abnormalities may have a normal karyotype *(69)*. FISH techniques are also useful, and may detect a small subset of cases not recognized by conventional cytogenetics. The clustering of breakpoints within the *mll* gene is well-suited to their detection by Southern-blot analysis *(63,70)*. Using *BamHI* digested DNA, a single *mll* cDNA probe spanning an 8.3 kb genomic fragment detects most of the common and uncommon 11q23 translocations as gene rearrangements.

The introns between exons 5 through 11 are very large and thus standard PCR methods cannot be used for detecting 11q23 translocations. However, the cDNA corresponding to exons 5 through 11 is <700 bp, allowing RT-PCR analysis. A panel of primers needs to be used to detect the 11q23 translocations because of the number of possible partner chromosomes. Multiplex RT-PCR approaches are most convenient *(71)*. RT-PCR methods are probably more useful for monitoring residual disease, once the partner chromosome involved is known, rather than for initial diagnosis (or screening).

AML with t(9;11) Approximately 20–30% of AMLs of the FAB M5 (and less commonly M4) type are associated with 11q23 translocations *(68,72)*. Of these, the t(9;11)(p22;q23) is the most common (Fig. 7). AMLs with the t(9;11) represent approx 2% of all AMLs *(2)*. AMLs with the t(9;11) may be either *de novo* or therapy-related. *De novo* neoplasms occur in both children and adults *(61)*. Patients with *de novo* AML with the t(9;11) tend to have a more favorable outcome than that of adult patients with other 11q23 abnormalities *(73)*. Therapy-related cases of AML have been reported in patients previously treated with chemotherapeutic agents that target topoisomerase II *(61,72)*. The majority of therapy-related AMLs are monocytic neoplasms with relatively little differentiation (FAB-M5a).

The t(9;11)(p22;q23) is a balanced and reciprocal translocation that disrupts the *mll* gene on 11q23 and the *AF-9* gene (also known as *LTG9* for leukemia translocation gene) on chromosome 9p22. The translocation results in the formation of a *mll-AF-9* fusion gene, located on the derivative chromosome 11, from which chimeric mRNA and protein are generated. The function of the normal *AF-9* gene is incompletely understood, but it is normally expressed in megakaryocytes and erythroid cells.

Secondary cytogenetic abnormalities can be detected in t(9;11)-positive AMLs. Of these secondary cytogenetic lesions, trisomy of chromosome 8 is most common.

AML with t(11;16) The t(11;16)(q23;p13.3) is a rare recurrent translocation that has been identified in therapy-related AMLs and MDS, occurring almost exclusively in patients pre-

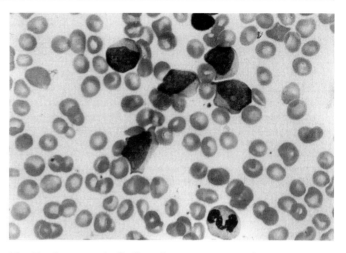

Fig. 7. Cytogenetic findings in AML. A case of *de novo* AML, FAB-M4, with the t(9;11)(p22;q23) shown by conventional cytogenetics. Peripheral blood smear stained with Wright-Giemsa, magnification ×1000.

viously treated with agents that inhibit topoisomerase II *(74,75)*. The t(11;16)(q23;p13.3) is a reciprocal translocation that disrupts the *mll* gene at 11q23 and the *CBP* gene (for cAMP response element or CREB-binding protein) at 16p13.3, resulting in the formation of a *mll-CBP* fusion gene located on the derivative chromosome 11 *(74,75)*. A *CBP-mll* fusion gene is also produced in most, but not all cases, and therefore is not thought to be leukemogenic. The normal CBP protein is a transcriptional adaptor/coactivator protein.

Other 11q23 Translocations in AML Other 11q23 translocations less commonly identified in AMLs include the t(6;11)(q27;q23), t(11;19)(q23;p13.3), t(11;19)(q23;p13.1), t(1;11)(p32;q23), t(1;11)(q21;q23), t(11;17)(q23;q21), and t(10;11)(p11;q23). In each of these translocations, the *mll* gene is disrupted and its 5' end is fused with the 3' end of the partner gene: *AF-6* in the t(6;11), *ENL* in the t(11;19)(q23;19p13.3), *ELL* in the t(11;19) (11q23;19p13.1), *AF-1p* in the t(1;11)(p32;q23), *AF-1q* in the t(1;11)(q21;q23), *AF-17* in the t(11;17), and *AF-10* in the t(10;11) *(67,76–80)*. The formation of these fusion genes, all located on the derivative chromosome 11, results in the generation of a novel chimeric protein.

Preliminary data in children and adolescents (<20 yr old but not infants) suggest that t(9;11)-positive AMLs may have a better prognosis than AMLs with other 11q23 translocations *(29,81)*. For example, children with AML associated with 11q23 translocations other than the t(9;11) more commonly present with extreme hyperleukocytosis, central nervous system (CNS) involvement, and skin lesions as compared with children with t(9;11)-positive AMLs *(73,81)*.

11q23 Rearrangements Identified in AMLs with Trisomy 11 In AMLs with trisomy 11, without cytogenetic evidence of 11q23 translocations, Caligiuri and colleagues *(69,82)* have shown *mll* gene rearrangements using Southern-blot analysis. Additional studies in these cases revealed a tandem duplication of a part of the *mll* gene. This duplication occurs in the area between exons 2 through 8 of the *mll* gene, and is in frame. This finding suggests that the tandem duplicated region is transcribed and translated, resulting in a duplicated mll protein.

11q23 Rearrangements Identified in AMLs with Normal Cytogenetics Caligiuri and colleagues *(69,83)* have also screened a number of cases of AML with normal conventional cytogenetics by Southern-blot analysis and have identified *mll* gene rearrangements in approx 10% of cases. The cases with *mll* gene rearrangements were classified as FAB M2, M4, and M1. All were shown to have a partial tandem repeat in the *mll* gene, similar to cases of AML with trisomy 11 *(69)*.

TRANSLOCATIONS INVOLVING NUCLEOPORIN GENES

t(6;9)(p23;q34) The t(6;9)(p23;q34) has been identified in approx 1–2% of cases of AML *(2,84)*. Most t(6;9)-positive neoplasms are morphologically classified as FAB-M4; a smaller subset of cases have been classified as FAB-M2, FAB-M1, or as a MDS *(84)*. Patients with AML and the t(6;9) are commonly of young age (<40 yr old) and have a poor prognosis *(84,85)*. Approximately 50% of patients affected achieve clinical remission with chemotherapy, but relapse is common. A subset of patients present with an aggressive MDS rather than AML; others present with overt AML with coexistent morphologic evidence of a MDS *(84)*.

The t(6;9) disrupts the *dek* gene at chromosome 6p23 and the *can* (*NUP214*) gene at chromosome 9q34, resulting in a *dek-can* fusion gene on the derivative 6 chromosome that encodes a chimeric mRNA and protein *(86)*. The breakpoints in the t(6;9) are consistent and clustered. The breakpoints in the *dek* gene occur in one intron, known as *icb-6* (for intron containing breakpoint on chromosome 6). The breakpoints in the *can* gene also cluster in one intron, known as *icb-9*. The *dek* gene is approx 40 kb in size and encodes a 43 kDa protein, located in the cell cytoplasm, and thought to be a transcription factor. The *can* gene is relatively larger (over 140 kb) and encodes a 214 kDa protein. The normal can protein is a component of the nuclear-pore complex (hence the name nucleoporin), involved in transport of mRNA and proteins between the cytoplasm and the nucleus *(87)*. The dek-can fusion protein, of predicted size of 165 kDa, has a nuclear distribution, suggesting it is a part of the transcription factor system *(88)*.

The t(6;9) is effectively detected by conventional cytogenetics, which also allows the detection of additional abnormalities that may occur with disease progression; trisomies of 8 and 13 are the most common additional abnormalities *(85)*. Southern-blot analysis can be used and genomic probes derived from the *dek* and *can* genes have been cloned. Soekerman et al. *(85)*, using two *dek* and two *can* probes and three restriction-enzyme digests, reported that Southern-blot analysis reliably detects the t(6;9). The clustering of breakpoints in *icb-6* of *dek* and *icb-9* of *can* also allows convenient detection by using RT-PCR methods (Fig. 8) *(85,89)*.

One case of acute undifferentiated leukemia with a normal karyotype has been shown to be associated with the *set-can* fusion gene *(90)*. The chromosome rearrangement resulting in this fusion gene may be either an insertion, inversion, or a small translocation that was unrecognized by conventional cytogenetics *(90)*. The breakpoint in the *can* gene, at 9q34, is identical to that in the t(6;9) and involves *icb-9*. The *set* gene is also located at chromosome 9q34 *(90,91)*. The *set* gene is relatively

DEK /CAN

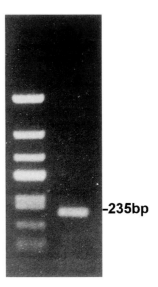

–235bp

RT - PCR

Fig. 8. RT-PCR analysis of dek-can fusion gene transcripts in a case of AML, FAB-M4, with the t(6;9)(p23;q34) shown by conventional cytogenetics. RT-PCR amplification demonstrated the presence of *dek-can* fusion gene transcripts. Ethidium-stained agarose gel. Lane 1, φX174-pUC19/*Hae*III size markers. Lane 2, AML.

small, approx 8 kb, and encodes a protein of 32 kDa. The breakpoint in the *set-can* fusion gene is 800 bp 3' to the *set* gene, in an exon *(90)*. The function of the *set* gene is unknown, but it is widely expressed in tissues, suggesting that it has a general cellular function.

t(7;11)(p15;p15) The t(7;11)(p15;p15) is a rare recurrent chromosomal translocation that occurs in AML. Morphologically, most AMLs with the t(7;11) exhibit granulocytic maturation and are classified as FAB-M2; cases classified as FAB-M4 and FAB-M5 also have been reported *(92)*. Coexistent myelodysplastic features are common *(92,93)*. The t(7;11) is not completely restricted to AML; rare t(7;11)-positive cases of CML have been reported *(92)*. The majority of patients with t(7;11)-positive AML have been Japanese, suggesting genetic predisposition for this type of AML *(93)*. Most patients are adults and the prognosis is not significantly different from patients with other types of AML *(92)*.

The t(7;11) disrupts the *HOXA9* gene at chromosome 7p15 and the *NUP98* gene at 11p15, resulting in the formation of the *NUP98-HOXA9* and *HOXA9-NUP98* fusion genes *(94,95)*. The *NUP98-HOXA9* fusion gene, located on the derivative chromosome 11, is thought to be involved in leukemogenesis, based on the predicted structure of the chimeric protein *(94,95)*. The reciprocal *HOXA9-NUP98* fusion gene is probably nonfunctional, and was not amplifiable by RT-PCR in a subset of cases tested *(95)*. The normal *HOXA9* gene is a member of the homeobox gene family, and is involved in development and differentiation. The *HOXA9* gene encodes a class I homeodomain protein that is expressed in hematopoietic cells and the kidney *(94,95)*. The normal *NUP98* gene is relatively small, with five exons, and encodes a component of the nuclear-pore complex that is 98 kDa. The NUP98 protein plays a role in bi-directional transport of RNA and proteins between the nucleus and the cytoplasm *(96)*. The *NUP98* gene is expressed in a variety of tissues *(96)*.

inv(11)(p15q22) The inv(11)(p15q22) has been identified in a very small number of *de novo* and therapy-related cases of AML *(97)*. This inversion disrupts the *DDX10* gene at chromosome 11q22 and the *NUP98* gene at 11p15, creating the *NUP98-DDX10* fusion gene, from which a leukemogenic chimeric protein is generated. A reciprocal *DDX10-NUP98* fusion gene is also created and may be expressed, but is not thought to be involved in neoplastic transformation *(97)*. The normal *DDX10* gene is large, spanning 200 kb, and is composed of at least 12 exons. This gene is a DEAD-box putative RNA helicase gene, that encodes a protein that may be involved in ribosomal assembly *(98)*. The *DDX10* gene is ubiquitously expressed in normal tissues. The normal *NUP98* gene encodes a nuclear-pore complex protein that is also ubiquitously expressed *(96)*.

TRANSLOCATIONS INVOLVING GENES OF THE ETS FAMILY

t(16;21)(p11;q22) The t(16;21)(p11;q22) is a relatively recently characterized chromosomal translocation that occurs in AML. Yao et al. *(99)* reported the first two cases in 1988. Since then, approx 50 neoplasms with this translocation have been reported *(100)*. Most neoplasms with the t(16;21) have been AMLs of all FAB types except M3. However, rare cases of CML in blast crisis and MDS with the t(16;21) have been described *(100,101)*. Patients with AML associated with the t(16;21) are generally young and have a poor prognosis. In a group of 19 cases reported by Kong et al. *(100)*, the median age was 22 yr and 100% of the patients died with a median survival of 16 mo. The t(16;21) is a reciprocal and balanced translocation that disrupts the *TLS/FUS* gene at chromosome 16p11 and the *erg* (*ets*-related gene) gene on chromosome 21q22 *(102,103)*. As a result two fusion genes are created, *TLS/FUS-erg* on the derivative chromosome 21 and *erg-TLS/FUS* on the derivative chromosome 16. Although both fusion genes may be expressed, only the *TLS/FUS-erg* fusion gene is consistently expressed in all cases, suggesting that this chimeric protein is involved in leukemogenesis *(102)*. Both the *TLS/FUS* and *erg* genes are oriented 5'→3'. The normal *TLS/FUS* gene encodes an RNA-binding protein that is highly homologous to the *ews* gene involved in Ewing's sarcoma. The *TLS/FUS* gene is also involved in another chromosomal translocation associated with myxoid liposarcoma, the t(12;16). The TLS/FUS protein plays a role in activating transcription. The normal *erg* gene, a member of the *ets* proto-oncogene superfamily, also encodes an RNA-binding protein and is a potent transcriptional activator *(104)*. At least four different transcripts of the *TLS/FUS-erg* have been identified. These transcripts result from variability in the breakpoints and alternative RNA splicing. In most cases, the breakpoint in the *erg* gene is tightly clustered in one intron. The breakpoints in the *TLS/FUS* gene are more variable *(100,103)*.

t(12;22)(p13;q11) The t(12;22)(p13;q11) is another rare translocation found in AMLs and rare cases of MDS and CML *(2,105)*. All FAB types of AML, except M3, have been reported

with the t(12;22). The t(12;22) is a reciprocal translocation involving the *TEL* gene at chromosome 12p13 and the *MN1* (meningioma) gene at chromosome 22q11 *(106)*. The translocation disrupts the *TEL* and *MN1* genes, resulting in the formation of *MN1-TEL* and *TEL-MN1* fusion genes. The *MN1-TEL* fusion gene is likely to encode the leukemogenic protein, based on the predicted structure of the fusion protein, which is consistent with an altered transcription factor. The *MN1-TEL* fusion gene also has been constantly expressed in the small number of neoplasms analyzed, unlike the *TEL-MN1* fusion gene *(106)*. The normal *TEL* gene is very large, exceeding 150 kb, and is a member of the *ets* gene family of transcription factors. The *TEL* gene is ubiquitously expressed in tissues. The normal *MN1* gene is less well-known. The gene was originally cloned from a t(4;22)(p16;q11) identified in a case of sporadic meningioma *(107)*. The gene spans 70 kb, has at least two exons separated by a large intron, and encodes a protein predicted to have 1319 amino acids. The breakpoints in the *MN1* gene appear to be clustered in the 5'-region of the intron *(107)*.

ADDITIONAL TRANSLOCATIONS IN AML

t(8;16)(p11;p13) The t(8;16)(p11;13) is a rare recurrent chromosomal abnormality, identified in <1% of all cases of AML *(2)*. The majority of AMLs with the t(8;16) exhibit monocytic differentiation and are morphologically classified as FAB M4 or M5 *(108)*. The blasts often exhibit evidence of erythrophagocytosis *(108)*. Both *de novo* and therapy-related AMLs with the t(8;16) have been reported. *De novo* cases commonly occur in children and adolescents (<18 yr of age) *(108)*. Therapy related AMLs occur in adults; the median age in one study was 58 years *(109)*. The t(8;16) is a reciprocal translocation, involving the *MOZ* (monocytic leukemia zinc-finger protein) located at chromosome 8p11 and the *CBP* located at 16p13 *(110)*. The translocation disrupts these genes, resulting in the formation of a *MOZ-CBP* fusion gene on the derivative chromosome 8, from which chimeric mRNA and protein are generated. A *CBP-MOZ* fusion gene is also created but is thought to be nonfunctional. The *MOZ* gene encodes a 225 kDa protein that is widely expressed in tissues. The protein has both zinc-finger and acetyltransferase domains, leading Borrow et al. *(110)* to suggest that the protein may mediate leukemogenesis by aberrant acetylation of chromatin. The *CBP* gene spans 190 kb and encodes a protein involved in transcriptional activation. Mutations in the *CBP* gene have been identified in a rare genetic syndrome, the Rubinstein-Taybi syndrome, characterized by mental retardation, dysmorphic cranial features, and digital abnormalities *(111)*.

Less common translocations that involve the 8q11 locus are reported in AMLs, such as the t(8;22)(p11;q13) and the t(8;19)(p11;q13) *(112,113)*. These translocations may also involve the *MOZ* gene.

t(9;22)(q34;q11) The t(9;22)(q34;q11) is rarely identified in apparently *de novo* cases of AML, in approx 1–2% of cases *(2,114)*. However, if the t(9;22) is identified, one must also consider the possibility of CML initially presenting in blast crisis. Successful therapy in some patients with t(9;22)-positive AML has resulted in the emergence of CML, in chronic phase.

The t(9;22) involves the c-*abl* gene at chromosome 9q34 and the *bcr* gene at chromosome 22q11. The translocation results in a *bcr-abl* fusion transcript and a novel fusion protein. Two different forms of the t(9;22) have been detected in AML, that result in either a 190 kDa or 210 kDa fusion protein *(115)*. In both translocations, the breakpoint in c-*abl* occurs in the same general area, in the proximal portion of the gene. In the p190^bcr-abl form, the breakpoint in *bcr* occurs in the first exon. In contrast, in the p210^bcr-abl form the breakpoint occurs in the 5.8 kb major breakpoint region of *bcr*. The detection of the p190^bcr-abl form of the t(9;22) in a case of AML is evidence to support the diagnosis of *de novo* AML. At least some of the cases with the p210^bcr-abl form of the t(9;22) are probably CML, first presenting as blast crisis.

flt3 GENE EXPRESSION AND DUPLICATION IN AML

The *flt3* (for fms-like tyrosine kinase 3) gene, located on chromosome 13q12, encodes a receptor kinase that is related to two other protein receptors, kit and fms. The flt3 protein (like kit and fms) is involved in the regulation of hematopoietic-cell proliferation and differentiation. The *flt3* gene is normally expressed in cells of the hematopoietic system, CNS, and gonads, and is abundantly expressed in AMLs *(116)*. The flt3 protein has a number of domains including extracellular, transmembrane, intracellular, and juxtamembrane domains. Internal tandem duplication of the *flt3* gene segments that encode for the intracellular and juxtamembrane domains have been identified almost exclusively in AMLs. In one study, these duplications were identified in 22/112 (20%) AMLs and in 1/37 (3%) cases of MDS *(117)*. Gene duplications involving the *flt3* gene were not identified in ALLs of immature B-cell or T-cell lineage nor were they found in mature B-cell neoplasms *(117)*.

GENE MUTATIONS IN AML

Gene mutations have been identified in AMLs, involving either proto-oncogenes or tumor-suppressor genes. Genes that are commonly affected in AMLs include the c-*ras* gene family, *Rb1*, and *p53*.

Gene Mutations Involving the c-ras Gene Family The c-H-*ras*, c-K-*ras*, and c-N-*ras* proto-oncogenes encode homologous 21 kDa proteins that are located at the inner surface of the plasma-cell membrane. The c-ras proteins all reversibly bind and hydrolyze GTP and are involved in signal transduction and cellular proliferation. The c-N-*ras* gene is situated on chromosome 1p11-p13, c-K-*ras* is located on chromosome 12p11-p12, and the c-H-*ras* gene is found at chromosome 11p15. Mutations of the c-*ras* genes represent one of the more frequent molecular abnormalities identified in AML. The c-N-*ras* gene is involved most often, in up to 25% of cases of AML *(118,119)*. Point mutations predominate, which are usually found in the first exon of the gene at codon 12 or 13. Less commonly, mutations have been identified at codon 61, in the promoter region of c-N-*ras*, and in the c-K-*ras* gene *(119,120)*. Loss of heterozygosity (LOH) of the short arm of chromosome 11 also has been reported in a small subset of AMLs *(121)*. Chromosome 11p is the site of the c-H-*ras* gene, but is also the site of other important genes that may be involved (for example, the *WT1* and *WT2* genes known to be involved in Wilms' tumor).

The Rb1 Tumor-Suppressor Gene The *Rb1* tumor-suppressor gene, located at chromosome 13q14, encodes a 110 kDa nuclear phosphoprotein that can bind to DNA as well as

form complexes with other proteins. The pRb protein is integrally involved in the transition of the cell cycle from the G_1 to S phase. Abnormalities in the *Rb1* gene have been identified in a subset of AMLs. In a study by Ahuja et al. *(122)* using Southern-blot analysis, 5/54 (9.3%) cases of AML had structural abnormalities of the *Rb1* locus, including 4/15 (26.7%) AMLs with monocytic differentiation (FAB M4 and M5). In most of these neoplasms, *Rb1* gene abnormalities correlated with absence of protein expression. *Rb1* gene abnormalities were also identified in 6/42 (14.3%) CMLs in myeloid blast crisis and 2/18 (11.1%) cases of MDS *(122)*.

The p53 Tumor-Suppressor Gene The *p53* tumor-suppressor gene, located at chromosome 17p13, is commonly mutated in a wide variety of human cancers, including AMLs. The normal *p53* gene encodes for a nuclear phosphoprotein that binds to DNA and can influence the expression of other genes. p53 protein appears to be involved in cell proliferation and apoptosis. Prokocimer and Rotter *(123)*, in their review of the literature, identified over 200 cases of AML in which the status of the *p53* gene was assessed. Point mutations were identified in approx 6% of cases. *p53* gene mutations have been identified in all morphologic types of AML, except FAB-M3, and are more common in cases with chromosome 17 alterations, such as complex translocations or monosomy *(124)*. The presence of *p53* gene mutations also correlates with older patient age, the presence of myelodysplasia, and poor prognosis *(125,126)*.

ANTIGEN-RECEPTOR GENE REARRANGEMENTS IN AMLs

Immunoglobulin heavy chain (*IgH*) and/or T-cell receptor (*TCR*) β- and γ-chain gene rearrangements have been detected in less than 5% of cases of AML using Southern-blot analysis *(127–130)*. However, a recent study of AMLs using PCR-based methods found a substantially higher number of cases with *IgH* gene rearrangements *(131)*. Many of the cases with antigen-receptor gene rearrangements have been primitive neoplasms, often TdT-positive and expressing one or more lymphoid-associated antigens, suggesting that these leukemias are arising from an early bone marrow-precursor cell with multilineage potential *(128)*. Kyoda et al. have provided data to suggest that AMLs with *IgH* gene rearrangements have a poorer prognosis than those without *IgH* gene rearrangements. However, additional studies will be required to resolve this issue.

ACUTE LYMPHOBLASTIC LEUKEMIA

ALLs are neoplasms composed of immature lymphoid cells that are derived from the bone marrow. Traditionally, these leukemias have been classified on the basis of their morphological features as L1, L2, or L3 according to FAB criteria *(5)*. More recently, it has been shown that these are neoplasms of immature B-cells or T-cells that are arrested at an early stage in lymphocyte maturation. Approximately 80–90% of ALLs are of immature B-cell phenotype, and include neoplasms once designated as non-B/non-T, null, and common ALL. Based on antigen expression, ALLs of B-cell lineage may be further subclassified into as many as five subgroups (pre-pre-B-ALL, early pre-B ALL, pre-B ALL, transitional B-ALL, or B-ALL) although subdivision into fewer subgroups based on the expression of CD10, cytoplasmic IgM, and surface immunoglobulin is the usual practice *(132)*. The remaining 10–20% of

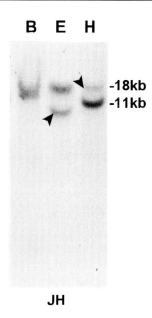

Fig. 9. Southern analysis of *IgH* rearrangement in B-cell ALL. A case of precursor B-cell ALL analyzed by Southern-blot hybridization using an *IgH* gene joining region probe (J$_H$). **(B)**, *Bam*HI; E, *Eco*RI, H, *Hin*dIII. Single nongermline bands consistent with gene rearrangements are identified in the *Eco*RI and *Hin*dIII digests. The dashes indicate the size of the germline bands: 18 kb for *Bam*HI and *Eco*RI and 11 kb for *Hin*dIII. Arrowheads indicate rearrangements.

ALLs are of T-cell lineage *(133)*. ALLs that are of T-cell lineage also may be further subclassified by their immunophenotype as pro-thymocyte, early thymocyte, mature thymocyte ALL, or mature T-ALL *(132)*.

The molecular findings in the majority of immature B-cell and T-cell ALLs are virtually indistinguishable from those of their lymphoblastic lymphoma counterparts. The Revised European-American Classification of Lymphoid Neoplasms and the recent proposal for an updated World Health Organization (WHO) Classification therefore designate these tumors as precursor B-cell or T-cell lymphoblastic leukemia/lymphoma *(134,135)*. Heritable syndromes predisposing to ALL and germline mutations in known tumor-suppressor genes are uncommon, implying that most cases probably arise from somatic mutations in immature lymphoid cells.

PRECURSOR B-CELL (EARLY PRE-B AND PRE-B) ALLS

Nearly all precursor B-cell ALLs carry *IgH* gene rearrangements (Fig. 9). In addition, 40–50% of ALLs also contain *Ig*κ gene rearrangements; approx 20–25% contain *Ig*λ gene rearrangements *(133,136)*. Lineage infidelity is common in ALLs and the *TCR* genes are frequently rearranged as well *(133,137)*. *TCR*-δ is rearranged or deleted (after rearrangement) in as many as 80% of cases. The *TCR*-γ and *TCR*-β genes are rearranged in 50–60%, and 20–30% of cases, respectively. As a result, either the *TCR* or *Ig* genes can be assessed to determine clonality, but evaluation of individual antigen receptor genes is less useful for lineage determination.

Standard cytogenetic studies demonstrate the presence of nonrandom chromosomal translocations in precursor B-cell ALL *(1,138,139)*. These translocations typically involve

known or candidate proto-oncogenes. In a subset of cases, tumor-suppressor genes have also been implicated. The molecular cytogenetic findings are summarized in Table 2. A number of the most frequent and best-characterized molecular abnormalities are discussed in the following subsections.

t(9;22)(q34;q11) The Philadelphia chromosome or t(9;22)(q34;q11), is among the most prevalent recurrent chromosomal translocations in precursor B-cell ALL, detected in approx 20% of adults and 5% of children with this disease *(1,140)*. This translocation brings together the c-*abl* (for Abelson leukemia virus) gene at chromosome 9q34 and the *bcr* (for breakpoint cluster region) locus at 22q11 (Figs. 10–12). This juxtaposition results in the formation of a chimeric mRNA transcript that encodes a fusion gene with increased tyrosine kinase activity. Two forms of the t(9;22) occur. In about 25–50% of adult cases of ALL, the translocation appears identical to that found in chronic myeloid leukemia (CML); a fusion protein with a molecular weight of 210 kDa is formed, known as p210. In the remaining 50–75% of adult cases and the majority of childhood cases of ALL, the breakpoint on chromosome 22 is 100 kb upstream of the *bcr* region, resulting in a smaller fusion protein with a molecular weight of 190 kDa. This p190 protein has enhanced tyrosine kinase activity and transforming capability compared to p210 *(141)*. For those translocations that form p210, the breakpoints in the *bcr* gene are clustered tightly enough to be detected using Southern-blot analysis. However, translocations that produce a p190 product have breakpoints scattered over a larger region that are therefore less amenable to evaluation by Southern blotting. Assays have been developed based on RT-PCR *(142)*, and may be used to detect either type of translocation. To enhance the clinical utility of this method, some investigators are developing multiplex RT-PCR assays to detect several important translocations simultaneously, including the t(9;22), t(1;19), and t(4;11) chromosomal reaarangements *(143)*.

t(1;19)(q23;p13) and t(17;19)(q22;p13) The t(1;19) (q23;q13) is found in approx 30% of precursor B-cell ALLs or 6% of all ALLs *(1,144,145)*. It is most prevalent in leukemias with a pre-B cell (cytoplasmic Igμ positive) immunophenotype. This translocation joins the *pbx1* gene on chromosome 1q23 to the *E2A* gene on chromosome 19p13 *(144,145)*. Thes *pbx1* gene is a member of the homeobox gene family. The *E2A* gene encodes an enhancer-binding transcription factor *(146)*. The result of the translocation is a fusion gene that encodes for a chimeric transcription factor. Because the sequences involved in the t(1;19) have been cloned and sequenced, it is amenable to Southern-blot analysis. Using an *E2A* probe and Southern-blot analysis, Kawamura and coworkers detected *E2A* rearrangements in 15/16 (94%) cases known to have the t(1;19) by conventional cytogenetic analysis *(147)*. Because the breakpoints are clustered, PCR-based methods can also be used for detection *(148)*. In addition, a MAb reactive with the fusion E2A-pbx1 protein has been developed that may be useful for diagnosis *(149)*.

In the t(17;19)(q22;p13) the *HLF* (for hepatic leukemia factor) gene located on chromosome 17 is joined to the *E2A* gene on chromosome 19p13 *(150)*. The translocation creates a fusion gene that encodes for a chimeric protein containing the

Table 2
Cytogenetic and Molecular Abnormalities in ALL

Chromosomal Translocations	*Genes*	*Comments*
B-Cell lineage		
t(9;22)(q34;q11)	*c-abl*	Tyrosine kinase
	bcr	Unknown function·
Involving E2A		
t(1;19)(q23;q13)	*PBX1*	Homeobox gene
	E2A	bHLH transcription factor
(17;19)(q22;p13)	*HLF*	bZIP transcription factor
	E2A	bHLH transcription factor
Involving *mll*		
t(11;v)(q23;v)	*mll*	*Drosophila trithorax* homology
	Variable	Many partner genes
		Infancy, high risk
Involving *TEL* and *KIP1*		
t(12;21)(p12;q22)	*TEL*	*ets*-like transcription factor
	aml1	*runt*-like transcription factor
Involving IL-3		
t(5;14)(q31;q32)	*IL-3*	Cytokine gene
	IgH	Ig heavy-chain enhancer
Involving c-*myc*		
t(8;14)(q24;q32)	*c-myc*	bHLH transcription factor
	IgH	Ig heavy-chain enhancer
t(2;8)(p12;q24)	*Igκ*	Igκ chain enhancer
	c-myc	bHLH transcription factor
t(8;22)(q24;q11)	*c-myc*	bHLH transcription factor
	Igλ	Igλ chain enhancer
Gene amplification		
Hyperdiploid karyotype		Favorable prognosis
DHFR		Associated with *p53* mutations
T-Cell lineage		
Involving TAL1, TAL2, and LYL1		
Interstitial deletions	*TAL1*	bHLH transcription factor
	SIL	Gene expressed T cells
		Up to 30% T-ALL
t(1;14)(p32;q11)	*TAL1*	bHLH transcription factor
	TCR-δ	TCR enhancer
t(1;7)(p33;q35)	*TAL1*	bHLH transcription factor
	TCR-β	TCR enhancer
t(7;9)(q34;q32)	*TCR-β*	TCR enhancer
	TAL2	bHLH transcription factor
t(7;19)(q34;q13)	*TCR-β*	TCR enhancer
	LYL1	bHLH transcription factor
del(9)(p21-22)	$P16^{INK4A}$	Cell-cycle inhibitor
	$P1^{INK4B}$	Cell-cycle inhibitor
Involving *HOX11*		
t(10;14)(q24;q11)	*HOX11*	Homeobox gene
	TCR-α/δ	TCR enhancer
t(7;10)(q34;q24)	*TCR-β*	TCR enhancer
	HOX11	Homeobox gene
Miscellaneous		
t(8;13)(p11;q11)	*FGFR1*	Growth-factor receptor
	ZNF198	Novel gene, Zn finger
t(8;14)(q24;q11)	*c-myc*	bHLH transcription factor
	TCR-δ	TCR enhancer
Involving *TTG1* and *TTG2*		
t(11;14)(p15;q11)	*TTG2*	LIM protein
	TCR-δ	TCR enhancer
t(11;14)(p13;q11)	*TTG2*	LIM protein
	TCR-δ	TCR enhancer

Table 2 *(Continued)*

Chromosomal Translocations	Genes	Comments
Involving *mll*		
t(11;v)(q23;v)	*mll*	*Drosophila trithorax* homology
	Variable	Many partner genes
Involving *TAN1*		
t(7;9)(q34;q34.3)	*TCR-β*	TCR enhancer
	TAN1	*Drosophila notch*-like
Involving *TCL1*		
t(14;14)(q11;q32.1),	*TCR-δ*	TCR enhancer
inv(14)(q11;q32.1)	*TCL1*	Homology to *MTCP1* of T-CLL
t(7;14)(q35;q32.1)	*TCR-β*	TCR enhancer
	TCL1	Homology to *MTCP1* of T-CLL

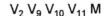

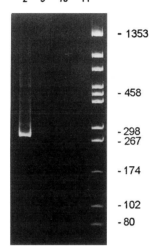

V_2 V_9 V_{10} V_{11} M

- 1353

- 458

- 298
- 267

- 174

- 102
- 80

Fig. 10. TCR-γ chain gene rearrangements in T-cell ALL. A case of T-cell ALL analyzed for *TCR-γ* chain gene rearrangements using PCR, four variable region (V) primers, and two joining region (J) primers. The four V primers, V2, V9, V10, and V11, used singly in each lane as indicated, are specific for each of four V region families. Both J primers are added to each lane. The lane designated M contains φX174-pUC19/*Hae*III size markers.

basic region/leucine zipper domain of the HLF protein fused to the transactivation domain of the E2A protein *(151)*.

11q23 Rearrangements Involving mll As outlined in the section on AML, a large number of partner genes (over 30 to date) on different chromosomes have been reported to be involved in translocations at the 11q23 locus. In most of these neoplasms, the breakpoints within the 11q23 locus are localized to a 9 kb region and involve the promiscuous *mll* proto-oncogene *(1,67)*. Translocations involving the 11q23 region usually result in the formation of fusion transcripts that code for chimeric proteins *(67)*. In ALLs, 11q23 abnormalities are detected as translocations involving the following partner chromosome loci: 9p11, 9p21-p22, 4q21, 19p13, 1q21, 1p32, 6q27, 12p13, 17q21, 17q25, 20q13, and Xq13 *(67)*. Of these the t(4;11), t(9;11), and t(11;19) are most prevalent. Although the vast majority of ALLs with 11q23 abnormalities are of immature B-cell lineage, a small subset of cases possess an immature T-cell immunophenotype. In infants with precursor B-cell ALL, 11q23 abnormalities account for approximately 80% of the cases *(152)*. Rearrangements of *mll* correlate with age less than

six mo, hyperleukocytosis, absence of the CD10 antigen, and frequent co-expression of myeloid antigens (especially the CD15 antigen) *(153)*. The *mll* gene has been cloned and probes are available that may be used to detect rearrangements or deletions using Southern-blot hybridization or FISH methods *(67,153)*. Deletions and inversions of the 11q23 locus also occur in a subset of ALLs. These cases, unlike leukemias with 11q23 translocations, do not have *mll* gene rearrangements and have a relatively better prognosis *(154)*.

The t(4;11)(q21;q23), which occurs in approx 2% of childhood ALLs and 5–6% of adult ALLs, confers a poor prognosis *(1)*. The gene located at 4q21 is named *AF4* or *FEL* (for four eleven leukemia). The t(9;11)(p22;q23) accounts for about 1% of all ALL cases *(2)*. In the t(9;11), the gene located at 9p22 is known as *AF9*. The t(11;19)(q23;p13.3) accounts for about 2% of all ALL cases *(2)*. In the t(11;19), the gene located on chromosome band 19p13 is named *ENL* (for eleven nineteen leukemia) *(67)*. Chimeric proteins are formed by all three translocations, which have nuclear-targeting sequences that may facilitate transcriptional regulation.

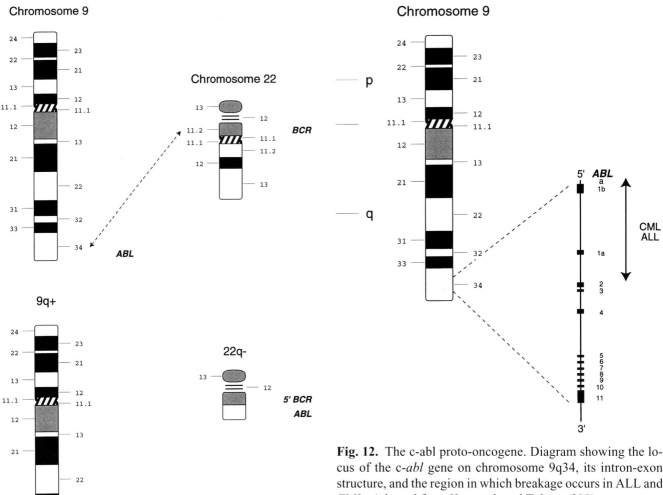

Fig. 11. Idiogram of the cytogenetic events in CML. Compare the normal chromosomes (top set) to the derivative chromosomes (bottom set) of the balanced and reciprocal translocation between the long arms of chromosomes 9 and 22, t(9;22)(q34;q11). The derivative 22q- is known as the Philadelphia chromosome. The *BCR* gene at 22q11 is divided and the *ABL* gene of 9q34 is joined to the remainder of *BCR* on chromosome 22.

t(12;21)(p12;q22) A number of unbalanced translocations and interstitial deletions occur in the 12p13 region in a wide range of hematopoietic neoplasms, including a subset of childhood ALLs *(155)*. Abnormalities of three genes identified at this locus may be mechanistically involved with the development of hematopoietic malignancies: rearrangements involving *TEL (ETV6)*, deletions of *KIP1,* or amplifications of *CCND2*, which encodes cyclin D2 *(156)*.

TEL is an *ets*-like gene on 12p that is a transcription factor. The t(12;21)(p12;q22) joins sequences from the *TEL* gene with

Fig. 12. The c-abl proto-oncogene. Diagram showing the locus of the c-*abl* gene on chromosome 9q34, its intron-exon structure, and the region in which breakage occurs in ALL and CML. Adapted from Kurzrock and Talpaz *(298)*.

those from the *aml1* gene on chromosome 21q. This translocation produces a fusion gene that encodes a chimeric protein containing the basic helix-loop-helix (bHLH) domain of *TEL* fused to the DNA-binding subunit of the aml1/CBFβ transcription-factor complex *(157)*. Although this translocation is detectable by routine cytogenetic studies in less than 5% of pediatric ALL cases, cryptic *TEL/aml1* fusions have been found using RT-PCR methods in 22–27% of pediatric ALL patients, representing the most frequent genetic lesion in childhood ALL *(157,158)*. Most but not all 12p cytogenetic abnormalities in childhood ALL involve *TEL (159)*. These cases are associated with a nonhyperdiploid DNA content and a favorable prognosis *(159)*.

KIP1 is a candidate tumor-suppressor gene that encodes the p27^{KIP1} cdk inhibitor of the cyclin E-cdk2 complex *(160)*. p27^{KIP1} belongs to a group of cdk inhibitors that possess ankryn-repeat motifs *(161)*. However, abnormalities of *KIP1* have not been demonstrated in childhood ALL *(162,163)*. Translocations and deletions involving the 12p13 locus may be detected using either Southern-blot analysis or FISH *(155,160)*.

t(5;14)(q31;q32) Involving IL-3 Some precursor B-cell ALLs are associated with eosinophilia and carry the t(5;14)(q31;q32) chromosomal rearrangement *(164,165)*. Meeker and coworkers determined that the breakpoints on chromosome 5 are tightly clustered within the promoter region of the *interleukin-3* (*IL-3*) gene, whereas the chromosome 14 breakpoints occur within the joining region of the *IgH* gene *(165,166)*. The translocation results in the head-to-head juxtaposition of the *IL-3* gene with the *IgH* gene-joining region. In all likelihood, this chromosomal translocation results in overexpression of *IL-3* mRNA, resulting in interleukin-3 (IL-3)-induced eosinophilia and stimulation of the leukemic clone presumably via an autocrine loop.

Other Proto-oncogenes and Tumor-Suppressor Genes *p53* gene mutations have been identified in a small subset of t(1;19) ALLs. In one study, 2/22 (9%) cases at diagnosis and three additional cases at the time of relapse had *p53* mutations. *p53* gene mutations appear to correlate with a worse prognosis *(147)*.

c-N-*ras* gene mutations have been reported in 6/33 (18%) null cell (precursor B-cell) ALLs *(167)*. Neri and coworkers reported that c-N-*ras* gene mutations preferentially involve codons 12 or 13 *(167)*. Kawamura and colleagues also identified a c-N-*ras* gene mutation in 1/22 (4.5%) cases of ALL that exhibit the t(1;19) chromosomal rearrangement *(147)*. c-K-*ras* and c-H-*ras* gene mutations are rare in precursor B-cell ALLs *(147,167)*.

p16^{INK4A} and *p15^{INK4B}* are two candidate tumor-suppressor genes whose products function to inhibit cyclin D-dependent kinases. Occasional immature B-cell ALLs with *p16^{INK4A}* and *p15^{INK4B}* homozygous deletions also have been described *(168–171)*. For example, out of 31 cases of B-lineage ALL, Hebert and colleagues found only 1 homozygous deletion and 4 possible hemizygous deletions of the *p16^{INK4A}* locus *(169)*. As these genes likely play a greater role in T-cell ALL, they are described in greater detail in that section.

Gene Amplification Childhood ALL patients with a hyperdiploid karyotype (defined as >50 chromosomes or a DNA index ≥1.16) have a favorable prognosis, presumably because their disease tends to be more responsive to chemotherapy **(172,173)**. Studies have shown that trisomy of both chromosomes 4 and 10 identify a subgroup of pediatric B-cell ALL patients with an extremely favorable 4-yr event-free survival and are likely to be cured with antimetabolite-based chemotherapy *(174)*. Increased copy number of genes on these chromosomes may contribute to leukemogenesis and to the greater responsiveness to chemotherapy.

Amplification of the *dihydrofolate reductase (DHFR)* gene, a known mechanism of resistance to methotrexate in cell lines, was demonstrated in 31% of 29 patients with ALL at the time of relapse *(175)*. The twofold to fourfold increase in *DHFR* gene copy number correlated with increased levels of *DHFR* mRNA and enzyme activity. Moreover, there was a statistically significant association between *p53* mutations and *DHFR* gene amplification, leading these investigators to postulate that mutations in the *p53* gene may lead to *DHFR* gene amplification as a result of defects in cell-cycle regulation.

B-CELL ALL

t(8;14), t(2;8), and t(8;22) Altogether, these three translocations occur in approx 6% of all ALLs, and in 85–90% of surface Ig-positive ALLs with FAB-L3 morphology *(1,139,176,177)*. These leukemias are counterparts to Burkitt's

lymphoma (BL). These subtypes are important to identify because they often present with retroperitoneal lymph-node or CNS involvement, are rapidly progressive, and may be more responsive to intensive chemotherapy protocols *(178,179)*.

The t(8;14)(q24;q32) juxtaposes the coding region of the c-*myc* gene on chromosome 8 with the enhancer for the *IgH* locus on chromosome 14, presumably bringing c-*myc* mRNA expression under control of the cis-elements that regulate *IgH* expression *(176)*. Investigators studying BL have found that the translocated, or deregulated, copy of c-*myc* may contain point mutations in the transactivation domain, suggesting possible expression of a mutant rather than a normal c-myc protein *(180)*. Two other variant translocations, t(2;8)(p12;q24) and t(8;22)(q24;q11), also place c-*myc* under control of an enhancer for one of the *Ig* light chain genes in an analogous fashion.

The c-*myc* gene on chromosome 8q24 encodes a transcription factor with a bHLH domain. The c-myc protein forms an activating heterodimeric complex with a protein called max *(181,182)*, which in turn is regulated by dimers formed between max and the c-myc-related proteins mad and mxi1 that antagonize the activity of the c-myc/max heterodimer *(183,184)*. Overexpression of c-*myc* is thought to upset the equilibrium between c-myc/max and c-myc/mad complexes, thereby leading to overexpression of other poorly characterized target genes in the pathway.

PRECURSOR T-CELL ALL Gene rearrangement studies of precursor T-cell ALLs have shown various patterns of *TCR* gene rearrangement (Fig. 10), corresponding to the stage of differentiation of the neoplasm. These may be divided into three groups (early-thymic, mid-thymic, and late-thymic) in accord with the maturation sequence of normal thymic T-cells *(185,186)*. ALLs are typically arrested at an earlier stage of differentiation than their lymphoblastic-lymphoma counterparts. Lineage infidelity occurs frequently in precursor T-cell precursor ALLs. *IgH* gene rearrangements occur in about 20% of cases *(187)*. However, *IgL* gene rearrangements are rare.

In a subset of early-thymic T-cell ALLs, only rearrangements of the *TCR-δ* gene or both the *TCR-δ* and *TCR-γ* genes are identified with the *TCR-β* gene in the germline configuration *(185)*. In the remaining early-thymic cases, and all of the mid-thymic and late-thymic ALLs, each of the *TCR* genes are rearranged. The *TCR-δ* gene is often deleted after rearrangement *(185)*. Although the *TCR-α* gene is difficult to analyze by Southern-blot analysis due to its large size, *TCR-α* gene transcripts have been detected in late-thymic T-cell ALLs using Northern-blot hybridization. These findings suggest a hierarchy of *TCR* gene rearrangements in normal developing T lymphocytes: the *TCR-δ* gene rearrangment occurs first, followed by rearrangement of the *TCR-γ* and the *TCR-β* genes, followed by rearrangement of the *TCR-α* locus *(185)*.

A number of nonrandom chromosomal translocations involving candidate proto-oncogenes have been described in precursor T-cell ALLs. Tumor-suppressor genes also may be involved. Some of the more common abnormalities are discussed in the following subsections.

Rearrangements Involving tal-1 The *tal-1* gene is rearranged in 25–30% of precursor T-cell ALLs *(188,189)*. It is found with a consistently greater frequency in childhood T-

ALL than in adult T-ALL *(190–192)*. The *tal-1* gene is located at chromosome 1p32. It encodes a protein with a bHLH domain that is a member of a family of transcription factors involved in growth regulation and differentiation. The *tal-1* gene is not normally expressed in T cells. As a consequence of interstitial deletions, chromosomal translocations, or possibly point mutations, *tal-1* comes under the influence of the regulatory elements of a gene that is expressed in T cells. This event results in the inappropriate expression of *tal-1*. Studies in transgenic mice suggest that hyperphosphorylation of the aberrantly expressed tal-1 protein may be leukemogenic *(193)*.

In most cases with *tal-1* gene rearrangements, small interstitial deletions in the *tal-1* locus result in the joining of the *tal-1* gene with a gene known as *SIL* that is normally expressed in T cells. This joining is thought to be due to illegitimate recombination mediated by the VDJ recombinase mechanism using heptamer-nonamer-like sequences flanking each gene *(188,194)*. In these cases, no abnormalities are detectable by standard cytogenetic analysis. In a small subset of cases the t(1;14)(p32;q11) is present. This translocation places the *tal-1* gene in continuity with the *TCR-δ* enhancer. A similar translocation, the t(1;7)(p33;q35), places the *tal-1* gene in continuity with the *TCR-β* enhancer. Immunohistochemical studies with a MAb that reacts with tal-1 protein have shown that its expression can occur independently of *tal-1* deletions or translocations *(195)*. Thus, mechanisms other than *tal-1* gene rearrangement, such as point mutations, may also be involved in protein expression. Gene rearrangements involving *tal-1*, both deletions and translocations, are identifiable by Southern-blot or PCR analyses.

del(9)(p21-22) Involving p15INK4B and p16INK4A

Approximately 10% of precursor ALLs, most often of T-cell lineage, have deletions of chromosome 9p21-p22 as demonstrated by conventional cytogenetics *(196,197)*. Recent studies have identified several closely related candidate tumor-suppressor genes at this locus: two cell-cycle inhibitors, *p16^{INK4A}* at 9p21 and *p15^{INK4B}* located 12 kb centromeric to the *p16^{INK4A}* exon 1β *(198)*. The *p16^{INK4A}* and *p15^{INK4B}* genes encode 16 kDa and 15 kDa proteins, respectively, that inhibit cdk4 and cdk6. Cdk4 and cdk6 are involved in regulating cell-cycle progression from the G_1 to the S phase, and their inhibition would be expected to provide a cell with a growth advantage, perhaps by resulting in the shortening the cell-generation time *(168)*.

Homozygous (and less frequently heterozygous) deletions of the *p16^{INK4A}* locus have been identified in precursor ALLs, with the vast majority of cases being of immature T-cell lineage *(168–171)*. *p16^{INK4A}* deletions have been identified in most cases with 9p21-p22 deletion as shown by conventional cytogenetics as well as in cases in which conventional cytogenetics are normal *(168)*. The *p15^{INK4B}* locus has a similar frequency of homozygous deletions in immature T-cell ALLs, although this locus has been analyzed less commonly *(168)*. *p16^{INK4A}* and *p15^{INK4B}* gene deletions, in addition to correlating strongly with immature T-cell lineage, correlate with a poorer survival and are uncommon in hyperdiploid ALLs *(168,169,172,173)*.

Recently, the breakpoints in *p16^{INK4A}* have been found to occur in two clusters (*bcrα* and *bcrβ*) that are located near heptamers whose sequences resemble those involved in VDJ

recombination *(199)*. Because all of the cases of T-cell ALL studied by Cayuela et al. *(199)* also contained short deletions, GC-rich tandem nucleotide additions, or clone-specific junctional sequences, the combined findings not only suggest tumor-suppressor gene inactivation by an illegitimate VDJ recombinational mechanism, but also bolster the hypothesis that this process is involved in normal T-cell differentiation and plays a role in the development of T-cell ALL.

t(10;14)(q24;q11) and t(7;10)(q34;q24) Approximately 5–10% of T-cell ALLs carry the t(10;14), involving the *hox11* gene situated on chromosome 10q24. T-cell ALLs with the t(7;10)(q34;q24) also involve the *hox11* gene. The *hox11* gene has been characterized as a homeobox gene, which is involved in transcriptional regulation *(200)*. It is not normally expressed in T-cells but is expressed in the adult livers and fetal spleens of animals *(200,201)*. Overexpression of this gene in the thymus of transgenic mice appears to correlate with the development of T-cell neoplasms *(202)*. In the majority of cases, the breakpoint on chromosome 10 is upstream of the *hox11* gene, placing it under the influence of a *TCR* enhancer, thereby resulting in deregulation and increased expression of the normal hox11 protein *(200)*. *TCR-α/δ* and *TCR-β* are located at 14q11 and 7q34, respectively. DNA probes to detect *hox11* gene rearrangements can be obtained and an antibody reactive with hox11 protein has been developed *(203)*. Immunohistochemical studies have shown that hox11 protein is maximally expressed at the transition from G_1 to S phases of the cell cycle *(203)*.

t(8;13)(p11;q11) Rare cases of precursor T-cell ALL/LBL are associated with peripheral blood or tissue eosinophilia and carry a t(8;13)(p11;q11) *(204–206)*. Clinical follow-up of these patients has shown that they have a high risk for developing myeloid hyperplasia, MDS, or AML. This translocation results in the joining of the *FGFR1* (fibroblast growth factor receptor 1) gene on chromosome 8p11 with the novel *ZNF198* gene on chromosome 13q11 *(207)*. The *ZNF198-FGFR1* fusion transcript encodes an approx 76 kDa polypeptide, localized predominantly to the cytoplasm. It is predicted to contain zinc-finger domains from the novel gene fused to the tyrosine kinase domain of *FGFR1* that probably results in zinc-finger-mediated homodimerization. Southern-blot analysis and RT-PCR methods may be used to detect this translocation.

Other Translocations Involving TCR Loci Other translocations have been identified in precursor T-cell ALLs by conventional cytogenetics, often involving the T-cell antigen receptor loci: *TCR-α/δ* at 14q11, *TCR-β* at 7q34, and *TCR-γ* at 7p15 *(1)*. These translocations, present in small subsets of precursor T-cell ALL, involve known or candidate proto-oncogenes brought into continuity with the antigen-receptor locus, with dysregulation and inappropriate overexpression of the proto-oncogene product. For example, the c-*myc* gene may be rearranged in T-cell ALLs, as a result of translocation to the *TCR-δ* locus *(208)*. This subgroup of leukemias are aggressive and frequently accompanied by extramedullary disease. Rearrangements joining the candidate proto-oncogene *tcl1* on chromosome 14q32 to the *TCR* locus at 14q11 have been described in acute as well as chronic T-cell leukemias arising in the immunodeficiency syndrome ataxia telangiectasia (AT) *(209)*.

The t(7;9)(q34;q32) activates the *tal-2* gene, a transcription factor with a bHLH motif bearing great sequence homology to *tal-1*. The *tal-2* gene is located on chromosome 9q32, and the t(7;9)(q34;q32) juxtaposes *tal-2* next to sequences from the *TCR-β* locus on chromosome 7q34 *(210)*. The t(7;19)(q34;p13) is another translocation in T-ALL that involves the *lyl-1* gene at chromosome 19p13. The *lyl-1* gene encodes another member of this subgroup of bHLH transcription factors that is inappropriately altered. The t(7;19)(q34;p13) results in its head-to-head juxtaposition of *lyl-1* with the *TCR-β* locus and truncation of its mRNA *(211)*.

t(11;14)(p15;q11) and t(11;14)(p13;q11) The *ttg-1* (T-cell translocation gene 1, also known as *RHOMB1 or RBTN1* for rhombotin 1) and *ttg-2 (RHOMB2 or RBTN2)* genes are candidate proto-oncogenes that are located at chromosome 11p15 and 11p13, respectively. The frequency of translocations in T-ALL with *ttg-1* is less than 1%, whereas it may be nearly 7% for *ttg-2 (212)*. These genes become juxtaposed with the *TCR-δ* locus at 14q11 via t(11;14)(p15;q11) or t(11;14)(p13;q11) translocations, respectively, due to erroneous VDJ joining *(212,213)*. These genes are not normally expressed in T-cells. The ttg-1 and ttg-2 proteins are members of a subset of nuclear-localizing zinc-finger proteins containing cysteine-rich LIM domains and likely function as regulators of transcription *(212,214)*. The *ttg-2* has been demonstrated to be essential in erythropoiesis using homologous recombination in mice *(215)*.

A translocation is thought to cause aberrant expression of the encoded protein. Dysregulation may occur either by putting the gene under the control of the *TCR-δ* enhancer or, in those cases lacking this enhancer on the translocated allele, by disturbing the negative regulatory region of the T-cell translocation gene's promoter *(216)*. The incidence of T-cell malignancies in transgenic mice is tied to the level of transgene expression *(217,218)*. Intriguingly, ttg-1 and ttg-2 also possess the ability to associate specifically with tal-1, tal-2 or lyl-1 in vivo, but not with other bHLH proteins, and a subgroup of T-cell ALL patients harbor both *ttg-2* and *tal-1* rearrangements *(219)*.

11q23 Rearrangements Involving mll Rearrangements involving the *mll* gene are uncommon in T-cell ALL, when compared to their frequency in precursor B-cell ALL or AML. Several cases of t(11;19)(q23;p13) have been reported, one of which was studied and shown to contain an *mll-ENL* fusion gene *(220,221)*. The t(X;11)(q13;q23) has been reported in a human T-ALL cell line *(222)*.

t(7;9)(q34;q34.3) The incidence of t(7;9)(q34;q34.3) ranges up to 5% of patients with T-cell ALL. This translocation juxtaposes sequences from the *tan1* gene on 9q with the *TCR-β* locus on 7q34, leading to the inappropriate expression of a truncated gene product in T lymphocytes *(223,224)*. The *tan1* gene is a mammalian homolog of the *Drosophila notch* gene that encodes a transmembrane protein *(211,223,225)*. This integral membrane protein is usually involved with signal transduction during cellular differentiation. The abnormal tan1 protein produced by the translocation aberrantly localizes to the nucleus and induces T-cell neoplasms when introduced into the bone marrow of mice *(224)*.

inv(14)(q11q32.3) The inv(14)(q11q32.3), commonly found in AT *(226)*, also has been reported in T-cell ALL *(227)*. It arises from interlocus VDJ recombination and may signify a propensity towards abnormal recombinational activity rather than being oncogenic in-and-of itself *(227)*.

Tumor-Suppressor Genes *p53* gene mutations are infrequent at diagnosis in patients with T-cell ALL *(228)*, but appear to be common in cell lines established at the time of relapse *(229)*. The *Rb1* tumor-suppressor gene has been reported to be inactivated in 11–29% of ALL that exhibit the Philadelphia chromosome rearrangement *(122)*. Inactivation of this tumor-suppressor gene has been suggested to play a role in ALL disease progression *(122)*.

CHRONIC MYELOID LEUKEMIA

CML primarily affects adults and is distinguished by a neutrophilic leukocytosis, basophilia, eosinophilia, anemia, and splenomegaly, among other findings. The bone marrow at diagnosis is usually hypercellular with granulocytic hyperplasia. The disease course frequently entails two or three separate phases: 1) an initial chronic phase that lasts at least 3–4 yr; 2) a transitional accelerated phase that lasts about 6 mo in which there is a progressive left shift in myeloid maturation, often associated with new cytogenetic abnormalities; and 3) a terminal blast crisis characterized by a proliferation of myeloid, lymphoid, or less commonly megakaryoblastic or erythroid blasts.

CML is a paradigm for the leukemias in several ways. It is a clonal disorder in which nearly all classical cases show cytogenetic evidence of a distinct chromosomal abnormality *(230)*, a small chromosome 22 called the Philadelphia chromosome after the city where it was discovered. Moreover, it was one of the first chromosomal translocations associated with human neoplasia to be characterized at the molecular cytogenetic level *(231,232)*. CML is now defined by the presence of the t(9;22)(q34;q11) and as a result, the definition of CML has been extended to include variant cases that lack cytogenetic evidence of the Philadelphia chromosome, but have molecular evidence of its constituent hybrid gene component, *bcr-abl* *(233,234)*.

PHILADELPHIA CHROMOSOME-POSITIVE CML The Philadelphia chromosome, which can be found in 90–95% of cases of CML, is the cytogenetic hallmark of this disease. Initially described as 22q- *(230)*, it was subsequently recognized as a partner in a reciprocal translocation, designated t(9;22)(q34;q11) *(235)*. Although it was once thought to be pathognomonic for CML, evidence of this translocation is also found in approx one-third of cases of ALL and in <1% of AMLs. The t(9;22)(q34;q11) in CML involves the translocation of sequences from the proto-oncogene c-*abl*, the cellular homolog of the transforming sequence of Abelson murine leukemia virus (v-*abl*), located on chromosome 9, to the *bcr* locus of chromosome 22q- (Fig. 11) *(231)*. Although a provocative cytogenetic study supported maternal origin for the Philadelphia chromosome and paternal origin for the derivative 9q+ based on inheritance patterns of polymorphic heterochromatin near the centromeres *(236)*, molecular studies have shown that neither gene is actually imprinted *(237,238)*. In addition, *bcr-abl* recombination occurs in variants of the classical Philadel-

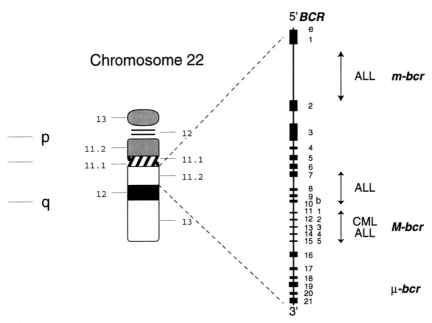

Fig. 13. The bcr gene. Diagram showing the *bcr* gene on chromosome 22q11, its intron-exon structure, and the regions in which breakage occurs (including the breakpoint cluster regions) for ALL and CML. Adapted from Heisterkamp et al. *(248)*.

phia chromosome that include complex translocations between chromosomes 9, 22, and another chromosome (usually chromosome 1 or 11) *(234)*.

c-abl The c-*abl* gene spans over 230 kb *(239,240)*. By convention the exons of c-*abl* are numbered 1b, 1a, and a2-a11 from 5'→3' (Fig. 12). The 5'-exons (1b and 1a) of c-*abl* undergo alternative splicing to exon a2. This normally yields 6 kb and 7 kb mRNA transcripts that encode two alternative type 1a and 1b p145[abl] proteins that differ in their N-terminal amino acid sequence *(241–243)*. The normal c-*abl* gene product resides at least in part in the nucleus *(244)* and contains regulatory *src*-homology domains SH2 and SH3, a tyrosine kinase domain, a DNA-binding domain, and actin-binding domains. It is probably involved in cell-cycle regulation *(245)* and its level of expression decreases with granulocytic differentiation *(246)*. In CML the breakpoint on chromosome 9 can occur over a 300 kb segment of the c-*abl* gene, upstream of exon 1b, between exons 1b and 1a, or between exons 1b and a2 *(247)*.

bcr The breakpoints on chromosome 22 are localized to a 5.8 kb region, originally called the breakpoint-cluster region or *bcr (232)*. It is now referred to as the major breakpoint-cluster region (M-*bcr*) because two additional breakpoint-cluster regions have since been described. Heisterkamp and colleagues *(248)* showed that this breakpoint-cluster region was part of a larger gene on chromosome 22 (Fig. 13), now known as *bcr*. It encompasses exons e12-e16 of *bcr* that historically are referred to as M-*bcr* exons b1-b5. In its entirety, the *bcr* gene consists of 21 exons that stretch over a region of 130 kb *(249–252)*. It encodes a protein (p160[bcr]) with dimerization, phospho-serine/threonine-rich SH2 binding, *DBL*-like (a guanine-nucleotide-releasing factor for the GTP-binding protein CDC24H), and GTPase activating protein for p21[RAC] (GAP[RAC]) domains *(253–258)*. The subcellular localization of bcr protein shifts from being predominantly cytoplasmic in interphase cells to being largely perichromosomal during mitosis *(259,260)*. The overall features suggest that bcr protein may be involved in signal-transduction pathways and cytoskeletal/chromatin organization. The *bcr* breakpoints in CML most frequently arise between M-*bcr* exons b2 and b3, or between M-*bcr* exons b3 and b4. A breakpoint either 5' or 3' of M-*bcr* is uncommon, occurring in less than 5% of cases.

bcr-abl and *p210*[bcr-abl]. The aforementioned translocations result in aberrant hybrid genes, *bcr-abl* on the 22q- (Philadelphia chromosome) and *abl-bcr* on the 9q+ derivative chromosome, respectively *(261)*. Despite the absolute position of the c-*abl* breakpoint, processing of the primary *bcr-abl* transcript generally produces a fusion mRNA with a b2-a2 junction, a b3-a2 junction, or occasionally both types due to alternative splicing *(115)*. Translation yields at least two very similar p210[bcr-abl] fusion protein variants that differ only slightly by the amino acids encoded by M-*bcr* exon 3 without affecting clinical outcome *(262,263)*.

Regardless of which molecular species is produced, p210[bcr-abl] is uniformly expressed in Philadelphia chromosome-positive CML, aberrantly localizes to the cytoplasm, and possesses enhanced tyrosine kinase activity and transforming capabilities *(115,233,246)*. Moreover, a CML-like syndrome can be induced in irradiated mice reconstituted with bone marrow-progenitor cells transfected with a retrovirus containing *bcr-abl* constructs *(264,265)*.

bcr-abl plays a crucial role in the initiation of CML *(266–268)*. The *bcr-abl* oncogene encoding p210[bcr-abl] combines N-terminal *bcr* and C-terminal c-*abl* sequences *(269)*. The *bcr* first exon is a critical component of the transforming capability exerted by *bcr-abl*. The serine/threonine kinase domain of the bcr protein is able to bind to the SH2 regulatory domain of c-abl and other putative signal transduction proteins such as the SH2 domain of the GRB2 (for growth factor receptor binding protein 2) adaptor protein *(255,270,271)*. Its coiled-coil oligomerization domain brings about tetramerization of bcr-abl

(258). The net effect is to initiate constitutive tyrosine kinase activity and activate the F-actin-binding domain contributed by c-abl. The c-ras-related signal-transduction proteins are likely substrates of p210$^{bcr-abl}$, resulting in disruption of these important signaling pathways (254,271–274). For example, p210$^{bcr-abl}$ binds GRB2 and CRKL (CT10 regulator of kinase-like adapter protein), each of which can bind SOS (son of sevenless; a guanine-nucleotide releasing factor) and then activate the c-ras signaling pathway (34,275). Activation of F-actin binding probably leads to aberrant subcellular localization by promoting attachment to the cytoskeleton, thereby interfering with translocation to the nucleus (245). The c-myc protein also has been implicated in bcr-abl-induced transformation (276,277). Other aspects concerning the pathogenesis of CML are beyond the scope of this chapter and are reviewed elsewhere (275,278,279).

Variant bcr-abl Transcripts A minor breakpoint cluster region (m-bcr) that occurs upstream of M-bcr between exons e1 and e2 produces an e1a2 transcript that encodes a smaller (p190$^{bcr-abl}$) fusion protein (280). The m-bcr is involved in nearly two-thirds of Philadelphia chromosome-positive ALLs, but only rarely in CML or AML. The rare cases of CML associated with p190$^{bcr-abl}$ share certain characteristics with chronic myelomonocytic leukemia, such as an absolute monocytosis and a decreased neutrophil:monocyte ratio (281).

A micro breakpoint-cluster region (μ-bcr) also has been found at the 3' end of the bcr gene, between exons e19 and e20, that encodes a larger (p230$^{bcr-abl}$) fusion protein (282–284). Those rare cases associated with p230$^{bcr-abl}$ show a greater degree of myeloid maturation and have been characterized as neutrophilic-CML or chronic neutrophilic leukemia (282–284).

Report of bcr-abl in Healthy Individuals bcr-abl transcripts have been detected at extraordinarily low levels by RT-PCR in healthy adults and children (285). This observation suggests that bcr-abl has to be expressed in the appropriate progenitor cells in order to gain a selective growth advantage and cause clinical disease (278).

abl-bcr In contrast to bcr-abl, the reciprocal chimeric abl-bcr gene on derivative chromosome 9q+ encodes a product that is not thought to play a pivotal role in the pathogenesis of CML because it is not expressed in almost 40% of cases (247). Although the fusion transcript has been detected in cases of CML by RT-PCR (247), the abl-bcr protein has not been found, perhaps due to technical limitations (278). It has been suggested that if abl-bcr is expressed, it might account for some of the differences in presentation or clinical outcome. Although one group of investigators advanced preliminary data that abl-bcr-positive patients might respond more favorably to interferon-α (IFN-α) therapy (286), this hypothesis has not been confirmed (287,288).

PHILADELPHIA CHROMOSOME-NEGATIVE CML Studies employing molecular techniques have identified bcr-abl recombinations in molecular variants that have seemingly unaltered chromosomes 9 or 22 at the cytogenetic level or a subtle alteration at 9q34 (289–292). These Philadelphia chromosome-negative bcr-positive CML cases have a clinical course comparable to that of cases that contain the Philadelphia chromosome. Mechanisms elucidated thus far include intersti-

tial insertion of c-abl next to M-bcr and multiple recombinations involving 9q34, 22, and another chromosome (289,293). Cases harboring masked or cryptic bcr-abl recombinations account for approx 5% of patients with CML.

Kurzrock and coworkers reported a small series of cases of chronic phase CML that lacked evidence of the t(9;22)(q34;q11) or bcr-abl, and whose presentation differed from Philadelphia chromosome-positive bcr-positive CML only by older age at onset and B symptoms (294). The clinical course of these patients was distinctive in that they did not enter blast crisis. Rather, their course was characterized by an increasing leukemia burden, organomegaly, involvement of extramedullary sites, and bone marrow failure without a marked increase in blasts (294).

Finally, a subset of cases have been historically classified as Philadelphia chromosome-negative CML (or atypical CML) on the basis of some shared morphologic features, but lack evidence of the t(9;22)(q34;q11) or bcr-abl. These cases probably represent myelodysplastic disorders such as chronic myelomonocytic leukemia (295). Interestingly, Cogswell and colleagues reported that 54% of patients who exhibit bcr-negative chronic-phase CML (atypical CML) with features suggestive of a variant of chronic myelomonocytic leukemia harbored mutations in the c-ras gene family (296).

ACCELERATED PHASE AND BLAST CRISIS At the microscopic level, additional cytogenetic changes may herald the onset of the accelerated phase or the blast phase of CML. The most frequently observed cytogenetic abnormalities include trisomy 8, iso-chromosome 17, an additional Philadelphia chromosome, or iso-chromosome 19 (297). A t(3;21)(q26;q22) translocation, monosomy 7, and loss of chromosome Y occur less commonly (298,299).

At the molecular level, a variety of low-frequency acquired events have been reported in association with transformation, suggesting that maturation arrest may occur as a result of the interruption of several pathways (268,278,300). Gene amplification of c-myc, located at 8q24, also has been implicated in progression of CML (301). Alterations of the p53 gene have been found in the myeloid and megakaryocytic variants of blast crisis, accounting for progression in around 25% of CML patients (300,302). Deletion of a single p53 allele is associated with CML displaying i(17q) and or no karyotypic changes, and this deletion event is presumably followed by inactivation of the remaining p53 allele through loss of expression, point mutation, or rarely rearrangement (302). Theories regarding the potential role of a second Philadelphia chromosome, such as increased gene expression or a new bcr-abl rearrangement, are intriguing but the evidence is inconclusive (298). Homozygous deletion of the p16^{INK4A} tumor-suppressor gene has been reported in 50% of CML patients with lymphoid blast crisis (303). Structural abnormalities of the Rb1 gene with absent protein expression were reported with a 11–29% incidence in lymphoid blast crisis of Philadelphia chromosome-positive CML (122). Some cases of CML in megakaryoblastic crisis may lack expression of pRb as well (304). As in AML, the t(3;21)(q26;q22) in CML encodes a novel aml1-evi1 fusion protein that is a chimeric transcription factor, which would be predicted to induce a differentiation block and stimulate proliferation *(299)*. In contrast, c-*ras* gene mutations are uncommon in this situation as compared to chronic-phase Philadelphia chromosome-negative CML; only one case was reported in 18 patients with Philadelphia chromosome-positive CML in blast crisis *(296)*. The apparent emergence of p190[bcr-abl] in p210[bcr-abl]-positive CML patients also has been put forth as a putative mechanism of transformation *(305)*. However, recent reports indicate that low-level co-expression of p190[bcr-abl] with p210[bcr-abl] may occur due to alternative splicing and is detectable by RT-PCR in most cases of CML with M-*bcr* breakpoints *(306–308)*.

JUVENILE CML AND CHILDHOOD PHILADELPHIA CHROMOSOME-POSITIVE CML Juvenile chronic myelogenous leukemia (JCML) is a biologically distinctive entity of monocytic lineage that differs clinically and pathologically from adult Philadelphia chromosome-positive CML, more closely resembling adult chronic myelomonocytic leukemia *(309)*. It affects children less than 4 yr of age and represents only 2% of all childhood leukemias *(310)*. Cases of JCML are Philadelphia chromosome-negative and lack the *bcr-abl* recombination *(311,312)*. The mononuclear blasts in this disorder express c-*myc* and c-*fos* mRNA at high levels, consistent with proliferative state and monocytic origin *(313)*. Mutations of the c-*ras* genes occur in a small number of cases *(314)*. In addition, rearrangement of the *IgH* gene has been reported, suggesting transformation of a stem cell with intermediate differentiation towards both the myelomonocytic and the B-cell lineages *(315)*.

There are also rare cases of childhood Philadelphia chromosome-positive CML that closely resemble adult CML clinically, phenotypically, and cytogenetically *(316–319)*. As in adult CML, a M-*bcr* breakpoints yield a p210[bcr-abl] fusion protein. However, in contrast to adult CML, b2-a2 transcripts b3-a2 transcript *(317)*.

MOLECULAR METHODS FOR DIAGNOSIS AND DETECTION OF MINIMAL RESIDUAL DISEASE The diagnosis of CML may be confirmed by conventional cytogenetic analysis *(230,235)* or by routine Southern-blot analysis using an M-*bcr*-specific probe and multiple-enzyme digests *(320)*. More sensitive techniques such as FISH *(321,322)*, or RT-PCR are also very popular because they permit molecular characterization and assessment of minimal residual disease following therapy *(323)*. FISH allows semiquantitative determination of the percentage of cells positive for the t(9;22) and variations of the RT-PCR technique also permit semiquantitative determinations. Cautious interpretation is advised because there is a high incidence of RT-PCR positivity in the first year post-bone marrow transplantation and a single positive result may not be predictive of relapse *(324)*. However, analysis of serial specimens is a better measure of the risk of relapse, permitting stratification of patients into risk groups *(324)*. A subset of patients on prolonged maintenance therapy who were in clinical remission and were cytogenetically negative, but were still RT-PCR positive, ultimately became RT-PCR-negative *(325)*.

CHRONIC LYMPHOID LEUKEMIAS

B-CELL CHRONIC LYMPHOCYTIC LEUKEMIA Virtually all cases of B-cell chronic lymphocytic leukemia (B-CLL) express surface Ig and have *IgH* and *IgL* gene rearrangements *(326)*. Either one or both *IgH* genes may be rearranged. In tumors with two rearranged bands, presumably one rearranged allele is nonfunctional and the other allele yields a functional rearrangement. More B-CLLs express *Igκ* than *Igλ*. Thus, in the majority of B-CLLs, the *Igκ* light chain gene is rearranged and the *Igλ* light chain is germline. In Igλ-positive tumors, both the *Igκ* and *Igλ* genes are rearranged, although the *Igκ* light-chain gene also may be subsequently deleted *(326)*. The *TCR* genes are usually in the germline configuration; less than 10% of B-CLLs have *TCR* gene rearrangements (lineage infidelity).

Biased use of *Ig* gene variable (V) segments has been described in B-CLL cases. The *VH1* gene family of the *IgH* gene and the *VIIIb* family of the *Igκ* gene are used in the formation of *Ig* gene rearrangements more often than can be explained by chance alone *(327,328)*. DNA sequence analysis of the V, diversity (D) and joining (J) segments involved in *IgH* and *Igk* gene rearrangement has shown a low frequency of somatic mutations *(328,329)*. These findings suggest that B-CLLs arise from B cells that have not been exposed to antigen selection *(327,328)*. However, a subset of B-CLLs do exhibit a significant frequency of somatic mutations in the V segments, particularly in cases with 13q14 chromosomal abnormalities and in cases that have undergone Ig heavy-chain switching and express either IgG or IgA *(327,330)*.

Low surface Ig expression is present in most cases of B-CLL. Surface Ig expression requires functional Ig protein and two other critical proteins, B29 (Igβ and CD79b) and mb-1 (Igα and CD79a), that are essential components of the B-cell antigen-receptor complex *(331)*. Thompson et al. *(332)* have shown that mutations in the *B29* gene and/or abnormalities of *B29* expression (at the mRNA level) are common in B-CLL. The diminished surface Ig on B-cell CLL cells may result in these cells being unresponsive to antigen binding, perhaps preventing initiation of growth signals or apoptosis cascades *(332)*.

Using conventional cytogenetic analysis, chromosomal abnormalities have been identified in approx 50% of cases of B-CLL, including trisomy 12, abnormalities of 13q14, deletions of 11q, and abnormalities of 14q32. Complex karyotypes are associated with a poor prognosis *(333)*. Trisomy 12 is most common, found in approx 10–20% of cases, and the 12q13-22 region is likely to be most important *(334–337)*. Trisomy 12 is usually identified in a subclone of neoplastic cells, and is not thought to be required for neoplastic transformation. Trisomy 12 is more commonly identified in B-CLL cases with atypical cytological features and may correlate with a poorer prognosis *(336)*. 13q14 abnormalities in B-CLL do not appear to have an impact on prognosis. However, B-cell CLLs with 11q deletions appear to be more aggressive and patients have shorter survival *(337,338)*. One problem encountered in conventional cytogenetic analysis is that B-CLLs are poorly proliferative, even with exposure to mitogens, and thus many cases are negative using this method. Chromosome abnormalities can be detected in B-CLL cases with a normal karyotype using other methods, such as FISH or CGH. For example, Bentz and colleagues compared conventional cytogenetics with CGH in 28 cases of B-CLL. In 13/28 (46%) cases, CGH detected chromosomal abnormalities involving a variety of chromosomes not detected by routine karyotyping. Loss of chromosome 17p most likely affecting p53 was most common, occurring in 9/28 (32%) cases of B-CLL *(339)*.

Conventional cytogenetic studies have rarely identified the t(14;18)(q32;q21) in B-CLL *(15)*. More commonly, Southern-blot hybridization studies have shown *bcl2* gene involvement, in 5–10% of cases of B-CLL. In these cases, the *bcl2* gene at 18q21 is involved in either the t(2;18)(p11;q21) or t(18;22)(q21;q11), involving the *Igκ* (chromosome 2p11) or *Igλ* (chromosome 22q11) gene loci *(340–342)*. The breakpoint on chromosome 18 usually occurs within the variant cluster region, 5' to the *bcl2* gene, but may also occur 3' to the *bcl2* gene, at a location intermediate between the major and minor breakpoint cluster regions *(340–342)*. Errors in the VDJ recombination process may be involved in the generation of the t(2;18) and t(18;22), as a heptamer-like recognition sequence is present upstream of the *bcl2* gene *(12)*. Conventional cytogenetic studies also have shown the presence of either the t(2;18)(p11;q21) or the t(18;22)(q21;q11) in small subset of B-cell CLLs *(342)*. Despite the infrequency of chromosomal translocations involving the *bcl2* gene in B-CLLs, the majority of cases express bcl2 protein. The bcl2 protein is known to inhibit apoptosis (programmed cell death). Because chemotherapeutic drugs act by inducing apoptosis, bcl2 expression in B-CLL appears to be a major mechanism for drug resistance *(18)*.

Other chromosomal translocations identified in B-CLL include the t(14;19) and t(11;14). In both translocations, proto-oncogenes are juxtaposed with the *IgH* gene at chromosome 14q32 *(5,13)*. As a result, the transcriptional control of the proto-oncogene is brought under the control of the *IgH*-enhancer elements resulting in constitutive expresson. The t(14;19)(q32;q13) involves the *bcl3* gene at chromosome 19q13 *(343)*. This translocation is rare in B-CLL, approx 15 cases have been reported. The *bcl3* gene encodes a protein of the IκB family and is involved in regulating the NF-κB family of transcription factor proteins. The t(14;19) is commonly associated with trisomy 12 *(343)*. The t(11;14)(q13;q32) involves the *bcl1* gene at chromosome 11q13. The t(11;14) has been reported in approx 5% of B-CLLs *(344)*. The *bcl1* locus on 11q13 encodes cyclin D1 protein, which is involved in progression of the cell cycle from G_1 to S phase. Although the t(11;14) may occur in rare cases of B-CLL, the t(11;14) is common in mantle cell lymphoma, being present in virtually all cases *(345)*. Because it may be difficult to distinguish B-CLL from mantle-cell lymphoma in peripheral blood, it seems likely that most previously reported cases of B-CLL with the t(11;14) were, in fact, mantle-cell lymphoma. The *bcl6* gene is not usually rearranged in B-cell CLL *(346)*. The c-*myc* proto-oncogene is not rearranged in typical cases of B-CLL, and when found, usually correlates with histological transformation *(347)*.

Various tumor-suppressor genes have been analyzed for mutations in B-CLL. Of these, the *RB* locus or another tumor-suppressor cell gene telomeric to the *Rb1* locus is deleted commonly in B-CLL. Liu et al. *(348)* and Dohner and colleagues *(349)* have reported 13q14 deletions using Southern-blot analysis or FISH in approx 45% of cases of B-CLL. Studies using FISH and CGH also have frequently shown *Rb1* and 13q dele-

tions *(339,349)*. Abnormalities of other suppressor-cell genes also have been reported in B-CLL. *p53* gene mutations, identified in approx 10% of cases, correlate with drug resistance *(350)*. Deletions of the *p16^{INK4A}* and *p15^{INK4B}* genes have been identified in 5–10% of B-CLLs *(351)*. Additional chromosome abnormalities have been identified, such as loss of 11q involving the ATM tumor-suppressor genes at 11q22*(339)*.

Diffuse and widespread microsatellite instability (MSI) has been identified in a subset of cases (<10%) of B-CLL *(352)*. This finding, also known as a mutator phenotype, often correlates with mutations in critical mismatch repair (MMR) genes. The clinical and prognostic importance of the mutator phenotype in B-CLL cases is uncertain.

RICHTER'S SYNDROME B-CLL also may transform into high-grade diffuse lymphoma; this phenomenon has been given the eponym Richter's syndrome *(353)*. The high-grade lymphoma most often resembles diffuse large-cell or large-cell immunoblastic lymphoma. In the majority of cases of Richter's syndrome, conventional cytogenetics or Southern-blot analysis have demonstrated that both the B-CLL and the high-grade lymphoma components have common chromosomal abnormalities and/or identical *Ig* gene rearrangements, indicating that both tumors arose from the same neoplastic clone *(353)*. However, in other patients, Southern-blot studies have shown different patterns of *Ig* gene rearrangement in the low and high-grade lymphoma components. Because the *Ig* genes frequently undergo somatic mutation and may also undergo reiterative *Ig* gene rearrangements, so-called Ig receptor editing *(354)*, these changes can alter restriction-enzyme sites and the size of the rearranged fragments *(355)*. Thus, in these cases both components may still represent origin from the same clone. The presence of common cytogenetic abnormalities or common DNA sequences within the rearranged immunoglobulin genes in both the B-CLL and the high-grade lymphoma have proven a common clonal origin for that at least some Richter's syndrome cases with dissimilar Southern-blot results *(355)*. However, in a subset of patients with Richter's syndrome, the high-grade lymphoma may arise as a second and independent B-cell clone *(352)*.

In many cases of Richter's syndrome, cytogenetic abnormalities not present in the B-CLL have been found in the high-grade lymphoma, a reflection of the genomic instability of the neoplastic cells at the time of histological transformation *(334,356)*. There is no consistent pattern of cytogenetic abnormalities. In one study, Brynes and colleagues *(356)* showed that trisomy 12 was not initially present in the low-grade component but was acquired at the time of transformation. Occasionally, specific translocations have been identified only in the high-grade component, such as the t(8;14)(q24;q32) *(357)*. *p53* gene mutations are also commonly found in the high-grade lymphomas of Richter's syndrome, as compared with low-grade B-CLL *(358)*.

B-CELL PROLYMPHOCYTIC LEUKEMIA As in B-CLL, the *IgH* and *IgL* genes are rearranged in B-cell prolymphocytic leukemia (PLL) *(326)*. The *TCR* genes are rarely rearranged. Unlike B-CLL, the *Ig* genes demonstrate a higher frequency of somatic mutation consistent with antigen selection *(327)*. The t(11;14)(q13;q32) has been reported in a subset of cases of B-cell PLL *(359)*. Those cases may represent transformed mackel cell lymphoma. Trisomy 12 has been detected in a subset of cases *(335,359)*. The t(14;18)(q32;q21) and *bcl2* gene rearrangements have not been identified *(340)*. Other known B-cell proto-oncogenes (such as *bcl3*, *bcl6*, and c-*myc*) are not rearranged. The *p53* tumor-suppressor gene is frequently mutated in B-cell PLL. Lens and colleagues *(360)* found mutations of the *p53* gene in 10/19 (53%) cases. Unlike other lymphoid neoplasms with *p53* gene mutations, which are usually single-base substitutions, approx half of the mutations in B-cell PLL were deletions or insertions *(360)*.

HAIRY-CELL LEUKEMIA Molecular genetic studies were essential in establishing the B-cell lineage of hairy-cell leukemia (HCL) *(326,361)*. These neoplasms have rearrangements of the *IgH* and *IgL* genes *(361)*. In contrast with most other B-cell lymphoid neoplasms, which express Igκ more often than Igλ, *Igλ* is expressed as often or more commonly than *Igκ* in HCL *(361)*. Accordingly, the *Igλ* gene is productively rearranged more commonly than in other B-cell neoplasm. The *TCR-β* gene is usually in the germline configuration although lineage infidelity has been reported *(37)*. The *Ig* genes commonly undergo somatic mutations, consistent with these tumors arising from cells influenced by antigen selection *(362)*. Trisomy 12 has been infrequently identified in HCL *(363)*. No specific chromosomal translocations are known and known B-cell proto-oncogenes (such as *bcl1*, *bcl2*, *bcl3*, *bcl6*, and c-*myc*) are not involved in HCL *(340)*. Tumor-suppressor genes have been infrequently analyzed in cases of HCL. In one study of seven cases, there was no evidence of either $p15^{INK4B}$ or $p16^{INK4A}$ gene deletions *(351)*.

HAIRY-CELL LEUKEMIA-VARIANT Relatively few cases of HCL-V have been analyzed using molecular methods. As expected in mature B-cell tumors, *IgH* and *IgL* gene rearrangements are found in HCL-V *(1)*. The *TCR* genes are usually in the germline configuration. Relatively few of the known B-cell proto-oncogenes have been assessed in HCL-V. Dyer and colleagues did not identify *bcl2* gene rearrangements in 12 cases studied *(340)*.

T-CELL CHRONIC LYMPHOCYTIC LEUKEMIA/T-CELL PROLYMPHOCYTIC LEUKEMIA T-cell chronic lymphocytic leukemia (CLL) and T-cell prolymphocytic leukemia are grouped together by most observers, as the immunophenotypic and molecular findings in neoplasms designated as either T-CLL or T-PLL are very similar. T-CLL/PLL are neoplasms of mature T-cell lineage. As a result, these neoplasms have rearrangements of the *TCR-β* and *TCR-γ* genes. The *TCR-δ* gene is usually deleted. Lineage infidelity is uncommon and thus the *Ig* genes are usually in the germline configuration *(326)*. A characteristic chromosomal abnormality, inv(14)(q11;q32), occurs in approx two-thirds of T-cell CLL/PLLs *(364)*. A subset of cases also has been described with chromosomal translocations, such as the t(14;14)(q11;q32) and the t(7;14)(q35;q32) *(364,365)*. These translocations juxtapose the *TCL1* gene at 14q32 with either the *TCR-γ/δ* or *TCR-β* genes *(365)*. The *TCL1* gene is then thought to come under the influence of the *TCR-α* regulatory elements, deregulating the *TCL1* gene. Increased levels of normal TCL1 protein provides the cell with a growth advantage *(365)*. Although its function is as yet unknown, the TCL1 protein has considerable sequence homology to the *MTCP-1* gene product on chromosome Xq28, which has been identified in a sub-set of T-CLL *(365,366)*. Trisomy 8 is common in T-CLL/PLL *(367)*. The t(X;14)(q28;q11) also has been identified in cases of T-cell PLL, occurring in patients with AT *(368,369)*.

LARGE GRANULAR LYMPHOCYTE LEUKEMIA

Immunophenotypic studies have shown T-cell and natural killer (NK)-cell subtypes of large granular lymphocyte leukemia (LGLL) *(370)*. The major difference between these subtypes is that T-cell LGLLs express the CD3 antigen and TCR, usually the *TCR-α/β* but rarely the *TCR-γ/δ*. NK cell LGLLs lack CD3 and the TCRs *(370)*. Molecular studies have shown that T-cell LGLLs have rearrangements of the *TCR-γ*, *TCR-α*, and *TCR-β* genes *(370,371)*. The *TCR-δ* gene is usually deleted. NK-cell LGLLs do not have *TCR* gene rearrangements. In both subtypes of LGLL, the *Ig* genes are usually in the germline configuration.

CONCLUSIONS

Molecular characterization of the abnormalities in leukemias has been and continues to be important for a number reasons. From the scientific viewpoint these studies help to identify the genes and the mechanisms involved in hematopoiesis and the pathogenesis of leukemia. Further progress may help to identify targets for rational drug design or gene therapy. From a more immediate clinical perspective, information gleaned from these studies has improved the accuracy of diagnosis, helped to predict therapeutic response, provided criteria for selecting high-risk patient groups who may benefit from intensive but highly toxic chemotherapy protocols or bone marrow transplantation, and aid in the detection of minimal residual disease before clinical relapse.

REFERENCES

1. Cline, M. (1994) The molecular basis of leukemia. *N. Engl. J. Med.* **330**:328–336.
2. Mitelman, F. and Heim, S. (1992) Quantitative acute leukemia cytogenetics. *Genes Chromosomes Cancer* **5**:57–66.
3. Rabbitts, T. (1991) Translocations, master genes, and differences between the origins of acute and chronic leukemias. *Cell* **67**:641–644.
4. Thandla, S. and Aplan, P. (1997) Molecular biology of acute lymphocytic leukemia. *Semin. Oncol.* **24**:45–56.
5. Bennett, J. M., Catovsky, D., Daniel, M. T., Flandrin, G., Galton, D. A., Gralnick, H. R., et al. (1985) Proposed revised criteria for the classification of acute myeloid leukemia. A report of the French-American-British Cooperative Group. *Ann. Internal Med.* **103**:620–625.
6. Douer, D., Preston-Martin, S., Chang, E., Nichols, P. W., Watkins, K. J., and Levine, A. M. (1996) High frequency of acute promyelocytic leukemia among Latinos with acute myeloid leukemia. *Blood* **87**:308–313.
7. Vyas, R. C., Frankel, S. R., Agbor, P., Miller, W. H., Jr., Warrell, R. P., Jr., and Hittelman, W. N. (1996) Probing the pathobiology of response to all-*trans*-retinoic acid in acute promyelocytic leukemia: premature chromosome condensation/fluorescence in situ hybridization analysis. *Blood* **87**:218–226.
8. Grignani, F., Fagioli, M., Alcalay, M., Longo, L., Pandolfi, P. P., Donti, E., et al. (1994) Acute promyelocytic leukemia: from genetics to treatment. *Blood* **83**:10–25.
9. Warrell, R. P., Jr., de The, H., Wang, Z. Y., and Degos, L. (1993) Acute promyelocytic leukemia. *N. Engl. J. Med.* **329**:177–189.

10. Bitter, M. A., Le Beau, M. M., Rowley, J. D., Larson, R. A., Golomb, H. M., and Vardiman, J. W. (1987) Associations between morphology, karyotype, and clinical features in myeloid leukemias. *Human Pathol.* **18**:211–225.

11. Kakizuka, A., Miller, W. H., Jr., Umesono, K., Warrell, R. P., Jr., Frankel, S. R., Murty, V. V., et al. (1991) Chromosomal translocation t(15;17) in human acute promyelocytic leukemia fuses *RARα* with a novel putative transcription factor, *PML. Cell* **66**:663–674.

12. de The, H., Lavau, C., Marchio, A., Chomienne, C., Degos, L., and Dejean, A. (1991) The *PML-RARα* fusion mRNA generated by the t(15;17) translocation in acute promyelocytic leukemia encodes a functionally altered RAR. *Cell* **66**:675–684.

13. Miller, W. H., Jr., Kakizuka, A., Frankel, S. R., Warrell, R. P., Jr., DeBlasio, A., Levine, K., et al. (1992) Reverse transcription polymerase chain reaction for the rearranged retinoic acid receptor a clarifies diagnosis and detects minimal residual disease in acute promyelocytic leukemia. *Proc. Natl. Acad. Sci. USA* **89**:2694–2698.

14. Huang, W., Sun, G. L., Li, X. S., Cao, Q., Lu, Y., Jang, G. S., et al. (1993) Acute promyelocytic leukemia: clinical relevance of two major PML-RARα isoforms and detection of minimal residual disease by retrotranscriptase/polymerase chain reaction to predict relapse. *Blood* **82**:1264–1269.

15. Gallagher, R. E., Willman, C. L., Slack, J. L., Andersen, J. W., Li, Y. P., Viswanatha, D., et al. (1997) Association of PML-RARα fusion mRNA type with pretreatment hematologic characteristics but not treatment outcome in acute promyelocytic leukemia: an intergroup molecular study. *Blood* **90**:1656–1663.

16. Li, Y. P., Andersen, J., Zelent, A., Rao, S., Paietta, E., Tallman, M. S., et al. (1997) RARα1/RARα2-PML mRNA expression in acute promyelocytic leukemia cells: a molecular and laboratory-clinical correlative study. *Blood* **90**:306–312.

17. Schad, C. R., Hanson, C. A., Paietta, E., Casper, J., Jalal, S. M., and Dewald, G. W. (1994) Efficacy of fluorescence in situ hybridization for detecting *PML/RARα* gene fusion in treated and untreated acute promyelocytic leukemia. *Mayo Clin. Proc.* **69**:1047–1053.

18. Biondi, A., Rambaldi, A., Alcalay, M., Pandolfi, P. P., Lo Coco, F., Diverio, D., et al. (1991) *RARα* gene rearrangements as a genetic marker for diagnosis and monitoring in acute promyelocytic leukemia. *Blood* **77**:1418–1422.

19. Dyck, J. A., Warrell, R. P., Jr., Evans, R. M., and Miller, W. H., Jr. (1995) Rapid diagnosis of acute promyelocytic leukemia by immunohistochemical localization of PML/RAR-alpha protein. *Blood* **86**:862–867.

20. Falini, B., Flenghi, L., Fagioli, M., Coco, F. L., Cordone, I., Diverio, D., et al. (1997) Immunocytochemical diagnosis of acute promyelocytic leukemia (M3) with the monoclonal antibody PG-M3 (Anti-PML). *Blood* **90**:4046–4053.

21. Lo Coco, F., Diverio, D., Pandolfi, P. P., Biondi, A., Rossi, V., Avvisati, G., et al. (1992) Molecular evaluation of residual disease as a predictor of relapse in acute promyelocytic leukaemia. *Lancet* **340**:1437–1438.

22. Miller, W. H., Jr., Levine, K., DeBlasio, A., Frankel, S. R., Dmitrovsky, E., and Warrell, R. P., Jr. (1993) Detection of minimal residual disease in acute promyelocytic leukemia by a reverse transcription polymerase chain reaction assay for the PML/RAR-alpha fusion mRNA. *Blood* **82**:1689–1694.

23. Zhao, L., Chang, K. S., Estey, E. H., Hayes, K., Deisseroth, A. B., and Liang, J. C. (1995) Detection of residual leukemic cells in patients with acute promyelocytic leukemia by the fluorescence in situ hybridization method: potential for predicting relapse. *Blood* **85**:495–499.

24. Licht, J. D., Chomienne, C., Goy, A., Chen, A., Scott, A. A., Head, D. R., et al. (1995) Clinical and molecular characterization of a rare syndrome of acute promyelocytic leukemia associated with translocation (11;17). *Blood* **85**:1083–1094.

25. Chen, S. J., Zelent, A., Tong, J. H., Yu, H. Q., Wang, Z. Y., Derre, J., et al. (1993) Rearrangements of the retinoic acid receptor α and promyelocytic leukemia zinc finger genes resulting from t(11;17)(q23;q21) in a patient with acute promyelocytic leukemia. *J. Clin. Invest.* **91**:2260–2267.

26. Redner, R. L., Rush, E. A., Faas, S., Rudert, W. A., and Corey, S. J. (1996) The t(5;17) variant of acute promyelocytic leukemia expresses a nucleophosmin-retinoic acid receptor fusion. *Blood* **87**:882–886.

27. Kalwinsky, D. K., Raimondi, S. C., Schell, M. J., Mirro, J., Jr., Santana, V. M., Behm, F., et al. (1990) Prognostic importance of cytogenetic subgroups in *de novo* pediatric acute nonlymphocytic leukemia. *J. Clin. Oncol.* **8**:75–83.

28. Swansbury, G. J., Lawler, S. D., Alimena, G., Arthur, D., Berger, R., Van den Berghe, H., et al. (1994) Long-term survival in acute myelogenous leukemia: a second follow-up of the Fourth International Workshop on Chromosomes in Leukemia. *Cancer Genet. Cytogenet.* **73**:1–7.

29. Nucifora, G. and Rowley, J. D. (1995) AML1 and the 8;21 and 3;21 translocations in acute and chronic myeloid leukemia. *Blood* **86**:1–14.

30. Martinez-Climent, J. A., Lane, N. J., Rubin, C. M., Morgan, E., Johnstone, H. S., Mick, R., et al. (1995) Clinical and prognostic significance of chromosomal abnormalities in childhood acute myeloid leukemia *de novo. Leukemia* **9**:95–101.

31. Nakamura, H., Kuriyama, K., Sadamori, N., Mine, M., Itoyama, T., Sasagawa, I., et al. (1997) Morphological subtyping of acute myeloid leukemia with maturation (AML- M2): homogeneous pink-colored cytoplasm of mature neutrophils is most characteristic of AML-M2 with t(8;21). *Leukemia* **11**:651–655.

32. Gao, J., Erickson, P., Gardiner, K., Le Beau, M. M., Diaz, M. O., Patterson, D., et al. (1991) Isolation of a yeast artificial chromosome spanning the 8;21 translocation breakpoint t(8;21)(q22;q223) in acute myelogenous leukemia. *Proc. Natl. Acad. Sci. USA* **88**:4882–4886.

33. Nisson, P. E., Watkins, P. C., and Sacchi, N. (1992) Transcriptionally active chimeric gene derived from the fusion of the AML1 gene and a novel gene on chromosome 8 in t(8;21) leukemic cells. *Cancer Genet. Cytogenet.* **63**:81–88.

34. Sawyers, C. (1997) Molecular genetics of acute leukaemia. *Lancet* **349**:196–200.

35. Larson, R. A., Williams, S. F., Le Beau, M. M., Bitter, M. A., Vardiman, J. W., and Rowley, J. D. (1986) Acute myelomonocytic leukemia with abnormal eosinophils and inv(16) or t(16;16) has a favorable prognosis. *Blood* **68**:1242–1249.

36. Maruyama, F., Yang, P., Stass, S. A., Cork, A., Freireich, E. J., Lee, M. S., et al. (1993) Detection of the AML1/ETO fusion transcript in the t(8;21) masked translocation in acute myelogenous leukemia. *Cancer Res.* **53**:4449–4451.

37. Nucifora, G., Birn, D. J., Erickson, P., Gao, J., LeBeau, M. M., Drabkin, H. A., et al. (1993) Detection of DNA rearrangements in the AML1 and ETO loci and of an AML1/ETO fusion mRNA in patients with t(8;21) acute myeloid leukemia. *Blood* **81**:883–888.

38. Downing, J. R., Head, D. R., Curcio-Brint, A. M., Hulshof, M. G., Motroni, T. A., Raimondi, S. C., et al. (1993) An AML1/ETO fusion transcript is consistently detected by RNA-based polymerase chain reaction in acute myelogenous leukemia containing the (8;21)(q22;q22) translocation. *Blood* **81**:2860–2865.

39. Kusec, R., Laczika, K., Knobl, P., Friedl, J., Greinix, H., Kahls, P., et al. (1994) AML1/ETO fusion mRNA can be detected in remission blood samples of all patients with t(8;21) acute myeloid leukemia after chemotherapy or autologous bone marrow transplantation. *Leukemia* **8**:735–739.

40. Jurlander, J., Caligiuri, M. A., Ruutu, T., Baer, M. R., Strout, M. P., Oberkircher, A. R., et al. (1996) Persistence of the AML1/ETO fusion transcript in patients treated with allogeneic bone marrow transplantation for t(8;21) leukemia. *Blood* **88**:2183–2191.

41. Jurlander, J., Caligiuri, M. A., and Bloomfield, C. D. (1997) Response. *Blood* **90**:3231.

42. Sacchi, N., Schiaffonati, L., Magnani, I., Pappalardo, C., Hughes, A. J., Jr., Darfler, M., et al. (1996) Detection and subcellular localization of an AML1 chimeric protein in the t(8;21) positive acute myeloid leukemia. *Oncogene* **12**:437–444.

43. Rubin, C. M., Larson, R. A., Bitter, M. A., Carrino, J. J., Le Beau, M. M., Diaz, M. O., et al. (1987) Association of a chromosomal 3;21 translocation with the blast phase of chronic myelogenous leukemia. *Blood* **70**:1338–1342.

44. Rubin, C. M., Larson, R. A., Anastasi, J., Winter, J. N., Thangavelu, M., Vardiman, J. W., et al. (1990) t(3;21)(q26;q22): A recurring chromosomal abnormality in therapy-related myelodysplastic syndrome and acute myeloid leukemia. *Blood* **76**:2594–2598.

45. Nucifora, G., Begy, C. R., Kobayashi, H., Roulston, D., Claxton, D., Pedersen-Bjergaard, J., et al. (1994) Consistent intergenic splicing and production of multiple transcripts between *AML1* at 21q22 and unrelated genes at 3q26 in (3;21)(q26;q22) translocations. *Proc. Natl. Acad. Sci. USA* **91**:4004–4008.

46. Roulston, D., Nucifora, G., Dietz-Band, J., Le Beau, M. M., and Rowley, J. D. (1993) Detection of rare 21q22 translocation breakpoints within the *AML1* gene in myeloid neoplasms by fluorescence *in situ* hybridization. *Blood* **82**:532a.

47. Xue, Y., Yu, F., Xin, Y., Lu, D., Zou, Z., Guo, Y., and Xie, X. (1997) t(8;20)(q22;p13): a novel variant translocation of t(8;21) in acute myeloblastic leukaemia. *Br. J. Haematol.* **98**:733–735.

48. Liu, P. P., Hajra, A., Wijmenga, C., and Collins, F. S. (1995) Molecular pathogenesis of the chromosome 16 inversion in the M4Eo subtype of acute myeloid leukemia. *Blood* **85**:2289–2302.

49. Le Beau, M. M., Larson, R. A., Bitter, M. A., Vardiman, J. W., Golomb, H. M., and Rowley, J. D. (1983) Association of an inversion of chromosome 16 with abnormal marrow eosinophils in acute myelomonocytic leukemia. A unique cytogenetic-clinicopathological association. *N. Engl. J. Med.* **309**:630–636.

50. Tobal, K., Johnson, P. R., Saunders, M. J., Harrison, C. J., and Liu Yin, J. A. (1995) Detection of *CBFβ/MYH11* transcripts in patients with inversion and other abnormalities of chromosome 16 at presentation and remission. *Br. J. Haematol.* **91**:104–108.

51. Horiike, S., Misawa, S., Nishida, K., Nishigaki, H., Tsuda, S., Taniwaki, M., et al. (1989) Myelodysplastic syndrome preceding acute myelomonocytic leukemia with dysplastic marrow eosinophilia and inv(16). *Acta Haematol.* **82**:161–164.

52. Heim, S., Christensen, B. E., Fioretos, T., Sorensen, A. G., and Pedersen, N. T. (1992) Acute myelomonocytic leukemia with inv(16)(p13q22) complicating Philadelphia chromosome positive chronic myeloid leukemia. *Cancer Genet. Cytogenet.* **59**:35–38.

53. Asou, N., Sanada, I., Tanaka, K., Hidaka, M., Suzushima, H., Matsuzaki, H., et al. (1992) Inversion of chromosome 16 and bone marrow eosinophilia in a myelomonocytic transformation of chronic myeloid leukemia. *Cancer Genet. Cytogenet.* **61**:197–200.

54. Marlton, P., Keating, M., Kantarjian, H., Pierce, S., O'Brien, S., Freireich, E. J., et al. (1995) Cytogenetic and clinical correlates in AML patients with abnormalities of chromosome 16. *Leukemia* **9**:965–971.

55. Dauwerse, J. G., Wessels, J. W., Giles, R. H., Wiegant, J., van der Reijden, B. A., Fugazza, G., et al. (1993) Cloning the breakpoint cluster region of the inv(16) in acute nonlymphocytic leukemia M4 Eo. *Human Mol. Genet.* **2**:1527–1534.

56. van der Reijden, B. A., Dauwerse, J. G., Wessels, J. W., Beverstock, G. C., Hagemeijer, A., van Ommen, G. J., et al. (1993) A gene for a myosin peptide is disrupted by the inv(16)(p13q22) in acute nonlymphocytic leukemia M4Eo. *Blood* **82**:2948–2952.

57. Claxton, D. F., Liu, P., Hsu, H. B., Marlton, P., Hester, J., Collins, F., et al. (1994) Detection of fusion transcripts generated by the inversion 16 chromosome in acute myelogenous leukemia. *Blood* **83**:1750–1756.

58. Shurtleff, S. A., Meyers, S., Hiebert, S. W., Raimondi, S. C., Head, D. R., Willman, C. L., et al. (1995) Heterogeneity in CBF beta/MYH11 fusion messages encoded by the inv(16)(p13q22) and the t(16;16)(p13;q22) in acute myelogenous leukemia. *Blood* **85**:3695–3703.

59. Arthur, D. C. and Bloomfield, C. D. (1983) Partial deletion of the long arm of chromosome 16 and bone marrow eosinophilia in acute nonlymphocytic leukemia: a new association. *Blood* **61**:994–998.

60. Ohyashiki, K., Ohyashiki, J. H., Kondo, M., Ito, H., and Toyama, K. (1988) Chromosome change at 16q22 in nonlymphocytic leukemia: clinical implication on leukemia patients with inv(16) versus del(16). *Leukemia* **2**:35–40.

61. Rubnitz, J., Behm, F., and Downing, J. (1996) 11q23 rearrangements in acute leukemia. *Leukemia* **10**:74–82.

62. Hilden, J. M., Smith, F. O., Frestedt, J. L., McGlennen, R., Howells, W. B., Sorensen, P. H., et al. (1997) MLL gene rearrangement, cytogenetic 11q23 abnormalities, and expression of the NG2 molecule in infant acute myeloid leukemia. *Blood* **89**:3801–3805.

63. Hunger, S., Tkachuk, D., Amylon, M., Link, M., Carroll, A., Welborn, J., et al. (1993) *HRX* involvement in *de novo* and secondary leukemias with diverse chromosome 11q23 abnormalities. *Blood* **81**:3197–3203.

64. Ziemin-van der Poel, S., McCabe, N. R., Gill, H. J., Espinosa, R., III, Patel, Y., et al. (1991) Identification of a gene, MLL, that spans the breakpoint in 11q23 translocations associated with human leukemias. *Proc. Natl. Acad. Sci. USA* **88**:10,735–10,739.

65. Tkachuk, D., Kohler, S., and Cleary, M. (1992) Involvement of a homolog of *Drosophila trithorax* by 11q23 chromosomal translocations in acute leukemias. *Cell* **71**:691–700.

66. Djabali, M., Selleri, L., Parry, P., Bower, M., Young, B. D., and Evans, G. A. (1992) A trithorax-like gene is interrupted by chromosome 11q23 translocations in acute leukaemias. *Nature Genet.* **2**:113–118.

67. Bernard, O. A. and Berger, R. (1995) Molecular basis of 11q23 rearrangements in hematopoietic malignant proliferations. *Genes Chromosomes Cancer* **13**:75–85.

68. Broeker, P. L., Super, H. G., Thirman, M. J., Pomykala, H., Yonebayashi, Y., Tanabe, S., et al. (1996) Distribution of 11q23 breakpoints within the *MLL* breakpoint cluster region in *de novo* acute leukemia and in treatment-related acute myeloid leukemia: correlation with scaffold attachment regions and topoisomerase II consensus binding sites. *Blood* **87**:1912–1922.

69. Caligiuri, M. A., Schichman, S. A., Strout, M. P., Mrozek, K., Baer, M. R., Frankel, S. R., et al. (1994) Molecular rearrangement of the *ALL-1* gene in acute myeloid leukemia without cytogenetic evidence of 11q23 chromosomal translocations. *Cancer Res.* **54**:370–373.

70. Thirman, M., Gill, H., Burnett, R., Mbangkollo, D., McCabe, N., Kobayashi, H., et al. (1993) Rearrangement of the MLL gene in acute lymphoblastic and acute myeloid leukemias with 11q23 chromosomal translocations. *N. Engl. J. Med.* **329**:909–914.

71. Repp, R., Borkhardt, A., Haupt, E., Kreuder, J., Brettreich, S., Hammermann, J., et al. (1995) Detection of four different 11q23 chromosomal abnormalities by multiplex-PCR and fluorescence-based automatic DNA-fragment analysis. *Leukemia* **9**:210–215.

72. Super, H. J., McCabe, N. R., Thirman, M. J., Larson, R. A., Le Beau, M. M., Pedersen-Bjergaard, J., et al. (1993) Rearrangements of the *MLL* gene in therapy-related acute myeloid leukemia in patients previously treated with agents targeting DNA- topoisomerase II. *Blood* **82**:3705–3711.

73. Mrózek, K., Heinonen, K., Lawrence, D., Carroll, A. J., Koduru, P. R. K., Rao, K. W., et al. (1997) Adult patients with *de novo* acute myeloid leukemia and t(9; 11)(p22; q23) have a superior outcome to patients with other translocations involving band 11q23: a cancer and leukemia group B study. *Blood* **90**:4532–4538.

74. Taki, T., Sako, M., Tsuchida, M., and Hayashi, Y. (1997) The t(11;16)(q23;p13) translocation in myelodysplastic syndrome fuses the *MLL* gene to the *CBP* gene. *Blood* **89**:3945–3950.

75. Rowley, J. D., Reshmi, S., Sobulo, O., Musvee, T., Anastasi, J., Raimondi, S., et al. (1997) All patients with the T(11;16)(q23;p133) that involves *MLL* and *CBP* have treatment-related hematologic disorders. *Blood* **90**:535–541.

76. Hillion, J., Le Coniat, M., Jonveaux, P., Berger, R., and Bernard, O. A. (1997) AF6q21, a novel partner of the *MLL* gene in t(6;11)(q21;q23), defines a forkhead transcriptional factor subfamily. *Blood* **90**:3714–3719.

77. Corral, J., Forster, A., Thompson, S., Lampert, F., Kaneko, Y., Slater, R., et al. (1993) Acute leukemias of different lineages have similar *MLL* gene fusions encoding related chimeric proteins resulting from chromosomal translocation. *Proc. Natl. Acad. Sci. USA* **90**:8538–8542.

78. Bernard, O. A., Mauchauffe, M., Mecucci, C., Van den Berghe, H., and Berger, R. (1994) A novel gene, *AF-1p*, fused to *HRX* in t(1;11)(p32;q23), is not related to *AF-4, AF-9* nor *ENL*. *Oncogene* **9**:1039–1045.

79. Prasad, R., Leshkowitz, D., Gu, Y., Alder, H., Nakamura, T., Saito, H., et al. (1994) Leucine-zipper dimerization motif encoded by the AF17 gene fused to *ALL-1 (MLL)* in acute leukemia. *Proc. Natl. Acad. Sci .USA* **91**:8107–8111.

80. Chaplin, T., Bernard, O., Beverloo, H. B., Saha, V., Hagemeijer, A., Berger, R., et al. (1995) The t(10;11) translocation in acute myeloid leukemia (M5) consistently fuses the leucine zipper motif of AF10 onto the HRX gene. *Blood* **86**:2073–2076.

81. Martinez-Climent, J., Espinosa, R., III, Thirman, M., Le Beau, M., and Rowley, J. (1995) Abnormalities of chromosome band 11q23 and the *MLL* gene in pediatric myelomonocytic and monoblastic leukemias. Identification of the t(9;11) as an indicator of long survival. *J. Pediatr. Hematol. Oncol.* **17**:277–283.

82. Caligiuri, M. A., Strout, M. P., Schichman, S. A., Mrozek, K., Arthur, D. C., Herzig, G. P., et al. (1996) Partial tandem duplication of *ALL1* as a recurrent molecular defect in acute myeloid leukemia with trisomy 11. *Cancer Res.* **56**:1418–1425.

83. Caligiuri, M., Strout, M., and Gilliland, D. (1997) Molecular biology of acute myeloid leukemia. *Semin. Oncol.* **24**:32–44.

84. Lillington, D. M., MacCallum, P. K., Lister, T. A., and Gibbons, B. (1993) Translocation t(6;9)(p23;q34) in acute myeloid leukemia without myelodysplasia or basophilia: two cases and a review of the literature. *Leukemia* **7**:527–531.

85. Soekarman, D., von Lindern, M., Daenen, S., de Jong, B., Fonatsch, C., Heinze, B., et al. (1992) The translocation (6;9)(p23;q34) shows consistent rearrangement of two genes and defines a myeloproliferative disorder with specific clinical features. *Blood* **79**:2990–2997.

86. von Lindern, M., Fornerod, M., van Baal, S., Jaegle, M., de Wit, T., Buijs, A., et al. (1992) The translocation (6;9), associated with a specific subtype of acute myeloid leukemia, results in the fusion of two genes, *dek* and *can*, and the expression of a chimeric, leukemia-specific *dek-can* mRNA. *Mol. Cell. Biol.* **12**:1687–1697.

87. Kraemer, D., Wozniak, R. W., Blobel, G., and Radu, A. (1994) The human CAN protein, a putative oncogene product associated with myeloid leukemogenesis, is a nuclear pore complex protein that faces the cytoplasm. *Proc. Natl. Acad. Sci. USA* **91**:1519–1523.

88. Fornerod, M., Boer, J., van Baal, S., Jaegle, M., von Lindern, M., Murti, K. G., et al. (1995) Relocation of the carboxyterminal part of *CAN* from the nuclear envelope to the nucleus as a result of leukemia-specific chromosome rearrangements. *Oncogene* **10**:1739–1748.

89. Nakano, H., Shimamoto, Y., Suga, K., and Kobayashi, M. (1995) Detection of minimal residual disease in a patient with acute myeloid leukemia and t(6;9) at the time of peripheral blood stem cell transplantation. *Acta Haematol.* **94**:139–141.

90. von Lindern, M., Breems, D., van Baal, S., Adriaansen, H., and Grosveld, G. (1992) Characterization of the translocation breakpoint sequences of two *DEK-CAN* fusion genes present in t(6;9) acute myeloid leukemia and a *SET-CAN* fusion gene found in a case of acute undifferentiated leukemia. *Genes Chromosomes Cancer* **5**:227–234.

91. von Lindern, M., van Baal, S., Wiegant, J., Raap, A., Hagemeijer, A., and Grosveld, G. (1992) *Can*, a putative oncogene associated with myeloid leukemogenesis, may be activated by fusion of its 3' half to different genes: characterization of the set gene. *Mol. Cell. Biol.* **12**:3346–3355.

92. Sato, Y., Abe, S., Mise, K., Sasaki, M., Kamada, N., Kouda, K., et al. (1987) Reciprocal translocation involving the short arms of chromosomes 7 and 11, t(7p-;11p+), associated with myeloid leukemia with maturation. *Blood* **70**:1654–1658.

93. Kwong, Y. L. and Chan, T. K. (1994) Translocation (7;11)(p15;p15) in acute myeloid leukemia M2: association with trilineage myelodysplasia and giant dysplastic myeloid cells. *Am. J. Hematol.* **47**:62–64.

94. Nakamura, T., Largaespada, D. A., Lee, M. P., Johnson, L. A., Ohyashiki, K., Toyama, K., et al. (1996) Fusion of the nucleoporin gene *NUP98* to *HOXA9* by the chromosome translocation t(7;11)(p15;p15) in human myeloid leukaemia. *Nature Genet.* **12**:154–158.

95. Borrow, J., Shearman, A. M., Stanton, V. P., Jr., Becher, R., Collins, T., Williams, A. J., et al. (1996) The t(7;11)(p15;p15) translocation in acute myeloid leukaemia fuses the genes for nucleoporin NUP98 and class I homeoprotein HOXA9. *Nature Genet.* **12**:159–167.

96. Radu, A., Moore, M. S., and Blobel, G. (1995) The peptide repeat domain of nucleoporin Nup98 functions as a docking site in transport across the nuclear pore complex. *Cell* **81**:215–222.

97. Arai, Y., Hosoda, F., Kobayashi, H., Arai, K., Hayashi, Y., Kamada, N., et al. (1997) The inv(11)(p15q22) chromosome translocation of de novo and therapy-related myeloid malignancies results in fusion of the nucleoporin gene, *NUP98*, with the putative RNA helicase gene, *DDX10*. *Blood* **89**:3936–3944.

98. Savitsky, K., Ziv, Y., Bar-Shira, A., Gilad, S., Tagle, D. A., Smith, S., et al. (1996) A human gene *(DDX10)* encoding a putative DEAD-box RNA helicase at 11q22-q23. *Genomics* **33**:199–206.

99. Yao, E., Sadamori, N., Nakamura, H., Sasagawa, I., Itoyama, T., Ichimaru, M., et al. (1988) Translocation t(16;21) in acute nonlymphocytic leukemia with abnormal eosinophils. *Cancer Genet. Cytogenet.* **36**:221–223.

100. Kong, X. T., Ida, K., Ichikawa, H., Shimizu, K., Ohki, M., Maseki, N., et al. (1997) Consistent detection of *TLS/FUS-ERG* chimeric transcripts in acute myeloid leukemia with t(16;21)(p11;q22) and identification of a novel transcript. *Blood* **90**:1192–1199.

101. Ferro, M. R., Cabello, P., Garcia-Sagredo, J. M., Resino, M., San Roman, C., and Larana, J. G. (1992) t(16;21) in a Ph positive CML. *Cancer Genet. Cytogenet.* **60**:210–211.

102. Ichikawa, H., Shimizu, K., Hayashi, Y., and Ohki, M. (1994) An RNA-binding protein gene, *TLS/FUS*, is fused to *ERG* in human myeloid leukemia with t(16;21) chromosomal translocation. *Cancer Res.* **54**:2865–2868.

103. Shimizu, K., Ichikawa, H., Tojo, A., Kaneko, Y., Maseki, N., Hayashi, Y., et al. (1993) An ets-related gene, *ERG*, is rearranged in human myeloid leukemia with t(16;21) chromosomal translocation. *Proc. Natl. Acad. Sci. USA* **90**:10,280–10,284.

104. Prasad, D. D., Ouchida, M., Lee, L., Rao, V. N., and Reddy, E. S. (1994) TLS/FUS fusion domain of TLS/FUS-erg chimeric protein resulting from the t(16;21) chromosomal translocation in human myeloid leukemia functions as a transcriptional activation domain. *Oncogene* **9**:3717–3729.

105. Hagemeijer, A., Hahlen, K., and Abels, J. (1981) Cytogenetic follow-up of patients with nonlymphocytic leukemia II. Acute nonlymphocytic leukemia. *Cancer Genet. Cytogenet.* **3**:109–124.

106. Buijs, A., Sherr, S., van Baal, S., van Bezouw, S., van der Plas, D., Geurts van Kessel, A., et al. (1995) Translocation (12;22)(p13;q11) in myeloproliferative disorders results in fusion of the *ETS*-like *TEL* gene on 12p13 to the *MN1* gene on 22q11. *Oncogene* **10**:1511–1519.

107. Lekanne Deprez, R. H., Riegman, P. H., Groen, N. A., Warringa, U. L., van Biezen, N. A., Molijn, A. C., et al. (1995) Cloning and characterization of *MN1*, a gene from chromosome 22q11, which is disrupted by a balanced translocation in a meningioma. *Oncogene* **10**:1521–1528.

108. Hanslip, J. I., Swansbury, G. J., Pinkerton, R., and Catovsky, D. (1992) The translocation t(8;16)(p11;p13) defines an AML subtype with distinct cytology and clinical features. *Leukemia Lymphoma* **6**:479–486.

109. Quesnel, B., Kantarjian, H., Bjergaard, J. P., Brault, P., Estey, E., Lai, J. L., et al. (1993) Therapy-related acute myeloid leukemia with t(8;21), inv(16), and t(8;16): a report on 25 cases and review of the literature. *J. Clin. Oncol.* **11**:2370–2379.

110. Borrow, J., Stanton, V. P., Jr., Andresen, J. M., Becher, R., Behm, F. G., Chaganti, R. S., et al. (1996) The translocation t(8;16)(p11;p13) of acute myeloid leukaemia fuses a putative acetyltransferase to the CREB-binding protein. *Nature Genet.* **14**:33–41.

111. Petrij, F., Giles, R. H., Dauwerse, H. G., Saris, J. J., Hennekam, R. C., Masuno, M., et al. (1995) Rubinstein-Taybi syndrome caused by mutations in the transcriptional co-activator CBP. *Nature* **376**:348–351.

112. Stark, B., Resnitzky, P., Jeison, M., Luria, D., Blau, O., Avigad, S., et al. (1995) A distinct subtype of M4/M5 acute myeloblastic leukemia (AML) associated with t(8:16)(p11:p13), in a patient with the variant t(8:19)(p11:q13): case report and review of the literature. *Leukemia Res.* **19**:367–379.

113. Lai, J. L., Zandecki, M., Fenaux, P., Preudhomme, C., Facon, T., and Deminatti, M. (1992) Acute monocytic leukemia with (8;22)(p11;q13) translocation. Involvement of 8p11 as in classical t(8;16)(p11;p13). *Cancer Genet. Cytogenet.* **60**:180–182.

114. Kurzrock, R., Shtalrid, M., Talpaz, M., Kloetzer, W. S., and Gutterman, J. U. (1987) Expression of *c-abl* in Philadelphia-positive acute myelogenous leukemia. *Blood* **70**:1584–1588.

115. Kurzrock, R., Gutterman, J., and Talpaz, M. (1988) The molecular genetics of Philadelphia chromosome-positive leukemias. *N. Engl. J. Med.* **319**:990–998.

116. Birg, F., Courcoul, M., Rosnet, O., Bardin, F., Pebusque, M. J., Marchetto, S., et al. (1992) Expression of the *FMS/KIT*-like gene *FLT3* in human acute leukemias of the myeloid and lymphoid lineages. *Blood* **80**:2584–2593.

117. Yokota, S., Kiyoi, H., Nakao, M., Iwai, T., Misawa, S., Okuda, T., et al. (1997) Internal tandem duplication of the *FLT3* gene is preferentially seen in acute myeloid leukemia and myelodysplastic syndrome among various hematological malignancies. A study on a large series of patients and cell lines. *Leukemia* **11**:1605–1609.

118. Bos, J. L., Verlaan-de Vries, M., van der Eb, A. J., Janssen, J. W., Delwel, R., Lowenberg, B., et al. (1987) Mutations in N-ras predominate in acute myeloid leukemia. *Blood* **69**:1237–1241.

119. Ahuja, H. G., Foti, A., Bar-Eli, M., and Cline, M. J. (1990) The pattern of mutational involvement of *RAS* genes in human hematologic malignancies determined by DNA amplification and direct sequencing. *Blood* **75**:1684–1690.

120. Thorn, J., Molloy, P., and Iland, H. (1995) SSCP detection of N-*ras* promoter mutations in AML patients. *Exp. Hematol.* **23**:1098–1103.

121. Ahuja, H. G., Foti, A., Zhou, D. J., and Cline, M. J. (1990) Analysis of proto-oncogenes in acute myeloid leukemia: loss of heterozygosity for the *Ha-ras* gene. *Blood* **75**:819–822.

122. Ahuja, H., Jat, P., Foti, A., Bar-Eli, M., and Cline, M. (1991) Abnormalities of the retinoblastoma gene in the pathogenesis of acute leukemia. *Blood* **78**:3259–3268.

123. Prokocimer, M. and Rotter, V. (1994) Structure and function of p53 in normal cells and their aberrations in cancer cells: projection on the hematologic cell lineages. *Blood* **84**:2391–2411.

124. Fenaux, P., Jonveaux, P., Quiquandon, I., Lai, J. L., Pignon, J. M., Loucheux-Lefebvre, M. H., et al. (1991) p53 gene mutations in acute myeloid leukemia with 17p monosomy. *Blood* **78**:1652–1657.

125. Fenaux, P., Preudhomme, C., Quiquandon, I., Jonveaux, P., Lai, J. L., Vanrumbeke, M., et al. (1992) Mutations of the p53 gene in acute myeloid leukaemia. *Br. J. Haematol.* **80**:178–183.

126. Kitagawa, M., Yoshida, S., Kuwata, T., Tanizawa, T., and Kamiyama, R. (1994) p53 expression in myeloid cells of myelodysplastic syndromes association with evolution of overt leukemia. *Am. J. Pathol.* **145**:338–344.

127. Cheng, G. Y., Minden, M. D., Toyonaga, B., Mak, T. W., and McCulloch, E. A. (1986) T cell receptor and immunoglobulin gene rearrangements in acute myeloblastic leukemia. *J. Exp. Med.* **163**:414–424.

128. Norton, J. D., Campana, D., Hoffbrand, A. V., Janossy, G., Coustan-Smith, E., Jani, H., et al. (1987) Rearrangement of immunoglobulin and T cell antigen receptor genes in acute myeloid leukemia with lymphoid-associated markers. *Leukemia* **1**:757–761.

129. Rovigatti, U., Mirro, J., Kitchingman, G., Dahl, G., Ochs, J., Murphy, S., et al. (1984) Heavy chain immunoglobulin gene rearrangement in acute nonlymphocytic leukemia. *Blood* **63**:1023–1027.

130. Ackland, S. P., Westbrook, C. A., Diaz, M. O., Le Beau, M. M., and Rowley, J. D. (1987) Evidence favoring lineage fidelity in acute nonlymphocytic leukemia: absence of immunoglobulin gene rearrangements in FAB types M4 and M5. *Blood* **69**:87–91.

131. Kyoda, K., Nakamura, S., Matano, S., Ohtake, S., and Matsuda, T. (1997) Prognostic significance of immunoglobulin heavy chain gene rearrangement in patients with acute myelogenous leukemia. *Leukemia* **11**:803–806.

132. Paietta, E. (1996) Immunobiology of Acute Leukemias. *In: Neoplastic Diseases of the Blood* (Wiernik, P. H., Caneloos, G. P., Dutcher, J. P., and Kyle, R. A., eds.), Churchill Livingstone, New York, pp. 226.

133. Felix, C. A., Poplack, D. G., Reaman, G. H., Steinberg, S. M., Cole, D. E., Taylor, B. J., et al. (1990) Characterization of immunoglobulin and T-cell receptor gene patterns in B-cell precursor acute lymphoblastic leukemia of childhood. *J. Clin. Oncol.* **8**:431–442.

134. Harris, N. L., Jaffe, E. S., Stein, H., Banks, P. M., Chan, J. K., Cleary, M. L., et al. (1994) A revised European-American classification of lymphoid neoplasms: a proposal from the International Lymphoma Study Group. *Blood* **84**:1361–1392.

135. Jaffe, E. S., Harris, N. L., Chan, J. K. C., Stein, H., and Vardiman, J. (1997) Society for Hematopathology program. Proposed World Health Organization Classification of neoplastic diseases of hematopoietic and lymphoid tissues. *Am. J. Surg. Pathol.* **21**:114–121.

136. Korsmeyer, S. J., Hieter, P. A., Ravetch, J. V., Poplack, D. G., Waldmann, T. A., and Leder, P. (1981) Developmental hierarchy of immunoglobulin gene rearrangements in human leukemic pre-B-cells. *Proc. Natl. Acad. Sci. USA* **78**:7096–7100.

137. Yano, T., Pullman, A., Andrade, R., Uppenkamp, M., de Villartay, J. P., Reaman, G., et al. (1991) A common V delta 2-D delta 2-D delta 3 T cell receptor gene rearrangement in precursor B acute lymphoblastic leukaemia. *Br. J. Haematol.* **79**:44–49.

138. Rabbitts, T. H. (1994) Chromosomal translocations in human cancer. *Nature* **372**:143–149.

139. Heim, S. and Mitelman, F. (1992) Cytogenetic analysis in the diagnosis of acute leukemia. *Cancer* **70**:1701–1709.

140. Preti, H. A., O'Brien, S., Giralt, S., Beran, M., Pierce, S., and Kantarjian, H. M. (1994) Philadelphia-chromosome-positive adult acute lymphocytic leukemia: characteristics, treatment results, and prognosis in 41 patients. *Am. J. Med.* **97**:60–65.

141. Kelliher, M., Knott, A., McLaughlin, J., Witte, O., and Rosenberg, N. (1991) Differences in oncogenic potency but not target cell specificity distinguish the two forms of the BCR/ABL oncogene. *Mol. Cell. Biol.* **11**:4710–4716.

142. Kawasaki, E., Clark, S., Coyne, M., Smith, S., Champlin, R., Witte, O., et al. (1988) Diagnosis of chronic myeloid and acute lymphocytic leukemias by detection of leukemia-specific mRNA sequences amplified in vitro. *Proc. Natl. Acad. Sci. USA* **85**:5698–5702.

143. Head, D. R., Raimondi, S. C., and Behm, F., et al. (1993) Multiplex reverse transcriptase polymerase chain reaction (RT-PCR) for the diagnosis and monitoring of reciprocal translocations in ALL. *Blood* **82**:37a.

144. Mellentin, J. D., Murre, C., Donlon, T. A., McCaw, P. S., Smith, S. D., Carroll, A. J., et al. (1989) The gene for enhancer binding proteins E12/E47 lies at the t(1;19) breakpoint in acute leukemias. *Science* **246**:379–382.

145. Nourse, J., Mellentin, J., Galili, N., Wilkinson, J., Stanbridge, E., Smith, S., et al. (1990) Chromosomal translocation t(1;19) results in synthesis of a homeobox fusion mRNA that codes for a potential chimeric transcription factor. *Cell* **60**:535–545.

146. Hunger, S. (1996) Chromosomal translocations involving the E2A gene in acute lymphoblastic leukemia: clinical features and molecular pathogenesis. *Blood* **87**:1211–1224.

147. Kawamura, M., Kikuchi, A., Kobayashi, S., Hanada, R., Yamamoto, K., Horibe, K., et al. (1995) Mutations of the p53 and *ras* genes in childhood t(1;19)-acute lymphoblastic leukemia. *Blood* **85**:2546–2552.

148. Hunger, S., Galili, N., Carroll, A., Crist, W., Link, M., and Cleary, M. (1991) The t(1;19)(q23;p13) results in consistent fusion of *E2A* and *PBX1* coding sequences in acute lymphoblastic leukemias. *Blood* **77**:687–693.

149. Sang, B. C., Shi, L., Dias, P., Liu, L., Wei, J., Wang, Z. X., et al. (1997) Monoclonal antibodies specific to the acute lymphoblastic leukemia t(1;19)-associated E2A/pbx1 chimeric protein: characterization and diagnostic utility. *Blood* **89**:2909–2914.

150. Inaba, T., Roberts, W. M., Shapiro, L. H., Jolly, K. W., Raimondi, S. C., Smith, S. D., et al. (1992) Fusion of the leucine zipper gene *HLF* to the *E2A* gene in human acute B-lineage leukemia. *Science* **257**:531–534.

151. Murre, C., McCaw, P., and Baltimore, D. (1989) A new DNA binding and dimerization motif in immunoglobulin enhancer binding, daughterless, MyoD, and myc proteins. *Cell* **56**:777–783.

152. Rubnitz, J., Link, M., Shuster, J., Carroll, A., Hakami, N., Frankel, L., et al. (1994) Frequency and prognostic significance of *HRX* rearrangements in infant acute lymphoblastic leukemia: a Pediatric Oncology Group study. *Blood* **84**:570–573.

153. Pui, C., Behm, F., Downing, J., Hancock, M., Shurtleff, S., Ribeiro, R., et al. (1994) 11q23/MLL rearrangement confers a poor prognosis in infants with acute lymphoblastic leukemia. *J. Clin. Oncol.* **12**:909–915.

154. Raimondi, S. C., Frestedt, J. L., Pui, C. H., Downing, J. R., Head, D. R., Kersey, J. H., et al. (1995) Acute lymphoblastic leukemias with deletion of 11q23 or a novel inversion (11)(p13q23) lack MLL gene rearrangements and have favorable clinical features. *Blood* **86**:1881–1886.

155. Raimondi, S. C., Williams, D. L., Callihan, T., Peiper, S., Rivera, G. K., and Murphy, S. B. (1986) Nonrandom involvement of the 12p12 breakpoint in chromosome abnormalities of childhood acute lymphoblastic leukemia. *Blood* **68**:69–75.

156. Höglund, M., Johansson, B., Pedersen-Bjergaard, J., Marynen, P., and Mitelman, F. (1996) Molecular characterization of 12p abnormalities in hematologic malignancies: deletion of KIP1, rearrangement of TEL, and amplification of CCND2. *Blood* **87**:324–330.

157. Shurtleff, S., Buijs, A., Behm, F., Rubnitz, J., Raimondi, S., Hancock, M., et al. (1995) TEL/AML1 fusion resulting from a cryptic t(12;21) is the most common genetic lesion in pediatric ALL and defines a subgroup of patients with an excellent prognosis. *Leukemia* **9**:1985–1989.

158. McLean, T., Ringold, S., Neuberg, D., Stegmaier, K., Tantravahi, R., Ritz, J., et al. (1996) TEL/AML-1 dimerizes and is associated with a favorable outcome in childhood acute lymphoblastic leukemia. *Blood* **88**:4252–4258.

159. Raimondi, S. C., Shurtleff, S. A., Downing, J. R., Rubnitz, J., Mathew, S., Hancock, M., et al. (1997) 12p abnormalities and the TEL gene (ETV6) in childhood acute lymphoblastic leukemia. *Blood* **90**:4559–4566.

160. Sato, Y., Suto, Y., Pietenpol, J., Golub, T. R., Gilliland, D. G., Davis, E. M., et al. (1995) *TEL* and *KIP1* define the smallest region of deletions on 12p13 in hematopoietic malignancies. *Blood* **86**:1525–1533.

161. Kawamata, N., Morosetti, R., Miller, C., Park, D., Spirin, K., Nakamaki, T., et al. (1995) Molecular analysis of the cyclin-dependent kinase inhibitor gene p27/*Kip1* in human malignancies. *Cancer Res.* **55**:2266–2269.

162. Stegmaier, K., Takeuchi, S., Golub, T., Bohlander, S., Bartram, C., and Koeffler, H. (1996) Mutational analysis of the candidate tumor suppressor genes *TEL* and *KIP1* in childhood acute lymphoblastic leukemia. *Cancer Res.* **56**:1413–1417.

163. Scriu, D., Erz, D., and Bartram, C. (1996) Germline configuration of the p27(Kip1) gene in childhood acute lymphoblastic leukemia (ALL). *Leukemia* **10**:345.

164. Hogan, T., Koss, W., Murgo, A., Amato, R., Fontana, J., and VanScoy, F. (1987) Acute lymphoblastic leukemia with chromosomal 5;14 translocation and hypereosinophilia: case report and literature review. *J. Clin. Oncol.* **5**:382–390.

165. Meeker, T., Hardy, D., Willman, C., Hogan, T., and Abrams, J. (1990) Activation of the interleukin-3 gene by chromosome translocation in acute lymphocytic leukemia with eosinophilia. *Blood* **76**:285–289.

166. Grimaldi, J. and Meeker, T. (1989) The t(5;14) chromosomal translocation in a case of acute lymphocytic leukemia joins the interleukin-3 gene to the immunoglobulin heavy chain gene. *Blood* **73**:2081–2085.

167. Neri, A., Knowles, D. M., Greco, A., McCormick, F., and Dalla-Favera, R. (1988) Analysis of RAS oncogene mutations in human lymphoid malignancies. *Proc. Natl. Acad. Sci. USA* **85**:9268–9272.

168. Okuda, T., Hirai, H., Valentine, V. A., Shurtleff, S. A., Kidd, V. J., Lahti, J. M., et al. (1995) Molecular cloning, expression pattern, and chromosomal localization of human CDKN2D/INK4d, an inhibitor of cyclin D-dependent kinases. *Genomics* **29**:623–630.

169. Hebert, J., Cayuela, J., Berkeley, J., and Sigaux, F. (1994) Candidate tumor-suppressor genes MTS1 (*p16^{INK4A}*) and MTS2 (*p15^{INK4B}*) display frequent homozygous deletions in primary cells from T- but not from B-cell lineage acute lymphoblastic leukemias. *Blood* **84**:4038–4044.

170. Fizzotti, M., Cimino, G., Pisegna, S., Alimena, G., Quartarone, C., Mandelli, F., et al. (1995) Detection of homozygous deletions of the cyclin-dependent kinase 4 inhibitor (p16) gene in acute lymphoblastic leukemia and association with adverse prognostic features. *Blood* **85**:2685–2690.

171. Ogawa, S., Hirano, N., Sato, N., Takahashi, T., Hangaishi, A., Tanaka, K., et al. (1994) Homozygous loss of the cyclin-dependent kinase 4-inhibitor (p16) gene in human leukemias. *Blood* **84**:2431–2435.

172. Look, A., Roberson, P., and Murphy, S. (1987) Prognostic value of cellular DNA content in acute lymphoblastic leukemia of childhood. *N. Engl. J. Med.* **317**:1666.

173. Trueworthy, R., Shuster, J., Look, T., Crist, W., Borowitz, M., Carroll, A., et al. (1992) Ploidy of lymphoblasts is the strongest predictor of treatment outcome in B-progenitor cell acute lymphoblastic leukemia of childhood: a Pediatric Oncology Group study. *J. Clin. Oncol.* **10**:606–613.

174. Harris, M., Shuster, J., Carroll, A., Look, A., Borowitz, M., Crist, W., et al. (1992) Trisomy of leukemic cell chromosomes 4 and 10 identifies children with B-progenitor cell acute lymphoblastic leukemia with a very low risk of treatment failure: a Pediatric Oncology Group study. *Blood* **79**:3316–3324.

175. Göker, E., Waltham, M., Kheradpour, A., Trippett, T., Mazumdar, M., Elisseyeff, Y., et al. (1995) Amplification of the dihydrofolate reductase gene is a mechanism of acquired resistance to methotrexate in patients with acute lymphoblastic leukemia and is correlated with p53 gene mutations. *Blood* **86**:677–684.

176. Croce, C. and Nowell, P. (1985) Molecular basis of human B cell neoplasia. *Blood* **65**:1–7.

177. Korsmeyer, S. (1992) Chromosomal translocations in lymphoid malignancies reveal novel proto-oncogenes. *Ann. Rev. Immunol.* **10**:785–807.

178. Raimondi, S. (1993) Current status of cytogenetic research in childhood acute lymphoblastic leukemia. *Blood* **81**:2237–2251.

179. Patte, C., Philip, T., Rodary, C., Zucker, J., Behrendt, H., Gentet, J., et al. (1991) High survival rate in advanced-stage B-cell lymphomas and leukemias without CNS involvement with a short intensive polychemotherapy: results from the French Pediatric Oncology Society of a randomized trial of 216 children. *J. Clin. Oncol.* **9**:123–132.

180. Bhatia, K., Huppi, K., Spangler, G., Siwarski, D., Iyer, R., and Magrath, I. (1993) Point mutations in the c-Myc transactivation domain are common in Burkitt's lymphoma and mouse plasmacytomas. *Nature Genet.* **5**:56–61.

181. Blackwood, E. and Eisenman, R. (1991) Max: a helix-loop-helix zipper protein that forms a sequence-specific DNA-binding complex with Myc. *Science* **251**:1211–1217.

182. Cole, M. (1991) Myc meets its Max. *Cell* **65**:715–716.

183. Ayer, D., Kretzner, L., and Eisenman, R. (1993) Mad: a heterodimeric partner for Max that antagonizes Myc transcriptional activity. *Cell* **72**:211–222.

184. Zervos, A., Gyuris, J., and Brent, R. (1993) Mxi1, a protein that specifically interacts with Max to bind Myc-Max recognition sites. *Cell* **72**:223–232.

185. de Villartay, J. P., Pullman, A. B., Andrade, R., Tschachler, E., Colamenici, O., Neckers, L., et al. (1989) Gamma/delta lineage relationship within a consecutive series of human precursor T-cell neoplasms. *Blood* **74**:2508–2518.

186. Weiss, L. M., Bindl, J. M., Picozzi, V. J., Link, M. P., and Warnke, R. A. (1986) Lymphoblastic lymphoma: an immunophenotype study of 26 cases with comparison to T cell acute lymphoblastic leukemia. *Blood* **67**:474–478.

187. Kitchingman, G., Rovigatti, U., Mauer, A., Melvin, S., Murphy, S., and Stass, S. (1985) Rearrangement of immunoglobulin heavy chain genes in T cell acute lymphoblastic leukemia. *Blood* **65**:725–729.

188. Brown, L., Cheng, J., Chen, Q., Siciliano, M., Crist, W., Buchanan, G., et al. (1990) Site-specific recombination of the *tal-1* gene is a common occurrence in human T cell leukemia. *EMBO J.* **9**:3343–3351.

189. Kikuchi, A., Hayashi, Y., Kobayashi, S., Hanada, R., Moriwaki, K., Yamamoto, K., et al. (1993) Clinical significance of *TAL1* gene alteration in childhood T-cell acute lymphoblastic leukemia and lymphoma. *Leukemia* **7**:933–938.

190. Aplan, P., Lombardi, D., Reaman, G., Sather, H., Hammond, G., and Kirsch, I. (1992) Involvement of the putative hematopoietic transcription factor SCL in T-cell acute lymphoblastic leukemia. *Blood* **79**:1327–1333.

191. Bash, R., Crist, W., Shuster, J., Link, M., Amylon, M., Pullen, J., et al. (1993) Clinical features and outcome of T-cell acute lymphoblastic leukemia in childhood with respect to alterations at the *TAL1* locus: a Pediatric Oncology Group study. *Blood* **81**:2110–2117.

192. Stock, W., Westbrook, C. A., Sher, D. A., et al. (1995) Low incidence of *TAL1* gene rearrangements in adult acute lymphoblastic leukemia. *Clin. Cancer Res.* **1**:459–463.

193. Baer, R. (1993) A family of basic helix-loop-helix proteins implicated in T cell acute leukaemia. *Semin. Cancer Biol.* **4**:341–347.

194. Aplan, P., Lombardi, D., Ginsberg, A., Cossman, J., Bertness, V., and Kirsch, I. (1990) Disruption of the human SCL locus by "illegitimate" V-(D)-J recombinase activity. *Science* **250**:1426–1429.

195. Chetty, R., Pulford, K., Jones, M., Mathieu-Mahul, D., Close, P., Hussein, S., et al. (1995) SCL/Tal-1 expression in T-acute lymphoblastic leukemia: an immunohistochemical and genotypic study. *Human Pathol.* **26**:994–998.

196. Chilcote, R., Brown, E., and Rowley, J. (1985) Lymphoblastic leukemia with lymphomatous features associated with abnormalities of the short arm of chromosome 9. *N. Engl. J. Med.* **313**:286–291.

197. Murphy, S., Raimondi, S., Rivera, G., Crone, M., Dodge, R., Behm, F., et al. (1989) Nonrandom abnormalities of chromosome 9p in childhood acute lymphoblastic leukemia: association with high-risk clinical features. *Blood* **74**:409–415.

198. Okuda, T., Shurtleff, S., Valentine, M., Raimondi, S., Head, D., Behm, F., et al. (1995) Frequent deletion of p16^{INK4A}/*MTS1* and p15^{INK4B}/*MTS2* in pediatric acute lymphoblastic leukemia. *Blood* **85**:2321–2330.

199. Cayeula, J.-M., Gardie, B., and Sigaux, F. (1997) Disruption of the Multiple Tumor suppressor gene *MTS1*/p16^{INK4A}/*CDKN2* by illegitimate V(D)J recombinase activity in T-cell acute lymphoblastic leukemias. *Blood* **90**:3720–3726.

200. Hatano, M., Roberts, C., Minden, M., Crist, W., and Korsmeyer, S. (1991) Deregulation of a homeobox gene, HOX11, by the t(10;14) in T cell leukemia. *Science* **253**:79–82.

201. Yamamoto, H., Hatano, M., Iitsuka, Y., Mahyar, N., Yamamoto, M., and Tokuhisa, T. (1995) Two forms of *Hox11* a T cell leukemia oncogene, are expressed in fetal spleen but not in primary lymphocytes. *Mol. Immunol.* **32**:1177–1182.

202. Hatano, M., Roberts, C., and Minden, M. (1991) Cell cycle progression, cell death and T cell lymphoma in *HOX11* transgenic mice. *Blood* **80**:355a.

203. Zhang, N., Gong, Z. Z., Minden, M., and Lu, M. (1993) The *HOX-11 (TCL-3)* homeobox proto-oncogene encodes a nuclear protein that undergoes cell cycle-dependent regulation. *Oncogene* **8**:3265–3270.

204. Abruzzo, L. V., Jaffe, E. S., Cotelingam, J. D., Whang-Peng, J., Del Duca, V., Jr., and Medeiros, L. J. (1992) T-cell lymphoblastic lymphoma with eosinophilia associated with subsequent myeloid malignancy. *Am. J. Surg. Pathol.* **16**:236–245.

205. Inhorn, R. C., Aster, J. C., Roach, S. A., Slapak, C. A., Soiffer, R., Tantravahi, R., et al. (1995) A syndrome of lymphoblastic lymphoma, eosinophilia, and myeloid hyperplasia/malignancy associated with t(8;13)(p11;q11): description of a distinctive clinicopathologic entity. *Blood* **85**:1881–1887.

206. Naeem, R., Singer, S., and Fletcher, J. A. (1995) Translocation t(8;13)(p11;q11-12) in stem cell leukemia/lymphoma of T-cell and myeloid lineages. *Genes Chromosomes Cancer* **12**:148–151.

207. Xiao, S., Nalabolu, S. R., Aster, J. C., Ma, J., Abruzzo, L., Jaffe, E. S., et al. (1998) *FGFR1* is fused with a novel zinc-finger gene, *ZNF198*, in the t(8;13) leukaemia syndrome. *Nature Genet.* **18**:84–87.

208. Erikson, J., Finger, L., Sun, L., ar-Rushdi, A., Nishikura, K., Minowada, J., et al. (1986) Deregulation of c-*myc* by translocation of the alpha-locus of the T-cell receptor in T-cell leukemias. *Science* **232**:884–886.

209. Narducci, M., Virgilio, L., Isobe, M., Stoppacciaro, A., Elli, R., Fiorilli, M., et al. (1995) *TCL1* oncogene activation in preleukemic T cells from a case of ataxia-telangiectasia. *Blood* **86**:2358–2364.

210. Xia, Y., Brown, L., Yang, C., Tsan, J., Siciliano, M., Espinosa R. I., et al. (1991) *TAL2*, a helix-loop-helix gene activated by the (7;9)(q34;q32) translocation in human T-cell leukemia. *Proc. Natl. Acad. Sci. USA* **88**:11,416–11,420.

211. Mellentin, J., Smith, S., and Cleary, M. (1989) *Lyl-1*, a novel gene altered by chromosomal translocation in T cell leukemia, codes for a protein with a helix-loop-helix DNA binding motif. *Cell* **58**:77–83.

212. Sánchez-García, I. and Rabbitts, T. (1993) LIM domain proteins in leukaemia and development. *Semin. Cancer Biol.* **4**:349–358.

213. Boehm, T., Baer, R., Lavenir, I., Forster, A., Waters, J., Nacheva, E., et al. (1988) The mechanism of chromosomal translocation t(11;14) involving the T-cell receptor C delta locus on human chromosome 14q11 and a transcribed region of chromosome 11p15. *EMBO J.* **7**:385–394.

214. McGuire, E., Hockett, R., Pollock, K., Bartholdi, M., O'Brien, S., and Korsmeyer, S. (1989) The t(11;14)(p15;q11) in a T-cell acute lymphoblastic leukemia cell line activates multiple transcripts, including *Ttg-1*, a gene encoding a potential zinc finger protein. *Mol. Cell. Biol.* **9**:2124–2132.

215. Warren, A., Colledge, W., Carlton, M., Evans, M., Smith, A., and Rabbitts, T. (1994) The oncogenic cysteine-rich LIM domain protein rbtn2 is essential for erythroid development. *Cell* **78**:45–57.

216. Royer-Pokora, B., Rogers, M., Zhu, T., Schneider, S., Loos, U., and Bolitz, U. (1995) The TTG-2/RBTN2 T cell oncogene encodes two alternative transcripts from two promoters: the distal promoter is removed by most 11p13 translocations in acute T cell leukaemia's (T-ALL). *Oncogene* **10**:1353–1360.

217. McGuire, E., Rintoul, C., Sclar, G., and Korsmeyer, S. (1992) Thymic overexpression of Ttg-1 in transgenic mice results in T-cell acute lymphoblastic leukemia/lymphoma. *Mol. Cell. Biol.* **12**:4186–4196.

218. Fisch, P., Boehm, T., Lavenir, I., Larson, T., Arno, J., Forster, A., et al. (1992) T-cell acute lymphoblastic lymphoma induced in transgenic mice by the *RBTN1* and *RBTN2* LIM-domain genes. *Oncogene* **7**:2389–2397.

219. Wadman, I., Li, J., Bash, R., Forster, A., Osada, H., Rabbitts, T., et al. (1994) Specific in vivo association between the bHLH and LIM proteins implicated in human T cell leukemia. *EMBO J.* **13**:4831–4839.

220. Huret, J., Brizard, A., Slater, R., Charrin, C., Bertheas, M., Guilhot, F., et al. (1993) Cytogenetic heterogeneity in t(11;19) acute leukemia: clinical, hematological and cytogenetic analyses of 48 patients—updated published cases and 16 new observations. *Leukemia* **7**:152–160.

221. Chervinsky, D., Sait, S., Nowak, N., Shows, T., and Aplan, P. (1995) Complex *MLL* rearrangement in a patient with T-cell acute lymphoblastic leukemia. *Genes Chromosomes Cancer* **14**:76–84.

222. McCabe, N., Kipiniak, M., Kobayashi, H., Thirman, M., Gill, H., Rowley, J., et al. (1994) DNA rearrangements and altered transcripts of the *MLL* gene in a human T-ALL cell line Karpas 45 with a t(X;11) (q13;q23) translocation. *Genes Chromosomes Cancer* **9**:221–224.

223. Ellisen, L., Bird, J., West, D., Soreng, A., Reynolds, T., Smith, S., et al. (1991) *TAN-1*, the human homolog of the Drosophila notch gene, is broken by chromosomal translocations in T lymphoblastic neoplasms. *Cell* **66**:649–661.

224. Aster, J., Pear, W., and Hasserjian, R. (1994) Functional analysis of the T*AN-1* gene, a human homolog of the Drosophila *notch*. *Cold Spring Harbor Symp. Quant. Biol.* **59**:125–136.

225. Boehm, T., Foroni, L., Kaneko, Y., Perutz, M., and Rabbitts, T. (1991) The rhombotin family of cysteine-rich *LIM*-domain oncogenes: distinct members are involved in T-cell translocations to human chromosomes 11p15 and 11p13. *Proc. Natl. Acad. Sci. USA* **88**:4367–4371.

226. Aurias, A., Dutrillaux, B., Buriot, D., and Lejeune, J. (1980) High frequencies of inversions and translocations of chromosomes 7 and 14 in ataxia telangiectasia. *Mut. Res.* **69**:369–374.

227. Boehm, T. and Rabbitts, T. (1989) The human T cell receptor genes are targets for chromosomal abnormalities in T cell tumors. *FASEB J.* **3**:2344–2359.

228. Jonveaux, P. and Berger, R. (1991) Infrequent mutations in the P53 gene in primary human T-cell acute lymphoblastic leukemia, *Leukemia* **5**:839,840.

229. Yeargin, J., Cheng, J., and Haas, M. (1992) Role of the p53 tumor suppressor gene in the pathogenesis and in the suppression of acute lymphoblastic T-cell leukemia. *Leukemia* **6**:85S–91S.

230. Nowell, P. C. and Hungerford, D. A. (1960) A minute chromosome in human chronic granulocytic leukemia. *Science* **132**:1497.

231. de Klein, A., van Kessel, A., Grosveld, G., Bartram, C., Hagemeijer, A., Bootsma, D., et al. (1982) A cellular oncogene is translocated to the Philadelphia chromosome in chronic myelocytic leukaemia. *Nature* **300**:765–767.

232. Groffen, J., Stephenson, J., Heisterkamp, N., de Klein, A., Bartram, C., and Grosveld, G. (1984) Philadelphia chromosomal breakpoints are clustered within a limited region, *bcr*, on chromosome 22. *Cell* **36**:93–99.

233. Ben-Neriah, Y., Daley, G. Q., Mes-Masson, A. M., Witte, O. N., and Baltimore, D. (1986) The chronic myelogenous leukemia-specific p210 protein is the product of the *bcr/abl* hybrid gene. *Science* **233**:212–214.

234. Bartram, C. R., de Klein, A., Hagemeijer, A., van Agthoven, T., Geurts van Kessel, A., Bootsma, D., et al. (1983) Translocation of *c-abl* oncogene correlates with the presence of a Philadelphia chromosome in chronic myelocytic leukaemia. *Nature* **306**:277–280.

235. Rowley, J. (1973) A new consistent chromosomal abnormality in chronic myelogenous leukaemia identified by quinacrine fluorescence and Giemsa staining. *Nature* **243**:290–293.

236. Haas, O., Argyriou-Tirita, A., and Lion, T. (1992) Parental origin of chromosomes involved in the translocation t(9;22). *Nature* **359**:414–416.

237. Melo, J. V., Yan, X. H., Diamond, J., and Goldman, J. M. (1994) Lack of imprinting of the *ABL* gene. *Nature Genet.* **8**:318–319.

238. Fioretos, T., Heisterkamp, N., and Groffen, J. (1994) No evidence for genomic imprinting of the human *BCR* gene. *Blood* **83**:3441–3444.

239. Bernards, A., Rubin, C., Westbrook, C., Paskind, M., and Baltimore, D. (1987) The first intron in the human *c-abl* gene is at least 200 kilobases long and is a target for translocations in chronic myelogenous leukemia. *Mol. Cell. Biol.* **7**:3231–3236.

240. Grosveld, G., Verwoerd, T., van Agthoven, T., de Klein, A., Ramachandran, K. L., Heisterkamp, N., et al. (1986) The chronic myelocytic cell line K562 contains a breakpoint in *bcr* and produces a chimeric *bcr/c-abl* transcript. *Mol. Cell. Biol.* **6**:607–616.

241. Konopka, J. B. and Witte, O. N. (1985) Detection of c-*abl* tyrosine kinase activity in vitro permits direct comparison of normal and altered abl gene products. *Mol. Cell. Biol.* **5**:3116–3123.

242. Shtivelman, E., Lifshitz, B., Gale, R. P., Roe, B. A., and Canaani, E. (1986) Alternative splicing of RNAs transcribed from the human abl gene and from the *bcr-abl* fused gene. *Cell* **47**:277–284.

243. Fainstein, E., Einat, M., Gokkel, E., Marcelle, C., Croce, C. M., Gale, R. P., et al. (1989) Nucleotide sequence analysis of human *abl* and *bcr-abl* cDNAs. *Oncogene* **4**:1477–1481.

244. Van Etten, R. A., Jackson, P., and Baltimore, D. (1989) The mouse type IV c-abl gene product is a nuclear protein, and activation of transforming ability is associated with cytoplasmic localization. *Cell* **58**:669–678.

245. McWhirter, J. and Wang, J. (1993) An actin-binding function contributes to transformation by the Bcr-Abl oncoprotein of Philadelphia chromosome-positive human leukemias. *EMBO J.* **12**:1533–1546.

246. Wetzler, M., Talpaz, M., Van Etten, R. A., Hirsh-Ginsberg, C., Beran, M., and Kurzrock, R. (1993) Subcellular localization of Bcr, Abl, and Bcr-Abl proteins in normal and leukemic cells and correlation of expression with myeloid differentiation. *J. Clin. Invest.* **92**:1925–1939.

247. Melo, J., Gordon, D., Cross, N., and Goldman, J. (1993) The *ABL-BCR* fusion gene is expressed in chronic myeloid leukemia. *Blood* **81**:158–165.

248. Heisterkamp, N., Stam, K., Groffen, J., de Klein, A., and Grosveld, G. (1985) Structural organization of the bcr gene and its role in the Ph' translocation. *Nature* **315**:758–761.

249. Mes-Masson, A. M., McLaughlin, J., Daley, G. Q., Paskind, M., and Witte, O. N. (1986) Overlapping cDNA clones define the complete coding region for the P210^{c-abl} gene product associated with chronic myelogenous leukemia cells containing the Philadelphia chromosome. *Proc. Natl. Acad. Sci. USA* **83**:9768–9772.

250. Hariharan, I. K. and Adams, J. M. (1987) cDNA sequence for human *bcr*, the gene that translocates to the *abl* oncogene in chronic myeloid leukaemia. *EMBO J.* **6**:115–119.

251. Hermans, A., Heisterkamp, N., von Linden, M., van Baal, S., Meijer, D., van der Plas, D., et al. (1987) Unique fusion of *bcr* and *c-abl* genes in Philadelphia chromosome positive acute lymphoblastic leukemia. *Cell* **51**:33–40.

252. Heisterkamp, N., Knoppel, E., and Groffen, J. (1988) The first *BCR* gene intron contains breakpoints in Philadelphia chromosome positive leukemia. *Nucleic Acids Res.* **16**:10,069–10,081.

253. Stam, K., Heisterkamp, N., Reynolds, F. H., Jr., and Groffen, J. (1987) Evidence that the *PHL* gene encodes a 160,000-dalton phosphoprotein with associated kinase activity. *Mol. Cell. Biol.* **7**:1955–1960.

254. Diekmann, D., Brill, S., Garrett, M., Totty, N., Hsuan, J., Monfries, C., et al. (1991) BCR encodes a GTPase-activating protein for p21^{rac}. *Nature* **351**:400–402.

255. Pendergast, A., Muller, A., Havlik, M., Maru, Y., and Witte, O. (1991) *BCR* sequences essential for transformation by the *BCR-ABL* oncogene bind to the *ABL* SH2 regulatory domain in a non-phosphotyrosine-dependent manner. *Cell* **66**:161–171.

256. Ron, D., Zannini, M., Lewis, M., Wickner, R. B., Hunt, L. T., Graziani, G., et al. (1991) A region of proto-*dbl* essential for its transforming activity shows sequence similarity to a yeast cell cycle gene, *CDC24*, and the human breakpoint cluster gene, *bcr*. *New Biol.* **3**:372–379.

257. Shou, C., Farnsworth, C. L., Neel, B. G., and Feig, L. A. (1992) Molecular cloning of cDNAs encoding a guanine-nucleotide-releasing factor for Ras p21. *Nature* **358**:351–354.

258. McWhirter, J. R., Galasso, D. L., and Wang, J. Y. (1993) A coiled-coil oligomerization domain of Bcr is essential for the transforming function of Bcr-Abl oncoproteins. *Mol. Cell. Biol.* **13**:7587–7595.

259. Dhut, S., Dorey, E. L., Horton, M. A., Ganesan, T. S., and Young, B. D. (1988) Identification of two normal *bcr* gene products in the cytoplasm. *Oncogene* **3**:561–566.

260. Wetzler, M., Talpaz, M., Yee, G., Stass, S. A., Van Etten, R. A., Andreeff, M., et al. (1995) Cell cycle-related shifts in subcellular localization of BCR: association with mitotic chromosomes and with heterochromatin. *Proc. Natl. Acad. Sci. USA* **92**:3488–3492.

261. Gale, R. and Canaani, E. (1984) An 8-kilobase *abl* RNA transcript in chronic myelogenous leukemia. *Proc. Natl. Acad. Sci. USA* **81**:5648–5652.

262. Kurzrock, R., Kloetzer, W. S., Talpaz, M., Blick, M., Walters, R., Arlinghaus, R. B., et al. (1987) Identification of molecular variants of p210^{bcr-abl} in chronic myelogenous leukemia. *Blood* **70**:233–236.

263. Zaccaria, A., Martinelli, G., Buzzi, M., Testoni, N., Farabegoli, P., Zuffa, E., et al. (1993) The type of *BCR/ABL* junction does not predict the survival of patients with Ph1-positive chronic myeloid leukaemia. *Br. J. Haematol.* **84**:265–268.

264. Daley, G., Van Etten, R., and Baltimore, D. (1990) Induction of chronic myelogenous leukemia in mice by the P210bcr/abl gene of the Philadelphia chromosome. *Science* **247**:824–830.

265. Kelliher, M. A., McLaughlin, J., Witte, O. N., and Rosenberg, N. (1990) Induction of a chronic myelogenous leukemia-like syndrome in mice with v-*abl* and *BCR/ABL. Proc. Natl. Acad. Sci. USA* **87**:6649–6653.

266. Gishizky, M. and Witte, O. (1992) Initiation of deregulated growth of multipotent progenitor cells by bcr-abl in vitro. *Science* **256**:836–839.

267. Witte, O. (1993) Role of the *BCR-ABL* oncogene in human leukemia: fifteenth Richard and Hinda Rosenthal Foundation Award Lecture. *Cancer Res.* **53**:485–489.

268. Wetzler, M., Talpaz, M., Estrov, Z., and Kurzrock, R. (1993) CML: mechanisms of disease initiation and progression. *Leukemia Lymphoma* **11**:47–50.

269. Shtivelman, E., Lifshitz, B., Gale, R. P., and Canaani, E. (1985) Fused transcript of *abl* and *bcr* genes in chronic myelogenous leukaemia. *Nature* **315**:550–554.

270. Muller, A., Pendergast, A., Havlik, M., Puil, L., Pawson, T., and Witte, O. (1992) A limited set of SH2 domains binds *BCR* through a high-affinity phosphotyrosine-independent interaction. *Mol. Cell. Biol.* **12**:5087–5093.

271. Pendergast, A., Quilliam, L., Cripe, L., Bassing, C., Dai, Z., Li, N., et al. (1993) *BCR-ABL*-induced oncogenesis is mediated by direct interaction with the SH2 domain of the GRB-2 adaptor protein. *Cell* **75**:175–185.

272. Druker, B., Okuda, K., Matulonis, U., Salgia, R., Roberts, T., and Griffin, J. (1992) Tyrosine phosphorylation of ras^{GAP} and associated proteins in chronic myelogenous leukemia cell lines. *Blood* **79**:2215–2220.

273. Egan, S. and Weinberg, R. (1993) The pathway to signal achievement. *Nature* **365**:781–783.

274. Simon, M. A., Dodson, G. S., and Rubin, G. M. (1993) An SH3-SH2-SH3 protein is required for p21^{Ras1} activation and binds to sevenless and Sos proteins in vitro. *Cell* **73**:169–177.

275. Sawyers, C. L. (1997) Signal transduction pathways involved in BCR-ABL transformation. *Baillieres Clin. Haematol.* **10**:223–231.

276. Sawyers, C., Callahan, W., and Witte, O. (1992) Dominant negative MYC blocks transformation by *ABL* oncogenes. *Cell* **70**:901–910.

277. Sawyers, C. (1993) The role of myc in transformation by BCR-ABL. *Leukemia Lymphoma* **11**:45–46.

278. Melo, J. (1996) The molecular biology of chronic myeloid leukaemia. *Leukemia* **10**:751–756.

279. Clarkson, B. D., Strife, A., Wisniewski, D., Lambek, C., and Carpino, N. (1997) New understanding of the pathogenesis of CML: a prototype of early neoplasia. *Leukemia* **11**:1404–1428.

280. Chissoe, S. L., Bodenteich, A., Wang, Y. F., Wang, Y. P., Burian, D., Clifton, S. W., et al. (1995) Sequence and analysis of the human *ABL* gene, the *BCR* gene, and regions involved in the Philadelphia chromosomal translocation. *Genomics* **27**:67–82.

281. Melo, J. V., Myint, H., Galton, D. A., and Goldman, J. M. (1994) p190$^{BCR-ABL}$ chronic myeloid leukaemia: the missing link with chronic myelomonocytic leukaemia? *Leukemia* **8**:208–211.

282. Saglio, G., Guerrasio, A., Rosso, C., Zaccaria, A., Tassinari, A., Serra, A., et al. (1990) New type of *Bcr/Abl* junction in Philadelphia chromosome-positive chronic myeloid leukemia. *Blood* **76**:1819–1824.

283. Wada, H., Mizutani, S., Nishimura, J., Usuki, Y., Kohsaki, M., Komai, M., et al. (1995) Establishment and molecular characterization of a novel leukemic cell line with Philadelphia chromosome expressing p230$^{BCR/ABL}$ fusion protein. *Cancer Res.* **55**:3192–3196.

284. Pane, F., Frigeri, F., Sindona, M., Luciano, L., Ferrara, F., Cimino, R., et al. (1996) Neutrophilic-chronic myeloid leukemia: a distinct disease with a specific molecular marker (*BCR/ABL* with C3/A2 junction). *Blood* **88**:2410–2414.

285. Biernaux, C., Loos, M., Sels, A., Huez, G., and Stryckmans, P. (1995) Detection of major *bcr-abl* gene expression at a very low level in blood cells of some healthy individuals. *Blood* **86**:3118–3122.

286. Yin, J. L., Williams, B. G., Arthur, C. K., and Ma, D. D. (1995) Interferon response in chronic myeloid leukaemia correlates with ABL/BCR expression: a preliminary study. *Br. J. Haematol.* **89**:539–545.

287. Shepherd, P., Suffolk, R., Halsey, J., and Allan, N. (1995) Analysis of molecular breakpoint and m-RNA transcripts in a prospective randomized trial of interferon in chronic myeloid leukaemia: no correlation with clinical features, cytogenetic response, duration of chronic phase, or survival. *Br. J. Haematol.* **89**:546–554.

288. Melo, J. V., Hochhaus, A., Yan, X. H., and Goldman, J. M. (1996) Lack of correlation between ABL-BCR expression and response to interferon-alpha in chronic myeloid leukaemia. *Br. J. Haematol.* **92**:684–686.

289. Bartram, C., Kleihauer, E., de Klein, A., Grosveld, G., Teyssier, J., Heisterkamp, N., et al. (1985) c-*abl* and *bcr* are rearranged in a Ph1-negative CML patient. *EMBO J.* **4**:683–686.

290. Bartram, C. (1985) *bcr* Rearrangement without juxtaposition of c-abl in chronic myelocytic leukemia. *J. Exp. Med.* **162**:2175–2179.

291. Morris, C., Reeve, A., Fitzgerald, P., Hollings, P., Beard, M., and Heaton, D. (1986) Genomic diversity correlates with clinical variation in Ph'-negative chronic myeloid leukaemia. *Nature* **320**:281–283.

292. Wiedemann, L., Karhi, K., Shivji, M., Rayter, S., Pegram, S., Dowden, G., et al. (1988) The correlation of breakpoint cluster region rearrangement and p210 phl/abl expression with morphological analysis of Ph-negative chronic myeloid leukemia and other myeloproliferative diseases. *Blood* **71**:349–355.

293. Dreazen, O., Klisak, I., Rassool, F., Goldman, J. M., Sparkes, R. S., and Gale, R. P. (1987) Do oncogenes determine clinical features in chronic myeloid leukaemia? *Lancet* **1**:1402–1405.

294. Kurzrock, R., Kantarjian, H. M., Shtalrid, M., Gutterman, J. U., and Talpaz, M. (1990) Philadelphia chromosome-negative chronic myelogenous leukemia without breakpoint cluster region rearrangement: a chronic myeloid leukemia with a distinct clinical course. *Blood* **75**:445–452.

295. Brunning, R. D. and McKenna, R. W. (1994) *Tumors of the Bone Marrow.* Armed Forces Institute of Pathology, Washington, DC, pp. 195–254.

296. Cogswell, P., Morgan, R., Dunn, M., Neubauer, A., Nelson, P., Poland-Johnston, N., et al. (1989) Mutations of the *ras* protooncogenes in chronic myelogenous leukemia: a high frequency of *ras* mutations in *bcr/abl* rearrangement-negative chronic myelogenous leukemia. *Blood* **74**:2629–2633.

297. Potter, A. M. and Watmore, A. (1992) Cytogenetics in myeloid leukemia. *In: Human Cytogenetics: A Practical Approach*, vol. II (Rooney, D. E. and Czepulkowski, B. H., eds.), Oxford University Press, New York, pp. 27–66.

298. Kurzrock, R. and Talpaz, M. (1996) Molecular biology of chronic leukemias. *In: Neoplastic Diseases of the Blood* (Wiernik, P. H., Caneloos, G. P., Dutcher, J. P., and Kyle, R. A., eds.), Churchill Livingstone, New York, pp. 81–104.

299. Mitani, K. (1997) Molecular mechanism of blastic crisis in chronic myelocytic leukemia. *Leukemia* **11**:503–505.

300. Ahuja, H., Bar-Eli, M., Arlin, Z., Advani, S., Allen, S., Goldman, J., et al. (1991) The spectrum of molecular alterations in the evolution of chronic myelocytic leukemia. *J. Clin. Invest.* **87**:2042–2047.

301. Jennings, B. (1995) A study of changes in methylation status and copy number at the c-*myc* locus during progression of chronic myeloid leukemia. *Br. J. Haematol.* **89**:37.

302. Feinstein, E., Cimino, G., Gale, R., Alimena, G., Berthier, R., Kishi, K., et al. (1991) p53 in chronic myelogenous leukemia in acute phase. *Proc. Natl. Acad. Sci. USA* **88**:6293–6297.

303. Sill, H., Goldman, J. M., and Cross, N. C. (1995) Homozygous deletions of the p16 tumor-suppressor gene are associated with lymphoid transformation of chronic myeloid leukemia. *Blood* **85**:2013–2016.

304. Towatari, M., Adachi, K., Kato, H., and Saito, H. (1991) Absence of the human retinoblastoma gene product in the megakaryoblastic crisis of chronic myelogenous leukemia. *Blood* **78**:2178–2181.

305. Dhingra, K., Talpaz, M., Kantarjian, H., Ku, S., Rothberg, J., Gutterman, J. U., et al. (1991) Appearance of acute leukemia-associated P190$^{BCR-ABL}$ in chronic myelogenous leukemia may correlate with disease progression. *Leukemia* **5**:191–195.

306. Saglio, G., Pane, F., Gottardi, E., Frigeri, F., Buonaiuto, M. R., Guerrasio, A., et al. (1996) Consistent amounts of acute leukemia-associated P190$^{BCR/ABL}$ transcripts are expressed by chronic myelogenous leukemia patients at diagnosis. *Blood* **87**:1075–1080.

307. van Rhee, F., Hochhaus, A., Lin, F., Melo, J., Goldman, J., and Cross, N. (1996) p190 BCR-ABL mRNA is expressed at low levels in p210-positive chronic myeloid and acute lymphoblastic leukemias. *Blood* **87**:5213–5217.

308. Melo, J. (1996) The diversity of BCR-ABL fusion proteins and their relationship to leukemia phenotype. *Blood* **88**:2375–2384.

309. Hess, J. L., Zutter, M. M., Castleberry, R. P., and Emanuel, P. D. (1996) Juvenile chronic myelogenous leukemia. *Am. J. Clin. Pathol.* **105**:238–248.

310. Freedman, M. H., Estrov, Z., and Chan, H. S. (1988) Juvenile chronic myelogenous leukemia. *Am. J. Pediatr. Hematol. Oncol.* **10**:261–267.

311. Nakamura, H., Sadamori, N., Ichimaru, M., Shigeno, K., Kinoshita, K., Ohyashiki, J. H., et al. (1988) Juvenile chronic myeloid leukemia: no rearrangement of the breakpoint cluster region. *Cancer Genet. Cytogenet.* **36**:227–229.

312. Toren, A., Mandel, M., Amariglio, N., Hakim, Y., Brok-Simoni, F., Rechavi, G., et al. (1991) Lack of *bcr* rearrangement in juvenile chronic myeloid leukemia. *Med. Pediatr. Oncol.* **19**:493–495.

313. Ross, D. W. and Dent, G. (1989) Juvenile chronic myeloid leukemia: oncogene characterization. *Pediatr. Pathol.* **9**:669–678.

314. Kalra, R., Paderanga, D., Olson, K., and Shannon, K. (1994) Genetic analysis is consistent with the hypothesis that NF1 limits myeloid cell growth through p21^{ras}. *Blood* **84**:3435–3439.

315. Mark, Z., Toren, A., Amariglio, N., Vonsover, A., Rechavi, G., and Brok-Simoni, F. (1995) Rearrangement of the immunoglobulin heavy chain gene in juvenile chronic myeloid leukaemia. *Br. J. Haematol.* **90**:353–357.

316. Valiente, A., Benitez, J., and Bernacer, M. (1990) Ph-positive chronic myeloid leukemia in a child. Rearrangement of the breakpoint cluster region. *Cancer Genet. Cytogenet.* **44**:277–278.

317. Aurer, I., Butturini, A., and Gale, R. P. (1991) *BCR-ABL* rearrangements in children with Philadelphia chromosome-positive chronic myelogenous leukemia. *Blood* **78**:2407–2410.

318. Fioretos, T., Heim, S., Garwicz, S., Ludvigsson, J., and Mitelman, F. (1992) Molecular analysis of Philadelphia-positive childhood chronic myeloid leukemia. *Leukemia* **6**:723–725.

319. Farhi, D. C., Luckey, C. N., and Siddiqui, A. M. (1995) Breakpoint cluster region, immunoglobulin, and T-cell receptor gene rearrangement analysis in juvenile chronic myelogenous leukemia. *Mod. Pathol.* **8**:389–393.

320. Grossman, A., Mathew, A., O'Connell, M., Tiso, P., Distenfeld, A., and Benn, P. (1990) Multiple restriction enzyme digests are required to rule out polymorphism in the molecular diagnosis of chronic myeloid leukemia. *Leukemia* **4**:63–64.

321. Tkachuk, D. C., Westbrook, C. A., Andreeff, M., Donlon, T. A., Cleary, M. L., Suryanarayan, K., et al. (1990) Detection of bcr-abl fusion in chronic myelogeneous leukemia by in situ hybridization. *Science* **250**:559–562.

322. Bentz, M., Cabot, G., Moos, M., Speicher, M. R., Ganser, A., Lichter, P., et al. (1994) Detection of chimeric *BCR-ABL* genes on bone marrow samples and blood smears in chronic myeloid and acute lymphoblastic leukemia by in situ hybridization. *Blood* **83**:1922–1928.

323. Cross, N. C., Feng, L., Chase, A., Bungey, J., Hughes, T. P., and Goldman, J. M. (1993) Competitive polymerase chain reaction to estimate the number of *BCR-ABL* transcripts in chronic myeloid leukemia patients after bone marrow transplantation. *Blood* **82**:1929–1936.

324. Pichert, G. and Ritz, J. (1993) Clinical significance of *bcr-abl* gene rearrangement detected by the polymerase chain reaction after allogeneic bone marrow transplantation in chronic myelogenous leukemia. *Leukemia Lymphoma* **10**:1–8.

325. Talpaz, M., Estrov, Z., Kantarjian, H., Ku, S., Foteh, A., and Kurzrock, R. (1994) Persistence of dormant leukemic progenitors during interferon-induced remission in chronic myelogenous leukemia. Analysis by polymerase chain reaction of individual colonies. *J. Clin. Invest.* **94**:1383–1389.

326. Medeiros, L. J., Bagg, A., and Cossman, J. (1994) Molecular genetics in the diagnosis and classification of lymphoid neoplasms. *In: Surgical Pathology of the Lymph Nodes and Related Organs,* 2nd ed. (Jaffe, E. S., ed.) W.B. Saunders, Philadelphia, pp. 58–97.

327. Oscier, D. G., Thompsett, A., Zhu, D., and Stevenson, F. K. (1997) Differential rates of somatic hypermutation in V(H) genes among subsets of chronic lymphocytic leukemia defined by chromosomal abnormalities. *Blood* **89**:4153–4160.

328. Kipps, T. J., Tomhave, E., Chen, P. P., and Carson, D. A. (1988) Autoantibody-associated kappa light chain variable region gene expressed in chronic lymphocytic leukemia with little or no somatic mutation Implications for etiology and immunotherapy. *J. Exp. Med.* **167**:840–852.

329. Aoki, H., Takishita, M., Kosaka, M., and Saito, S. (1995) Frequent somatic mutations in D and/or JH segments of Ig gene in Waldenstrom's macroglobulinemia and chronic lymphocytic leukemia (CLL) with Richter's syndrome but not in common CLL. *Blood* **85**:1913–1919.

330. Matolcsy, A., Casali, P., Nador, R. G., Liu, Y. F., and Knowles, D. M. (1997) Molecular characterization of IgA- and/or IgG-switched chronic lymphocytic leukemia B cells. *Blood* **89**:1732–1739.

331. van Noesel, C. J. and van Lier, R. A. (1993) Architecture of the human B-cell antigen receptors. *Blood* **82**:363–373.

332. Thompson, A. A., Talley, J. A., Do, H. N., Kagan, H. L., Kunkel, L., Berenson, J., et al. (1997) Aberrations of the B-cell receptor B29 (*CD79b*) gene in chronic lymphocytic leukemia. *Blood* **90**:1387–1394.

333. Juliusson, G., Oscier, D. G., Fitchett, M., Ross, F. M., Stockdill, G., Mackie, M. J., et al. (1990) Prognostic subgroups in B-cell chronic lymphocytic leukemia defined by specific chromosomal abnormalities. *N. Engl. J. Med.* **323**:720–724.

334. Escudier, S. M., Pereira-Leahy, J. M., Drach, J. W., Weier, H. U., Goodacre, A. M., Cork, M. A., et al. (1993) Fluorescent in situ hybridization and cytogenetic studies of trisomy 12 in chronic lymphocytic leukemia. *Blood* **81**:2702–2707.

335. Dohner, H., Pohl, S., Bulgay-Morschel, M., Stilgenbauer, S., Bentz, M., and Lichter, P. (1993) Trisomy 12 in chronic lymphoid leukemias—a metaphase and interphase cytogenetic analysis. *Leukemia* **7**:516–520.

336. Matutes, E., Oscier, D., Garcia-Marco, J., Ellis, J., Copplestone, A., Gillingham, R., et al. (1996) Trisomy 12 defines a group of CLL with atypical morphology: correlation between cytogenetic, clinical and laboratory features in 544 patients. *Br. J. Haematol.* **92**:382–388.

337. Neilson, J. R., Auer, R., White, D., Bienz, N., Waters, J. J., Whittaker, J. A., et al. (1997) Deletions at 11q identify a subset of patients with typical CLL who show consistent disease progression and reduced survival. *Leukemia* **11**:1929–1932.

338. Dohner, H., Stilgenbauer, S., James, M. R., Benner, A., Weilguni, T., Bentz, M., et al. (1997) 11q deletions identify a new subset of B-cell chronic lymphocytic leukemia characterized by extensive nodal involvement and inferior prognosis. *Blood* **89**:2516–2522.

339. Bentz, M., Huck, K., du Manoir, S., Joos, S., Werner, C. A., Fischer, K., et al. (1995) Comparative genomic hybridization in chronic B-cell leukemias shows a high incidence of chromosomal gains and losses. *Blood* **85**:3610–3618.

340. Dyer, M. J., Zani, V. J., Lu, W. Z., O'Byrne, A., Mould, S., Chapman, R., et al. (1994) *BCL2* translocations in leukemias of mature B cells. *Blood* **83**:3682–3688.

341. Adachi, M., Tefferi, A., Greipp, P. R., Kipps, T. J., and Tsujimoto, Y. (1990) Preferential linkage of bcl-2 to immunoglobulin light chain gene in chronic lymphocytic leukemia. *J. Exp. Med.* **171**:559–564.

342. Tashiro, S., Takechi, M., Asou, H., Takauchi, K., Kyo, T., Dohy, H., et al. (1992) Cytogenetic 2;18 and 18;22 translocation in chronic

lymphocytic leukemia with juxtaposition of *bcl-2* and immunoglobulin light chain genes. *Oncogene* 7:573–577.

343. McKeithan, T. W., Takimoto, G. S., Ohno, H., Bjorling, V. S., Morgan, R., Hecht, B. K., et al. (1997) *BCL3* rearrangements and t(14;19) in chronic lymphocytic leukemia and other B-cell malignancies: A molecular and cytogenetic study. *Genes Chromosomes Cancer* 20:64–72.

344. Newman, R. A., Peterson, B., Davey, F. R., Brabyn, C., Collins, H., Brunetto, V. L., et al. (1993) Phenotypic markers and *BCL-1* gene rearrangements in B-cell chronic lymphocytic leukemia: a Cancer and Leukemia Group B study. *Blood* 82:1239–1246.

345. Medeiros, L. J., Van Krieken, J. H., Jaffe, E. S., and Raffeld, M. (1990) Association of *bcl-1* rearrangements with lymphocytic lymphoma of intermediate differentiation. *Blood* 76:2086–2090.

346. Bastard, C., Deweindt, C., Kerckaert, J. P., Lenormand, B., Rossi, A., Pezzella, F., et al. (1994) *LAZ3* rearrangements in non-Hodgkin's lymphoma: correlation with histology, immunophenotype, karyotype, and clinical outcome in 217 patients. *Blood* 83:2423–2427.

347. Rechavi, G., Katzir, N., Brok-Simoni, F., Holtzman, F., Mandel, M., Gurfinkel, N., et al. (1989) A search for *bcl1, bcl2,* and *c-myc* oncogene rearrangements in chronic lymphocytic leukemia. *Leukemia* 3:57–60.

348. Liu, Y., Hermanson, M., Grander, D., Merup, M., Wu, X., Heyman, M., et al. (1995) 13q deletions in lymphoid malignancies. *Blood* 86:1911–1915.

349. Dohner, H., Pilz, T., Fischer, K., Cabot, G., Diehl, D., Fink, T., et al. (1994) Molecular cytogenetic analysis of *RB-1* deletions in chronic B-cell leukemias. *Leukemia Lymphoma* 16:97–103.

350. Newcomb, E. W. (1995) p53 gene mutations in lymphoid diseases and their possible relevance to drug resistance. *Leukemia Lymphoma* 17:211–221.

351. Haidar, M. A., Cao, X. B., Manshouri, T., Chan, L. L., Glassman, A., Kantarjian, H. M., et al. (1995) p16$^{\text{ink4a}}$ and p15$^{\text{ink4b}}$ gene deletions in primary leukemias. *Blood* 86:311–315.

352. Gartenhaus, R., Johns, M. M., III, Wang, P., Rai, K., and Sidransky, D. (1996) Mutator phenotype in a subset of chronic lymphocytic leukemia. *Blood* 87:38–41.

353. Foon, K. A., Thiruvengadam, R., Saven, A., Bernstein, Z. P., and Gale, R. P. (1993) Genetic relatedness of lymphoid malignancies Transformation of chronic lymphocytic leukemia as a model. *Ann. Internal Med.* 119:63–73.

354. Gay, D., Saunders, T., Camper, S., and Weigert, M. (1993) Receptor editing: an approach by autoreactive B cells to escape tolerance. *J. Exp. Med.* 177:999–1008.

355. Cherepakhin, V., Baird, S. M., Meisenholder, G. W., and Kipps, T. J. (1993) Common clonal origin of chronic lymphocytic leukemia and high-grade lymphoma of Richter's syndrome. *Blood* 82:3141–3147.

356. Brynes, R. K., McCourty, A., Sun, N. C., and Koo, C. H. (1995) Trisomy 12 in Richter's transformation of chronic lymphocytic leukemia. *Am. J. Clin. Pathol.* 104:199–203.

357. Asou, N., Osato, M., Horikawa, K., Nishikawa, K., Sakitani, O., Li, L., et al. (1997) Burkitt's type acute lymphoblastic transformation

associated with t(8;14) in a case of B cell chronic lymphocytic leukemia. *Leukemia* 11:1986–1988.

358. Matolcsy, A., Inghirami, G., and Knowles, D. M. (1994) Molecular genetic demonstration of the diverse evolution of Richter's syndrome (chronic lymphocytic leukemia and subsequent large cell lymphoma). *Blood* 83:1363–1372.

359. Brito-Babapulle, V., Pittman, S., Melo, J. V., Pomfret, M., and Catovsky, D. (1987) Cytogenetic studies on prolymphocytic leukemia. I. B-cell prolymphocytic leukemia. *Hematol. Pathol.* 1:27–33.

360. Lens, D., De Schouwer, P. J., Hamoudi, R. A., Abdul-Rauf, M., Farahat, N., Matutes, E., et al. (1997) p53 abnormalities in B-cell prolymphocytic leukemia. *Blood* 89:2015–2023.

361. Korsmeyer, S., Greene, W., Cossman, J., Hsu, S., Jensen, J., Neckers, L., et al. (1983) Rearrangement and expression of immunoglobulin genes and expression of Tac antigen in hairy cell leukemia. *Proc. Natl. Acad. Sci. USA* 80:4522–4526.

362. Wagner, S. D., Martinelli, V., and Luzzatto, L. (1994) Similar patterns of V$_{\text{K}}$ gene usage but different degrees of somatic mutation in hairy cell leukemia, prolymphocytic leukemia, Waldenstrom's macroglobulinemia, and myeloma. *Blood* 83:3647–3653.

363. Cuneo, A., Bigoni, R., Balboni, M., Carli, M. G., Piva, N., Fagioli, F., et al. (1994) Trisomy 12 in chronic lymphocytic leukemia and hairy cell leukemia: a cytogenetic and interphase cytogenetic study. *Leukemia Lymphoma* 15:167–172.

364. Brito-Babapulle, V., Pomfret, M., Matutes, E., and Catovsky, D. (1987) Cytogenetic studies on prolymphocytic leukemia. II. T cell prolymphocytic leukemia. *Blood* 70:926–931.

365. Fu, T., Virgilio, L., Narducci, M., Facchiano, A., Russo, G., and Croce, C. (1994) Characterization and localization of the TCL-1 oncogene product. *Cancer Res.* 54:6297–6301.

366. Stern, M., Soulier, J., Rosenzwajg, M., Nakahara, K., Canki-Klain, N., Aurias, A., et al. (1993) *MTCP-1:* a novel gene on the human chromosome Xq28 translocated to the T cell receptor alpha/delta locus in mature T cell proliferations. *Oncogene* 8:2475–2483.

367. Mossafa, H., Brizard, A., Huret, J. L., Brizard, F., Lessard, M., Guilhot, F., et al. (1994) Trisomy 8q due to i(8q) or der(8) t(8;8) is a frequent lesion in T- prolymphocytic leukaemia: four new cases and a review of the literature. *Br. J. Haematol.* 86:780–785.

368. Fisch, P., Forster, A., Sherrington, P. D., Dyer, M. J., and Rabbitts, T. H. (1993) The chromosomal translocation t(X;14)(q28;q11) in T-cell pro- lymphocytic leukaemia breaks within one gene and activates another. *Oncogene* 8:3271–3276.

369. Thick, J., Mak, Y. F., Metcalfe, J., Beatty, D., and Taylor, A. M. (1994) A gene on chromosome Xq28 associated with T-cell prolymphocytic leukemia in two patients with ataxia telangiectasia. *Leukemia* 8:564–573.

370. Semenzato, G., Zambello, R., Starkebaum, G., Oshimi, K., and Loughran, T. P., Jr. (1997) The lymphoproliferative disease of granular lymphocytes: updated criteria for diagnosis. *Blood* 89:256–260.

371. Pelicci, P. G., Allavena, P., Subar, M., Rambaldi, A., Pirelli, A., Di Bello, M., et al. (1987) T cell receptor (α, β, γ) gene rearrangements and expression in normal and leukemic large granular lymphocytes/natural killer cells. *Blood* 70:1500–1508.

20 Molecular Genetic Applications to the Diagnosis of Non-Hodgkin's Lymphoma

GREGORY J. TSONGALIS, PHD AND WILLIAM N. REZUKE, MD

INTRODUCTION

The hematological malignancies can be broadly categorized into the malignant lymphomas. which include the two major categories, non-Hodgkin's lymphoma and Hodgkin's disease; the acute and chronic lymphoid leukemias, which may be of B-cell or T-cell type; acute myelogenous leukemia (AML); the myelodysplastic syndromes; and the myeloproliferative disorders. NHL accounts for 5% of new cancer cases annually with 57,000 new cases expected to be diagnosed in 1999 *(1)*. The goal of this chapter is to focus on the hematopathological approach to the diagnosis of B-cell and T-cell lymphomas for which molecular genetic methods, specifically Southern blotting and polymerase chain reaction (PCR), are most commonly employed.

In general, precise diagnosis of hematological malignancies often requires a multiparameter approach, which correlates morphological evaluation of traditional hematoxylin- and eosin-stained tissue sections or Wright-stained smears with a variety of special studies. These special studies may include any combination of cytochemical and histochemical stains, immunopathological studies, molecular genetic techniques, and cytogenetic techniques. Although many of these studies are quite sensitive and specific, final interpretation of any study must always be made in the context of traditional morphological findings.

NON-HODGKIN'S LYMPHOMA

Non-Hodgkin's lymphoma is a heterogeneous group of disorders that occurs as a result of neoplastic transformation of B and T lymphocytes at different stages of B-cell and T-cell development *(2,3)*. The wide variety of lymphoid malignancies reflects the varying stages of lymphocyte development and the complexity of the immune system. The clinical and pathological characteristics of the lymphoid malignancies are summa-

rized in a comprehensive manner in the Revised European American Lymphoma (REAL) classification *(4,5)* and the proposed World Health Organization (WHO) classification.

Historically, the diagnosis of lymphoma prior to 1980 was based on traditional morphology. Our understanding of the immune system and ability to diagnose and classify lymphoid malignancies improved significantly in the 1980s. This was largely due to the development of immunopathological methods, which employ a wide variety of monoclonal antibodies (MAbs) to study cell-surface antigens *(6,7)* (Figs. 1A and B). Traditional morphological findings, in conjunction with immunopathological studies, are now the cornerstone of diagnosis in lymphoid malignancies. In the mid-1980s, the availability of molecular genetic methods further enhanced our ability to diagnose and classify lymphoid malignancies *(8–13)*. These methods are extremely powerful tools, which are used in select situations.

The major application of molecular genetic methods in the evaluation of lymphoid neoplasms involves the determination of B-cell and T-cell clonality. These methods are considered to be the gold standard for determining clonality and are utilized primarily when clonality cannot be determined immunopathologically. For B-cell neoplasms, clonality can often be determined immunopathologically by demonstrating the presence of monoclonal surface immunoglobulin *(6)*. For T-cell malignancies, there is no immunopathological equivalent to monoclonal surface immunoglobulin, although aberrant loss of T-cell antigen expression is considered to be presumptive evidence of T-cell malignancy *(6)*. Thus, in T-cell malignancies, molecular genetic studies for the determination of clonality, are especially important.

Other applications of molecular genetics to the assessment of lymphoid malignancies include determination of B-cell or T-cell lineage, detection of chromosomal translocations and detection of minimal residual disease. The latter application is becoming increasingly important in evaluating patients before and after bone marrow transplantation *(14)*. The detection of a specific chromosomal translocation may help define a specific

From: *The Molecular Basis of Human Cancer* (W. B. Coleman and G. J. Tsongalis, eds.), © Humana Press Inc., Totowa, NJ.

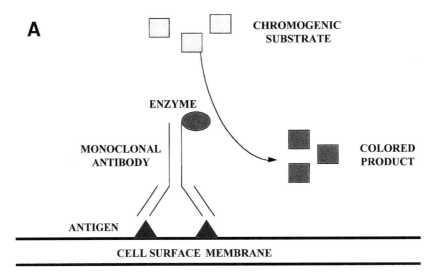

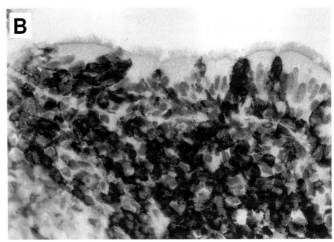

Fig. 1. Immunopathological detection of cell surface antigens. **(A)** Diagram illustrating the basic principle of immunopathological methods. An enzyme is linked to a monoclonal antibody that recognizes a specific cell-surface membrane antigen. A chromogenic substrate is added and is enzymatically converted to a colored product that is visualized microscopically. **(B)** Bronchial biopsy with involvement by a low grade B-cell lymphoma of mucosa-associated lymphoid tissue (MALT). An immunoperoxidase study for the B-cell antigen, CD20, illustrates infiltration of the submucosa and overlying epithelium (arrows) by neoplastic B-cells (immunoperoxidase stain).

type of malignancy. For example, the detection of a clonal *bcl2* rearrangement indicates the presence of a chromosomal translocation involving chromosomes 14 and 18, t(14;18), which is commonly associated with non-Hodgkin's lymphomas of follicular center cell origin and the detection of a clonal *bcl1* rearrangement indicates the presence of a t(11;14), which is common to mantle cell lymphoma *(15)*.

NORMAL B-CELL DEVELOPMENT

According to current concepts of the normal development of the humoral immune system, all B lymphocytes arise from pluripotent stem cells in the bone marrow and then subsequently migrate to secondary lymphoid organs such as lymph node follicles and Peyer's patches in the gastrointestinal tract. The stages of B-cell differentiation in the bone marrow occur largely independent of the presence of antigen whereas the stages of differentiation in secondary lymphoid organs require the presence of antigen for transformation *(2,16)*. Fig. 2 shows the normal stages of B-cell development, which occur in an orderly

fashion beginning with a progenitor B-cell, which matures to a terminally differentiated plasma cell. A variety of recognized changes occur at different maturational stages both at the molecular level and with regard to the presence of specific cellular antigens. At the molecular level, the genes that code for the immunoglobulin heavy- and light-chain proteins undergo sequential rearrangements early in B-cell development (Fig. 2). Initially, the immunoglobulin μ heavy chain located on chromosome 14q32 rearranges and is followed by κ light-chain rearrangement on chromosome 2p12 and λ light-chain rearrangement on chromosome 22q11 *(17)*. Subsequent transcription and translation of the μ heavy-chain gene results in the appearance of cytoplasmic μ heavy-chain protein, which defines the pre-B-cell stage of development. The immature, mature, and activated B-cell stages are characterized by the presence of an intact surface immunoglobulin receptor, which consists of two heavy- and two light-chain proteins (Fig. 3A).

As illustrated in Fig. 2, a variety of cellular antigens can be detected at different stages of B-cell development and the

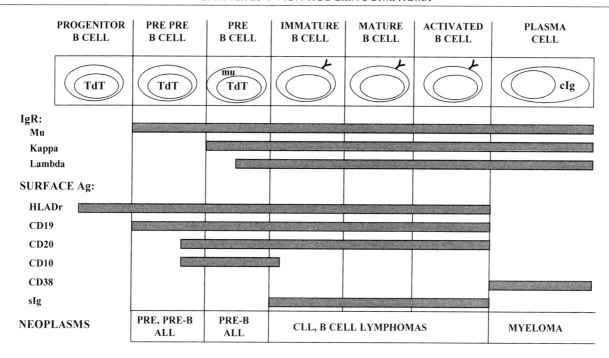

	PROGENITOR B CELL	PRE PRE B CELL	PRE B CELL	IMMATURE B CELL	MATURE B CELL	ACTIVATED B CELL	PLASMA CELL
	TdT	TdT	mu TdT				cIg
IgR:							
Mu							
Kappa							
Lambda							
SURFACE Ag:							
HLADr							
CD19							
CD20							
CD10							
CD38							
sIg							
NEOPLASMS	PRE, PRE-B ALL	PRE-B ALL	CLL, B CELL LYMPHOMAS				MYELOMA

Fig. 2. Normal B-cell development. Normal stages of B-cell development indicating both molecular and cellular antigen changes that occur beginning with the progenitor B-cell through maturation to a terminally differentiated plasma cell. TdT, terminal deoxynucleotidyl transferase; μ, cytoplasmic μ heavy chain; cIg, cytoplasmic immunoglobulin; IgR, immunoglobulin rearrangement; sIg, surface immunoglobulin.

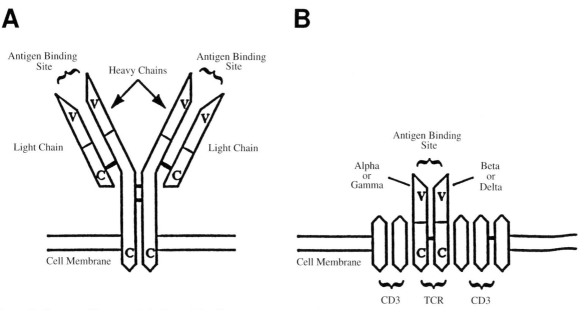

Fig. 3. Schematic diagram of immunoglobulin and T-cell receptors. **(A)** The immunoglobulin protein is a heterodimer composed of two heavy and two light chains, each of which has variable (V) and constant (C) regions. **(B)** The T-cell receptor (TCR) is also a heterodimer composed of either one α and one β chain or one γ and one δ chain. Each of the TCR proteins has variable (V) and constant (C) regions. CD3 is a complex of 5 proteins associated with the TCR.

majority are referred to by CD (cluster designation) numbers. The earliest antigens expressed on B-cells are terminal deoxynucleotidyl transferase (TdT) and human leukocyte antigen type DR (HLA-DR). Neither of these antigens are B-lineage specific. B-cell-associated antigens, CD19, CD20, and CD10, are subsequently expressed. As a B-cell matures to a terminally differentiated plasma cell, the majority of B-cell associated antigens are lost and the CD38 antigen appears.

The fundamental theory of lymphoid neoplasia is that disorders of lymphoid cells represent arrested at various stages in the normal differentiation scheme *(18)*. For example, pre-B-cell acute lymphoblastic leukemia (ALL) mimics normal precursor B-cells showing expression for TdT, HLA-Dr, CD10, CD19, CD20, and cytoplasmic μ heavy chains (Fig. 2). Other examples of neoplastic counterparts to normal precursors include chronic lymphocytic leukemia (CLL)/small lymphocytic lymphoma at

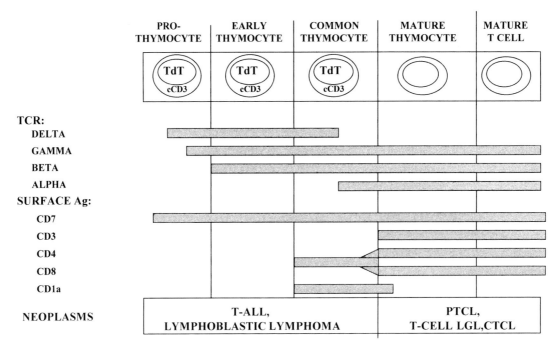

Fig. 4. T-cell development. Normal stages of T-cell development indicating both molecular and cellular antigen changes that occur beginning with the pro-thymocyte through differentiation to a mature T-cell. TdT, terminal deoxynucleotidyl transferase; cCD3, cytoplasmic CD3; TCR, T-cell receptor rearrangements; Ag, antigen.

the immature B-cell stage, follicular center-cell lymphoma at the activated B-cell stage, and multiple myeloma at the terminally differentiated B-cell or plasma-cell stage.

NORMAL T-CELL DEVELOPMENT

T lymphocytes also arise from pluripotent stem cells in the bone marrow. In contrast to B-cell development in which the earliest stages of maturation occur in the bone marrow, progenitor T-cells migrate from the bone marrow to the thymus where the early stages of T-cell development occur *(3,19)*. Subsequently, mature T-cells circulate in the peripheral blood and seed peripheral lymphoid tissues, which include paracortical areas of lymph nodes and periarteriolar sheaths of the spleen.

Figure 4 shows the normal stages of T-cell development in the thymus, which, analogous to B- cell development, occur in an orderly fashion. T lymphocytes possess a surface-membrane protein complex referred to as the T-cell receptor, which is structurally similar to the immunoglobulin receptor *(8,10,20)* (Fig. 3B). The genes that code for the T-cell receptor undergo sequential rearrangements early in T-cell development. There are four T-cell receptor genes (α, β, γ, and δ), which code for two types of T-cell receptors that exist as heterodimers: the α–β receptor and the γ–δ receptor. The majority of T-cells (98–99%) possess the α–β receptor with the remaining 1–2% possessing the γ–δ receptor *(20)*. The α- and δ-chain genes are located on chromosome 14q11, the β-chain gene on chromosome 7q34 and the γ-chain gene on chromosome 7p15 *(17)*. The first T-cell receptor gene to rearrange is δ, which is followed sequentially by γ, β, and α genes.

Analogous to developing B-cells, a variety of cellular antigens can be detected at different stages of T-cell development

(Fig. 4). The earliest antigens expressed are TdT and CD7. The CD3 antigen, which is part of the protein complex associated with the T-cell receptor (Fig. 3B), is present early primarily in the cytoplasm and manifests on the cell surface at a later stage. The common thymocyte stage is defined by expression of CD1a, the common thymocyte antigen, and is frequently associated with co-expression of the CD4 (helper/inducer) and CD8 (cytotoxic/suppressor) antigens. As T-cells reach the mature stage, they express either CD4 or CD8, but not both. Similar to B-cell neoplasms, T-cell neoplasms occur due to maturation arrest at various stages of T-cell development *(18)*. For example, lymphoblastic lymphoma frequently mimics normal common thymocytes showing expression of TdT, CD1a, cytoplasmic CD3, CD7, and co-expression of CD4 and CD8 (Fig. 4). Other examples of neoplastic counterparts to normal precursors include peripheral T-cell lymphoma, cutaneous T-cell lymphoma (mycosis fungoides), and the T-cell type of lymphoproliferative disorder of granular lymphocytes, which are all neoplasms of mature T-cells *(4)*.

B-CELL IMMUNOGLOBULIN AND T-CELL-RECEPTOR GENE REARRANGEMENTS

The B-cell immunoglobulin and T-cell receptors are involved in the process of antigen recognition by normal B and T lymphocytes. These receptors are structurally similar being heterodimer proteins linked by disulfide bonds and are composed of both variable (V) and constant (C) regions *(17)* (Fig. 3). The variable regions of these proteins are similarly involved in antigen recognition. The constant region of the immunoglobulin heavy-chain protein defines the nine immunoglobulin classes (IgG1, IgG2, IgG3, IgG4, IgA1, IgA2, IgM, IgD, and IgE) *(16)*. The genes that code for the B-cell and T-cell recep-

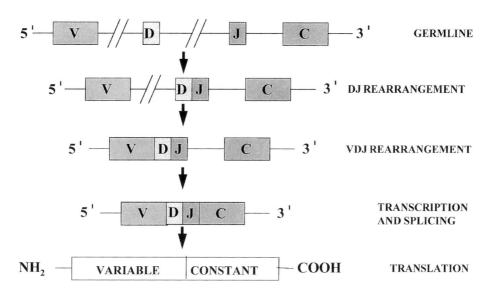

Fig. 5. The sequential steps involved in immunoglobulin and T-cell receptor gene rearrangements. The germline configuration of these genes undergoes a series of rearrangements that result in the transcription and translation of immunoglobulin or T-cell recptor. V, variable segments; D, diversity segments; J, junctional segments; C, constant segments.

IMMUNOGLOBULIN HEAVY CHAIN GENE
CHROMOSOME 14q32

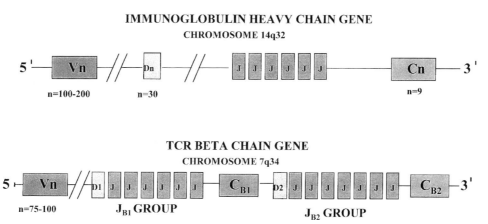

TCR BETA CHAIN GENE
CHROMOSOME 7q34

Fig. 6. Schematic diagram of the IgH chain and the T-cell receptor β-chain supergene families. To detect B-cell heavy chain or T-cell-receptor chain gene rearrangements by Southern-blot analysis, probes that recognize consensus joining (J) or constant (C) segments are used.

tors are also structurally similar and consist of a large number of exons referred to as a supergene family, which undergo a similar process of DNA recombination leading eventually to the formation of functional receptor proteins *(8,16,17,20,21)*.

A general scheme of B-cell immunoglobulin and T-cell receptor gene rearrangements is shown in Fig. 5. The germline configuration refers to nonrearranged DNA. The exons that code for the variable regions of the immunoglobulin and T-cell receptors are referred to as variable (V) segments, diversity (D) segments, and junctional (J) segments, and those that code for the constant regions are referred to as (C) segments. The process of gene rearrangement first involves the selective apposition of one D segment with one J segment by deletion of the intervening coding and noncoding DNA sequences resulting in a DJ rearrangement. By a similar process of rearrangement, a V segment, located in the 5'-direction becomes apposed to D and J to form a VDJ rearrangement. Transcription to mRNA

then occurs even though the VDJ segments are not yet directly apposed to C segments, which are remotely located in the 3'-direction. Subsequent splicing of the mRNA with deletion of noncoding sequences results in apposition of VDJ with C to form a VDJC mRNA, which can then be translated into an immunoglobulin or T-cell receptor protein. The genes coding for the immunoglobulin heavy-chain protein and T-cell receptor β and δ proteins include V, D, J, and C segments. The genes coding for the κ and λ light chain proteins and the T-cell receptor α and γ proteins include only V, J, and C segments without D segments *(8,17,21)*.

The complex process of DNA recombination or rearrangement allows for tremendous diversity of both the humoral and cell-mediated immune systems and the ability to detect a wide array of antigens *(8,16,17,20,21)*. The large number of V, D, J, and C segments results in many combinations that can be transcribed and translated to millions of different antigen recep-

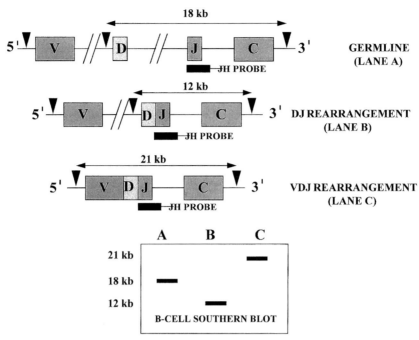

Fig. 7. Schematic diagram illustrating the Southern-blot approach for detecting B-cell gene rearrangements. Arrowheads identify restriction-enzyme cleavage sites.

tors. A detailed diagram of the B-cell heavy chain and the T-cell receptor β-chain supergene families is shown in Fig. 6. The immunoglobulin heavy-chain gene consists of at least 100 V segments, approx 30 D segments, 6 J segments, and 9 C segments. The T-cell receptor β-chain gene includes 75–100 V segments, and two tandem DJC complexes referred to as D1J1C1 and D2J2C2. Each DJC complex contains one D segment and one C segment. The first DJC complex contains six J segments (J_{B1} group) and the second DJC complex contains seven J segments (J_{B2} group) *(8,17,21)*.

SOUTHERN BLOTS AND THE DETERMINATION OF B- AND T-CELL CLONALITY

To establish a diagnosis of B-cell or T-cell malignancy, the ability to prove that a neoplastic population of B-cells or T-cells is monoclonal in origin is of central importance. A monoclonal, or simply, clonal-cell population refers to a population of cells that share similar characteristics and are all derived from a single precursor cell. In lymphoid malignancies, clonality can be defined in several different ways. Clonality may be suggested based on traditional morphology if a monomorphous-cell population is present, immunopathologically by showing the presence of monoclonal surface immunoglobulin (in the case of B-cell neoplasms), cytogenetically by demonstrating a recurrent chromosomal alteration such as recurrent translocation, and by molecular genetic methods demonstrating the presence of a clonal B or T-cell gene rearrangement. In B- and T-cell neoplasms, the primary application of molecular genetics is to prove clonality in cases that are not morphologically malignant, and in which clonality cannot be proven immunopathologically. Southern-blot analysis is a very sensitive and specific method for determining clonality and may

detect a monoclonal population that comprises as little as 1–5% of the total cell population *(7,8,17)*.

For Southern-blot analysis, DNA is first extracted and purified from the cells that are to be analyzed. Fresh or frozen specimens are most suitable for Southern-blot analysis of hematological disorders and these include cell suspensions prepared from peripheral blood, bone marrow aspirates, and body fluids, as well as cell suspensions or cryostat sections prepared from tissues such as lymph node or spleen. Separate samples of purified DNA are then digested with three different restriction enzymes suitable for the probe being used *(22–24)*. Restriction enzymes cleave DNA at specific sites by recognizing specific base-pair sequences. The digested DNA fragments are then electrophoresed using agarose gels, which separate the DNA fragments according to molecular size. These DNA fragments are then transferred to a nylon membrane and hybridized with a specific DNA probe. DNA-probe detection systems include radioactive labeling with ^{32}P, chemiluminescence, and colorimetric *(23–25)*.

DNA probes, which are commonly used for detection of monoclonal B-cell populations, are J_H, which recognizes the heavy-chain J segments, and Jκ, which recognizes the κ light-chain J segments. DNA probes commonly used for the detection of monoclonal T-cell populations recognize the two groups of β-chain J segments or the two β-chain C segments. Figure 6 shows the specific sites of recognition in the immunoglobulin heavy-chain and T-cell receptor β-chain genes in the germline configuration.

The Southern-blot approach for detecting B-cell gene rearrangements is shown schematically in Figu.7. In reactive or polyclonal lymphocyte populations, the primary band identified with J_H probe is the germline band (Lane A). Thousands of

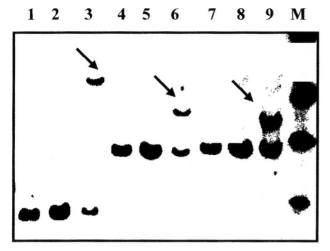

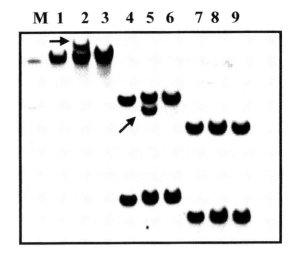

Fig. 8. Assessment of B-cell clonality by Southern blot. Evaluation for B-cell clonality with Southern blots using the J6 probe (DAKO Corp., Carpenteria, CA) and restriction enzymes *Bgl*II (Lanes 1–3), XbaI (Lanes 4–6), and *Bam*HI/*Hin*DIII (Lanes 7–9). Each restriction enzyme has a control lane identifying the germline configuration (Lanes 1,4,7). Clonal B-cell gene rearrangements are identified in a case of B-cell non-Hodgkin's lymphoma (Lanes 3,6,9) with novel bands present in each lane (arrows). Only the germline configuration is identified in a lymph node biopsy showing reactive hyperplasia (Lanes 2,5,8). M, marker lane.

Fig. 9. Assessment of T-cell clonality by Southern blot. Evaluation of T-cell clonality with Southern blots using the TCRBC probe probe (DAKO Corp., Carpenteria, CA) and restriction enzymes *Bam*HI (Lanes 1–3), *Eco*RI (Lanes 4–6), and *Hin*DIII (Lanes 7–9). Each restriction enzyme has a control lane identifying the germline configuration (Lanes 1,4,7). Clonal T-cell gene rearrangements are identified in a case of T-cell non-Hodgkin's lymphoma (Lanes 2,5,8) with novel bands present in lanes 2 and 5 (arrows). Only the germline configuration is identified in a lymph-node biopsy showing reactive hyperplasia (Lanes 3,6,9). M, marker lane.

different rearrangements are actually present in this lane, but individually, the rearrangements are too small to be detected. In a monoclonal B-cell population, all B-cells are derived from a single precursor cell and have identical gene rearrangements, which will be detected by Southern blots as a novel band. If the monoclonal B-cell population has a DJ rearrangement, numerous intervening coding and noncoding DNA sequences are deleted resulting in a smaller fragment of DNA detected by the J_H probe (Lane B). If the monoclonal B-cell population has a VDJ rearrangement, a restriction-enzyme cleavage site is also deleted resulting in a larger fragment of DNA detected by the J_H probe (Lane C).

Southern blots using FITC-labeled DNA probes are shown in Figs. 8 and 9. Figure 8 (Lanes 3,6,9) shows the presence of a clonal B-cell heavy-chain gene rearrangement, which was detected with a JH probe in a case of B-cell, non-Hodgkin's lymphoma. Figure 9 (Lanes 2,5) shows the presence of a clonal T-cell gene rearrangement, which was detected with the TCRBC probe in a case of T-cell, non-Hodgkin's lymphoma. In each set of blots, a marker lane (Lane M) consisting of pre-digested fragments of lambda-phage DNA is present to establish restriction-fragment sizes. With each enzyme digest, a control lane consisting of normal placental DNA is run to identify the germline configuration. A novel band refers to any band occurring in a lane other than: 1) a germline band; 2) a cross-hybridization band, which occurs due to hybridization of the probe to partially homologous DNA sequences in other areas of the genome; or 3) a partial digest band, which occurs due to incomplete digestion of DNA by a restriction enzyme. A diagnosis of a clonal B-cell or T-cell gene rearrangement is established according to the guidelines established by Cossman et al. *(22)*, which require the identification of at least two novel bands

that may be present either in two separate enzyme digests or may both be present in the same enzyme digest.

PCR AND THE DETERMINATION OF B- AND T-CELL CLONALITY

The PCR technique has become a popular method for evaluating the presence or absence of B- and T-cell clonality in lymphoid neoplasms *(26–43)*. This powerful methodology for DNA analysis allows for the evaluation of minute quantities of DNA by in vitro amplification. Analogous to Southern-blot methods, the application of PCR to detect B-cell and T-cell clonality involves evaluation of gene rearrangements in those segments of DNA, which code for the variable regions of the immunoglobulin and T-cell receptors. Each V segment of DNA has a unique DNA sequence that contributes to the great diversity of the immunoglobulin and T-cell receptor-antigen recognition sites. In addition, short sequences of DNA are shared by nearly all of the V segments, which can be recognized by a primer referred to as a consensus V region primer. In a similar fashion, short sequences of DNA shared by nearly all of the J segments can be recognized by a consensus J region primer *(26–43)*.

A diagram illustrating the application of PCR to detect B-cell heavy-chain gene rearrangements using V_H and J_H consensus primers is shown in Fig. 10. An ethidium bromide-stained PCR gel is shown in Fig. 11 for IgH gene rearrangements. In order to successfully amplify a segment of DNA by PCR, the primers must recognize DNA sequences within a short segment of DNA. In the germline configuration, because V and J segments are widely separated, no significant DNA product is obtained following amplification by PCR (Fig. 10, Lane A and Fig. 11, Lane 3). If a VDJ rearrangement occurs, the proximity

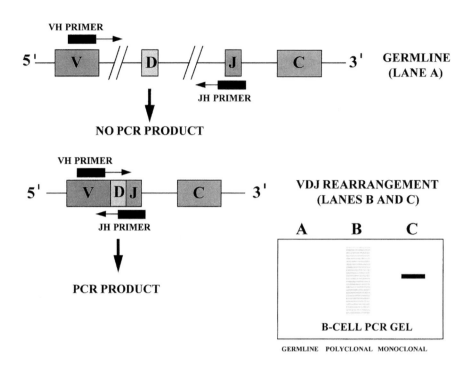

Fig. 10. Schematic diagram illustrating the polymerase chain reaction (PCR) approach for detecting B-cell gene rearrangements.

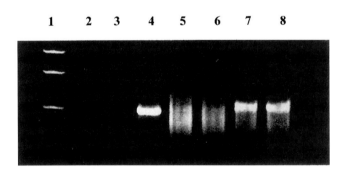

Fig. 11. Assessment of IgH gene rearrangement. Immunoglobulin heavy-chain gene rearrangement patterns shown in a PCR gel after ethidium-bromide staining. In the germline configuration, no PCR product is obtained (Lane 3). Polyclonal B-cell populations have a characteristic smear pattern (Lanes 5 and 6). Monoclonal B-cell populations are characterized by a single distinct band (Lanes 4, 7, and 8). Lane 1, molecular size marker; Lane 2, blank control.

of the V and J segments allows for the production of an amplified DNA product. Polyclonal B-cell or T-cell populations have large numbers of rearrangements that differ in size, resulting in a smear pattern (Fig. 10, Lane B and Fig. 11, Lanes 5 and 6). In contrast, monoclonal B-cell or T-cell cell populations contain identical rearrangements that result in the formation of a distinct band (Fig. 10, Lane C and Fig. 11, Lanes 4, 7, and 8).

Although the Southern-blot method is considered to be the gold standard for demonstrating clonality in lymphoid neoplasms, PCR offers distinct advantages *(26,44–46)*. Southern blotting is costly and labor-intensive, requiring 7–10 d to obtain a result; PCR can be performed at a lower cost in just 1–2 d. The Southern-blot method also requires a relatively large amount (at least 30 µg) of high-quality intact DNA, which in most cases can only be obtained from fresh or frozen tissue samples. In contrast, the amplification of DNA by PCR requires only short segments of DNA, allowing this type of analysis to be performed on small concentrations of DNA and on DNA that is of low quality or only partially intact (such as DNA extracted from paraffin-embedded tissues) *(47–49)*. Finally, although Southern blotting may detect a 1–5% clonal lymphoid population, PCR may detect as small as a 0.1% clonal lymphoid population *(28)*.

Despite the many advantages of PCR in evaluating for B-cell and T-cell clonality, the technique is associated with a higher percentage of false-negative results than Southern blotting *(44,45)*. This high false-negative rate likely occurs because of the inability of consensus V primers to recognize complementary DNA sequences in all of the V segments and because of the inability of V and J primers to recognize genetic alternations, such as partial rearrangements (DJ rearrangements), chromosomal translocations, and somatic mutations involving the antigen-receptor gene loci *(26,50)*.

CHROMOSOMAL TRANSLOCATIONS IN NON-HODGKIN'S LYMPHOMA

A number of specific, nonrandom chromosomal translocations have been described in association with different subtypes of non-Hodgkin's lymphoma. These translocations can be demonstrated by traditional cytogenetic methods as well as by molecular genetic methods, which include Southern blotting, PCR, and fluorescence *in situ* hybridization (FISH). Because the demonstration of cytogenetic abnormalities in lymphoid neoplasms with traditional cytogenetic methods is technically difficult, especially in low-grade neoplasms, which

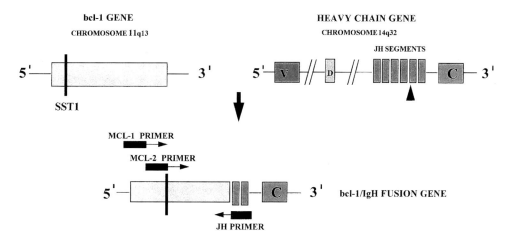

Fig. 12. Schematic diagram of the t(11;14) translocation involving the bcl1 and IgII chain genes.

are associated with a low mitotic rate, molecular approaches currently are the methods of choice. The majority of cases of non-Hodgkin's lymphoma can be accurately classified based primarily on morphological and immunopathological characteristics. However, in select cases the demonstration of a specific chromosomal translocation may help confirm a diagnosis. For example, the demonstration of a t(8;14) in a lymphoma, which is morphologically and immunopathologically suspicious for Burkitt's lymphoma (BL) would confirm this diagnosis *(15)*. More importantly, the ability to detect specific chromosomal translocations in lymphomas by highly sensitive methods such as PCR provides a means to potentially monitor patient therapy and to follow patients for evidence of minimal residual disease.

Chromosomal translocations in both leukemia and lymphoma often involve the transposition of a proto-oncogene from one chromosome to another. Proto-oncogenes are defined as normal cellular genes that are involved in the regulation of cellular processes such as growth and proliferation, and have the potential to contribute to neoplastic transformation when they are structurally or functionally altered, as occurs with a chromosomal translocation *(51)*. Proto-oncogenes can be categorized as promoters of cell growth and proliferation, tumor-suppressor genes that normally inhibit growth and proliferation, and genes that regulate programmed cell death or apoptosis *(51,52)*.

C-MYC AND BL

BL is a clinically aggressive non-Hodgkin's lymphoma characterized at the molecular level by a reciprocal translocation involving the c-*myc* proto-oncogene, which normally resides on chromosome 8 *(53–60)*. The t(8;14), t(2;8), or t(8;22) translocations result in the juxtaposition of c-myc from chromosome 8 to the heavy- or light-chain immunoglobulin loci on chromosomes 14, 2, or 22 with resultant deregulation of the c-*myc* gene. Endemic BL have been shown to carry the t(8;14) translocation, which includes a breakpoint upstream of the c-*myc* gene juxtaposing to one of the joining regions of IgH. Sporadic cases, meanwhile, possess breakpoints within the first exon or intron of the c-*myc* gene *(60)*. Constitutive expression

of c-*myc* subsequently results due to its newly formed association with the IgH enhancer. The basic helix-loop-helix (bHLH) c-myc structure functions as a transcription factor that regulates genes involved in the cell cycle *(59)*. The c-myc protein is a sequence specific transactivator that requires heterodimerization with Max before binding to a CAC(G/A)TG motif can occur *(61–63)*. It is now known that overexpression of c-*myc* can lead to increased transcription of several target genes through increased interactions with the rhabdoid tumor suppressor gene INI1 and the SWI/SNF multiprotein transcription complexes *(61)*.

BCL1 AND MANTLE-CELL LYMPHOMA

Mantle-cell lymphoma (MCL) is a distinct B-cell lymphoma that is associated with a moderately aggressive clinical course *(4)*. It is characterized morphologically by a proliferation of small to medium-sized lymphoid cells with slightly irregular nuclear contours in a diffuse or a nodular/mantle zone pattern *(5,64,65)*. In addition, MCL has been shown to manifest as a blastoid variant. MCL is characterized genetically by the translocation t(11;14)(q13;32) resulting in the juxtaposition of the proto-oncogene *bcl1* from chromosome 11 to the immunoglobulin heavy-chain gene on chromosome 14 *(64)* (Fig. 12). This results in the overexpression of the *cyclin D1* (also known as *PRAD-1* or *bcl1*) gene that is involved in the control of cell-cycle progression at the G_1/S checkpoint *(66–68)*. The identification of this translocation can aid in the precise characterization of cases as MCL because this entity is less favorable prognostically and tends to be less responsive to chemotherapy compared to other small B-cell lymphocytic disorders *(65,69,70)*.

The molecular identification of translocation t(11;14) can be achieved by PCR analysis in the majority of the 30–40% of MCL cases thought to contain this genetic alteration *(70,71)*. This is in part due to the clustering of breakpoints within the major translocation cluster (MTC) region of the *bcl1* gene *(72–74)* (Fig. 13). PCR analysis consists of using primers to a consensus IgH-joining sequence and to regions within the MTC (Fig. 13). Lack of a t(11;14) PCR-amplified product, when internal PCR controls for housekeeping genes demonstrate a

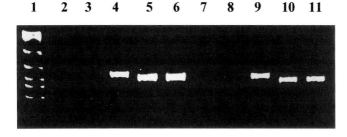

Fig. 13. Analysis of t(11;14) PCR products by gel electrophoresis. Lane 1, molecular size marker; lane 2, blank control; lane 3, negative control; lane 4, MCL-1 positive control; lanes 5 and 6, MCL-1 positive patient; lane 7, blank control; lane 8, MCL-2 negative control; lane 9, MCL-2 positive control; lanes 10 and 11, MCL-2 positive patient. Ethidium-bromide staining.

product, indicates the absence of this translocation. A single amplified PCR product that results from the primer sequences being in close proximity to one another indicates the presence of this translocation (Fig. 13).

BCL2 AND FOLLICULAR LYMPHOMA

Apoptosis or programmed cell death is part of normal homeostasis and is the body's way of maintaining a delicate balance between cell proliferation and cell death. The proto-oncogene *bcl2* normally resides on chromosome 18 and is involved in blocking apoptosis *(52)*. In healthy adults, expression of *bcl2* is limited to long-lived cells, which include some subsets of normal T and B lymphocytes. In follicular lymphoma, *bcl2* becomes overexpressed after being translocated from chromosome 18 to the heavy-chain locus on chromosome 14. The overexpression of *bcl2* is likely one step in the process of lymphomagenesis with elevated levels of *bcl2* extending the life-span of neoplastic cells *(51,52,75)*. The t(14;18) has been reported in up to 80–90% of cases of follicular lymphoma and less frequently in other types of hematopoietic and nonhematopoietic malignancies *(75)*. Figure 14 schematically shows the reciprocal translocation involving the *bcl2* locus on chromosome 18q21 and the IgH locus on chromosome 14q32. The *bcl-2* gene contains 3 exons including exon 1, which is a noncoding exon (upper panel, Fig. 14). The majority of chromosomal breaks occur in two regions referred to as the major breakpoint-cluster region (mbr) where 50–75% of the breaks occur, and the minor breakpoint cluster region (mcr) where 20–40% of the breaks occur *(52,75,76)*. The mbr is located in exon 3 and the mcr is located downstream in the 3' direction from exon 3. The breakpoints in the heavy-chain locus involve the J_H segments. The t(14;18) results in a *bcl2*/IgH fusion gene as depicted in the middle and lower panels of Fig. 14.

Detection of *bcl2*/IgH gene rearrangements can be performed by both Southern blotting and PCR. PCR is especially suited for analyzing for *bcl-2*/IgH rearrangements because the *bcl2* and JH breakpoints are located within a short segment of DNA *(76,77)*. Analysis by PCR is performed using two separate primer combinations to analyze for breaks at both the major and minor breakpoint cluster regions: a combination of mbr and J_H primers and a combination of mcr and J_H primers (Fig. 15). If a t(14;18) and hence a *bcl2*/IgH rearrangement has not

occurred, no PCR product will be obtained following amplification. Only when the primers are in close proximity to one another will a PCR-amplified product be detected.

BCL6 AND DIFFUSE LARGE-CELL LYMPHOMA

Reciprocal translocations in non-Hodgkin's lymphomas are traditionally associated with overexpression of a proto-oncogene with subsequent deregulated cell-cycle progression. The *bcl6* gene, located on chromosome 3q27, has been identified in the t(3;14) translocation found in diffuse large cell lymphoma *(78)* (Fig. 16). All of the breakpoints observed thus far are located within the first exon or intron of the *bcl6* gene *(79,80)*. Up to 40% of large-cell lymphoma cases have been shown to contain this translocation *(78,81)*. Both Southern blot and reverse-transcriptase (RT-) PCR have been utilized in the detection of this translocation *(81,82)*. It is thought that the bcl6 protein functions as a DNA-binding transcription factor, which is involved in differentiation and development *(82)*. Unlike other translocations, it appears that the *bcl6* status is an independent prognostic marker of survival and disease progression that is associated with a significant survival advantage *(78,82)*.

T(2;5) IN ANAPLASTIC LARGE-CELL LYMPHOMA

Anaplastic large-cell lymphoma (ALCL) is an aggressive but very treatable form of non-Hodgkin's lymphoma characterized in most cases morphologically by the presence of large anaplastic cells which express the CD30 (Ki-1) antigen. At the molecular level, ALCL is characterized by the translocation t(2;5)(p23;q35) *(83)*. This translocation results in the juxtapositioning of the nucleolar phosphoprotein (NPM) gene (5q35) to the anaplastic lymphoma kinase (ALK) gene (2p23) (Fig. 17) *(84)*. The t(2;5) translocation has been identified in up to 73% of ALCL cases *(85)*.

DETECTION OF MINIMAL RESIDUAL DISEASE

Minimal residual disease (MRD) refers to the presence of a residual clone of malignant T-cells in a patient that cannot be detected by standard pathological and radiological staging approaches and may eventually result in disease relapse *(86,87)*. For example, at presentation patients with acute leukemia have a tumor burden consisting of 10^{12} leukemic cells, which is readily detectable by microscopic examination of the bone marrow. Following induction chemotherapy, the tumor burden is reduced by several orders of magnitude resulting in clinical remission (defined as less than 5% bone marrow blasts). However, an undetectable residual tumor burden of 10^8 or 10^9 leukemic cells may still remain *(14)*. Traditional morphological assessment of the bone marrow cannot distinguish a patient with MRD of 10^9 leukemic cells from a patient with no leukemic cells.

The presence of MRD in patients with leukemia and lymphoma has been assessed by a variety of approaches including traditional morphology, immunophenotypic analysis by flow cytometry, cell-culture methods, conventional cytogenetics, and by molecular methods that include FISH, Southern blotting, and PCR *(14)*. Each of these methods has advantages and disadvantages. With the exception of PCR, the approaches listed lack sensitivity and are capable of detecting approx a 1%

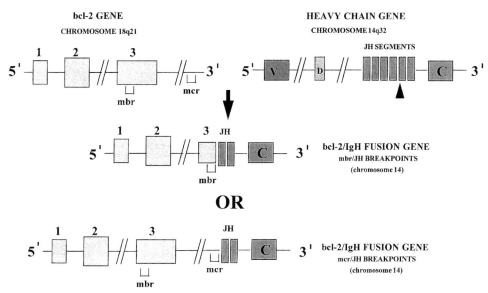

Fig. 14. Chromosomal translocations involving *bcl2*. Schematic diagram showing the translocation of *bcl2* from chromosome 18 (shaded boxes) to the heavy chain gene (IgH) on chromosome 14 (open boxes) resulting in a *bcl2*/IgH fusion gene. For *bcl2*, most breaks occur in either the major breakpoint cluster (mbr) or minor breakpoint cluster (mcr) regions. Breakpoints in the heavy-chain gene involve JH segments (arrowhead). The translocation may involve mbr and JH breakpoints (middle panel) or mcr and JH breakpoints (lower panel).

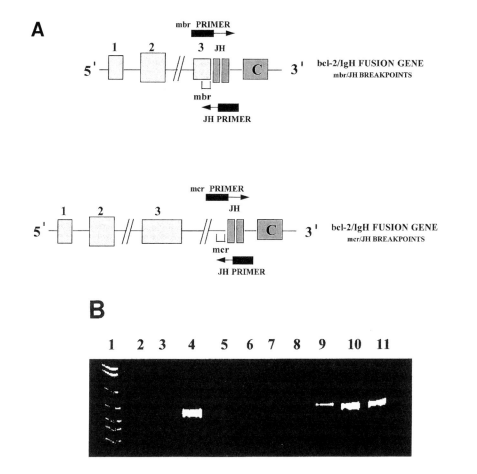

Fig. 15. PCR analysis of chromosomal translocations involving *bcl2*. **(A)** Analysis for *bcl2*/IgH gene rearrangements by PCR involves two separate primer combinations: mbr and JH primers (upper panel) and mcr and JH primers (lower panel). **(B)** Analysis of t(14;18) PCR products by gel electrophoresis and staining with ethidium bromide. Lane 1, molecular-size marker; lane 2, blank control; lane 3, negative control; lane 4, mcr positive control; lanes 5 and 6, mcr negative patient; lane 7, blank control; lane 8, mbr negative control; lane 9, mbr positive control; lanes 10 and 11, mbr positive patient.

t(3:14)(q27;q32)

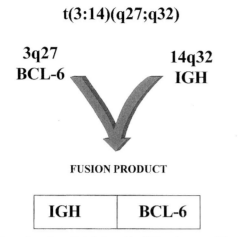

Fig. 16. Translocation t(3;14) found in diffuse large-cell lymphoma.

t(2:5)(p23;q35)

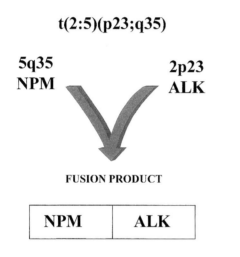

Fig. 17. Translocation t(2;5)(p23;q35) found in anaplastic large-cell lymphoma.

malignant-cell population. In contrast, PCR is significantly more sensitive and has the capability of detecting one malignant cell among 10^5–10^6 normal cells *(86–89)*. In order to evaluate for the presence of MRD by PCR, the malignant cell must have a unique set of DNA sequences that allow for distinction from normal cells. Evaluation for the presence of chromosomal translocations such as t(14;18) (q32;q21) in follicular, non-Hodgkin's lymphoma are ideal for detecting MRD *(88)*. An alternative approach in B-cell and T-cell malignancies involves detection of immunoglobulin and T-cell receptor-gene rearrangements. A variety of PCR-based strategies have been devised based on the premise that each clone of malignant B-cells or T-cells has a unique VDJ rearrangement that can be used as a molecular marker to probe for the presence of MRD *(14)*.

The ability to detect MRD more precisely would be expected to improve clinical management by optimizing therapy *(14,83,84)*. In some diseases, the presence of significant MRD may be a predictor of disease relapse, requiring more aggressive therapeutic approaches such as bone marrow transplantation. In contrast, patients with little or no residual MRD may require less intensive therapy, thus reducing patient exposure to potentially toxic drugs.

CONCLUSION

Molecular genetic techniques are powerful tools that have greatly enhanced our ability to precisely diagnose and classify hematological diseases. In lymphoid neoplasms, the ability to prove or disprove the presence of B-cell or T-cell clonality by either immunopathological or molecular genetic approaches is often central to establishing a correct diagnosis. In both myeloid and lymphoid neoplasms, the identification of a specific chromosomal abnormality may be useful in confirming a diagnosis in cases that are otherwise inconclusive. This same chromosomal abnormality may subsequently be used as a marker to evaluate patients for response to therapy and for evidence of minimal residual disease. As our understanding of the basic molecular alterations involved in the pathogenesis of hematological diseases continues, it is likely that future therapies for hematological diseases will become more refined.

REFERENCES

1. Landis, S. H., Murray, T., Bolden, S., and Wingo, P. A. (1999) Cancer statistics, 1999. *CA Cancer J. Clin.* **49**:8–31.
2. Bertoli, L. F. and Burrows, P. D. (1988) Normal B-lineage cells: Their differentiation and identification. *Clin. Lab. Med.* **8**:15–30.
3. Denning, S. M. and Haynes, B. F. (1988) Differentiation of human T cells. *Clinics Lab. Med.* **8**:1–14.
4. Harris, N. L., Jaffe, E. S., Stein, H., Banks, P. M., Chan, J. K. C., Cleary, M. L., et al. (1994) A revised European-American classification of lymphoid neoplasms: a proposal from the International Lymphoma Study Group. *Blood* **84**:1361–1392.
5. Chan, J. K. C., Banks, P. M., Cleary, M. L., Delsol, G., De Wolf-Peeters, C., Falini, B., et al. (1995) A revised European-American classification of lymphoid neoplasms proposed by the International Lymphoma Study Group. *Am. J. Clin. Pathol.* **103**:543–560.
6. Jaffe, E. S. (1990) The role of immunophenotypic markers in the classification of non-Hodgkin's lymphomas. *Semin. Oncol.* **17**:11–19.
7. Rezuke, W. N., Abernathy, E. C., and Tsongalis, G. J. (1997) Molecular diagnosis of B and T cell lymphomas: fundamental principles and clinical applications. *Clin. Chem* **43**:1814–1823.
8. Cossman, J., Uppenkamp, M., Sundeen, J., Coupland, R., and Raffeld, M. (1988) Molecular genetics and the diagnosis of lymphoma. *Arch. Pathol. Lab. Med.* **112**:117–127.
9. Griesser, H., Feller, A., Lennert, K., Minden, M., and Mak, T. W. (1986) Rearrangement of the β chain of the T cell antigen receptor and immunoglobulin genes in lymphoproliferative disorders. *J. Clin. Invest.* **78**:1179–1184.
10. Cossman, J. and Uppenkamp, M. (1988) T cell gene rearrangements and the diagnosis of T cell neoplasms. *Clinics. Lab. Med.* **8**:31–44.
11. Pugh, W. C. and Stass, S. A. (1988) Immunoglobulin gene rearrangements and its implications for the study of B-cell neoplasia. *Clinics Lab. Med.* **8**:45–64.
12. Aisenberg, A. (1993) Utility of gene rearrangements in lymphoid malignancies. *Ann. Rev. Med.* **44**:75–84.
13. Gill, J. I. and Gulley, M. L. (1994) Immunoglobulin and T cell receptor gene rearrangement. *Hematol. Oncol. Clin. North Am.* **8**:751–767.
14. Campana, D. and Pui, C-H. (1995) Detection of minimal residual disease in acute leukemia: Methodologic advances and clinical significance. *Blood* **85**:1416–1434.
15. Medeiros, L. J., Bagg, A., and Cossman, J. (1992) Application of molecular genetics to the diagnosis of hematopoietic neoplasms. *In*: *Neoplastic Hematopathology* (Knowles, D. M., ed.), Williams and Wilkins, Baltimore, MD, pp. 263–298.

16. Cooper, M. D. (1987) B lymphocytes: Normal development and function. *N. Engl. J. Med.* **317**:1452–1456.

17. Sklar, J. (1992) Antigen receptor genes: Structure, function, and techniques for analysis of their rearrangements. *In: Neoplastic Hematopathology* (Knowles, D.M., ed.), Williams and Wilkins, Baltimore, MD, pp. 215–244.

18. Foon, K. A. and Todd, R. F. (1986) Immunologic classification of leukemia and lymphoma. *Blood* **68**:1–31.

19. Spits, H., Lanier, L. L., and Phillips, J. H. (1995) Development of human T and natural killer cells. *Blood* **85**:2654–2670.

20. Royer, H. D. and Reinherz, E. L. (1987) T lymphocytes: Ontogeny, function, and relevance to clinical disorders. *N. Engl. J. Med.* **317**:1136–1142.

21. Gill, J. I. and Gulley, M. L. (1994) Immunoglobulin and T cell receptor gene rearrangement. *Hematol. Oncol. Clin. North Am.* **8**:751–770.

22. Cossman, J., Zehnbauer, B., Garrett, C. T., Smith, L. J., Williams, M., Jaffe, E. S., et al. (1991) Gene rearrangements in the diagnosis of lymphoma/leukemia. Guidelines for use based on a multi-institutional study. *Am. J. Clin. Pathol.* **95**:347–354.

23. Farkas, D. H. (1992) The Southern blot: application to the B and T cell gene rearrangement test. *Lab. Med.* **23**:723–729.

24. Beishuizen, A., Verhoeven, M. J., Mol, E. J., and van Dongen, J. J. M. (1994) Detection of immunoglobulin kappa light chain gene rearrangement patterns by Southern blot analysis. *Leukemia* **8**:2228–2236.

25. Hodges, K. A., Kosciol, C. M., Rezuke, W. N., Abernathy, E. C., Pastuszak, W. T., and Tsongalis, G. T. (1996) Chemiluminescent detection of gene rearrangements in hematologic malignancy. *Ann. Clin. Lab. Sci.* **26**:114–118.

26. Medeiros, L. J. and Weiss, L. M. (1994) The utility of the polymerase chain reaction as a screening method for the detection of antigen receptor gene rearrangements. *Human Pathol.* **25**:1261–1263.

27. Macintyre, E. A. (1989) The use of the polymerase chain reaction in hematology. *Blood Rev.* **3**:201–210.

28. Weiss, L. M. and Spagnolo, D. V. (1993) Assessment of clonality in lymphoid proliferations. *Am. J. Pathol.* **142**:1679–1682.

29. McCarthy, K. P., Sloane, J. P., Kabarowski, J. H. S., Matutes, E., and Wiedemann, L. M. (1991) The rapid detection of clonal T-cell proliferations in patients with lymphoid disorders. *Am. J. Pathol.* **138**:821–828.

30. Ben-Ezra, J. (1992) Variable rate of detection of immunoglobulin heavy chain V-D-J rearrangement by PCR: A systematic study of 41 B-cell non-Hodgkin's lymphomas and leukemias. *Leukemia Lymphoma* **7**:289–295.

31. Diss, T. C., Peng, H., Wotherspoon, A. C., Isaacson, P. G., and Pan, L. (1993) Detection of monoclonality in low-grade B-cell lymphomas using the polymerase chain reaction is dependent on primer selction and lymphoma type. *J. Pathol.* **169**:291–295.

32. Segal, G. H., Jorgensen, T., Masih, A. S., and Braylan, R. C. (1994) Optimal primer selection for clonality assessment by polymerase chain reaction analysis. Low grade B-cell lymphoproliferative disorders of nonfollicular center cell type. *Human Pathol.* **25**:1269–1275.

33. Slack, I. N., McCarthy, K. P., Wiedemann, L. M., and Sloane, J. P. (1993) Evaluation of sensitivity, specificity, and reproducibility of an optimized method for detecting clonal rearrangements of immunoglobulin and T-cell receptor genes in formalin-fixed, paraffin-embedded sections. *Diagnostic Mol. Pathol.* **2**:223–232.

34. Algara, P., Caridad, S., Martinez, P., Sanchez, L., Villuendas, R., Garcia, P., et al. (1994) Value of PCR detection of TCRγ gene rearrangments in the diagnosis of cutaneous lymphocytic infiltrates. *Diagnostic Mol. Pathol.* **3**:275–282.

35. Achille, A., Scarpa, A., Montresor, M., Scardoni, M., Zamboni, G., Chilosi, M., et al. (1995) Routine application of polymerase chain reaction in the diagnosis of monoclonality of B-cell lymphoid proliferations. *Diagnostic Mol. Pathol.* **4**:14–24.

36. Fodinger, M., Buchmayer, H., Schwarzinger, I., Simonitsch, I., Winkler, K, Jager, U., et al. (1996) Multiplex PCR for rapid detec-

tion of T-cell receptor gamma chain gene rearrangements in patients with lymphoproliferative diseases. *Br. J. Haematol.* **94**:136–139.

37. Lozano, M. D., Tierens, A., Greiner, T. C., Wickert, R. S., Weisenburger, D. D., and Chan, W. C. (1996) Clonality analysis of B-lymphoid proliferations using the polymerase chain reaction. *Cancer* **77**:1349–1355.

38. Abdel-Reheim, F. A., Edwards, E., and Arber, D. A. (1996) Utility of a rapid polymerase chain reaction panel for the detection of molecular changes in B-cell lymphoma. *Arch. Pathol. Lab. Med.* **120**:357–363.

39. Lombardo, J. F., Hwang, T. S., Maiese, R. L., Millson, A., and Segal, G. H. (1996) Optimal primer selection for clonality assessment by polymerase chain reaction analysis: Intermediate and high grade B-cell neoplasms. *Human Pathol.* **27**:373–380.

40. Diaz-Cano, S. (1996) PCR-based alternative for diagnosis of immunoglobulin heavy chain gene rearrangement. *Diagnostic Mol. Pathol.* **5**:3–9.

41. Ritter, J. H., Wick, M. R., Adesokan, P. N., Fitzgibbon, J.F ., Zhu, X., and Humphrey, P. A. (1997) Assessment of clonality in cutaneous lymphoid infiltrates by polymerase chain reaction analysis of immunoglobulin heavy chain gene rearrangements. *Am. J. Clin. Pathol.* **108**:60–68.

42. Ashton-Key, M., Diss, T. C., Du, M. Q., Kirkham, N., Wotherspoon, A., and Isaacson, P. G. (1997) The value of the polymerase chain reaction in the diagnosis of cutaneous T-cell infiltrates. *Am. J. Surg. Pathol.* **21**:743–747.

43. Tsongalis, G. J. Stevenson, A. J., Hodges, K. A., and Rezuke, W. N. (1998) Clonal analysis of B-cell lymphoproliferative disorders. *Eur. J. Lab. Med.* **3**:142–145.

44. Sioutos, N., Bagg, A., Michaud, G. Y., Irving, S. G., Hartmann, D. P., Siragy, H., et al. (1995) Polymerase chain reaction versus Southern blot hybridization. Detection of immunoglobulin heavy-chain gene rearrangements. *Diagnostic Mol. Pathol.* **4**:8–13.

45. Lehman, C. M., Sarago, C., Nasim, S., Comerford, J., Karcher, D. S., and Garrett, C. T. (1995) Comparison of PCR with Southern hybridization for the routine detection of immunoglobulin heavy chain gene rearrangements. *Am. J. Clin. Pathol.* **103**:171–176.

46. Tbakhi, A. and Tubbs, R. R. (1996) Utility of the polymerase chain reaction in detecting B cell clonality in lymphoid neoplasms. *Cancer* **77**:1223–1225.

47. Kuppers, R., Zhao, M., Rajewsky, K., and Hansmann, M. L. (1993) Detection of clonal B cell populations in paraffin-embedded tissues by polymerase chain reaction. *Am. J. Pathol.* **143**:230–239.

48. Inghirami, G., Szabolcs, M. J., Yee, H. T., Corradini, P., Cesarman, E., and Knowles, D. M. (1993) Detection of immunoglobulin gene rearrangement of B cell nonHodgkin's lymphomas and leukemias in fresh, unfixed and formalin fixed, paraffin-embedded tissue by polymerase chain reaction. *Lab. Invest.* **68**:746–757.

49. Reed, T. J., Reid, A., Wallberg, K., O'Leary, T. J., and Frizzera, G. (1993) Determination of B cell clonality in paraffin-embedded lymph nodes using the polymerase chain reaction. *Diagnostic Mol. Pathol.* **2**:42–49.

50. Segal, G. H., Jorgensen, T., Scott, M., and Braylan, R. C. (1994) Optimal primer selection for clonality assessement by polymerase chain reaction analysis: II. Follicular lymphomas. *Human Pathol.* **25**:1276–1282.

51. Gaidano, G. and Dalla-Favera, R. (1992) Protooncogenes and tumor suppressor genes. *In: Neoplastic Hematopathology* (Knowles, D.M., ed.), Williams and Wilkins, Baltimore, MD, pp. 245–261.

52. Korsmeyer, S. J. (1992) Bcl-2 initiates a new category of oncogenes: regulators of cell death. *Blood* **80**:879–886.

53. Cory, S. (1986) Activation of cellular oncogenes in hemopoietic cells by chromosome translocation. *Adv. Cancer Res.* **47**:189–234.

54. Adams, J. M., Gerondakis, S., Webb, E., Mitchell, J., Bernard, O., and Cory, S. (1982) Transcriptionally active DNA region that rearranges frequently in murine lymphoid tumors. *Proc. Natl. Acad. Sci. USA* **79**:6966–6970.

55. Adams, J. M., Gerondakis, S., Webb, E., Corcoran, L. M., and Cory S. (1983) Cellular myc oncogene is altered by chromosome trans-

location to an immunoglobulin locus in murine plasmacytomas and is rearranged similarly in human Burkitt lymphomas. *Proc. Natl. Acad. Sci. USA* **80**:1982–1986.

56. Taub, R., Kirsch, I., Morton, C., Lenoir, G., Swan, D., Tronick, S. Aaronson, S., and Leder, P. (1982) Translocation of the c-myc gene into the immunoglobulin heavy chain locus in human Burkitt and murine plasmacytoma cells. *Proc. Natl. Acad. Sci. USA* **79**:7837–7841.

57. Dalla-Favera, R., Martinotti, S., Gallo, R. C., Erikson, J., and Croce, C. M. (1983) Translocation and rearrangements of the c-myc oncogene locus in human undifferentiated B cell lymphomas. *Science* **219**:963–967.

58. Bernard, O. Cory, S., Gerondakis, S., Webb, E., and Adams, J. M. (1983) Sequence of the murine and human cellular myc oncogenes and two modes of myc transcription resulting from chromosome translocation in B lymphoid tumors. *EMBO J.* **2**:2375–2383.

59. Cory, S., Vaux, D. L., Strasser, A., Harris, A. W., and Adams, J. M. (1999) Insights from Bcl-2 and myc: Malignancy involves abrogation of apoptosis as well as sustained proliferation. *Cancer Res.* **59**:1685s–1692s.

60. Yano, T., Sander, C. A., Clark, H. M., Dolezal, M. V., Jaffe, E. S., and Raffeld, M. (1993) Clustered mutations in the second exon of the myc gene in sporadic Burkitt's lymphoma. *Oncogene* **8**:2741–2748.

61. Cheng, S. W. G., Davies, K. P., Yung, E., Beltran, R. J., Yu, J., and Kalpana, G. V. (1999) C-myc interacts with INI1/hSNF5 and requires the SWI/SNF complex for transactivation function. *Nature Genet.* **22**:102–105.

62. Facchini, L. M. and Penn, I. Z. (1998) The molecular role of myc in growth and transformation: recent discoveries lead to new insights. *FASEB J.* **12**:633–651.

63. Henriksson, M. and Luscher, B. (1996) Proteins of the myc network: essential regulators of cell growth and differentiation. *Adv. Cancer Res.* **68**:109–182.

64. Williams, M. E., Westermann, C. D., and Swerdlow, S. H. (1990) Genotypic characterization of centrocytic lymphoma:frequent rearrangement of the chromosome 11 bcl-1 locus. *Blood* **76**:1387–1391.

65. Fiel-Gan, M. D., Almeida, L., Rose, D. C., Takano, A., Rezuke, W. N., Coleman, W. B., et al. (1999) Proliferative fraction, bcl-1 gene translocation, and p53 mutation status as markers in mantle cell lymphoma. *Int. J. Mol. Med.* **3**:373–379.

66. Rosenberg, C. L., Wong, E., Petty, E. M., Bale, A. E., Tsujimoto, Y., Harris, N. L., et al. (1991) PRAD-1, a candidate bcl-1 oncogene: mapping and expression in centrocytic lymphoma. *Proc. Natl. Acad. Sci. USA* **88**:9638–9642.

67. Seto, M., Yamamoto, K., Iida, S., Akao, Y., Utsumi, K. R., Kubonishi, I., et al. (1992) Gene rearrangement and overexpression of PRAD-1 in lymphoid malignancy with t(11;14)(q13;q32) translocation. *Oncogene* **7**:1401–1406.

68. Motokura, T., Bloom, T., Kim, H. G., Juppner, H., Runderman, J. V., Kronenberg, H. M, et al. (1991) A novel cyclin encoded by bcl-1 linked candidate oncogene. *Nature* **350**:512–515.

69. Argatoff, L. H., Connors, J. M., Klasa, R. J., Horsman, D. E., and Gascoyne, R. D. (1997) Mantle cell lymphoma: A clinicopathologic study of 80 cases. *Blood* **89**:2067–2078.

70. Chibbar, R., Leung, K., McCormick, S., Ritzkalla, K., Strickler, J., Staggs, R., et al. (1998) bcl-1 gene rearrangements in mantle cell lymphoma: A comprehensive analysis of 118 cases, including B-5 fixed tissue, by polymerase chain reaction and Southern transfer analysis. *Mod. Pathol.* **11**:1089–1097.

71. Molot, R. J., Meeker, T. C., Wittwer, C. T., Perkins, S. L., Segal, G. H., Masih, A. S., et al. (1994) Antigen expression and polymerase chain reaction amplification of mantle cell lymphomas. *Blood* **83**:1626–1631.

72. Williams, M. E., Swerdlow, S. H., Rosenberg, C. L., and Arnold, A. (1992) Characterization of chromosome 11 translocation breakpoints at the bcl-1 and PRAD1 loci in centrocytic lymphoma. *Cancer Res.* **52**:5541s–5544s.

73. Williams, M. E., Meeker, T. C., and Swerdlow, S. H. (1991) Rearrangement of the chromosome 11 bcl-1 locus in centrocytic lymphoma: analysis with multiple breakpoint probes. *Blood* **78**:493–498.

74. Williams, M. E., Swerdlow, S. H., and Meeker, T. C. (1993) Chromosome t(11;14)(q13;q32) breakpoints in centrocytic lymphoma are highly localized at the bcl-1 major translocation cluster. *Leukemia* **7**:1437–1440.

75. Crisan, D., Chen, S-T., and Weil, S. C. (1994) Polymerase chain reaction in the diagnosis of chromosomal breakpoints. *Hematol. Oncol. Clin. North Am.* **8**:725–750.

76. Banks, P. M., Chan, J., Cleary, M. L., Delsol, G., De Wolf-Peeters, C., and Gatter, K. (1992) Mantle cell lymphoma. A proposal for unification of morphologic, immunologic, and molecular data. *Am. J. Surg. Pathol.* **16**:637–640.

77. Ngan, B-Y., Nourse, J., and Cleary, M. L. (1989) Detection of chromosomal translocation t(14;18) within the minor cluster region of *bcl-2* by polymerase chain reaction and direct genomic sequencing of the enzymatically amplified DNA in follicular lymphomas. *Blood* **73**:1759–1762.

78. Baron, B. W., Stanger, R. R., Hume, E., Sadhu, A., Mick, R., Kerckaert, J. P., et al. (1995) Bcl6 encodes a sequence specific DNA binding protein. *Genes Chromosomes Cancer* **13**:221–224.

79. Kerckaert, J. P., Deweindt, C., Tilly, H., Quief, S., Lecocq, G., and Bastard, C. (1993) LAZ3, a novel zinc-finger encoding gene, is disrupted by recurring chromosome 3q27 translocations in human lymphomas. *Nature Genet.* **5**:66–70.

80. Ye, B. H., Rao, P. H., Chaganti, R. S. K., and Dalla-Favera, R. (1993) Cloning of bcl-6, the locus involved in chromosome translocations affecting band 3q27 in B cell lymphoma. *Cancer Res.* **53**:2732–2735.

81. Kawamata, N., Nakamura, Y., Miki, T., Sato, E., Isobe, Y., Furusawa, S., et al. (1998) Detection of chimaeric transcripts of the immunoglobulin heavy chain and bcl6 genes by reverse transcriptase polymerase chain reaction in B cell non-Hodgkin's lymphomas. *Br. J. Haematol.* **100**:484–489.

82. Muramatsu, M., Akasaka, T., Kadowaki, N., Ohno, H., Yamabe, H., Edamura, S., et al. (1996) Rearrangement of the bcl6 gene in B cell lymphoid neoplasms: comparison with lymphomas associated with bcl2 rearrangement. *Br. J. Haematol.* **93**:911–920.

83. Mason, D. Y., Bastard, C., Romokh, R., Dastugue, N., Huret, J. L., Kristoffersson, U., et al. (1990) CD30-positive large cell lymphomas ("Ki-1 lymphoma") are associated with a chromosomal translocation involving 5q35. *Br. J. Haematol.* **74**:161–168.

84. Morris, S. W., Kirstein, M. N., Valentine, M. B., Dittmer, K. G., Shapiro, D. N., Saltman, D. L., et al. (1994) Fusion of a kinase gene, ALK, to a nucleolar protein gene, NPM, in non-Hodgkin's lymphoma. *Science* **263**:1281–1284.

85. Lamant, L., Meggetto, F., Al Saati T., Brugieres, L., de Paillerets, B. B., Dastugue, N., et al. (1996) High incidence of the t(2;5)(q35) translocation in anaplastic large cell lymphoma and its lack of detection in Hodgkin's disease. Comparison of cytogenetic analysis, reverse transcriptase polymerase chain reaction, and P-80 immunostaining. *Blood* **87**:284–291.

86. Negrin, R. S. and Blume, K. G. (1991) The use of the polymerase chain reaction for the detection of minimal residual malignant disease. *Blood* **78**:255–258.

87. Sklar, J. (1991) Polymerase chain reaction: The molecular microscope of residual disease. *J. Clin. Oncol.* **9**:1521–1524.

88. Corradini, P., Astolfi, M., Cherasco, C., Ladetto, M., Voena, C., Caracciolo, D., et al. (1997) Molecular monitoring of minimal residual disease in follicular and mantle cell non-Hodgkin's lymphomas treated with high-dose chemotherapy and peripheral blood progenitor cell autografting. *Blood* **89**:724–731.

89. Wu, G. Q., Sharp, J. G., Wu, G., Vose, J., Greiner, T. C., and Chan, W. C. (1997) The detection of minimal lymphoma by molecular and combined culture-molecular methods. *Br. J. Haematol.* **99**:873–881.

FUTURE DIRECTIONS VII

21 Cancer Genetic Counseling

Katherine Schneider, MPH, Kristen Shannon, MS, Anu Chittenden, MS, Elaine Hiller, MS, MD and Stephanie Kieffer, MS

INTRODUCTION

Our fundamental understanding of carcinogenesis has expanded dramatically over the past five years. Of foremost importance has been the discovery of genes that, when mutated in the germline, confer high risks of specific malignancies. The translation of these laboratory findings into clinical practice has led to the creation of a new medical subspecialty termed cancer genetic counseling. Cancer genetic counseling is defined as a communication process concerning an individual's risk of developing specific inherited forms of cancer. This risk may be higher than or similar to the general population risks of cancer. Cancer genetic counseling can, but does not always, lead to genetic testing. The genetic counseling process involves: 1) obtaining detailed family, medical, and lifestyle histories; 2) documentation of cancer-related diagnoses; 3) pedigree analysis; 4) risk assessment and counseling; 5) general discussion of options for early detection and prevention; and 6) provision of genetic testing when appropriate. This chapter provides an overview of cancer genetic counseling, including a general description of the providers and patients involved, the cancer genetic-counseling process in a high-risk clinical setting and a predisposition-testing program, the provision of genetic counseling for selected hereditary-cancer syndromes, and case examples to highlight some of the complexities inherent to this process.

THE PROVIDERS AND THE PATIENTS

CANCER GENETIC COUNSELING PROVIDERS

Cancer genetic counselors are typically Masters-level health care professionals who have training and expertise in genetic risk assessment and counseling. Cancer genetic counselors can elicit extensive family cancer histories and assess the likelihood of an inherited gene mutation contributing to cancer development, while providing emotional support to patients and

From: *The Molecular Basis of Human Cancer* (W. B. Coleman and G. J. Tsongalis, eds.), © Humana Press Inc., Totowa, NJ.

their families. They are familiar with cancer genetics principles and can accurately interpret DNA results. Cancer genetic counselors are also able to discuss the medical and emotional implications of testing and deal effectively with family issues as they arise.

Utilizing a multidisciplinary team of providers is the most effective way to care for patients at increased risk for cancer, either in a high-risk cancer clinic setting or a predisposition-testing program *(1)*. Providers may include: a genetic counselor, oncologist, geneticist, gynecologist, surgeon, pathologist, radiologist, nurse, social worker, psychologist, and/or nutritionist. Each member of the team contributes his/her own expertise to the proper assessment and medical management of the patient and this input from providers in different disciplines is extremely valuable. Although it is optimal for the multidisciplinary team to be housed in the same clinic, the establishment of a provider network can work just as effectively.

CANCER GENETIC COUNSELING PATIENTS Patients presenting for cancer genetic counseling or predisposition testing have either had cancer themselves or have close relatives who have developed cancer. According to the American Cancer Society (ACS), about one in every three Americans will be diagnosed with cancer in their lifetime, with the current number of cancer survivors in the United States exceeding 8 million people *(2)*. It is estimated that about 10–15% of cancer cases are due to a dominantly inherited gene mutation *(3)*. As shown in Table 1, appropriate candidates for cancer genetic counseling are patients who have significant family histories of cancer, specifically taking into account the number of affected relatives, types of cancer in the family, and ages at diagnosis *(4)*. A clear example is a woman with two sisters who were both diagnosed with breast cancer in their thirties. This woman and her sisters are appropriate candidates for cancer genetic counseling. Conversely, a woman whose only family history of cancer is a mother who developed breast cancer at age 75 would not be considered high risk and does not need a referral to a high-risk clinic. Some patients, however, may find it beneficial

Table 1
Appropriate Candidates for Cancer Genetic Counseling

- Individual with a personal or family history of a known hereditary cancer syndrome such as familial adenomatous polyposis, neurofibromatosis, or retinoblastoma
- Individual with several relatives with the same or related cancer diagnoses
- Individual with a family history of cancer present in two or more generations
- Individual with a personal or family history of cancers occurring at unusually young ages
- Individual with a personal or family history of rare or less-commonly diagnosed cancers (e.g., male breast cancer)
- Individual with a personal history of multiple primary tumors or bilateral disease
- Individual of Eastern European Jewish ancestry with a personal or family history of breast, ovarian, or colorectal cancer

to meet with a cancer genetic counselor to alleviate their fears that they are at high risk for developing a specific malignancy.

The level of interest and understanding of the genetic counseling process varies substantially among patients. Some patients have requested a referral to a high-risk clinic or are self-referred, whereas others have been referred by their physicians. The physician referrals may follow a routine visit or accompany the decision-making process regarding prophylactic surgery or appropriate screening for cancer. Although patients are sometimes referred within days after being diagnosed with cancer, this is not an optimal time for these discussions. Patients may be motivated to come to a high-risk clinic because of a recent cancer diagnosis in the family, concerns about their children's risks of developing cancer, or interest in learning about cancer prevention or early detection. Patients will often be accompanied by their affected relative or other at-risk relatives. Although this may provide extra support for the patient, it can also complicate the counseling aspects of the encounter, because motivations and concerns can differ among various family members.

GENETIC COUNSELING IN A HIGH-RISK CLINIC

The genetic counseling process actually begins with the telephone intake prior to the patient's appointment in the clinic. Some programs have a clinic coordinator who will initially sketch out the patient's family history and may request additional information or documentation prior to the visit. This family history is meant to quickly assess clinic eligibility, and thus, need not be a comprehensive pedigree. As an alternative approach, some clinics ask that patients complete a family-history questionnaire and mail it back to the clinic prior to the scheduled appointment. Obtaining family history information beforehand gives the clinic coordinator the opportunity to assess eligibility (pre-determined by the clinic) and allows the high-risk clinic visit to focus more on the interpretation of the pedigree.

The cancer genetic counseling session typically consists of the following components: 1) contracting and assessing motivation; 2) collecting and discussing family history; 3) assessing risks and medical management strategies; 4) teaching basic genetic concepts; and 5) discussing genetic testing options.

CONTRACTING AND ASSESSING MOTIVATION The initial part of the session, known as contracting, sets the parameters of the patient's clinic visit. This includes outlining the visit from the specifics of the genetic counseling session to the general flow of the clinic. The role of each clinic provider is described, so that the patient knows what to expect from each encounter. Patients should also be informed about the clinic's confidentiality practices (how much information will be placed in the medical record) as well as plans for follow-up (will the patient or referring physician be sent a letter summarizing the visit). Many programs separate the initial genetic counseling visit from subsequent testing visits, which patients need to know from the outset. It is also important that patients be told about the eligibility criteria, if any, for acceptance in the testing program and the costs of the counseling and laboratory analysis, which are not uniformly covered by insurance companies. The patient, in turn, is given a chance to express his/her motivation for the visit and state the questions he/she hopes will be answered by the conclusion of the clinic visit. This allows the providers to tailor the visit to best suit the patient's needs. The genetic counselor addresses these needs and questions within the limits of his/her training and refers to other clinic providers outside of those limits. This introductory part of the genetic-counseling session can be the most important as it builds trust and begins a rapport between patient and counselor (5).

COLLECTING AND DISCUSSING CANCER HISTORY The first and most important step in assessing a patient's hereditary cancer risk is the taking of a careful and detailed family history. Some aspects of collecting and analyzing pedigree information in the cancer setting differ from other genetic counseling endeavors. The goal of gathering a cancer history is to be able to assess whether or not the patient has increased lifetime risks of specific inherited forms of malignancy and, when possible, to generate a quantitative estimate of these risks. Meeting this goal involves confirming the verbal information given by the patient, with documentation.

General Suggestions A pedigree taken for cancer risk assessment should span at least three generations (1). At minimum, the pedigree should include all first- and second-degree relatives of the patient and selected third-degree relatives (6). One useful rule of thumb is to gather information about all first-degree relatives for each person with cancer. Pedigrees may need to be expanded for cancer syndromes that pose higher cancer risk for only one gender (breast-ovarian cancer syndrome, familial prostate cancer syndrome). Patients tend to report only the cancers that they believe are relevant, so it is important to ask questions about specific cancerous and pre-cancerous tumors. By far, the major limitation of taking a complete family history is the patient's knowledge of more distant relatives. Always obtain information about both sides of the family, even when there is a strong suspicion about which side of the family has an inherited predisposition to cancer.

Specific Information to Obtain Table 2 lists sample questions for affected and unaffected members of a family (7). For each affected member of the family, as much detail as possible should be obtained regarding the cancer diagnosis. This information includes the exact location of the tumor, the stage at

Table 2
Sample Questions for Affected and Unaffected Relatives[a]

Affected Relatives	*Unaffected Relatives*
Diagnosis	**Ages and dates**
What type of cancer was diagnosed?	Is your relative living or deceased?
Do you know the exact diagnosis? (i.e., pathologic diagnosis)	If living, what is your relative's current age?
Where was your relative diagnosed and/or treated?	If deceased, what year and at what age did your relative die?
Did the relative develop any other types of cancer?	If deceased, what was his/her cause of death?
If the relative has a second cancer, do you know if the second cancer spread from the original tumor?	
Ages and dates (approx)	**Cancer screening**
How old was your relative at diagnosis?	Did your relative ever undergo cancer surveillance?
What year was the cancer diagnosed?	If yes, what kind of screening was done and what were the results (and dates) of most recent tests?
Is your relative still living?	Did your relative ever have prophylactic surgery?
If yes, how old is he/she now? If no, what year and at what age did your relative die?	
Environmental exposures	
What was your relative's occupation?	
Did your relative smoke cigarettes?	
Was your relative exposed to any other harmful agents that might have caused the cancer?	

[a] Adapted from Schneider *(7)*.

diagnosis, and how the cancer was treated. If there was a second primary malignancy or bilateral disease in paired organs, this is very important information. Distinguishing primary from metastatic sites of disease may be difficult in some cases, but is highly relevant for assessing familial risk. It may be helpful to consider the interval between the cancer diagnoses. Pre-cancerous conditions (colonic adenomatous polyps) should also be ascertained, as should benign, but possibly related, conditions (lipomas). Because early age of onset is a distinguishing feature of inherited cancers, special attention should be paid to ages and dates of cancer diagnoses and treatment, as well as current ages or ages at death. This information may also be useful when requesting written confirmation in the form of medical records. Asking about treatment may help verify the diagnosis.

The patient should also be asked about other shared cancer risk factors in the family, such as environmental and occupational exposures. These may help to explain an apparent clustering of cancer in some families. Additional specific risk factors should be explored that may be pertinent to each diagnosis; smoking for lung or bladder cancer, sun exposure for melanoma, or in utero diethylstilbestrol (DES) exposure for vaginal cancer. It is equally important to ask about family members, who are unaffected, that is cancer-free. Their current ages (if living) or ages and causes of death (if deceased) should be ascertained. The ratio of affected to unaffected family members plays a significant role in risk assessment, as do the ages of unaffected family members. The interpretation of a family history involving two close relatives with cancer may be entirely different for a very small family with few at-risk individuals compared to a large family with many elderly, cancer-free individuals.

Even if the patient is an exceptionally good historian, the cancer history at this stage may be incomplete. Obtaining a complete and accurate history can be challenging. For example, it is not uncommon for patients to be estranged from certain relatives or for the cancer diagnoses in the family to be shrouded in secrecy. Coming for cancer counseling and risk assessment often represents the beginning of a process that includes talking with relatives, gathering records, and sometimes challenging family taboos and belief systems about cancer.

Importance of Documentation Because the risk assessment and options for genetic testing are based on the pattern of cancer in the family, it is important that this information be accurate. Unfortunately, patient's recall of the family cancer history may be quite inadequate *(8)*. Thus, it is important to obtain written confirmation of the type of cancer diagnosed and the age at which the cancer was diagnosed. The best source of confirmation is a pathology report; other sources include discharge summary reports, physician notes, or death certificates. For families suggestive of a hereditary-cancer syndrome, it is common practice to document cancers in the patient (if affected), all first-degree relatives, and any key diagnoses in other relatives that could alter the likelihood of a specific hereditary cancer syndrome; for example, a sarcoma in a family suspected to have Li-Fraumeni syndrome. Unless the family is participating in a research study, it is not necessary to document every case of cancer in the family.

The clinic will need to set a policy regarding the amount of documentation needed and at what point it will be required. Some programs require that medical records documentation be received prior to the clinic visit or brought to the genetic counseling visit, whereas other programs require documentation before drawing blood for DNA analysis. If the patient is not able to document the cancer history, then it is important to include a disclaimer that the risk assessment is based on verbal recollection only, and to encourage the patient to re-contact the center if information becomes available.

Table 3
Features Suggestive of a Hereditary-Cancer Syndrome

- Similar or related types of cancer in multiple family members
- Ages of cancer diagnoses are younger than is typical
- Pattern of cancer follows vertical transmission in two or more generations
- Presence of rare cancers in more than one family member
- Presence of two separate cancers in same individual
- Presence of physical features consistent with syndrome
- Absence of known environmental risk factors

Use of Pedigree as a Teaching Tool After collecting the detailed cancer history, the genetic counselor can point out specific features of the pedigree that support a hereditary or nonhereditary basis for the cancers in the family. The features of inherited cancer syndromes, shown in Table 3, can be reviewed with the patient *(7)*. The idea is to emphasize the overall pattern of cancer rather than the importance of a single feature.

ASSESSING CANCER RISK AND MANAGEMENT OPTIONS The purpose of obtaining a detailed personal and family history of cancer is to provide an accurate cancer risk assessment and to help develop a personalized cancer-surveillance plan *(9)*. Families can be categorized as having a high, moderate, or low probability of having a hereditary cancer syndrome.

High-Risk Families High-risk families have patterns of cancer that are suggestive or consistent with one of the known hereditary-cancer syndromes. In some ways, risk assessment in high-risk families is the most straightforward. Based on the pattern of cancer, the family is assumed to carry an inherited gene mutation that predisposes to specific forms of cancer. The patient's lifetime risk of cancer can therefore be estimated by his or her position in the pedigree; current age; and published estimates of age-specific penetrance of the gene(s) in question *(10)*. Because associated cancer risks are rarely 100%, patients are presented with lifetime estimates that they will develop specific forms of cancer. These concepts of probability, rather than absolute risk, can be confusing and overwhelming to patients. Studies looking at risk perception have found that patients interpret their risks based on many factors, including their own cancer experiences, personality traits, and fear of developing cancer *(11)*.

Patients who are known or suspected of being at 25 or 50% risk for carrying an inherited gene mutation may be asked to undergo more involved and more frequent screening for cancer. The surveillance may be similar to that offered to the general population, but initiated at a younger age. Patients may also be asked to consider risk-reduction strategies, such as chemoprevention or prophylactic surgery. Patients are also encouraged to recognize early warning signs of cancer and seek medical attention promptly. Patients with one of the rare cancer syndromes should be given written information so that their providers, in turn, can be alerted of the full spectrum of benign and malignant tumors in the syndrome *(9)*.

Moderate-Risk Families In moderate-risk families, there are certain features that are suggestive of an inherited cancer syndrome as well as some features that make this less likely.

Thus, estimating a patient's cancer risk becomes a matter of using empirical data or a range of risk. This makes risk assessment and counseling perhaps more difficult to provide. An example is a family with two sisters and a maternal aunt who all had breast cancer around age 60. There are three possible explanations for this pattern of cancer: 1) the family has a familial *BRCA1* or *BRCA2* mutation with later than usual ages of onset; 2) the family has a mutation in a lower penetrance gene that has not yet been identified; or 3) the family has a chance clustering of a relatively common disease.

Because of the possibility that there is an inherited component to the family's pattern of cancer, moderate-risk patients are encouraged to follow surveillance guidelines similar to that of high risk patients. However, emphasis might be given to the specific cancer(s) seen in the family rather than the entire spectrum of malignancies occurring in the syndrome. For example, the patient with three relatives who developed breast cancer in their sixth decade of life will be suggested to have increased monitoring for breast cancer, but it is unlikely that she will be suggested to initiate ovarian-cancer surveillance, unless genetic testing subsequently reveals a *BRCA1* or *BRCA2* mutation.

Low-Risk Families Given the prevalence of cancer, especially in older people, some patients may be at a low risk for an inherited predisposition to cancer, despite having their family histories of cancer. This is true of patients who have a single relative who has developed cancer and patients whose relatives have developed cancer at age 65 or older. These patients can be reassured about the low likelihood of an inherited etiology and given standard information about cancer surveillance and risk avoidance *(10)*. The ACS is an excellent resource for written materials that discuss general cancer risks and management recommendations (www.cancer.org).

TEACHING BASIC GENETIC CONCEPTS An important component of the genetic counseling session is to introduce basic genetic concepts. Providing basic genetic concepts hopefully diminishes the patient's feeling that cancer in the family is random and unavoidable. This discussion should include definitions of basic genetic terminology (such as chromosomes, genes and DNA) and explanations for relevant genetic concepts, including autosomal dominant inheritance (50% risk of carrying gene mutation if parent affected), variable expressivity (severity of disease varies even within a family), and incomplete penetrance (cancer risks are less than 100%). The concept that not all individuals who inherit an altered gene will develop cancer may lead to a discussion of more complicated cancer genetics concepts, such as Knudsen's two-hit hypothesis and carcinogenesis *(12)*, which describes cancer as the end result of multiple genetic changes within a cell. The issue of somatic vs germline gene mutations may also arise for cancer patients who have undergone DNA tumor analysis. The discussion of basic genetic concepts can be cursory or detailed, depending on the patient's level of interest and understanding.

DESCRIBING GENETIC TESTING OPTIONS The appropriateness of genetic testing for cancer susceptibility varies among the different hereditary cancer syndromes. In our experience, interest in genetic testing remains low for hereditary cancer syndromes in which: 1) gene-mutation carriers are reli-

Table 4
Genetic Tests Currently Available on a Clinical or
Research Basis^a

Gene	Clinical basis	Research basis
APC	Yes	No
BRCA1	Yes	Yes
BRCA2	Yes	Yes
hMLH1	Yes	Yes
hMSH2	Yes	Yes
hMSH6	Yes	Yes
NF1	Yes	Yes
PTEN	Yes	Yes
p16^{INK4A}	Yes	Yes
P53	Yes	Yes
Rb1	Yes	No
RET	Yes	No
VHL	Yes	No
WT1	No	Yes

^{a}Compiled from: Offit (23) and from GeneTests (*http://www. genetests.org*).

ably detected by physical exam (such as neurofibromatosis or familial melanoma), 2) occurrences of cancer are rarely familial (such as Wilms' tumor), and/or 3) there are no effective early detection or prevention strategies available (such as Li-Fraumeni syndrome). In contrast, interest in genetic testing tends to increase if: 1) the recommended surveillance is burdensome and expensive (e.g., familial adenomatous polyposis and von Hippel Lindau syndrome), 2) there are potentially effective early-detection or risk-reduction strategies available, and/or 3) it is rarely possible to detect gene-mutation carriers by other means (breast-ovarian cancer syndrome and hereditary nonpolyposis colon cancer).

GENETIC COUNSELING IN A PREDISPOSITION-TESTING PROGRAM

The testing process begins with ascertaining eligibility for testing, continues with the provision of genetic counseling prior to testing and at results disclosure, and concludes with providing follow-up services and support as needed.

ASCERTAINING ELIGIBILITY Because only 5–10% of cancer cases have an underlying inherited component (a germline mutation in a cancer-susceptibility gene), testing is not appropriate for all patients with cancer. Determining eligibility for a specific genetic test relies on a thorough assessment of personal and family history of cancer. Table 4 lists the major genetic tests that are available on a clinical or research basis. Because of the rapidly developing field, the list of available tests changes frequently. GeneTests, The National Cancer Institute, and National Society of Genetic Counselors are excellent resources for identifying laboratories that perform specific genetic tests and genetic testing and counseling programs.

In general, genetic testing is appropriate for families deemed at high or moderate risk for carrying a gene mutation associated with a specific hereditary-cancer syndrome. Some institutions have set eligibility criteria for offering testing to a family (10% risk of carrying a mutation in a specific gene). The appropriate classification of a family is imperative, because testing involves

a significant emotional and financial investment on the part of the patient and his/her family. Once it has been determined that a family is eligible for genetic testing, the next issue is to determine which family member to test first. Often the individual who has sought information about genetic testing is the unaffected sibling or child of the person with cancer. Ideally, the first person to be tested is the person most likely to carry the gene mutation, for instance, a relative who developed cancer at an unusually young age or who developed an uncommon type of cancer. At times, individuals who seek testing are not satisfied with this approach, because of their eagerness to get an answer for themselves. It may be useful to point out that their results are most meaningful if a mutation has already been identified in a relative with cancer. However, testing an affected relative first is not always possible; the affected relative may not be available or interested in testing. In these cases, testing can be offered to an individual who has not had cancer with the caveat that only a positive result provides conclusive information. In the absence of a known mutation, a negative result does not provide the reassurance that the patient has the general population risk of cancer, because the underlying inherited factor in the family has not yet been established.

PRE-TEST GENETIC COUNSELING The primary goal of the pre-test counseling session is to give people sufficient information to make an informed decision about whether or not to proceed with testing (13). The pre-test counseling session should include the following issues: 1) the prior risks of finding a mutation; 2) possible test results, including accuracy and limitations; 3) the medical and psychosocial implications of these results to the patient and his/her relatives; 4) the risks and benefits of learning this information (14,15). The amount of time spent discussing each topic will vary depending on the patient's prior knowledge about testing, number of questions, and any special issues that are of concern to the patient or genetic counselor.

Logistics of Testing It is important for patients to have a clear understanding about the logistics of the testing process. This includes answering questions about: 1) the testing program, including the number of in-person sessions involved and whether the testing program is conducted using a research protocol; 2) the laboratory analysis, including cost of test, accuracy rate of the laboratory analysis, and approximate date when results will be available; and 3) the results disclosure, in particular how results will be disclosed and whether results will be stored in the patient's medical record (13).

The Possible Results and Prior Risks of Carrying Mutation The possible results and the individual's *a priori* risk of carrying a germline mutation in a cancer susceptibility gene depend on whether or not there is a known mutation in the family.

Known Mutation in the Family In a family with a known mutation, the individual's prior risk of carrying the mutation are determined by his/her placement in the pedigree. The *a priori* risk of carrying a familial mutation may be higher if the person being tested has personally developed cancer, but will not be 100%, because of the possibility that the cancer occurred sporadically. Conversely, the risk of having a gene mutation may be lower if the individual remains cancer-free beyond the age at which the cancers typically occur. For example, a man who is 35 yr old and has no colonic polyps is extremely unlikely to have inherited the *APC* mutation known to be in his family. In a family with a known mutation, test results are straightforward. The presence of a germline mutation (a positive result) confers increased risks of cancer, whereas the absence of the mutation (a negative result) typically means the person has the general-population risks of cancer. Results are definitive and should have close to 100% accuracy rates if the laboratory is reputable and has the correct information about the familial mutation.

Family Not Known to Have Mutation Estimation of the individual's prior risk of carrying a germline mutation in a cancer-susceptibility gene is based on the likelihood that the family has such a mutation as well as his/her placement in the pedigree. In families not known to have a mutation, there are three possible results, which need to be thoroughly explored in the pre-test session: 1) a mutation is present, 2) mutation is absent, or 3) the result is inconclusive.

The first possibility is that the testing detects a mutation. If the analysis reveals a frameshift mutation or a previously reported deleterious missense mutation, then this is a positive result that has clinical significance.

The second possibility is that testing determines the absence of mutation. A negative result in a family not known to carry a specific gene mutation provides limited information. This is because the underlying cause of the cancer in the family has not been established. The family history of cancer may be due to a mutation in a different cancer-susceptibility gene or the cancer may not be due to a single Mendelian gene. The result may reduce the likelihood that the family has an inherited predisposition to cancer, but individuals should be cautioned that these results do not rule out a hereditary factor in the family. A negative result has the potential of becoming more meaningful if a relative is subsequently found to have a specific gene mutation. Only in this circumstance can the person's result be considered a true negative. One of the complexities of a negative result is the determination of what other testing may be appropriate. For example, a person of Ashkenazi Jewish ancestry, who is negative for the three common *BRCA1* and *BRCA2* mutations, may decide to have full gene sequencing.

The third possibility is that the results of testing are inconclusive. The laboratory analysis, if performed by DNA sequencing, may reveal a novel DNA variation. Generally, this is a change in a single DNA nucleotide (missense mutation), which may or may not disrupt protein function and thus, could turn out to be a functional mutation or a normal variant of no clinical significance. Other family members should not be offered clinical testing unless the inconclusive result is determined to be a functional mutation. To date, there is no standard functional assay for most cancer-susceptibility gene mutations, which means that clarifying an inconclusive result is difficult. The laboratory may request blood samples from additional members of the family to determine if the variant is tracking with the cancer diagnoses. Family members asked to donate samples for such a linkage study need to be aware that this is more of a research effort than a clinical test. Reporting inconclusive results often leads to a very complicated and unsatisfying counseling session.

Major Risks and Benefits of Testing When there are proven strategies to prevent or cure inherited forms of cancer, the emphasis on risks vs benefits of testing will dissipate. Until that time, a discussion of the risks and benefits is a key part of the pre-test genetic counseling session. The four major benefits of genetic testing are: 1) ending the uncertainty about one's gene status, 2) possibly learning negative results, 3) possibly impacting medical management decisions, and 4) clarifying cancer risk for other family members with a positive result. The four major risks of testing for cancer susceptibility include: 1) the possibility of remaining uncertainty, 2) discrimination and stigma, 3) psychological sequelae, and 4) strain on family relationships.

Ending the Uncertainty About One's Gene Status This psychological benefit may be an important factor in decisions about testing. One breast cancer testing program found that individuals who chose not to be tested had greater adverse psychological reactions than those who had undergone testing, regardless of the results *(16)*.

Possibility of Learning Negative Results In a family with a known mutation, a negative result reduces that person's cancer risks to that of the population and also means that his/her offspring cannot inherit the familial mutation. This may be of significant psychological benefit and some medical benefit as well, because of the less stringent surveillance recommendations.

Positive Result May Influence Medical Management Decisions The extent to which medical management decisions are important depends on the cancer syndrome. Individuals may be advised to begin cancer-surveillance practices at an earlier age and continue doing them at more frequent intervals than their counterparts in the general population (breast-ovarian cancer syndrome). In addition, some at-risk individuals may have the option of prophylactic surgery (familial adenomatous polyposis), which provides a substantial reduction of cancer risk.

Positive Result May Clarify Cancer Risks for Other Family Members A positive result increases the cancer risks for first-degree relatives (siblings and children). The initial positive result in the family or in a specific branch of the family also affects other relatives, including aunts, uncles, and cousins, and allows them to have informative genetic testing.

The Possibility of Remaining Uncertainty There is an element of uncertainty that remains after disclosure of the test results. A positive result confers increased risks, but does not give definitive information about when (or if) the cancer will occur, the exact site of cancer, how advanced the stage of cancer will be, or how well the person will respond to treatments. Conversely, a negative result does not mean that the person will never develop cancer.

Discrimination and Stigma People seem most concerned about possible health insurance discrimination. Health insurance discrimination can take many forms, including cancellation of policy, higher monthly premiums, or refusal to cover cancer-related illnesses. The people who are most vulnerable to health-insurance discrimination are those living in states without any legal protections from utilizing this information, those who have never had cancer, and those who are self-insured or are working in small firms (with less than 50 employers). Some states have passed legislation prohibiting such discrimination and similar legislation is being drafted on the national level. Possible discrimination by other third parties, especially employers, life insurers, and adoption agencies, have also sparked concern. As with any genetic condition, there are also concerns about stigmatization, particularly among cultures for which such information could affect marriageability and status in the community.

Psychological Sequelae of Results Individuals receiving positive results may exhibit depression, anxiety, and anger *(17–19)*. Although the majority of patients eventually cope satisfactorily with their results, a subset will require follow-up interventions with a mental-health professional. Although considered good news, a negative result can require a period of adjustment and may engender intense feelings of survivor guilt *(17)*.

Strain on Family Relationships Some family members will receive positive results and others will be negative. Even within a family, there will be differences regarding being tested, communication of results, styles of coping, and subsequent decisions about medical management. All of these factors can cause family relationships to be strained, either temporarily or long-term. Uptake rates in predisposition testing research programs have been well below earlier attitude surveys, which predicted uptake rates greater than 70% *(18,20)*. However, these findings are not unexpected given the experiences of testing programs for other adult-onset disorders, notably Huntington's disease (HD). There are a multitude of reasons why people decide not to have predisposition testing for cancer susceptibility. The major reasons for declining testing are: 1) a lack of interest in obtaining genetic information; 2) uncertainty that results would change their screening practices in any way; 3) fear that results could be positive; concerns about possible insurance discrimination; 4) cost of commercially available tests (which can range from $300–3,000); and 5) inappropriate timing because of seriously ill family members or other stressors *(21)*.

Counseling Issues in Pre-Test Session Special circumstances require tact and sensitivity, such as testing terminally ill patients or finding positive results in an individual whose parent had previously declined testing. Each patient has an established pattern of communication within their family, as well as set styles for making decisions and coping with major life stressors. Recognizing these patterns may be helpful in providing care and may lead to the identification of patients who require additional psychological support. Predisposition-testing programs need to have a plan for identifying and handling patients who are psychologically vulnerable *(22)*. During the testing process, patients should be referred to a mental-health professional if there are concerns about: 1) the possibility of suicide upon learning results; 2) overall ability to cope with the results; 3) evidence of significant, untreated depression, anxiety, or other psychosis; 4) lack of social support; 5) an intense grief reaction triggered by the testing process; and 6) major life stres-

sors, such as cancer-related death of relative or loss of job. The program should consider deferral of drawing blood for analysis or disclosing results if the patient's safety is an issue.

RESULTS DISCLOSURE VISIT The primary goal of the results disclosure session is to disclose the genetic-test results and provide immediate information and emotional support as needed. Patients should be encouraged to bring someone with them to the results-disclosure session. More detailed explanations of the implications or limitations of results are important, but should follow the patient's initial reaction to the news.

Psychological Reactions to Results Patients will react differently upon learning their results. There may be open displays of grief, anger, or joy. Others may be quieter in their response, either because they are still processing the information or they are numb with shock. Because of the emotional impact of learning their results, patients may not be able to listen to much of the remaining discussion. For this reason, it may be more useful to review the information in a later follow-up visit or telephone conversation. Positive results can engender feelings of depression and anxiety, although in the pilot HD testing program, no suicide attempts or hospitalizations were reported and levels of depression returned to baseline levels by 1 yr postdisclosure *(17)*. The overwhelming majority of patients receiving genetic test results for cancer susceptibility also seem to cope adequately with the information *(18)*. Positive results may also lead to increased feelings of control, greater motivation to pursue cancer monitoring, relief from uncertainty, closer identification with affected relatives, and greater fear of cancer *(18)*. Definitive negative results (in a family with a previously identified mutation) can invoke feelings of relief and joy and decrease levels of depression, anxiety, and cancer worry. Patients may also experience intense survivor guilt, isolation from affected or mutation-positive family members, and regret about major life decisions *(17)*. Results that are indeterminate (like a variant of unknown significance or a negative result in a family not known to have a mutation) can lead to conflicting emotions, including relief that the result is not positive, sadness that the result is not good news, and frustration that there is still no definitive explanation for the cancer in the family.

Review of Implications During this session, the focus can be on the patient's actual result (whether positive or negative) rather than detailing all possibilities. It will also be possible to tailor the information to the patient's situation. For example, a discussion of the implications of a positive *BRCA1* or *BRCA2* result will vary depending on the patient's gender and whether he/she has children and/or has ever had cancer. Although patients have already been told this information, it may seem as though they are hearing this information for the first time, because now it is more relevant. Discussions about medical management will need to involve physicians specializing in cancer-risk management as well as primary-care physicians. Patients with positive results may need to consider increasing the type and frequency of surveillance. They should also be reminded that the purpose of monitoring is to detect the cancer at an early stage, not cancer prevention *per se*. Patients with indeterminate results are asked to continue increased monitoring practices. Patients should also be informed of the warning signs of cancer, because cancers are often detected by the patients themselves. Patients with a true negative result may be able to decrease surveillance; however, some express reluctance to do so.

Counseling Issues in Results Disclosure Session The results disclosure session often engenders high emotions of one sort or another. Although displays of grief are not inappropriate, the counselor should assess whether the patient is displaying a more extreme demonstration of anxiety or sadness that requires additional psychological support. Patients rarely require immediate psychological intervention. For all patients, it is a good policy to query about their plans for the remainder of the day and to determine that the patient has at least one person that he/she can call upon for support if need be. This can be a partner, relative, friend, or therapist.

POST-TEST GENETIC COUNSELING Follow-up services are an important component of predisposition testing programs. This can include the management of cancer risks as well as an ongoing assessment of the individual's emotional reactions. Provision of follow-up services may involve the utilization of a network of health care specialists, including primary care physicians, oncologists, breast surgeons, and mental-health professionals.

Review of Implications of Results The focus of the discussion may focus on solidifying a plan for being monitored or making decisions about chemoprevention or prophylactic surgery. This is also the time to review implications of the results to other family members, particularly offspring and siblings, and discuss possible strategies for making them aware of this information.

Counseling Issues in Follow-Up Visit The emotional response to testing seems to be most intense in the first few weeks or months after learning results, but tends to dissipate over time. However, specific issues and concerns may arise in the future, as the patient's children become older or when another relative is diagnosed with cancer. It is important for patients to be aware of resources that are available to them if and when they need additional information in the future. Relationships among family members may become strained, either temporarily or permanently, as individuals make different decisions about testing and perhaps receive different test results. In addition, patients may feel an obligation to share the information with relatives with whom they are not particularly close. Other relatives may not welcome the opportunity to be tested and may resent the individual initially found to have the gene mutation.

GENETIC COUNSELING FOR SELECTED CANCER SYNDROMES

HEREDITARY BREAST-OVARIAN CANCER SYNDROME The majority of cancer genetic counseling articles focus on hereditary breast-ovarian cancer syndrome, because of the availability of genetic testing and amount of media attention on the opportunities and dilemmas facing at-risk families.

Contracting and Assessing Motivation Contracting with patients at increased risk for hereditary breast-ovarian cancer syndrome involves explaining how many providers the patient will be seeing and how many visits the counseling process takes. Ascertaining the patient's motivation for seeking cancer ge-

netic-counseling may be useful in terms of tailoring information that is most relevant; for example, if the patient has adult daughters, is seriously considering prophylactic surgery, or has reached menopause and wants to take hormone-replacement therapy.

Collecting and Discussing Cancer History The likelihood of finding a germline *BRCA1* or *BRCA2* mutation is increased if: 1) three or more women have developed ovarian or premenopausal breast cancer, 2) at least one female relative has developed both breast and ovarian cancer, and/or 3) at least one male relative has developed breast cancer *(23)*. Identification of a family with hereditary breast-ovarian cancer syndrome depends on the number of relatives who have developed breast or ovarian cancer and the ages at which the diagnoses occurred. Documentation of cancer diagnoses is important, particularly for cases of ovarian cancer, which may, in fact, be cancer of the cervix, uterus, or colon. It is also important to separate cases of two separate primaries from recurrent or metastatic disease. Additional cancers that have been reported in families with hereditary breast-ovarian cancer syndrome are colon and prostate cancer (in *BRCA1* families) and pancreatic and ocular melanoma (in *BRCA2* families) *(23)*. In collecting information about unaffected female members of the family, it is useful to find out whether any relatives have had their breasts and/or ovaries surgically removed and why this was done (prophylactically or for cancer). It may also be useful to find out the most recent dates and results of any breast and/or ovarian screening and whether other family members have expressed interest in having genetic testing.

As patients describe their personal and/or family histories of breast and ovarian cancer, they may re-experience feelings of grief, loss, anxiety, or anger. It is important to be sensitive to the emotional overtones while collecting family history information and recognize that these feelings may contribute to the patient's own perception of cancer risk or cancer survival.

Assessing Cancer Risk and Management Options There are various options available for estimating the risk that a patient (or family) harbors a *BRCA1* or *BRCA2* mutation. Complex statistical models, like Berry et al. *(24)*, require information on relationship of all family members (affected and unaffected), ages at diagnosis for affected individuals, and ages at exam for unaffected individuals *(24)*. The Berry computer model uses Bayes' theorem to determine the probability of a *BRCA1* or *BRCA2* mutation based on family data and published data on age-specific incidence rates and frequencies of mutations. Although useful in determining thresholds for testing, these estimates do not serve the individual patient very well. Most individuals feel that it is all or nothing; that is, they either have a mutation or they do not. This is where direct mutational analysis comes into play.

Risks of specific cancers associated with inherited *BRCA1* and *BRCA2* mutations continue to be refined. Original estimates were based on retrospective studies of families selected because of the occurrence of early-onset breast or ovarian cancer and most likely represent overestimates. More recent estimates have provided a lower boundary for the risks associated with mutations in these two genes, and future studies may give even lower estimations of risk. Table 5 gives the current ranges

Table 5
Specific Cancer Risks for Men and Women with a Germline *BRCA1*
or *BRCA2* Mutation Compared to General Population Risks[a]

	Breast cancer before age 85	Ovarian cancer before age 85	Other cancers before age 85
Women with 2 <u>normal</u> *BRCA1/2* genes	11%	1–2%	Pancreatic, ~1% Colon, 5–6%
Women with an <u>altered</u> *BRCA1* gene	55–85%	20–60%	Colon, up to 8%
Women with an <u>altered</u> *BRCA2* gene	55–85%	10–20%	Pancreatic, somewhat increased
Men with 2 <u>normal</u> *BRCA1/2* genes	Very low	N/A	Pancreatic , ~1%
Men with an <u>altered</u> *BRCA1* gene	Not increased	N/A	Colon, up to 8% Prostate, slightly increased
Men with an <u>altered</u> *BRCA2* gene	6–10%	N/A	Pancreatic, somewhat increased

[a]Compiled from Ford et al. *(25)* and Struewing et al. *(26).*

used in counseling individuals known to have a *BRCA1* or *BRCA2* gene mutation *(25–27)*. There exist various limitations of these current estimates. First, the estimates do not take into consideration the influence of environmental factors (exposures, dietary habits). In addition, the estimates do not account for other hereditary factors (modifying genes). Finally, the estimates do not distinguish among specific mutations. There is some data, and more to come, that suggest that different mutations confer different risks (some mutations are associated with lower risk).

The guidelines for the medical management of a patient with a *BRCA1* or *BRCA2* mutation are still being refined. Patients should be cautioned that none of these detection methods are 100% reliable. Female patients with a *BRCA1* or *BRCA2* mutation are typically suggested to have the following *(28)*: 1) monthly breast self-exams beginning at age 18; 2) clinical breast exams by a doctor or nurse at least twice a year, beginning at age 25–30; 3) mammograms yearly beginning at age 25–30; 4) pelvic examinations done at least annually; 5) trans-vaginal ultrasound done twice a year. The use of ultrasound to view the ovaries is being studied as a way to improve early detection of ovarian cancer; 6) CA-125 blood test for postmenopausal women.

Risk-reduction strategies, none of which offer complete protection, include chemopreventive agents, such as Tamoxifen and oral contraceptives, as well as prophylactic surgery. Women appear to be having prophylactic oophorectomies more frequently than prophylactic mastectomies, because the surgery tends to be less disfiguring and because ovarian cancer, in general, is more difficult to detect and successfully treat.

Offering and Providing Genetic Testing The *BRCA1* gene lies on chromosome 17q21 and the *BRCA2* gene is located on chromosome 13p12. The length of the *BRCA1* and *BRCA2* genes, 22 exons and 27 exons, respectively, makes the genetic analysis both difficult and expensive *(23)*. *BRCA1* and *BRCA2*

testing is currently available in both research and clinical settings.

COWDEN SYNDROME Cowden syndrome is one of the multiple hamartoma syndromes that is associated with increased risks of breast and thyroid cancer. Multiple hamartomas are benign hyperplastic disorganized growths that can occur in any organ system. Cowden syndrome follows an autosomal dominant pattern of inheritance. Although thought to be a rare syndrome, Cowden syndrome is almost certainly under-recognized by clinicians.

Contracting and Assessing Motivation At the outset of the visit, it is important to determine the extent of information the patient has about Cowden syndrome. For patients who have already been diagnosed with Cowden syndrome, the clinic visit involves a review of cancer risks as well as an update on molecular advances. For patients who have not been diagnosed, the emphasis will be on making the diagnosis of Cowden syndrome, through physical examination and careful review of the patient's personal and family medical history. Some patients, who have struggled with the seemingly unrelated medical problems associated with Cowden syndrome, will welcome the diagnosis as an explanation. Others, especially those initially referred for *BRCA1* or *BRCA2* testing, may be much less enthusiastic about learning they have a syndrome that includes benign growths and thyroid cancer.

Collecting and Discussing Cancer History The diagnostic criteria for Cowden syndrome are listed in Table 6 *(29)*. The key feature of Cowden syndrome is the presence of facial trichilemmomas. The pattern of disease should also include benign and malignant thyroid and breast disease. Patients should be asked if they have any unusual skin growths that are currently present or were removed. A physician, optimally a dermatologist or geneticist, needs to carefully examine the patient's skin (particularly the face), and review the pathology report of any growth or mole that was removed. To assess physi-

Table 6
Cowden Syndrome Operational Criteria[a]

Pathognomonic criteria
- Facial trichilemmomas
- Acral keratoses
- Papillomatous lesions
- Mucosal lesions

Major criteria:
- Breast cancer
- Thyroid cancer (especially papillary)
- Macrocephaly (97th percentile)
- Lhermitte-Duclos disease

Minor criteria:
- Thyroid lesions (goiter)
- Mental retardation (IQ<75)
- Gastrointestinal hamartomas
- Fibrocystic disease of the breast
- Lipomas
- Fibromas
- Genitourinary tumors or malformations

Operational diagnosis:
- The pathognomonic criteria
- Two major criteria
- One major and 3 minor criteria
- Four minor criteria

[a]Compiled from Eng (30).

Table 7
Diagnostic Criteria for Classic and Variant Forms of Li-Fraumeni Syndrome[a]

Classic Li-Fraumeni syndrome criteria
(must meet all of the following criteria)
- Proband with sarcoma under age 45
- First-degree relative with LFS component tumor[b] under age 45
- First- or second-degree realtive with any cancer under age 45,

OR
- A sarcoma at any age

Variant Li-Fraumeni syndrome criteria
- Individual with three separate primary cancers with the first cancer diagnosed under age 45

OR
(must meet all of the following criteria)
- Proband with any childhood cancer or sarcoma or brain tumor or adrenocortical carcinoma under age 45
- First/second-degree relative(s) with component LFS tumors[b] at any age
- first/second-degree relative(s) with any cancer under age 60

[a] Adapted from Eng et al. (32).
[b]Li-Fraumeni syndrome component tumors include sarcoma, breast cancer, brain tumor, leukemia, adrenal-gland cancer.

cal features of relatives (such as head size and shape), patients can be asked to bring in pictures of their family members. It is not uncommon for patients to have been given conflicting diagnoses or information, which need to be clarified. Making the diagnosis, as with any genetic disease, needs to be handled with sensitivity and tact. Providers need to make sure that all the patients' questions are satisfactorily answered, without overwhelming them with medical facts.

Assessing Cancer Risk and Management Options Cowden disease is a fairly new cancer syndrome, so cancer risks are not yet well-established. Current estimates include a lifetime breast-cancer risk in women of between 30–50% and a lifetime risk of thyroid cancer for both males and females of between 3–10% (30). Women with Cowden syndrome also have a higher chance of having fibrocystic breast disease, which may make the breasts more difficult to evaluate. Cancer risk surveillance for Cowden syndrome includes monitoring for breast and thyroid cancer via annual physicals (thyroid exam) beginning in the teens. Monitoring for Cowden syndrome includes (30): 1) annual thyroid examinations, 2) annual clinical breast exams for women beginning in their twenties, 3) mammography beginning around age 30 or younger if there are young cases of breast cancer in the family, 4) annual skin examinations.

Offering and Providing Genetic Testing The gene responsible for Cowden disease is *PTEN*, a tumor suppressor gene, located at 10q23 (31). Most, but not all, of the individuals with documented Cowden syndrome will have an identifiable mutation in the *PTEN* gene. Genetic testing for Cowden syndrome is currently performed clinically.

LI-FRAUMENI SYNDROME Li-Fraumeni syndrome is a very rare cancer family syndrome. Fewer than 300 Li-Fraumeni syndrome families have been reported worldwide.

Contracting and Assessing Motivation Counseling may range from making the initial suggestion that the family has Li-Fraumeni syndrome to providing predisposition testing for a family with a known germline *p53* mutation. Learning the patient's level of understanding about Li-Fraumeni syndrome and motivation for the visit (such as worry about their children, interest in testing) allows the session to be tailored to best fit the patient's needs.

Collecting and Discussing Cancer History The malignancies seen in Li-Fraumeni syndrome include soft-tissue sarcomas, osteosarcomas, adrenal gland carcinomas, breast cancer, leukemia, and brain tumors. Gastrointestinal cancers have also been reported as have other cancers. Diagnostic criteria for classic and variant forms of Li-Fraumeni syndrome are listed in Table 7 (32). Ages of diagnosis are important to confirm, as are all rare tumors reported in first- or second-degree relatives. The occurrence of multiple primary tumors in patients is a key determinant of the syndrome. Individuals with multiple primary tumors (that is individuals with two, three, or more separate cancers) need to be distinguished from individuals with a single primary tumor and one or more metastatic tumors. The majority of Li-Fraumeni syndrome families have remarkable family histories of cancer. This aids in the classification of the family, but may make the counseling aspects more difficult. A discussion about the pattern of cancer in the family may be emotionally charged, because of the number of cancer related illnesses and deaths in close relatives.

Assessing Cancer Risk and Management Options Li-Fraumeni syndrome is a highly penetrant, autosomal dominant condition. Risks of cancer in Li-Fraumeni syndrome are 50%

Table 8
Diagnostic Criteria for Hereditary Non-Polyposis Colon Cancer[a]

Amsterdam Criteria	*Bethesda Criteria*
(must meet all criteria)	*(must meet 1 criteria)*
• Colorectal cancer diagnosis in 3+ relatives one of whom is a first-degree relative of the other two • Colorectal cancer present in at least 2 generations • One diagnosis of colorectal cancer must be before age 50	• Family meets Amsterdam Criteria • Individual has 2 HNPCC-related cancers[b] • Individual has colorectal cancer and a first-degree relative with an HNPCC-related cancer[b] or a colorectal adenoma; one of the cancers diagnosed before age 45, or the adenoma diagnosed before age 40 • Individual with colorectal or endometrial cancer diagnosed before age 45 • Individual with adenomas diagnosed before or at age 40

[a]Compiled from: International Collaborative Group on HNPCC, Amsterdam Criteria, 1991. International Collaborative Group on HNPCC, Bethesda Criteria, 1996.

[b]HNPCC-related cancers: colorectal, endometrial, ovarian, gastric, hepatobiliary, small-bowel, and transitional-cell carcinoma of renal pelvis or ureter.

by age 30, and 90% by age 50. One-third of the malignancies occur in children under age 18. The risk for developing a second cancer may be as high as 50%. For women, the highest risk of cancer is that of the breast (which sometimes occurs in their twenties). Men who escape childhood and adolescent cancers may have lower lifetime risks of cancer *(32,33)*.

Individuals in Li-Fraumeni syndrome families speak of the helplessness they feel regarding their at-risk status. This stems from both the fear that cancer could occur in virtually any organ and the paucity of effective early detection or prevention strategies available to them. Although no surveillance measures have been shown to be effective in reducing morbidity or mortality, recommended surveillance in childhood include annual physical exams (including manual exams of the chest and abdomen) and neurological exams, urinalysis, and white blood count (WBC). In addition, physicians are urged to pay greater attention to lingering childhood aches and illnesses, particularly headaches, bone pain, and abdominal discomfort. For adults, surveillance should include annual physical exams (including skin, rectal, and neurological exams), and for women, monthly breast self-exams, and twice yearly clinical breast exams. There is controversy regarding the use of routine mammograms in women with Li-Fraumeni syndrome, because of possible radiation-sensitivity associated with *p53* mutations. Although some centers advocate the use of breast ultrsonography instead, others continue to recommend mammograms, because it continues to be the most effective breast-screening technique *(32,33)*.

Offering and Providing Genetic Testing About two-thirds of Li-Fraumeni syndrome families have a germline mutation in the *p53* gene. *p53* is a tumor-suppressor gene located at 17p13 *(34)*. Because of the extremely high risk of diverse tumor types (for which there is little surveillance available), interest in predisposition testing has remained low. Testing is primarily available at major medical centers and is typically offered to adults only. There have been very few requests for prenatal testing, although it is technically feasible.

HEREDITARY NON-POLYPOSIS COLON CANCER
Colon cancer is the third most common cancer in the United

States and is the most common of the hereditary tumors affecting both men and women. Approximately 5% of colon cancer is believed to be due to a highly penetrant, dominant mutation in a cancer-susceptibility gene. Hereditary non-Polyposis Colon Cancer (HNPCC) is the most common of the hereditary colon cancer syndromes.

Contracting and Assessing Motivation Patients may not be aware that their family is affected by HNPCC, but the vast majority already know that they are at increased risk for developing colon cancer and have been advised to initiate colon cancer screening by their physicians. Patients are often referred to a high-risk clinic to discuss genetic-testing options, motivated by concern on behalf of themselves and their children or a desire to avoid colonoscopy procedures if they are not at-risk. Part of the contracting involves a discussion of the extra-colonic malignanices associated with HNPCC and reminding patients that monitoring should not be placed on hold while gene analysis, which can take months or years, is being completed.

Collecting and Discussing Cancer History HNPCC is characterized by early onset of colon cancer (or colonic polyps), a tendency toward right-sided tumors, and other associated cancers of the uterus, ovary, stomach, urinary tract, small intestine, and bile duct *(35)*. A diagnosis of HNPCC can be made using the Amsterdam Criteria, developed in 1991 by the International Collaborative Group *(36)*. In a subsequent meeting, the Bethesda Criteria were adopted to include the extracolonic tumors seen in HNPCC kindreds *(37)*. Table 8 presents both the Amsterdam and Bethesda Criteria. Even if the family does not meet the Amsterdam or Bethesda Criteria, the patient may have increased risks for developing colon cancer.

There are two variants of HNPCC that should be considered: Turcot syndrome and Muir-Torre syndrome. Kindreds with Turcot Syndrome must demonstrate a pattern of cancer consistent with HNPCC as well as a diagnosis of glioblastoma in at least one individual *(38)*. Muir-Torre syndrome is characterized by a sebaceous adenoma, sebaceous epithelioma, or sebaeceous carcinoma and an internal malignancy, such as cancer in the large or small intestine *(39)*.

Colon cancer in the United States is exceedingly common and there are a variety of nonhereditary risk factors (including diet, alcoholism, inflammatory-bowel disease) that can lead to colon cancer. This can create two separate issues. First, it means that the patient may have an increased risk of colon cancer, separate from his/her risk for developing an inherited form of cancer. Second, the presence of any of these risk factors may mistakenly foster the patient's belief that he/she carries the inherited susceptibility to cancer.

Assessing Cancer Risk and Management Options Individuals with HNPCC have about 70–80% risks of colorectal cancer by age 65 and also have increased risks of extracolonic tumors, including stomach and pancreatic cancer. Women have about a 30% lifetime risk of endometrial cancer and may also have increased risks of ovarian and breast cancer (23,40). Options for cancer surveillance in individuals with HNPCC (or their at-risk relatives) include (41): 1) colonoscopy every 1–3 yr beginning at age 20–25, 2) pelvic examination annually beginning at age 25-35, 3) mammography annually beginning at age 40, 4) transvaginal ultrasound annually beginning at age 25–35.

Colectomy may be discussed with patients diagnosed with colon cancer; however, at-risk patients are not being advised to consider prophylactic colectomy. Undergoing a hysterectomy and oophorectomy may be discussed as an option to reduce the risk of uterine and ovarian cancer in women with HNPCC.

Patients may have very different attitudes about the cancer risks and effectiveness of monitoring depending on whether their relatives were successfully diagnosed and treated or died from their disease. Patients may be focused on the risk of a specific cancer, because of the family's experience, and may need to be gently reminded about other cancer risks, especially uterine cancer in women. As an extreme example, a woman may be vigilant about having colonoscopies, because her mother died from advanced-stage colon cancer, but may be ignoring the small lump in her breast.

Offering and Providing Genetic Testing At this point in time, we know that a germline mutation in any of the five following genes can cause HNPCC: *MSH2, MLH1, PMS2, PMS1,* and *MSH6* (42,43). About 60% of families with HNPCC are found to have a germline mutation in the *MSH2* or *MLH1* gene. The *MSH6, PMS1,* and *PMS2* genes represent a small number of cases of HNPCC. The genetic basis for the remainder of HNPCC cases has yet to be identified (23). One of the major genetic counseling challenges is the high percentage of families, perhaps 30%, that carry missense mutations in one of these genes that are of unknown clinical significance. As the HNPCC genes are better characterized and functional tests become available, this problem should abate.

FAMILIAL ADENOMATOUS POLYPOSIS COLI Familial adenomatous polyposis coli (FAP) is a rare hereditary colon cancer syndrome that accounts for less than 1% of total cases of colon cancer. However, the associated risk of colon cancer in individuals with FAP is virtually 100%, unless the colon is surgically removed. This makes Familial Adenomatous Polyposis (FAP) one of the few fully penetrant hereditary-cancer syndromes and one in which early identification of at-risk individuals carries clear medical benefit (44).

Contracting and Assessing Motivation Individuals with classic features of FAP are often interested in the option of genetic testing to determine which of their relatives are at risk and which are not. Often, parents will come to the clinic on behalf of their young children. Programs need to decide if they will accept young children for *APC* testing or if they will only test children old enough to have some understanding of why the test is being done. If the clinic patient is not the person in the family with FAP, then he/she needs to be told, up front, that the testing process needs to begin with an affected relative and that he/she will not be tested that day.

Collecting and Discussing Cancer History FAP is characterized by hundreds to thousands of colonic polyps in late teens or early twenties. Typically, an individual needs to have greater than 100 adenomatous polyps in the colon to make diagnosis (this can be compared to individuals with HNPCC, who rarely have more than 50 polyps in their colon). Making the diagnosis of FAP involves review of colonoscopy and pathology reports for one or more affected relatives. Polyps may also arise in other parts of the gastrointestinal tract, including the Ampulla of Vater. Cases of pediatric hepatoblastoma have also been reported in FAP families (44,45).

There exists an attenuated form of FAP, in which the number of colonic polyps is far fewer and average age of onset is later (46). Families with attenuated FAP may be difficult to distinguish from those with HNPCC, although it is an important distinction to make, because of the different surveillance recommendations. Patients with attenuated FAP are not routinely advised to undergo prophylactic colectomy (23).

There are two variants of classic FAP: Turcot syndrome and Gardner syndrome. In Turcot syndrome, there is a pattern of early-onset colonic polyposis as well as brain tumors, specifically medulloblastoma. These features are somewhat different from the HNPCC form of Turcot syndrome (38). In Gardner syndrome, individuals have colonic polyposis and a greater likelihood of desmoid tumors (usually along the digestive tract), osteomas, and dermoid cysts (23).

While the focus of collecting a family history is on the individuals with colonic polyposis, the patient should also be asked about extra-colonic tumors in relatives. However, these variants are highly variable in expression; some individuals in families have all the features, some have only a few.

Assessing Cancer Risk and Management Options If the colon is not removed in patients with FAP, there is a 100% likelihood that colon cancer will develop by age 50. By age 25, most individuals have the characteristic feature of polyps carpeting the colon. Individuals with FAP also have about a 10–12% risk of developing duodenal cancer. Approximately 50% of individuals with FAP will have congenital hypertrophy of the retinal epithelium, which consists of pigmented lesions in the retina that can be detected by fundoscopic examination (23,44). Medical-management options for individuals with FAP include: 1) annual flexible sigmoidoscopy beginning at age 10–11; 2) prophylactic colectomy, when polyps are detected (usually by age 25); and 3) surveillance for extracolonic adenomatous polyps (upper gastrointestinal tract) (23).

Offering and Providing Genetic Testing The gene responsible for FAP is the *APC* gene located on 5q21. Approximately 97% of the mutations in *APC* have been observed in the 5′-end of the gene *(46)*. Approximately one-third of FAP cases are due to *de novo* germline mutations *(46)*. There are special challenges with offering genetic testing to children or adolescents. Minors who undergo predisposition testing need to be given age appropriate information and emotional support and the genetic-counseling process usually involves discussions with both the patient and his/her parents.

MULTIPLE ENDOCRINE NEOPLASIA TYPE 2 Multiple endocrine neoplasia type 2 (MEN2) holds a special place among hereditary-cancer syndromes, because to date it is the only one caused by a germline mutation in a proto-oncogene. Genetic testing for MEN2 has become the clinical standard of care, which again differs from the recommendations in hereditary-cancer syndromes.

Contracting and Assessing Motivation Patients with MEN2 may be referred to a high-risk clinic with an initial diagnosis of medullary thyroid carcinoma (MTC) or for review of information in a family known to carry an *RET* mutation. Because our knowledge about hereditary-cancer syndromes continues to evolve, it is useful to provide a review of current information, even for patients who have received genetic counseling in the past. This can be done quite successfully in a family meeting, with the option of personalized genetic counseling to address more sensitive issues.

Collecting and Discussing Cancer History A family history of sporadic MTC can be a challenge for providers. A very thorough pathology review can shed light on whether a sporadic case has significance for other family members. In the absence of C-cell hyperplasia and/or a multifocal tumor, approx 5% are inherited *(47)*.

The family history should include questions that target the various features associated with MEN2. The patient may report that no one in the family has been diagnosed with a benign or malignant endocrine tumor. Because endocrine tumors may be under-diagnosed, it is important to ask about medical histories that could suggest the presence of MEN2-related tumors, including presence of severe kidney stones, which could indicate hyperparathyroidism; strokes in nonelderly persons (during childbirth) or childhood deaths, which could indicate pheochromocytomas; and large goiters or noticeable lumps in the neck, which could indicate MTC. Medical records in all of these situations would assist in determining the degree of cancer risk to other family members.

Assessing Cancer Risk and Management Options Individuals who carry a germline mutation in the c-*ret* gene have about a 70% chance of developing some type of endocrine problem by age 70 *(47)*. There are three forms of MEN2: 1) MEN2A, 2) MEN2B, and 3) familial medullary thyroid carcinoma (FMTC). Thyroidectomies are recommended for individuals carrying a c-*ret* mutation, regardless of which form of MEN2 they have. In the absence of a thyroidectomy or when genetic testing is not feasible or is inconclusive, close biochemical screening is warranted. This involves annual pentegastrin-stimulated calcitonin, 24-h urine catecholamines, and serum calcium and parathyroid hormone between the ages of 6 and 35. Screening may be discontinued after age 35 if there is no evidence of MEN2 *(48)*.

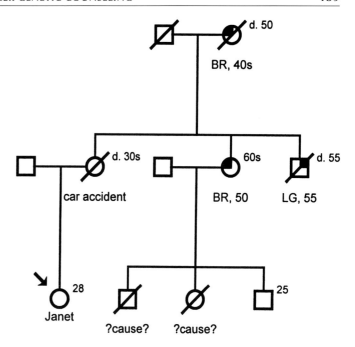

Fig. 1. Initial family history collected. Initial family history of cancer reveals two female relatives with perimenopausal breast cancer and a male relative with lung cancer. History is suggestive of hereditary breast cancer, but requires documentation.

MEN2A This by far the most common form of MEN2. Individuals with MEN2A have increased chances of developing MTC, adrenal gland tumors (pheochromocytomas), and parathyroid tumors *(48)*.

MEN2B This form of MEN2 is characterized by MTCs, pheochromocytomas, and less commonly, parathyroid hyperplasia. MEN2B tends to have an earlier onset of MTC than MEN2A, with some cases being reported as young as age five. There can also be developmental abnormalities, such as ganglioneuromatosis, myelinated corneal nerves, and marfanoid habitus *(48)*.

FMTC Individuals with FMTC have increased risks for developing MTC, but do not seem predisposed to developing the other problems associated with MEN2A and MEN2B. In addition, the onset of MTC seems to occur later. Diagnosing FMTC, which seems to be the rarest form of MEN2, is a matter of excluding MEN2A and MEN2B *(48)*.

Offering and Providing Genetic Testing The underlying cause of MEN2 is a germline mutation in the c-*ret* proto-oncogene located at 10q11.2. Mutations have been identified in 90% of families studied. Many different mutations have been reported in families with MEN2A or FMTC. The underlying cause of MEN2B is a point mutation in codon 918 (exon 16). In cases of isolated MTC, up to 24% may be due to a c-*ret* mutation *(48,49)*. Patients known or suspected to have MEN2 are routinely referred for *RET* testing. This, however, does not guarantee that patients have a clear understanding of the implications of a positive result for themselves or their family. Genetic testing for affected and unaffected members of MEN2 families is considered standard of care, so the cost of testing is generally covered by insurance. This may make the decision

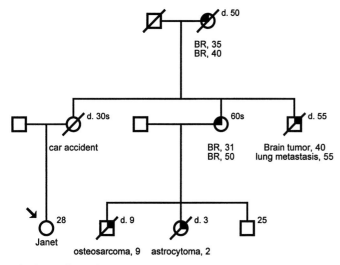

Fig. 2. Pedigree for Scenario A. Documented cancer history is consistent with Li-Fraumeni syndrome.

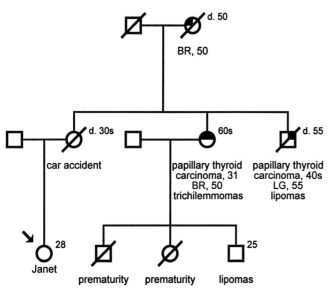

Fig. 3. Pedigree for Scenario B. Documented cancer history is consistent with Cowden syndrome.

about whether or not to have testing less complex than for other inherited cancer-susceptibility syndromes.

GENETIC COUNSELING CASE EXAMPLES

In addition to the challenges of obtaining an accurate family history and providing appropriate cancer-risk estimates, individuals may have significant difficulties coping with their at-risk status or communicating with other family members. This section presents five cases that illustrate specific counseling issues that can arise during a cancer genetic-counseling session. These cases are not based on specific patients, but have been compiled from multiple patient interactions.

IMPORTANCE OF CONFIRMING FAMILY HISTORY

Case Presentation Janet comes to your high-risk clinic with the following history. She has a maternal aunt who developed breast cancer at age 50 and is now in her 60s and a maternal uncle diagnosed with lung cancer at age 55 who died a few months later. Janet's aunt had three children, one son who is

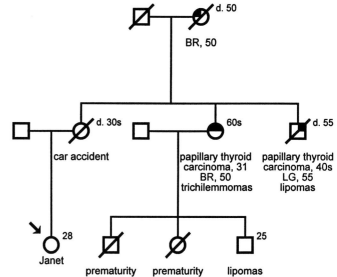

Fig. 4. Pedigree illustrating Scenario C. Documented cancer history not suggestive of a hereditary-cancer syndrome.

alive and well at age 25 and a son and daughter who are both deceased, cause of death unknown. Janet's uncle had no children. Janet thinks that her maternal grandmother had breast cancer in her 40s and died at age 50. Janet's mother never had cancer, but died in her 30s in a car accident. Pedigree is shown in Figure 1. This history shows two women in two generations who developed perimenopausal breast cancer. Thus, it may be appropriate to offer the family *BRCA1* and *BRCA2* analysis, following documentation of the cancer diagnoses. However, gathering this additional information might lead to different conclusions, as demonstrated in Scenarios A–C.

Scenario A Perhaps Janet's maternal aunt had bilateral breast cancer at ages 31 and 50 and Janet's maternal grandmother had bilateral breast cancer at ages 35 and 40. Janet learned that her maternal uncle died from lung metastases at age 55, having been diagnosed with a brain tumor at age 40. Lastly, it turns out that Janet's two cousins, who are deceased, were affected with childhood cancers; one with an osteogenic sarcoma at age 9 and one with an astrocytoma at age 2. A revised pedigree is shown in Fig. 2. This constellation of cancers fits with a diagnosis of Li-Fraumeni syndrome and it would be more appropriate to test the family for a *p53* germline mutation than a *BRCA1* or *BRCA2* mutation.

Scenario B Another possibility, shown in Fig. 3, is that Janet's aunt had papillary thyroid carcinoma (PTC) at age 31 and breast cancer at age 50. Upon further evaluation, Janet's aunt is also noted to have facial trichilemmomas. Janet's aunt had two children born prematurely, who died during infancy and has one living son who is noted to have lipomas. Janet's maternal uncle died from lung cancer at age 55, but had a history of PTC and lipomas. Janet's maternal grandmother was diagnosed with advanced-stage breast cancer at age 50. This pattern of cancer is consistent with Cowden syndrome, associated with germline mutations in the *PTEN* gene. If this is the case, then Janet should be carefully evaluated for signs of Cowden syndrome and her family can consider *PTEN* testing.

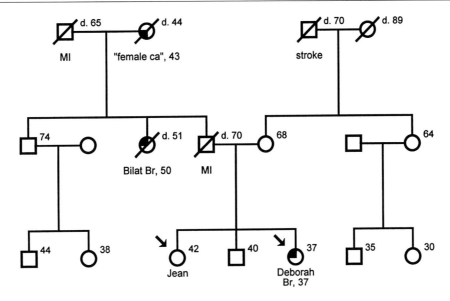

Fig. 5. Family history of hereditary breast/ovarian cancer syndrome.

Scenario C Finally, it is possible that medical-records documentation will not reveal a pattern of cancer that is suggestive of a hereditary cancer syndrome (Fig. 4). In further conversations with relatives, Janet learns that her maternal aunt had never had breast cancer, but rather had two benign breast biopsies at ages 48 and 50. Janet's aunt had three children, two of whom were born prematurely and did not survive. Janet's uncle, a heavy smoker, was diagnosed with lung cancer at age 55. Janet's grandmother did have breast cancer, but not until age 75. Based on this history, Janet's family would be extremely unlikely to have a mutation in a dominant breast-cancer susceptibility gene and Janet could follow general guidelines for cancer monitoring.

Outcome Janet was told that more information was needed before she could be given an accurate risk assessment. Specifically, she was asked to find out more information about her cousins, including the cause of death and age at death. The first step is for Janet to query the relatives who are likely to have more information about the diagnosis, that is the person affected with cancer or their first-degree relatives. The second step is for Janet to ask the relatives (or, if deceased, their next-of-kin) if they would be willing to send written documentation of the diagnosis to the high-risk clinic. Janet will be scheduled for a second clinic visit when the requested documentation is received or when it becomes clear that it will not be possible to document the family further due to lost medical records or estrangement in the family.

ISSUES RAISED BY THE OPTION OF BRCA1 TESTING

Case Presentation Jean comes to you because her younger sister, Deborah, was diagnosed with breast cancer three weeks earlier. Jean expresses her concern about being next and wants monitoring recommendations. Although she has always been aware of the family history of breast cancer, she feels especially vulnerable now that her sister has been diagnosed. Her sister is the first female relative in her generation to develop breast cancer. The family history, as shown in Fig. 5, is consistent with hereditary breast/ovarian cancer syndrome. Jean is given

monitoring suggestions and is told that her family is eligible for *BRCA1* and *BRCA2* testing. Jean's sister, Deborah, agrees to be tested and is found to have a *BRCA2* mutation. Jean has now returned to the high-risk clinic to have pre-test counseling and blood drawn for DNA analysis.

Counseling Issues During the session, the genetic counselor asks a standard set of questions to elicit Jean's current psychological state and whether she has a history of psychological problems. Jean replies that she is feeling somewhat unhappy right now, which she attributes to problems with her current job. Jean says that she was diagnosed with depression several years ago, but is not currently in therapy or taking medication. Two years ago, she made a suicide attempt after breaking up with her boyfriend, but denies any thoughts of suicide at this time. Jean insists that she is prepared to learn that she has the familial *BRCA2* mutation. However, she becomes quite tearful when talking about the treatment her sister is undergoing. Jean also admits that she becomes hysterical even thinking about the possibility that she will get breast cancer. The genetic counselor then asks Jean to imagine how she will react upon hearing that she does or does not have the gene mutation. Jean says that she will probably fall apart if her result is positive and will probably feel horribly guilty about her sister's diagnosis if the result is negative. In fact, she is not sure that she will tell anyone her results, because she has little contact with other family members and has few close friends. At the end of the discussion, Jean still wishes to proceed with testing. However, the genetic counselor is concerned about Jean's ability to cope with the genetic-testing results at this time in her life. Prior to blood being drawn, the genetic counselor discusses the situation with other members of the program staff, including the oncologist and psychologist.

Outcome The program personnel unanimously agree to defer Jean's participation in the testing program and the genetic counselor shares this decision with Jean. This decision is made based on Jean's history of untreated depression, fairly recent suicide attempt, lack of social support, and the stressful events

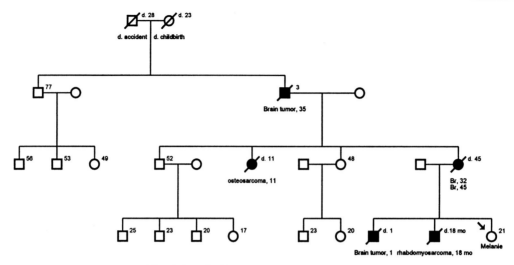

Fig. 6. Family history of Li-Fraumeni syndrome.

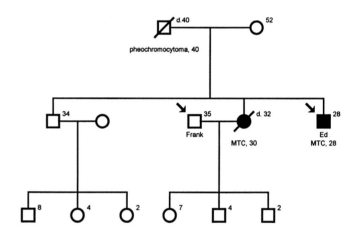

Fig. 7. Family history of multiple endocrine neoplasia type 2A (MEN2A).

going on in Jean's life right now. Although Jean is not happy with this outcome, she acknowledges that she would have a hard time dealing with a positive result and accepts the program staff's decision. Jean agrees to begin seeing a therapist and says that she will re-contact the program in a few months to resume testing. When Jean is telephoned three months later, she says that she has not yet contacted a therapist, but still plans to do so. About a year later, Jean re-contacts the testing program and asks to resume testing. She comes to her pre-test session with her boyfriend, who seems very supportive of her. Jean says that she has been in therapy and on anti-depressants for about four months. At the session, Jean seems to be doing quite well; she has changed jobs and her sister has completed her breast-cancer treatments and is in remission. She proceeds to be tested and learns that she does carry the familial gene mutation. Jean is saddened by this result, but is able to satisfactorily cope with the information.

UNCOVERING FAMILY SECRETS

Case Presentation Melanie comes to you to discuss her family history of cancer (Fig. 6). The family history is consistent with Li-Fraumeni syndrome, making the assessment of cancer risks straight-forward. However, the counseling issues in this case turn out to be much more difficult.

Counseling Issues During the genetic-counseling session, Melanie reveals that she only recently learned about the history of cancer in her family. When going through her mother's belongings after her death, Melanie had uncovered two baby books that she had never seen before. This discovery led to the realization that her mother had had two sons, who died of cancer during infancy. Melanie had never been told of their existence, as this had occurred prior to Melanie's birth. When Melanie probed her relatives for more information, she was further astounded to learn that she had an aunt who had cancer and died at age 11 and that her grandfather had not died in World War II as she had always been told, but rather from a brain tumor in his 30s. Melanie's grief over the recent death of her mother was compounded by her anger that her mother had never told her the truth about the family's history of cancer. She

felt the need to grieve for the two brothers she never knew she had and expressed the desire to obtain more detailed information about them (which unfortunately did not seem readily available). Melanie was extremely anxious about the risks of cancer for herself and her future offspring.

Outcome The emotional issues raised in this case were extraordinary and could not be dealt with in one genetic counseling session. The majority of the initial session was spent reviewing the information that Melanie had gathered and exploring her feelings about uncovering these family secrets. Melanie was encouraged to see a therapist so that she could continue to work through her feelings of grief, anger, and fear. A second genetic counseling session was scheduled a few weeks later to discuss the inheritance pattern and cancer risks associated with Li-Fraumeni syndrome.

FAMILY PRESSURES AND TIMING ISSUES

Case Presentation Frank comes to your high-risk clinic, because his wife developed MTC at age 30 and died six months ago from complications. Frank's primary motivation for coming to clinic is to learn whether his children are at increased risk for developing MTC. Frank is accompanied by his brother-in-law, Ed, who was diagnosed with MTC two weeks ago.

Counseling Issues As shown in Fig. 7, this family history is suggestive of MEN2. Although Frank wants to know as much as he can about MEN2, including the inheritance pattern and spectrum of problems in the syndrome, Ed remains quiet. During the discussion, the genetic counselor explains that genetic testing for MEN2 is available and that individuals found to have a c-*ret* mutation are recommended to have prophylactic thyroidectomies. Frank immediately asks to set up an appointment for his young children to be tested. Frank is told that c-*ret* testing first needs to be performed on a family member who has MEN2, but that his children can be tested once the specific c-*ret* mutation has been established for the family. Genetic testing is then offered to Ed, who is the only living member of his family with MEN2. He flatly refuses to be tested, stating that he already has MTC, so he does not see a benefit to having this information. Frank becomes forceful in pressuring Ed to be tested, which only seems to enrage Ed.

Outcome The genetic counselor asks to speak privately with Ed about the option of genetic testing, explaining to Frank that it is standard protocol to discuss testing on a one-on-one basis. After Frank leaves the room, Ed seems more comfortable asking questions about MEN2 and explaining why he does not want to have *RET* testing. Ed reveals that he is feeling overwhelmed about his cancer diagnosis, which has occurred less than a year after his sister died from the same disease and just two months prior to the date of his wedding. It becomes clear that Ed is not opposed to testing *per se*, but that the timing of the request is problematic. The genetic counselor assures Ed that this is not a decision that he needs to make right away and they agree to speak by phone in a few months and consider setting up a second counseling session. Frank agrees with this follow-up plan, once the rationale behind it is explained. After two telephone conversations, Ed asks to schedule a second genetic-counseling session. The genetic counselor meets with Ed, and his wife, to discuss *RET* testing. Ed has had no further health problems and seems much more interested in obtaining information about MEN2. He agrees to have c-*ret* testing and is found to have a deleterious mutation. He willingly shares this information with other family members as well as his brother-in-law, who promptly makes an appointment for his children to be tested.

HOW TO DISTINGUISH ATTENUATED FAP FROM HNPCC

Case Presentation Elaine, age 30, comes to the high-risk clinic because she is concerned about her family history of cancer. In taking the family history, she relates that her paternal grandmother had uterine cancer at age 58 and that her father, an only child, died at age 58 from colon cancer (Fig. 8). On autopsy, her father was found to have 70 polyps throughout his colon. Since then, Elaine and her siblings have undergone colonoscopy. Elaine has been found to have 50 polyps in her colon and has undergone a partial colectomy. Her brother, Charlie, has been found to have 40 colonic polyps. The differential diagnosis includes HNPCC and the attenuated form of FAP.

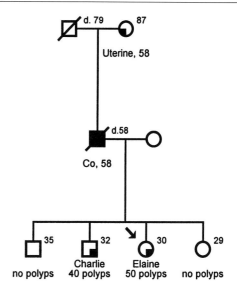

Fig. 8. Family history of multiple colonic polyps.

Counseling Issues At the clinic's request, Elaine has gathered medical records information on all her affected relatives and brought them to her appointment. When Elaine is told that her family history could represent HNPCC or FAP, she expresses frustration and anger that a definitive diagnosis cannot be made. Part of Elaine's anger stems from her fear about additional cancer risks. During Elaine's recent physical exam, her physician had mentioned that she may be at risk for developing extra-colonic tumors. This news was a complete surprise to her. She has come to high risk clinic in hopes of learning that this is not the case; however, she ends up having this information confirmed. Elaine is especially upset at the potential increased risk of uterine cancer (if the family has HNPCC), because she and her husband have decided to wait five years before having children. She wonders aloud if this still seems like a wise course to take, although she is not sure that they can afford to have a baby any earlier. Although Elaine expresses interest in genetic testing to obtain a definitive answer, she is concerned about the potential impact this information could have on her future insurability.

Outcome The genetic counselor discusses the potential impact that genetic information could have on Elaine's ability to obtain health or life insurance. Elaine is told that her genetic test result would remain completely confidential within the testing program and would not be placed in her medical record without her consent. She is also told that a positive result is likely to have little impact, given that she already has a significant risk factor for developing colon cancer (polyposis). Elaine decides that her need to obtain a definitive diagnosis outweighs her concerns about insurance and elects to undergo testing.

Elaine is found to have a truncated APC protein, which indicates that she has a germline *APC* mutation. This confirms that she has the attenuated form of FAP. Genetic testing is now available to her siblings and two of them elect to have testing. Elaine's grandmother also chooses to have genetic testing and does not have the truncation. Thus, her uterine cancer does not appear to be related to the cases of colon cancer or polyps in the family. As time passes, Elaine becomes less anxious about the risks of extra-colonic tumors, especially as her screening tests remain normal. She understands that she may need to have a total colectomy in the future. Elaine and her husband decide to follow their original plan and wait several years before starting their family, now that the risk of uterine cancer is not a factor. Lastly, the genetic counselor reminds Elaine that her future child(ren) could also develop attenuated FAP. The *APC* mutation may have come from Elaine's paternal grandfather or may represent a new genetic event in Elaine's father. In either case, Elaine will have a 50% chance of passing the familial *APC* mutation to each child.

REFERENCES

1. Schneider, K. A. and Marnane, D. (1997) Cancer risk counseling: how is it different? *J. Genet. Counseling* **6**:97–110.
2. Parker, S. L., Tong, T., Bolden, S., and Wingo, P. A. (1997) Cancer statistics, 1997. *CA: Cancer J. Clin.* **47**:5–27.
3. Easton, D. and Peto, J. (1990) The contribution of inherited predisposition to cancer incidence. *Cancer Surveys* **9**:395–416.
4. Raffel, L. (1998) Genetic counseling and genetic testing for cancer risk assessment. *Clin. Obstet. Gynecol.* **41**:141–156.
5. Peters, J. A. (1994) Familial cancer risk, Part II: breast cancer risk counseling and genetic susceptibility testing. *J. Oncol. Mgmt.* **Nov/Dec**:18–26.
6. Lynch, H., Lynch, J., and Fusaro, R. (1985) Clinical importance of familial cancer. *In: Familial Cancer: First International Research Conference on Familial Cancer* (Mueller, H. and Weber, W., eds.), Karger Publishers, New York, pp. 6–12.
7. Schneider, K. A. (1995) *Counseling About Cancer: Strategies for Genetic Counselors*, National Society of Genetic Counselors.
8. Love, R., Alida, E., and Josten, D. (1985) The accuracy of patient reports of a family history of cancer. *J. Chronic Disease* **38**:289–293.
9. Peters, J. and Stopfer, J. (1996) Role of the genetic counselor in familial cancer. *Oncology* **10**:159–166.
10. Offit, K. and Brown, K. (1994) Quantitating familial cancer risk: a resource for clinical oncologists. *J. Clin. Oncol.* **12**:1724–1736.
11. Richards, M. R. M., Hallowell, N., Green, J. M., Murton, F., and Statham, H. (1995) Counseling families with hereditary breast and ovarian cancer: a psychosocial perspective. *J Genet. Counseling* **4**:219–233.
12. Geller, G., Botkin, J. R., Green, M. J., Press, N.., Biesecker, B. B., Wilford, B., et al. (1997) Genetic testing for susceptibility to adult-onset cancer: The process and content of informed consent. *JAMA* **277**:1467–1474.
13. Knudson, A. G. (1971) Mutation and cancer: A statistical study of retinoblastoma. *Proc. Natl. Acad. Sci. USA* **68**:820–823.
14. Holtzman, N. A. and Watson, M. S. (1998) *Promoting Safe and Effective Genetic Testing in the United States: Final Report of the Task Force on Genetic Testing*. Johns Hopkins University Press, Baltimore.
15. McKinnon, W. C., Baty, B. J., Bennett, R. L., Magee, M., Neufeld-Kaiser, W. A., Peters, K. F., et al. (1997) Predisposition genetic testing for late-onset disorders in adults: a position paper of the National Society of Genetic Counselors. *JAMA* **278**:1217–1220.
16. Lerman, C., Hughes, C., Lemon, S. J., Main, D., Snyder, C., Durham, C., et al. (1998) What you don't know can hurt you: adverse psychologic effects in members of BRCA1-linked and BRCA2-linked families who decline genetic testing. *J. Clin. Oncol.* **16**:1650–1654.
17. Wiggins, S., Whyte, P., Huggins, M., Adam, S., Theilmann, J., Bloch, M., et al. (1992) The psychological consequences of predictive testing for Huntington's disease. Canadian Collaborative Study of Predictive Testing. *N. Engl. J. Med.* **327**:1401–1405.
18. Lynch, H. T., Lemon, S. J., Durham, C., Tinley, S. T., Connolly, C., Lynch, J. F., et al. (1997) A descriptive study of BRCA1 testing and reactions to disclosure of test results. *Cancer* **79**:2219–2228.
19. Bloch, M., Adam, S., Wiggins, S., Huggins, M., and Hayden, M. R. (1992) Predictive testing for Huntington disease in Canada: the experience of those receiving an increased risk. *Am. J. Med. Genet.* **42**:499–507.
20. Struewing, J. P., Lerman, C., Kase, R. G., Giambarresi, T. R., and Tucker, M. A. (1995) Anticipated uptake and impact of genetic testing in hereditary breast and ovarian cancer families. *Cancer Epidemiol. Biomark. Prevent.* **4**:169–173.
21. Schneider, K. A., Patenaude, A. F., and Garber, J. E. (1995) Testing for cancer genes: Decisions, decisions. *Nature Med.* **1**:302–303.
22. Botkin, J. R., Croyle, R. T., Smith, K. R., Baty, B. J., Lerman, C., Goldgar, D. E., et al. (1996) A model protocol for evaluating the behavioral and psychosocial effects of BRCA1 testing. *J. Natl. Cancer Inst.* **88**:872–882.
23. Offit, K. (1998) *Clinical Cancer Genetics: Risk Counseling and Management*. Wiley-Liss, New York.
24. Berry, D. A., Parmigiani, G., Sanchez, J., Schildkraut, J., and Winer, E. (1997) Probability of carrying a mutation of breast-ovarian cancer gene BRCA1 based on family history. *J. Natl. Cancer Inst.* **89**:227–238.
25. Ford, D., Easton, D. F., Bishop, D. T., Narod, S. A., and Goldgar, D. E. (1994) Risks of cancer in BRCA1-mutation carriers. Breast Cancer Linkage Consortium. *Lancet* **343**:692–695.
26. Struewing, J. P., Hartge, P., Wacholder, S., Baker, S. M., Berlin, M., McAdams, M., et al. (1995) The risk of cancer associated with specific mutations of BRCA1 and BRCA2 among Ashkenazi Jews. *N. Engl. J. Med.* **336**:1401–1408.
27. Wooster, R., Neuhausen, S. L., Mangion, J., Quirk, Y., Ford, D., Collins, N., et al. (1994) Localization of a breast cancer susceptibility gene, BRCA2, to chromosome 13q12-13. *Science* **265**:2088–2090.
28. Burke, W., Daly, M., Garber, J., Botkin, J., Kahn, M. J. E., Lynch, P., et al. (1997) Recommendations for follow-up care of individuals with an inherited predisposition to cancer. II. BRCA1 and BRCA2. *JAMA* **277**:997–1003.
29. Nelen, M. R., Padberg, G. W., Peeters, E. A. J., Lin, A. Y., van den Helm, B., Frants, R. R., et al. (1996) Localization of the gene for Cowden disease to chromosome 10q22-23. *Nature Genet.* **13**:114–116.
30. Eng, C. (1997) Cowden Syndrome. *J. Genet. Counseling* **6**:181–192.
31. Liaw, D., Marsh, D. J., Li, J., Dahia, P. L., Wang, S. I., Zheng, Z., et al. (1997) Germline mutations of the PTEN gene in Cowden disease, an inherited breast and thyroid cancer syndrome. *Nature Genet.* **16**:64–67.
32. Eng, C., Schneider, K., Fraumeni, J. F., Jr, and Li, F. (1997) Third international workshop on collaborative interdisciplinary studies of p53 and other predisposing genes in Li-Fraumeni syndrome. *Cancer Epidemiol. Biomark. Prevent.* **6**:379–383.
33. Varley, J. M., Evans, D. G. R., and Birch, J. M. (1997) Li-Fraumeni syndrome: a molecular and clinical review. *Br. J. Cancer* **76**:1–14.
34. Malkin, D., Li, F. P., Strong, L. C., Fraumeni, J. F. J., Nelson, C. E., Kim, D. H., et al. (1990) Germ-line p53 mutations in a familial syndrome of breast cancer, sarcomas, and other neoplasms. *Science* **250**:1233–1238.
35. Aarnio, M., Mecklin, J. P., Aaltonen, L. A., Nystrom-Lahti, M., and Jarvinen, H. J. (1995) Life-time risk of different cancers in hereditary non-polyposis colorectal cancer (HNPCC) syndromes. *Int. J. Cancer* **64**:430–433.
36. Vasen, H. F. A., Mecklin, J. P., Khan, P. M., and Lynch, H. T. (1991) The International Collaborative Group on Hereditary Non-Polyposis Colorectal Cancer (ICG-HNPCC). *Dis. Colon Rectum* **34**:424–425.
37. Rodriguez-Bigas, M. A., Boland, C. R., Hamilton, S. R., Henson, D. E., Jass, J. R., Khan, P. M., et al. (1997) A National Cancer Institute Workshop on Hereditary Nonpolyposis Colorectal Cancer Syndrome: meeting highlights and Bethesda guidelines. *J. Natl. Cancer Inst.* **89**:1758–1762.

38. Hamilton, S. R., Liu, B., Parsons, R. E., Papadopoulos, N., Jen, J., Powell, S. M., et al. (1995) The molecular basis of Turcot's syndrome. *N. Engl. J. Med.* **332**: 839–847.
39. Schwartz, R. A., Goldberg, D. J., Mahmood, F., DeJager, R. L., Lamber,W. C., Najem, A. Z., et al. (1989) The Muir-Torre syndrome: a disease of sebaceous and colonic neoplasms. *Dermatologica* **178**:23–28.
40. Lynch, H. T., Smyrk, T., and Lynch, J. (1997) An update of HNPCC (Lynch syndrome). *Cancer Genet. Cytogenet.* **93**:84–99.
41. Burke, W., Petersen, G., Lynch, P., Botkin, J., Daly, M., Garber, J., et al. (1997) Recommendations for follow-up care of individuals with an inherited predisposition to cancer. I. Hereditary nonpolyposis colon cancer. *JAMA* **277**:915–919.
42. de la Chapelle, A. and Peltomake, P. (1995) Genetics of hereditary colon cancer. *Ann. Rev. Genet.* **29**:329–48.
43. Edelmann, W., Yang, K., Umar, A., Heyer, J., Lau, K., Fan, K., et al. (1997) Mutation in the mismatch repair gene Msh6 causes cancer susceptibility. *Cell* **91**:467–477.
44. Peterson, G. M. and Brensinger, J. D. (1996) Genetic testing and counseling in familial adenomatous polyposis. *Oncology* **10**: 89–94.
45. Giardiello, F. M., Brensinger, J. D., Luce, M. C., Petersen, G. M., Cayouette, M. C., Krush, A. J., et al. (1997) Phenotypic expression of disease in families that have mutations in the 5' region of the adenomatous polyposis coli gene. *Ann. Intern. Med.* **126**:514–519.
46. Lynch, H. T., Smyrk, T., McGinn ,T., Lanspa, S., Cavalieri, J., Lynch, J., et al. (1995) Attenuated familial adenomatous polyposis (AFAP): a phenotypically and genotypically distinctive variant of FAP. *Cancer* **76**:2427–2433.
47. Neumann, H. P., Eng, C., Mulligan, L. M., Glavac, D., Zauner, I., Ponder, B. A., et al. (1995) Consequences of direct genetic testing for germline mutations in the clinical management of families with multiple endocrine neoplasia, type II. *JAMA* **274**:1149–1151.
48. Eng, C. and Ponder, A. J. (1997) Multiple endocrine neoplasia type 2 and medullary thyroid carcinoma. *In: Clinical Endocrinology,* 2nd rd. (Grossman, A., ed.), Blackwell Scientific Publications, London, pp. 637–652.
49. Eng, C., Clayton, D., Schuffenecker, I., Lenoir, G., Cote, G., Gagel, R. F., et al. (1996) The relationship between specific RET proto-oncogene mutations and disease phenotype in multiple endocrine neoplasia type 2. International RET mutation consortium analysis. *JAMA* **276**:1575–1579.

22 Molecular Genetic Diagnosis of Inherited Cancer Predisposition

ELIZABETH M. PETTY, MD AND BEVERLY M. YASHAR, PHD

OVERVIEW

The discovery of specific genes involved in human malignancy has grown at an exciting and unprecedented pace during the last decade of the 20th century. These discoveries were sparked by the 1990 launch of the Human Genome Project, whose goal to sequence the entire human genome (some 30,000–100,000 genes) was finished in draft form by the spring of 2000 *(1,2)*. Additionally, the explosion of innovative molecular genetic technology in the last quarter of the century, including development of recombinant DNA methods in the 1970s and the advent of the polymerase chain reaction (PCR) in 1985, has allowed investigators to characterize cancer genes more rapidly. Many of the laudable scientific advances in characterizing novel cancer genes have been, and continue to be, translated into clinically useful diagnostic and prognostic tests.

Some of the most widely applied types of clinical molecular testing in oncology involve the actual analysis of a specific DNA sequence or its resulting protein product. This chapter will largely focus on these DNA-based or RNA-based methods of molecular genetic testing for diagnostic and predictive testing of inherited cancer syndromes. However, it is important to note that other genetic tests have demonstrated significant utility in the investigation, detection, and management of human malignancy. Available genetic tests useful in oncology vary considerably, from those based on analysis of single nucleotide changes at the DNA level to those looking at large structural chromosome rearrangements. Traditionally, cytogenetic analysis of blood or bone marrow cells to detect particular translocations have been important in the diagnosis and management of various hematological malignancies *(3,4)*. For instance, identification of the so-called Philadelphia chromosome, which represents a translocation between the long arms of chromosomes 9 and 22 and creates a novel fusion gene (*bcr-abl*) involved in the oncogenesis of chronic myelogenous leukemia

(CML), is useful in establishing the diagnosis *(3,5)*. Molecular genetic tests, rather than cytogenetic studies, that specifically detect new fusion genes such as *bcr-abl* caused by translocations, are rapidly becoming more commonplace than routine cytogenetics in the analyses of these malignancies. In addition to being cost-effective, one strength of using highly sensitive PCR-based techniques to help evaluate malignancy is that the same test can be easily employed before, during, and after therapy to detect minimal residual disease that requires further intervention or treatment *(6,7)*. In some instances, genetic testing looks not at a specific gene, but rather at loss or gain of a specific genetic region in solid tumor tissue. Loss of heterozygosity (LOH) analysis detects changes in the copy number of one or more alleles in the tumor tissue compared to matched normal DNA samples from the same individual *(8)*. This type of genetic analysis provides a means of identifying novel tumor-suppressor genes. It also demonstrates clinical utility by helping to determine the prognosis of some malignancies. A prime example of this is demonstrated by the detection of chromosome 18q loss in colon cancer *(9)*. This finding is associated with a worse prognosis than for tumors that do not exhibit 18q loss that are otherwise at the same clinical stage. Alternatively, regions of genomic amplification associated with increased expression of an oncogene may be detected in some tumors and serve as prognostic markers. Thus, a wide array of different types of genetic tests have been employed in the analysis and management of malignant disease.

To date, the major impact of modern molecular genetics in clinical oncology has been in the improvement of our ability to predict, diagnose, and classify human malignancy *(10–12)*. Despite this, the actual number of proven, cost-effective and clinically useful molecular genetic diagnostic tests available at the start of the 21st century is relatively limited. Until recently, one of the largest roadblocks in the rapid and efficient translation of molecular genetic information into the development of sensitive, robust clinical DNA-based tests for cancer was secondary to limitations in the technology for cost-effective mutation screening. With innovative and increasingly automated

From: *The Molecular Basis of Human Cancer* (W. B. Coleman and G. J. Tsongalis, eds.), © Humana Press Inc., Totowa, NJ.

molecular genetic technology being developed, it is likely that these limitations will be significantly reduced. Armed with tremendous new knowledge about various cancer genes and significant advances in technology to manipulate and analyze DNA, RNA, and proteins, we are poised with the real potential to develop molecular genetic tests not only for clinical predictive and diagnostic testing, but also for more specific prognostic testing and potentially, as a rapid means of directing the development of specific gene therapies. With a deeper understanding of genetic mechanisms underlying the pathogenesis of cancer, the widespread use of DNA or molecular-based testing may become a practical reality for the rapid diagnosis and focused management of several types of malignancies, both inherited and sporadic. Future progress should provide new tools for predicting genetic risk and therapeutic responses, hopefully leading to a significant shift in medical therapy towards disease prevention. It is anticipated that our knowledge in this area will continue to skyrocket, ushering in a new era of molecular genetics in clinical oncology that will significantly alter the practice of oncology in the next century, especially in the areas of predictive-risk analysis, preventive management strategies, and anticipatory guidance. One of the biggest challenges of this millennium will be understanding, appropriately applying, and accurately interpreting the plethora of anticipated molecular diagnostic tests. A critical first step in using these tests effectively is understanding basic genetic principles as applied to clinical molecular genetic diagnostic tests.

INTRODUCTION TO CLINICAL DIAGNOSTICS

Most of the predictive clinical cancer-gene tests currently available have been developed for testing in families with clear inherited cancer-predisposition syndromes rather than general population-based mutation screening efforts. The main purpose of this chapter is to provide readers with basic information regarding the application of predictive molecular genetic tests for these syndromes and to help individuals learn to critically evaluate and appropriately utilize these molecular genetic tests. Rather than focusing on specific diseases and currently available tests, the emphasis will be on helping the reader consider not only what test might be most appropriate, but also when testing might be most appropriate. The fields of predictive and presymptomatic molecular genetic testing for late-childhood or adult-onset disorders such as cancer are relatively new areas in clinical medicine.

Presymptomatic testing implies that an asymptomatic individual who has a positive genetic test for a disease gene will, at some time in their life, develop symptoms of the disease if they live as long as their average anticipated life-span. Predictive testing implies that the test result will enable one to make a calculated prediction about the likelihood of an asymptomatic individual developing the disease over the course of their anticipated life-span. Therefore, simply stated, presymptomatic testing implies that one will get the disease if one has the mutation, whereas predictive testing helps determine only the likelihood that one will develop the disease. In general, because of the incomplete penetrance of most cancer gene mutations, genetic testing of asymptomatic individuals is most properly referred to as predictive testing and that term will be used in the

Table 1
Potential Uses of Molecular Diagnostic Testing in Clinical Oncology

Diagnostic
- Confirm or establish a specific clinical diagnosis
- Define clinical stage of tumor

Predictive
- Provide calculated risk assessment, anticipatory guidance, and preventive management in high-risk families and populations

Prognostic
- Determine genotype/phenotype correlations
- Increase understanding about disease course
- Monitor minimal residual disease

Therapeutic
- Develop specific molecular based interventions
- Determine course of therapy based on molecular phenotype

context of this chapter. Sometimes the term susceptibility testing is used in discussions of predictive testing. Susceptibility testing also implies that one is able to calculate an individual's risk of developing the disease for which they have inherited the gene. In general, however, susceptibility testing refers to testing for genetic mutations that have a very low penetrance and/or diseases that do not follow clear Mendelian inheritance patterns. It is important to bear in mind that the degree of penetrance will vary for each disease gene in question, and likely for different mutant alleles within a disease gene. Therefore, it is absolutely essential that both the patient and health-care provider fully understand that predictive genetic tests are probabilistic rather than deterministic in nature. The test results only help determine the specific probability or odds that an individual will develop a specific type of cancer by a certain age.

The early uses of molecular diagnostic testing for cancer, beginning in the 1990s, have been limited largely to predictive diagnostic testing in families at highest risk of developing cancer, but the potential and anticipated future uses are even broader (Table 1). Not only will molecular genetic testing likely be used to predict one's risk for developing cancer, but increasingly molecular genetic tests will be used to assess prognosis, classify tumor types, monitor disease progression, and guide appropriate therapeutic interventions, perhaps in the form of specific gene therapy. Unlike other inherited genetic diseases where mutation detection will generally only be performed once in a given patient, it is anticipated that DNA-based cancer-detection assays may frequently require multiple determinations; initially to establish a diagnosis and subsequently to monitor therapy and to detect early relapse. It is widely anticipated that for many malignancies, DNA-based mutation detection may soon be an extremely valuable tool for the pathologist because it may provide the most accurate and rapid means of establishing a precise diagnosis and prognostic classification of malignancy. New PCR-based assays are continually being developed for the detection of specific cancer cells. Precise DNA diagnosis may carry important implications for therapy and therapeutic trails. One of the most rapidly growing areas in genetic testing is in predictive genetic testing to determine those individuals who are at highest risk for developing a specific kind of malignancy.

This chapter will address issues that need to be considered prior to predictive genetic testing, familiarize readers with the basic strengths and weakness of widely used clinical molecular genetic tests, and provide readers new to genetics with a basic framework as to when, how, and why to consider genetic testing. It is not meant to be fully comprehensive or to provide specific details about any one genetic test, because both the discovery of cancer genes and the emerging technology to study these genes are evolving. The main purpose of this chapter is to give the reader insight into molecular genetic testing and to suggest appropriate approaches to applying molecular genetic testing that can be used in assessing one's inherited genetic contribution to cancer. The chapter is divided into three major sections, with the first section designed to help the reader think genetically and consider genetic events, genetic testing, and genetic counseling when confronting questions about cancer risks in the clinical or research setting. The second briefly reviews several types of molecular genetic tests and some of their general applications for use in the prediction of cancer risk. The final part of this chapter focuses on clinical applications of molecular diagnostic tests and appropriate uses and interpretations of genetic tests, including a discussion of important issues in genetic counseling and education as related to molecular genetic testing.

CLINICAL MOLECULAR DIAGNOSTICS AND CANCER GENETICS: BASIC CONCEPTS

As recently as a few decades ago, the concept that cancer is a genetic disease was relatively novel and discussed largely among research scientists, not clinical oncologists, despite several pieces of clinical evidence suggesting the familial nature of some cancers. Today, it is widely recognized by scientists, health-care professionals and, thanks to recent widespread publicity, the public, that malignancies arise and progress secondary to the accumulation of many different genetic events. Some of these genetic alterations can be passed on through the germline (egg and sperm cells) from generation to generation, and others arise in somatic cells during the life of an individual. The development of cancer is hypothesized to be a clonal, multistep process involving several genes and other environmental and hormonal factors *(8,13)*. Continued identification of novel genes involved in oncogenesis should help to elucidate their interrelated roles in the pathway of the malignant transformation of a normal cell. Ultimately, such knowledge will facilitate earlier detection, molecular-based classification of lesions, and improved medical management. The growing recognition of the importance of genetic make-up as a key risk factor for the development of cancer has stimulated significant interest among professionals and the public alike to learn more about how this genetic information can be used to predict, prevent, treat, and ultimately eradicate inherited human malignancy.

Genes play critical roles in the development of malignancy in individuals of all ages. The genetic influence on the expression of the disease, the phenotype, is often modified by associated environmental agents. The extent of genetic and environmental contributions vary depending on the specific malignancy being considered. In most cases of sporadic cancer it is likely that genetic and environmental factors interact to influence the phenotypic expression of cancer. Examples of sporadic cancers where known environmental risk factors make a significant contribution to development of the disease would include lung cancer and skin cancer. However, in most cancers the environmental factors are not well-defined and are poorly understood. To help determine if cancer is inherited and genetic testing is potentially indicated, it is necessary to get a detailed family history, consider the ethnic background of the individual, and to review all relevant medical records (including pathology reports, laboratory studies, and clinical summaries) of the patient. In some cases, it is necessary to fully evaluate and review medical records of other family members. Only a small percentage (<10%) of cancers are thought to be due to these inherited cancer pre-disposition syndromes *(13)*. Thus, only occasionally, a comprehensive family history will reveal a Mendelian-inheritance pattern (autosomal dominant) that suggests a discrete and significant single-gene contribution for a cancer-predisposition syndrome that has specific cancer-related risks associated with it. Sometimes, however, even when a strong genetic contribution exists within a family, a clear Mendelian pattern of inheritance will not be elucidated by pedigree review due to a number of factors, including the relatively small size of the family, the lack of accurate medical histories of relatives, incomplete penetrance of the gene, variable expression of the gene, and the occurrence of other sporadic cancers (phenocopies or common sporadic cancer that mimic an inherited cancer in families). These other factors often make it extremely difficult to ascertain a particular inherited-cancer syndrome even when it is present. Even if a clearly recognizable inherited cancer predisposition is strongly suggested by pedigree review, it may be difficult to determine which gene is the culprit gene that merits further diagnostic investigation due to the genetic heterogeneity that is seen in many of these syndromes, including early-onset breast/ovarian cancer and familial colon cancer.

In most cases of cancer, examination of the family history will not reveal any recognizable inherited predisposition because the vast majority of malignancies are sporadic with no clear single germline genetic event underlying their development. In fact, in up to 25% of individuals, a familial clustering of cancer may be ascertained by pedigree analysis that currently does not fit any recognizable Mendelian cancer-predisposition syndrome. Determining the genetic contribution of cancer for these individuals is quite complex. Providing DNA diagnostic tests for cancers that are multifactorial (meaning that environmental and other epigenetic factors make a strong contribution to development of the disease in combination with the underlying genetic constitution of an individual) or polygenic (meaning that the interaction of several genetic factors, including various modifying genes, contribute to the disease phenotype) remains challenging in both clinical and research settings. At present, our knowledge about cancer genetics and our ability to test for complex genetic interactions are not sophisticated enough to test for multifactorial and polygenic cancers. In this chapter the focus will be on the molecular diagnosis of inherited-cancer syndromes that have a relatively straightforward Mendelian-inheritance pattern, because these are the most clearly understood at present and they have significant implications for patients. It is important to remember that some of the same types of tests discussed here may have broader future uses for common cancers where the family history of the disease is not as significant, but where the ethnic background of an individual may suggest that they are at higher risk of carrying a germline mutation or even in sporadic tumors when we have a better understanding of phenotype and genotype correlations, including those of premalignant lesions.

To understand some of the important issues that need to be considered when applying molecular genetic tests, some basic concepts in cancer genetics must be understood. Cancer arises when cells escape normal growth regulation and differentiation, allowing cells to proliferate rapidly, invade surrounding tissue, and metastasize to distant sites. Activating mutations in growth-promoting genes (proto-oncogenes), inactivating mutations in growth controlling-genes (tumor-suppressor genes), and aberrant function of mismatch control (or DNA-damage recognition and repair genes) all have demonstrated roles in carcinogenesis (8,14,15). Tumor-suppressor genes have exhibited a prominent role in the majority of inherited solid-tumor malignancies. Mutations in any of these genes, however, may contribute to tumorigenesis.

Several different types of mutations implicated in tumorigenesis can be detected through molecular genetic testing. In the simplest sense, a mutation is simply an alteration of the DNA sequence. Such an alteration may be a benign variant (polymorphism) or a disease-causing alteration. Polymorphism literally means many forms and it is important to realize that, on average, every 1 in 500 bp of DNA varies between us. When talking about polymorphisms within a DNA sequence, it generally indicates a variation in the sequence, which is seen in >1% of the population that has no known negative impact on the individual. A disease-causing mutation means that the mutation occurs in an area of the genome where the critical function of a gene is altered, which causes or predisposes the carrier of the mutation to a disease. It is extremely important to distinguish accurately a polymorphism from a disease susceptibility or causing mutation as the implications are obviously quite different for the individual who has the alteration.

There are several different types of disease-causing mutations. Mutations may involve the coding regions (exons) of genes or the noncoding regions (such as promoters, regulatory elements, and splice sites) of genes. Many of the currently available clinical molecular tests only screen the coding regions of genes for mutations and, therefore, will miss any mutations that are not located within coding exons. It is therefore important to understand which parts of the gene are examined in any given molecular diagnostic test. Mutations are often classified by, and referred to by, the type of DNA change that has taken place (such as a single base pair change or substitution). Nucleotide or base-pair substitutions can be further subdivided into missense (meaning it changes the amino acid) or nonsense (meaning it creates a stop codon that prevents further translation of the gene) mutations. Although nonsense mutations often lead to aberrant, nonfunctional protein products due to a premature stop codon, the effect of missense mutations are

often less predictable. The actual biological effect of a missense mutation will depend on many factors, including how drastic the amino acid change is or how important that specific amino acid is in the ultimate structure and normal function of the protein. For instance, if the mutation involves an important conserved amino acid within a critical binding site, it will have a more profound effect than a mutation in a poorly conserved, redundant area of the gene. For instance, missense mutations in the c-*ret* proto-oncogene that predispose to medullary thyroid cancer most often occur in one of the five highly conserved cysteine rich regions, rather than in other areas of the gene (16). Although mutations can occur virtually anywhere in the human genome, regions rich in CpG dinucleotides are known as mutation hot spots due to their propensity for methylation and subsequent deamination changing the nucleotide base to create a missense mutation (17). Regions of CpG mutation hot spots have been reported in many genes including the *p53* gene (18). Germline mutations in *p53* cause the Li-Fraumeni cancer predisposition syndrome, which is characterized by various tumors including sarcomas, lymphomas, brain tumors, adrenocortical tumors, and breast adenocarcinomas (19).

Other types of mutations that have been described in cancer genes include small deletions or insertions that have variable effects depending on a variety of factors, including whether or not they are in frame (meaning they maintain reading frame for creation of an amino acid sequence) or if they change the reading frame, known as a frame-shift mutation. Frame-shift mutations are more likely to lead to major problems in translating a normally functional protein product due to the generation of new stop codons that prohibit creation of a full-length protein product. A variety of other mutations may arise and predispose one to cancer, including: 1) large deletions or insertions of additional DNA; 2) duplications of DNA sequence; 3) inversions of a segment of the DNA sequence; 4) alternative splice-site mutations, which cause different parts of the DNA sequence to be spliced together generating a different protein; 5) repeat expansions of tandemly arrayed short sequences of DNA; and 6) mutations in noncoding regions of the gene that may affect the processing of the gene. In most known cancer genes, many different types of mutations have been identified. Generally these mutations span, at a minimum, the entire coding region of the gene as seen in the early-onset breast/ovarian cancer genes, *BRCA1* and *BRCA2* (20–22; see also http://www.nhgri.nih.gov/Intramural_research/Lab_Transfer/Bic). Sometimes mutations may be localized within certain regions or particular exons of the gene as seen in *p53* (18) or c-*ret*, which is associated with medullary thyroid carcinoma (MTC) and multiple endocrine neoplasia type 2 (MEN2) (16).

The consequences of mutations can vary considerably. The effect of a mutation may cause no protein product to be made. It may create an abnormal protein product that is completely dysfunctional or that has a novel function to transform a normal cell into a frankly malignant cell. Mutations may affect amino acid sequence but not gene expression, produce an abnormal protein product, affect the level of gene expression, destroy all gene expression, reduce gene expression, or even cause increased aberrant gene expression. Given this, it is often difficult to predict the effect of any particular DNA change on the ultimate function of the gene let alone on the potential disease course or prognosis of any one individual. Thus, molecular genetic testing results that report a specific DNA alteration must always be interpreted in context of what is previously know about genotype/phenotype correlations of that particular mutation with consideration of the family history always in mind.

Clearly, basic molecular genetic principles are critically important concepts for today's health-care professionals to fully understand, especially given the fact that molecular genetics and familial risk factors are increasingly and appropriately emphasized in medical care. Given an understanding of the genetic mechanisms underlying malignancy, a clinician is much better equipped to provide accurate diagnostic, prognostic, and therapeutic measures for individual patients and other family members at risk. Preventive-screening programs, medical management based on genetic predisposition, specific genetic counseling, provision of accurate recurrence risks, patient education, and referral to appropriate support resources for patients and their at-risk relatives can be appropriately provided once the genetic basis of a disease is suspected or proven. Increasingly, the widespread utility of precise DNA diagnostic tests to predict disease will allow for earlier intervention to alleviate or modify the expression of a disease.

One example of this would be familial adenomatous polyposis (FAP), classically a highly penetrant autosomal dominant condition due to mutations in the adenomatous polyposis coli gene (*APC*) located on the long arm of chromosome 5 *(23,24)*. In its most typical form, the majority of individuals who have inherited one copy of the mutated gene from an affected parent will develop colon cancer in early to mid-adulthood after having multiple polyps that develop earlier, often in adolescence. Sometimes the colon cancer is associated with other noncolonic features such as desmoid tumors, osteomas, eye findings, and skin lesions. Individuals in these families benefit from genetic counseling and education to fully understand their risk of developing colon cancer, to undergo predictive genetic testing, if desired, and to allow specific presymptomatic intervention as needed. Currently, in over 80% of affected individuals, causative mutations can be identified, allowing highly accurate specific mutation testing for other family members. Specific preventive-management strategies, consisting of serial colonoscopies or total colectomies, are utilized to greatly reduce the risk of cancer in mutation carriers. Individuals who are found not to have the mutation seen in other affected family members are not only spared the worry of developing early-onset colon cancer, but also do not have to undergo the regular surveillance and surgical intervention at an early age that mutation carriers must face. Thus, it is very cost-effective to genetically test individuals at a relatively early age in a highly penetrant late-adolescent/early adult-onset disorder such as FAP. In addition to clearly inherited highly penetrant mutations in the *APC* gene responsible for FAP, recent recognition of a relatively common polymorphism associated with a hypermutable tract of DNA in the *APC* gene in Ashkenazi Jewish individuals has been demonstrated to confer an increased risk of colon cancer in individuals with the polymorphism *(25)*. Although individuals with this polymorphism are at increased

risk of colon cancer, it is likely that their risk is significantly lower than those individuals with a highly penetrant familial *APC* mutation. Understanding the relative risks for colon cancer associated with various DNA changes is critical for both physicians and patients as they may have profound effects on preventive-management strategies. Interestingly, a recent survey analyzing the appropriate use of *APC* mutation testing highlighted the continued need for involvement of professionals with expertise in genetics to provide appropriate genetic counseling and use of genetic *APC* testing for patients *(26)*.

Predictive molecular genetic testing can now be offered for a handful of inherited-cancer syndromes. Testing can be used in a variety of situations to serve various purposes, including molecular diagnostic confirmation of a disease process to facilitate more appropriate medical management and accurate recurrence-risk counseling, and predictive testing to more accurately determine one's risk of developing cancer. It is important to remember that genetic testing is an evolving process, with the development of increasingly more sensitive, specific, and cost-effective methods. The specific details of any one genetic test for a disease will not be addressed here, because it is likely that the methods and applications will continue to change, perhaps even moving largely to microchip and microarray technology to look at not only mutations in one gene but expression levels of many different genes through one microarray assay in the near future. Genetic testing-laboratory databases designed for health-care professionals are maintained online as detailed later in this chapter. Clinicians and researchers wanting to learn more about DNA testing can utilize online databases, consultation with local genetic centers, and information provided by national disease-associated organizations to ascertain current information about specific genetic testing for any disease in consideration.

MOLECULAR GENETIC DIAGNOSTIC TESTS: SPECIFIC EXAMPLES AND TECHNICAL CONSIDERATIONS

GENERAL CONSIDERATIONS The most appropriate type of genetic testing for a specific situation varies widely from an indirect method of analysis such as linkage analysis, direct mutation testing by screening DNA sequences for unknown mutations or doing a specific DNA test to look for a known mutation, to functional analyses of gene expression by looking at resultant gene-expression levels, protein products, or biochemical byproducts *(27–30)*. Each of the tests have their own strengths and weaknesses. The specificity and sensitivity of any one test may vary considerably from another genetic test for the same disorder. In cancer-predisposition syndromes where there is little or no genetic heterogeneity and the spectrum of potential mutations is well-understood (such as in the familial medullary thyroid carcinoma [FMTC] and MEN2 syndromes where mutations in the cystine rich exons of the c-*ret* proto-oncogene have been clearly implicated as causative), highly specific and sensitive mutation detection is available *(16)*. Additionally, in FMTC and MEN2A (a subtype of MEN2), there is a relatively clear benefit for the individual in knowing whether or not they have inherited this disease gene as presymptomatic management, including a total thyroidectomy and regular screening, will help significantly reduce the risk of early morbidity and mortality due to thyroid cancer *(16,29)*. For some disorders, such as hereditary non-polyposis colon cancer (HNPCC), an adult-onset autosomal dominant disease where genetic heterogeneity exists, clinicians may have to chose between a number of different types of available genetic-testing methods, identifying the most appropriate sensitive, specific, and cost-effective test for any one individual or family.

In HNPCC, defects in any one of at least four different mis-match repair (MMR) genes (*hMSH2* on chromosome, *hMLH1* on chromosome, *hPMS1* on chromosome 2, and *hPMS2* on chromosome 7) can cause the same clinical and pathological type of colorectal cancer *(23,24)*. Although one could feasibly screen each of these genes for particular mutations, it may be more cost-effective first to determine whether or not one of these genes is likely the culprit gene. Interestingly, mutations in these genes cause replication errors in DNA throughout the genome. The replication errors (termed RER) can be detected in tumors where the underlying genetic defect is in one of these DNA MMR genes *(23,24)*. Therefore, screening tumor DNA for the RER phenotype may be a more cost-effective approach in some individuals to initially determine if further specific mutational analysis of the MMR genes might be beneficial in a family.

In many cases where a disease gene has been cloned, the resulting DNA test often may be the most appropriate test to offer a patient; however, this is not always the case. Consider, for instance, a disease like multiple exostosis syndrome (an autosomal dominant disorder associated with abnormal benign bony growth during childhood) where approx 3% of affected individuals will go on to develop a chondrosarcoma in adult-hood *(31)*. The vast majority of affected individuals have an easily recognizable disorder in childhood based on physical examination. Genetically it is a heterogenous disorder, with at least three different loci implicated in causing the disease. Offering a genetic test to a clinically affected individual pre-senting for management of their symptoms provides no par-ticular clinical benefit to the patient, especially given the current lack of any genotype/phenotype correlations that could offer insight into the patient's prognosis. Such DNA testing, how-ever, would be quite appropriate to explore in an adult with multiple hereditary exostosis who is interested in prenatal test-ing of a pregnancy to determine whether or not the fetus has inherited the disease gene so that personal decisions regarding the continuation of the pregnancy can be made if desired.

It is critically important to remember that genetic testing encompasses more than a simple laboratory analysis; it needs to include pre-testing counseling and education, provision of informed consent, accurate interpretation of the test results and their implications, follow-up conveyance of test results, and post-testing education, management, and support. This is espe-cially true when DNA-based testing is used to more accurately determine a healthy individual's genetic risk as in preconceptual testing to determine carrier status of parents for a given inherited disease, or in predictive testing of an asymp-tomatic individual who, by virtue of their family history and/or their ethnicity, is at risk of having inherited a particular muta-tion and seeks to learn whether or not they have indeed inher-

Table 2
Examples of General Types of Molecular Diagnostic Tests

Indirect gene analysis
- Linkage studies
- Loss of heterozygosity studies
- Gene-amplification detection

Direct DNA mutation testing
- Scan for unknown mutations
- Direct analysis of known (previously reported) mutations

Functional assays of gene
- Analysis of a protein product
- Analysis of yeast or cellular gene expression

ited the mutation in question. In the future, it is likely that this type of predictive testing will be readily available for a wide variety of malignancies and the reasons for requesting this in-formation will be equally broad.

The types of molecular testing currently available can be divided into three main groups: indirect DNA analysis, direct mutation detection, and RNA-based functional assays as sum-marized in table (Table 2). Technically, the analysis of protein products and functional assays could also be considered a form of indirect testing as the specific disease-causing DNA muta-tion is not identified. However, given that the functional assays currently used in cancer diagnosis demonstrate a gene-specific abnormal product, it seems they are best left in their own clas-sification. It is anticipated that functional-based genetic tests will be some of the most widely applied genetic diagnostic methods in the near future as they may be more readily applied to large population-based screening in disease such as breast cancer where no predominant mutations have been identified in the cloned cancer genes. Because the field of genetic testing in cancer is an evolving, rapidly growing field, it is anticipated that the exact methods and actual scope of molecular genetic-based cancer genetic testing will undoubtedly be different at the time this is being published from the time it was written. Thus, the goal of this section is to introduce the reader to some basic concepts and the general utility of the currently available methods.

INDIRECT MUTATION ANALYSIS

Linkage Analysis Molecular genetic diagnoses are largely dependent on knowing the specific genetic region involved in a given disorder. Localization of a disease gene to a well-de-fined genomic region often enables a form of diagnostic testing based on genetic linkage in a family. Linkage analysis is an indirect method for tracking the inheritance of a disease gene by analyzing the transmission of intragenic or flanking markers linked to a specific disease gene through members in a family to determine if an individual inherited the genetic region or haplotype that segregates with the disease from an affected parent *(32–34)*. The power and reliability of linkage analysis is based in part on knowing the genetic distance, or the recombi-nation rate, of the genetic markers traced through the family from the disease gene. The recombination rate is determined by analyzing the rate of crossing over between genetic regions in chromatids during meiosis. Obviously, the closer the markers are to the disease gene and the more markers that are used, the more robust this type of testing will be. For cloned genes, intragenic markers may be utilized to decrease the possibility of recombination between the mutation and the markers studied. The results of linkage analysis are computer-analyzed using sophisticated analytical software that calculates the likelihood that a person inherited a disease gene from an affected parent. For accurate linkage analysis in the diagnosis of a disease, there must be a precise clinical diagnosis and no, or limited, genetic heterogeneity.

Predictive linkage analysis can be offered to individuals who have a clear family history of cancer and multiple affected members. Before one can determine that an individual within a given kindred has inherited a disease haplotype, it is essential that there is clear evidence of linkage in that family to the disease locus being tested. If there is no genetic heterogeneity, linkage analysis can be used in relatively small families, but for linkage analysis where significant genetic heterogeneity exists, it is essential to study many family members in order to determine the likelihood that the correct gene is being tracked in the family. Generally to establish linkage with odds of approx 1,000 to 1 (a LOD score of 3.0), analysis of at least 10 individuals are needed (32–34). In cases where fewer individuals are available, a computer generation of probability for risk of developing cancer is calculated.

Although the exact methods for linkage analysis are beyond the scope of this chapter, it is important to note that this type of genetic-linkage testing is dependent on many variables, which must be considered in the computer analysis including allele frequencies for the markers used (which may vary in different ethnic populations), the penetrance of the disorder for the ages of the individuals in the analysis (known as the liability classes), and prior probability that this family's cancer is caused by a mutation in the particular gene being studied (34). Inherent potential problems in linkage analysis include problems or errors in typing due to nonpaternity, formation of new alleles, misclassification or diagnosis of affected individuals who may have a sporadic phenocopy of the disease, and misclassification of nonexpressing gene carriers as unaffected. At present, given the genetic heterogeneity of many inherited cancer syndromes and the increasingly available cost-effective specific mutation-detection methods, it is doubtful that genetic-linkage testing will be clinically robust for the vast majority of individuals with cancer. It may remain very useful, however, for a small subset of individuals, perhaps for individuals in large kindreds with clear inherited-cancer syndromes where no specific mutation can be identified or when the specific disease gene has been mapped but not yet been cloned or characterized.

DIRECT MUTATION DETECTION

Screening for Unknown Mutations DNA-based detection of unknown mutations is a complex task and methods to do this are evolving rapidly to improve the specificity, sensitivity, and cost-effectiveness of tests (27–29,35,36). The type of test employed depends largely on the size of the genetic region or gene being studied, whether or not there is a hot spot of mutations in a particular region, the kinds of mutations that have been identified, and the type of template available for analysis. Increasingly, tests are being designed for maximal automation.

In any of the readily available methods for mutation screening, it is important to remember that the absence of detecting a mutation does not rule out the possible existence of a disease-causing mutation in that gene. With most available methods, mutations may be missed because the entire gene (including coding and noncoding regions and regulatory elements) is not generally studied due to current technical limitations and costs of the available technology. Also, none of the techniques currently used are 100% sensitive. Further development of automated methods including continued development and utilization of DNA microchip and microarray assays may increase the likelihood of more extensive and comprehensive mutation screening in the near future.

Several methods for mutation screening have been developed over the last decade of the 20th century that are largely rooted in PCR methodology. PCR involves designing synthetic oligonucleotides (primers) flanking a specific DNA region or sequence of interest and subjecting a DNA sample and primers to thermocycling to synthesize many new copies of that DNA sequence for further analysis often by electrophoresis (size separation in a gel). The DNA substrate for starting material can be minutely small, even one nucleus, and be derived from any nucleated tissue. Briefly described below are just some of the methods that are currently being employed in both research and clinical settings. More extensive reviews of the applications of these techniques can be found in standard molecular genetic laboratory manuals (37). When ordering a test from a laboratory, it is important to know what method of mutation detection is being used and, specifically, what the reported sensitivity and specificity of the test is in that particular laboratory.

Direct Automated Sequencing High-throughput, automated sequencing is a first-line reliable, rapid, and cost-effective method to detect unknown or previously unidentified mutations. It is used to screen for mutations in many research and clinical laboratories. Several methods of sequencing are currently available with one of the most commonly used automated forms based on a combination of dideoxy-sequencing and PCR reactions, known as cycle-sequencing (38,39). Full-scale sequencing of the coding regions of large transcripts such as that seen in *BRCA1* or *BRCA2* is available. In other cancer genes that clearly demonstrate hot spots for mutations, such as the *p53* gene or c-*ret* proto-oncogene, sequencing specific exons is an excellent predictive clinical diagnostic test. If a sequence abnormality is detected, however, it is still absolutely necessary to determine if the sequence alteration is truly a disease-causing mutation rather than a benign polymorphism. Analysis of the DNA variation in nonaffected individuals can help establish whether or not the mutation represents a benign polymorphic variant, but unless the sequence can be predicted to cause a significant disruption in the resulting gene product, is shown to segregate with a disease phenotype within a family, or if abnormal functional assays can be determined, there may still be questions regarding the significance of a particular base-pair change. Oftentimes sequencing is used as a second step in actual mutation detection after the mutation containing region is sub-localized in the gene by one of the following or other related PCR-based methods for mutation screening.

Advances in microarray and solid microchip-hybridization technology for analyzing sequences using hybridization of a target sequence from a patient to millions of arrays of small oligonucleotides, fixed on a small solid support representing the entire normal sequence of a gene and potentially all the known sequence mutations of the putative culprit gene, may become an optimal way for screening sequences at a much more rapid pace than current automated methods (40–43). Research demonstrating the utility of this method in analysis of BRCA1 mutations has been reported and commercial companies are developing this technology with anticipation of widespread use for molecular diagnostics (40).

Single-Stranded Conformation Polymorphism and Heteroduplex Analysis Single-stranded conformation polymorphism (SSCP) analysis is one widely used PCR-based method of detecting conformational changes in single-stranded DNA (ssDNA) sequences, which are caused by a change in the underlying nucleotide sequence. The mobility of ssDNA during electrophoresis is affected by both its linear size or length (number of nucleotides) and its shape or conformation (folding of the ssDNA) (44). Alterations in this mobility reflects a change in the DNA sequence of the gene, either a benign polymorphism or a disease-causing mutation. For this type of analysis a relatively small PCR product from the genetic region of interest is labeled, denatured to ssDNA, and electrophoresed through a nondenaturing gel (45–47). Modifications of this technique have demonstrated that variations in the gel composition and analysis at different temperatures can greatly influence the sensitivity of this technique (44,45). The technique is most robust when the target DNA sample is less than 300 bp in length. In general, PCR-based SSCP analysis is relatively easy to perform with standard molecular genetic laboratory equipment, but is variable in sensitivity anywhere from 60–99% dependent on gel and electrophoresis conditions (45,46). This technique has demonstrated utility in screening BRCA1 and BRCA2 mutations but is often combined with other techniques such as concurrent analysis of heteroduplexes.

Heteroduplexes are new complexes of double-stranded DNA (dsDNA) that form from two ssDNAs that have some difference in their DNA sequence. These heteroduplexes migrate at a different rate through the gel than homoduplexes (dsDNA from ssDNA with exactly the same sequence). By itself, heteroduplex detection is a relatively simple PCR-based detection method that is based solely on the slower migration of heteroduplexes vs homoduplexes through a polyacrylamide gel. Samples are amplified, denatured, renatured to allow the formation heteroduplexes, if the ssDNA strands in the sample do not match exactly, and analyzed by mobility through a polyacrylamide gel (48). This method has been used to detect both small deletions/insertions as well as single-base changes. There is wide variability in the reported sensitivity of the mutation-detection rate. Both of these methods, SSCP and heteroduplex analysis, either singly or combined, are widely used in laboratories to screen for mutations, but they do not define the specific DNA mutation, only provide a clue that a mutation is present. Further sequencing of the aberrant band(s) must be done in order to identify the specific mutation. It is likely that these kinds of screening methods may be phased out as more

specific and sensitive sequencing technology is developed and made cost-effective.

Restriction Endonuclease Fingerprinting Restriction endonuclease fingerprinting is a modified method of SSCP that was originally designed to detect all mutations in an approx 1 kb segment of DNA (49). It has been applied to detection of mutations in several genes including the p53. In this method a region of genomic DNA is amplified by PCR and then cleaved in separate reactions by different groups of restriction enzymes. The digested DNA fragments are then end-labeled and electrophoresed through a nondenaturing gradient gel as in SSCP analysis. A ladder of single-stranded fragments are then produced and analysis of differences of both restriction-digest patterns and SSCP mobility shifts between patients and controls can be analyzed. As with the other methods described earlier, the detection of a mutation in this manner does not identify whether or not this is a benign polymorphism or a disease-causing mutation. Another related method known as dideoxy fingerprinting, which combines modified sequencing and SSCP components, has demonstrated usefulness in screening p53 for mutations (50).

Denaturing Gradient Gel Electrophoresis Denaturing gradient gel electrophoresis (DGGE) is another PCR-based method that is based on the difference in migration of dsDNA through a unique polyacrylamide gel containing a gradient of chemical-denaturing agents (51–53). Migration is dependent on the nucleotide sequence and composition of the dsDNA. The specific place in the gradient where the strands separate (denature) will depend on its nucleotide composition. Therefore, single-base mutations in DNA sequence can potentially alter the denaturing behavior of the dsDNA, alter its migration through the gel, and subsequently be detected as an abnormally migrating band when compared to normal samples treated in the same fashion. Many modifications of the general DGGE procedure have taken place to improve its sensitivity. One method widely employed is to use PCR to artificially add a GC-rich region on the DNA sample (52). This GC-clamp, which has a very high denaturing domain, enables a more uniform, sensitive detection of other mutations within the genetic region of interest. Other modifications of DGGE are development of a temperature-based gradient gel electrophoresis, rather than a chemically based denaturing system.

Chemical-Mismatch Cleavage Analysis Unlike the aforementioned PCR-based techniques for mutation detection, chemical-mismatch cleavage will theoretically detect close to 100% of the mutations in a gene and will also localize the specific mutation, obliterating the need for further sequence analysis (54). In addition, longer stretches of DNA can be analyzed at one time (roughly on the order of up to 1 kb). The basic principle behind this technique is relatively simple. Mutations are detected by a series of chemical reactions that cleave one strand of DNA. It is based on the concept that alkylating chemicals covalently link to single-stranded nucleotides. Generally hydroxylamine is used to link to ss cytosine and osmium tetroxide is used to link to thymine. Following exposure to piperidine, alkylated residues are cleaved. Therefore, if a DNA heteroduplex is formed with one normal strand and one mutated strand, after exposure to the alkylating chemicals and piperidine, a single-stranded cleavage will occur at the point of the mutation. Analysis of the resulting product on a sequencing gel will detect the exact site and type of mutation. Although this form of mutation detection is quite accurate and useful for screening relatively large DNA fragments, it is relatively complex to perform and involves working with several hazardous substances. An alternative method to detect single base-pair mutations is based on the cleavage of heteroduplexes by the use of enzymes such as bacteriophage T4 resolvases or endonucleases (55,56).

Analysis of Large Rearrangements by Southern Analysis Southern blotting followed by hybridization using a gene-specific probe is still a good, reliable, and relatively inexpensive way to screen for genetic changes that are due to large gene rearrangements or abnormalities such as large deletions, gene duplications, or inversions. Large rearrangements have been described in several genetic disorders, but they have not been widely reported as a germline mutational mechanism in inherited cancer-predisposition syndromes. One exception, however, is in the gene on chromosome 3 that is responsible for the autosomal dominant von Hippel Lindau (VHL) cancer-predisposition syndrome where renal carcinomas may develop (57–59). In VHL, approx 15% of the causative mutations are large rearrangements that can be detected by Southern-blot analysis (60). In this method, restriction digests of genomic DNA are transferred to a nylon membrane by Southern blotting, and hybridized to a gene-derived probe. Detection of a novel band on the blot reveals an alteration of the gene.

Direct DNA Detection of Known Mutations Once a gene is identified and specific mutations are isolated, sensitive DNA testing can often be conducted to specifically detect previously reported mutations within the gene. In some disorders where one mutation in a given gene accounts for all cases of the disease, such as the single base-pair mutation in the beta hemoglobin gene, which causes sickle-cell anemia, the resultant DNA testing is relatively straightforward. Although there are no known inherited cancer-predisposition syndromes that are the result of only one particular mutation, there are some cancers where a significant number can be accounted for by a handful of mutations. An example of this are the mutations in the specific *BRCA1* and *BRCA2* genes that account for the majority of inherited breast/ovarian cancer in Ashkenazi Jewish women.

In this case, a DNA test is based simply on the hybridization of complementary strands of DNA where the nucleotide adenine always pairs up with thymidine and guanine pairs up with cytosine. One way of doing this test is a dot-blot or slot-blot where DNA from a patient is blotted onto a nylon membrane or other solid support, denatured, and hybridized with a labeled synthetic allele specific oligonucleotide (ASO), which is complimentary to either the mutant or normal sequence (61). DNA from a homozygous affected individual would only hybridize with the mutant probe, a homozygous normal individual would hybridize only with the normal probe, and a heterozygous individual would hybridize with both probes. A reverse dot-blot or slot-blot works much the same way except that the synthetic DNA strands representing the wild-type and mutated sequences are fixed to the membrane and patient DNA samples are labeled and used to probe the membrane. The advantage of the reverse

dot-blot is that it can be used repeatedly and can contain a number of different mutations. This type of clinical testing is amenable to DNA diagnosis of a disease where a relatively few number of mutations account for the vast majority of disease. In this type of testing, DNA samples from patients can be screened rapidly for disease-causing mutations that have been previously identified in other individuals.

Other DNA diagnostic methods to analyze known mutations include designing specific PCR primers to amplify only mutant or wild-type sequence or using restriction enzymes that will cut only mutant or wild-type sequence. These methods are based on the finding that one mutation, or a limited number of mutations, cause a specific disease within the population or within a specific ethnic group. This type of testing is widely applied to screening for three common breast-cancer gene mutations in the *BRCA1* and *BRCA2* genes that have been identified in approx 2.5% of the general Ashkenazi Jewish population, and in nearly three quarters of Ashkenazi Jewish women with breast cancer (62). With advancing microchip technology, it is anticipated that hybridization assays based on reverse dot blots will be a very cost-effective method of screening for hundreds of different specific mutations in one or more genes with one relatively simple and inexpensive test.

FUNCTIONAL DETECTION OF MUTATIONS Because there are a plethora of different mutations that may cause cancer, even within a single gene, it is becoming apparent that direct mutational screening may not be the most sensitive and cost-effective way to rapidly detect mutations for many cancer genes. For this reason, techniques that look beyond the actual gene sequence to its protein product or its functional biochemical or cellular properties are being developed and applied as potential alternatives to actual DNA testing for many disorders. Just as the mutation that causes sickle-cell anemia causes a specific protein abnormality that can be detected by protein electrophoresis, many mutations that give rise to cancer may also produce abnormal proteins, which can be detected by protein analysis or electrophoresis. In cancers associated with Li-Fraumeni syndrome where mutations of the *p53* gene are responsible, functional assays in yeast along with DNA sequencing have been utilized to detect at-risk family members (63). It is likely that further functional assays and protein-based studies will be developed for cancer detection and monitoring. The main advantages of functional assays are that they detect only mutations that cause an aberrant or dysfunctional protein product.

Protein Truncation Test The protein truncation test (PTT), which is also known as in vitro transcription and translation assays or (IVTT), is a method for analysis of aberrant proteins that has been diagnostically useful and commercially applied in the analysis of several genes associated with solid tumors including the *APC*, *BRCA1*, and *BRCA2* (64). The majority of mutations identified in these genes are predicted to create a truncated protein product that can be assayed for diagnostic purposes. PTTs are relatively simple to perform and are based on the in vitro transcription and translation of the gene (65). In brief, the gene region is amplified by PCR with modified primers, which contain a T7 promoter along with an eukaryotic translation sequence. Coupling of the PCR product with a reticulocyte lysate system (commercially available) allows in vitro translation. The translation products can then be analyzed on a polyacrylamide gel. This procedure is relatively quick and has immediate clinical relevance as the effect of the DNA mutation is detected and its approximate position is revealed.

Yeast Functional Assays The use of yeast-expression assays as a system for the functional testing of mutations causing human disease is being explored in research laboratories for several different genes and is being applied clinically for detection of some cancer-gene mutations. The basic principle of these assays is that many human disease genes can be expressed in yeast or other cells and be detected by altering the yeast or cellular phenotype. Functional mutations of the *p53* have been identified in yeast assays *(63,66)*. Currently, this type of testing is being offered commercially for detection of *p53* mutations in the molecular diagnostics of breast cancer in individuals where Li-Fraumeni syndrome is present in the family or individual patient.

CLINICAL APPLICATIONS IN PREDICTIVE GENETIC TESTING

Historically, a genetic disease has been defined by a single gene mutation that is inherited through the germ line following the laws of Mendelian inheritance. For inherited conditions with complete penetrance, carriers will manifest the full symptoms of the genetic disease. For most of the known cancer-susceptibility syndromes, however, the degree of penetrance is reduced compared to other common genetic syndromes. In fact, inheritance alone does not guarantee that a carrier will develop cancer. The risk of oncogenesis for inherited cancer syndromes is dependent on the form of the mutant allele and is modified by other genes and poorly understood dietary, lifestyle, and environmental factors. The incomplete penetrance of the known inherited cancer syndromes means that the results of molecular tests that screen for the presence of a mutation are not diagnostic but rather predictive. Genetic testing can detect a specific change in a unique DNA sequence, in a region of the chromosome or in the product of a cancer-susceptibility gene, and provide a concrete result that diagnoses the form of the inherited cancer-susceptibility gene. The clinical application of the test requires translation of these molecular results into an estimate of the risk of developing cancer at some future time. This is quite distinct from a traditional diagnostic test, which is ordered when a patient exhibits clinical symptoms that suggest a specific disorder. Commonly, the results of a diagnostic test are used to provide an explanation for the physiological symptoms of a patient. In contrast, predictive genetic tests are usually ordered on a healthy individual who, on the basis of family history, is at risk of developing cancer. For these individuals the test results are not deterministic; rather, they define the probability that inheritance of a germline mutation will result in the development of a specific cancer syndrome at a later point in the life of the individual. The benefits of having this predictive information are often strong, but in many cases the attendant risks are equally great and not yet fully understood. The decision to order a predictive genetic test requires consideration of unique medical, psychological, and societal concerns.

Table 3
Critical Components of Predictive Molecular Diagnostic Testing

Pre-test
- Obtain and confirm a detailed family history
- Review newest literature on suspected cancer syndrome and evaluate available tests
- Provide education about the disease process
- Provide risk estimates of gene inheritances and cancer susceptibility
- Discuss test specifics: benefits and risks
- Provide counseling
- Discuss management options including alternative approaches

Test
- Obtain and document informed consent
- Ensure that test is properly performed, documented, and shipped or delivered to the appropriate laboratory

Post-test
- Convey and interpret results in person
- Provide post-test education and counseling in person
- Ensure appropriate follow-up medical management and support
- Make referrals

This section is focused on clarifying some of these complex issues.

WHEN IS GENETIC TESTING INDICATED?

Guidelines for Cancer Genetic Tests The identification of new genes has become a fairly common occurrence in cancer genetics. Almost concurrent with these discoveries has been the introduction of commercially available predictive genetic tests. It is essential to ensure that the commercialization of cancer genetic testing does not become a driving force that mandates the decision to offer these tests to patients *(67)*. A patient's decision to undergo cancer genetic testing must be moderated by careful evaluation of the benefits and the potential risks this knowledge can present. For each inherited cancer syndrome there are unique clinical issues and specific test limitations. Given the state of flux of cancer genetics and predictive genetic testing as well as individualized psychosocial considerations, only the most general guidelines are appropriate for defining when a predictive genetic test should or should not be offered. Critical components of predictive molecular diagnostic testing are outlined in Table 3. The American Society of Clinical Oncologists (ASCO) recommends that predictive cancer testing only be offered when there is: 1) a strong family history of cancer, 2) the genetic test is one that can be adequately interpreted and 3) the results of the test will influence the medical management of the patient and/or family member *(68)*.

Presently only a handful of tests fulfill ASCO criteria, however, as our understanding of other cancer-susceptibility syndromes expands, more tests will satisfy these requirements. The current list of predictive genetic tests that are appropriate cancer-susceptibility screening tools will be outdated by the time this book becomes available. Thus, the evaluation of whether or not it is appropriate to offer testing for an inherited cancer syndrome to an individual must be based on not only the family history, but also on the most current information on the

Table 4
Which Cancers are Appropriate to Consider for Molecular Diagnostic Testing?

	Group one	Group two	Group three
Inheritance?	Family history consistent with inherited cancert	Family history consistent with inherited cancer	Family history not consistent with inherited cancer
Predictive value of genetic test?	Strong	Moderate	Questionable
Value in knowing carrier status?	Clear	Possible	Unknown
Syndrome (Gene)[a]	• FAP (*APC*) • MEN2A (c-*ret*) • MEN2B (c-*ret*) • Retinoblastoma (*Rb1*) • von Hippel Lindau (*VHL*)	• HNPCC (*hMSH2, hMLH1, hPMS1, hPMS2*) • Early-onset breast/ovarian cancer (*BRCA1, BRCA2*) • Li-Fraumeni (*p53*) • ?Familial melanoma (*p16^{INK4A}*)	• ? Familial melanoma (*p16^{INK4A}*) • Hereditary telangiectasia (*ATM*)

[a]Potential classifications as of February, 1998.

molecular basis of the syndrome, the clinical significance of the test and the potential efficacy of early diagnosis, existing surveillance and management regimes. These fundamental criteria are the basis for the test categories in Table 4. This table is based on ASCO guidelines and is meant to provide a framework within which the specifics of a predictive genetic test can be considered, but should not be used to make absolute determinations of when testing will be useful. It is anticipated that modifications to these criteria, groupings, and representative syndromes will need to be made as we gain more experience in utilizing predictive genetic tests. Ultimately the decision to undergo cancer genetic testing must be shaped by the specific concerns of the individual. The merits of a specific predictive test should be decided on an individual basis for each patient and their families.

Predictive tests for cancers in Group One have the greatest potential positive value. The patterns of cancer inheritance in the family are a key component in achieving a successful test outcome, so analysis of the pedigree should be consistent with a well-defined hereditary syndrome. The cancer-susceptibility test should be one which has proven predictive value. Attainment of this criteria is dependent on clear establishment of the molecular basis for the syndrome, linkage of cancer susceptibility to a specific gene(s), and a clear understanding of what constitutes a disease-causing mutation. This body of information results in a genetic test with high sensitivity and specificity. Genetic testing for inherited cancers in this group should be considered a standard of medical care. Finally there should be clear benefits in determining the carrier status of an individual. The medical care of both carrier and noncarrier of a susceptibility mutation should be influenced by the test results. As of 1998, inherited cancer syndromes for which predictive genetic tests fulfill Group One criteria include FAP, MEN2A, MEN2B, retinoblastoma, and VHL Syndrome.

Moderate confidence in the predictive value of the test provides the distinction between Group One and Group Two. In Group Two, the inherited cancer syndrome should be linked to a cancer-susceptibility gene(s), but not all cases of these inherited cancers can be explained by mutations in these genes. This allelic and genetic heterogeneity reduces the predictive value of the test. To maximize the usefulness of Group Two predic-

tive genetic tests, these tests should only be offered to individuals from families where the patterns of inheritance are consistent with a hereditary-cancer syndrome. The predictive power of the test will also be increased if a mutation is identified in an affected family member prior to screening unaffected individuals. As for Group One cancers, a negative test result for a known family mutation can have considerable medical and psychological value and a positive test result may result in the initiation of earlier surveillance or consideration of preventative options. However, the clinical benefits of early detection and the efficacy of the current surveillance and management protocols for these cancer syndromes are less certain. Genetic testing in this category is not yet considered a standard of medical care; the data on the clinical value and reliability of these tests are often based on research studies and their predictive values have not yet been firmly established. The cancer syndromes that are currently part of this group include HNPCC, early-onset breast/ovarian cancer, and Li-Fraumeni Syndrome.

The use of cancer genetic tests that fall into Group Three can be contraindicated for a number of reasons. An individual with a family history that is weakly suggestive of an inherited cancer syndrome should not be generally offered a predictive genetic test. Genetic tests should also not be offered for inherited-cancer syndromes when the predictive value of the test has not been clearly demonstrated. This may be due to a weak association between the suspected cancer-susceptibility gene and the syndrome or where the significance of mutations in the cancer-susceptibility gene are not clear. These tests are also contraindicated where there is no clear value in knowing the carrier status of an individual (no early intervention or therapies exist).

These categories serve to outline critical factors that influence the value of a predictive genetic test. These simplified groupings are not exclusive and some tests may not be easily categorized. Screening for *p16^{INK4A}* mutations is the predictive genetic test currently in use for familial melanoma (69). Individuals from a family with a strong history of this cancer in which there has been a previously identified mutation in the *p16^{INK4A}* gene fulfill the criteria for a Group Two cancer and may benefit from this test. However not all the mutations in the *p16^{INK4A}* gene are associated with melanoma susceptibility, nor is $p16^{INK4A}$ the only gene that can increase the susceptibility to inherited melanoma. In fact, mutations in another gene, *CDK4*, which interacts with $p16^{INK4A}$, have been identified in some families *(70)*. In other families, no mutations in either gene can be detected, suggesting that other as-of-yet unidentified genes may be involved in hereditary melanoma. For this reason familial melanoma testing can also be challenged regarding its current benefit and for some individuals may be categorized as a Group Three cancer. In addition, in families where DNA tests have not been done but where melanoma segregates as a dominant trait, thorough, noninvasive, regular cutaneous examinations can allow for early detection and removal of lesions to prevent significant morbidity and early mortality. Individuals who may feel anxiety with an uninformative or moderately predictive test result may feel that the potential benefits are not sufficiently strong to validate testing as they would continue getting the same cutaneous screening even after the DNA test.

ASCO recommends that genetic testing only be offered for cancer syndromes that fulfill Group One or Group Two criteria. These guidelines however are not universally accepted. Numerous geneticists feel that genetic tests in which the risks and benefits are uncertain (Group Two criteria) should currently only be offered on a research basis *(11,67,71,73;* see also http://cancernet.nci.nih.gov/genetics/breast.htm). Discussion about limiting the availability of predictive genetic tests of the early-onset breast/ovarian cancer genes *BRCA1* and *BRCA2* has focused on the possibility that commercial companies are acting irresponsibly by offering the test not only to women who have a strong family history of breast/ovarian cancer, but also to women who have a family history that includes one first-degree or second-degree relative who was diagnosed with breast cancer before the age of 40 or two relatives who were diagnosed with breast cancer before the age of 50. There is debate as to whether there is sufficient evidence that screening the *BRCA1* and *BRCA2* genes in these families will be optimally informative *(67,73)*. Women who have a risk of breast cancer that is greater than that of the general population may not be counseled properly or offered the appropriate medical management if an uninformative test result is wrongly interpreted as a negative result. The failure to understand the limitations of testing could generate a health-care risk as predictive genetic testing becomes a more common medical practice.

Pedigree Analysis In deciding if it is appropriate to offer cancer genetic testing to a patient, it is essential to determine if there is a pattern of cancers in their family that is consistent with a familial form rather than due to sporadically occurring cancers. The risk of developing cancer in the general population is quite high; one in three individuals will develop some form of cancer over their lifetimes *(74)*. On the basis of this risk it is expected that many families will contain members who have been diagnosed with cancer.

There are several key features that suggest familial cancer patterns. The vast majority of known inherited-cancer syndromes are inherited as autosomal dominant conditions (Table 5). This means that within a pedigree the characteristic pattern of inheritance is vertical: 1) there should be members of each generation who have developed similar types of cancers; 2) the affected family members should be first-degree relatives to

Table 5
General Features of Inherited Cancer-Predisposition Syndromes

Mendelian inheritance patterns
- Most are autosomal dominant
- Multiple family members in several generations have cancer
- Affected individuals include first- and second-degree relatives

Early ages of specific cancer diagnoses compared to the general population

Unusual constellation of tumor(s)
- Multiple primaries in a single individual
- Bilateral cancers in paired organs

Association with other nonmalignant manifestations

each other (parent-to-child and siblings); and 3) there should be no disparity in the ratio of affected males and females (both can transmit the trait with equal probability to children of either sex). In addition, autosomal dominant inheritance generally implies that affected children have affected parents and none of the offspring of an unaffected parent have developed cancer *(75)*. Secondly, cancers due to an inherited-cancer syndrome are usually diagnosed before age 50, with inherited forms of ovarian cancer and prostate cancer being notable exceptions. Finally, the appearance of multiple primary tumors in a single individual or the appearance of bilateral cancer in paired organs is more common in inherited cancers than in sporadic ones. Modifications to these general rules are dependent on the form of the cancer being considered; male breast cancer rarely occurs in early-onset breast/ovarian cancer and thus fathers are generally unaffected carriers and, obviously, prostate and ovarian cancer will not occur in gene carriers who are females or males, respectively. Additionally the incomplete penetrance of this cancer syndrome means that carriers of a susceptibility gene will not always develop cancer. Analysis can also be confounded by small family size, uncertain family histories, and sporadic cancers of the same type as those characteristic of the inherited susceptibility gene.

The construction of a pedigree is a key step in defining the inheritance of cancers within a family. The pedigree should span three generations and include detailed information about siblings, parents, maternal and paternal aunts and uncles, and grandparents. It is best to generate a graphic record of the family health history that diagrams the relationships between family members *(76)*. For each individual it is important to gather as detailed a medical history as possible; questions should focus on the types of cancer, the location(s) of the primary site(s), were there single or multiple primary sites, what was the age at first diagnosis? If appropriate, questions should also determine whether the primary sites were unilateral or bilateral, and if there were secondary metastases, at what age and where did they occur *(77)*? Because a patient's recall of this detailed medical information may be inaccurate, it is important to confirm the diagnoses with written pathology reports and other medical records. It is also essential to include within the pedigree the ages of family members who are unaffected. Finally the pedigree should make note of any inherited disorders that could predispose individuals to a variety of malignancies (Fanconi anemia, xeroderma pigmentosum, Bloom syndrome, or ataxia telangiectasia [AT]) as these conditions could confuse analysis of the family history.

For some of the better-characterized cancer syndromes like FAP, HNPCC, and early-onset breast/ovarian cancer, specific guidelines for distinguishing families with inherited cancers have been developed *(68,78–80)*. As more information on inherited-cancer syndromes is accumulated it is anticipated that these guidelines may be modified and additional ones will be proposed for other inherited cancer syndromes. The rapid pace of change in this field demands a high degree of vigilance in keeping aware of the newest developments. Careful construction and analysis of a pedigree is the critical first step in maximizing the benefits and minimizing the limitations of predictive genetic testing. For families in which the pedigree reveals a clustering of affected individuals that suggest an inherited syndrome but where it is not yet appropriate to perform a DNA test, there is the option of banking DNA samples. Specimens are collected from affected individuals and other key family members and then stored indefinitely in a qualified DNA bank. This service, offered by a number of genetic-testing laboratories, will help to guarantee that the results of a future test will be informative when testing becomes available by ensuring the availability of DNA from an affected individual.

The early identification of a mutation in a cancer-susceptibility gene can decrease cancer mortality and morbidity by altering the medical management of carriers. There is also a potential economic benefit in defining carriers and noncarriers of susceptibility genes because routine syndrome-specific screening procedures will not be necessary for individuals who are not at risk. However, it is the opinion of many in the genetics community that none of the currently available genetic tests should be offered as general-population screens *(10,67,68,81–83)*. This is based on the number of potential risks associated with testing and the fact that in the absence of information about a familial mutation, none of the currently available genetic tests have the appropriate sensitivity and specificity to ensure that a negative test result is truly informative. The negative impact of false results is too large to justify offering testing to asymptomatic individuals with no family history of cancer. Thus, many geneticists currently feel that predictive genetic testing should be limited to individuals who have a family history suggesting that they are at risk for an inherited-cancer syndrome. However, it should be noted that many others have differing views and, in fact, some physicians and laboratories currently routinely offer genetic screening for *BRCA1* and *BRCA2* mutations in Ashkenazi Jewish women with no significant family history, but for whom population studies have determined that 2.5% of women are mutation carriers.

Evaluating Predictive Genetic Testing The methodology being used in predictive genetic tests is relatively new and often is being simultaneously developed, introduced, and altered. Not all labs offering these tests have equal experience in performing and evaluating these tests. A limited survey of labs offering molecular genetic testing in 1997 found that although some labs reported performing these tests at a high volume

(>31,500 annually), others perform as few as four tests per year *(84)*. At the present time, the decision to order a molecular test is not routine for most clinicians and often the interpretation of these results is more complex than that of a standard medical test. Because the results of the predictive test will be utilized by a healthy individual who is at-risk to make a decision with long-term consequences that can affect not only their own health but that of the rest of the family, it is essential that the accuracy and validity of both the test, the result, and the interpretation are established before the test is ordered. Knowing the predictive value of the genetic test will help to determine how much confidence can be placed in the results of the test *(75,85)*.

An effective test should have a strong positive predictive value. This value estimates the probability that a person with a positive test result (a mutation has been detected in a cancer-susceptibility gene) has or will develop the disease. Conversely, the negative predictive value, the probability that a person with a negative result does not have the disease should also be high. The predictive value of a test is defined by both its sensitivity and its clinical or diagnostic specificity. The utility of a test is increased with higher levels of sensitivity and specificity. The sensitivity of the test marks its ability to detect affected individuals, the frequency with which the test yields a positive result when the disease is actually present. Thus a test that has low sensitivity will be unable to detect all the disease-related mutations in the cancer-susceptibility gene. Specificity refers to the ability of the test to exclude those who are unaffected. It is measured by the frequency with which the test yields a negative result when the disease is absent. For rare inherited-cancer syndromes like FAP, with an estimated population frequency of 1 in 8000, the number of affected individuals who could undergo testing is quite small. As a consequence, our abilities to calculate the positive predictive value of these test with statistically significant confidence can be limited.

Generally a test is offered clinically when it has been optimized for maximal effectiveness and is able to definitively diagnosis the presence of disease *(85)*. Although there are no specific criteria that define when this analytical standard has been obtained, it is generally accepted that a test should have a high degree of precision (the results of repeated testing on the same specimen are identical), be accurate (correctly identify positive and negative results), and be performed reliably in many lab settings. Traditionally great emphasis has been placed on testing the quality of the testing process and ensuring that there are standardized protocols, reagents, and diagnostic criteria. Predictive genetic tests were originally developed as components of research protocols. The intent was not to generate diagnostic tools to be used in clinical practice but rather to create investigative probes. The translation of these probes into clinical practice has been rapid and genetic testing is now routinely available from both research and commercial labs. However, there is often minimal oversight of the components used in genetic testing; there are no mandated standardized mechanisms that ensure that the appropriate quality of procedures specific to genetic tests is maintained. In research labs that offer genetic tests, the testing protocols are peer-reviewed and it is generally expected that labs in research institutions that offer testing have been evaluated by an institutional review board.

Table 6
Consequences of Genetic Testing

Benefits	Risks
Refined risk analysis	**Medical uncertainties**
• Improved risk awareness	• Wide risk estimate ranges
• More accurate knowledge	• Medical-management options vary
Psychological gain	**Emotional distress**
• Relief from uncertainty	• Individual
• Future planning	• Family
Diagnosis at earlier stage of life	**Potential discrimination**
• Directed medical surveillance	• Insurance
• Educated decision-making	• Employment
• Preventive medical intervention or management	• Societal

There are no formal mechanisms that monitor compliance to this review process and no standard criteria by which the test protocols in these research labs are appraised.

Genetic testing is also available through clinical laboratories; the number of clinical labs offering genetic tests has grown dramatically in the 1990s. Testing in clinical labs is regulated by the federal Clinical Laboratory Improvement Amendments (CLIA) (86). CLIA regulations provide standard requirements for certification of lab personnel and directors and the attainment of proper levels of quality control. The particulars of these requirements are tailored to the type of lab in which the tests are being performed. At present CLIA has only set the standards for labs that offer cytogenetic testing; there are no standards specific for labs that offer predictive genetic tests. Many laboratories participate in quality programs for genetic testing through the College of American Pathologists (CAP) and the American College of Medical Genetics Molecular Genetics proficiency testing program (87). However participation is voluntary and there is no assurance that the standards for genetic tests in commercial labs are properly controlled. There is considerable interest in establishing standards among diagnostic labs and it is anticipated that in the next several years there will be stringent guidelines for the standardization, regulation, and certification of labs that offer predictive genetic tests (http://www.cap.org/html/advocacy.html).

Medical, Social, and Ethical Issues There is great appeal in possessing knowledge about one's genes. It is hoped that the ability to foretell one's medical future can be accompanied by the power to change it. However, there are ramifications in knowing the composition of one's genes that can extend beyond the health concerns of the individual. By virtue of inheritance, genetic information also impacts the family. Additionally, it has the potential to affect an individual's position in society. Genetic testing is in its infancy, and although the anticipated benefits of this information are strong in the absence of long-standing experience with this type of knowledge, there is great concern that that it may also contain the power to harm. The factors that will be considered important in the decision to order a test will vary from patient to patient and from family to family. The role of the health-care professional who

offers a predictive genetic test must be expanded beyond offering the test to ensure that the decision-making process by an individual who undergoes a predictive genetic test has been preceded by a careful analysis of the individualized benefits and risks that the possession of this knowledge offers (Table 6).

One of the clearest benefits of a predictive genetic test is the ability to determine the risk of cancer susceptibility. If a mutation in a cancer-susceptibility gene has been identified in a family, then either a positive or a negative test result is informative. A negative test result frees an at-risk individual from the worry of an increased risk of developing cancer based on the specific inherited syndrome in the future, whereas a positive test result definitively demonstrates that the cancer-susceptibility gene has been inherited and provides a calculated measure of the risk of developing the inherited-cancer syndrome. For highly penetrant inherited cancer syndromes like MEN2 or FAP, one can be fairly confident about the risk conferred by mutations in the cancer-susceptibility genes *RET* and *APC*, respectively (13). However, in other cancer syndromes like early-onset breast/ovarian cancer, the validity of the risk calculation is still being defined (83). This uncertainty is one of the limitations of current genetic testing; however, predictive genetic testing is generally viewed as beneficial if the diagnosis of an increased risk of a cancer susceptibility at an earlier stage in life can be accompanied by the initiation of effective clinical management.

Case Example The family in Fig. 1 first came to the attention of their physician when individual III-4, a 24-yr-old male, was diagnosed with multiple polyps of the colon at age 22. At that time the polyps were excised, a follow-up colonoscopy two yr later identified numerous additional polyps and at age 24 he had a total colectomy. One of his three sisters (III-1) has a similar medical history. Multiple colon polyps were first detected at age 24 and a colectomy was performed at age 28. Their father was diagnosed with multiple colon polyps at age 45 and died from colon cancer at age 55. There were also reports of two paternal aunts who had died of unknown forms of cancer; medical records were not available on these individuals. This pedigree suggests that this family is affected with the inherited colon-cancer syndrome FAP. Affected individuals develop adenomatous polyps in the colon in early adolescence. These can grow in number to hundreds or thousands of polyps, which, if untreated, have an almost certain chance of becoming cancerous, usually by age 40 (88; see also http://www.ncbi.nlm.nih.gov/OMIM/). This syndrome is caused by a truncating mutation of the APC gene on chromosome 5q. Identification of a mutation in the APC gene is diagnostic for this cancer and because the penetrance is close to 100%, individuals who carry a mutated APC gene will almost certainly develop colon polyps. However there is great variation in expression and the individuals in a single family, all carrying the same mutation, may manifest the symptoms of this condition differently (89). Genetic test results can not predict the course of the disease, when polyps will develop, or when they will become cancerous. Yearly endoscopy screening starting at around age 10 is recommended for all at risk family members. A total colectomy is preventative and is the recommended treatment for this syndrome. This is usually performed soon after polyps are first diagnosed.

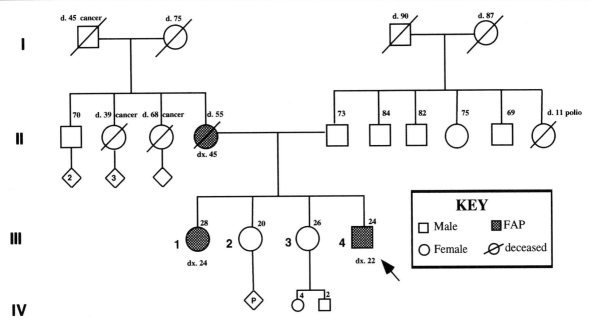

Fig. 1. Pedigree analysis of a family affected by an inherited colon cancer syndrome suggestive of familial adenomatous polyposis (FAP).

For individual III-4, screening his *APC* gene for a susceptibility mutation will confirm his diagnosis, but will not affect his future medical management. At present, this test is fairly accurate and is able to detect mutations in about 80% of those individuals who have the disease. FAP is inherited as an autosomal dominant condition and on the basis of his family history, both of his currently healthy sisters (III-2 and III-3) and their children are also at risk for developing FAP. Information about their APC genes will determine whether or not they need to screen for colon polyps with yearly endoscopies.

The repercussions of testing III-4 are far-reaching in this family. If a mutation is identified in this individual's *APC* gene, then it will be possible to screen the rest of the family and determine their risk status definitively. A negative test result for these individuals will save them from the anxiety of not knowing whether or not they will develop the disease and spare them the discomfort of repeated screenings. Those with a positive test result can initiate preventive measures at the appropriate time in their lives. There are clear benefits to this test from the perspectives of medical management and the emotional security of these at-risk family members. However there are also risks. Genetic information affects both the individual and their family. The future medical care of multiple family members is dependent on the test results. If individual III-3 does not carry the FAP-susceptibility mutation, then neither she nor her children are at risk of developing inherited colorectal cancer, a result that negates the need to suffer uncomfortable yearly colonoscopies. However, if she is found to have inherited the mutation, then her children are at risk of developing colorectal cancer.

Case Discussion The consensus opinion is that testing of minors for adult-onset cancers is not encouraged unless clear medical benefits result from such testing. Testing of children at risk for FAP is clearly beneficial because a positive test will allow them to take advantage of effective preventative therapies, whereas a negative test result will spare them repeated

invasive medical surveillance. It is recommended that predictive genetic testing is not performed before the earliest age at which health benefits can be gained. For FAP, the test should not be performed before the age of 8–9 yr when colorectal polyps first began to appear. However predictive testing of children is not appropriate for adult-onset inherited-cancer syndromes for which there are no effective treatments. Prenatal testing is also an option that could be pursued in this family if it is established that there is a parent who carries the cancer-susceptibility gene. The decision to test a fetus for susceptibility to an adult-onset cancer syndrome should be preceded by a thoughtful consideration of how this genetic information (both positive and negative) would impact the course of the pregnancy. It is essential to discuss with parents what the perceived value is of possessing this genetic information many years before surveillance or treatment would be initiated. Additionally, consideration should be given to future advances in cancer health care. Although it is not possible to predict specific changes in preventative and medical management, it is inevitable that there will be improvement.

The value of predictive genetic testing is less apparent for inherited-cancer syndromes for which no therapies are currently available or where the effectiveness of available therapies is still being determined. This is of particular concern for women who are at risk for early-onset breast/ovarian cancer. None of the currently available screening options—mammography, ovarian ultrasound or serum markers—have been clearly shown to be 100% effective in preventing early morbidity and mortality. Based on this uncertainty, women who are at risk for early-onset breast/ovarian cancer may choose the preventative option of prophylactic mastectomy or oophorectomy, chemoprevention strategies, increased surveillance and/or lifestyle modifications. This decision may be guided by the results of a *BRCA1/BRCA2* predictive genetic test. One of the few studies to look at the effectiveness of the procedures found that the gains in life expectancy for patients who elect these drastic procedures were small. For prophylactic mastectomy, there was a gain of 2.9–5.3 yr, whereas for prophylactic oophorectomy there was a gain of 0.3–1.7 yr in the life expectancy *(90)*. Moreover, prophylactic surgery does not completely eliminate the risk of cancer because residual breast and ovarian tissue still present a risk.

Genetic conditions are generally viewed as stigmatizing. For individuals at risk for an inherited-cancer syndrome, predictive genetic testing can influence the psychological burden of their genetic inheritance. An informative negative test result provides the obvious benefit of freeing them from the risk of cancer susceptibility and can increase their feelings of control. These emotions may be accompanied by guilt if other close family members are found to carry the susceptibility mutation and regret over previous life decisions made on the basis of their previous at risk status. The emotional benefits for patients who receive a positive test can be equally mixed. Similar feelings of control may be experienced following the knowledge that a cancer-susceptibility gene has been inherited; this information can motivate more rigorous pursuit of screening and early detection regimes. Possessing this knowledge can enable them to plan for the future. This information can also serve as a source of extreme distress; some individuals may find it difficult to live with the knowledge that they will develop a condition for which there is no guaranteed cure and limited therapies. Feelings of anxiety, depression, and vulnerability are not uncommon in carriers of gene mutations that result in adult-onset disorders *(91–93)*. The facts of inheritance can also create emotional and psychological burdens for multiple members within a family because identification of an inherited cancer-susceptibility gene places family members at risk of inheritance. The fear of having passed a cancer-susceptibility gene onto children and grandchildren can become a source of guilt for the person in whom it was identified. The psychological ramifications of predictive genetic test results should be discussed with an at-risk individual as part of the decision-making process. Anticipating the impact of a positive, a negative, or an uninformative test results on the individual's present and future health and emotional stability is an essential component of the decision-making process.

The enormous potential benefit of cancer-susceptibility testing in early diagnosis and treatment is accompanied by the fear that this information may be misused by providing the basis for discrimination against individuals who carry cancer-susceptibility genes. It is feared that the current mechanisms for ensuring the privacy of an individual's genetic legacy are inadequate and at-risk carriers could suffer employment and health- and life-insurance discrimination. Scenarios illustrating these potential risks are found in scientific journals and many anecdotal stories can be found in the lay press.

There are no established policies regulating the privacy of genetic information. Few limits have been placed on the access of an employer to the information in a worker's medical records. The concern is that information from a predictive genetic test could be used to generate a genetic profile of an individual and their family that could be used to limit their employability and potential opportunities for advancement and compensation. Similar fears surround the discussion of genetic discrimination

by medical- and life-insurance companies. Insurance standards have not been established to determine if a genetic condition can be classified as a pre-existing condition, and although at present genetic tests are not required as part of the underwriting process, genetic-testing results are being used as part of the decision-making process in the insurance industry. There is concern that discrimination against individuals who carry genes that predispose them to the development of cancer could lead to the revoking or denying of coverage for health and life insurance *(94,95;* see also http://www.napbc.org). In a limited survey of insurance companies in the United States, some insurers reported that they would deny health and life insurance to individuals who have HNPCC or their relatives *(96)*. Concern about this potential risk has prompted legislation at both the state and federal levels. In 1995, the Equal Employment Opportunity Commission released an interpretation of the 1990 Americans with Disabilities Act stating that a person may not be denied employment because he or she carries a disease-susceptibility gene. The Health Insurance Portability and Accountability Act of 1996 expressly recognizes genetic information as protected medical information that can not be used by an employer-based group health plan to deny coverage when a person moves from job to job. At least 26 states have enacted laws to limit the use of genetic information by health insurers *(97)*. However the existing laws do not provide any privacy protections and do not prohibit group health plans from increasing rates, excluding all coverage for a particular condition, or imposing lifetime caps on benefits *(95)*.

This flurry of legislation demonstrates the depth of concern over the ethical, legal, and societal issues posed by genetic testing. It remains to be seen how this legislation will be incorporated into business and clinical practices. Confidentiality of a patient's medical information plays an important role in the relationship between a patient and their physician *(94)*. Clinicians offering genetic tests should consider how they will ensure the privacy of a patient's genetic information. In the absence of laws to protect the privacy of genetic information, the risk that the results of a cancer-susceptibility test could become public information may force an individual who believes that they can benefit from genetic testing to decline it because of the fear of discrimination. It is the responsibility of the health-care professional offering the genetic test to ensure that patients are sufficiently educated about the risks and benefits of testing to make an informed decision.

INFORMATION AND COUNSELING COMPONENTS OF GENETIC TESTING

Basic Risk Analysis The results of cancer genetic tests provide a molecular profile of a cancer-susceptibility gene. Although identification of a mutation in one of these genes (a positive test result) defines the precise form of the gene or allele, the certainty with which these molecular changes can be translated into a statistical prophesy is far less exact. For some of the inherited-cancer syndromes, including VHL and FAP, there is a high degree of confidence in defining the risk of cancer on the basis of a mutation in the susceptibility gene. For other syndromes like early-onset hereditary breast/ovarian cancer, there is less confidence about the predictive value of the molecular test. The accuracy of the risk estimate is influenced by a number of factors, including the depth of knowledge about the molecular basis of the cancer syndrome, the degree of penetrance of the molecular change, differences in the effectiveness of the genetic tests, and the statistical strength of the epidemiological models, which translate the molecular results into risk estimates. Continuing advances in genetic research, genetic technology, and genetic epidemiology will facilitate the development of more precise tests that a physician or healthcare professional can confidently interpret. However until the field of predictive cancer testing has sufficiently matured, it is essential that the interpretation of a predictive cancer test takes into consideration the efficacy and validity of the predicted risk estimate.

Case Example Like all of the molecular genetic tests currently available, the molecular genetic test for the VHL is relatively new. VHL has been recognized as a clinical entity for almost 70 years. In 1964, it was recognized as an inherited-cancer syndrome; in 1993, the VHL gene was identified on chromosome 3p25-p26; and as of 1998, four laboratories are offering genetic testing of the *VHL* gene. A woman with a family history (an affected father and sister) of this autosomally dominant inherited cancer syndrome wants predictive testing. At the time that she has requested testing, she does not have any manifestations of the syndrome, but is at risk of developing a variety of cysts and tumors, including retinal, cerebellar, spinal, and medullary hemangioblastomas, pheochromocytomas, and renal-cell carcinoma *(98,99)*. Because there is a wide array of organ systems with the potential to develop cancer, recommended screening regimes include a number of clinical laboratory tests, imaging tests, and ophthalmoscopic tests be performed at periodic intervals throughout most, if not all, of this patient's life. Based on Mendelian inheritance, this patient has a 50% risk of inheriting the VHL cancer-susceptibility gene from her father. If a susceptibility mutation in the *VHL* gene has been previously identified in this family, a molecular test that screens for this specific mutation will lower her risk of inheritance to essentially zero or increase it to essentially 100%. The potential benefits of this test are dramatic. A negative test result can eliminate the risk of developing cancer and save her from undergoing a lifetime of rigorous and costly screening procedures, whereas a positive result will aid in the early detection of the associated cancers and can reduce the mortality and morbidity associated with this cancer syndrome.

Case Discussion Currently VHL testing is performed in two steps; in the first stage, the *VHL* gene is screened for rearrangements by Southern-blot analysis, a method that has a 15% likelihood of detecting a mutation. In the second stage, direct sequencing of the three exons in this gene increases the mutation detection rate to near 90%. It is essential to ensure that the interpretation of the results of the genetic test takes into consideration its technical limitations. When there is no molecular information on the form of the *VHL* gene from another affected family member, then an at-risk family member with a negative test result has a substantially reduced risk of developing VHL, but this risk does not equal zero. On the basis of a modified Bayesian analysis, which utilizes the genetic test result to modify the prior Mendelian risk, the risk of developing VHL is decreased to 16%, a substantial improvement over her initial

**Table 7
Modification of Mendelian Risk Estimate
Through DNA Testing[a]**

Probability	Patient is a carrier of the mutation	Patient is not a carrier of a mutation
Prior (Mendelian)	0.5	0.5
Conditional (DNA test)	0.2	1.0
Joint	$0.5 \times 0.2 = .10$	$0.5 \times 1.0 = 0.5$
Posterior	$.10/.10 + .50 = .16 = 16\%$	$0.5/.10 + .50 = .83 = 83\%$

[a] Based on Bayes Theorem.

risk based on Mendelian inheritance of 50% (Table 7) *(100)*. This type of technical shortcoming is not limited to testing of the VHL gene, but is a limitation of a number of currently available clinical tests. It is therefore recommended that a genetic test for an inherited cancer syndrome is performed first on a family member who has been diagnosed with the syndrome. A positive result in this individual sets a baseline for the test, and increases the sensitivity to close to 100% because the susceptibility gene in other at-risk family members can then be screened for only the specific mutation. If a mutation is not found in this gene, then these individuals can be reassured that a negative result is due to the failure to inherit the susceptibility gene and not due to the limitations of the test itself.

One of the anticipated benefits of continuing research on the molecular basis of cancer susceptibility will be a more detailed understanding of the variable expression that is characteristic of many of the cancer syndromes. Based on correlations between the genotype (mutant form of a susceptibility gene) and the phenotype (the clinical features that carriers exhibit) interpretation of the results of a genetic test may predict both the clinical course of the condition in an affected individual and anticipate the specifics of patient surveillance and medical management. VHL is an example of one of the inherited cancer conditions in which progress has been made in explaining some of the clinical variability of the disease based on the type and position of the mutation in the gene. Individuals with VHL who develop pheochromocytomas often have missense mutations in the gene, whereas individuals with VHL gene mutations that generate truncated forms of the protein are at a decreased risk for developing pheochromocytomas *(58)*. In interpreting a VHL test result, it is important to know not only if a mutation has been detected, but also to consider the type of mutation (missense or nonsense) and its position within the coding sequence of the gene. A positive test result predicts that a carrier has close to a 100% risk of developing cancer, whereas investigating the specific form of the mutation can define some of the medical-management guidelines for individuals who carry the mutation.

Complex Risk Analysis Analysis of most cancer genes indicate that no one mutation accounts for a high percentage of the disease-causing mutations. Therefore, unlike other genetic conditions like sickle-cell anemia in which one mutation in a gene accounts for the disease phenotype, mutations in cancer genes can be located in multiple sites in coding and noncoding portions of the gene and can alter the function of the gene through a variety of inactivating mechanisms *(13)*. Complicating the analysis is the fact that many of the inherited-cancer syndromes can be caused by mutations in different genes that belong to a group of functionally related genes. This genetic and allelic heterogeneity poses a number of challenges to the analysis of a genetic-test result.

A vivid illustration of the complexities in the analysis of a predictive genetic test is derived from considering screening for early-onset breast/ovarian cancer. Breast cancer is the most common malignancy among women, affecting approx one in eight women over the course of their lifetime *(101,102)*. The first insights into the molecular basis of the inherited form of breast cancer were provided by the cloning of the *BRCA1* gene in 1994, and in 1995 *BRCA2*, a second susceptibility gene, was cloned *(20,22)*. In the intervening five yr over 1000 mutations have been identified within these two genes, these mutations are scattered throughout the coding regions of *BRCA1* and *BRCA2* (http://www.nhgri.nih.gov/Intramural_research/ Lab_Transfer/Bic). The large sizes of the *BRCA1* and *BRCA2* genes (24 and 27 exons, respectively) make direct mutation analysis extremely labor-intensive and quite expensive. It is estimated that as many as 10–15% of the cancer-susceptibility mutations in these genes are not detectable by the existing laboratory techniques, which screen only the coding regions of the genes *(11,103)*. Furthermore, mutations in *BRCA1* are estimated to account for less than 45% of the hereditary cases of breast cancer and mutations in *BRCA2* could account maximally for 35%. It has been suggested that as many as four additional susceptibility genes play a role in early-onset breast/ ovarian cancer syndrome.

The newness of the molecular data on BRCA1 and BRCA2, coupled with the extensive allelic heterogeneity of these genes has made it difficult to define the degree of increased risk for a woman who carries one of the *BRCA1* or *BRCA2* gene mutations. Within the current pool of mutations, the Ashkenazi mutations in *BRCA1* (185delAG and 5382insC) and *BRCA2* (6174delT) are the most commonly identified *(62,67)*. They have been associated with disease in multiple families and the evidence is compelling that an individual who carries these mutations has an increased risk of developing early-onset breast/ovarian cancer over that in the general population. There are other groups of mutations that are predicted to alter the function of the BRCA1 and BRCA2 proteins, but that have been identified in only a few families. Nonetheless, these mutations increase the risk of early-onset breast/ovarian cancer in carriers *(104,105)*. Finally there are recurrent familial forms of the *BRCA1* and *BRCA2* gene that contain missense mutations. The mechanisms by which these gene changes could alter the function of the *BRCA1* or *BRCA2* genes is not immediately apparent; thus, it is difficult to determine if these changes are causative of disease or are inherited sequence polymorphisms. There are a limited number of genetic epidemiological studies that have assessed the empiric risk of cancer for a woman who carries one of these mutations. Initially the lifetime risk of breast cancer in a woman with one of the more common *BRCA1* or

BRCA2 mutations was estimated from 76–87% *(106–109)*. A more recent study has estimated that the risk of breast cancer among carriers is closer to 56% *(62)*. Neither of these estimates is considered to be a definitive measure of the empiric risk. Both numbers are thought to be overestimate risk because families with breast-cancer history were over-represented in the study population.

These examples illustrate the evolving face of empiric risk analysis for cancer susceptibility. With the increasing sophistication of epidemiological methods, it is anticipated that the risk estimates will become sufficiently refined to consider the specific risks associated with different mutations in a gene and will be able to consider the effects of risk modifiers that include dietary, hormonal, environmental, and additional genetic factors. The lack of precision in defining the susceptibility risk for a *BRCA1* or *BRCA2* mutation carrier is one of the failings of the current state of genetic testing for not only early-onset breast/ ovarian cancer but also a number of inherited-cancer syndromes. However, this failing does not mean that test results are flawed, rather it cautions careful interpretation that incorporates these uncertainties rather than ignoring them.

IMPORTANT ASPECTS OF THE GENETIC-TESTING SESSION Most cancer genetic testing is currently being performed in a multi-disciplinary clinic where care is coordinated by a health-care team consisting of medical and surgical oncologists, oncology nurses, clinical geneticists, genetic counselors, psychologists, and social workers. The interweaving of the expertise of these specialists assists at-risk individuals in dealing with the immediate and long-term consequences of knowing that they have an increased susceptibility to cancer. In this setting, genetic testing is a time-intensive process that encompasses medical assessment, patient education, genetic counseling, risk assessment, laboratory testing, analysis, interpretation, psychosocial assessment and support, and on-going medical management. The increasing public awareness of inherited-cancer syndromes and the relative paucity of clinical genetic professionals will likely result in an increase in the number of cancer genetic tests that are performed by clinicians and related health-care professionals in primary health-care settings. As predictive genetic tests move into the main stream of health care, it is important that the provision of a predictive genetic test continues to be accompanied by genetic education and both pre-test and post-test counseling. These elements are essential in ensuring that a patient's decision to undergo genetic testing is grounded in an understanding of the genetic, medical, psychological, and societal consequences of the test.

The first step in testing is to ensure that the test is medically appropriate. A detailed family history should be obtained, confirmed, and evaluated with respect to the possible inherited-cancer syndrome. This should be followed by a pre-test education for the at-risk individual that presents comprehensive information about the disease process, including details on the natural history of the condition, the basis for its inheritance, and the risks to other family members. A thorough discussion of the most current medical options for surveillance and prevention and their efficacy should also be provided. At-risk individuals should be provided with a pre-test assessment of their risk of inheriting the susceptibility gene and the attendant risks of developing cancer. Discussions about the testing process should include explicit information about potential benefits and risks, strengths, and limitations, and the possibility of positive, negative, and uninformative test results and how each would alter the risk estimates. Discussions of the issues surrounding the confidentiality of genetic information and the risk of genetic discrimination in employment or in obtaining or maintaining insurance are also important aspects of the testing process. Details of the actual test process should also be discussed, including specimen collection, turnaround time, and cost. Patients should be aware that their insurance may not cover the expenses of the test and/or the education/counseling session. The pre-test session should also consider how the test results will be disclosed, who they can be released to, and how the privacy of this information will be protected. This information must be presented in a nonjudgmental and balanced manner, in language that is understandable to the patient and takes into consideration how much information a patient is able to absorb. Individuals considering testing should understand that predictive genetic testing is not a necessity, but rather an option that can be accepted or rejected.

The attainment of autonomy, a central value in the patient-clinician relationship, in the decision-making process requires that patients be reasonably informed of risks before deciding to undergo a medical procedure (94). Pretest education in predictive cancer testing should be structured to ensure that the patient can give an informed consent to the test (110). To obtain this consent, the clinician must educate and counsel in a manner that facilitates voluntary, informed decision making. There are numerous obstacles to obtaining this consent: 1) the imbalance of power between an emotionally vulnerable patient and a clinician who represents the authority of the medical profession, 2) the variability of personal experience and knowledge with cancer, and 3) the difficulty of translating a probabilistic risk analysis into a decision (111). Because genetic information carries personal, family, and social burdens, each individual who is considering a genetic test will weigh the risks and the benefits of the test uniquely. It is essential that the clinician educate a patient about the risks, benefits, and limitations of the test in a manner that enables the patient to incorporate their personal value system into the decision process. If an individual does decide to undergo a predictive genetic test, then it is also recommended that an explicit informed consent is obtained. Many companies offering predictive genetic testing require that a test request is accompanied by a signed consent form. There is some variation in the information that is contained in these forms. Usually they describe the DNA test in general terms and lay out the test benefits, limitations, reliability, and cost. Additional clauses may discuss issues of privacy of the samples and the results. Before a patient signs the form, each clause should be discussed specifically. However not all companies require explicit informed consent before testing. Health-care providers offering predictive genetic tests may need to develop their own forms to ensure that a patient can give informed consent. These forms should describe in general terms the DNA basis of the predictive test and the technical limitations, possible positive, negative, and uninformative test outcomes, and issues of privacy protection (Table 8).

Table 8
General Components of Informed Consent for Predictive Molecular Diagnostic Testing

- Explicit agreement to participate in testing
- General description of type of test including the technical limitations
- Consideration of all possible test results and interpretations
- Appropriate level of understanding about the test and its implications
- Definition of privacy protection of test samples and results
- Knowledge about future use, storage, or disposal of samples

Pretest counseling is an important component of the testing process. This provides the opportunity to explore the patient's perceptions, concerns, and beliefs about cancer etiology, what they feel their risks are, and their motives for requesting the test. At-risk individuals should be encouraged to consider the effects of positive, negative, and uninformative test results on their emotional state and on their relationships with family members, friends, and co-workers. It is appropriate as part of this session to consider who they will share their test results with and the impact that they perceive this will have on these relationships.

The results of a genetic test should always be disclosed in a face-to-face session. This post-test session provides the opportunity to discuss the interpretation of the result and to consider specifically the appropriate medical management and where it can best be obtained. In addition, in this session the patient should be given time to address all issues that are raised by the results of the test, both medical and psychological. Follow-up for the patient and other family members should be scheduled as appropriate. In the post-test session, patients should be provided with appropriate educational resources and referrals to the relevant support services (psychologists and social workers) and organizations (support groups).

GENETIC-TEST MECHANICS To optimize the benefits of genetic testing, it is essential to obtain detailed information about the lab, its procedures, and the mechanics of specimen collection and shipping. A practical first step is to obtain a listing of labs that perform genetic tests for inherited-cancer susceptibility genes. An up-to-date listing is available through GeneTests on the Internet (at http://www.genetests.org/). This online site is maintained by the University of Washington and is accessible to all health-care professionals following a simple registration. This database lists both diagnostic and research testing labs, along with some information about the molecular form of the available tests and contact numbers. There is variation from lab to lab in the specific genes being studied (both *BRCA1* and/or *BRCA2* can be tested in families with early-onset breast/ovarian cancer, but not all labs test both), the type of testing being offered (FAP gene testing is available by either direct sequencing, protein truncation, or linkage analysis), and the region of the gene that is being scanned. These molecular details often change quite rapidly and it is important to confirm these specifics before ordering a test (Table 9). Labs should also be able to provide information on the sensitivity and specificity of their methods, their quality control, and quality-assurance standards and accreditation. There are great discrepancies

Table 9
Molecular Diagnostic Tests: General Specimen Requirements

DNA-based studies (mutational analysis, linkage analysis)
Fresh nucleated cells shipped at ambient temperature
- Whole blood in EDTA or ADC tubes
- Fresh tissue specimens in tissue-culture media
- Cheek swabs/brush of buccal cells
Other archival, pathologic, or stored specimens
- Dried blood spots
- Paraffin-embedded tissue

RNA-based studies (functional assays)
Fresh nucleated cells separated and shipped overnight on ice
Tissue that was immediately frozen in liquid nitrogen

Cytogenetic studies
Fresh nucleated cells shipped at room temperature
- Whole blood in sodium heparin tubes
- Tissue or bone marrow in tissue-culture media

from lab to lab in the costs, the turnaround time and the billing requirements. The reporting formats also vary so it is necessary to clarify in which form the results will be reported, the type of information that will be included in the report, to whom the results be released, and how the confidentiality of these results will be assured. Each lab has specific handling and shipping requirements; it is important to clarify the type and amount of sample (blood or tumor cells) that is needed, the type of tube they should be shipped in, and the shipping temperature. DNA samples generally should be shipped in an ADC (yellow top) or EDTA (purple top) tube at room temperature. Samples for chromosome analyses should be shipped in heparin tubes (green top) at room temperature, and RNA samples should be shipped as nucleated cell pellets on dry ice. The requirements for all specimens including other pathology specimens need to be checked with the specific lab performing the test. Specimens for genetic tests often must be shipped with specific detailed information and paperwork. Often the samples must be accompanied with details about insurance, clinical and genetic information, and special request and consent forms. Finally it is important to clarify what the maximum allowable time is between collection and receipt of the sample in the lab. Because some labs only accept samples on certain days it is essential to clarify how and when the sample should be shipped. Acquiring this detailed information is critical to the success of the testing process.

GENETIC-TEST RESOURCES The fast pace of research in cancer medical genetics means that information is constantly at risk of becoming outdated. Before ordering a genetic test, it is important to ensure that the resources being utilized are the most up-to-date. Consultation with health-care professionals with genetics expertise, medical geneticists, genetic counselors, or oncologists is one means of gathering this information. These specialists can also be helpful in identifying resources for at-risk patients. Another means of gathering up-to-date information is the Internet. No single site is sufficiently comprehensive to provide all the necessary information, but the combination of the wide variety of available sites can be a valuable resource. Some useful sites include Online Mendelian Inheritance in Man (OMIM) (at http://www.ncbi.nlm.nih.gov/

omim/searchomim.html) and GeneClinics (at http://www.geneclinics.org/), regularly updated databases of inherited disorders with information on clinical presentation, molecular basis, cytogenetics, mapping, and population genetics. OMIM also has direct links to the National Library of Medicine's MEDLINE database, DNA sequence databases, the Genome Database, and, in some instances, color images of relevant physical findings. Many key features about the genetics of specific syndromes mentioned in this chapter can be expanded with specific references in OMIM. The National Cancer Institute has a genetics information center (at http://cancernet.nci.nih.gov/p_genetics.html) and The Human Genome Project under the auspices of the United States Department of Energy offers a number of useful links to other sites on the Net (at http://www.orn./gov/techresources/human_genome/publicat/publications.html. The web pages of a number of genetic support groups also are useful resources. The Alliance of Genetic Support Groups (at http://medhlp.netusa.net/www/agsg.htm) maintains up-to-date listings of these groups and includes contact resources (telephone numbers and addresses). The Journal of the American Medical Association (JAMA) web site (at http://www.ama-assn.org/jama) and NetSight on the Medsite navigator Web site (at http://www.Medsite Navigator.com) contains an extensive list of potentially useful sites, and the Genetics Education Center at the University of Kansas Medical Center maintains an up-to-date listing of clinical genetic computer resources (at http://www.kumc.edu/GEC/prof/geneprof.html).

CONCLUSION

With the discovery of culprit genes critical to the development of cancer in an individual, new molecular tests are being developed to analyze the genotype associated with cancer prior to the development of malignancy. Predictive molecular testing for cancer has rapidly growing applications in clinical practice. This area of molecular genetic testing for cancer-predisposition syndromes is a relatively new, growing, and exciting area of medicine. In a minority of human malignancies, the identification of a few predisposing genes has clearly paved the way for relatively specific genetic testing. Today, in large kindreds where early cancer segregates in an autosomal dominant fashion, mutational analysis of the putative culprit gene may provide predictive risks for family members.

Analysis of most cancer genes to date, however, indicates that no one mutation accounts for a high percentage of the disease-causing mutations, and that new mutations continue to be identified. Furthermore, in many types of cancer, different mutations in potentially a handful of different genes may act independently or in concert with one another to promote oncogenesis. This makes the process of molecular-based diagnosis quite challenging at present from both a clinical and technical standpoint. Indeed, many types of cancer are excellent examples of a disease where there is strong evidence for genetic heterogeneity and at any given locus, significant allelic heterogeneity within a gene, incomplete penetrance, and variable expression. Currently, the diagnosis of cancer is most often based on histopathological analysis of the tissue involved, but with continued advances in the area of cancer genetics, it is

Table 10
Assessment of a Genetic Test

What genetic test is being considered?
- What is its predictive value?
- What is the sensitivity?
- What is the specificity?

What type of laboratory is performing the test (clinical vs research)?
- Are there appropriate standards for quality assurance and quality control?
- What specific gene is being studied
- What regions of the gene are being analyzed?
- What type of molecular test is being done?
- What is the cost and the turnaround time?

How are the results interpreted?
- What is the cancer risk of a positive result?
- What is the risk of cancer following a negative result?

How will the results of this test influence?
- Medical management of the patient?
- Family planning issues?
- Psychosocial concerns of the patient?

widely anticipated that diagnostic tests will become more molecular-based. Many different types of alterations in genes associated with cancer will be identified. Some of these alterations will be benign polymorphism that have no clinical relevances while others may be mutations directly involved in malignant tumorigenesis. Thus, each genetic alteration identified must be carefully characterized to determine if it is a benign genetic polymorphism or a disease causing mutation so that clinically relevant tests can be appropriately developed and accurately interpreted. The last major hurdle, and likely the most critically important one, is developing the educational and counseling resources to enable all health-care providers and patients to fully understand the implications and limitations of such testing so that it can be used in an informed, reliable, and educated framework. Before offering a genetic test, clinicians should assess the value of the specific test in context of benefit to their patient. Some of the questions a clinician should ask are listed in Table 10.

Continued modification of molecular genetic technology to create a cost effective means of delivering a sensitive, specific test that provides accurate results in a timely, affordable fashion will also facilitate more available genetic tests. With this technology, however, many new questions and concerns are raised about how to responsibly, ethically, and cost-effectively apply this new information. The general public, our patients, students, and practicing physician colleagues are constantly being bombarded by an often-glamorized media blitz catering to our societal interests in health-care issues where genetics and cancer are high-interest topics. After all, cancer is second only to heart disease as the cause of mortality for adults in our country. Clearly, for the most part, this media attention provides an avenue for education. However, sometimes false hope and enthusiasm may be instilled in the minds of patients and physicians alike. As physicians and scientists, we have the power to help regulate the appropriate translation of basic science

research to direct patient care by fostering collaborations between basic-research scientists, clinical-research investigators, and interfacing with private industry biotechnology developers and governmental lobbyist groups. As such we have the responsibility to critically analyze the health-care costs and benefits of new applied technology, from economic, intellectual, and psychosocial perspectives. We have a responsibility to use the technology wisely.

REFERENCES

1. Collins, F. S. (1997) Sequencing the human genome. *Hosp. Pract.* **32**:35–54.
2. Green, E. D., Cox, D. R., and Myers, R. M. (1995) The human genome project and its impact on the study of human disease. *In: The Metabolic and Molecular Basis of Inherited Disease*, 7th ed. (Scriver, C. R., Beaudet, A. L., Sly, W. S., and Valle, D., eds.), McGraw-Hill, New York, pp. 401–436.
3. Glassman, A. B. (1997) Cytogenetics. An evolving role in the diagnosis and treatment of cancer. *Clin. Lab. Med.* **17**:21–37.
4. Solomon, E., Borrow, J., and Goddard, A. D. (1991) Chromosome aberrations and cancer. *Science* **254**:1153–1160.
5. Saglio, G., Pane, F., Martinelli, G., and Guerrasio, A. (1997) BCR/ABL transcripts and leukemia phenotype: an unsolved puzzle. *Leukemia Lymphoma* **26**:281–286.
6. Crisan, D., Chen, S. T., and Weil, S. C. (1994) Polymerase chain reaction in the diagnosis of chromosomal breakpoints. *Hematol. Oncol. Clin. North Am.* **8**:725–750.
7. Hochhaus, A., Reiter, A., Skladny, H., Reichert, A., Saussele, S., and Hehlmann, R. (1998) Molecular monitoring of residual disease in chronic myelogenous leukemia patients after therapy. *Cancer Res.* **144**:36–45.
8. Knudson, A. G. (1993) Antioncogenes and human cancer. *Proc Natl Acad Sci USA* **90**:10,914–10,921.
9. Shibata, D., Reale, M. A., Lavin, P., Silverman, M., Fearon, E. R., Steele, G., et al. (1996) The DCC protein and prognosis in colorectal cancer. *N. Engl. J. Med.* **335**:1727–1732.
10. Caldas, C. and Ponder, B. (1997) Cancer genes and molecular oncology in the clinic. *Lancet* **349**:16–18.
11. Ponder, B. (1997) Genetic testing for cancer risk. *Science* **278**:1050–1054.
12. Garber, J. and Schrag, D. (1996) Testing for cancer susceptibility. *JAMA* **275**:1928–1929.
13. Fearon, E. (1997) Human cancer syndromes: clues to the origin and nature of cancer. *Science* **278**:1043–1050.
14. Fearon, E. R. and Vogelstein, B. (1994) A genetic model for colorectal tumorigenesis. *Cell* **61**:759–767.
15. Hartwell, L. H. and Kasten, M. D. (1994) Cell cycle control and cancer. *Science* **266**:1821–1828.
16. Heshmati, H. M., Gharib, H., van Heerden, J. A., and Sizemore, G. W. (1997) Advances and controversies in the diagnosis and management of medullary thyroid carcinoma. *Am. J. Med.* **103**:60–69.
17. Cooper, D. N., Krawczak, M., and Antonarakis, S. E. (1995) The nature and mechanisms of human gene mutation. *In: The Metabolic Basis of Inherited Disease*, 7th ed. (Scriver, C. R., Beaudet, A. L., Sly, W. S., and Valle, D., eds.), McGraw Hill, New York, pp. 259–291.
18. Greenblatt, M. S., Bennett, W. P., Hollstein, M., and Harris, C. C. (1994) Mutations in the p53 tumor suppressor gene: clues to cancer etiology and molecular pathogenesis. *Cancer Res.* **54**:4855–4878.
19. Strong, L. C., Williams, W. R., and Tainsky, M. A. (1992) The Li-Fraumeni Syndrome: from clinical epidemiology to molecular genetics. *Am. J. Epidemiol.* **135**:190–199.
20. Miki, Y., Swenson, J., and Shattuck-Eidens, D. (1994) A strong candidate for the breast and ovarian cancer susceptibility gene BRCA1. *Science* **266**:66–71.
21. Futreal, P. A., Liu, Q., Shattuck-Eidens, D., Cochran, C., Harshman, K., Tavtigian, S., et al. (1994) BRCA1 mutations in primary breast and ovarian carcinomas. *Science* **266**:120–122.

22. Wooster, R., Bignell, G., Lancaster, J., Swift, S., Seal, S., Manglon, J., et al. (1995) Identification of the breast cancer susceptibility gene BRCA2. *Nature* **378**:789–792.

23. Boland, C. R. and Meltzer, S. J. (1997) Cancer of the colon and gastrointestinal tract. *In: Emery and Rimoin's Principles and Practice of Medical Genetics* (Emery, A. H. snd Rimoin, D. L., eds.), Churchill Livingstone, New York, pp. 1579–1598.

24. Kinzler, K. W. and Vogelstein, B. (1995) Colorectal tumors. *In: The Metabolic and Molecular Basis of Inherited Disease,* 7th ed. (Scriver, C. R., Beaudet, A. L., Sly, W. S., and Valle, D., eds.), McGraw-Hill, New York, pp. 643–663.

25. Laken, S. J., Petersen, G. M., Gruber, S. B., Oddoux, C., Ostrer, H., Giardiello, F. M., et al. (1997) Familial colorectal cancer in Ashkenazi due to a hypermutable tract in APC. *Nature Genet.* **17**:79–83.

26. Giardiello, F. M., Brensinger, J. D., Petersen, G. M., Luce, M. C., Hylind, L. M., Bacon, J. A., et al. (1997) The use and interpretation of commercial APC gene testing for familial adenomatous polyposis. *N. Engl. J. Med.* **336**:823–827.

27. McPherson, R. (1995) Molecular basis of genetic disease and molecular methods. *Clin. Lab. Med.* **15**:779–794.

28. Ben-Ezra, J. (1995) Amplification methods in the molecular diagnosis of genetic diseases. *Clin. Lab. Med.* **15**:795–815.

29. Sidransky, D. (1997) Nucleic acid-based methods for the detection of cancer. *Science* **278**:1054–1058.

30. Merajver, S. D. and Petty, E. M. (1996) Risk assesment and presymptomatic diagnosis of hereditary breast cancer. *North Am. Clin. Lab. Med.* **16**:139–167.

31. Wuyts, W., VanHul, W., DeBoulle, K., Hendrickx, J., Bakker, E., Vanhoenacker, F., et al. (1998) Mutations in the EXT1 and EXT2 genes in hereditary multiple exostoses. *Am. J. Human Genet.* **62**:346–354.

32. Bale, A. E. and Petty, E. M. (1995) Linkage analysis of human disease. *In: Molecular Endocrinology: Basic Concepts and Clinical Correlations* (Weintraub, B. D., ed.), Raven Press, New York, pp. 23–32.

33. Ott, J. (1991) *Analysis of Human Genetic Linkage.* The Johns Hopkins University Press, Baltimore, MD.

34. Terwilliger, J. D. and Ott, J. (1994) *Handbook of Human Genetic Linkage.* The Johns Hopkins University Press, Baltimore, MD.

35. Grompe, M. (1993) The rapid detection of unknown mutations in nucleic acids. *Nature Genet.* **5**:111–117.

36. Cotton, R. G. (1993) Current methods of mutation detection. *Mut. Res.* **285**:125–144.

37. Dracopoli, N. C., Haines, J. L., Korf, B. R., Moir, D. T., Morton, C. C., Seidman, C. E., Seidman, J. G., and Smith, D. R. (eds.) (1994) *Current Protocols in Human Genetics.* John Wiley & Sons, Inc., New York.

38. Shuldiner, A. R., LeRoith, D., and Roberts, C. T. (1995) DNA sequence analysis. *In: Molecular Endocrinology: Basic Concepts and Clinical Correlations* (Weintraub, B. D., ed.), Raven Press, New York, pp. 13–21.

39. Thierfelder, L. (1998) Mutation detection by cycle sequencing. *In: Current Protocols in Human Genetics* (Dracopoli, N. C., Haines, J. L., Korf, B. R., Moir, D. T., Morton, C. C., Seidman, C. E., et al., eds.), John Wiley & Sons, Inc., New York, pp. 7.7.1–7.7.6.

40. Hacia, J. G., Brody, L.C., Chee, M. S., Fodor, S. P. A., and Collins, F. S. (1996) Detection of heterozygous mutations in BRCA1 using high density oligonucleotide arrays and two-color fluorescence analysis. *Nature Genet.* **14**:441–447.

41. Cronin, M. T., Fucini, R. V., Kim, S. M., Masino, R. S., Wespi, R. M., and Miyada, C. G. (1996) Cystic fibrosis mutation detection by hybridization to light-generated DNA probe arrays. *Human Mut.* **7**:244–255.

42. Chee, M., Yang, R., Hubbell, E., Berno, A., Huang, X. C., Stern, D., et al. (1996) Accessing genetic information with high-density DNA arrays. *Science* **274**:610–614.

43. Pease, A. C., Solas, D., Sullivan, E. J., Cronin, M. T., Holmes, C. P., and Fodor, S. P. A. (1994) Light-generated oligonucleotide arrays for rapid DNA sequence analysis. *Proc. Natl. Acad. Sci. USA* **91**:5022–5026.

44. Warren, W., Hovig, E., Smith-Sorensen, B., Borresen, A. L., Fujimura, F. K., Liu, Q., et al. (1998) Detection of mutations by single-strand conformation polymorphism (SSCP) analysis and SSCP-hybrid methods. *In: Current Protocols in Human Genetics* (Dracopoli, N. C., Haines, J. L., Korf, B. R., Moir, D. T., Morton, C. C., Seidman, C. E., et al., eds.), John Wiley & Sons, Inc, New York, pp. 7.4.1–7.4.23.

45. Fan, E., Levin, D. B., Glickman, B. W., and Logan, D. M. (1993) Limitations in the use of SSCP analysis. *Mut. Res.* **288**:85–92.

46. Hayashi, K. (1991) PCR-SSCP: a simple and sensitive method for detection of mutations in the genomic DNA. *PCR Methods Appl.* **1**:34–38.

47. Sekiya, T. (1993) Detection of mutant sequences by single-strand conformation polymorphism analysis. *Mut. Res.* **288**:79–83.

48. White, M. B., Carvalho, M., Derse, D., O'Brien, S. J., and Dean, M. (1992) Detecting single base pair substitutions as heteroduplex polymorphisms. *Genomics* **12**:301–306.

49. Liu, Q. and Sommer, S. (1995) Restriction endonucleases fingerprinting (REF): a sensitive method for screen mutations in long contiguous segments of DNA. *BioTechniques* **18**:470–477.

50. Blaszyk, H., Hartmann, A., Schroeder, J. J., McGovern, R. M., Sommer, S. S., and Kovach, J. S. (1995) Rapid and efficient screening for p53 gene mutations by dideoxy fingerprinting (ddF). *BioTechniques* **18**:256–260.

51. Cariello, N. F. and Skopek, T. R. (1993) Mutational analysis using denaturing gradient gel electrophoresis and PCR. *Mut. Res.* **288**:103–112.

52. Fodde, R. and Losekoot, M. (1994) Mutation detection by denaturing gradient gel electrophoresis (DGGE). *Human Mut.* **3**:83–94.

53. Borresen-Dale, A. L., Hovig, E., and Smith-Sorensen, B. (1998) Mutational analysis using denaturing gradient gel electrophoresis. *In: Current Protocols in Human Genetics* (Dracopoli, N. C., Haines, J. L., Korf, B. R., Moir, D. T., Morton, C. C., Seidman, C. E., et al., eds.), John Wiley & Sons, Inc, New York, pp. 7.5.1–7.5.13.

54. Smooker, P. M. and Cotton, R. G. (1993) The use of chemical reagents in the detection of DNA mutations. *Mut. Res.* **288**:65–77.

55. Youil, R., Kemper, B. W., and Cotton, R. H. (1995) Screening for mutations by enzyme mismatch cleavage with T4 endonuclease VII. *Proc. Natl. Acad. Sci. USA* **92**:87–91.

56. Mashal, R. D., Koontz, J., and Sklar, J. (1995) Detection of mutations by cleavage of DNA heteroduplexes with bacteriophage resolvases. *Nature Genet.* **9**:177–183.

57. Zbar, B., Kishida, T., Chen, F., Schmiddt, L., Maher, E. R., Richards, F. M., et al. (1996) Germline mutations in the von Hippel-Lindau disease (VHL) gene in families from North America, Europe and Japan. *Human Mut.* **8**:348–357.

58. Crossey, P. A., Richards, F. M., Foster, K., Green, J. S., Prowse, A., Latif, F., et al. (1994) Identification of intragenic mutations in the von Hippel-Lindau disease tumor suppressor gene and correlation with disease phenotype. *Human Mol. Genet.* **3**:1303–1308.

59. Chen, F., Kishida, T., Yao, M., Hustad, T., Glavac, D., Dean, M., et al. (1995) Germline mutations in the von Hippel-Lindau disease tumor suppressor gene: correlations with phenotype. *Human Mut.* **5**:66–75.

60. Jarcha, J. (1998) Restriction fragment length polymorphism analysis. *In: Current Protocols in Human Genetics* (Dracopoli, N. C., Haines, J. L., Korf, B. R., Moir, D. T., Morton, C. C., Seidman, C. E., et al., eds.), John Wiley & Sons, Inc, New York, pp. 2.7.1–2.7.11.

61. Handelin, B. and Shuber, A. P. (1998) Simultaneous detection of multiple point mutations using allele-specific oligonucleotides. *In: Current Protocols in Human Genetics* (Dracopoli, N. C., Haines, J. L., Korf, B. R., Moir, D. T., Morton, C. C., Seidman, C. E., et al., eds.), John Wiley & Sons, Inc, New York, pp. 9.4.1–9.4.8.

62. Struewing, J., Hartge, P., Wacholder, S., Baker, S., Berlin, M., McAdams, M., et al. (1997) The risk of cancer associated with specific mutations of *BRCA1* and *BRCA2* among Ashkenazi Jews. *N. Engl. J. Med.* **336**:1401–1408.

63. Ishioka, C., Frebourg, T., Yan, Y. X., Vidal, M., Friend, S. H., Schmidt, S., et al. (1993) Screening patients for heterozygous p53 mutations using a functional assay in yeast. *Nature Genet.* **5**:124–129.

64. Hogervorst, F. B. L., Cornelis, R. S., Bout, M., vanVliet, M., Oosterwijk, J. C., Olmer, R., et al. (1995) Rapid detection of BRCA1 mutations by the protein truncation test. *Nature Genet.* **10**:208–212.

65. denDunnen, J. T. (1998) Protein truncation test. In: *Current Protocols in Human Genetics* (Dracopoli, N. C., Haines, J. L., Korf, B. R., Moir, D. T., Morton, C. C., Seidman, C. E., et al., eds.), John Wiley & Sons, Inc, New York, pp. 9.11.1–9.11.18.

66. Korf, B. R. and Pagon, R. A. (1998) Overview of molecular genetic diagnosis. In: *Current Protocols in Human Genetics* (Dracopoli, N. C., Haines, J. L., Korf, B. R., Moir, D. T., Morton, C. C., Seidman, C. E., et al., eds.), John Wiley & Sons, Inc, New York, pp. 9.1.1–9.1.9.

67. Collins, F. (1996) BRCA1: lots of mutations, lots of dilemmas. *N. Engl. J. Med.* **334**:186–188.

68. Anonymous (1996) Statement of the American Society of Clinical Oncology: genetic testing for cancer susceptibility. *J. Clin. Oncol.* **14**:1730–1736.

69. Dracopoli, N. C. and Fountain, J. W. (1996) CDKN2 mutations in melanoma. *Cancer Surv.* **26**:115–132.

70. Fitzgerald, M. G., Harkin, D. P., Silva-Arrieta, S., MacDonald, D. J., Lucchina, L. C., Unsal, H., et al. (1996) Prevalence of germline mutations in p16, p19ARF, and CDK4 in familial melanoma: analysis of a clinic-based population. *Proc. Natl. Acad. Sci. USA* **93**:8541–8545.

71. Anonymous (1994) Statement of The American Society of Human Genetics on genetic testing for breast and ovarian cancer predisposition. *Am. J. Human Genet.* **55**:i–iv.

72. Anonymous (1994) Statement on use of DNA testing for presymptomatic identification of cancer risk. National Advisory Council for Human Genome Research. *JAMA* **271**:785–780.

73. Editorial (1997) BRCA Genes - Bookmaking, fortune telling, and medical care. *N. Engl. J. Med.* **336**:1448–1449.

74. National Institutes of Health (1998) *SEER Cancer Statistics Review NCI. 1973–1991.*

75. Gelehrter, T., Collins, F., and Ginsburg, D. (1998) *Principles of Medical Genetics.* Williams & Wilkins, Baltimore, MD.

76. Bennett, R., Steinhaus, K., Uhrich, S., O'Sullivan, C., Resta, R., Lochner-Doyle, D., et al. (1995) Recommendations for standardized human pedigree nomenclature. *J. Genet. Counseling* **4**:267–279.

77. Schneider, K. (1994) *Counseling About Cancer: Strategies for Genetic Counselors.* Graphic Illusions, Dennisport, MA.

78. Hoskins, K., Stopfer, J., Calzone, K., Merajver, S., Rebbeck, T., Garber, J., et al. (1995) Assessment and counseling for women with a family history of breast cancer (A guide for clinicians). *JAMA* **273**:577–585.

79. Petersen, G. and Brensinger, J. (1996) General testing and counseling in familial adenomatous polyposis. *Oncology* **10**:89–94.

80. Wihawer, S. (1997) Colorectal cancer screening: clinical guidelines and rationale. *Gastroenterology* **112**:594–642.

81. Hubbard, R. and Lewontin, R.C. (1996) Sounding Board: pitfalls of genetic testing. *N. Engl. J. Med.* **334**:1192–1194.

82. Kahn, P. (1996) Coming to grips with genes and risk. *Science* **274**:496–498.

83. Healey, B. (1997) BRCA Genes: bookmaking, fortunetelling, and medical care. *N. Engl. J. Med.* **336**:1448.

84. McGovern, M., Keenlyside, R., Benach, M., and Desnick, R. (1997) Quality assurance practices in molecular genetic testing laboratories in the United States. *Am. J. Human Genetics* **61**:A57.

85. Garrett, C. and Sell, S. (1995) Summary and perspective: Assessing test effectiveness: the identification of good tumor markers. In: *Cellular Cancer Markers* (Garrett, C. and Sell, S., eds.), Humana Press, Totowa, NJ, pp. 455–477.

86. Medicare, Medicaid and CLIA Programs: Regulations Implementing the Clinical Laboratory Improvement Amendments of 1988 (CLIA) (Health Care Financing Administration, HHS, Federal Regulation). *Federal Register* **57** FR 7002, February 28, 1992.

87. American College of Medical Genetics (1993) *American College of Medical Genetics: Standards and Guidelines: Clinical Laboratory Genetics.* Bethesda, MD.

88. Burt, R. W. (1995) Polyposis syndromes. In: *Textbook of Gastroenterology.* (Yamada, T., Alpers, D. H., Owyang, C., Powell, D. W., and Silverstein, F. E., eds.), J.B. Lippincott, Philadelphia, PA, pp. 1944–1966.

89. Fearon, E. R., Cho, K. R., Nigro, J. M., Kern, S. E., Simons, J. W., Ruppert, J. M., et al. (1990) Identification of a chromosome 18q gene that is altered in colorectal cancers. *Science* **247**:49–55.

90. Schrag, D., Kuntz, K., Garber, J., and Weeks, J. (1997) Decision analysis: effects of prophylactic mastectomy and oophorectomy on life expectancy among women with BRCA1 or BRCA2 gene mutations. *N. Engl. J. Med.* **336**:1465–1471.

91. Bloch, M., Adam, S., Wiggins, S., Huggins, M., and Hayden, M. (1992) Predictive testing for Huntington disease in Canada: the experience of those receiving an increased risk. *Am. J. Med. Genet.* **42**:499–507.

92. Wiggins, S., Whyte, P., and Huggins, M. (1992) The psychological consequences of predictive testing for Huntington's disease. *N. Engl. J. Med.* **327**:1401–1405.

93. Lerman, C. and Croyle, R. (1994) Psychological issues in genetic testing for breast cancer susceptibility. *Arch. Int. Med.* **154**:609–616.

94. Ad Hoc Committee on Genetic Testing/Insurance Issues, (1995) Background Statement: Genetic Testing and Insurance. *Am. J. Human Genet.*, **56**, 327–331.

95. Rothenberg, K., Fuller, B., Rothstein, M., Duster, T., Ellis-Kahn, M., Cunningham, R., et al. (1997) Genetic information and the workplace: legislative approaches and policy challenges. *Science* **275**:1755–1757.

96. Birmingham, K. (1997) Insurers admit genetic discrimination. *Nature Med.* **3**:710.

97. Reilly, P. R., Boshar, M. F., and Holtzman, S. H. (1997) Ethical issues in genetic research: disclosure and informed consent. *Nature Genet.* **15**:16–20.

98. Maher, E., Yates, J., Harries, R., Benjamin, C., Harris, R., Moore, A, et al. (1990) Clinical features and natural history of von Hippel-Lindau disease. *Q. J. Med.* **77**:1151–1163.

99. Choyke, P., Glenn, G., Walther, M., Patronas, N., Linehan, W., and Zbar, B. (1995) von Hippel-Lindau disease: genetic, clinical, and imaging features. *Radiololgy* **194**:629–642.

100. Young, I. (1996) Risk Estimation in Genetic Counseling. In: *Emery & Rimoin's Principles and Practice in Medical Genetics* (Emery, A. H. and Rimoin, D. L., eds.), Churchill Livingstone, New York, pp. 521–533.

100a. Rothenberg, F., Fuller, B., Rotherstein, M., Duster, T., Ellis Kahn, M. J., Cunningham, R., Fine, B., Hudson, K., King, M. C., Murphy, P., Swergold, G., and Collins, F. (1997) Genetic information and the workplace: legislative approaches and policy changes. *Science* **275**(5307):1755–1757.

101. (1996) Cancer facts and figures. *ACS*, (Abstract)

102. Silverberg, E., Boring, C. C., and Squires, T. S. (1990) Cancer statistics. *CA Cancer J. Clin.* **40**:9–26.

103. Calzone, K. (1997) Predisposition testing for breast and ovarian cancer susceptibility. *Sem. Oncol. Nurs.* **13**:82–90.

104. Shattuck-Eidens, D., McClure, M., and Simard, J. (1995) A collaborative study of 80 mutations in the BRCA1 breast and ovarian cancer susceptibility gene: implications for presymptomatic genetic testing and screening. *JAMA* **273**:535–541.

105. Greene, M. (1997) Genetics of breast cancer. *Mayo Clin. Proc.* **72**:54–65.

106. Easton, D., Bishop, D., Ford, D., and Crockford, G. (1993) Breast Cancer Linkage Consortium. Genetic linkage analysis in familial breast and ovarian cancer: results from 214 families. *Am. J. Human Genet.* **52**:678–701.

107. Ford, D., Easton, D., Bishop, D., Narod, S., and Goldgar, D. (1994) Breast Cancer Linkage Consortium. Risks of cancer in BRCA1 mutation carriers. *Lancet* **343**:692–695.

108. Wooster, R., Neuhausen, S. L., Mangion, J., Quirk, Y., Ford, D., Collins, N., et al. (1994) Localization of a breast cancer susceptibility gene, BRCA2, to chromosome 13q12-13. *Science* **265**:2088–2090.

109. Easton, D. F., Ford, D., and Bishop, D. T. (1995) Breast and ovarian cancer incidence in BRCA1-mutation carriers. Breast Cancer Linkage Consortium. *Am. J. Human Genet.* **56**:265–271.

110. Elias, S. and Annas, G. (1994) Generic consent for genetic screening. *N. Engl. J. Med.* **330**:1611–1613.

111. Geller, G., Botkin, J., Green, M., Press, N., Biesecker, B., Wilfond, B., et al. (1997) Genetic testing for susceptibility to adult-onset cancer (The process and content of informed consent). *JAMA* **277**:1467–1474.

23 Novel Molecular Targets for Cancer Drug Discovery

JOHN K. BUOLAMWINI, PHD

INTRODUCTION

Conventional cancer chemotherapy leaves much to be desired because the drugs in current use are highly cytotoxic and lack selectivity between cancer cells and normal cells. Therefore, there is a need for novel cancer therapies that will selectively eliminate neoplastic cells without toxicity to normal tissues. Recent advances in cancer cell biology, made possible by advances in recombinant DNA technology, offer new hope for achieving selective cancer chemotherapy. Many molecular mechanisms and genes involved in neoplastic transformation, tumor progression, tumor angiogenesis, and metastasis have been elucidated, providing a plethora of potential molecular targets for specific anticancer therapy *(1–6)*. In addition to the discovery of novel molecular targets, advances in recombinant DNA technology have also facilitated investigation of the potential of these targets for drug design and development, including the functional expression or production of the targets. Production of target molecules enables high-throughput screening assays of natural and synthetic molecule libraries. Production of sufficient quantities of target proteins facilitates X-ray crystallography, which provides the three-dimensional structure of the target molecule and reveals the nature of interactions between target molecules and their ligands/inhibitors at the atomic level. These advances potentially contributes valuable information for rational structure-based drug design *(7)*. Interesting and creative approaches to selectively killing cancer cells while sparing normal cells are emerging, like the use of engineered adenoviruses such as ONYX-015, which is currently in clinical trials (Onyx Pharmaceuticals). This adenovirus selectively replicates in and kills cells that have lost p53 function (>50% of all human cancers). ONYX-015 cannot replicate in cells with normal p53 function and therefore lacks cytotoxicity against normal cells.

This chapter provides a general overview of current research efforts towards identification and exploitation of novel molecular targets in the development of more selective and less toxic small-molecule anticancer drugs. Recent developments towards exploitation of novel molecular targets in clinical treatment of human cancer based on gene therapy *(8)*, antibody treatment *(9)*, and antisense oligonucleotide approaches *(10)* will not be reviewed.

NOVEL CANCER MOLECULAR TARGETS AND DRUG DISCOVERY

Malignant transformation is a multi-step process involving genetic changes of proto-oncogenes *(11)* and/or tumor-suppressor genes *(12)*. Activation of proto-oncogenes by mutation, gene amplification, and/or overexpression in combination with the loss of tumor suppressor gene function leads to neoplastic transformation. Tumors emerge from cell populations when the normal balance between cell survival and cell loss by apoptosis (programmed cell death) is shifted in favor of the former. Apoptosis research has been extensive, and many genes have been discovered that either promote or prevent it *(13)*. The numerous potential molecular targets that have been uncovered can be grouped into three broad categories: (1) cell surface and cytoplasmic mitogenic signal-transduction targets, (2) nuclear targets, and (3) extracellular matrix (ECM) targets. The first category is made up primarily of growth factor receptor kinases and nonreceptor kinases. The second category comprises cell-cycle progression, apoptosis, and cell longevity targets. The third category consists of ECM enzymes and adhesion molecules and their receptors involved in tissue remodeling, tumor metastasis, invasion, and angiogenesis. Table 1 gives a summary of the major targets organized into these categories, and lists known representative inhibitors for these categories.

CELL-SURFACE AND CYTOPLASMIC SIGNAL TRANSDUCTION PATHWAYS TARGETS

Several components of signal transduction pathways that relay mitogenic signals to the cell nucleus in the initiation or

From: *The Molecular Basis of Human Cancer* (W. B. Coleman and G. J. Tsongalis, eds.), © Humana Press Inc., Totowa, NJ.

Table 1
Major Potential Novel Molecular Targets and Prototype Small Molecule Inhibitors

Category	Common cancers	Typical Inhibitor
Oncogenic Growth-Factor Receptors		
EGFR	Breast, ovarian, lung	Anilinoquinazolines
HER-2	Breast, ovarian	Benzylidene tyrphostins
PDGFR	Gliomas	3–arylquinolines
Non-Receptor Tyrosine Kinases		
c-src	Colon, pancreatic	Dihydropyrimidinoquinolinones
c-lck	T-lymphomas	Phenylcarboxamide imminochromenes
c-abl	CML	Phenylaminipyrimidines (STI571)
Oncogenic Serine/Threonine Kinases		
PKC	Breast cancer, gliomas, thyroid cancer, melanoma	7–hydroxystaurosporin, Safingol
Oncogenic GTP-Binding Proteins		
c-ras	Pancreatic, lung, colorectal, Myeloid leukemia	SCH44342 (FTase inhibitor)
Oncogenic Cyclins		
A	Liver	None
B	Breast (?)	None
D1	Lymphoma, breast, esophagus, bladder, lung	None
D2	Colon, testicular, CLL	None
D3	Retinoblastoma, lymphoma, ALL	None
E	Breast, leukemia, lung, stomach, Kidney, prostate, lung	None
Cyclin-Dependent Kinases		
cdk1, cdk2, cdk4	Gliomas, soft tissue sacrcomas	Flavopiridol, olomoucine, UCN-01
p53 Antagonists		
mdm2	Sarcomas	None
bcl2	B-cell lymphoma, prostate, breast, colorectal, lung	None
Cell Longevity Targets		
Telomerase	Most human cancers	Anthraquinones
Angiogenesis and Metastasis Targets		
VEGFR-2/flk-1	General	Quinoxalines
bFGFR	General	Oxindoles, thioindoles
MMPs	General	Batimastat, marimastat
uPA/uPAR	Melanoma, colon, non-small cell lung, stomach, breast and ovarian cancers	Amiloride analogs (uPA inhibitors)
CAM	Colorectal	RDG peptides (for integrins)

promotion of cell proliferation represent targets for chemotherapy, including growth factor receptor tyrosine kinases (RTKs), nonreceptor tyrosine kinases, and serine/threonine kinases. One of the best-characterized signal-transduction systems in mammalian cells involves tyrosine phosphorylation, which may be the primary effector of signal transduction in multicellular organisms *(14)*. Stimulation of RTKs by their endogenous ligands (growth factors) causes their dimerization and initiates tyrosine phosphorylation of the receptors to begin the mitogenic signal-transduction cascade. A comprehensive review of growth factors, their receptors and signaling cascades/networks, and their inhibitors has been published *(15)*. Monomeric or dimeric growth factors bind to the extracellular domain of their specific receptor causing receptor homodimerization or heterodimerization, which triggers receptor autophosphorylation of tyrosine residues in the intracellular domain of the receptor. In the most studied branch of this signaling pathway (Fig. 1), the phosphorylation allows the bind-

ing to the intracellular domain of RTKs by the Grb2 adapter protein via its SH2 (src homology 2) domain. The bound Grb2 is now activated to bind, via its SH3 (src homology 3) domain, to the guanine nucleotide exchange factor, the sos (for son of sevenless) protein, and translocate it to the cell membrane where it binds to the c-ras GTP-binding protein. This causes c-ras to undergo a molecular switch involving the release of GDP and the binding of GTP in its place, thereby activating ras. Activated c-ras then triggers several different cascades *(16)*, the most studied being the mitogen-activated protein (MAP) kinase cascade that ends with activated ERK kinase. This cascade begins with the activation of c-raf-1 kinase by c-ras. Activated c-raf-1 kinase (MAP kinase kinase kinase) then initiates the MAP kinase cascade by phosphorylating MEK kinase, which in turn phosphorylates the ultimate MAP kinase in the cascade, ERK. Activated ERK translocates into the cell nucleus where it propagates the mitogenic signal by way of phosphorylating and activating the appropriate transcription factors to

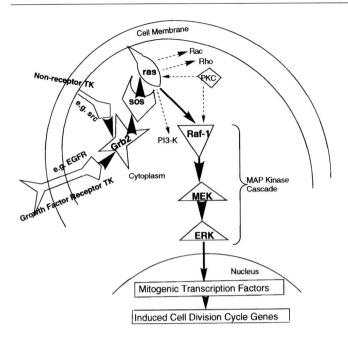

Fig. 1. Schematic representation of receptor and non-receptor mitogenic signaling pathways. Bold-lettered items are those in the classical or major receptor and non-receptor tyrosine kinase mitogenic signaling pathways. Bold arrows point to or from targets in the pathways, while broken arrows indicate cross-talk.

induce the expression of genes necessary for initiating and driving the cell-division cycle *(14,17)*. Several other upstream regulators and downstream effectors of c-ras have been identified *(16,18–20)*.

The mutational activation or overexpression of RTKs have been implicated in many human cancers, especially breast, ovarian, and nonsmall cell lung cancers (NCLCs) *(14,21)*, and this makes them potential novel molecular targets for cancer chemotherapy *(22–24)*. The most widely explored growth-factor RTKs, in terms of novel anticancer drug discovery, are epidermal growth-factor receptor (EGFR), c-erbB2/HER-2 receptor, platelet-derived growth-factor receptor (PDGFR), vascular endothelial growth-factor receptor (VEGFR), and fibroblast growth factor receptor (FGFR). The roles of growth-factor receptors and their ligands involved in autocrine or paracrine loops in the development of various tumors have been discussed *(21)*, as well as strategies to target them for therapeutic purposes *(22)*. EGFR, HER-2, and PDGFR are being explored primarily as anti-proliferative molecular targets, whereas VEGFR and FGFR are being explored primarily as anti-angiogenesis targets. Many reviews have appeared on drug-discovery efforts targeting the proliferative RTKs *(23–30)*. Strategies for the discovery of tyrosine kinase inhibitors with anticancer activity have been presented by Fry et al. *(26)*, which include the production of the target kinases, primary screening for potency and specificity, investigation of cellular effects, and in vivo evaluation for anticancer activity. Cytoplasmic serine/threonine kinases such as the protein kinase C (PKC) family, and the MAP kinases are also important in oncogenic signaling, and are being investigated as novel targets for cancer discovery and development.

Type 1 Growth Factor Receptor Tyrosine Kinases The type 1 growth-factor RTK family, also known as the erbB or HER family, comprises four well characterized members *(31)*. The first member is designated EGFR, c-erbB1, or HER1 (epidermal growth-factor receptor); the second member c-erbB2 or HER-2/neu; the third member c-erbB3 or HER3; and the fourth member c-erbB4 or HER-4 *(17)*. The amino acid sequence identity among these four type 1 RTKs is 40–60% in the extracellular domain and 60–80% in the intracellular domain *(32)*. Several ligands have been identified for all the type 1 RTK family members except HER2, for which no direct high-affinity specific ligand has yet been found *(33)*. The specific ligands for EGFR are EGF and transforming growth factor-α (TGFα), whereas the major high-affinity ligand for HER3 and HER4 is heregulin, also known as neu differentiation factor or neuregulin 1 *(33)*. Signaling via these receptors involves homodimerization or heterodimeization upon ligand binding. One or more of these RTKs has been shown to be activated by mutation (resulting in ligand-independent activation), or to be overexpressed in certain tumors, including breast, ovarian, and non-SCLCs *(14,21,31)*. RTK overexpression is associated with expression of a neoplastic phenotype, and has been implicated in resistance to chemotherapy *(32)*. Thus, RTKs constitute a family of potential molecular targets for cancer chemotherapy *(23,24)*. Undoubtedly, the type 1 RTK family is the most widely explored group in the search for novel targets for cancer therapeutics. Several antibody products directed against the EGFR are in phase I/II clinical trials for solid tumors including breast, lung, kidney, colon, and esophageal cancers *(34)*. Numerous small-molecule organic compounds have been synthesized and evaluated as inhibitors of EGFR and/or c-erbB2 tyrosine kinases *(24,25,29,30)*. These inhibitors are being designed as (1) substrate analogs, (2) ligands to bind in the ATP-binding site, or (3) compounds incorporating both substrate analog and ATP-binding site ligand moieties *(25)*. Among these, the tyrphostin substrate analogs introduced by Levitzki and coworkers *(35)*, and represented by Compound 1, were the first seriously investigated EGFR inhibitors (Fig. 2). Extensive structure-activity relationships (SAR) data have been acquired for the benzylidene malonitrile tyrphostins as selective EGFR inhibitors *(36–38)*. These SAR studies have led to the proposal of a tyrphostin pharmacophore for EGFR inhibitors, consisting of a 3,4–dihydroxyphenyl (catechol) ring and a *cis* cyano (nitrile) group that is coplanar with the ring *(36–38)*.

Beyond the tyrphostins, many new and more interesting selective EGFR inhibitors have been reported (Fig. 2), the most important of which include substituted anilinoquinazolines *(26,27)* and their bicyclic and tricyclic analogs, such as PD 153035 (Compound 2), dianilinopyrimidines (Compound 3), dianilinophthalimides such as CGP52411 (Compound 4), which are simplified staurosporin analogs *(30)*, and benzoylacetylene derivatives such as DAP-720 (Compound 5). The in vitro IC$_{50}$s of most of these inhibitors are in the 1–800 nM range *(28)*. PD 153035 (Compound 2) is highly potent, and is the most specific EGFR kinase inhibitor ever reported *(26,27)*, with an IC$_{50}$ value of 5 picomolar, which makes it four to five orders of magnitude more potent than all earlier reported tyrosine kinase inhibitors *(28)*. A new series of tyrosine kinase

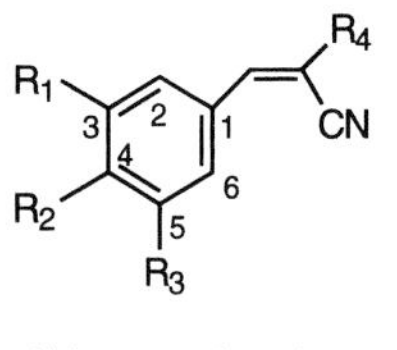

1 (benzylidenetyrphostins)

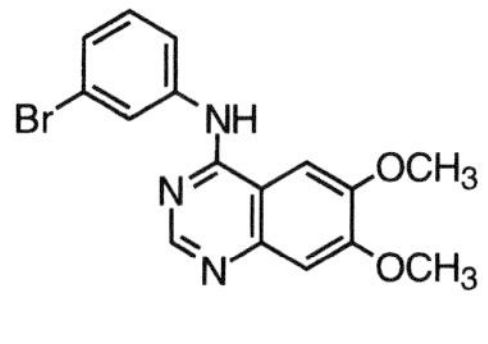

2 (PD 153035, anilinoquinazoline)

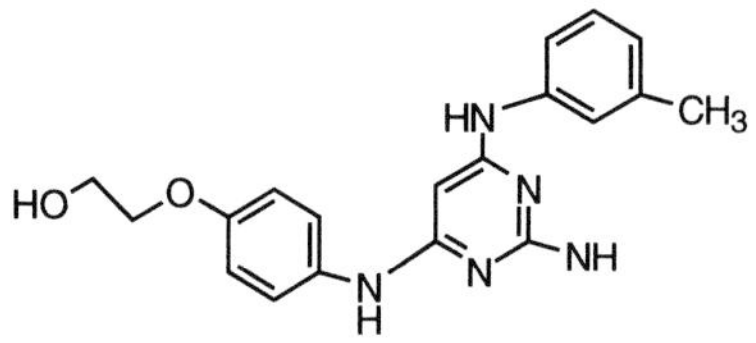

3 (dianilinopyrimidine)

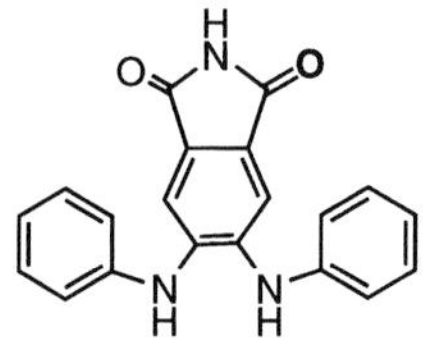

4 (CGP524)

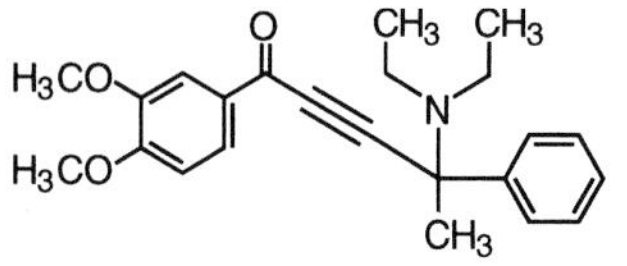

5 (DAP-720, a benzoylacetylene)

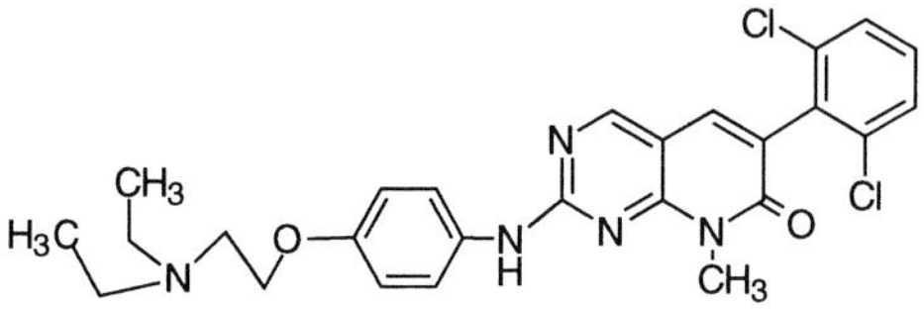

6 (aminopyrido[2,3-*d*]pyrimidinone)

Fig. 2. Inhibitors of EGFR function. Compound 1, benzylidenetyrphostins. Compound 2, PD 153035, an anilinoquinazoline. Compound 3, dianilinopyrimidine. Compound 4, CGP524. Compound 5, DAP-720, a benzoylacetylene. Compound 6, an aminopyrido[2,3–d]pyrimidinone.

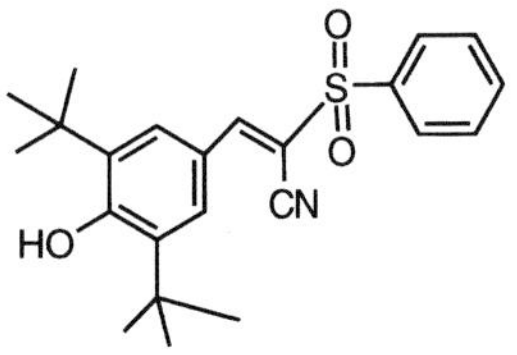

7

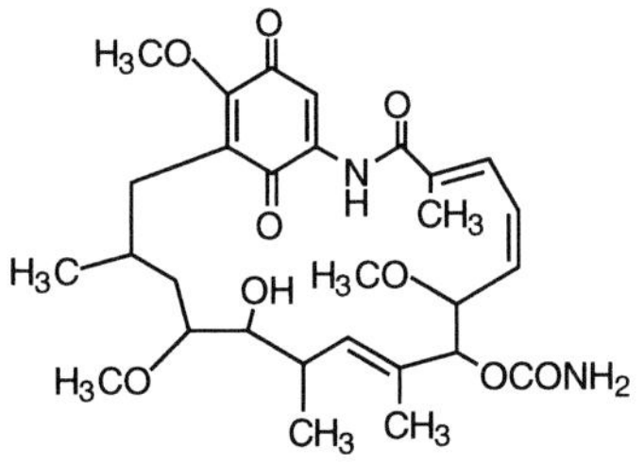

8 (Geldanamycin)

Fig. 3. Inhibitors of HER-2 function. Compound 7 and 8 (Geldanamycin).

inhibitors, 2–substituted aminopyrido[2,3–*d*]pyrimidinones (Compound 6), were reported recently *(39)* that showed in vivo anticancer activity against ovarian and colon cancers, and selective inhibitory activity against several tyrosine kinases, including EGFR, PDGF and c-src.

HER-2, the human homolog of the mouse *neu* gene, was discovered recently *(40,41)*, and has attained importance as a major oncogene in metastatic breast cancer. The HER-2 gene encodes a 185 kDa transmembrane protein, p185^{HER-2} *(41)*, which is homologous to the EGFR, differing from it mainly in the kinase domain. HER-2 is activated indirectly by heterodimerization with one of the other RTK family members to which a ligand binds. It is proposed that even though HER-2 does not have a specific high-affinity ligand, it interacts with the ligands of the other HER receptors through low-affinity binding. In this case, the ligands have to work in a dimeric manner, with the high-affinity binding to their cognate recep-

tor, and at the same time participate in low-affinity binding to HER-2 to trigger heterodimerization *(33)*. HER-2 is over-expressed in as many as 40% human primary breast cancers *(42,43)* and 25% of human breast cancer cell lines *(44)*. The overexpression of HER-2 causes malignant transformation *(45)* and progression of mammary and ovarian cancers, and is associated with poor survival of breast-cancer patients *(42,46)*. Overexpression of HER-2 is also associated with tamoxifen-resistance in steroid-receptor positive breast cancer *(47)*. The exciting early clinical success in breast-cancer patients treated with the humanized HER-2 antibody, Herceptin (Genentech, Inc.), has propelled this novel molecular target into the forefront of anticancer drug-discovery research. Structural modifications of the benzylidene tyrphostins described earlier have afforded potent inhibitors of HER-2 kinase activity *(37)*. Methylation of the 3–hydroxyl group (R$_1$) and substitution with *S*-arylalkyl at the 5–position (R$_2$) resulted in potent compounds

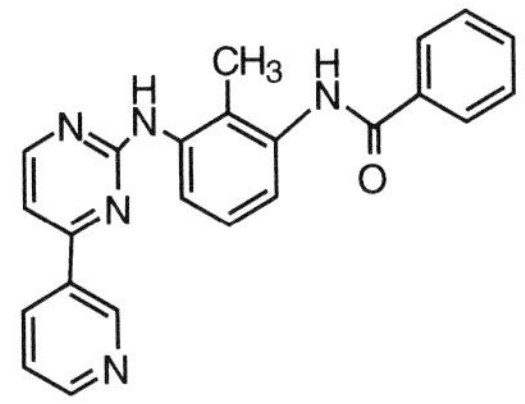

Fig. 4. Inhibitors of PDGF tyrosine kinase activity. Compound 9, 10 (CGP 57148), and 11.

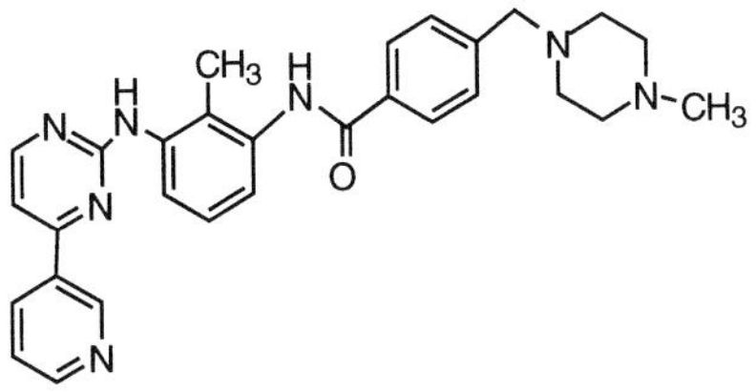

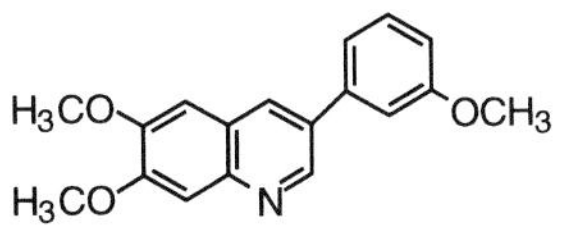

with up to 60–fold selectivity towards the HER-2 RTK relative to EGFR in vitro *(38,48)*. The HER-2–selective inhibitors were also potent antiproliferative agents *(38,48)*. Tyrphostin analogs such as Compound **7** (Fig. 3), are the most selective HER-2 inhibitors reported to date. Molecular dynamics *(49)* and homology modeling *(50)* studies of p185^{HER-2}, as well as comparative molecular field analysis of HER-2 kinase inhibitors *(51)*, set the stage for computer-aided rational drug-design approaches to HER-2 inhibitor discovery. Interestingly, the ansamycin geldanamycin (Compound **8**), through its interaction with the heat shock protein HSP90, depletes the HER-2 gene product from cells, making this class of compounds indirect inhibitors of HER-2 *(52,53)* (Fig. 3).

PDGF RTK PDGF receptor deregulation has been most commonly shown in gliomas *(21)*. The cellular effects of PDGFR include proliferation, actin rearrangement, and chemotaxis, as well as protection against apoptosis *(54)*. Signaling via PDGFR is quite complex. Some of its growth-promoting effects involve c-ras activation, whereas others are c-ras-independent *(54)*. Although it is considered here as a proliferative growth-factor receptor, it is also involved in angiogenesis *(21)*, albeit less so than VEGFR and bFGFR. The progress made in the discovery of chemical inhibitors of the PDGF RTK has been reviewed recently *(28)*. 2–Phenylaminopyrimidines such as Compound **9** (Fig. 4) have selective inhibitory activity against PDGFR relative to EGFR and bFGFR, and have demonstrated antitumor activity in mice. The N^4–methylpiperazinyl-1–methyl derivative of Compound 9, CGP57148 (Compound **10**), has similar activity to Compound 9 against PDGFR. 3–Aryl-substituted quinoxalines and quinolines (Compound **11**) have shown selective activity against PDGFR with IC$_{50}$ values as low as 1.0 nM *(28)*. 2–Substituted aminopyrido[2,3–d]pyrimidinones (Compound **6**) are also active against PDGFR kinase with IC$_{50}$s in the 0.07–10 μM range *(39)*.

Nonreceptor Tyrosine Kinases Non-RTKs are also involved in mitogenic signal transduction. The prominent oncogenic nonreceptor protein tyrosine kinases involved in human cancer are the c-src gene product pp60^{src}, implicated in colon *(21)* and pancreatic *(55)* cancers; the c-src family member c-lck gene product p56^{lck} *(56)*, involved in T-cell lymphomas *(57)*;

and the bcr-abl gene product p210$^{bcr-abl}$, implicated in most chronic myelogenous leukemias (CMLs) *(21)*.

Many small molecule inhibitors of c-src proto-oncogene kinase activity have been identified. Many growth-factor RTK inhibitors also show inhibitory activity against c-src. Interestingly, in the 2–substituted aminopyrido[2,3–d]pyrimidinones series *(39)*, the compound evaluated most, Compound **6** (Fig. 2), was 5–10–fold more selective towards pp60^{src} than the RTKs. Other small-molecule pp60^{src}-specific inhibitors have been reviewed *(28)*. These pp60^{src}-specific inhibitors include 5,10–dihydropyrimidino[4,5–b]quinolin-4(1H)-ones (Compound **12**) and 3–(N-phenyl)carboxamide-2–iminochromene derivatives (Compound **13**), and are shown in Fig. 5. Compound 13 also exhibits inhibitory activity against the non-RTK p56^{lck}. Recently, the X-ray crystal structure of the v-src SH2 domain bound to a peptide ligand was used in the *de novo* structure-based design of novel nonpeptide small molecule N-(4–benzylox-3–acetamidobenzyl)benzamide-4–phosphate (Compound **14**) inhibitors (Fig. 6) that bind to the pp60^{src} SH2 domain *(58)*. The 2–phenylaminopyrimidine derivative, CGP 57148 (STI571, Fig. 4), in addition to inhibiting PDGFR kinase, also inhibits p210$^{bcr-abl}$ tyrosine kinase activity in vitro and in vivo at submicromolar concentrations *(59)* and is successful in treating CML. Another key non-RTK for which specific inhibitors have been discovered is p56^{lck} *(28)*. These inhibitors are shown in Fig. 6. The dihydroxystyrene salicylic acid (Compound **15**), the 7,8–dihydroxyisoquinoline derivative (Compound **16**), and 4–amino-5–(4–methylphenyl)-7–(t-butyl)pyrazolo[3,4–d]pyrimidine (Compound **17**), exhibit potent kinase inhibitory activities against p56^{lck} *(28)*.

Serine/Threonine Kinases The PKC isozyme family is an important serine/threonine kinase family in mammalian signal-transduction pathways *(60)*. The development of specific inhibitors targeting serine/threonine kinases, including protein kinase A (PKA), PKC, MAP kinases, and cell-cycle related kinases, as probes and potential drugs, has been reviewed *(61)*. PKC isozymes are very much involved in cell growth regulation and tumor promotion. They are the molecular targets of the well-known tumor-promoting phorbol esters, which cause their activation *(62,63)*. Their endogenous activator is diacylglycerol, which is produced through the phosphoinositide

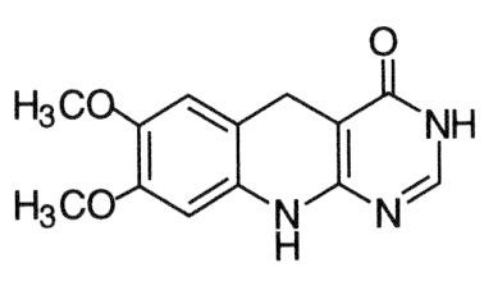

12 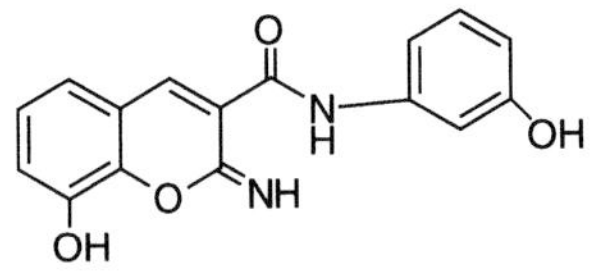   **13**

Fig. 5. Inhibitors of pp60[src] activity. Compounds 12 and 13.

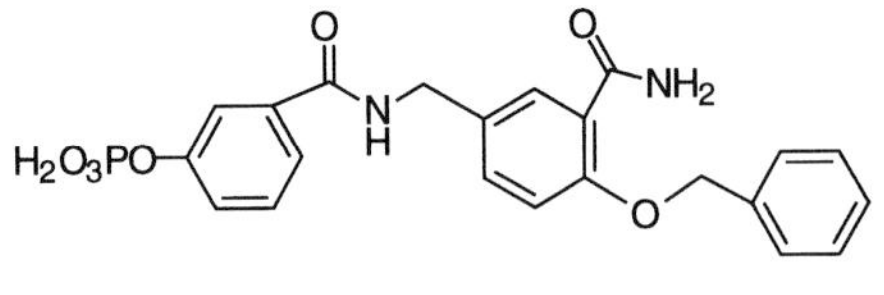

14 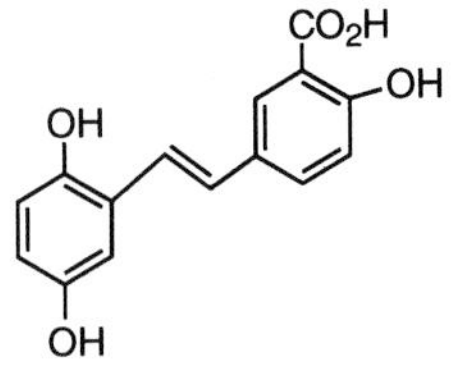   **15**

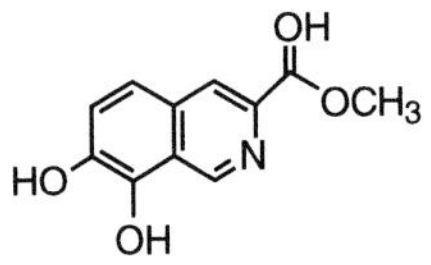

16 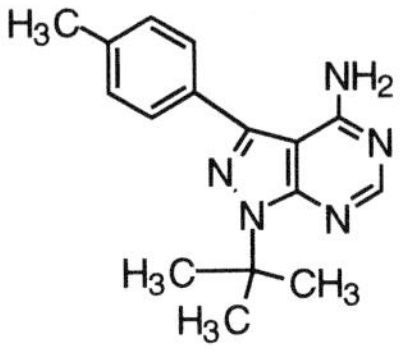   **17**

Fig. 6. Inhibitors of p56[lck] function. Compounds 14–17.

cycle, wherby it is generated by the activation of phopholipase C-β *(64)*. The effects of PKC such as proliferation and hypertrophy are mediated, at least in part, by ERK through the interaction of PKC with c-raf-1 and c-ras *(19)*, as shown in Fig. 1. The PKC family is unusually large, containing 12 isozymes, the classical ones being PKC α, βI, βII, and γ. The novel PKCs include δ, ε, η, and θ, whereas the atypical PKCs are exemplified by PKCλ and ζ *(65)*. Some isozymes are calcium-dependent and some are not *(66)*. PKCs are involved in signal transduction from cell-membrane receptors, after their activation by diacylglycerol (65). The potential of PKC as a novel target for cancer therapy has been reviewed quite extensively *(65,67–70)*. Isozyme-specific inhibitors of PKCs are regarded as potentially useful in chemotherapy. The antiproliferative effect of PKC inhibitors is cell-context dependent *(65)*. Many PKC inhibitors, albeit not isozyme specific, have been identified (Fig. 7), prominent among which are the indolocarbazole derivative 7–hydroxystaurosporin (UCN-01, Compound 18), and safingol (Compound 19), which inhibit PKC's kinase activity at concentrations as low as 1.0 nM *(65,67,69,71)*. Extensive medicinal chemistry has been done on PKC inhibitors, especially the modification of staurosporin in attempts to obtain more selective compounds *(61)*. Computer-aided drug-design methods have also been applied to the discovery of novel PKC modulators *(72–74)*. The availability of the X-ray crystal structure of PKCδ complexed with phorbol 13–acetate has been valuable in this regard, leading to the recent design of novel γ-lactam PKC activators *(74)*. PKC overexpression has been observed in estrogen receptor-negative breast cancer, thyroid cancer, gliomas, and melanoma *(70)*. PKC overexpression is also implicated in angiogenesis *(70)*. PKC inhibitors have been shown to be apoptosis-inducers, making them potentially useful for enhancing the efficacy of current cancer chemotherapy *(69)*. Furthermore, the involvement of aberrant PKC expression in multidrug resistant tumors, especially the PKCα isoform *(65,70)* makes PKC inhibitors attractive for combating multidrug resistance. Several PKC inhibitors are being evaluated in clinical trials for combination therapy with conventional chemotherapeutic agents. One such inhibitor is safingol (Compound 19), which is being evaluated in combination therapy with doxorubicin *(69)*. This combination appeared to be well-tolerated, with blood levels similar to the concentrations showing PKC inhibitory activity, and without any deleterious pharmacokinetic interactions or significant toxicity. The phase I clinical trials of PKC inhibitors or activators (modulators) as single agents or in combination with current anticancer therapy, have been reviewed recently *(70)*. Phase I clinical trials with the PKC modulator Bryostatin 1 (Compound 20), a macrocyclic lactone, have indicated a dose-limiting toxicity of myalgia, other toxicities included phlebitis and headache *(69,70)*. The specificity of current PKC modulators is still questionable, because many also inhibit other serine/threonine kinases, especially cyclin-dependent kinases. Nevertheless, it appears that PKC inhibitors may find clinical use as modulators of conventional chemotherapy and inducers of apoptosis *(15,69,70)*.

The Grb2 Adapter Protein The Grb2 adapter protein *(75)* is a key player in mitogenic signal transduction, involved in both receptor and non-RTK signaling. Inhibiting Grb2 represents an attractive means to simultaneously abrogate mitogenic signals from various protein tyrosine kinases of both receptor and nonreceptor type. This will be especially useful in cancers

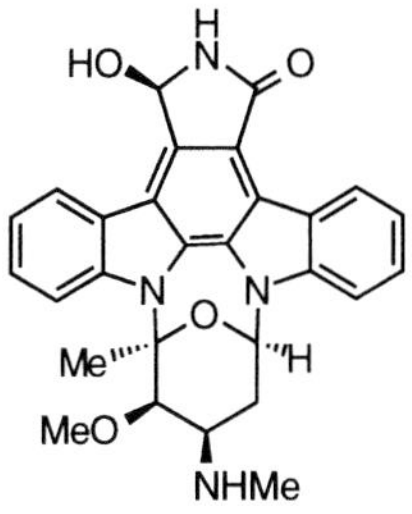

18 (UCN-01) 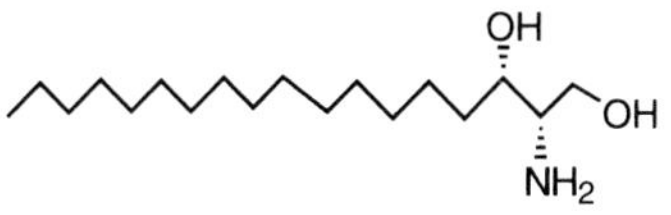   **19** (Safingol, L-threo-dihydrosphingosine)

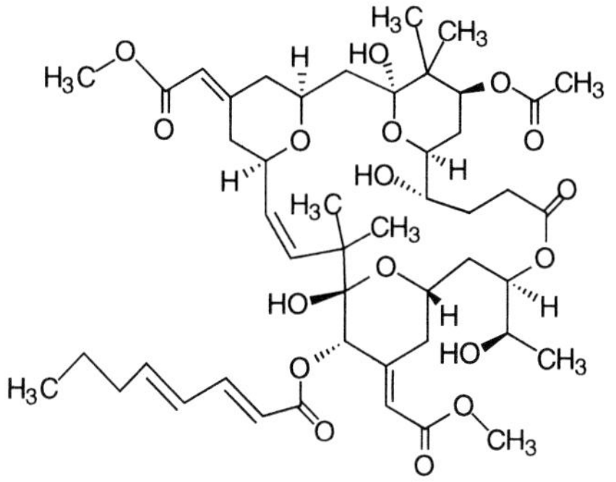

20 (Bryostatin 1)

Fig. 7. Inhibitors of PKC. Compound 18, UCN-01. Compound 19, Safingol, L-threo-dihydrosphingosine. Compound 20, Bryostatin 1.

involving activation and/or overexpression of multiple tyrosine kinases *(76)*. The potential of inhibiting the Grb2 adapter function to abrogate mitogenic signaling from bcr-abl non-RTK for CML therapy has been discussed *(18)*. There are two types of domains on the Grb2 protein that it uses to perform its adapter function: the SH2 and SH3 domains *(18,77)*. The SH2 domain is used to bind to the phosphotyrosine region of the phosphorylated tyrosine kinase, whereas the SH3 domain is used to bind to a proline-rich region on the sos protein to form a ternary complex that is then able to cause c-ras activation *(18)*. X-ray crystallographic data show a small pocket for the SH2 domain and a large surface for the SH3 domain *(76)*. In terms of small molecule drug design, SH2 site-specific ligands could be designed. Drugs designed against Grb2 may also work on other SH2 domain containing molecular targets such as src, Shc, and others *(76)*. At the present time most SH2 domain small-molecule inhibitors in development are phosphotyrosine mimics, but only a limited structure-activity relationship has been developed *(76)*.

Ras GTP-Binding Protein Targeting c-ras appears to be one of the great success stories in the new emerging paradigms for cancer chemotherapy *(78,79)*. At least in breadth, the c-ras proto-oncogene family is probably second only to the growth-factor RTK family as the most pursued novel anticancer drug discovery target. The c-ras family is a major hub in cellular growth and differentiation signaling pathways, with several immediate upstream regulators and downstream effectors *(80)*. In humans, the c-ras GTP-binding protein family is made up of three members, c-K-ras, c-H-ras, and c-N-ras *(81)*, which play a critical role in mitogenic signal-transduction pathways that lead to cell proliferation and differentiation *(82)*. The 21 kDa

c-ras protein (p21^{ras}), is a GTP-binding protein that acts as a molecular switch. In the inactive state, p21^{ras} is bound to GDP. Activation of p21^{ras} occurs by the binding of a GTP molecule that replaces the GDP molecule. This p21^{ras} GTP binding is stimulated by binding of the sos nucleotide exchange factor. The three-dimensional crystal structure of the ras-sos complex has been reported recently *(83)*, showing the regions of interaction between the large sos protein (149 kDa) and the much smaller p21^{ras} protein. Mutations in c-ras occur in about 30% of human cancers, being highly prevalent in pancreatic (90%), lung (40%), colorectal (50%), and myeloid leukemias (30%), but rarely present (<5%) in breast, ovarian, or cervical cancers (84). Nonetheless, the function of c-ras protein may play a major role in the latter cancers because they often harbor activated growth-factor tyrosine kinase mutations or amplifications that send mitogenic signals through c-ras *(14)*. Oncogenic mutations cause ras to be permanently activated and continuously stimulate its downstream effectors, leading to mitogenic activity without the need for upstream mitogenic signals. Therefore, c-ras proto-oncogene-directed drugs should, in principle, be acting at points of intervention between c-ras and its downstream effectors.

A comprehensive treatment of the significance of c-ras in neoplasia, and approaches to target c-ras for cancer chemotherapy has been published *(78)*. Drug discovery efforts have focused on (1) antagonists of protein-protein interaction and (2) inhibitors of the post-translational modification of the c-ras protein. The first approach has led to the discovery of peptides that inhibit ras-GAP (GTPase-activating protein) interaction, but none have been reported for disruptors of ras-sos or ras-raf interactions *(78)*. The large surfaces involved in protein-pro-

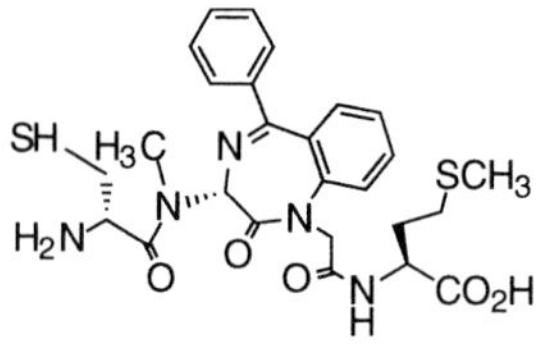

21 (BZA-2B, CAAX-based, IC$_{50}$ 0.85 nM) 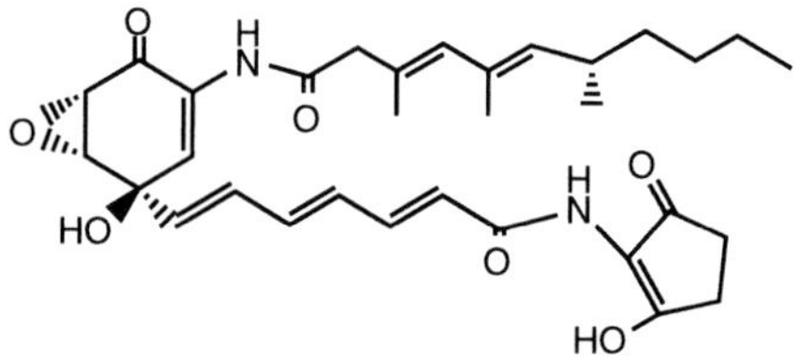 **22** (Manumycin, natural product, IC$_{50}$ 5μM)

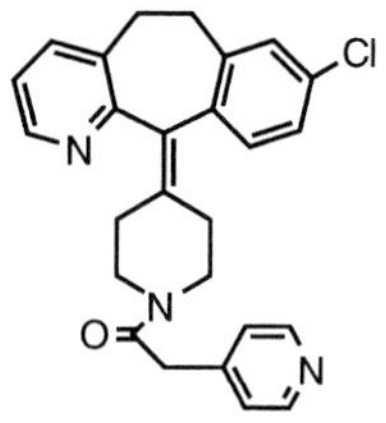

23 (SCH44342, synthetic compound, IC$_{50}$ 250 nM) 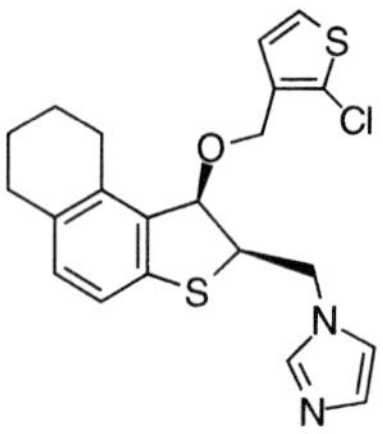   **24** (dihydrobenzothiophene)

Fig. 8. Inbibitors of c-ras farnesyltransferase activity. Compound 21, BZA-2B, CAAX-based, IC$_{50}$ 0.85 nM. Compound 22, Manumycin, natural product, IC$_{50}$ 5 μM. Compound 23, SCH44342, synthetic compound, IC$_{50}$ 250 nM. Compound 24, dihydrobenzothiophene.

tein interactions make it difficult to find effective small-molecule inhibitors of these. The availability of the X-ray structure of the ras-sos complex *(83)* should facilitate the design of inhibitors of this interaction. It has been suggested that this structural information can be used to design inhibitors by making or identifying nucleotide analogs that will bind to the altered nucleotide-binding site in the ras-sos complex to stabilize it, mimicking the action of dominant negative alleles of c-*ras*, or by designing hydrophobic compounds that will bind to the core hydrophobic region of the ras-sos binding interface *(83)*.

Anticancer drug discovery based on the inhibition of posttranslational modification of c-ras protein has been a great success, especially the discovery of c-ras inhibitors targeted against the ras farnesyltransferase (FTase) enzyme *(78,79,85,86)*. Upon translation, c-ras proteins need to be anchored to the cell membrane before they can perform their signal-transduction functions *(87,88)*. This occurs by the attachment of a farnesyl moiety to the cystein in the CAAX amino acid sequence at the C-terminus of c-ras (where C is cysteine, A is any aliphatic amino acid, and X is any amino acid), catalyzed by FTase *(87,88)*, using farnesyl pyrophosphate as a substrate. The farnesyl pyrophosphate is generated by the mevalonate biosynthetic pathway, which also produces cholesterol, starting with the action of hydroxymethylglutaryl CoA (HMG CoA) reductase on hydroxymethylglutaryl CoA, to form mevalonate, which then gets coverted ultimately to farnesyl pyrophosphate and geranylgeranyl pyrophosphate, both of which are used in the prenylation of proteins by FTase and geranylgeranyltransferase (GGTase), respectively *(78,79)*. Blocking the action of HMG CoA, which will preclude the synthesis of farnesyl pyrophosphate, can indirectly inhibit c-ras function. The cholesterol-lowering drug lovastatin, a HMG CoA reductase inhibitor, has been shown to inhibit c-ras function *(79,89)*. Geranylgeranylation of proteins also aids in their anchoring to the cell membrane. The CAAX motif found in c-

ras proteins is specific for FTase, whereas GGTase is more promiscuous, able to add the geranylgeranyl moiety to CAAL, XXCC, XCXC, and CCXX motifs *(78)*. There are more than 40 other cellular proteins that are farnesylated other than c-ras, including lamins A and B, transducin, RhoB, and RhoE *(79)*. Ras-related proteins that are geranylgeranylated include Rac and Rho. An undersirable effect of some FTase inhibitors is their inhibition of GGTase as well. Many FTase-selective inhibitors have been discovered, and constitute the most popular agents for targeting the c-*ras* oncogene for cancer chemotherapy *(79,86,90)*. Ras-FTase inhibitors are being obtained in several ways. There are those designed based on the CAAX motif of c-ras, those designed after the farnesyl moiety, those that are designed bisubstrate inhibitors (selectivity for FTase over GGTase up to 2000–fold), and those obtained from random screening of natural products and synthetic compound libraries *(86)*. Representative ras-FTase inhibitors are shown in Fig. 8 *(86)*.

The SAR data derived from structure optimization of SCH44342 (Compound 23) have been used to generate a three-dimensional pharmacophore with the Catalyst computer program (Molecular Simulations), which was used in database searching to identify new structural classes of FTase inhibitors *(91)*. From those new compounds, the dihydrobenzothiophene series was subjected to SAR studies to obtain Compound 24 (Fig. 8), the most active against FTase inhibitor in the series (IC$_{50}$ 0.2 μM), and the most selective relative to GGTase (84–fold). The selectivity of this series may need much improvement before they can be useful therapeutic agents.

The fact that other proteins are also farnesylated raises doubts about selectivity in using ras farnesylation inhibitors. Surprisingly, FTase inhibitors have not shown toxicity towards normal cells *(79)*. Some c-ras related proteins, which are geranylgeranylated rather than farnesylated, can perform some of the functions of c-ras to compensate for the loss of c-ras function in normal cells *(79)*. Some concern has been expressed that c-ras inactivation might be counter-productive in cells where c-ras activation is required for induction of apoptosis *(86)*. Although encouraging results have been obtained with FTase inhibitors, there still remain questions with regard to the actual mechanism by which they effect their anticancer activity, including whether or not they have targets other than c-ras *(79)*.

The c-ras-related GTP-binding proteins Rac and Rho, have also been proposed as potential drug-discovery targets for ras-mediated cancers *(92)*. These proteins are said to be key players in actin cytoskeletal reorganizations in the cytoplasm. A recent report *(20)* shows that Rho suppresses p21^{WAF1} by an unclear mechanism to allow c-ras to drive cells into S phase. This ras-Rho connection needs further investigation, and may open new therapeutic opportunities.

Ras-targeted drugs may find use as single agents, or as adjuvant chemotherapeutic agents, particularly for radiosensitization of tumors with c-*ras* mutations, which are often resistant to radiation therapy. Inhibitors of c-ras function may also be combined with growth-factor RTK inhibitors for greater efficacy, because oncogenic c-ras is known to drive growth factor and growth factor receptor signaling, even to the extent of promoting angiogenesis through VEGF *(79)*. New inhibitors are needed for c-K-*ras* mutant cancers (the most common human mutant ras cancers), which tend to be the most difficult to erradicate with the present FTase inhibitors *(79)*. The ras-FTase inhibitor R115777 (Fig. 8) is currently in a National Cancer Institute phase I clinical trial for advanced cancers (NCI Cancernet website, http://cancernet.nci.gov/cgi-bin/cancer-phy).

MAP Kinases as Potential Targets There are several MAP kinase cascades that have been uncovered in cellular signal-transduction pathways. They include the ERK cascade, the JNK cascade, and other less well-defined cascades *(93)*. It should also be noted that there are cross talks between many of the cascades, creating a complex network *(93)*. The ERK kinase cascade is probably the most important of these with regard to receptor and non-RTK mitogenic signaling, especially from c-ras, and harbors potential oncogenic members. The cascade starts with c-raf-1, which is activated by c-ras, and in turn activates MEK. Next, MEK activates the ultimate MAP kinase in the cascade, ERK. It has been suggested that c-raf-1 also ties mitogenic signal transduction to cell-cycle activation by interaction with Cdc25A phosphatase *(94)*. MEK and c-raf-1 are the noted oncogenic members in this cascade *(11)*. While antisense oligonucleotide strategies are being pursued for c-raf-1 modulation *(95)*, a selective small-molecule inhibitor of MEK, the flavone PD 98059 *(24)*, which is also able to inhibit cell growth and reverse c-ras transformation, has been reported *(96)*. The structure of PD 98059 is shown in Fig. 9.

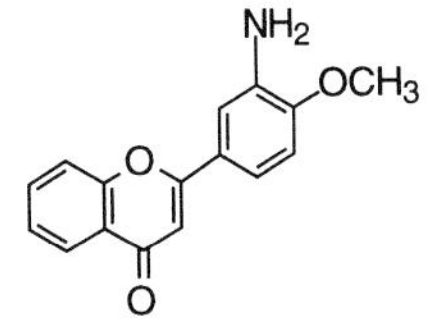

CELL NUCLEAR TARGETS

Oncogenic Transcription Factors as Potential Novel Anticancer Targets Many oncogenic transcription factors involved in cell proliferation and differentiation, such as c-*myc*, *ets*, c-*fos*, c-*jun*, *rel*/NF-κB, and c-*myb*, have been identified *(11,97,98)*. Their activation in cancers mainly involve chromosomal translocations, and they are predominately associated

25 (PD 98059)

Fig. 9. PD 98059 inhibits MEK activity.

with leukemias. The structure-function relationships, and the conceptual approaches to structure-based targeting of oncogenic transcription factors for anticancer drug design and development have been reviewed recently *(98)*. That review pointed out the large breadth of information available on the molecular structure and biochemical pathways of transcription-factor function, and considered the conceptual frame work for computer-aided structure-based drug design, but did not offer any examples. A recent report that c-*myc* activates telomerase in human mammary epithelial cells and normal human diploid fibroblasts *(99)*, is interesting in that it offers a different way in which to view the role of this transcription factor in oncogenesis. It also supports the potential of c-*myc* as an anticancer target. No small-molecule inhibitors against oncogenic transcription factors have been reported, but that is certainly an area to explore for future cancer therapeutics.

Cell-Cycle Targets After being activated as part of the RTK-initiated or non-RTK-initiated mitogenic signaling cascades, MAP kinases translocate to the nucleus where they activate transcription factors that cause the expression of genes to initiate the cell-division cycle. The cell cycle progresses from the G_1 to S to G_2/M phases. In the last decade, exciting cell-cycle research has shown that serine/threonine kinases, termed cyclin-dependent kinases (cdks), are key regulatory molecules that work as binary complexes with various activating cyclins (regulatory units), to drive the progression of the cell division cycle through the different phases *(100,101)*. Different cdks, individually or as groups, bind to different cyclins or subsets of cyclins as follows: cdk1 (Cdc2) binds cyclins A and B1–B3; cdk2 binds cyclins A, D1–D3, and E; cdk4, cdk5 and cdk6 all bind cyclins D1–D3; and cdk7 binds cyclin H *(102)*. The cdks are also regulated by phosphorylation/dephosphorylation; for example, phosphorylation of Thr161 in cdk1 is required for optimal activity, whereas phosphorylation of Thr14 and Tyr15 tends to inhibit activity. The phosphatase Cdc25 dephosphorylates Thr14 and Tyr15 to generate active cdks. Several genes encoding protein products that function as cdk inhibitors to regulate their activity have been identified *(103)*. The best known of these cdk inhibitors is the gene product p21^{WAF1} *(104–107)*, which is induced by p53, resulting in cell cycle arrest in G_1. Other cdk inhibitors related to p21^{WAF1} are p27^{KIP1} *(108)* and p57^{KIP2} *(109)*. Another important family of endogenous cdk inhibitory proteins are the p16$^{INK4/MST1}$ and related *INK4* gene products *(108)*, which have been ascribed a tumor-suppressor function *(110,111)*. The targets of activated cyclin-cdk complexes include the retinoblastoma tumor suppressor gene product (pRb) and related proteins, as well as the E2F transcription-factor family *(112–114)*. Insights into the inter-

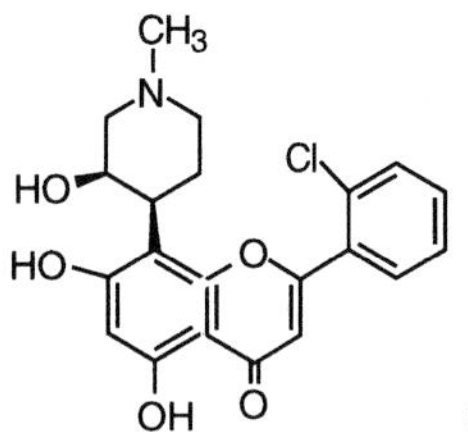

26 (Flavopyridol) 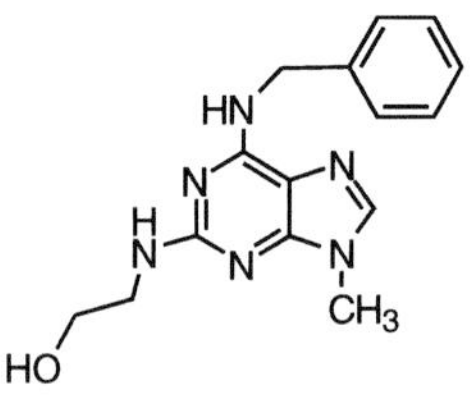   **27** (Olomoucin) 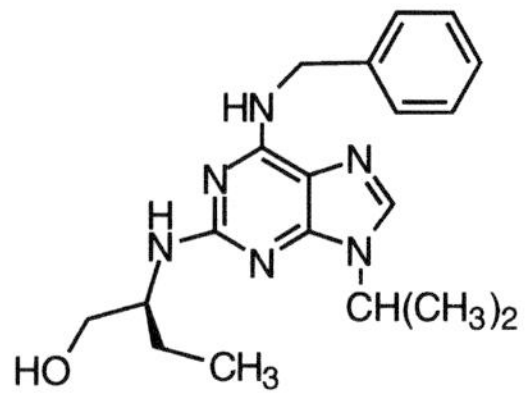   **28** (Roscovitine)

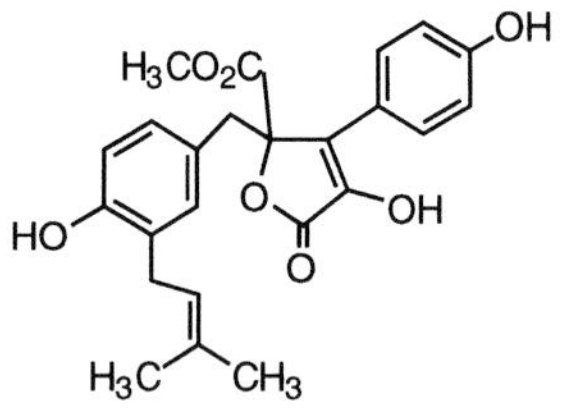

29 (Butyrolactone 1) 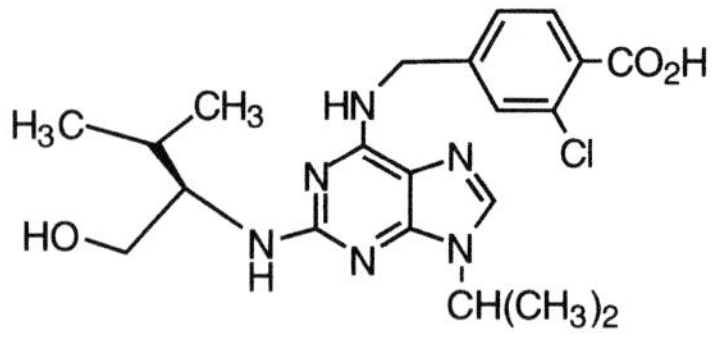   **30** (Purvalanol B)

Fig. 10. Inhibitors of cdks. Compound 26, Flavopyridol. Compound 27, Olomoucin. Compound 28, Roscovitine. Compound 29, Butyrolactone 1. Compound 30, Purvalanol B.

actions of cdk inhibitors with cdks as provided by recent X-ray crystallographic studies have been reviewed recently *(115)*. Cdk inhibitors inactivate cdks either by preventing their binding to cyclin or by binding to the cyclin-cdk complexes.

Oncogenic Potential of Cyclins and cdks The inappropriate expression and/or mutations of cyclins and cdks, and the common cancers in which these occur, as well as drug-discovery efforts targeting them for cancer therap, have been reviewed *(116)*. The oncogenic properties of the G_1 cyclins *(101,108)* have been demonstrated *(2,114)*, with overexpression of cyclin D1 being linked to the promotion of transformation in some instances *(117–119)*, but associated with suppression of cell proliferation in other instances *(120–123)*. In B-lineage lymphomas, cyclin D1 overexpression is reported to promote malignancy in cooperation with c-*myc (124,125)*. Gene amplification and overexpression of one or more of the D cyclins (D1, D2, and D3) have been reported in several tumor types including lymphomas, leukemias, esophageal, bladder, and breast (cyclin D1 overexpression is said to occur in more than 50% of breast cancers *(126)*, non-SCLCs, and colon cancers, as well as retinoblastomas *(2)*. Amplification of cyclin E has also been reported, especially in breast cancers *(127,128)*, where alterations in cyclin E expression show a strong correlation with tumor aggressiveness *(2)*. To that extent, G_1 cyclins are potential novel molecular targets for cancer therapy and prevention in a subset of tumor types. It has also been reported that cyclin D1 overexpression was associated with elevated levels of dihydrofolate reductase enzyme in a human fibrosarcoma cell line, with implications for a role of this cyclin in drug resistance to antifolate anticancer agents such as methotrexate *(129)*. On a more general level, alteration of cell-cycle regulatory genes may affect the response to some anticancer drugs. Oncogenic amplification and overexpression of cdks have been reported in cancers such as gliomas and soft-tissue sarcomas *(130)*. The G_1 cyclins and cdks are, therefore, potential antiproliferative drug-discovery targets.

Small Molecule Inhibitors of cdks Unlike the cyclins, for which no chemical inhibitors have yet been reported, cdks are among the potential novel anticancer targets being investigated intensively for small-molecule anticancer-drug development *(61,102,131)*. Most of the small-molecule cdk inhibitors discovered to date interact with the ATP-binding site in the kinase domain of the cdks. The lack of inhibitors that interfere with the binding between cyclins and cdks, and the availability of many potent inhibitors of cdk catalytic function, is illustrative that it is more difficult to design small molecules that will competitively antagonize protein-protein binding often involving large surface areas, than it is to design drugs that inhibit enzyme active sites, which contain small-molecule substrate and co-substrate binding sites. Several groups of cdk inhibitors with surprisingly high selectivity for different cdks or classes of cdks, have been identified, and are being investigated with much enthusiasm for use in cancer chemotherapy *(102,131)*.

The cdk-selectivity among these molecules, both within the cdk family and relative to non-cdk kinases has been reviewed *(131)*. Their selectivity is attributed to their ability to bind in the ATP-binding sites of the cdks and interact with regions in the vicinity of the ATP-binding site that do not interact with the bound ATP (as revealed by X-ray crystallographic studies), and are not conserved in amino acid sequence among the cdks *(131)*. This offers the opportunity for structure-based design of more specific inhibitors. Among the chemical inhibitors of cdks (Fig. 10), the most prominent are flavopyridol (Compound 26), olumoucine (2–(2–hydroxyethylamino)-6–benzylamino-9–methylpurine (Compound 27) and its analog roscovitine (2–(1–D,L-2–hydroxymethylpropylamino)-6–benzylamino-9–isopropylpurine (Compound 28), UCN-01 (Compound 18) and butyrolactone 1 (Compound 29). Flavopiridol is a flavone derivative that inhibits cdk2 and cdk4, and causes cell-cycle arrest in G_1 independent of functional p53 or pRb *(132)*, as well as cell cycle arrest at G_2, attributed to the alteration of the phosphorylation state of cdk1, and/or inhibition of the kinase activity of cyclin B-cdk1 complex *(133)*. Flavopiridol inhibits the growth of human tumor xenografts originating from lung, colon, stomach, breast, and brain, and is currently in clinical trials as one of the most promising compounds in the National Cancer Institute's anticancer drug-development pipeline *(133)*. The ability to induce apoptosis independent of p53 function, is an attractive property of the cdk inhibitors. This property may be related to their ability to inhibit PKC, especially flavopiridol and UCN-01 *(69)*. In human phase I clinical trials, the dose-limiting toxicity of flavopiridol was diarrhea, while other less severe side effects such as malaise, fever, minimal nausea, and vomiting were also observed. More encouraging, was the absence of leukopenia, anemia, or thrombocytopenea *(69)*.

Purine derivatives that exhibit high selectivity towards cdks relative to other protein kinases have been reported *(134)*. Among these purine-derivative cdk inhibitors, olumoucine (Compound 27) and its analog roscovitine (Compound 28) have emerged as clinical candidates, with a potential for use in the treatment of gastric cancers *(135)*. New powerful technologies of drug discovery and design are being applied to develop more specific and potent purine inhibitors of cdks, as reported recently *(136)*. The report describes the use of combinatorial chemistry to explore the effects of a diverse array of substituents at the purine ring 2–, 6– and 9–positions, and high-throughput screening in 24 purified protein kinase systems. This led to the discovery of highly specific purine inhibitors of human cdk1–cyclin B, cdk2–cyclin A, cdk2–cyclin E, cdk5–p35, as well as yeast (*Saccharomycis cerevisiae*) Cdc28p. The most potent of these was purvalanol B (Compound 30), with an IC_{50} of 6 nM, 1000–fold more potent than olomoucine against cdk2–cyclin A complex. The binding interactions of these inhibitors at the ATP-binding site of the cdks were also determined by X-ray crystallography *(136)*. In addition, the cellular effects of the compounds in mammalian cells were characterized employing the genomics technique of high density oligonucleotide-probe arrays. The results indicate that even though two closely related chemicals may show the same in vitro activity, their cellular effects may vary widely; this is not surprising, because metabolic and cellular distribution (pharmacokinetic) phenomena may differ widely, even for very closely related compounds. The ligand-receptor interactions revealed by the X-ray crystallographic data should aid molecular-modeling applications in the design of new cdk inhibitors.

The staurosporin derivative (Compound 18), UCN-01 (137), previously identified as a PKC inhibitor *(69)*, is one of the drugs under development by the NCI *(133)*. It causes cell-growth arrest in G_1 by a mechanism involving dephosphorylation of the Rb gene product and cdk2, and the induction of p21^{WAF1} *(88)*. Butyrolactone 1 (Compound 29), an inhibitor of cdk2 and Cdc2 kinases, and 9–hydroxyellipticine are less-explored cdk inhibitors in comparison to those discussed earlier *(102)*.

p53 and Apoptosis Targets The p53 tumor suppressor gene can rightly be regarded as the single most important factor driving cancer research in the last decade. Crowned as the *Science* molecule of the year in 1993 *(138)*, p53's involvements in cell-cycle arrest and apoptosis have been investigated extensively. The p53 gene product is a nuclear phosphoprotein, which is a transcription factor that functions primarily to cause cell

cycle arrest at the G_1 checkpoint or apoptosis, in response to DNA damage *(139,140)*. p53 is also thought to play a role in DNA repair in addition to other functions *(141)*, and is considered the guardian of the genome *(142)*. The cell cycle arrest function of p53 is achieved through transcriptional induction of the cdk inhibitor p21^{WAF1} *(104–107)*, and/or the GADD45 gene product *(143)*. On the other hand, p53–induced apoptosis can be caused by its transcriptional induction of the bax gene product *(144)*, which competes with the anti-apoptotic bcl2 gene product, or by transcription-independent mechanisms *(13,141,145)*. Cell cycle arrest and apotosis, as well as DNA repair, are the mechanisms by which p53 performs its tumor-suppressor functions. Mutant p53 loses its tumor-suppressor function; most frequently the DNA-binding ability is lost, probably due to a conformational change. Restoration of function may be achieved by introduction of wild-type p53 or by a change to the functional conformation. The first approach has been successful, and many examples have been reported for the experimental therapeutics of cancer, in the form of gene therapy approaches with the wild-type p53 gene. Recent reports have demonstrated the second approach of successfully changing the conformation of a mutant p53 to restore its DNA-binding activity. Small molecules have been identified that are able to change the conformation of mutant p53 to restore its function. Many anticancer agents have been shown to work through induction of apoptosis in the presence of functional p53 *(146,147)*. In addition, the loss of p53 function correlates with drug resistance and aggressiveness in many cancers, including epithelial ovarian malignances *(148)* and breast cancers *(149)*. It has been pointed out that the curable cancers (90–95% cure rates), namely, testicular teratomas, and childhood lymphoblastic leukemias all contain wild-type p53 *(140)*. It has also been shown in the NCI anticancer screen that the large majority of compounds were generally more active in cells with wild-type p53 than those with mutant p53 *(150)*. However, not all classes of compounds showed this correlation. The most striking deviation from this general correlation were the antitubulin agents, including paclitaxel (Taxol^R), the activity of which appeared not to be dependent on p53 status *(150)*. It has been reported that p53 mutations, surprisingly, sensitize normal fibroblast cells to the cytotoxic effects of paclitaxel, but cause resistance to the same drug in corresponding cancer cells (151). It should also be noted that in some cancer types such as lung cancer, there appears to be no correlation between p53 status and chemosensitivity *(151)*. Therefore, not only is the relationship between p53 status and chemosensitivity tissue-specific and perhaps chemotherapeutic agent-specific, but it may also be different between normal and cancer cells *(151)*.

An important oncogenic molecular target in the p53 pathway(s) is the product of the human *mdm2* gene. The *mdm2* gene, a zinc finger protein, is transcriptionally induced by p53 as a negative-feedback control loop to regulate p53 function *(152–154)*. The oncogenic expression of the mdm2 protein *(155)* is thought to suppress normal p53 function *(156)*, by both protein-protein interaction and direct interference with the basal transcriptional machinery *(157)*. The suppression of p53 by mdm2 could be a potential intervention site for anticancer-drug action. Not only does mdm2 repress p53, but it also inactivates pRb *(158)*, and stimulates the E2F1/DP-1 transcription factors *(159)*. This results in the promotion of the G_1 to S phase transition *(160)*. Amplification of the *mdm2* gene occurs in some cancers that express normal p53, such as sarcomas *(155)*. The *INK4a* tumor-suppressor gene product, p19^{Arf}, has been shown recently to interact with mdm2 and neutralize its inhibition of p53 *(161)*. These observations demonstrate the potential of the mdm2 protein as a novel molecular target for cancer therapy. In this light, assays for identifying inhibitors of mdm2–p53 interaction will be useful for drug discovery. One such assay is purported to identify agents that disrupt mdm2 binding to p53 without interfering with p53 binding to DNA (Chene, P. and Hochkeppel, H.-K., *International Patent Application* WO 97/11367162), but no examples of such inhibitors identified using the assay have been reported. Recently, enzyme-linked immunosorbent assay (ELISA) and electrophoretic gel-mobility assays in combination with phage-display methods were used to identify 12–15mer peptides that inhibit p53–MDM2 binding with IC_{50} values as low as 0.1 μ*M (162,163)*. The availability of the crystal structure of MDM2 bound to the transactivation domain of p53 *(164)* may be useful for structure-based design of inhibitors of MDM2 p58 interaction. Antisense oligonucleotides against MDM2 have been used to prove the anticancer potential of MDM2 inhibitors *(165)*.

The anti-apoptotic proto-oncogene *bcl2 (166)* is also a potential anticancer molecular target. The *bcl2* gene cooperates with c-*myc* to cause oncogenic transformation *(167)*, and is especially important in B-cell lymphomas (168). Overexpression of *bcl2* has been observed in prostate, breast, colorectal cancers, SCLCs, and non-SCLCs *(169)*. There are other bcl2 family proteins that have anti-apoptotic effects, such as bcl-xL, that may also serve as potential chemotherapy targets *(169)*. These along with bcl2, and the possible ways to search for inhibitors have been reviewed *(169)*. Peptidyl blockers of the dimerization of the bcl2 family members have been designed, but have lower affinities than their protein competitors *(170)*. Assays are available for testing compounds as bcl2 inhibitors. These inhibitors may target bcl2 dimerization, ion-channel activity, or phosphorylation state. To date, no such inhibitors have been reported *(169)*. One concern to keep in mind in attempts to use bcl2 inhibitors in cancer therapy may be their adverse effects in patients with ischemic cardiac disease, where the anti-apoptotic effects of bcl2 are beneficial *(169)*.

A new and interesting potential anti-apoptosis molecular target is *survivin*, the downregulation of which has been shown to increase apoptosis and to inhibit the growth of transformed cells *(171)*. This protein is reported to be expressed in the most common human cancers but not in normal adult tissues *(171)*. Work on this target is still in very early stages, and it will be interesting to see how research on *survivin* pans out. Though no small-molecule inhibitors of these antiapoptosis targets have been reported, that will certainly be a worthwhile research area.

CELL LIFESPAN/LONGEVITY TARGETS There is currently much interest in the enzyme telomerase as an enzyme that prolongs the proliferation lifespan of cells in which it is expressed *(172)*. Telomerase is a ribonucleoprotein DNA polymerase that lengthens telomeres, which are specialized nucleotide sequences at the ends of chromosomes consisting of long

Fig. 11. Inhibitor of telomerase activity. Compound 31, an anthraquinone.

tandem repeats of the sequence TTAGGG *(173)*. It has been shown that telomere length in cells progressively shorten with each cell division, until critical length is achieved beyond which the cells cannot continue to multiply. This places a cap on how many cell-division cycles can be attained for any cell capable of division, even immortalized cell lines. Telomerase maintains telomere length by using its integral RNA as a template to add TTAGGG tracks to telomeres, and has been shown to be induced in actively dividing cells and cancer cells, but not in otherwise normal cells *(172,174)*. Telomerase activity is said to be elevated in 86% of all cancers studied *(175)*. This has prompted the investigation of the enzyme as a potential cancer therapeutic target. In addition to its potential as a powerful diagnostic marker for detecting cancer, telomerase may also serve as a viable target for selective cancer chemotherapy *(176,177)*. The status of research on exploiting telomerase for therapeutic application has been reviewed *(175)*. A few classes of small molecule inhibitors of telomerase activity have been identified using mainly the telomerase repeat amplification protocol (TRAP) assay *(172)*, and are being investigated for cancer chemotherapy. Telomerase inhibitors designed as G-quadruplex interactive compounds have advanced the fastest *(175)*. These include porphyrins and anthraquinones *(178)*. A recent series of anthraquinone telomerase inhibitors with IC_{50} values of 4–11 μ*M* were shown to be antiproliferative against human cancer cell lines *(178)*. Compound 31 (Fig. 11) exhibited cytotoxicity against human ovarian carcinoma cell line A2780 with an IC_{50} of 16 nM. Nucleotide analogs, which when incorporated into telomeric sequences prevent the formation of G-quadruplexes, like the 7–deaza-nucleotide analogs of ATP and GTP, as well as AZT triphosphate, have also exhibited telomerase-inhibitory activity *(5)*. The occurrence of telomerase in renewable tissues such as the liver, appears to pose a potential toxicity problem *(174)*. This notwithstanding, encouraging results have been obtained at the preclinical level that will facilitate the entry of telomerase inhibitors into clinical trials.

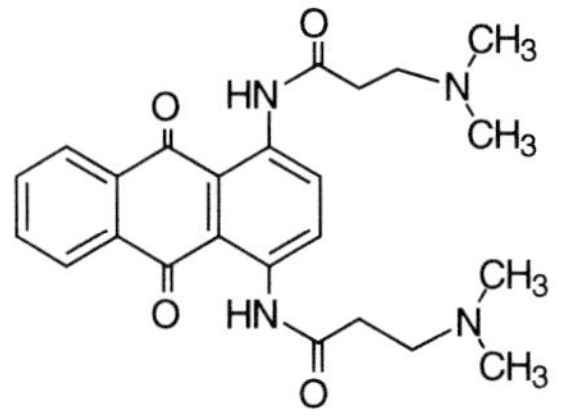

TUMOR ANGIOGENESIS AND METASTASIS MOLECULAR TARGETS Angiogenesis has been shown to be critical for cancer establishment and metastasis, as well as other diseases, including rheumatoid arthritis (RA) and diabetic retinopathy *(179–181)*. Angiogenesis occurs in two stages: the initial stage called vasculogenesis consists of differential expansion and coalescence of endothelial-cell precursors into a network of homogenous-sized vessels. The second stage, which is considered the real angiogenesis, involves remodeling of the

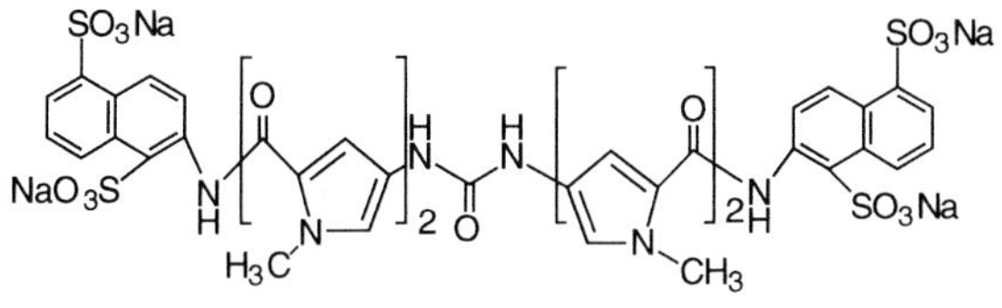

32 (FCE 27266)

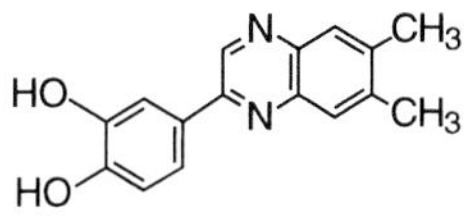

33 (SU1493)

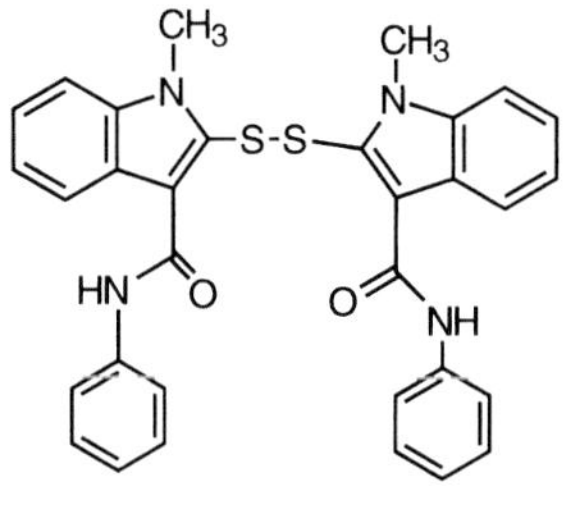

34 (PD145709)

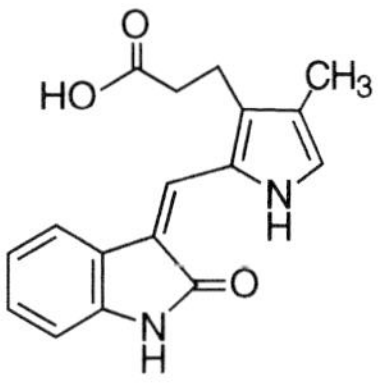

35 (SU5402)

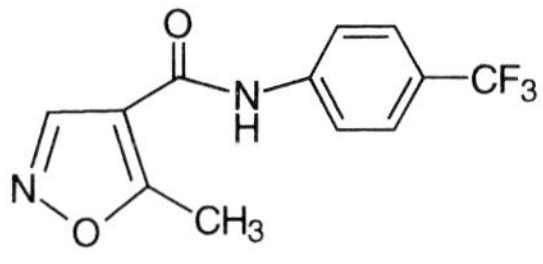

36 (SU101, Leflunomide)

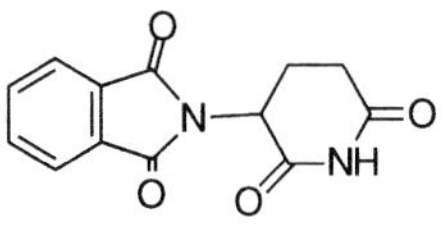

37 (Thalidomide)

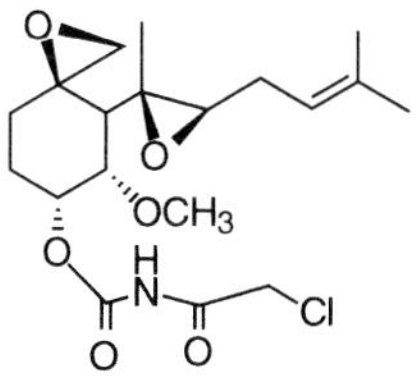

38 (AG-1470)

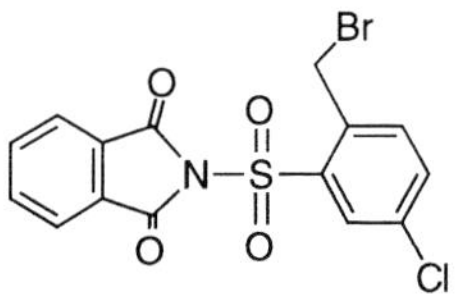

39 (SCH 13929)

Fig. 12. Inhibitors of angiogenesis. Compound 32, FCE 27266. Compound 33, SU1493. Compound 34, PD145709. Compound 35, SU5402. Compound 36, SU101, Leflunomide. Compound 37, Thalidomide. Compound 38, AG-1470. Compound 39, SCH 13929.

initial network into sprouting and branching blood vessels and the recruitment of associated supporting cells such as smooth muscle cells *(182,183)*. VEGF and its receptor VEGFR2 are implicated in vasculogenesis *(182,183)*, whereas VEGFR1 receptor is more involved in the second stage. The involvement of growth factors and their RTK in angiogenesis has been summarized recently *(184)*. The most prominent angiogenic growth-factor RTKs are VEGFR2 (flk-1), bFGFR, and PDGFRb *(21,185)*. It has also been shown that bFGF can induce mdm2 protein expression by a p53–independent mechanism to prolong cell survival and resistance to cisplatin *(186)*. One other important angiogenic factor is angiogenin, a polypeptide that can both induce or suppress angiogenesis, but does not appear to be mitogenic towards endothelial cells *(185)*.

Recent reports of the highly effective elimination of tumors in mice by the anti-angiogenic molecules angiostatin and endostatin, peptidyl compounds that antagonize the angiogenic actions of angiogenin, and the subsequent human clinical trials that have begun as a result, have focused much attention on angiogenic targets for novel cancer chemotherapy *(63)*. Many small-molecule angiogenesis inhibitors have been discovered (Fig. 12) *(184)*. They include suramin and its analogs such as FCE 27266 (Compound 32), nonspecific agents that block the growth-stimulatory activity of many growth factors (including VEGF, PDGF, and bFGF) by inhibiting binding to their cognate receptors. FCE 27266 inhibits the binding of bFGF, PDGFb, and VEGF to cells, with IC_{50} values of 145, 45, and 15 μM, respectively *(184)*. Other compounds acting on angiogenesis molecular targets include steroids (general inhibitors of growth factors), VEGFR-2 (flk-1)-selective inhibitors affecting receptor autophosphorylation, such as the quinoxaline, SU1493 (Compound 33); bFGF receptor kinase inhibitors, such as the thioindole compound, PD145709 (Compound 34) *(187)* and the oxindole compound, SU5402 (Compound 35) *(50)*; and the PDGFβ receptor kinase inhibitor, leflunomide (SU 101, Compound 36), which has been shown to be an effective inhibitor of PDGFβ-promoted glioma tumor growth in vivo *(188)*.

The availability of the X-ray crystal structure of bFGF RTK domain in complex with the oxindole inhibitors *(50)* should pave a way for structure-based design of novel bFGF receptor tyrosine kianse inhibitors. Many other small molecules of diverse structural classes have exhibited anti-angiogenic activity (Fig. 12), but their mechanism of action is still unclear. These include the once notorious teratogen, thalidomide (Compound 37), and the fumagilins such as AG-1470 (Compound 38) *(184)*, and the number will continue to grow, as will points of intervention in tumor angiogenesis. Interestingly, the small molecule SCH 13929 (Compound 39) has been shown to interact with, and competitively inhibit the binding of PDGF to its receptors, and inhibits its biological functions in vitro and in vivo *(189)*. The structure of Compound 39 is similar in some way to thalidomide, and probably might provide a clue to the mecha-

Table 2
Some Small Molecule Anti-angiogenic Agents in Clinical Trials[a]

Compound	Trial Phase	Sponsor	Mechanism	Cancers
Suramin	II/III	Park-Davis	Nonspecific	Pancreas, non- small cell lung, breast
SU5416 (oxindole derivative)	II	Sugen, Inc.	VEGFR-2 blocker	-
Thalidomide[b]	II	Entremed	Unknown	-
Marimastat[c]	III	British Biotech	MMP inhibitor	-
Bay 12–9566	III	Bayer	MMP inhibitor	Lung, prostate
AG3340	III	Agouron	MMP inhibitor	Lung, prostate
CGS27023A	I	Norvatis	MMP inhibitor	-
COL-3	I	Collagenex Pharmaceuticals	Antibiotic MMP inhibitor	-

[a]The information in this table was compiled from Nelson (63) and from the NCI Cancer Trials Web Site (http:/207.121.187.155/NCI_CANCER_...S/zones/PressInfo?Angio/table.html).
[b]Compound 37 (Fig.12).
[c]Compound 41(Fig. 13).

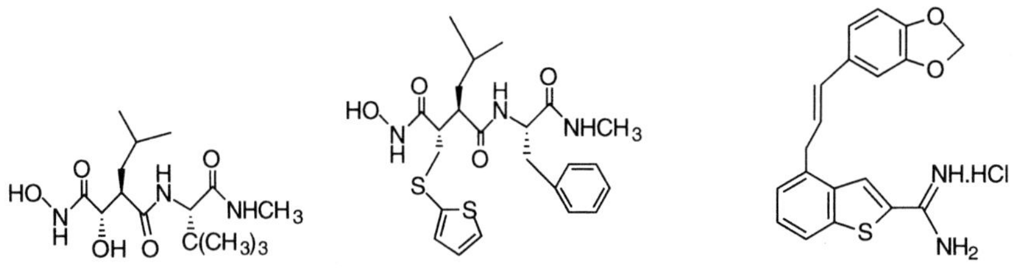

40 (Barimastat)   **41** (Marimastat)   **42** (B623, IC$_{50}$, 70 nM)

Fig. 13. Inhibitors of matrix metalloproteinases. Compound 40, Barimastat. Compound 41, Marimastat. Compound 42, B623.

nism of thalidomides anti-angiogenesis action, which is at present unknown.

Matrix metalloproteinases (MMPs) and urokinase (uPA) have come under intense study because of their involvement in tumor invasion and angiogenesis, which culminate in cancer progression and metastasis (190,191). MMPs are a large family of zinc-binding proteins that can be divided into five classes based on substrate preference as follows: (1) type 1 collagenases, comprising MMP-1, MMP-8, and MMP-13; (2) type IV collagenases, including MMP-2 and MMP-9, (3) stromelysins, comprising MMP-3, MMP-7, MMP-10, and MMP-11; (4) elastases, including MMP-12; and (5) membrane-type MMPs (190). Another classification of MMPs divides them into four families based on similarities of their domain structures (192). MMP-2 and MMP-9 are particularly notorious in tumor metastasis, invasion and angiogenesis (193). The MMPs are tightly regulated by endogenous inhibitors known as TIMPs (tissue inhibitors of metalloproteinases). uPA is a serine protease formed initially as a high molecular weight uPA (HMWuPA) that is cleaved into an amino terminal fragment (ATF) and low molecular-weight uPA (LMWuPA). LMWuPA causes proteolytic degradation and activation of TGF-β. In addition, it also converts plasminogen to plasmin, the active product that has proteolytic activity that affects various ECM components. The ATF binds to the uPA receptor (uPAR), causing cell migration and osteoblast proliferation (190). uPA also has an endog-

enous-inhibitor, plasminogen-activator inhibitor. uPA and uPAR have been shown to cooperate with MMPs, especially MMP-9, to cause tumor-cell intravasation (194). There is much optimism regarding therapeutic agents targeting MMPs (Table 2) and uPA/uPAR (195).

Several small-molecule MMP inhibitors have been discovered (Fig. 13) and exhibit different selectivities towards the different MMPs with nanomolar to picomolar potencies (192). Notable among these are batimastat (Compound 40) and its more water-soluble analog, marimastat (Compound 41), which are hydroxamate-based inhibitors currently undergoing clinical trials. The clinical results appear promising, except for the troubling side effects of musculoskeletal pain and stiffness. Several MMP inhibitors are in advanced clinical trials as shown in Table 2.

The potential role of uPA-receptor antgonists in metastatic disease has been summarized recently (191). Antibody and peptide inhibitors have been identified, but small-molecule inhibitors are still lacking, with only amiloride analogs such as B623 (Fig. 13) being reported as potent uPA enzyme inhibitors that block tumor invasion in vivo (184). Studies using the available uPA-receptor antagonists indicate the potential utility of such antagonists in patients with malignant melanoma, colon, non-SCLCs, stomach, breast, and ovarian cancers (191). Just like MMP inhibitors, minimal residual disease will be the logical context in which to use these antagonists, and the consequent long-term treatment will require that side effects be minimal.

Another group of ECM-interacting molecules relevant to cancer invasion, and gaining attention is the cell-adhesion class of molecules. Adhesion molecules mediate cell-matrix and cell-cell interactions, and are implicated in tumor invasion and organ-specific metastasis *(196)*. The adhesion molecules identified include integrins (the largest class), which are transmembrane heterodimeric proteins composed of α and β subunits, functioning as receptors for matrix proteins such as fibronectin, vitronectin, laminin, and collagen. The integrin $\alpha_6\beta_4$ promotes the invasiveness of MDA-MB-435 breast-cancer cells by activating phosphoinositol 3–OH kinase *(197)*. Other groups of cell-adhesion molecules (CAMs) include cadherins, selectins, mucins, hyaluronan (CD44), the Ig superfamily that is made up of the MHC antigens, CD2, CD4, and CD8, and other Igs such as ICAM-1, ICAM-2, VCAM-1, CEA, C-CAMs, and DCC *(196,199)*, and gangliosides *(200)*. The potential for CAMs as pharmaceutical targets in cancer chemotherapy has been reviewed recently *(198,199)*. Current anti-adhesion-molecule cancer therapy is dominated by the use of neutralizing antibodies, immunotoxins, and soluble proteins. Synthetic peptides designed to antagonize adhesion interactions, especially those incorporating a RGD (Arg-Gly-Asp) motif, are also being investigated with some success in preventing metastasis *(184,196,199)*. The potential of targeting gangliosides for cancer therapy has also been discussed *(200)*. Antibodies that recognize the ganglioside disialoglycosphingolipid have been used to obtain partial regression of melanomas. Anti-adhesion metastasis suppression has been extensively studied with melanoma, lymphomas, colon, and breast cancers metastasizing to the liver and/or lungs *(196)*. The evidence indicates a real potential for exploiting cell-adhesion interactions in treating metastatic disease, but more research into the specific functions and interactions CAMs is needed for their rational targeting in cancer therapy. Many anti-angiogenesis and anti-metastasis compounds are currently in various stages of clinical trials as shown in Table 2.

CONCLUSION

As described in the preceding sections, and summarized in Table 1, many molecular targets have been identified that hold promise for novel cancer chemotherapy that will be relatively nontoxic and cancer-selective. Drug discovery efforts to harness these targets have advanced significantly, as well as understanding of the targets and their function. There are still several targets for which no small-molecule inhibitors are yet known. The fact that different cancers harbor different targets (or combinations thereof) implies that therapy will have to be tailored according to individual cancer profiles of these targets, i.e., customized strategies will have to be adopted, as well as cocktails of inhibitors in some cases, for optimal therapy.

The redundancy in the signal-transduction pathways had brought into question the viability of targeting them for cancer chemotherapy. However, the initial fears have been allayed, as it now appears clear that with the appropriate compounds, signal-transduction pathways may provide some of the most promising targets for achieving selective and nontoxic anticancer

therapy. However, it is not known whether agents directed at signal-transduction pathway targets will produce cytostatic or cytocidal effects on target cells. If the action of these compounds is cytostatic, then the drugs will need to be administered over long periods of time to be effective, and should have minimal toxicity. It has also been suggested that the present models, and the endpoints that are used to evaluate the preclinical and clinical efficacy of newer compounds, may not be appropriate because these models were developed for the old cytotoxic paradigm of cancer chemotherapy. That issue has to be addressed to allow for the proper evaluation of the efficacy of the new agents. Individualized therapy regimens based on tumor profiles of the plethora of potential molecular targets will have to be devised to allow the efficient use of the new agents. Some agents, especially the MMP inhibitors, are being touted not for aggressive chemotherapy, but for residual disease elimination. These questions not withstanding, much progress is being made towards developing novel therapeutics based on the novel targets, as exemplified by many clinical trials based on antibodies to the EGFR or HER-2, and the approval of Herceptin antibody for the treatment of metastatic breast cancers expressing the HER-2 oncogene (Genentech). Small-molecule drug discovery is catching up, as agents targeting EGFR, BCR-ABL c-*ras* oncogene or MMPs may soon find clinical use. Although the number of potential novel molecular targets for cancer drug discovery covered in this chapter does not represent all possible targets, it is evident we are inundated with more targets than the present drug-discovery resources can cope with. Even so, the search for novel cancer therapeutic targets continues, utilizing functional genomics and proteomics in combination with bioinformatics *(150,201,202)*. The sequencing of the human genome will help accelerate this. Certainly, decisions have to be made as to which targets are more valid to pursue, and need more resource allocation to enable the harnessing of the seemingly unlimited potential for the development of more tolerable cancer chemotherapy. Routine methods for the molecular profiling of tumors to obtain mutant gene fingerprints need to be developed and integrated into cancer diagnosis and treatment. Much work is also still needed to elucidate the precise mechanisms by which these targets perform their roles in oncogeneseis to allow for better rational drug design and therapy. Finally, issues of drug resistance will emerge eventually, and will have to be addressed as well.

ACKNOWLEDGMENTS

The author acknowledges Ms. Tomoko Mineno for interpretation of journal articles written in Japanese, and Dr. Larry A. Walker for reading through the manuscript and for useful suggestions.

REFERENCES

1. Workman, P. (1994) The potential for molecular oncology to define new drug targets. *In: New Molecular Targets for Cancer Chemotherapy* (Kerr, D.J. and Workman, P., eds.), CRC Press, Boca Raton, FL, pp. 1–44.
2. Karp, J.E. and Broder, S. (1995) Molecular foundations of cancer: new targets for intervention. *Nature Med.* **1**:309–320.
3. Oliff, A., Gibbs, J.B., and McCormick, F. (1996) New molecular targets for cancer therapy. *Sci. Am.* **275**:144–149.

4. Kuwano, N. (1997) Novel molecular targets for anticancer drugs. *Jpn. J. Cancer Chemother.* **24**:2187–2189.

5. Aszalos, A. and Eckhardt, S. (1997) Molecular events as targets of anticancer drug therapy. *Pathol. Oncol. Res.* **3**:147–158.

6. Akinaga, S. (1998) Molecular target therapy of cancer. D. Cancer genes and cancer regulating genes. *Kagaku Ryo no Ryoiki* **14**:33–40.

7. Kuntz, I.D. (1992) Structure-based strategies for drug design and discovery. *Science* **257**:1078–1082.

8. Chong, C. and Vile, R. (1997) Gene therapy for cancer. *Drugs Future* **22**:857–874

9. Jurcic, J.G., Scheinberg, D.A., and Houghton, A.N. (1997) Monoclonal antibody therapy of cancer. *Cancer Chemother. Biol. Response Modif.* **17**:195–216.

10. Mukhopadhyay, T. and Roth, J.A. (1996) Antisense regulation of oncogenes in cancer. *Crit. Rev. Oncol.* **7**:151–190.

11. Hunter, T. (1997) Oncoprotein networks. *Cell* **88**:573–582.

12. Weinberg, R.A. (1991) Tumor suppressor genes. *Science* **254**:1138–1146.

13. White, E. (1996) Life, death and the pursuit of apoptosis. *Genes Dev.* **10**:1–15.

14. Ullrich, A. and Schlessinger, J. (1991) Signal transduction by receptors with tyrosine kinase activity. *Cell* **61**:203–212.

15. Sauseville, E.A. and Longo, D.L. (1994) Growth factors and growth factor inhibitors. *In: Cancer Therapeutics: Experimental and Clinical Agents* (Teicher, B., ed.), Humana Press, Totowa, NJ, pp. 337–370.

16. Katz, M.E. and McCormick, F. (1997) Signal transduction from multiple ras effectors. *Curr. Opin. Gene. Dev.* **7**:75–79.

17. Fantl, W.J., Johnson, D.E., and Williams, L.T. (1993) Signaling by receptor tyrosine kinases. *Ann. Rev. Biochem.* **62**:453–481.

18. Gishizky, M.L. (1995) Tyrosine kinase induced mitogenesis: breaking the link with cancer. *Ann. Rep. Med. Chem.* **30**:247–253

19. Marais, R., Light, Y., Mason, C., Paterson, H., Olson, M.F., and Marshall, C.J. (1998) Requirement of ras-GTP-raf complexes for activation of Raf-1 by protein kinase C. *Science* **280**:109–112.

20. Olson, M.F., Paterson, H.F., and Marshall, C.J. (1998) Signals from ras and rho GTPases interact to regulate expression of p21$^{Waf1/Cip1}$. *Nature* **394**:295–299.

21. Kolibaba, K.S. and Druker, B.J. (1997) Protein tyrosine kinases and cancer. *Biochim. Biophys. Acta* **1333**:F217–F248.

22. Lofts, F. J. and Gullick, W. J. (1994). Growth factor receptors as targets. *In: New Molecular Targets for Cancer Chemotherapy.* (Kerr, D.J. and Workman, P., Eds.), CRC Press, Boca Raton, FL, pp. 45–66.

23. Levitzki, A. (1994) Protein tyrosine kinase inhibitors. *In: New Molecular Targets for Cancer Chemotherapy* (Kerr, D.J. and Workman, P., eds.), CRC Press, Boca Raton, FL, pp. 67–79.

24. Levitzki, A. and Gazit A. (1995) Tyrosine kinase inhibition: an approach to drug development. *Science* **267**:1782–1788.

25. Burke, T.R. (1992) Protein tyrosine kinase inhibitors. *Drugs Future* **17**:119–131.

26. Fry, D.W., Kraker, A.J., Connors, R.C., Elliot, W.L., Nelson, J.M., Showalter, H.D.H., et al. (1994) Strategies for the discovery of novel tyrosine kinase inhibitors with anticancer activity. *Anti-Cancer Drug Design* **9**:331–351.

27. Fry, D.W., Kraker, A.J., McMichael, Ambroso, L.A., Nelson, J.M., Leopold, Connors, R.C. and Bridges, A.J. (1994) A specific inhibitor of epidermal growth factor receptor tyrosine kinase. *Science* **265**:1093–1095.

28. Fry, D.W. (1996) Recent advances in tyrosine kinase inhibitors. *Ann. Rep. Med. Chem.* **31**:151–160.

29. Traxler, P. and Lydon, N. (1995) Recent advances in protein tyrosine kinase inhibitors. *Drugs Future* **20**:1261–1274.

30. Traxler, P., Furet, P., Met, H., Buchdunger, E., Meyer, T., and Lydon, N. (1997) Design and synthesis of novel tyrosine kinase inhibitors using a pharmacophore model of the ATP-binding site of the EGF-R. *J. Pharm. Belg.* **52**:88–96.

31. Aaronson, S. A. (1991) Growth factors and cancer. *Science* **254**:1146–1152.

32. Rajkumar, T. and Gullick, W.J. (1994) Type I growth factors in human breast cancer. *Breast Cancer Res. Treat.* **29**:3–9.

33. Tzahar, E. and Yarden, Y. (1998) The ErbB-2/HER2 oncogenic receptor of adenocarcinomas: from orphanhood to multiple stromal ligands. *Biochim. Biophys. Acta* **1377**:M25–M37.

34. *Facts About Cancer* (1997). Pharmaceutical Research and Manufacturers of America.

35. Yaish, P., Gazit, A. Gilom, C., and Levitzki, A. (1988) Blocking of EGF-dependent cell proliferation by EGF receptor kinase inhibitors. *Science* **242**:933–935.

36. Gazit, A., Yaish, P., Gilon, C., and Levitzki, A. (1989) Tyrphostins 1: synthesis and biological activity of protein tyrosine kinase inhibitors *J. Med. Chem.* **32**:2344–2352

37. Gazit, A., Osherov, N., Posner, I., Yaish, P., Poradosu, E., Gilon, C., et al. (1991) Tyrphostins 2: heterocyclic and α-substituted benzomalonitrile tyrphostins as potent inhibitors of EGF receptor and *ErbB2/neu* tyrosine kinases. *J. Med Chem.* **34**:1896–1907.

38. Gazit, A., Osherov, N., Posner, I., Bar-Sinai, Gilon, C., and Levitzki, A. (1993) Tyrphostins 3: structure-activity relationship studies of α-substituted benzylidenemalonitrile 5–S-aryltyrphostins. *J. Med. Chem.* **36**:3556–3564.

39. Klutchko, S.R., Hamby, J.M., Boschelli, D.H., Wu, Z., Jraker, A.J., Amar, A.M., et al. (1998) 2–Substituted aminopyrido[2,3–d]pyrimidin-7(8H)-ones. Structure-activity relationships against selected tyrosine kinases and in vitro and in vivo anticancer activity. *J. Med. Chem.* **41**:3276–3292.

40. Coussens, L., Yang-Feng, T., Liao, Y.-C., Chen, E., Gray, A., McGarth, J., et al. (1985) Tyrosine kinase receptor with extensive homology to EGF receptor shares chromosomal location with neu oncogene. *Science* **230**:1132–1139.

41. Yamamoto, T., Ikawa, S., Akiyama, T., Semba, K., Nomura, N., Miyajima, N., et al. (1986) Similarity of protein encoded by the human c-erbB-2 gene to epidermal growth factor receptor. *Nature* **319**:230–234.

42. Slamon, D.J., Clark, G.M., Wong, S.G., Levin, W.J., Ullrich, A., and McGuire, W.L. (1987) Human breast cancer: correlation of relapse with the amplification of *HER-2/neu* oncogene. *Science* **235**:177–172.

43. Isola, J.J., Holi, K., Oksa, H., Teramoto, Y., and Kallioniemi, O.-P. (1994) Elevated erbB-2 oncoprotein levels in preoperative and follow-up serum samples define an aggressive disease course in patients with breast cancer. *Cancer* **73**:652–658.

44. Kraus, M.H., Popescu, N.C., Amsbaugh, S.C., and King, C.R. (1987) Overexpression of EGF receptor-related proto-oncogene erbB-2 in human mammary tumor cell lines by different mechanisms. *EMBO J.* **6**:605–610.

45. Di Fiore, P.P., Pierce, J.H., Kraus, M.H., Sergatto, O., King, C.R., and Aaronson, S.A. (1987) erbB-2 is a potent oncogene when overexpressed in NIH/3T3 cells. *Science* **237**:178–182.

46. Slamon, D.J., Godolphin, W., Jones, L.A., Holt, J.A., Wong, S.G., Keith, D.E., et al. (1989) Studies of *HER-2/neu* proto-oncogene in human breast and ovarian cancer. *Science* **244**:707–712.

47. Borg, A.K., Baldetorp, B., Ferno, M., Killander, D., Olsson, H., Ryden, S., et al. (1994) *ERBB2* amplification is associated with tamoxifen resistance in steroid-receptor positive breast cancer. *Cancer Lett.* **81**:137–144.

48. Osherov, N., Gazit, A., Gilon, C., and Levistzki, A. (1993) Selective inhibition of epidermal growth factor and HER2/Neu receptors by tyrphostins. *J. Biol. Chem.* **268**:11,134–11,142.

49. Garnier, N., Genest, D., Hebert, E., and Genest, M. (1994) Influence of a mutation in the transmembrane domain of the p185$^{c\text{-}erbB2}$ oncogene-encoded protein studied by molecular dynamics stimulations. *J. Biomol. Struct. Dyn.* **11**:983–1002.

50. Mohammadi, M., McMahon, G., Sun, L., Tang, C., Hirth, P., Yeh, B.K., et al. (1997) Structures of the tyrosine kinase domain of fibroblast growth factor receptor in complex with inhibitors. *Science* **276**:955–960.

51. Buolamwini, J.K. (1998) A comparative molecular field analysis study of benzylidene malonitrile tyrphostins as HER2/neu

autophosphorylation inhibitors. *Proc. Am. Assoc. Cancer Res.* **39**:175a.

52. Miller, P., DiOrio, C., Moyer, M., Schnur, R.C., Bruskin, A., Cullen, W., et al. (1994) Depletion of the erbB-2 gene product p185 by the benzoquinone ansamycins. *Cancer Res.* **54**:2724–2730.

53. Schnur, R.C., Corman, M.L., Gallaschun, R.J., Cooper, B.A., Dee, M.F., Doty, T.L., et al. (1995) Inhibition of the oncogene product p185 erbB-2 in vitro and in vivo by geldanamycin and dihydrogeldanamycin derivatives. *J. Med. Chem.* **38**:3806–3812.

54. Heldin, C.-H., Ostman, A., and Ronnstrand, L. (1998) Signal transduction via platelet-derived growth factor receptors. *Biochim. Biophys. Acta* **1378**:F79–F113.

55. Lutz, M.P., Eber, I.B.S., Flossmann-Kast, B.B.M., Vogelmann, R., Luhrs, H., Friess, H., et al. (1998) Overexpression and activation of the tyrosine kinase src in human pancreatic carcinoma. *Biochem. Biophys. Res. Commun.* **243**:503–508.

56. Bolen, J.B. and Veillet, A.A. (1989). Function for the *lck* proto-oncogene. *Trends Biochem. Sci.* **14**:404–407.

57. Cheung, R.K. and Dosch, H.M. (1991) The tyrosine kinase lck is critically involved in the growth transformation of human B lymphocytes. *J. Biol. Chem.* **266**:8667–8670.

58. Lunney, E.A., Para, K.S., Rubin, J.R., Humblet, C., Fergus, J.H., Marks, J.S., et al. (1997) Structure-based design of a novel series of ligands that bind to the pp60^{src} SH2 domain. *J. Am. Chem. Soc.* **119**:12,471–12,476.

59. Buchdunger, E., Zimmerman, J., Mett, H., Meyer, T., Muller, M., Druker, B.J., et al. (1996) Inhibition of the Abl protein-tyrosine kinase *in vitro* and *in vivo* by a 2–phenylaminopyrimidine derivative. *Cancer Res.* **56**:100–104.

60. Nishizuka, Y. (1984) The role of protein kinase C in cell surface signal transduction and tumor promotion. *Nature* **308**:693–698.

61. Lee, J.C. and Adams, J.L. (1995) Inhibitors of serine/threonine kinases. *Curr. Opin. Biotech.* **6**:657–661.

62. Castagna, M., Takai, Y., Kaibuchi, K., Sano, K., Kikkawa, U., and Nishizuka, Y. (1982) Direct activation of calcium-activated phospholipid-dependent protein kinase by tumor-promoting phorbol esters. *J. Biol. Chem.* **257**:7847–7851.

63. Nelson, N.J. (1998) Inhibitors of angiogenesis enter phase III testing. *J. Natl. Cancer Inst.* **90**:960–963.

64. Exton, J.H. (1997) Cell signaling through guanine-nucleotide-binding regulatory proteins (G proteins) and phospholipases. *Eur. J. Biochem.* **243**:10–20.

65. Basu, A. (1993) The potential of protein kinase C as a target for anticancer treatment. *Pharmacol. Ther.* **59**:257–280.

66. Dekker, L.V. and Parker, P.J. (1994) Protein kinase C: a question of specificity. *Trends Biochem. Sci.* **19**:73–77.

67. Grescher, A. and Dale, I.L. (1989) Protein kinase C: a novel target for rational anticancer drug design? *Anti-Cancer Drug Design* **4**:93–105.

68. Philip, P.A. and Harris, A.L. (1995) Potential for protein kinase C inhibitors in cancer therapy. *Cancer Treatment Res.* **78**:3–27.

69. Schwartz, G.K. (1996) Protein kinase C inhibitors as inducers of apoptosis for cancer treatment. *Exp. Opin. Invest. Drugs* **5**:1601–1615.

70. Capronigro, F., French, R.C., and Kaye, S.B. (1997) Protein kinase C: a worthwhile target for anticancer drugs? *Anti-Cancer Drugs* **8**:26–33.

71. Harris, W., Hill, C.H., Lewis, E.J., Nixon, J.S., and Wilkinson, S.E. (1993) Protein kinase C inhibitors. *Drugs Future* **18**:727–735.

72. Wang, S., Milne, G.W.A., Nicklaus, M.C., Marquez, V.E., Lee, J., and Blumberg, P.M. (1994) Protein kinase C: modeling of the binding site and prediction of binding constants. *J. Med. Chem.* **37**:1326–1338.

73. Wang, S., Zaharevitz, D.W., Sharma, R., Marquez, V.E., Milne, G.W.A., Lewin, N.E., et al. (1994) Discovery of novel, structurally diverse protein kinase C agonists through computer 3D-database pharmacophore search. Molecular modeling studies. *J. Med. Chem.* **37**:4479–4489.

74. Qiao, L., Wang, S., George, C., Lewin, L.E., Blumberg, P.M., and Kozikowski, A.P. (1998) Structure-based design of a new class of protein kinase C modulators. *J. Am. Chem. Soc.* **120**:6629–6630.

75. Lowenstein, E.J., Daly, R.J., Batzer, A.G., Li, W, Margolis, B., Lammers, R., et al. (1992) The SH2 and SH3 domain-containing protein GRB2 links receptor tyrosine kinases to ras signaling. *Cell* **70**:431–442.

76. Botfield, M.C. and Green, J. (1995) SH2 and SH3 domains: choreographers of multiple signaling pathways. *Ann. Rep. Med. Chem.* **30**:227–237.

77. Mayer, B.J. and Gupta, R. (1998) Functions of SH2 and SH3 domains. *Curr. Topics Microbiol. Immunol.* **228**:1–22.

78. Sebolt-Leopold, J.S. (1994) A case for ras targeted agents as antineoplastics. *In: Cancer Therapeutics: Experimental and Clinical Agents* (Teicher, B., ed.), Humana Press, Totowa, NJ, pp. 395–415.

79. Cox, A.D. and Der, C.J. (1997) Farnesyl transferase inhibitors and cancer treatment: Targeting simply ras? *Biochim. Biophys. Acta* **1333**:F51–F71.

80. Bourne, H.R., Sanders, D.A., and McCormick, F (1990) The GTPase superfamily: a conserved switch for diverse cell functions. *Nature* **348**:125–132.

81. Barbacid, M. (1987) *Ras* genes. *Ann. Rev. Biochem.* **56**:779–827.

82. Mulcahy, L.S., Smith, M.R., and Stacey, D. (1985) Requirement for ras proto-oncogene function during serum-stimulated growth in NIH 3T3 Cells. *Nature* **313**:241–243.

83. Boriack-Sjodin, P.A., Margait, S.M., Bar-Sagi, D., and Kuriyan, J. (1998) The structural basis of the activation of ras by sos. *Nature* **394**:337–343.

84. Bos, J.L. (1988) Ras oncogenes in human cancer: a review. *Cancer Res.* **49**:4682–4689.

85. Ayral-Kaloustian, S. and Skotnicki, J.S. (1996) Ras farnesyltransferase inhibitors. *Ann. Rep. Med. Chem.* **31**:171–180.

86. Leonard, D.M. (1997) Ras farnesyltransferase: a new therapeutic target. *J. Med. Chem.* **40**:2971–2990.

87. Jackson, J.H., Cochrane, C.G., Bourne, J.R., Solski, P.A., Buss, J.E., and Der, C.J. (1990) Farnesol modification of Kirsten-ras exon 4B protein is essential for transformation. *Proc. Natl. Acad. Sci. USA* **87**:3042–3046.

88. Kato, K., Cox, A.D., Hisaka, M.M., Graham, S.M., Buss, J.E., and Der, C.J. (1992) Isoprenoid addition to ras protein is the critical modification for its membrane association and transformation activity. *Proc. Natl. Acad. Sci. USA* **89**:6403–6407.

89. Akiyama, T., Yoshida, T., Tsujita, T., Shimizu, M., Mizukami, T., Okabi, M., et al. (1997) G1 phase accumulation induced by UCN-01 is associated with dephosphorylation of Rb and CDK2 proteins as well as induction of CDK inhibitor p21Cip1/WAF1/Sdi1. *Cancer Res.* **57**:1495–1501.

90. Bolton, G.L., Sebolt-Leopold, J.S., and Hodges, J.C. (1994) *Ras* oncogene directed approaches in cancer chemotherapy. *Ann. Rep. Med. Chem.* **29**:165–174.

91. Kaminsky, J.J., Rane, D.F., Snow, M.E., Weber, L., Rothofsky, M.L., Anderson, S.D., et al. (1997) Identification of novel farnesyl protein transferase inhibititors using three-dimensional database searching methods. *J. Med. Chem.* **40**:4103–4112.

92. Symons, M. (1995) The Rac and Rho pathway as a source of drug targets for Ras-mediated malignancies. *Curr. Opin. Biotech.* **6**:668–674.

93. Stein, B. and Anderson, D. (1996) The MAP kinase family: new "MAPs" for signal transduction pathways targets. *Ann. Rep. Med Chem.* **31**:289–298.

94. Galaktionov, K., Jessus, C., and Beach, D. (1995) Raf-1 interaction with Cdc25A phosphatase ties mitogenic signal transduction to cell cycle activation. *Genes Dev.* **9**:1046–1058.

95. Monia, B.P. (1997) First- and second-generation antisense inhibitors targeted to human c-*raf* kinase: in vitro and in vivo studies. *Anti-Cancer Drug Design* **12**:327–339.

96. Dudley, D.T., Pang, L., Decker, S.J., Bridges, A.J., and Saltiel, A.R. (1995) A synthetic inhibitor of the mitogen-activated protein kinase cascade. *Proc. Natl. Acad. Sci. USA* **92**:7686–7689.

97. Latchman, D.S. (1996) Transcription-factor mutations in disease. *N. Engl. J. Med* **334**:28–33.

98. Papavassiliou, A.G. (1997) Transcription factor-based drug design in anticancer drug development. *Mol. Med.* **3**:99–810.

99. Wang, J., Xie, L.Y., Allan, S., Beach, D., and Hannon, G.J. (1998) Myc activates telomerase. *Genes Dev.* **12**:1769–1774.

100. Draetta, G. (1990) Cell cycle control in eukaryotes: molecular mechanisms of cdc2 activation. *Trends Biol. Sci.* **15**, 378–383.

101. Sherr, C.J. (1993) Mammalian G1 cyclins. *Cell* **73**:1059–1065.

102. Coleman, K.G., Lyssikatos, and Yang, B.V. (1997) Chemical inhibitors of cyclin-dependent kinases. *Ann. Rep. Med. Chem.* **32**:171–179.

103. Morgan, D.O. (1995) Principles of CDK regulation. *Nature* **374**:131–134.

104. Xiong, Y., Zhang, H., and Beach, D. (1992) D-type cyclins associated with multiple protein kinases and the DNA replication and repair factor PCNA. *Cell* **71**:505–514.

105. Xiong, Y., Hannon, G.J., Zhang, H., Casso, D., Kobayashi, R., and Beach, D. (1993) p21 is a universal inhibitor of cyclin kinases. *Nature* **366**:701–704.

106. Harper, J.W., Adami, G.R., Wei, N., Keyomarsi, K., and Elledge, S.J. (1993) The p21 cdk-interaction protein, Cip1 is a potent inhibitor of G1 cyclin-dependent kinases. *Cell* **75**:805–816.

107. El-Deiry, W.S., Tokino, T., Velculescu, V.E., Levy, D.B., Parsons, R., Lin, D.M., et al. (1993) WAF1, a potential mediator of p53 tumor suppression. *Cell* **75**:817–825.

108. Hunter, T. and Pines, J. (1994) Cyclins and cancer II: Cyclin D and cdk inhibitors come of age. *Cell* **79**:573–582.

109. Lee, M.H., Renisdottir, I., and Massague, J. (1995) Cloning of p57KIP2, a cyclin-dependent kinase inhibitor with unique domain structure and tissue distribution. *Genes Dev.* **9**:639–649.

110. Guan, K.-L., Jenkins, C.W., Li, Y., Nichols, M.A., Wu, X., O'Keefe, C.L., et al. (1994). Growth suppression by p18, a p16$^{INK4/MST1-}$ and p14$^{INK4B/MST2-}$related CDK6 inhibitor, correlates with wild-type pRb function. *Genes Dev.* **8**:2939–2952.

111. Nobori, T.K., Mlura, K., Wu, D.J., Lois, A., Takabayashi, K., and Carson, D.A. (1994) Deletion of cyclin-dependent kinase 4 inhibitor gene in multiple human cancers *Nature* **368**:753–756.

112. Lees, E.M. and Harlow, E. (1995) Cancer and the cell cycle. *In: Cell Cycle Control* (Hutchison, C. and Glover, D.M., eds.), IRL Press, New York, pp. 228–263.

113. Weinberg, R.A. (1995) The retinoblastoma protein and cell cycle control. *Cell* **81**:323–330.

114. Draetta, G. and Pagano, M. (1996) Cell cycle control and cancer. *Ann. Rep. Med. Chem.* **31**:241–248.

115. Pines, J. (1997) Cyclin-dependent kinases: the age of crystals. *Biochim. Biophys. Acta* **1332**:M39–M42.

116. Imoto, M. (1998) Molecular target therapy of cancer: A. Cell cycle. *Kagaku Ryo no Ryoiki* **14**:13–19.

117. Filmus, J., Robles, A.I., Shi, W., Wong, M.J., Colombo, L.L., and Conti, C.J. (1994) Induction of cyclin D1 overexpression by activated *ras. Oncogene* **9**:3627–3633.

118. Daksis, J.I., Lu, R.Y., Facchini, L.M., Marhin, W.W., and Penn, L.J.Z. (1994) Myc induction of cyclin D1 overexpression in the absence of *de novo* protein synthesis and links mitogen-stimulated signal transduction to the cell cycle. *Oncogene* **9**:3635–3645.

119. Sherr, C.J. (1994) G1 phase progression: cycling on cue. *Cell* **79**:551–555.

120. Han, E.K.-H., Sgambato A., Jiang, W., Zhang, Y.-J., Santella, R.M., Doki, Y., et al. (1995) Stable over-expresssion of cyclin D1 in a human mammary epithelial cell line prolongs the S-phase and inhibits growth. *Oncogene* **10**:953–961.

121. Han, E.K.-H., Begemann, M., Sgambato, A., Sohn, J.-W., Doki, Y., Xing, W.Q., et al. (1996) Increased expression of cylin D1 in a murine mammary epithelial cell line induces p27, inhibits growth and enhances apoptosis. *Cell Growth Diff.* **7**:699–710.

122. Atadja, P., Wong, H., Veilette, C., and Riabowol, K. (1995) Overexpression of cylin D1 blocks proliferation of normal diploid fibroblasts. *Exp. Cell Res.* **217**:205–216.

123. Chen, X., Bargonetti, J., and Prives, C. (1995) p53 through p21 (WAF1/CIP1), induces cyclin D1 synthesis. *Cancer Res.* **55**:4257–4263.

124. Lovec, H., Grzeschiczek, A., Kowalski, M.-B., and Moroy, T. (1994) Cyclin D1/*bcl-1* cooperates with myc genes in the generation of B-cell lymphoma in transgenic mice. *EMBO J.* **13**:3487–3495.

125. Bodrug, S.E., Warner, B.J., Bath, M.L., Linderman, D.J., Harris, A.W., and Adams, J.M. (1994) Cyclin D1 transgene impedes lymphocyte maturation and collaborates in lymphomagenesis with the myc gene. *EMBO J.* **13**:2124–2130.

126. Bernards, R. (1997) E2F: a nodal point in cell cycle regulation. *Biochim. Biophys. Acta* **1333**:M33–M40.

127. Dutta, A., Chandra, R., Leiter, L., and Lester, S. (1995) Cyclins as markers of tumor proliferation: Immunocytochemical studies in breast cancer. *Proc. Natl. Acad. Sci. USA* **92**:5386–5390.

128. Keyomarsi, K. and Pardee, A.B. (1993) Redundant cyclin overexpression and gene amplification in breast cancer cells. *Proc. Natl. Acad. Sci. USA* **90**:1112–1116.

129. Hochhauser, D., Schnieders, B., Ercikan-Abali, E., Gorlic, R., Muise-Helmericks, R., Li, W.-W., et al. (1996) Effect of cyclin D1 overexpression in a human fibrosarcoma cell line. *J. Natl. Cancer Inst.* **88**:1269–1275.

130. Costello, J.F., Plass, C., Arap, W., Chapman, V.M., Held, W.A., Berger, M.D., et al. (1997) Cyclin-dependent kinase 6 (CDK6) amplification in human gliomas identified by using two-dimensional separation of genomic DNA. *Cancer Res.* **57**:1250–1254.

131. Meijer, L. (1996) Chemical inhibitors of cyclin dependent kinases. *Trends Cell Biol.* **6**:393–397.

132. Carlson, B.A., Dubay, M.M., Sausville, E.A. Brizuella, L., and Worland, P.J. (1996) Flavopiridol induces G1 arrest with inhibition of cyclin-dependent kinase (CDK) 2 and CDK4 in human breast carcinoma cells. *Cancer Res.* **56**:2973–2978.

133. Christain, M.C., Puda, J.M., Ho, P.T.C., Arbuck, S.G., Murgo, A.J., and Sausville E.A. (1997) Promising new agents under development by the division of cancer treatment, diagnosis, and centers of the National Cancer Institute. *Semin. Oncol.* **24**:219–140.

134. Vesely, J., Havlicek, L., Strand, M., Blow, J.J., Doella-Deana, A., Pinna, L., et al. (1994). Inhibition of cyclin-dependent kinase by purine analogues. *Eur. J. Biochem.* **224**:771–786.

135. Iseki, H., Ko, T.C., Xue, X.Y., Seapan, A., Hellmich, M.R., and Townsend, C.W. (1997) Cyclin-dependent kinase inhibitors block proliferation of human gastric cancer cells. *Surgery* **122**:187–194.

136. Gray, N.S., Wodika, L., Thunnissen, A.-M.W.H., Norman, T.C., Kwon, S., Espinoza, F.H., et al. (1998) Exploiting chemical libraries, structure, and genomics in the search for kinase inhibitors. *Science* **281**:533–538.

137. Takahashi, I., Kobayashi, E., Asano, K., Yoshida, M., and Nakano, H. (1987) UCN-01, A selective inhibitor of protein kinase C from Streptomyces. *J. Antibiot.* **40**:1782–1784.

138. Culotta, E. and Koshland, D.E. (1993) Molecule of the year: p53 sweeps cancer research. *Science* **262**:1958–1961.

139. Bates, S. and Vousden, K.H. (1996) p53 in signaling checkpoint arrest or apoptosis. *Curr. Opin. Genet. Dev.* **6**:12–19.

140. Levine, A.J. (1997) p53, the cellular gate keeper for growth and division. *Cell* **88**:323–331.

141. Harris, C.C. (1996) Structure and function of the p53 tumor suppressor gene: clues for rational cancer therapeutic strategies. *J. Natl. Cancer Inst.* **88**:1442–1455.

142. Lane, D.P. (1992) p53 guardian of the genome. *Nature* **358**:15–16.

143. Kastan, M.B., Zhan, Q., El-Deiry, W.S., Carrier, F., Jacks, T., Walsh, W.V., et al. (1992) A mammalian cell cycle checkpoint pathway utilizing p53 and GADD45 is defective in ataxia-telagiectasia. *Cell* **71**:587–597.

144. Miyashita, T. and Reed, J.C. (1995) Tumor suppressor p53 is a direct transcriptional activator of the bax gene. *Cell* **80**:293–299.

145. Caelles, C., Helmberg, A., and Karin, M. (1994) p53–dependent apoptosis in the absence of transcriptional activation of p53–targeted genes. *Nature* **370**:220–223.

146. Lowe, S.W., Ruley, H.E., Jacks, T., and Housman, D.E. (1993) p53–dependent apoptosis modulates the cytotoxicity of anticancer agents. *Cell* **74**:957–968.

147. Kerr, D.J. and Workman, P., (eds.) (1994) *New Molecular Targets for Cancer Chemotherapy.* CRC Press, Boca Raton, FL.
148. Buttitta, F., Marchetti, A., Gadducci, A., Pellegrini, S., Morganti, M., Carnicelli, V., et al. (1997) p53 alterations are predictive of chemoresistance and aggressiveness in ovarian carcinomas: a molecular and immunohistochemical study. *Br. J. Cancer* **75**:230–235.
149. Aas, T., Borressen, A.-L., Geisler, S., Smith-Sorensen, B., Johnsen, H., Varhaug, J.E., et al. (1996) Specific p53 mutations are associated with de novo resistance to doxorubicin in breast cancer patients. *Nature Med.* **2**:811–814.
150. Weinstein, J.N., Myers, T., O'Connor, P.M., Friend, S.H., Fornace, A.J., Kohn, K.W., et al. (1997) An information-intensive approach to the molecular pharmacology of cancer. *Science* **275**:343–349.
151. Wu, G.S. and El-Deiry, W.S. (1996) p53 and chemosensitivity. *Nature Med.* **2**:255–256.
152. Barak, Y., Juven, T., Haffner, R., and Oren, M. (1993) mdm-2 expressionis induced by wild-type p53 activity. *EMBO J.* **12**:461–468.
153. Wu, X., Bayle, J.H., Olson, D., and Levine, J. A. (1993) The p53–mdm-2 autoregulatory feedback loop. *Genes Dev.* **7**:1126–1132.
154. Chen, J., Lin, J., and Levine, A.J. (1995) Regulation of transcription function of the p53 tumor suppressor by the mdm-2 oncogene. *Mol. Med.* **1**:142–152.
155. Oliner, J.D., Kinzler, K.W., Meltzer, P.S., George, P.L., and Vogelstein, B. (1992) Amplification of a gene encoding a p53–associated protein in human sarcomas. *Nature* **358**:80–83.
156. Finlay, C.A. (1993) The mdm-2 oncogene can overcome wild-type p53 suppression of transformed cell growth. *Mol. Cell. Biol.* **13**:301–306.
157. Thut, C.J., Goodrich, J.A., and Tjian, R. (1997) Repression of p53–mediated transcription by MDM2: a dual mechanism. *Genes Dev.* **11**:1974–1986.
158. Martin, K., Trouche, D., Hagemeier, C., Sorensen, T.S., La Thangue, N.B., and Kouzarides, T. (1995) Stimulation of E2F1/DP1 transcriptional activity by MDM2 oncoprotein. *Nature* **375**:691–694.
159. Xiao, Z.-X., Chen, J., Levin, A.J., Modjtahedi, N., Xing, J., Sellers, W.R., et al. (1995) Interaction of the retinoblastoma protein and the oncoprotein MDM2. *Nature* **375**:694–698.
160. Marechal, V. (1997) Mdm2, p53 et cycle cellulaire: quand le mieux est l'ennemi du bien. *Path. Biol.* **45**:824–832.
161. Pomerantz, J., Shreiber-Argus, N., Liegeois, N.J., Silverman, A., Alland, L., Chin, L., et al. (1998) The Ink4a tumor suppressor gene product, p19Arf interacts with MDM2 and neutralizes MDM2's inhibition of p53. *Cell* **92**:713–723.
162. Bottger, V., Bottger, A., Howard, S.F., Picksley, S.M., Chene, P., Garcia-Echeverria, C., et al. (1996) Identification of novel mdm2 binding peptides by phage display. *Oncogene* **13**:2141–2147.
163. Bottger, A., Bottger, V., Garcia-Echeverria, C., Chene, P., Hochkeppel, H.-K., Sampson, W., et al. (1997) Molecular characterization of the mdm2–p53 interaction *J. Mol. Biol.* **269**:744–756.
164. Kussie, P.H., Gorina, S., Marachal, V., Elenbaas, B., Moreau, J., Levin, A.J., et al. (1996). Crystal structure of the MDM2 oncoprotein bound to the transactivation domain of the p53 tumor suppressor. *Science* **274**:948–953.
165. Chen, L., Agrawal, S., Zhou, W., Zhang, R., and Chen, Z. (1998) Synergistic activation of p53 by inhibition of MDM2 expression and DNA damage. *Proc. Natl. Acad. Sci. USA* **95**:195–200.
166. Bissonnette, R., Echeverri, F., Mahboubi, A., and Green, D.R. (1992) Apoptotic cell death induced by c-myc is inhibited by Bcl-2. *Nature* **359**:552–554.
167. Gauwerky, C.E., Haluska, F.G., Tsujimoto, Y., Nowell, P.C., and Croce, C.M. (1988) Evolution of B-cell malignancy: pre-B-cell leukemia resulting from MYC activation in a B-cell neoplasm with a rearranged *BCL2* gene. *Proc. Natl. Acad. Sci. USA* **85**:8548–8552.
168. Korsmeyer, S.J. (1992) Bcl-2 initiates a new category of oncogenes: regulators of cell death. *Blood* **80**:879–886.
169. Oltersdorf, T. and Fritz, L.C. (1998) The Bcl-2 family: targets for the regulation of apoptosis. *Ann. Rep. Med. Chem.* **33**:253–262.
170. Diaz, J.-L., Oltersdorf, T., Horne, W., McConnell, M., Wilson, G., Weeks, S., et al. (1997) A common binding site mediates heterodimerization and homodimerization of Bcl-2 family members. *J. Biol. Chem.* **272**:11,350–11,355.
171. Ambrosini, G., Adida, C., Sirugo, G., and Altieri, D.C. (1998) Induction of apoptosis and inhibition of cell proliferation by *survivin* gene targeting. *J. Biol. Chem.* **273**:11,177–11,182.
172. Kim, N.W., Piatyszek, M.A., Prowse, K.R., Harley, C.B., West, M.D., Ho, P.L.C., et al. (1994) Specific association of human telomerase activity with immortal cells and cancer. *Science* **266**:2011–2015.
173. Blackburn, E.H. (1992) Telomerases. *Ann. Rev. Biochem.* **61**:113–129.
174. Burger, A.M., Bibby, M.C., and Double, J.A. (1997) Telomerase activity in normal and malignant mammalian tissues: feasibility of telomerase as a target for cancer chemotherapy. *Br. J. Cancer* **75**:516–522.
175. Sharma, S., Raymond, E., Soda, H., and Von Hoff, D.D. (1997) Telomerase and telomere inhibitors in preclinical development. *Exp. Opin. Invest. Drugs* **6**:1179–1185.
176. Hamilton, S.E. and Corey, D.R. (1996) Telomerase: anti-cancer target or just a fascinating enzyme? *Chem. Biol.* **3**, 863–867.
177. Parkinson, E.K. (1996) Do telomerase antagnists represent a novel anticancer strategy? *Br. J. Cancer* **73**:1–4.
178. Perry, P.J., Gowan, S.M., Reszka, A.P., Polucci, P., Jenkins, T.C., Kelland, L.R., et al. (1998) 1,4– and 2,6–disubstituted amidoanthracene-9,10–dione derivatives as inhibitors of human telomerase. *J. Med. Chem.* **41**:3253–3260.
179. Folkman, J. (1995) Angiogenesis in cancer, vascular rheumatoid and other diseases. *Nature Med.* **1**:27–31.
180. Folkman, J. (1995) Clinical applications of research on angiogenesis *N. Engl. J. Med.* **333**:1757–1763.
181. Folkman, J. (1996) Fighting cancer by attacking its blood supply. *Sci. Am.* **275**:150–154.
182. Hanahan, D. (1997) Signaling vascular morphogenesis and maintenance. *Science* **277**:48–50.
183. Risau, W. (1997) Mechanisms of angiogenesis. *Nature* **386**:671–674.
184. Powell, D., Skotnicki, J., and Upeslacis, J. (1997) Angiogenesis inhibitors. *Ann. Rep. Med. Chem.* **32**:161–170.
185. Folkman, J. and Klagsbrun, M. (1987) Angiogenic factors. *Science* **235**:442–447.
186. Shaulian, E., Resnitzky, D., Shifman, O., Blandino, G., Amsterdam, A., Yayon, A., et al. (1997) Induction of mdm2 and enhancement of cell survival by bFGF. *Oncogene* **15**:2717–2725.
187. Fry, D.W. and Nelson, J.M. (1995) Inhibition of fibroblast growth factor-mediated tyrosine phosphorylation and protein synthesis by PD 145709, a member of the 2–thioindole class of tyrosine kinase inhibitors. *Anti-Cancer Drug Design* **10**:604–622.
188. Shawver, L.K., Schwartz, D.P., Mann, E., Chen, H., Tsai, J., Chu, L., et al. (1997) Inhibition of platelet-derived growth factor-mediated signal transduction and tumor growth by N-[4–(Trifluoromethyl)phenyl]-5–methylisoxazole-4–carboxamide. *Clin. Cancer Res.* **3**:1167–1177.
189. Mullins, D.E., Hamud, F., Reim, R., and Davis, H.R. (1994) Inhibition of PDGF receptor binding and PDGF-stimulated biological activity in vitro and of intimal lesion formation in vivo by 2–bromomethyl-5–chlorobenzen sulfonylphthalimide. *Arteriosclerosis Thrombosis* **14**:1047–1055.
190. Rabbani, S.A. (1998) Metalloproteases and urokinase in angiogenesis and tumor progression. *In Vivo* **12**:135–142.
191. Weidle, U.H. and Konig, B. (1998) Urokinase receptor antagonists: novel agents for the treatment of cancer. *Exp. Opin. Invest. Drugs* **7**:391–404.
192. Summers, J.B. and Davidsen, S.K. (1998) Matrix metalloproteinase inhibitors and cancer. *Ann. Rep. Med Chem.* **33**:131–140.
193. Mazzieri, R., Masiero, L., Zanetta, L., Monea, S., Onisto, M., Garbisa, S., et al. (1997) Control of type IV collagenase activity by

components of the urokinase-plasmin system: a regulatory mechanism with cell-bound reactants. *EMBO J.* **16**:2319–2332.

194. Kim, J., Wu, W., Kovalski, K., and Ossowski, L. (1998) Requirement of specific proteases in cancer cell intravasation as revealed by a novel semi-quantitative PCR-based assay. *Cell* **94**:335–362.

195. Edwards, D.R. and Murphy, G. (1998) Proteases: invasion and more. *Nature* **394**:527–528.

196. Huang, Y.-W., Baluna, R., and Vitetta, E.S. (1997) Adhesion molecules as targets for cancer therapy. *Histol. Histopathol.* **12**:467–477.

197. Shaw, L.M., Rabinovitz, I., Wang, H.H.-F., Toker, A., and Mercurio, A.M. (1997). Activation of phosphoinositol 3–OH kinase by the α6β4 integrin promotes carcinoma invasion. *Cell* **91**:949–960.

198. Engleman, V.W., Kellogg, M.S., and Rogers, T.E. (1996) Cell adhesion integrins as pharmaceutical targets. *Ann. Rep. Med. Chem.* **31**:191–200.

199. El-Hariry, I. and Pignatelli, M. (1997) Adhesion molecules: opportunities for modulation and a paradigm for novel therapeutic approaches in cancer. *Exp. Opin. Invest. Drugs* **6**:1465–1478.

200. Fish, R.G. (1996) Role of gangliosides in tumor progression: a molecular target for cancer therapy? *Med. Hypothesis* **46**:140–144.

201. Myers, T.G., Anderson, N.L., Waltham, M., Li, G., Buolamwini, J.K., Scudiero, D.A., et al. (1997) A protein expression database for the molecular pharmacology of cancer. *Electrophoresis* **18**:647–653.

202. Gelbert, L.M. and Gregg, R.E. (1997) Will genetics really revolutionize the drug discovery process? *Curr. Opin. Biotech.* **8**:669–674.

24 Gene Therapy in the Treatment of Human Cancer

Jesús Gómez-Navarro, MD, Guadalupe Bilbao, MD, and David T. Curiel, MD

INTRODUCTION

It is well-established that most cancers result from a series of accumulated, acquired genetic lesions. To a larger and larger extent, the genetic lesions associated with malignant transformation and progression in a wide variety of human cancers are being identified. In this regard, gene therapy is emerging as a new method of preventive and therapeutic intervention against cancer targeted at the level of cellular gene expression *(1)*. In this approach, altering the complex cancerous pathophysiologic state is achieved by delivering nucleic acids into cells. These nucleic acids may be genes, portions of genes, oligonucleotides, or RNA. In conventional therapeutics, as in pharmacotherapy, altering a cell or tissue phenotype is accomplished by altering cell physiology or metabolism at the level of protein expression. In contrast, in gene therapy this is accomplished by changing the pattern of expression of genes whose products may thus achieve the desired effect on the cellular phenotype.

In the treatment of human disease, gene therapy strategies may offer the potential to achieve a much higher level of specificity of action than conventional drug therapeutics by virtue of the highly specific control and regulatory mechanisms of gene expression that may be targeted. Additionally, interceding at an earlier, upstream step in disease pathogenesis (targeting proto-oncogenes, tumor-suppressor genes, etc.) may offer greater potential to induce fundamental changes in phenotypic parameters of disease, with a more favorable clinical outcome. The eventual availability of gene-transfer systems, or vectors, for permanent or long-term genetic modification of cells and tissues can allow definitive therapeutic or preventive interventions. Furthermore, gene transfer may be accomplished in a limited regional context, producing a high concentration of therapeutic molecules in the local area. Thus, undesired systemic effects of those therapeutic molecules are avoided.

From: *The Molecular Basis of Human Cancer* (W. B. Coleman and G. J. Tsongalis, eds.), © Humana Press Inc., Totowa, NJ.

Lastly, using the body to produce therapeutic proteins, potentially in only certain tissues, has practical advantages of its own *(2)*. Briefly, limitations associated with manufacture, stability, and duration of effect after administration of drugs based on synthetic peptides are completely avoided. From the same pharmacological point of view, designer drugs based on small molecules, currently under intensive investigation, can hardly be at this point a therapeutic alternative as substitutes for the protein products of tumor-suppressor genes.

In the treatment of human malignant tumors, several obstacles explain the limits of currently available treatments for achieving, in most cases of advanced disease, definitive cures (Table 1). It is apparent that new chemotherapy drugs, higher drug doses, cytokines, novel modalities of radiotherapy, and more ambitious and sophisticated surgeries can achieve incremental improvements in cancer treatment. But these therapies do not address critical biological obstacles, and thus probably will not bring the much-needed radical advances in the implementation and results of cancer treatment. Gene therapy, in contrast, offers certainly the potential for overcoming some of those fundamental barriers (Table 1).

A number of strategies have been developed to accomplish cancer-gene therapy. These approaches include: 1) mutation compensation; 2) molecular chemotherapy; and 3) genetic immunopotentiation. For mutation compensation, gene-therapy techniques are designed to correct the molecular lesions that are etiologic of malignant transformation, or to avoid the contribution by tumor-supporting normal cells. For molecular chemotherapy, methods have been developed to achieve selective delivery or expression of a toxin gene in cancer or tumor stromal cells to induce their eradication. Also, attempts have been made to deliver genetic sequences that protect normal bone marrow cells from the toxic effects of standard chemotherapeutic drugs, thus allowing the administration of higher drug doses without reaching otherwise limiting myelosuppression. Genetic immunopotentiation strategies attempt to achieve active immunization against tumor-associated antigens by gene-transfer methodologies. Both tumor cells and cellular

Table 1
Potential Contributions of Gene Therapy Against the Obstacles for Curing Cancer

Obstacles to curing cancer imposed by tumor cells	Potential contribution of gene transfer
Tumors are genetically unstable, and therefore extraordinarily adaptable to environmental changes	Gene transfer of DNA repair genes or cell-cycle checkpoint genes that restore DNA stability
Tumors are heterogeneous in many respects, including genetic mutations, expression of oncoproteins, immunogenicity, response to environmental changes, etc.	Targeting of genetically homogeneous tissues, such as the tumor vasculature; genetic immunopotentiation
Tumor genetic instability and heterogeneity contribute to the ability of tumors to express or acquire, resistance to cellular toxins and to many other therapeutically mediated cellular insults	Transfer of genes that sensitize tumor cells to chemotherapy or radiotherapy
Tumors often exhibit a low cellular-growth fraction and are thereby less susceptible to mitotic toxins and to gene-transfer vectors that require dividing cells	Use of vectors that do not require cellular division for gene delivery and expression (adenovirus, herpesvirus, lentivirus, chimeric systems); repeated administration of nonimmunogenic vectors
Progressive tumors form metastases distant from the primary tumor site, necessitating systemic therapy to eradicate the tumor	Use of targetable, injectable vectors (tropism-modified viruses, cellular vehicles); genetic immunopotentiation
Tumors do not express specific tumor antigens or immune cost-imulatory molecules, and tumors often downregulate immune recognition, induce tumor tolerance, and inhibit the immune response	Transfer of genes encoding costimulatory molecules and cytokines; genetic modification of APCs; induction of inflammatory reactions that activate antigen presentation; transfer of genes blocking tumor-secreted inhibitors of the immune response
The spontaneous behavior of human tumors is somewhat different from that of malignant cells in vitro, and from that of experimental tumors in animal models	Development of better animal models, including tumor models in transgenic mice
Tumors are typically diagnosed at an advanced stage, when local and distant metastases have already been established and the patient carries a significant tumor burden	Development of amplification vector systems (replicative viral vectors); use of targetable, injectable vectors; genetic immuno-potentiation
The understanding and treatment of cancer requires the contribution of very diverse fields of basic knowledge, biotechnology, and medical practice	De facto multidisciplinary recruitment of gene therapy researchers

components of the immune system have been genetically modified to this end. Importantly, each of these approaches has been rapidly translated into human gene-therapy clinical trials (Table 2).

To accomplish any gene therapy approach, certain basic criteria must be met to allow an effective genetic intervention. In this regard, gene-therapy approaches are based on the fundamental ability to deliver therapeutic nucleic acids into relevant target cells. Further, the delivered genes must be expressed at an appropriate level and for an adequately prolonged period of time. Finally, the delivery and expression of the therapeutic genes must not be deleterious to the surrounding normal tissue, nor to the individual as a whole (3). In practice, two general approaches have been employed to meet these gene vector criteria: an ex vivo approach and an in vivo approach. In the former method, target cells are removed from the body and transduced with the genetic vector extracorporally, followed by reimplantation. This approach has allowed reasonably efficacious transduction of target cells and has also allowed for a safety characterization of modified cells, prior to delivery into the patient. Unfortunately, the number and types of parenchymal cells that can be modified in this manner are quite limited.

An alternate approach to achieve therapeutic gene delivery has been the in vivo administration of vectors into target parenchymal cells directly in their natural body location. In this regard, both viral and nonviral vectors of diverse types have been employed to achieve in situ transduction of relevant target parenchymal cells (Table 3). In general, a fundamental recog-

nition in many of these studies, including many clinical trials, has been the disparity noted between the in vitro and in vivo gene-transfer efficiencies of these vector systems, and the suboptimal tumor transduction that presently available vector systems can achieve. In addition, the promiscuous tropism of current vectors may potentially allow for genetic modification of a number of normal tissues besides target cells. Furthermore, this nonselective gene transfer impedes the administration of vectors to tumor cells by the systemic route. Thus, important limitations of current approaches used for implementation of gene therapy for cancer have been noted. Although many potentially effective strategies exist to effect the molecular treatment of cancer, gene-delivery issues currently limit the definitive evaluation of these methods.

We examine below the lessons learned from the results of the first attempts to apply gene therapy in human cancer. This will show both the rationale of gene therapy and the problems encountered in its development. We emphasize in our discussion the general biological concepts of each therapeutic strategy, and suggest comprehensive reviews for readers interested in detailed discussions. Finally, we illustrate prospects for overcoming the obstacles to gene therapy by novel methods that are currently being refined.

MUTATION COMPENSATION

Gene-therapy techniques based on mutation compensation are designed to rectify either the molecular lesions in the can-

Table 2
Clinical Trials of Gene Therapy for the Treatment of Cancer[a]

Strategy	Clinical trials	Molecular mechanism of anticancer effect
Mutation compensation	7	Inhibition of expression of dominant oncogenes
	33	Augmentation of deficient tumor-suppressor genes
	2	Abrogation of autocrine growth-factor loops using single chain antibodies
Molecular chemotherapy	35	Selective delivery of toxin or toxin gene to cancer cells
	11	Chemoprotection of normal tissues during high-dose chemotherapy
Genetic immunopotentiation	78	In vitro transduction-augmentation of tropism or cell-killing capacity of tumor-infiltrating lymphocytes; genetic modification of irradiated tumor cells
	98	In vivo transduction-administration of costimulatory molecules or cytokines; immunization with virus encoding tumor-associated antigens
Viral-mediated oncolysis	9	Tumor-cell lysis by viral vector replication

[a]Registered in the NIH Office of Recombinant DNA Activities in the first half of 1998 (http://www.nih.gov/od/orda/protocol.htm).

Table 3
Gene-Transfer Systems Used Clinically Against Cancer[a]

Type	Vector system	Duration of expression	Distinguishing features
Nonviral	Liposomes	Transient	Repetitive and safe administration feasible, inefficient gene delivery, transient expression
	Naked DNA or RNA (injection, gene gun, electroporation)	Transient	Easy preparation, inefficient gene delivery, transient expression
	Molecular conjugates	Transient	Flexible design, inefficient gene delivery, transient expression, unstable in vivo
Viral	Retrovirus	Prolonged	Integrates into the chromosome of dividing cells, unstable in vivo
	Adenovirus	Transient	Highly efficient in vivo, production in high titer, tropism can be modified, induces potent inflammation and immunity, replicative vectors available
	Poxvirus (vaccinia)	Transient	Extensive clinical experience with parent virus, large insert capacity, induces potent inflammation and immunity
	Adeno-associated virus	Prolonged	Nonpathogenic, low insert capacity, difficult to scale-up
	Herpes simplex virus	Transient	Highly efficient in vivo, large insert capacity, cytotoxic, replicative vectors available
	Chimeric vectors	Prolonged	Combines features of component genetic vectors
	Lentivirus	Prolonged	Integrates into the chromosome of both dividing and nondividing cells, well-characterized production system not yet established

[a]Registered in the NIH Office of Recombinant DNA Activities in the first half of 1998 (http://www.nih.gov/od/orda/protocol.htm)

cer- cell etiologic of malignant transformation, or associated changes in stromal cells that support cancer progression. Many chromosomal changes and mutated genes associated with cancer have been identified, although the exact order of their activation and their precise roles in the progression of cancer have been defined only in a minority of tumor types. However, the elucidation of the molecular basis of carcinogenesis progresses steadily and supports the consideration of genetic approaches for cancer therapy. The genetic lesions involved in the pathogenesis of the malignant transformation may be thought of as a critical compilation of two general types: aberrant expression of dominantly acting proto-oncogenes or loss of expression of tumor-suppressor genes. In addition to changes in the individual cancer cells, the contribution of both its local microenvironment and the host are critical during cancer progression. Angiogenesis, cellular mobility, invasion, and metastasis are examples of processes controlled by multiple genes that are involved in carcinogenesis. Gene-therapy approaches have been proposed to achieve correction of each of these lesions and processes (Table 4).

THERAPEUTIC MODALITIES The knowledge on the major role that growth factors, signaling molecules, cell-cycle regulators, and determinant factors of angiogenesis, invasiveness, and metastasis play in neoplastic progression has positive implications for gene therapy. That is, it is possible to abrogate the malignant phenotype by correcting the underexpression of tumor-suppressor genes or overexpression of proto-oncogenes. The inactivation of tumor-suppressor genes contributes to the neoplastic phenotype by abrogating critical cell-cycle checkpoints and DNA-repair mechanisms. To approach this loss of function, the logical intervention is replacement of the deficient function with its wild-type counterpart gene. For dominantly acting proto-oncogenes, it is the aberrant expression of the corresponding gene product that elicits the associated neo-

Table 4
Mutations Compensation Strategies Used Clinically Against Cancer[a]

Target	Strategy	Vector	Tumor type
p53	Replacement of tumor-suppressorgene	Adenovirus	Nonsmall cell lung cancer, head and neck squamous-cell carcinoma, hepatic metastases of colon cancer, hepatocellular carcinoma, prostate cancer, breast cancer
Rb1 (Retinoblastoma)	Replacement of tumor-suppressorgene	Adenovirus	Bladder cancer
BRCA1	*Replacement of tumor-suppressorgene*	*Retrovirus*	*Ovarian cancer*
c-erBb2	Inhibition of promoter by E1A	Cationic liposome complex	Breast and ovarian cancers overexpressing e rbB-2
IGF-1	Blockade by antisense	Cationic liposome complex	Glioblastomas
c-K-ras	Blockade by antisense	Retrovirus	Nonsmall cell lung cancer
c-myc	Blockade by antisense	Retrovirus	Breast and prostate cancers
TGF-β	Blockade by antisense	Plasmid and electroporation	Glioblastoma
erBb-2	scFv (single-chain intra-cellular antibody)	Adenovirus	Ovarian cancer

[a]Registered in the NIH Office of Recombinant DNA Activities in the first half of 1998 (http://www.nih.gov/od/orda/protocol.htm).

plastic transformation. In this context, the molecular therapeutic intervention is designed to ablate expression of the dominant proto-oncogene. Inhibition of oncogenic function can be attempted at three levels. First, transcription of the proto-oncogene can be inhibited. This approach uses triplex-forming, antisense oligonucleotides or other sequences that bind transcriptional start sites in the genomic DNA. Second, translation of the proto-oncogene messenger RNA can be blocked, also using antisense sequences, which function by promoting RNAse degradation of the message. Third, mobilization of the nascent oncoprotein can be blocked or its function can be inhibited when in its final cell location. These strategies involve the use of intracellular antibodies that intercept and interfere with the processing of the oncoprotein, or the heterologous expression of mutant proteins that can inhibit the function of the native oncoprotein, respectively.

Replacement of Tumor-suppressor Genes Mutations of more than two dozen tumor-suppressor genes have been described in numerous cancers. Their functions are diverse and include structure and signaling of intercellular junctions and receptors (APC, DCC, DPC4, NF1), components and regulation of the transcription apparatus (VHL, Rb1, WT1, p53), and DNA mismatch (hMLH1, hMHS2, hPMS1, hPMS2) or excision repair (XPA, XPB, XPC, XPD, XPG). Of these, p53, Rb1, and BRCA1 are currently being administered in clinical trials as replacements for their mutated counterparts (Table 4).

The most common genetic alteration found in human cancer involves the p53 tumor-suppressor gene, affecting approx 50% of all cancers. Besides its high frequency, correction of mutations of p53 may be particularly relevant due to the central role of p53 as guardian of the genome and regulator of apoptosis (4). In this regard, p53-dependent apoptosis modulates the cytotoxic effects of common antitumor agents such as ionizing radiation and chemotherapy (5). An additional mechanism of action of p53 could be inhibition of angiogenesis (6,7). The logical intervention for approaching loss of function of this

tumor-suppressor gene has been replacement of the deficient function with its wild-type counterpart (8). This general strategy allows phenotypic correction (usually with subsequent apoptosis) both in vitro and in vivo in a variety of tumors. In particular, several authors have shown, in murine models employing human cancer xenografts, that intratumoral delivery of the wild-type p53 gene via recombinant viruses can prolong host survival by inducing apoptosis in tumor cells (9). Importantly, nontransformed cells can tolerate exogenous administration of p53, thereby providing an optimal therapeutic index for this intervention. It must be emphasized that restoration of wild-type p53 expression in cells with a mutant or deleted gene has been shown to be sufficient to cause apoptosis or growth arrest, despite the presence of multiple additional genetic abnormalities in the tumor cell. This fact has established the rationale for human clinical gene-therapy trials designed to achieve mutation compensation through restoration of p53 in several cancers. In a pioneering study, Roth et al. administered intratumoral injections of a p53-encoding retrovirus to patients with nonsmall cell lung cancer (SCLC) (10). Nine patients with refractory, mutant p53-containing tumors entered the study. Vector sequences were evident in eight of the treated tumors. In addition, apoptosis was observed in six out of seven evaluated tumors. Three patients experienced tumor regression, and in the other three there was stabilization; none presented toxicity related to the treatment. A second trial is evaluating adenovirus-mediated delivery of p53 with or without the chemotherapeutic drug cisplatin. These studies suggest that replacement of p53 is a clinically feasible genetic intervention that can induce tumor regressions in vivo.

Replacement of Rb1 and BRCA1 has shown similar preclinical experimental results, and is also undergoing clinical testing. Attempts to restore wild-type Rb1 have been described for prostate, retinoblastoma, osteosarcoma, breast, bladder, and non-SCLCs (11). Of note, and perhaps not surprisingly, some Rb1-deficient tumors have shown persistent tumorigenicity and proliferation after successful restoration and expression of wild-type *Rb1*, a phenomenon referred to as tumor-suppressor resistance *(12)*. Thus, restoration of the *Rb1* tumor-suppressor gene in certain tumors may not effect complete reversion of the malignant phenotype. *BRCA1* is rarely affected in spontaneous tumors, and its function has not been completely characterized. Its clinical use has therefore been somewhat controversial *(13)*.

Inhibition of Gene Transcription In addition to mutations that cause the loss of normal tumor-suppressor functions, most tumors exhibit dysregulated proto-oncogenes. In particular, dominant proto-oncogenes implicated in cancer and used as targets in clinical trials include genes encoding: 1) growth factors, such as insulin-like growth factor 1 (IGF-1), and transforming growth factor β1 (TGFβ1); 2) growth factor receptors, such as c-erbB2; 3) proteins involved in cell signaling, such as K-ras; 4) transcription factors, such as c-myc. Modulation of genes encoding cell-cycle regulatory proteins, although being tested in vitro, has not been employed in human clinical trials to date. In addition, genes involved in a variety of phenotypic characteristics dependent on multiple genes have been described. Examples of these processes are angiogenesis, the development of metastasis, and resistance to chemotherapy.

One possible method of ablating a dominant proto-oncogene is by inhibiting its promoter regulatory DNA sequence. It has been shown, for instance, that the K1 mutant of the viral SV40 large T antigen inhibits the human c-*erbB2* promoter in human ovarian-cancer cells. Moreover, liposome-mediated K1 gene transfer decreases the p185 c-erbB2 protein level by K1 expression in these cancer cells, and significantly prolongs survival in an in vivo orthotopic animal model *(14)*. Although not a human gene, the *E1A* gene of adenovirus serotype 5 exhibits tumor-suppressor functions in cancer cells overexpressing the proto-oncogene c-*erbB2*. Apparently, E1A inhibits transcription of the human c-*erbB2* promoter and accordingly suppresses the tumorigenicity and metastatic potential induced by the proto-oncogene. Studies have shown that both cationic liposomes and an adenoviral vector can efficiently deliver *E1A* into ovarian tumor cells in mice, resulting in suppression of tumor growth and significantly longer survival of treated animals *(15)*. These findings are the basis for two human gene-therapy clinical trials, currently ongoing, that study the intraperitoneal and intratumoral administration, respectively, of a cationic lipid complex containing the *E1A* gene in patients with breast or ovarian cancer, and other solid tumors overexpressing c-*erbB2*.

Antisense The most universally employed methodology to achieve proto-oncogene ablation is the utilization of antisense molecules, DNA or RNA oligonucleotides with sequence complementary to that of a nucleic acid target. These molecules are designed to specifically target coding (sense) sequences to achieve blockade of the encoded genetic information. Intervention approaches used along this pathway have included the use of triplex DNA to achieve functional ablation of transcriptional activation through blockade of binding sites of transcription factors. This approach has been developed in in vitro model systems for targeting the c-*myc*, c-*ras*, and c-*erbB2* proto-oncogenes. Targeting is also achieved at levels of gene expression distal to transcription. Specific antisense binding to transcribed RNA sequences may interrupt the flow of genetic

information through several mechanisms including RNase degradation, and less probably impaired transport, and translational arrest. These interventions may be accomplished by simple antisense oligonucleotides as well as by antisense molecules that possess catalytic activity to accomplish cleavage of target sense sequences, so called ribozymes *(16,17)*.

A variety of experimental models, both in vitro and in vivo, have demonstrated the potential utility of the antisense approach as an anti-cancer therapeutic *(18–21)*. Evidence for a specific effect of antisense molecules has been particularly compelling in selected cases, and these molecules are currently undergoing clinical tests. These include antisense sequences against IGF-1 in glioma *(22)*, c-K-*ras* in lung cancer *(23–27)*, c-*myc* in breast *(28)* and in prostate cancer *(29)*, and TGF-β in glioma *(30–32)* (Table 4). The specificity of antisense molecules has been convincingly shown in the case of c-K-*ras*. Antisense oligonucleoside methylphosphonates directed against either normal human c-H-*ras* and c-H-*ras* mutated at a single base in codon 61 have been examined for their efficacy and specificity as inhibitors of c-*ras* expression. Mixed cultures of cells expressing both forms of c-*ras* were treated with the antisense oligomer complementary to the normal c-H-*ras* or with the antisense oligomer complementary to the point-mutated c-H-*ras*. Each of the antisense oligomers specifically inhibited expression of only the form of c-*ras* to which it was completely complementary and left the other form of the gene unaffected. Thus, in general the antisense approach offers the potential to achieve targeted disruption of specific genes in human cancer.

Despite the potentially novel therapeutic strategies offered by the antisense approach, this methodology in practice is associated with severe limitations (19,33). These practical constraints have limited wide employment of this technology in protocols of human anticancer gene therapy. Most disturbingly, there are no universal rules dictating the efficacy of a given antisense oligonucleotide for achieving specific gene inhibition. An array with 1,938 oligonucleotides ranging in length from monomers to 17-mers has been built to measure the potential of the oligonucleotides for heteroduplex formation with rabbit β-globin mRNA *(34)*. The oligonucleotides were complementary to the first 122 bases of the mRNA. Surprisingly, very few oligonucleotides gave significant heteroduplex yield and no obvious features in the mRNA sequence or the predicted secondary structure could explain this variation. In fact, despite the utility of antisense inhibition in selected contexts, attempts to achieve antisense blockage of great many cancer-related genes have failed. In addition, delivery of the antisense molecules has been highly problematic. The tumor environment is deleterious to these unstable molecules, and it is often difficult to maintain effective intracellular levels. To circumvent this problem, a number of design modifications of the antisense molecules have been developed to enhance their in vivo stability. In addition, a number of vector approaches have been explored for effective cellular delivery. Despite these various maneuvers, the overriding limitations to the employment of this still-promising therapeutic modality remain the idiosyncratic efficacy of specific antisense for a given target gene and the suboptimal delivery of antisense molecules.

Single-Chain Antibodies Dominant proto-oncogenes have also been targeted at the level of the protein level. Techniques have been developed to allow the derivation of recombinant molecules that possess antigen-binding specificities expropriated from immunoglobins *(35)*. In this regard, single-chain immunoglobin (scFv) molecules retain the antigen-binding specificity of the immunoglobin from which they were derived, but lack other functional domains characterizing the parent molecule. The encoded scFv may be expressed in the target cell and localized to specific, targeted subcellular compartments by incorporating appropriate signal molecules. Based on this, a novel approach to proto-oncogene suppression has been developed in our laboratory. It was hypothesized that if an antibody directed against c-erbB2 could be localized to the endoplasmic reticulum (ER) of cancer cells, the nascent, newly synthesized c-erbB2 protein would be entrapped within the ER and therefore be unable to achieve its normal cell surface localization. It was further hypothesized that this intracellular entrapment would prevent the c-erbB2 protein, a transmembrane receptor, from interacting with its ligand, thus abrogating the autocrine growth-factor loop driving malignant transformation in c-*erbB2* overexpressing cell lines. We constructed a gene encoding an anti-c-*erbB2* scFv with a signal-peptide sequence that dictates its localization to the ER. The construct was cloned into an eukaryotic-expression vector and transfected into the c-*erbB2* overexpressing ovarian-carcinoma cell line SKOV3. We showed that intracellular expression of the anti-c-erbB2 results in the following cellular effects: 1) downregulation of cell surface c-erbB2 protein expression, 2) marked inhibition of cellular proliferation, 3) marked reduction in survival of neoplastic cell clones, and 4) selective cytotoxicity in tumor cells expressing the proto-oncogene target *(36)*. Furthermore, scFv-mediated c-erbB2 protein ablation induced additional phenotypic alterations in tumor cells, including chemosensitization and radiosensitization *(37)*. The ability to accomplish selective abrogation of c-*erbB2* expression has been shown to be effective in the eradicaton of primary human ovarian-cancer cells *(38)*. This suggests the feasibility of a novel therapeutic approach for tumor-cell eradication by utilizing intracellular immunoglobulins to achieve targeted disruption of dominant proto-oncogenes, thereby accomplishing reversion of the malignant phenotype, chemosensitization, radiosensitization, or initiation of cell death. This novel method of proto-oncogene knockout may offer significant practical advantages compared to antisense methodologies, such as the use of monoclonal antibodies (MAbs) already developed against cancer as parental antibodies, and the use of DNA-based methods for delivery implicit in the scFv strategy. To this end, we have translated the strategy into an approved human clinical-gene therapy protocol for ovarian carcinoma *(39)*. The feasibility of this strategy against the proto-oncogenes c-*ras* and c-*myc* has also been shown in animal models *(40)*.

Transdominant Molecules Alternatively, proto-oncogenes can be inactivated at the protein level by the heterologous expression of mutant proteins that inhibit the function of the native version of oncoproteins, the so called dominant-negative mutation strategy. For instance, transdominant mutants of c-H-*ras* have been shown in vitro to possess potent suppressive

effect on pancreatic cell lines with c-*ras* mutations. The feasibility of efficient delivery and production of adequate levels of mutant protein in vivo remains to be determined.

TUMOR PHENOMENA DEPENDENT ON MULTIPLE GENES

Angiogenesis The development of new blood vessels is a critical factor in the growth, progression, and metastatic spread of both solid and hematopoietic tumors. Despite heterogeneity in many other respects, all tumors share at least one universal feature: they depend absolutely on the vasculature to maintain their viability and to sustain their growth and dissemination. Extensive experimental data supports this contention *(41–44)*. Furthermore, numerous clinical studies have shown the correlation between the development of intratumoral microvessels and the prognosis of individual cases in a variety of cancers *(45–47)*. Vessel targeting, therefore, should be useful for the treatment of most kinds of cancer *(48–51)*. Importantly in this regard, the genetic stability of endothelial cells should essentially eliminate the appearance of resistance to molecular therapeutic interventions targeted to the endothelium *(52)*. This hypothesis has indeed recently been confirmed in a cancer animal model of treatment with the natural inhibitor of angiogenesis endostatin *(53)*. An additional advantage of targeted killing of endothelial cells is the highly amplified killing effect over large numbers of tumor cells when deprived from its vascularization.

In the last decade, antiangiogenic drugs targeted to the proliferating endothelium of tumors (and in other diseases) have been applied in the clinical setting and have entered clinical trials. In addition, the association of chemotherapy or radiotherapy with antiangiogenic agents has been shown to produce an enhanced antitumor effect in preclinical models. Notably, combined treatments can achieve cures that are not observed with either treatment alone *(54)*. Thus, molecular therapeutic interventions against the tumor and its vasculature are not only strongly appealing in theoretical grounds for their use in a variety of clinical contexts, but their utility is also rapidly being tested clinically *(55)*. Based on this, genetic modification of the endothelium of tumor vasculature has been proposed as an alternative therapeutic modality *(56)*. With this genetic strategy, the problems of previously explored approaches can be potentially overcome. For instance, local production of high levels of therapeutic proteins can be induced, thus obviating or diminishing the difficulties associated with systemic toxicity, and also pharmacological issues, such as large-scale manufacture, bioavailability, and cost of ordinary drugs. In addition, the ability to continuously release the gene-encoded product may be relevant in certain cases, such as for the appropriate antiangiogenic effect of interferon γ (IFN-γ).

Both suppression of angiogenic cellular signals and augmentation of natural inhibitors of angiogenesis have proved to be feasible strategies in in vivo tumor models. Examples of effective genetic interventions for the suppression of angiogenesis factors are the downregulation of vascular endothelial growth factor (VEGF) by antisense molecules, as shown in models of glioma *(57,58)*, and the blockade of VEGF-receptor (VEGFR) function by delivery of mutant versions of one of its cognate-membrane receptors, Flk-1 *(59–61)*, or of a secreted soluble version of its other receptor, sFlt-1 *(62,63)*. Conversely, the replacement or supplementation of inhibitors of angiogenesis has been attempted using viral vectors that encode soluble platelet factor 4 *(64)* and angiostatin. However, no one of these strategies has been clinically tested, and major issues remain unresolved. Most obvious is the probable need to assure long-term expression of the therapeutic antiangiogenic genes to keep the tumor deprived of its growth-enabling vascularization. In addition, the current lack of targetable, injectable vectors impedes the application of anti-angiogenesis gene-based strategies to multiple foci of tumor that characterize disseminated cancer. Lastly, different combinations of endothelial growth factors and its receptors are altered in different tumors, and may even change in single tumors during different stages of progression. Thus, despite its powerful rationale, the successful clinical implementation of antiangiogenesis gene therapy will require major developments.

Invasion and Metastasis Increasingly, genes and proteins involved in phenotypic aspects of tumors, other than disordered proliferation, are being described and identified as potentially useful therapeutic targets. In this regard, besides angiogenesis, one fundamental component of the metastatic cascade is the local invasion of the extracellular matrix (ECM) by tumor cells. Studies in animal models have begun to show that modulation by gene transfer of molecules involved in degradation of ECM, cellular motility, and cellular adhesion has the potential for inhibiting tumor-cell spread *(65)*.

Urokinase-type plasminogen activator (uPA) is a protease involved in the processes of tissue remodeling, tumor invasion, and cell migration in vitro. Plasminogen activators are thought to degrade ECM proteins and cellular-basement membranes and to allow local tumor invasion and access to the vascular system for metastasis *(66)*. The inhibitors of plasminogen activation, PA-1 and PA-2, have also been described in association with different types of cancer. The levels of both uPA and its receptor uPAR are elevated in ovarian, prostate, glioma, and other tumor cells and correlate with the clinical stage of disease *(67)*. Furthermore, it has been shown that inhibition of uPA receptor expression by antisense oligonucleotides can abrogate human glioblastoma spread in an in vitro model *(68)*. In addition, in an in vivo model of uveal melanoma, an adenoviral vector was used for the transfer of plasminogen activator inhibitor type 1 *(PAI-1)* cDNA *(69)*. Intraocular injection of the vector resulted in a 50% reduction in the number of animals developing liver metastases and a reduction in the metastatic tumor burden in animals that eventually developed metastases. These results support disruption of uPA function through gene transfer as an experimental strategy for preventing metastases and prolonging host survival.

Glioblastomas are known to express the CD44 cell-adhesion molecule (CAM). Human glioma-cell adhesion and invasion in vitro may in part be mediated by the interaction of CD44 with ECM proteins. To suppress the growth and invasive effects of CD44 expression on primary brain tumors, a hammerhead ribozyme against CD44 was designed, and showed significant in vivo cleavage activity against cellular CD44 transcripts following transient transfection into a glioma cell line. These results suggest that CD44-directed downregulation may

be a useful gene therapeutic maneuver. Therefore, abrogation of molecules involved in tumor cell adhesion may inhibit invasion and represent a novel approach to limiting the spread of locally aggressive tumors.

Obstacles to Mutation Compensation Although the strategies currently used for restoration and ablation of mutant genes have offered in-depth insights into the molecular biology involved in carcinogenesis and tumor progression of cancer, they face critical problems that impede their clinical application. Human tumors are remarkably heterogeneous in the patterns of expression of relevant proto-oncogenes. Thus, therapeutic targeting of a single molecular abnormality may have only an inconsequential impact on the clinical management of the disease, both for the population and for individual patients. In addition, several mutated genes produce molecules with transdominant effects, requiring the blocking of their effects and not only the mere supplementation with a wild-type version of the gene. Furthermore, because these strategies modulate intracellular responses, nearly every tumor cell must be targeted for these approaches to be clinically effective. The current state of development of gene therapy vectors, both viral and nonviral, makes this feat unachievable within nontoxic margins of vector dose. Clearly, breakthrough developments in vector technology are needed for these obstacles to be overcome. Also, approaches such as molecular chemotherapy or immune-system augmentation that exhibit an amplified regional or systemic effect hold the promise of tackling, by their own design, some of the aforementioned limitations.

MOLECULAR CHEMOTHERAPY

A number of distinct approaches to accomplish molecular chemotherapy for cancer have been developed. These include: 1) the administration of toxin genes to eliminate tumor cells and the stromal cells that support them, 2) the administration of drug resistance genes to protect the bone marrow from myelosuppression induced by chemotherapy, and 3) the administration of genes that enhance the effect of conventional anticancer treatments. Initially, the approach of molecular chemotherapy was designed to achieve selective eradication of carcinoma cells via expression of a toxin gene. This is similar to conventional chemotherapy, where pharmacological agents are employed. However, in the latter approach, the drug's toxicity is often expressed both in malignant and nonmalignant cells. Therefore, in order to effect a reduction in burden of neoplastic cells, the patient's normal tissues and organs have to be exposed to potentially harmful quantities of the drug. Molecular chemotherapy is designed to circumvent this limitation by selectively targeting toxin delivery or expression to cancer cells on the basis of more specific tissue or transformation-associated markers, and thus reduce the potential for nonspecific toxicity. Commonly, a nontoxic prodrug is administered that requires activation in genetically modified cells to be transformed into a toxic metabolite that ultimately leads to cell death *(70–74)*.

TOXIN GENES

Thymidine Kinase The most common molecular chemotherapy system utilized to date to accomplish cell killing has been the herpes simplex virus thymidine kinase (HSV-*tk*) gene

Table 5
Prodrug/enzyme Combinations for Molecular Chemotherapy

Enzyme (origin)	In vitro Prodrug[a]	bystander effect[b]	Target cell	Distinguishing features	References
Carboxylesterase (rabbit liver)	CPT-11 (irinotecan)	+++	Dividing cells	Prodrug already in clinical use	(91,189)
Carboxypeptidase G2 (bacterial)	CMDA	+++	Dividing and non-	Does not require cell cycling dividing cells	(190)
Cytochrome P-450 isoenzyme (rat liver)	Cyclophosphamide, Isophosphamide	Yes	Dividing cells	Brain intratumor administration allows generation of toxic metabolites that usually do not cross blood-brain barrier	(191)
Cytosine deaminase (E. coli)	5-Fluorocytosine	++ (Independent of cell contact)	Dividing and possibly nondividing cells	Intense sensitization	(93,192–194)
Deoxycytidine kinase (human)	Cytosine Arabinoside	+ (Dependent on cell contact)	Dividing cells an immune response	Human origin of gene avoids	(92,195)
Nitroreductase (E. coli)	CB1954	+++ (Independent of cell contact)	Dividing and	Does not require cell cycling nondividing cells	(196–199)
Purine nucleoside phosphorylase (DeoD gene of E. coli)	MeP-dR	+++	Dividing and non dividing cells	Most intense bystander effect	(200)
Xantine-6-guaninephosphoribosyl transferase (gpt gene of E. coli)	thioxanthine, 6-thioguanine	++ (Independent of cell contact)	Dividing cells	gpt is also a drug resistance gene	(201–203)
Thymidine kinase (herpes simplex virus)	Ganciclovir		Dividing cells	Most extensively used in clinical trials	(69)
Thymidine kinase (varicella zoster virus)	BVDU	++ (Dependent on cell contact)	Dividing cells	–	(204)

[a]BVDU: (E)-5-(2-bromovinyl)-2'-deoxyuridine; CB1954: 5-(aziridin-1-yl)-2,4-dinitrobenzamide; CMDA: 4-[(2-chloroetyl)(2-mesyloxyethyl)amino]benzoyl-L-glutamic acid; Mep-dR: 9-(beta-D-2-deoxyerythropentofuranosyl)-6-methylpurine.
[b]Transduced cells needed for complete cell-growth inhibition in cell-mixing experiments: +++, 10% or less; ++, from 10–50%; +, more than 50%.

given in combination with the prodrug ganciclovir (GCV) *(75)*. The selectivity of the HSV-*tk* system is based on the fact that, contrary to normal mammalian thymidine kinase, HSV-*tk* preferentially monophosphorylates GCV, rendering it toxic to the cell. GCV is then further phosphorylated by cellular kinases to triphosphates that are incorporated into cellular DNA. The incorporation of the triphosphate form of GCV causes inhibition of DNA synthesis and of RNA polymerase, leading to cell death *(70)*. Thus, tumor cells (or any other cell undergoing mitosis) transduced to express the HSV-*tk* gene have enhanced sensitivity to cell killing after exposure to GCV. Somewhat unexpectedly, normal cells transduced with HSV-*tk* after intravenous *(76)* or intrahepatic *(77)* administration of adenoviral HSV-*tk* vector have also shown high sensitivity to GCV, leading to liver degeneration and low survival in mice. The absence of toxicity of GCV after intravenous administration of a control adenovirus, or subcutaneous administration of an adenovirus encoding HSV-*tk*, suggests that the toxicity is specifically liver-associated. The relationship between toxicity and the proliferative status of liver parenchymal cells remains to be determined.

Toxicity and efficacy of the transfer of HSV-*tk* is currently being tested in more than two dozen human clinical trials, including tumors of the ovary, brain, prostate, head and neck, mesothelioma, multiple myeloma, leukemia, and liver metastasis of colon cancer (for an updated list of protocols, visit the Office of Recombinant DNA activities website at http://www.nih.gov/od/orda/protocol.htm).

Bystander Effect Although the benefits of selectively eradicating tumor cells are obvious, an important limitation associated with molecular chemotherapy is the inability to target 100% of the tumor cells with the toxin gene. However, this may prove not to be as severe a limitation as initially believed due to a phenomenon known as bystander effect, whereby eradication of HSV-*tk* transduced cells elicits a killing effect upon the surrounding nontransduced tumor cells. That not all of the tumor cells need to contain the HSV-*tk* gene for obtaining complete eradication of the tumor was an observation of early experiments employing the relatively inefficient retroviral vectors in brain tumors *(78,79)*. This occurrence was later confirmed in a variety of other tumor-model systems *(80,81)*. Our

Table 6
Targeting of Cancer Gene Therapy[a]

Principle	Basis	Strategies	Examples of applications
Selective delivery (transductional targeting)	Anatomically directed administration	Intratumoral, intravascular, or body compartment injection of vector	Injection of a plasmid encoding the immunostimulatory molecule B7 in foci of malignant melanoma *(97)*; intra-arterial infusion of a plasmid encoding VEGF in an ischemic vascular tree *(205)*; intraperitoneal administration of adenovirus expressing the suicide gene HSV-*tk* in ovarian cancer *(206)*
	Target-cell physiology	Exploit cell-cycle differences (gene transfer by retroviruses occurs only in dividing cells)	Brain tumors (tumors are surrounded by neural cells, which are nonmitotic) *(207)*
		Exploit cell-cycle differences (Herpes-virus deleted for *tk* or other genes replicates only in cells undergoing division)	Injection of virus is followed by lytic replication in liver metastasis *(208)* and brain tumors *(209)* (tumors are surrounded by cells that are nonmitotic)
		Exploit differences between transformed and normal cells (Adenovirus deleted for *E1B* gene replicates selectively in *p53*-defective tumor cells)	Injection of virus is followed by lytic replication in head and neck tumor cells *(210)*
	Specific receptors in target cells	Pseudotyped retroviruses (built with heterologous envelope proteins that confer novel tropism);Retroviruses with genetically, chemically, or immuno-	Retrovirus with the genome and core of Murine Leukemia Virus and the envelope protein of Vesicular Stomatitis Virus have logically modified envelope proteins wider tropism *(163)*; Retrovirus with modified envelope protein that includes a fragment of erythropoyetin *(211)* or a single-chain variable region directed against known epitopes such as MHC class I molecules *(212)* or CEA *(213)*
		Adenovirus (genetic modifications in	The modification of the adenovirus fiber is feasible
		the fiber; immunologically mediated attachment of cellular ligands) *(126,214)*. antibody fragments in ovarian tumors *(174)*	Adenovirus with folate *(180)* or the fibroblast growth factor (FGF) attached to the virus via anti-knob Fab
		Molecular conjugates that combine a DNA-binding domain and a cellular ligand	Asialoglycoprotein-based conjugates target hepatocytes *(177)*; adenovirus enhances transduction efficiency of conjugates *(215)* transferrin-based conjugates target leukemic cells *(216)*
		Liposomes modified with antibodies specific against cellular receptors	Liposomes coupled with antibodiy G22-MCA against glioma cells have higher transduction efficiency *(217)*
Selective expression (transcriptional targeting)	Tumor-specific promoters	A suicide gene is administered under the control of a promoter sequence that is active on tumor cells	Adenoviruses expressing *tk* under the alpha-fetoprotein promoter in hepatoma *(218)*, or *DF3* (MUC1) in breast cancer *(219)*. Also shown with cells stably expressing the CD gene under the CEA promoter in colon cancer *(220)*, and with cells transfected with the SLPI promoter, which is expressed in several carcinomas, to direct transcription of HSV-*tk* *(221)*. Same principle shown with promoter of c-*erbB2*, overexpressed in breast and pancreatic tumors *(222)*
	Tissue-specific promoters	A suicide gene is administered under the control of a promoter sequence that is active in a particular tissue	Tyrosinase (melanocytes) directs expression of HSV-*tk* into malignant melanoma *(223)* and other melanocytes; surfactant protein-A drives HSV-*tk* expression in lung-cancer cell lines *(224)*

[a]CD, cytosine deaminase; SLPI, secretory leukoprotease inhibitor; *tk*, thymidine kinase; VEGF, vascular endothelial growth factor.

laboratory established the necessary biological properties to elicit bystander-mediated cell killing in a murine model of ovarian cancer *(82)*. As a result, a human gene-therapy clinical trial has been initiated *(83)*.

In this regard, the basic biological mechanisms that underlie the bystander effect have been partially characterized. Both local and distant bystander effects have been described in in vitro and in vivo models. The local amplification of toxin gene expression includes the transfer of toxic metabolic products of GCV through intercellular gap junctions *(84,85)*, and, less probably, phagocytosis by live tumor cells of apoptotic vesicles from dead cells *(80,86)*. Both the local and distant bystander effects, observed in vivo in distant foci of untreated tumors, are accompanied by the regional induction of cytokines *(87)* and an immune cellular response against the tumor *(88–91)*. As mentioned, almost two dozen clinical trials have been rapidly developed that aim to exploit the toxin gene and bystander effects to achieve antitumor activity.

Other Toxins In addition to the HSV-*tk*/GCV system, several additional combinations of enzyme/prodrug have been developed to improve the efficacy of molecular chemotherapy (Table 5). Features of these combinations might overcome the limitations of HSV-*tk*/GCV. For example, some of them induce toxic effects not only in cycling but also in noncycling cells (carboxypeptidase G2, nitroreductase, purine nucleoside phosphorylase). With others, the bystander effect is stronger (purine nucleoside phosphorylase) or does not require cell contact (cytosine deaminase, nitroreductase) (Table 5).

The combination of cytosine deaminase (CD) and 5-fluorocytosine (5-FC) has been the first of these alternative systems to be tested clinically *(92)*. Studies in vitro and in vivo have shown that transfer of the microbial CD gene sensitizes cells to the innocuous antifungal drug 5-FC. This effect is induced by metabolizing 5-FC into the toxic antitumor agent, 5-fluorouracil (5-FU) *(93)*. By administering high doses of the nontoxic 5-FC, intratumoral activity of the enzyme can provide increased intratumoral concentrations of the active drug, without its accompanying systemic toxicity. Potential weaknesses of the system are its dependence on cellular proliferation, and its complex metabolism, which facilitates acquired resistance by tumor cells.

With some exceptions, single drugs in standard chemotherapy do not cure cancer. Historically, effective treatments were developed when drugs with different mechanisms of action were used in combination. Extending this concept to molecular chemotherapy, several combinations of enzyme/ prodrug have been shown to induce synergistic killing effects in vitro *(94,95)*. Combination protocols have achieved higher rates of tumor regression and cure in animal models *(96,97)*. The application of classical principles for designing drug combinations would recommend the use of prodrug/enzymes that target both dividing and nondividing cells, that elicit different mechanisms of bystander effect, and that have nonoverlapping toxicities.

GENE TARGETING Therapies based on gene transfer have been shown to be remarkably successful in in vitro and in vivo animal model systems. However, overriding limitations have consistently been made apparent in pre-clinical experiments

and in the first human gene-therapy clinical trials. Most current difficulties in obtaining clinically relevant benefits have come from the insufficient efficiency of current gene vectors in transducing target organs, tumors or immune cells, and their inability to access in a selective manner target cells distributed systemically.

With molecular chemotherapy, the specificity of tumor eradication is based on selective toxin expression in the neoplastic cells. Targeting in this context is critical for the reasons mentioned earlier. First, highly efficient transduction of tumor cells is needed to achieve therapeutic levels of toxin production. Second, transduction of normal cells should be avoided to reduce toxicity. Initially, these goals were pursued by anatomically directing the injection of gene-transfer vectors to the site or compartment where tumor was located, and occasionally exploiting also the natural tropism of retroviral vectors for dividing cells. The diversification of available vectors, the continuing effort to develop vectors for systemic administration, and safety requirements, all led to the design of more precise targeting maneuvers. There are two general types: 1) transductional targeting, whereby the toxin is specifically delivered to the tumor by means of a targeted gene delivery vector; and 2) transcriptional targeting, whereby tumor or target tissue-specific transcriptional activators are employed to selectively express the toxin gene exclusively within the tumor (Table 6).

The ability to alter the binding tropism of viral vectors is based on an understanding of the basic biology of viral entry. Modification of tropism involves altering initial binding to target cells via either genetic or immunological methods. In this regard, two distinct effects must be achieved: 1) ablation of the endogenous binding specificity, and 2) preservation of the efficient, post-binding, cellular-entry mechanisms. Implicit in this strategy is the assumption that the virus can accomplish distal steps in its entry pathway after internalization via the heterologous cellular pathway. Sufficient understanding of both retroviral and adenoviral entry exists to allow the development of strategies to modify vector tropism. However, structural requirements during retroviral binding and entry have impeded successful exploitation of this knowledge *(98)*. In contrast, the adenoviral particle has been more permissive for genetic and immunologically based changes towards tropism modification. Studies suggest that the requirements of this strategy may be met in the context of adenovirus-based vectors. This would allow the derivation of a vector with cell-specific gene-delivery capacity and, in contrast to retrovirus, endowed also with in vivo stability. Such adenoviral vector would thus be suitable for application in the context of targeted gene delivery to disseminated diseases.

Although extensively tested *(99)*, the use of transcriptional regulatory sequences for restricting the expression of therapeutic genes to the target tissue or tumor has shown inconsistent results in different vectors, with mounting evidence that *cis* elements located in the viral genome can alter both tissue specificity and activity of the promoter *(100)*. Further limitations come from the prohibitively large size of regulatory sequences in the context of current vectors. However, novel gene transfer systems with larger capacity are being developed and could overcome this limitation, such as adenoviral vectors *(101)*, recombinant herpes virus *(102)*, and human artificial chromosomes *(103)*. For detailed reviews, general references on vector targeting for cancer gene therapy *(104–107)* and on targeting of particular vector systems *(98,108)* are available.

DRUG-RESISTANCE GENES In a second molecular chemotherapy approach, the host tolerance to higher doses of standard chemotherapeutic drugs is increased by transducing bone marrow cells, known to be highly sensitive to chemotoxicity, with genes that confer drug resistance *(109,110)*. In this context, retroviral vectors have been the vectors of choice for the in vitro derivation of stably transduced cells, due to their capacity for integration in chromosomal DNA. It has been shown that when mice transplanted with bone marrow cells containing a transferred multiple drug-resistance *(mdr1)* gene were treated with the cytotoxic drug taxol, a substantial enrichment for transduced bone marrow cells was observed. This demonstration of positive selection established the ability to amplify clones of transduced hematopoietic cells in vivo and suggested possible applications in human therapy. In a clinical trial, the bone marrow hematopoietic cells of refractory ovarian-cancer patients will be transduced ex vivo with a retroviral vector encoding the *mdr1* gene. After treatment for systemic disease with high-dose chemotherapy, the modified progenitor cells containing the *mdr1* gene will be transplanted into the recipient and the patients will receive cyclic chemotherapy with taxol. Thus, it is expected that a treatment cycle-dependent enrichment of the marrow with hematopoietic cells resistant to the myeloablative effects of the chemotherapeutic drugs will be observed *(111)*. Some potential problems with this strategy exist. These include: 1) the failure to demonstrate that higher chemotherapy doses translate into improved patient survival; 2) very low transduction efficiency of the target human hematopoietic cells with retrovirus vectors; 3) the dose-limiting effects determined by other nonhematological toxicities; and 4) the fact that cancer cells in the marrow could be transduced with the drug-resistance gene, which could rapidly give rise to clones of treatment-resistant tumor cells.

CHEMOSENSITIZATION AND RADIOSENSITIZATION A third approach of molecular chemotherapy seeks to modulate the level of expression of a variety of genes that influence the sensitivity of the cell to toxic stimuli, including conventional chemotherapeutic drugs and radiotherapy. Genetic chemosensitization can be achieved by modulating apoptosis, inhibiting tumor-cell resistance, or enhancing intratumoral production of cytotoxic drugs. To facilitate apoptosis, genes such as *p53* may be administered to tumor cells to enhance the mechanisms of apoptosis induced by chemotherapeutic agents *(112)*. Our group has shown that downregulation of bcl2 protein levels by an intracellular anti-bcl2 single-chain antibody increases drug-induced cytotoxicity *(113)*. Analogously, genetic downregulation of cellular factors related to chemoresistance has been shown to enhance chemosensitivity. Again, we have been able to show that single-chain, antibody-mediated abrogation of the c-erbB2 oncoprotein can significantly mitigate intrinsic chemoresistance in c-*erbB2* overexpressing ovarian cancer cells and allows for augmented sensitivity to the DNA-damaging drug

cisplatin *(37)*. Alternatively, genes can be administered intratumorally that enhance metabolic conversion of conventional chemotherapeutic agents. Studies have shown that transfer of a liver cytochrome P450 gene (*CYP2B1*) into human breast-cancer cells greatly sensitized these cells to the cancer chemotherapeutic agent cyclophosphamide as a consequence of the acquired capacity for intratumoral drug activation. This effect produced a substantially enhanced antitumor activity *in vivo (114)*. Lastly, combinations of conventional chemotherapeutic agents and molecular chemotherapy can serve the established rule of administering cytotoxic drugs with different mechanisms of action and toxicities. For example, one clinical trial evaluates the association of adenovirus-mediated transduction of ovarian-cancer cells with the HSV-*tk* gene followed by administration of acyclovir and the chemotherapeutic drug topotecan (http://www.nih.gov/od/orda/protocol.htm).

Several drugs are proven radiosensitizers, a fact that is commonly exploited in the clinic. One of these drugs is 5-FU, which is the product of the CD suicide gene. In this regard, molecular chemotherapy based on CD has been shown to enhance the effects of radiation therapy in animal models of gliosarcoma *(115)* and cholangiocarcinoma *(116)*. Thus, strategies to alter both chemosensitivity and radiosensitivity by gene transfer appear to have potentially wide applicability in many tumor contexts.

OBSTACLES TO MOLECULAR CHEMOTHERAPY

With all its promise, molecular chemotherapy also bears some practical limitations. To date, the strategy of molecular chemotherapy has been mainly used in loco-regional disease models. In these *in situ* schemas, a vector encoding the toxin gene is administered intratumorally or into an anatomic compartment containing the tumor mass. The goals of this delivery method are to achieve high local vector concentration in order to favor tumor transduction and to limit vector dissemination. However transduction efficiencies of presently available vectors have been shown to be inadequate. Even in closed-compartment delivery contexts, it has not been possible to modify a sufficient number of tumor cells to achieve a relevant tumoral response in clinical models *(117–121)*. Furthermore, although transduction with HSV-*tk* followed by ganciclovir treatment reduces tumor burden and prolongs survival in various model systems, including those utilizing intratumoral and intraperitoneal administration, the required increased doses of viral vector needed for obtaining quantitative tumor-cell transduction is associated with limiting toxicity. In fact, substantial toxicity and experimental animal death has been noted *(76,77,120)*. Thus, the small therapeutic index of currently available vectors in the context of *in situ* administration is a critical limiting factor for the purpose of gene therapy of cancer. Furthermore, and most importantly, a well-known limitation of conventional chemotherapy is also to be expected with the use of molecular chemotherapy, that is, the appearance of drug-resistant tumor subpopulations (Table 1). In conclusion, vector limitations and well-known barriers to classical cytotoxic maneuvers impede the full exploitation of the promise of a more selective eradication of carcinoma cells via expression of toxin or protective genes.

GENETIC IMMUNOPOTENTIATION

The development of clinically evident tumors implies the obvious failure of the host immune system to recognize and eliminate tumor antigen(s). Genetic immunopotentiation strategies attempt to achieve active immunization against tumor-associated antigens by gene-transfer methodologies applied either to tumor cells or to cellular components of the immune system. To this end, recent insights into the pathophysiology of tumor escape from the immune-system surveillance offer guidance for designing new therapeutic strategies (122) (Table 6).

In contrast to the evidence for tumor escape, there is another rare clinical observation that indicates the potential for an effective therapeutic maneuver against cancer based on the genetic modulation of the host-immune system. This is the reproducible observation in clinical trials of immunotherapy against renal cancer and melanoma of dramatic spontaneous remissions of untreated patients with bulky, solid metastatic cancer, in a measurable proportion of cases (123). This unexplained observation suggest that the immune system can occasionally recognize and reject large volumes of tumor, and supports the undertaking of ambitious approaches for genetic immunopotentiation against cancer.

TUMOR ESCAPE Factors that can explain the failure of the immune system in the cancer patient include: 1) an inadequate immunogenicity of the tumor or 2) a deficiency of the immune system to recognize, respond, and reject the tumor. Reduced tumor immunogenicity can be related to the absence of either tumor-specific antigens or major histocompatibility complex (MHC) I molecules on the tumor cells, which are essential for presentation of cellular antigens to effector CD8$^+$ T lymphocytes. Alternatively, it may well be that the lack of costimulatory molecules, such as B7, in tumor cells establishes immune tolerance or ignorance, which keeps the tumor from being treated as foreign or dangerous. Immune-system deficiencies, in turn, can be either generalized or regional, including in the last case the active suppression by the tumor of host antigen-presenting and effector cells in the local microenvironment.

Tumor Antigens Tumor cells have been shown to express tumor antigens, which are cell determinants that can be recognized as extraneous by the immune system, at least in in vitro and syngeneic animal studies. Protective immunity in early animal studies was shown to depend on CD8$^+$ cytolytic T lymphocytes (CTL). To be recognized by T lymphocytes, tumor antigens should be intracellularly associated with MHC class I or class II molecules and then presented to cells of the immune system on the tumor-cell surface. Some clones of tumor-infiltrating lymphocytes (TIL) can lyse the majority of cancer cell lines of certain types, such as melanoma HLA-A2+, which suggests that there are antigens shared by tumors of the same histology from different individuals. It has been argued that this fact supports the development of universal vaccines against certain tumors.

There are five general categories of tumor antigens. First, antigens coded by genes that are silent in normal cells and expressed almost uniquely in tumors, such as the MAGE family of antigens in melanomas. Second, antigens resulting from mutations in normal proteins, such as p53, MUC-1, MUM-1,

cdk4, and β-catenin. Third, differentiation antigens, present normally in the tissue from which the tumor originates, such as MART-1, gp75, gp100, and tyrosinase, again in melanoma and melanocytes. Fourth, antigens encoded by normal genes that are dysregulated in tumor tissues, such as c-*erbB2*. Five, antigens encoded by genomes of oncogenic viruses, such as the human papillomavirus (HPV) E6 and E7 gene products. Notably, the role of CTL against these antigens in the rejection of human tumors has not been demonstrated in any case.

To identify tumor-associated antigens, mice have been immunized with tumor cells, and the resultant MAbs have been used to isolate the corresponding peptides from the surface of human melanoma cells. Due to the methodology used, which identifies any cognate antibody ligands, many of these antigens are not related with the neoplastic phenotype and are not necessarily immunogenic in humans. As mentioned, the activation of T lymphocytes (the cellular immune response) is more important than the humoral response for inducing tumor lysis and regression in experimental models. Therefore, the search for relevant antigens is currently based in the analysis of reactive circulating or tumor-infiltrating T lymphocytes isolated from patients with tumors (124,125). More than a dozen specific peptides recognizable by CTL have been identified to date. Unfortunately, after vaccination of melanoma patients with these peptides only sporadic responses have been observed. More importantly, in cases showing tumor regression, it has not been possible to correlate response with in vitro CTL responses. These results suggest that the existence of tumor-specific antigens does not assure the development of an effective immune response against tumors.

A theoretical barrier for antitumor vaccination, probably related to the observation just mentioned, can be deduced from the initial experiments done with tumor transplants in mice. It was observed that some tumors induced by carcinogenic agents were clearly immunogenic when transplanted into basically identical syngeneic animals. Paradoxically, primary tumors were not rejected in the original donor animals. In addition, lethally irradiated tumor cells were still capable of immunizing naïve animals against later exposure to tumorigenic doses of the cells. However, late vaccination of a tumor-bearing host could lead to rejection of a second fresh tumor-cell challenge, but the original tumor was usually not rejected. Conceivably, tumor antigens can be recognized, in the murine model, only after previous exposure or a change in the circumstances of exposure of the immune system to the tumor cells. Thus, the mere presence of antigens in tumors may be not enough for inducing an efficient antitumor immune response in the natural tumor site, which probably involves the attraction and activation of tumor-specific T cells at the site of established tumors.

Major Histocompatibility Complex MHC class I products, strongly expressed on normal tissues, are occasionally absent or downregulated in tumors of varying histology, in comparison with their respective normal counterpart tissues. Sometimes this downregulation occurs more significantly in metastatic lesions, or in later steps in tumor progression (126). Supporting the potential role of changes in MHC levels in tumor escape, it has been shown in co-cultures of cancer-cells and CD8$^+$ lymphocytes that cancer cell clones can arise that escape from lysis by autologous lymphocytes *(127,128)*, and that this phenomenon correlates with a marked decrease in the expression of MHC class I molecules. By itself, this observation could explain the local failure of the immune system to develop a strong antitumoral response in the clinical context. Thus, provision of MHC I expression in previously negative tumor cells could restore locally the functionality of the cytotoxic cellular immune response. In this regard, it is also interesting that IFN-y and tumor necrosis factor (TNF) induce in several tumor cell lines an increase in the expression of MHC class I and, under experimental conditions, can restore the antitumor lytic functions of the cytotoxic cellular immune response *(129)*.

The molecular basis of tumor escape has been further documented in a fascinating clinical case. A recurrent lesion was studied six yr after resection of the primary tumor, a malignant melanoma. The new lesion had concomitantly lost both a tumor-associated antigen and the protein TAP-1. This protein normally carries peptides from the cytoplasm to the endoplasmic reticulum, where they are associated with MHC class I molecules prior to their transport to the cell surface. Transfer of genes encoding the lost antigen and TAP-1 into tumor cells grown from the recurrent lesion restored sensitivity of the tumor cells to CTL *(130)*. Thus, tumor-associated antigen expression and presentation may not be sufficient, but is clearly needed for development of an efficient cellular immune response.

Costimulatory Signals and Antigen Presenting Cells In effect, rejection of the tumor by CTLs requires not only the presence of tumor antigens and their appropriate display in association with MHC class I molecules (signal 1) but also an array of costimulatory signals, provided by antigen-presenting cells (APCs) (signal 2). These cells, derived from the bone marrow, are critical for the activation of CTL, which happens through the interaction of molecules of the B7 family, present on APCs, and the CD28 receptor on T cells. This interaction occurs in the lymph nodes and requires the previous activation of the APCs in an inflammatory environment *(131)*. Once activated, T cells expand and are then able to migrate, seek, and destroy tumor cells that express the appropriate antigen in a MHC context. A critical observation for understanding tumor immunology and tumor escape is that the interaction of CTL and tumor cells in the absence of activated APCs results in a state of antigen-specific T-cell dormancy referred to as anergy *(132)*. The molecular basis of this phenomenon is unclear. In this regard, it has been speculated that a factor secreted by the tumor cell alters the lymphocyte TCR-CD3 surface complex, resulting in impaired intracellular signal transduction *(133)*. Thus, several ingredients of an effective immune response may be absent in the relationship between the tumor and cells of the immune system in normal conditions, favoring the development of weak and ineffectual responses and lack of tumor eradication.

Immune-System Exhaustion The simplest explanation for tumor escape is that the rapid growth and spread of the tumor overwhelms the effector mechanisms of immune responses. However, there is evidence against the exhaustion hypothesis as the explanation for the growth of cancer cells in immuno-

competent animals. Elegant experiments in T-cell receptor (TCR) transgenic mice have shown that, even when essentially all T cells recognize a given antigen, tumors expressing the antigen are not rejected, whereas skin cells expressing the same antigen are rejected. Therefore, systemic T-cell exhaustion or antigen-specific anergy is not responsible for the growth of the antigenic cancer cells, at least in this experimental model *(134)*.

Immunosuppression The immune-system deficiency present in the tumor microenvironment may be related to the local production of immunosuppressive gene products by tumor cells or infiltrating leukocytes. Candidate molecules thought to mediate this local immunosuppression are TGF-β, interleukin-10 (IL-10), VEGF, and Fas ligand (FasL).

TGF-β is secreted by a variety of malignant tumors and their supporting stroma. In addition to effects on cellular proliferation and theECM, TGF-β elicits potent growth-inhibitory effects on B and T lymphocytes through suppression of the generation of cytotoxic T and natural killer (NK) cells, downregulation of high-affinity IL-2 receptors, and inhibition of cytokine synthesis in peripheral T-lymphocytes. Tumor cells induced experimentally to produce TGF-β, though retaining expression of MHC class I molecules and tumor-specific antigens, do not stimulate primary CTL responses in vitro and are not effective in vivo for directly stimulating primary CTL or in priming for CTL responses *(135)*. Furthermore, TGF-β-producing tumors grow progressively in transiently immunosuppressed mice without losing the tumor antigen. More direct evidence has been obtained by using antisense molecules against TGF-β. Rats that were implanted with glioma tumor cells transfected with an antisense plasmid survived significantly longer than controls, and had effector cells in lymph nodes with increased lytic activity, as determined by in vitro cytotoxicity assays *(32)*. Thus, TGF-β produced by tumors may promote escape from immune surveillance through local immunosuppression.

IL-10 has potent anti-inflammatory and immunosuppressive properties. It blocks the release of mediators of inflammation by macrophages, and reduces the presentation of costimulatory molecules by APCs and tumor cells to lymphocytes. Its presence has been detected in several tumors, and especially high serum levels have been detected in advanced tumor stages *(122)*. One common clinical observation in the treatment of disseminated cancer is the diverse response of different metastatic lesions to a single cycle of antitumoral treatment. Recently, the function of APCs in regressing and nonregressing lesions has been compared. APCs from regressing lesions were significantly more potent inducers of allogeneic T lymphocytes than APCs from progressing lesions. Furthermore, antigen presenting cells from progressing lesions were able to induce anergy in vitro in CD4+ lymphocytes. IL-10 could be detected in the culture media of cells isolated from progressing lesions, but not in the culture media of cells from regressing lesions, where the stimulating cytokines IL-2, IFN-γ, and IL-12 were detected. These results show that mediators produced in some metastatic foci induce a change in APC function whereby tumor tolerance, instead of costimulation against the tumor is induced, silencing the antitumoral immune response *(136)*.

Recently, human cancer cell lines have been shown to release a soluble factor(s) that very remarkably inhibits maturation of precursors of dendritic cells (DC), one kind of APC, without affecting the function of relatively mature DCs *(137)*. This local immunosuppressive activity was determined to be, at least in large part, due to VEGF. Thus, VEGF may have a broader role in tumor development than its fundamental role in angiogenesis would suggest, with interference in maturation of DCs being a novel mechanism of tumor promotion of this vascular growth factor.

An additional mechanism of tumor escape from the immune system is the expression by tumor cells of FasL. When FasL on tumor surface binds to Fas, present in the cellular membrane of cytotoxic T lymphocytes, a series of events is triggered in the lymphocyte by Fas that lead to apoptosis *(138)*. Thus, the expression of FasL by tumors may protect them against T cell-mediated immune rejection. For instance, this mechanism has been demonstrated to be operating in all samples analyzed from seven patients with melanoma, as shown by the presence of FasL in the tumors and concomitant evidence of apoptosis in TILs *(139)*. The presence of immunosuppressive factors such as FasL and others in tumors clearly suggests the need to complement any immunotherapy strategy with maneuvers explicitly addressing the intratumoral presence of inhibitors of the immune-system response.

GENETIC MODIFICATION OF IMMUNE EFFECTOR CELLS The growing knowledge of tumor immunobiology has guided the development of strategies for genetic immunotherapy against cancer *(124)*. Two types of general interventions have been applied to increase the ability of the patient to mount an efficient antitumor immune response. First, cells of the immune system have been modified to augment their capacity for recognizing and rejecting tumor antigens. Second, the tumor cells themselves can be altered to increase their immunogenicity. Gene therapy offers the possibility of genetically modifying both types of cells, and, importantly, this intervention can be restricted regionally, thus avoiding the intolerable toxicity that characterizes most biologic-response modifiers when administered systemically.

Tumor Infiltrating Lymphocytes Several therapeutic maneuvers have been based in trying to modify the cells of the immune system. TILs are derived from mononuclear cells (MNCs) obtained from leukocytes infiltrating resected specimens of solid tumors. In the early 1990s, it was hypothesized that TILs could be an enriched source of NK cells and CTLs specific for tumor antigens, and could also have tropism towards systemic tumor foci. On this basis, technology for their expansion in culture was developed and TILs were the first immune cells to be genetically modified and applied in a human gene-therapy clinical trial against cancer *(140)*. It was soon observed that although TILs do include CTL and activated NK cells, only a few of these cells in these mixed populations are specific against the tumor from which they are isolated. An additional problem encountered with this approach involves the poor localization of TILs into tumors after their reintroduction into patients.

Three strategies have been applied to improve treatments based on TILs *(141)*. First, the IL-2 gene has been transferred into TILs to increase lymphocyte number and survival when in the host. Second, to boost antitumoral efficacy the gene for TNF has been transferred into TILs ex vivo previous to reinfusion. Thirdly, to improve localization into tumor foci, several novel cellular receptors have been engineered in lymphocytes by genetic and immunological means. However, localization of TILs in tumor biopsies is modest, which may account for the rarity of clinical responses observed in patients subjected to TIL-based treatment. Further, the IL-2 treatment that is typically included to maintain the requisite number and functionality of TILs results in notable toxicity to patients. Targeted lymphocytes expressing chimeric T-cell receptors against tumor antigens have been developed with the aim of improving that barely exploitable tropism, and are currently undergoing clinical testing in melanoma, colorectal, and ovarian cancer.

GENETIC MODIFICATION OF TUMOR CELLS An alternative strategy for trying to augment the antitumor immune response is to genetically modify tumor cells, or to manipulate their components, to facilitate the start of a robust immune response. Thus, it has been hypothesized that a formerly tolerant host may revert its immune status, characterized by tolerance or anergy, and ultimately experience tumor rejection. In other words, it is hypothesized that the host can be vaccinated against the tumor by exposing tumor antigens to the immune system in a more favorable context *(142–144)*. Most clinical experience with antitumor vaccines to date has been obtained in melanoma patients. For years, irradiated tumor cells, either autologous or allogeneic, have been administered in combination with different adjuvants, such as bacillus calmette-guerin (BCG). Later, the molecular definition of tumor-associated antigens allowed the testing of vaccines based on individual antigenic determinants delivered to the patient in the form of peptides or DNA. More recently, tumor cells themselves have been genetically modified to increase their immunogenicity by transfer of a variety of genes, including cytokines such as granulocyte-macrophage colony-stimulating factor (GM-CSF), costimulating molecules (such as B7), and MHC molecules. A common requirement, not adequately accomplished routinely yet, is to introduce the gene of interest in tumor explants or cultured cells with high efficiency.

Cytokine Gene Transfer The utility of antitumor vaccines based on whole tumor cells has been poor when analyzed in randomized clinical trials. However, it has been argued that the genetic modification of tumor cells with cytokine genes could augment the immune response against the tumor *(145)*. In fact, this maneuver could overcome the defects mentioned earlier, which are related to escape of the tumor from immune surveillance. One possible intervention is to induce, by intratumoral gene transfer, the secretion of cytokines that, once secreted by the tumor cell, can activate directly the response of CTLs, and increase the awareness of the immune-system cells to tumor cells in the tumor microenvironment. Cytokines tested to increase the antitumor immune response include: IL-1, IL-2, IL-

4, IL-6, IL-7, IL-10, IL-12, IFN-γ, TNF, G-CSF, and GM-CSF. In some cases, intense inflammatory infiltrates have been observed surrounding cytokine-secreting tumor cells, with the type of infiltrate varying with the particular cytokine. In animal models, immune-mediated tumor regressions are consistently observed with this strategy. Also, specific immunity mediated by CTLs against subsequent exposures to unmodified tumor cells is commonly observed in treated animals. More than 20 clinical trials are evaluating the effect of treatment with autologous or allogeneic tumor cells modified by cytokine genes. Preliminary results, reported in a trial using IL-2-secreting tumor cells, reveal poor tumor responses and a low frequency of CTLs specific against the tumor *(146)*. These results may not be surprising, given the recognized complexity of immunological phenomena and the one-sidedness of the single-gene interventions being tested.

Induction of MHC Expression and Transfer of Allogeneic MHC Recognition of a tumor-associated antigen by CTLs requires its simultaneous presentation with MHC class I molecules on the surface of tumor cells. However, numerous tumors exhibit decreased MHC class I antigen expression. IFN-γ stimulates the expression of MHC molecules by tumor cells, rendering the cells more recognizable by the immune system. Studies in vitro have confirmed that transfer of the gene for IFN-γ into tumor cells increases their MHC expression, and these results are the foundation for currently ongoing clinical trials *(147)*. Interestingly, transfer of allogeneic MHC genes into tumor cells results in the generation of CTLs that are reactive against the treated MHC-expressing tumor mass, but also against nonmodified tumor cells, producing widespread tumor regression *(148)*. Clinical trials have been performed by transferring the gene of human leukocyte antigen (HLA)-B7 by intratumoral injection into tumors that do not express the molecule *(149,150)*. A theoretical risk of this strategy is the inhibition of the antitumor activity of NK cells, which recognize and attack specifically MHC class I-negative cells.

Costimulatory Molecules Costimulatory signals promote clonal expansion of antigen-specific T cells and their differentiation into effector and memory cells. The efficacy of increased costimulation of T lymphocytes for antitumor immunotherapy has been shown in mice vaccinated with tumor cells expressing genes encoding several costimulatory molecules. For instance, tumor cells transfected with B7-1 (also known as CD80, a ligand of CD28 in lymphocytes and distinct from HLA-B7) potently stimulate an immune response, which is not observed with unmodified cells. When injected into syngeneic animals, cells expressing B7-1 are rejected, whereas unmodified cells are not. Furthermore, B7-1 expressing cells induce a potent immune response against unmodified cells in distant regions. The reason is probably that the presence of B7-1 increases the activation of T lymphocytes, but the cytolytic activity of differentiated CTLs does not depend on B7-1. These results in animals led to the development of clinical trials in which tumors from patients are cultured, genetically modified, irradiated, and finally reintroduced into the same patient as vaccines. This strategy, although time-consuming, technically demanding, and costly, could be effective even when no tumor antigens have been

identified. Experimental studies with mice have identified one potential problem with this treatment strategy. In immunized mice, an immune response could be observed against freshly injected subcutaneous tumors, whereas no response was observed against concomitant primary, established tumors, due to a lack of mobilization of activated T lymphocytes to the primary tumor site. Immune ignorance of primary tumor sites can therefore severely limit the utility of strategies based on costimulatory molecules.

Other important accessory molecules include the intercellular adhesion molecules ICAM-1, ICAM-2, ICAM-3 and the lymphocyte functional antigen (LFA-1). Many tumors do not express ligands of the ICAM family efficiently, thus decreasing their ability to costimulate or be targets of the immune response. Again, the transfer of the corresponding gene could conceivably be useful to augment the effect of antitumor vaccines, and that seems to have been the case in several animal models *(151,152)*. CD40, present in APCs, and its ligand in lymphocytes, CD40L, form a third system of costimulatory molecules of unclear importance with respect to the systems mentioned earlier.

Vaccination with Tumor-Associated Antigens Antitumor vaccines have also been developed based on tumor-associated antigens. Using TILs able to induce regression of tumors as a source, genes encoding the cognate tumor antigens have been isolated and cloned *(153)*. Patients could be vaccinated with these tumor-associated antigens combined with adjuvants that increase their immunogenicity. The rationale for this type of treatment is that existing T lymphocytes with antitumor specificity can be activated and specifically stimulated by the vaccine. Immunization could then be done: 1) by direct administration of the peptides, 2) by viral vectors encoding the antigens, 3) by cellular lysates obtained after infection of tumor specimens with vaccinia vectors encoding the antigens, or 4) by naked DNA.

One limitation of vaccines based on peptides is that it is improbable that these peptides could efficiently replace other nonimmunogenic peptides already present and associated with MHC molecules in the surface of tumor cells in the patient. Furthermore, extracellular proteins are presented to the immune system via MHC class II molecules, which activate CD4+ helper lymphocytes but not cytotoxic CD8+ lymphocytes. In contrast, DNA vaccines are better stimulators of CTL by leading to expression of antigens from within cells, where they are associated with MHC class I molecules and presented in the appropriate manner in the cell surface. Particularly attractive candidate antigens especially are those shared by multiple tumors, such as the melanoma antigens MAGE-1, MART-1, and gp100, which are currently being used in several ongoing clinical trials.

OBSTACLES TO GENETIC IMMUNOPOTENTIATION
The main advantage of genetic immunopotentiation is the possibility of enlisting physiological mechanisms for a potentially vast amplification of the therapeutic maneuver. To this end, even modest levels of gene transfer can potentially be followed by clonal expansion and systemic spread of effector immune cells and mediators. Thus, efficiency of gene transfer here is not

critical, given the relatively low amounts of cells and gene products needed to obtain a potentially powerful response from the immune system. There are, however, other more important obstacles that perhaps explain the poor results obtained to date by tumor immunotherapy in humans. Antigenic heterogeneity and plasticity, redundancy of immune-system regulation, and well-established tolerance to natural tumors are the more evident barriers.

Antigenic Heterogeneity and Plasticity During the last two decades numerous reports have confirmed both in vitro and in vivo that expression of tumor cellular antigens in different tumor types is heterogeneous, with variability being found not only between different patients with the same tumors, but between different regions of a single tumor and even in single cell clones (154,155). Moreover, this variability changes with time. This fact, first confronted by MAb therapists, may clearly limit the impact of vaccines against single tumor-associated antigens, and even those based on cultured, homogeneous populations of tumor cells.

Redundant Phenomenology of the Immune System The destructive power of the immune system, occasionally needed in its entire exuberance, obligingly requires a complex network of balances and counterbalances to control the pathways of activation and termination of the immune response. Interventions directed to supplement or inhibit single mediators will most probably obtain partial physiological and therapeutic results in the best case, may frequently yield no result at all, and occasionally will produce effects opposed to those desired. Increasingly, combinations of cytokines are being used to try to control the complexity of the immune response against tumors. Current therapeutic interventions for inducing organ-graft tolerance successfully prolong organ survival by blocking multiple effector cells and mediators of the adaptive and innate immune systems. Similarly, it is conceivable that breaking the tumor tolerance will require a strategy of multiple interventions including several target cells and cytokines.

Lack of Immune Response or Tumor Tolerance Current knowledge in tumor immunobiology establishes that T cells able to recognize tumor-associated antigens can be found in vivo and are inducible (with some difficulties) in vitro. Thus, the lymphocyte repertoire against these epitopes has not been deleted. However, either tolerance to these (tumor) self-antigens has been induced or, in the absence of costimulatory signals, peripheral T cells simply have ignored these antigens (156). This phenomenon should obviously be an early event in tumor progression (157), and may be totally missed in most animal models employed to date, which are based on tumor grafts. In this regard, studies with transgenic mice that develop spontaneous tumors have shown that vaccination with tumor cells transduced with cytokines fail to inhibit tumor onset and progression, whereas the same cells are able to immunize nontransgenic mice subsequently grafted with tumors (158). Thus, the failure of naturally established tumors to efficiently present antigens, and to attract and activate tumor-specific T cells at the tumor site, may impede successful vaccination against cancer antigens. Furthermore, ignorance by the immune system can abort most of the immunotherapy maneuvers being tested.

NOVEL STRATEGIES TO OVERCOME CURRENT LIMITATIONS

As we have reviewed earlier, gene transfer therapies are remarkably successful in in vitro and in vivo animal model systems. In effect, we already know: 1) that the malignant phenotype can be reverted in tumor cell lines by eliminating or adding certain genes; 2) that tumors can be eradicated by delivery of cytotoxic genes followed by treatment with appropriate prodrugs; and 3) that tumors can be cured in murine models by making the tumor cells either more immunogenic or by making the immune system cells more responsive, via the expression of cytokines, or costimulatory and immunogenic molecules. However, overriding limitations have been made apparent in preclinical experiments and in the first human gene-therapy clinical trials against cancer (http://www.nih.gov/od/orda/protocol.htm). Most difficulties in obtaining clinically relevant benefits come from the inefficiency of current gene vectors in transducing tumor or immune cells and their inability to access in a selective way target cells distributed systemically. In this regard, each of these limitations specially undermines the implementation of one particular gene-therapy strategy.

MUTATION COMPENSATION REQUIRES QUANTITATIVE GENE TRANSFER For mutation compensation strategies to work successfully, it seems that every tumor cell would have to be corrected in its genetic defect to achieve a therapeutic outcome. Thus, quantitative transduction of therapeutic genes into the tumor after in situ administration of the gene-therapy vector is an essential requirement. To this end, a variety of vector-amplification strategies are being explored, including replicative (159) and integrative viral systems (160).

Replicative Vector Systems One method to circumvent suboptimal tumor transduction of therapeutic genes in vivo would be the use of conditionally replicative viral vectors. In this context, a replication-competent virus would be employed to replicate selectively within transduced tumor cells, leaving normal tissues unaffected. Production of progeny virions from the transduced tumor cells would then facilitate infection of neighboring cells. Thus, the intratumoral viral inoculum would increase, improving the tumor transduction efficiency. In addition, the use of viruses that display a lytic life-cycle would allow virus-mediated oncolysis. This effect would occur irrespective of the delivered transgene. In either case, an amplification of the antitumor effect would be achieved (159,161).

For in vivo models of this strategy, a virus with in vivo stability and the capacity for conditional replication within tumor cells is mandated. In this regard, recombinant adenoviruses and herpesviruses have the potential to provide the required properties. Not only do they display high efficiency and stability in vivo, but also their replication can be controlled. In the case of adenoviruses, adenoviral replication can be restricted to tumor cells by placement of genes needed for viral replication under the control of tumor or tissue-specific transcriptional control elements, such as the promoter of the prostate-specific antigen for use in prostate cancer (162).

Alternatively, mutant adenoviruses have been developed that exhibit selective replication in cells lacking functional *p53*. Because *p53* is absent in many tumors, a selectively replicative system based on this lytic virus has been proposed for cancer-therapy purposes *(163)*. However, extensive studies in a variety of cell lines and animal-tumor models have to date failed to confirm the selective properties of the virus to replicate only in *p53* mutant tumor cells. Further refinements in these replicative vectors are anticipated. For example, our group is developing defective adenoviral vectors that replicate selectively under the stimulus of the cytokine IL-6, or under the controlled addition of second vectors carrying replication-enabling DNA sequences *(164,165)*.

Herpesviruses have also been developed that replicate conditionally in dividing or tumor cells. This selectivity is based on several possible mutations engineered in the viral genome that prevent it from replicating unless the infected cell provides for a substituting molecular activity *(166)*. These properties have established brain tumors, which are surrounded by nonmitotic cells, as an ideal therapeutic model for testing replication-conditional herpes vectors. Notably, human clinical trials have already begun to test both adenovirus and herpesvirus-based replicative vector systems.

Prolonged Transgene Expression: Integrative Vector Systems Lack of stability in vivo has confined the use of retroviruses to the ex vivo modification of target cells. For in situ gene delivery, vectors with high efficiency and stability in vivo are needed. Of vectors with both characteristics, adenoviruses have been most extensively characterized and used (Table 3). In addition to a significant inflammatory and immune response, an additional basis for the limited transgene expression associated with adenoviral vectors derives from their nonintegrative nature, such that vector sequences are not retained in the host genome and are not inherited by progeny cells. In this regard, after adenoviral-mediated gene transfer, the recombinant genome is present epi-chromosomally in target cells. Thus, with the proliferation of transduced cells, vector sequences are lost, with the consequence of limited duration of transgene expression. For utility in mutation compensation, and in other gene-therapy strategies, it is desirable to develop methods to achieve integration of adenoviral vector-delivered transgene sequences in infected cells. As a novel approach to meet this need, we have developed a chimeric viral vector system that exploits favorable aspects of both adenoviral and retroviral vectors. In this schema, adenoviral vectors induce target cells to function as transient retroviral producer cells in vivo. The progeny retroviral vector particles can then effectively achieve stable transduction of neighboring cells *(160)*. Thus, the principle of combining selected features of available vectors into novel chimeric vectors is already governing the development of virus-based gene-transfer systems *(167)*.

Lentiviruses are retroviruses that, in contrast to other members of the family, can infect both dividing and nondividing cells. This fundamental feature has driven significant efforts for its development, although practical issues related to production and safety have limited its widespread use. Efficiency of transduction of most potential cellular targets by lentiviral vectors and in vivo utility have just begun to be described *(168)*.

Prolonged Transgene Expression: Immune Tolerance to Viral Vectors Gene delivery via adenoviral vectors has been associated with the induction of characteristically intense inflammatory and immunological responses when employed *in vivo*. A number of specific cellular and humoral immune-effector mechanisms, together with nonspecific defense mechanisms, eliminate the infecting virus *(169–171)*. This process has been associated with attenuation of expression of the transferred therapeutic gene, based primarily on loss of the vector transduced cells. Based on an understanding of the biology of this phenomenon, specific strategies have been developed to mitigate this process *(172)*.

Maneuvers to minimize the immune response against viral vectors include manipulations of both the vector and the host. Firstly, recombinant viral vectors are genetically engineered to delete viral genes encoding highly immunogenic or cytotoxic viral proteins. However, these new generations of modified viral vectors are more difficult to propagate and are not devoid of immunogenic properties. Alternatively, different serotypes and adenoviruses of other species have been proposed to minimize the stimulus for an immune response. Secondly, vectors have been modified to express immunomodulatory molecules. It has been hypothesized that this could create a locally privileged environment for the vector. Some of these engineered molecules are viral genes that interfere with the apparatus of antigen presentation, such as the adenoviral glycoprotein 19K or the HSV immediate early protein ICP47. Others are recombinant molecules designed to abrogate antigen presentation, such as antisense oligonucleotides or single-chain antibodies against MHC class I and II proteins, or to block costimulation, such as CTL4IgG *(172)*.

Interventions against the immune system of the host have been adopted from common practices in the field of organ transplantation. In this regard, virally transduced cells have been considered to behave, to some extent, as allogeneic cell transplants. Thus, drugs are employed that inhibit the cellular immune response, such as anti-CD4 antibodies, cyclosporine, dexamethasone, and FK 506. In addition, drugs that decrease the humoral immune response, such as cyclophosphamide and deoxyspergualin, have been used. Recently, several groups have shown transient and more specific immune blockade with inhibitors of T-cell costimulation, such as anti-CD40 ligand, CTL4IgG, and anti-LFA-1. Unfortunately, the required chronic administration of these immunosuppressive drugs affect systemic immune function and results potentially in a number of complications, such as infection and malignancy. This makes them less attractive in principle for clinical application, although short-term treatment in cancer patients should be feasible. Lastly, induction of tolerance to adenovirus vectors by oral ingestion of adenoviral antigens has been described, but this approach needs further characterization. Thus, although inflammatory and immunological issues have limited the overall utility of adenoviral vectors for gene-therapy applications, many of the newly developed strategies appear promising and may ultimately overcome these limitations.

MOLECULAR CHEMOTHERAPY REQUIRES TARGETING In molecular chemotherapy strategies, other problems take precedence. Less than optimal transduction levels may require the employment of higher magnitudes of gene vectors leading to target-cell cytotoxicity. Thus, for direct *in situ* infection of selected organs, improvements in basic gene-transfer efficiency may be required. In addition, and more specifically, the promiscuous tropism of the vector may potentially allow ectopic transduction of nontumor cells with toxic genes. Therefore, strategies to enhance the efficiency of the vector as well as methods to enhance the specificity of target-cell transduction would be necessary to render gene delivery optimal for gene-therapy purposes. In this regard, studies have demonstrated the feasibility of creating tropism-modified retroviral and adenoviral vectors to achieve cell-specific targeting, as described earlier. To this end, immunological and genetic strategies for retargeting vectors to nonviral specific cellular receptors have been designed. Modifications of the adenovirus vector to alter native viral tropism in order to achieve selective transduction of target disease cells have proved to be feasible *(173–176)*, in contrast with the more structurally demanding characteristics of retroviruses. Notably, targeting maneuvers have shown in selected cases the additional ability to enhance the transduction efficiency of the recombinant adenoviral vector by orders of magnitude, by binding and entering into the cell via heterologous cellular-receptor pathways.

Immunological Targeting To test our immunological schema of adenoviral targeting, we chose to target the folate receptor, which is overexpressed on the surface of a variety of malignant cells, including ovarian carcinoma cells. We conjugated the Fab fragment of an antibody against the adenoviral fiber with a folate moiety. When this Fab-folate conjugate was complexed with an adenoviral vector carrying a reporter gene, we observed redirection of the adenoviral vector via the folate receptor at high efficiency. Furthermore, when complexed with an adenoviral vector carrying the HSV-*tk* gene, we obtained specific killing of cells overexpressing the folate receptor *(174)*. Thus, retargeting of adenovirus by bispecific conjugates based on anti-adenovirus antibody fragments and cellular receptor-specific cognate ligands was shown to be feasible. Similar strategies have been developed by other researchers *(173)*. Importantly, this flexible strategy permits the rapid derivation and testing of targeted adenoviral vectors. In this regard, we have recently shown that recombinant adenovirus can be targeted specifically to a variety of cell types, including ovarian-cancer cell lines, by exploiting the heterologous cellular pathway of basic fibroblast growth-factor receptor (bFGFR). Here, the levels of gene transduction by retargeted adenovirus were even greater than those achievable by adenovirus alone. Therefore, an adenoviral vector targeted to the bFGFR would allow higher or at least similar levels of gene delivery than nontargeted virus and lower nonspecific toxicity. This suggests that the small therapeutic index of currently available vectors in the context of in situ administration could be improved using targeted adenovirus for the purpose of gene therapy of cancer. In fact, recent experiments in our laboratory have confirmed that Fab-bFGFR targeted adenovirus achieved enhanced in vivo expression of a reporter gene in an intraperitoneal tumor model of ovarian carcinoma in nude mice *(177)*.

Genetic Targeting Strategies to derive a tropism-modified recombinant virus, most advanced with retroviruses and adenoviruses, have been directed towards modification of viral-surface proteins to accomplish incorporation of heterologous cell-binding ligands. This approach has capitalized on the extensive knowledge on the endogenous cell-binding ligands of both types of viral vectors. As with immunological strategies, retrovirus particles have been generally less tolerant to binding-modification maneuvers. In contrast, with adenovirus several groups have been able to localize novel ligands in the cell-binding knob portion of the viral fiber *(178–180)* and in the penton base protein. Engineered adenoviruses demonstrate improved transduction efficiencies in cells that are otherwise refractory to adenoviral gene transfer, such as endothelium and leukocytes. The achievement of these goals, even in a limited context, predicts that further analysis could identify, for particular target tissues, optimal ligands from the standpoints of cell binding and internalization. The possibility of employing therapeutic adenovirus vectors to selectively transduce cells in the context of disseminated disease clearly exists.

Definition of New Targets Ideally, new vectors will be administered by intravenous injection and will effect gene transfer specifically in systemically distributed target cells. Genetic and immunological targeting strategies allow for consideration of such a targetable/injectable vector. A systematic method for identification of ligands that can be incorporated into vectors for selective delivery to target cells is therefore needed. In addition to traditional ways of identifying single cellular receptors one-by-one, a high-throughput method has been developed based on the technology of phage-display libraries. In this approach, tens of millions of short peptides can be rapidly surveyed for tight binding to a cellular receptor using an epitope library. The library is a vast mixture of filamentous phage clones, each displaying one peptide sequence on the virion surface. The survey, originally performed by using the binding protein to affinity-purify phage that display tight-binding peptides *(181)*, can also be accomplished in vivo by propagating isolated phage from target organs after intravenous injection of the phage-random library *(182)*. After propagation of isolated phage in *Escherichia coli*, the amino acid sequences of the peptides displayed on the phage are then determined by sequencing the corresponding coding region in the phage DNAs. Thus, peptides with selective tropism for target organs can be isolated and ultimately used as binding motifs in engineered viral vectors.

GENETIC IMMUNOPOTENTIATION IS REQUIRED TO BREAK IMMUNE TOLERANCE TO TUMORS Modification of gene vectors to obtain amplification and targeting represent critical goals of the strategies of mutation compensation and molecular chemotherapy. In contrast, for genetic immunopotentiation strategies, it may well be that a sophisticated vector is not needed to facilitate the otherwise inefficient transfer of DNA into cells.

Polynucleotide Immunization The possibility exists for eliciting potent, prolonged, and specific immune responses through the intramuscular injection of fragments of nucleic-acid encoding tumor-associated antigens *(183)*. This so called polynucleotide-immunization approach offers several advantages with respect to classic protein immunization. First, synthesis of the antigen in eukaryotic cells in vivo is more likely to result in a protein that is correctly folded and with its antigenic domains adequately presented. Second, polynucleotide immunization elicits a CD8$^+$ cytotoxic T-lymphocyte response in addition to a humoral response. Third, long-term expression of the encoded antigen may favor long-lived immunity. Finally, safety concerns related to virus-derived vaccines are obviated. Polynucleotides in the form of both DNA and RNA can be used. For example, plasmid DNA encoding carcinoembryonic antigen, a nontransforming tumor-associated antigen, is being tested in a clinical protocol for colorectal-cancer patients. Transforming tumor-associated antigens, such as c-erbB2, may be encoded with RNA constructs that avoid the risk of integration of a potentially oncogenic sequence and are expressed only transiently. Once the antigen is expressed in myofibers, its presentation to the effector cells occurs through some unknown mechanism. Nonetheless, this reaction results in antibody production, T-cell proliferation, lymphokine release, generation of CTL, and delayed hypersensitivity reactions. Encouraging results in animal models have been followed by clinical trials for both immune protection and therapeutic applications. Although tumors are antigenically heterogeneous, the hypothesis is that immune responses against the polynucleotide-encoded antigens can break immune tolerance for the tumor via a single epitope, which, in turn, would alert the immune system to the existence of the tumor as a foreign entity, provoking a systemic response.

Danger vs Tolerance The classical paradigm of tumor immunology considers the responses of the immune system to follow a model of discrimination between self and nonself antigens. However, an alternative model has been proposed, according to which the key fact for initiating an efficient immune response is the detection by the host of danger (for instance, the beginning of either an inflammatory reaction or tissue damage) (156). This new model considers the location and kinetics of antigen presentation to the immune system as an alternative signal that can modulate the immune response (170). Thus, the presentation of the (tumor) antigen in the lymph-node environment by APCs activated in the tumor would be critical for an efficient response (131). This model can change the emphasis applied in immunotherapy strategies. Whereas in the classical model importance is given to the identification of tumor antigens and elaboration of vaccines based on these antigens, new goals potentially more relevant could be to orchestrate inflammatory processes in tumor foci, to activate dendritic cells and other APCs, and to drive the migration of T lymphocytes towards the tumor. In other words, the aim should be to recruit not only the adaptive immune response but also and most importantly the cells (macrophages, neutrophils, NK cells) and mediators (cytokines, chemokines) of the innate immune system (156).

Enhanced Antigen Presentation Many tumors are ignored by the immune system. Thus, tumor antigen-specific T lymphocytes, which are present in the immune repertoire, are not activated and migrate systemically without showing any special tropism towards its cognate antigens in the tumor. This has been attributed to a lack of functional DCs in tumors (184). Indeed, DCs infiltrating several tumors lack B7-1 and B7-2

molecules, which reveals a nonstimulatory status and impedes the encounter by T lymphocytes of the required signal 2 for antigen-specific activation. However, when DCs are exposed ex vivo to tumor antigens and these DCs are then reinfused, CTL activation ensues. In animal models, this intervention achieves a protective effect against subsequent exposure to tumors and also can induce a therapeutic effect in tumors already present (185). This strategy is currently being explored in patients (186,187). Multiple vectors are being tested for delivering tumor antigens into DCs, including viral vectors, naked DNA, RNA, tumor lysates, and peptides. It is probable that methods that maximize exposure of DCs to a variety of tumor antigens may have an advantage by overcoming the expected emergence of antigen-loss variants as well as natural immunovariation of tumors. Such a principle has been powerfully accomplished in animal studies by generating fusions of DCs and tumor cells (188). This strategy has been tested in transgenic animals tolerant to the antigen MUC1, and refractory to vaccination with irradiated MUC-1-positive cells. Immunization with the dendritic cell fusions that express MUC1 resulted in the rejection of established metastases and no apparent autoimmunity against normal tissues. These findings demonstrate that tolerance to tumor-associated antigens can be reversed, and suggest that immunization with hybrids of dendritic and carcinoma cells may be a powerful methodology for whole cell vaccination against cancer.

CONCLUSION

The delineation of the molecular basis of cancer allows for the possibility of specific intervention at the molecular level for therapeutic purposes. To this end, three main approaches have been developed: mutation compensation, molecular chemotherapy, and genetic immunopotentiation. For each of these conceptual approaches, human clinical protocols have entered testing in phase I and II to assess dose escalation, safety, and toxicity issues, and more recently to evaluate efficacy, respectively. However, major problems remain to be solved before these approaches can become effective and commonplace strategies for cancer. Principle among these is the basic ability to deliver therapeutic genes quantitatively, and specifically, not only into tumor cells but also into tumor supporting tissues and effector cells of the immune system. As vector technology fulfills these stringent requirements, it is anticipated that the promising results already observed in pre-clinical studies will translate quickly into the clinic for amelioration of life-threatening tumor diseases.

ACKNOWLEDGMENTS

The authors are supported by National Institute of Health grants CA68245-01, RO1-CA 72532-01, DAMD-17-94-J4398, RO1 CA 74242, Department of Defense grant PC970193, and grants from the Susan G. Komen Breast Cancer Foundation, the American Lung Association, and the Cure for Lymphoma Foundation.

REFERENCES

1. Verma, I. M. and Somia, N. (1997) Gene therapy: promises, problems and prospects *Nature* **389**:239–242.

2. Blau, H. and Springuer, M. L. (1995) Gene therapy: a novel form of drug delivery. *N. Engl. J. Med.* **333**:1204–1207.

3. Anderson, W. F. (1992) Human gene therapy. *Science* **256**:808–813

4. Harris, C. C. and Hollstein, M. (1993) Clinical implications of the p53 tumor-suppressor gene *N. Engl. J. Med.* **329**:1318–1327.

5. Lowe, S. W., Ruley, H. E., Jacks, T., and Housman, D. E. (1993) p53-dependent apoptosis modulate the cytotoxicity of anticancer agents. *Cell* **74**:957–967.

6. Xu, M., Kumar, D., Srinivas, S., Detolla, L. J., Yu, S. F., Stass, S. A., et al. (1997) Parenteral gene therapy with p53 inhibits human breast tumors in vivo through a bystander mechanism without evidence of toxicity *Human Gene Ther.* **8**:177–185.

7. Bouvet, M., Ellis, L. M., Nishizaki, M., Fujiwara, T., Liu, W., Bucana, C. D., et al. (1998) Adenovirus-mediated wild-type p53 gene transfer down-regulates vascular endothelial growth factor expression and inhibits angiogenesis in human colon cancer. *Cancer Res.* **58**:2288–2292.

8. Friedmann, T. (1992) Gene therapy of cancer through restoration of tumor-suppressor functions? *Cancer* **70**:1810–1817.

9. Nielsen, L. L. and Maneval, D. C. (1998) p53 tumor suppressor gene therapy for cancer *Cancer Gene Ther.* **5**:52–63.

10. Roth, J. A., Nguyen, D., Lawrence, D. D., Kemp, B. L., Carrasco, C. H., Ferson, D. Z., et al. (1996) Retrovirus-mediated wild-type p53 gene transfer to tumors of patients with lung cancer. *Nature Med.* **2**:985–991.

11. Xu, H. J., Zhou, Y., Seigne, J., Perng, G. S., Mixon, M., Zhang, C., et al. (1996) Enhanced tumor suppressor gene therapy via replication-deficient adenovirus vectors expressing an N-terminal truncated retinoblastoma protein *Cancer Res.* **56**:2245–2249.

12. Zhou, Y., Li, J., Xu, K., Hu, S. X., Benedict, W. F., and Xu, H. J. (1994) Further characterization of retinoblastoma gene-mediated cell growth and tumor suppression in human cancer cells. *Proc. Natl. Acad. Sci. USA* **91**:4165–4169.

13. Editorial (1997) No stranger to controversy. *Nature Genet.* **17**:247–248.

14. Xing, X., Matin, A., Yu, D., Xia, W., Sorgi, F., Huang, L., et al. (1996) Mutant SV40 large T antigen as a therapeutic agent for HER-2/neu- overexpressing ovarian cancer *Cancer Gene Ther.* **3**:168–174.

15. Yu, D., Matin, A., Xia, W., Sorgi, F., Huang, L., and Hung, M. C. (1995) Liposome-mediated in vivo E1A gene transfer suppressed dissemination of ovarian cancer cells that overexpress HER-2/neu. *Oncogene* **11**:1383–1388.

16. Kashani-Sabet, M. and Scanlon, K. J. (1995) Application of ribozymes to cancer gene therapy. *Cancer Gene Ther.* **2**:213–223.

17. Feng, M., Cabrera, G., Deshane, J., Scanlon, K. J., and Curiel, D. T. (1995) Neoplastic reversion accomplished by high efficiency adenoviral-mediated delivery of an anti-ras ribozyme. *Cancer Res.* **55**:2024–2028.

18. Zhang, W. W. (1996) Antisense oncogene and tumor suppressor gene therapy of cancer. *J. Mol. Med.* **74**:191–204.

19. Gibson, I. (1996) Antisense approaches to the gene therapy of cancer—'Recnac.' *Cancer Metastasis Rev.* **15**:287–299.

20. Alama, A., Barbieri, F., Cagnoli, M., and Schettini, G. (1997) Antisense oligonucleotides as therapeutic agents *Pharmacol. Res.* **36**:171–178.

21. Orr, R. M. and Monia, B. P. (1998) Antisense therapy for cancer. *Curr. Res. Mol. Ther.* **1**:102–108

22. Trojan, J., Johnson, T. R., Rudin, S. D., Ilan, J., and Tykocinski, M. L. (1993) Treatment and prevention of rat glioblastoma by immunogenic C6 cells expressing antisense insulin-like growth factor I RNA. *Science* **259**:94–97.

23. Mukhopadhyay, T., Tainsky, M., Cavender, A. C., and Roth, J. A. (1991) Specific inhibition of K-ras expression and tumorigenicity of lung cancer cells by antisense RNA. *Cancer Res.* **51**:1744–1748.

24. Chang, E. H., Miller, P. S., Cushman, C., Devadas, K., Pirollo, K. F., Ts'o, P. O., et al. (1991) Antisense inhibition of ras p21 expression that is sensitive to a point mutation. *Biochemistry* **30**:8283–8286.

25. Zhang, Y., Mukhopadhyay, T., Donehower, L. A., Georges, R. N., and Roth, J. A. (1993) Retroviral vector-mediated transduction of K-ras antisense RNA into human lung cancer cells inhibits expression of the malignant phenotype. *Human Gene Ther.* **4**:451–460.

26. Georges, R. N., Mukhopadhyay, T., Zhang, Y., Yen, N., and Roth, J. A. (1993) Prevention of orthotopic human lung cancer growth by intratracheal instillation of a retroviral antisense K-ras construct. *Cancer Res.* **53**:1743–1746.

27. Alemany, R., Ruan, S., Kataoka, M., Koch, P. E., Mukhopadhyay, T., Cristiano, R. J., et al. (1996) Growth inhibitory effect of anti-K-ras adenovirus on lung cancer cells. *Cancer Gene Ther.* **3**:296–301.

28. Watson, P. H., Pon, R. T., and Shiu, R. P. (1991) Inhibition of c-myc expression by phosphorothioate antisense oligonucleotide identifies a critical role for c-myc in the growth of human breast cancer. *Cancer Res.* **51**:3996–4000.

29. Balaji, K. C., Koul, H., Mitra, S., Maramag, C., Reddy, P., Menon, M., et al. (1997) Antiproliferative effects of c-myc antisense oligonucleotide in prostate cancer cells: a novel therapy in prostate cancer. *Urology* **50**:1007–1015.

30. Paulus, W., Baur, I., Huettner, C., Schmausser, B., Roggendorf, W., Schlingensiepen, K. H., et al. (1995) Effects of transforming growth factor-beta 1 on collagen synthesis, integrin expression, adhesion and invasion of glioma cells. *J. Neuropathol. Exp. Neurol.* **54**:236–244.

31. Jachimczak, P., Hessdorfer, B., Fabel-Schulte, K., Wismeth, C., Brysch, W., Schlingensiepen, K. H., et al. (1996) Transforming growth factor-beta-mediated autocrine growth regulation of gliomas as detected with phosphorothioate antisense oligonucleotides. *Int. J. Cancer* **65**:332–337.

32. Fakhrai, H., Dorigo, O., Shawler, D. L., Lin, H., Mercola, D., Black, K. L., et al. (1996) Eradication of established intracranial rat gliomas by transforming growth factor beta antisense gene therapy. *Proc. Natl. Acad. Sci. USA* **93**:2909–2914.

33. Stein, C. A. (1996) Antitumor effects of antisense phosphorothioate c-myc oligodeoxynucleotides: a question of mechanism. *J. Natl. Cancer Inst.* **88**:391–393.

34. Milner, N., Mir, K. U., and Southern, E. M. (1997) Selecting effective antisense reagents on combinatorial oligonucleotide arrays. *Nature Biotechnol.* **15**:537–541.

35. Marasco, W. A. (1997) Intrabodies: turning the humoral immune system outside in for intracellular immunization *Gene Ther.* **4**:11–15.

36. Deshane, J., Loechel, F., Conry, R. M., Siegal, G. P., King, C. R., and Curiel, D. T. (1994) Intracellular single-chain antibody directed against erbB2 down- regulates cell surface erbB2 and exhibits a selective anti- proliferative effect in erbB2 overexpressing cancer cell lines. *Gene Ther.* **1**:332–337.

37. Barnes, M. N., Deshane, J., Siegal, G.P., Alvarez, R. D., and Curiel, D. T. (1996) Novel gene therapy strategy to accomplish growth factor modulation induces enhanced tumor cell chemosensitivity. *Clin. Cancer Res.* **2**:1089–1095.

38. Deshane, J., Cabrera, G., Grim, J. E., Siegal, G. P., Pike, J., Alvarez, R. D., et al. (1995) Targeted eradication of ovarian cancer mediated by intracellular expression of anti-erbB-2 single-chain antibody. *Gynecol. Oncol.* **59**:8–14.

39. Alvarez, R. D. and Curiel, D. T. (1997) A phase I study of recombinant adenovirus vector-mediated delivery of an anti-erbB-2 single-chain (sFv) antibody gene for previously treated ovarian and extraovarian cancer patients. *Human Gene Ther.* **8**:229–242.

40. Cochet, O., Kenigsberg, M., Delumeau, I., Virone-Oddos, A., Multon, M. C., Fridman, W. H., et al. (1998) Intracellular expression of an antibody fragment-neutralizing p21 ras promotes tumor regression. *Cancer Res.* **58**:1170–1176.

41. Folkman, J. (1990) What is the evidence that tumors are angiogenesis dependent? *J. Natl. Cancer Inst.* **82**:4–6.

42. Folkman, J. (1995) Angiogenesis in cancer, vascular, rheumatoid and other disease *Nature Med.* **1**:27–31.

43. Bouck, N., Stellmach, V., and Hsu, S. C. (1996) How tumors become angiogenic *Adv. Cancer Res.* **69**:135–174.

44. Parangi, S., O'Reilly, M., Christofori, G., Holmgren, L., Grosfeld, J., Folkman, J., et al. (1996) Antiangiogenic therapy of transgenic

mice impairs de novo tumor growth. *Proc. Natl. Acad. Sci. USA* **93**:2002–2007.

45. Craft, P. S. and Harris, A. L. (1994) Clinical prognostic significance of tumour angiogenesis. *Ann. Oncol.* **5**:305–311.

46. Fox, S. B. (1997) Tumour angiogenesis and prognosis. *Histopathol.* **30**:294–301.

47. Weidner, N. (1998) Tumoural vascularity as a prognostic factor in cancer patients: the evidence continues to grow. *J. Pathol.* **184**:119–122.

48. Folkman, J. (1972) Anti-angiogenesis: new concept for therapy of solid tumors. *Ann. Surg.* **175**:409–416.

49. Denekamp, J. and Hobson, B. (1982) Endothelial-cell proliferation in experimental tumours. *Br. J. Cancer* **46**:711–720.

50. Denekamp, J. (1993) Review article: angiogenesis, neovascular proliferation and vascular pathophysiology as targets for cancer therapy. *Br. J. Radiol.* **66**:181–196.

51. Bicknell, R. (1994) Vascular targeting and the inhibition of angiogenesis. *Ann. Oncol.* **5**:45–50.

52. Kerbel, R. S. (1991) Inhibition of tumor angiogenesis as a strategy to circumvent acquired resistance to anti-cancer therapeutic agents. *Bioessays* **13**:31–36.

53. Boehm, T., Folkman, J., Browder, T., and O'Reilly, M. S. (1997) Antiangiogenic therapy of experimental cancer does not induce acquired drug resistance. *Nature* **390**:404–407.

54. Kakeji, Y. and Teicher, B. A. (1997) Preclinical studies of the combination of angiogenic inhibitors with cytotoxic agents. *Invest. New Drugs* **15**:39–48.

55. Gradishar, W. J. (1997) An overview of clinical trials involving inhibitors of angiogenesis and their mechanism of action. *Invest. New Drugs* **15**:49–59.

56. Kong, H. L. and Crystal, R. G. (1998) Gene therapy strategies for tumor antiangiogenesis. *J. Natl. Cancer Inst.* **90**:273–286.

57. Saleh, M., Stacker, S. A., and Wilks, A. F. (1996) Inhibition of growth of C6 glioma cells in vivo by expression of antisense vascular endothelial growth factor sequence. *Cancer Res.* **56**:393–401.

58. Cheng, S. Y., Huang, H. J., Nagane, M., Ji, X. D., Wang, D., Shih, C. C., et al. (1996) Suppression of glioblastoma angiogenicity and tumorigenicity by inhibition of endogenous expression of vascular endothelial growth factor. *Proc. Natl. Acad. Sci. USA* **93**:8502–8507.

59. Millauer, B., Wizigmann-Voos, S., Schnurch, H., Martinez, R., Moller, N. P., Risau, W., et al. (1993) High affinity VEGF binding and developmental expression suggest Flk-1 as a major regulator of vasculogenesis and angiogenesis. *Cell* **72**:835–846.

60. Millauer, B., Shawver, L. K., Plate, K. H., Risau, W., and Ullrich, A. (1994) Glioblastoma growth inhibited in vivo by a dominant-negative Flk-1 mutant. *Nature* **367**:576–579.

61. Millauer, B., Longhi, M. P., Plate, K. H., Shawver, L. K., Risau, W., Ullrich, A., et al. (1996) Dominant-negative inhibition of Flk-1 suppresses the growth of many tumor types in vivo. *Cancer Res.* **56**:1615–1620.

62. Kong, H. L., Hecht, D., Song, W., Kovesdi, I., Hackett, N. R., Yayon, A., et al. (1998) Regional suppression of tumor growth by in vivo transfer of a cDNA encoding a secreted form of the extracellular domain of the flt-1 vascular endothelial growth factor receptor. *Hum. Gene Ther.* **9**:823–833.

63. Goldman, C. K., Kendall, R. L., Cabrera, G., Soroceanu, L., Heike, Y, Gillespie, G. Y., et al. (1998) Paracrine expression of a native soluble vascular endothelial growth factor receptor inhibits tumor growth, metastasis, and mortality rate. *Proc. Natl. Acad. Sci. USA* **95**:8795–8800.

64. Tanaka, T., Kanai, F., Lan, K. H., Ohashi, M., Shiratori, Y., Yoshida, Y., et al. (1997) Adenovirus-mediated gene therapy of gastric carcinoma using cancer- specific gene expression in vivo. *Biochem. Biophys. Res. Commun.* **231**:775–779.

65. Huang, Y. W., Baluna, R., and Vitetta, E. S. (1997) Adhesion molecules as targets for cancer therapy. *Histol. Histopathol.* **12**:467–477.

66. Conese, M. and Blasi, F. (1995) The urokinase/urokinase-receptor system and cancer invasion. *Baillieres. Clin. Haematol.* **8**:365–389.

67. Kuhn, W., Pache, L., Schmalfeldt, B., Dettmar, P., Schmitt, M., Janicke, F., et al. (1994) Urokinase (uPA) and PAI-1 predict survival in advanced ovarian cancer patients (FIGO III) after radical surgery and platinum-based chemotherapy. *Gynecol. Oncol.* **55**:401–409.

68. Mohanam, S., Chintala, S. K., Go, Y., Bhattacharya, A., Venkaiah, B., Boyd, D., et al. (1997) In vitro inhibition of human glioblastoma cell line invasiveness by antisense uPA receptor. *Oncogene* **14**:1351–1359.

69. Ma, D., Gerard, R. D., Li, X. Y., Alizadeh, H., and Niederkorn, J. Y. (1997) Inhibition of metastasis of intraocular melanomas by adenovirus-mediated gene transfer of plasminogen activator inhibitor type 1 (PAI- 1) in an athymic mouse model. *Blood* **90**:2738–2746.

70. Moolten, F. L. (1994) Drug sensitivity ("suicide") genes for selective cancer chemotherapy. *Cancer. Gene Ther.* **1**:279–287.

71. Deonarain, M. P., Spooner, R. A., and Epenetos, A. A. (1995) Genetic delivery of enzymes for cancer therapy. *Gene. Ther.* **2**:235–244.

72. Martin, L. A. and Lemoine, N. R. (1996) Direct cell killing by suicide genes *Cancer Metastasis Rev.* **15**:301–316.

73. Rigg, A. and Sikora, K. (1997) Genetic prodrug activation therapy. *Mol. Med. Today* **3**:359–366.

74. Niculescu-Duvaz, I., Spooner, R., Marais, R., and Springer, C. J. (1998) Gene-directed enzyme prodrug therapy. *Bioconjug. Chem.* **9**:4–22.

75. Moolten, F. L. and Wells, J. M. (1990) Curability of tumors bearing herpes thymidine kinase genes transferred by retroviral vectors. *J. Natl. Cancer Inst.* **82**:297–300

76. Brand, K., Arnold, W., Bartels, T., Lieber, A., Kay, M. A., Strauss, M., et al. (1997) Liver-associated toxicity of the HSV-tk/GCV approach and adenoviral vectors. *Cancer Gene Ther.* **4**:9–16

77. van der Eb, M. M., Cramer, S. J., Vergouwe, Y., Schagen, F. H., van Krieken, J. H., van der Eb, A. J., et al. (1998) Severe hepatic dysfunction after adenovirus-mediated transfer of the herpes simplex virus thymidine kinase gene and ganciclovir administration. *Gene Ther.* **5**:451–458.

78. Culver, K. W., Link, C. J., Akdemir, N., and Blaese, R. M. (1993) In vivo gene transfer of the herpes simplex-thymidine kinase (hs-tk) gene for the treatment of solid tumors. *Proc. Ann. Meet. Am. Soc. Clin. Oncol.* **12**:A286.

79. Takamiya, Y., Short, M. P., Ezzeddine, Z. D., Moolten, F. L., Breakefield, X. O., and Martuza, R. L. (1992) Gene therapy of malignant brain tumors: a rat glioma line bearing the herpes simplex virus type 1-thymidine kinase gene and wild type retrovirus kills other tumor cells. *J. Neurosci. Res.* **33**:493–503.

80. Freeman, S. M., Abboud, C. N., Whartenby, K. A., Packman, C. H., Koeplin, D. S., Moolten, F. L., et al. (1993) The bystander effect: tumor regression when a fraction of the tumor mass is genetically modified. *Cancer Res.* **53**:5274–5274.

81. Pope, I. M., Poston, G. J., and Kinsella, A. R. (1997) The role of the bystander effect in suicide gene therapy. *Eur. J. Cancer* **33**:1005–1016.

82. Rosenfeld, M. E., Feng, M., Michael, S. I., Siegal, G. P., Alvarez, R. D., and Curiel, D. T. (1995) Adenoviral-mediated delivery of the herpes simplex virus thymidine kinase gene selectively sensitizes human ovarian carcinoma cells to ganciclovir. *Clin. Cancer. Res.* **1**:1571–1580

83. Alvarez, R. D. and Curiel, D. T. (1997) A phase I study of recombinant adenovirus vector-mediated intraperitoneal delivery of herpes simplex virus thymidine kinase (HSV-TK) gene and intravenous ganciclovir for previously treated ovarian and extraovarian cancer patients. *Human Gene Ther.* **8**:597–613.

84. Mesnil, M., Piccoli, C., Tiraby, G., Willecke, K., and Yamasaki, H. (1996) Bystander killing of cancer cells by herpes simplex virus thymidine kinase gene is mediated by connexins. *Proc. Natl. Acad. Sci. USA* **93**:1831–1835.

85. Mesnil, M., Piccoli, C., and Yamasaki, H. (1997) A tumor suppressor gene, Cx26, also mediates the bystander effect in HeLa cells. *Cancer Res.* **57**:2929–2932.

86. Hamel, W., Magnelli, L., Chiarugi, V. P., and Israel, M. A. (1996) Herpes simplex virus thymidine kinase/ganciclovir-mediated apoptotic death of bystander cells. *Cancer Res* **56**:2967–2702.

87. Freeman, S. M., Ramesh, R., Shastri, M., Munshi, A., Jensen, A. K., and Marrogi, A. J. (1995) The role of cytokines in mediating the bystander effect using hsv-tk xenogeneic cells. *Cancer Lett.* **92**:167–174

88. Vile, R. G., Nelson, J. A., Castleden, S., Chong, H., and Hart, I. R. (1994) Systemic gene therapy of murine melanoma using tissue specific expression of the HSVtk gene involves an immune component. *Cancer Res.* **54**:6228–6234.

89. Gagandeep, S., Brew, R., Green, B., Christmas, S. E., Klatzmann, D., Poston, G. J., et al. (1996) Prodrug-activated gene therapy: involvement of an immunological component in the "bystander effect." *Cancer Gene Ther.* **3**:83–88.

90. Vile, R. G., Castleden, S., Marshall, J., Camplejohn, R., Upton, C., and Chong, H. (1997) Generation of an anti-tumour immune response in a non-immunogenic tumour: HSVtk killing in vivo stimulates a mononuclear cell infiltrate and a Th1-like profile of intratumoural cytokine expression. *Int. J. Cancer* **71**:267–274.

91. Kianmanesh, A. R., Perrin, H., Panis, Y., Fabre, M., Nagy, H. J., Houssin, D., et al. (1997) A "distant" bystander effect of suicide gene therapy: regression of nontransduced tumors together with a distant transduced tumor. *Human Gene Ther.* **8**:1807–1814.

92. Crystal, R. G., Hirschowitz, E., Lieberman, M., Daly, J., Kazam, E., Henschke, C., et al. (1997) Phase I study of direct administration of a replication deficient adenovirus vector containing the E. coli cytosine deaminase gene to metastatic colon carcinoma of the liver in association with the oral administration of the pro-drug 5-fluorocytosine. *Human Gene Ther.* **8**:985–1001.

93. Mullen, C. A., Kilstrup, M., and Blaese, R. M. (1992) Transfer of the bacterial gene for cytosine deaminase to mammalian cells confers lethal sensitivity to 5-fluorocytosine: a negative selection system. *Proc. Natl. Acad. Sci. USA* **89**:33–37.

94. Bridgewater, J. A., Springer, C. J., Knox, R. J., Minton, N. P., Michael, N. P., and Collins, M. K. (1995) Expression of the bacterial nitroreductase enzyme in mammalian cells renders them selectively sensitive to killing by the prodrug CB1954. *Eur. J. Cancer* **31A**:2362–2370.

95. Blackburn, R. V., Galoforo, S. S., Corry, P. M., and Lee, Y. J. (1998) Adenoviral-mediated transfer of a heat-inducible double suicide gene into prostate carcinoma cells. *Cancer Res.* **58**:1358–1362.

96. Rogulski, K. R., Kim, J. H., Kim, S. H., and Freytag, S. O. (1997) Glioma cells transduced with an Escherichia coli CD/HSV-1 TK fusion gene exhibit enhanced metabolic suicide and radiosensitivity. *Human Gene Ther.* **8**:73–85.

97. Aghi, M., Kramm, C. M., Chou, T. C., Breakefield, X. O., and Chiocca, E. A. (1998) Synergistic anticancer effects of ganciclovir/thymidine kinase and 5-fluorocytosine/cytosine deaminase gene therapies. *J. Natl. Cancer Inst.* **90**:370–380.

98. Gunzburg, W. H., Fleuchaus, A., Saller, R., and Salmons, B. (1996) Retroviral vector targeting for gene therapy. *Cytokines Mol. Ther.* **2**:177–184.

99. Miller, N. and Whelan, J. (1997) Progress in transcriptionally targeted and regulatable vectors for genetic therapy. *Human Gene Ther.* **8**:803–815.

100. Shi, Q., Wang, Y., and Worton, R. (1997) Modulation of the specificity and activity of a cellular promoter in an adenoviral vector. *Human Gene Ther.* **8**:403-410.

101. Kochanek, S., Clemens, P. R., Mitani, K., Chen, H. H., Chan, S., and Caskey, C. T. (1996) A new adenoviral vector: Replacement of all viral coding sequences with 28 kb of DNA independently expressing both full-length dystrophin and beta-galactosidase. *Proc. Natl. Acad. Sci. USA* **93**:5731–5736.

102. Marconi, P., Krisky, D., Oligino, T., Poliani, P. L., Ramakrishnan, R., Goins, W. F., et al. (1996) Replication-defective herpes simplex virus vectors for gene transfer in vivo. *Proc. Natl. Acad. Sci. USA* **93**:11,319–11,320.

103. Harrington, J. J., Van Bokkelen, G., Mays, R. W., Gustashaw, K., and Willard, H. F. (1997) Formation of de novo centromeres and construction of first-generation human artificial microchromosomes. *Nature Genetics* **15**:345–355.

104. Douglas, J. T. and Curiel, D. T. (1995) Targeted gene therapy. *Tumor Targeting* **1**:67-84.

105. Harris, J.D. and Lemoine, N.R. (1996) Strategies for targeted gene therapy. *Trends Genet.* **12**:400–405.

106. Dachs, G. U., Dougherty, G. J., Stratford, I. J., and Chaplin, D. J. (1997) Targeting gene therapy to cancer: a review. *Oncol. Res.* **9**:313–325.

107. Vile, R. G., Sunassee, K., and Diaz, R. M. (1998) Strategies for achieving multiple layers of selectivity in gene therapy. *Mol. Med. Today* **4**:84–92.

108. Cosset, F. L. and Russell, S. J. (1996) Targeting retrovirus entry. *Gene Ther.* **3**:946–956.

109. Sorrentino, B. P., Brandt, S. J., Bodine, D., Gottesman, M., Pastan, I., Cline, A., et al. (1992) Selection of drug-resistant bone marrow cells in vivo after retroviral transfer of human MDR1. *Science* **257**:99–103.

110. Rafferty, J. A., Hickson, I., Chinnasamy, N., Lashford, L. S., Margison, G. P., Dexter, T. M., et al. (1996) Chemoprotection of normal tissues by transfer of drug resistance genes. *Cancer Metastasis Rev.* **15**:365–383.

111. Deisseroth, A. B., Holmes, F., Hortobagyi, G., and Champlin, R. (1996) Use of safety-modified retroviruses to introduce chemotherapy resistance sequences into normal hematopoietic cells for chemoprotection during the therapy of breast cancer: a pilot trial. *Human Gene Ther.* **7**:401–416.

112. Dorigo, O., Turla, S. T., Lebedeva, S., and Gjerset, R. A. (1998) Sensitization of rat glioblastoma multiforme to cisplatin in vivo following restoration of wild-type p53 function. *J. Neurosurg.* **88**:535–540.

113. Piche, A., Grim, J., Rancourt, C., Gomez-Navarro, J., Reed, J. C., and Curiel, D. T. (1998) Modulation of Bcl-2 protein levels by an intracellular anti-Bcl-2 single-chain antibody increases drug-induced cytotoxicity in the breast cancer cell line MCF-7. *Cancer Res.* **58**:2134–2140.

114. Chen, L., Waxman, D. J., Chen, D., and Kufe, D. W. (1996) Sensitization of human breast cancer cells to cyclophosphamide and ifosfamide by transfer of a liver cytochrome P450 gene *Cancer Res.* **56**:1331–1340.

115. Rogulski, K. R., Zhang, K., Kolozsvary, A., Kim, J. H., and Freytag, S. O. (1997) Pronounced antitumor effects and tumor radiosensitization of double suicide gene therapy *Clin. Cancer Res.* **3**:2081–2088.

116. Pederson, L. C., Buchsbaum, D. J., Vickers, S. M., Kancharla, S. R., Mayo, M. S., Curiel, D. T., et al. (1997) Molecular chemotherapy combined with radiation therapy enhances killing of cholangiocarcinoma cells in vitro and in vivo. *Cancer Res.* **57**:4325–4332.

117. Mujoo, K., Maneval, D. C., Anderson, S. C., and Gutterman, J. U. (1996) Adenoviral-mediated p53 tumor suppressor gene therapy of human ovarian carcinoma *Oncogene* **12**:1617–1623.

118. Smythe, W. R., Hwang, H. C., Elshami, A. A., Amin, K. M., Eck, S. L., Davidson, B. L., et al. (1995) Treatment of experimental human mesothelioma using adenovirus transfer of the herpes simplex thymidine kinase gene. *Ann. Surg.* **222**:78–86.

119. Elshami, A. A., Kucharczuk, J. C., Zhang, H. B., Smythe, W. R., Hwang, H. C., Litzky, L. A., et al. (1996) Treatment of pleural mesothelioma in an immunocompetent rat model utilizing adenoviral transfer of the herpes simplex virus thymidine kinase gene. *Human Gene Ther.* **7**:141–148.

120. Yee, D., McGuire, S. E., Brunner, N., Kozelsky, T. W., Allred, D. C., Chen, S.-H., et al. (1996) Adenovirus-mediated gene transfer of herpes simplex virus thymidine kinase in an ascites model of human breast cancer. *Human Gene Ther.* **7**:1251–1257.

121. Zhang, L., Wikenheiser, K. A., and Whitsett, J. A. (1997) Limitations of retrovirus-mediated HSV-tk gene transfer to pulmonary adenocarcinoma cells in vitro and in vivo. *Human Gene Ther.* **8**:563–574.

122. Wojtowicz-Praga, S. (1997) Reversal of tumor-induced immuno-suppression: a new approach to cancer therapy. *J. Immunother.* **20**:165–177.

123. Young, R. C. (1998) Metastatic renal-cell carcinoma: what causes occasional dramatic regressions? *N. Engl. J. Med.* **338**:1305–1306.

124. Tuting, T., Storkus, W. J., and Lotze, M. T. (1997) Gene-based strategies for the immunotherapy of cancer. *J. Mol. Med.* **75**:478–491.

125. Rosenberg, S. A. (1997) Cancer vaccines based on the identification of genes encoding cancer regression antigens. *Immunol. Today* **18**:175–182.

126. Vegh, Z., Wang, P., Vanky, F., and Klein, E. (1993) Selectively down-regulated expression of major histocompatibility complex class I alleles in human solid tumors. *Cancer Res.* **53**:2416–2420.

127. Kono, K., Halapi, E., Hising, C., Petersson, M., Gerdin, E., Vanky, F., et al. (1997) Mechanisms of escape from CD8+ T-cell clones specific for the HER-2/neu proto-oncogene expressed in ovarian carcinomas: related and unrelated to decreased MHC class 1 expression *Int. J. Cancer* **70**:112–119.

128. Kawakami, Y., Nishimura, M. I., Restifo, N. P., Topalian, S. L., O'Neil, B. H., Shilyansky, J., et al. (1993) T-cell recognition of human melanoma antigens. *J. Immunother.* **14**:88–93.

129. Abdel-Wahab, Z. A., Osanto, S., Darrow, T. L., Barber, J. R., Vervaert, C. E., Gangavalli, R., et al. (1994) Transduction of human melanoma cells with the gamma interferon gene enhances cellular immunity. *Cancer Gene Ther.* **1**:171–179

130. Maeurer, M. J., Gollin, S. M., Martin, D., Swaney, W., Bryant, J., Castelli, C., et al. (1996) Tumor escape from immune recognition: lethal recurrent melanoma in a patient associated with downregulation of the peptide transporter protein TAP-1 and loss of expression of the immunodominant MART-1/Melan- A antigen. *J. Clin. Invest.* **98**:1633–1641.

131. Mondino, A., Khoruts, A., and Jenkins, M. K. (1996) The anatomy of T-cell activation and tolerance. *Proc. Natl. Acad. Sci. USA* **93**:2245–2252.

132. Lombardi, G., Sidhu, S., Batchelor, R., and Lechler, R. (1994) Anergic T cells as suppressor cells in vitro. *Science* **264**:1587–1589.

133. Mizoguchi, H., O'Shea, J. J., Longo, D. L., Loeffler, C. M., McVicar, D. W., and Ochoa, A. C. (1992) Alterations in signal transduction molecules in T lymphocytes from tumor-bearing mice. *Science* **258**:1795–1798.

134. Wick, M., Dubey, P., Koeppen, H., Siegel, C. T., Fields, P. E., Chen, L., et al. (1997) Antigenic cancer cells grow progressively in immune hosts without evidence for T cell exhaustion or systemic anergy. *J. Exp. Med.* **186**:229–238.

135. Torre-Amione, G., Beauchamp, R. D., Koeppen, H., Park, B. H., Schreiber, H., Moses, H. L., et al. (1990) A highly immunogenic tumor transfected with a murine transforming growth factor type beta 1 cDNA escapes immune surveillance. *Proc. Natl. Acad. Sci. USA* **87**:1486–1490.

136. Enk, A. H., Jonuleit, H., Saloga, J., and Knop, J. (1997) Dendritic cells as mediators of tumor-induced tolerance in metastatic melanoma. *Int. J. Cancer* **73**:309–316.

137. Gabrilovich, D. I., Chen, H. L., Girgis, K. R., Cunningham, H. T., Meny, G. M., Nadaf, S., et al. (1996) Production of vascular endothelial growth factor by human tumors inhibits the functional maturation of dendritic cells. *Nature Med.* **2**:1096–1103.

138. Nagata, S. and Golstein, P. (1995) The Fas death factor. *Science* **267**:1449–1456.

139. Hahne, M., Rimoldi, D., Schroter, M., Romero, P., Schreier, M., French, L. E., et al. (1996) Melanoma cell expression of Fas (Apo-1/CD95) ligand: implications for tumor immune escape. *Science* **274**:1363–1366.

140. Rosenberg, S. A., Aebersold, P., Cornetta, K., Kasid, A., Morgan, R. A., Moen, R., et al. (1990) Gene transfer into humans—immunotherapy of patients with advanced melanoma, using tumor-infiltrating lymphocytes modified by retroviral gene transduction. *N. Engl. J. Med.* **323**:570–578.

141. Hwu, P. and Rosenberg, S. A. (1994) The genetic modification of T cells for cancer therapy: an overview of laboratory and clinical trials. *Cancer Detect. Prevent.* **18**:43–50.

142. Hodi, F. S. and Dranoff, G. (1998) Genetically modified tumor cell vaccines *Surg. Oncol. Clin. N. Am.* **7**:471–485.

143. Pardoll, D. M. (1998) Cancer vaccines. *Nature Med.* **4**:525-531.

144. Hellstrom, I. and Hellstrom, K. E. (1998) Tumor vaccines: a reality at last? *J. Immunother.* **21**:119–126.

145. Foa, R., Guarini, A., Cignetti, A., Cronin, K., Rosenthal, F., and Gansbacher, B. (1994) Cytokine gene therapy: a new strategy for the management of cancer patients. *Nature Immunol.* **13**:65–75.

146. Belli, F., Arienti, F., Sule-Suso, J., Clemente, C., Mascheroni, L., Cattelan, A., et al. (1997) Active immunization of metastatic melanoma patients with interleukin-2-transduced allogeneic melanoma cells: evaluation of efficacy and tolerability. *Cancer Immunol. Immunother.* **44**:197–203.

147. Abdel-Wahab, Z., Weltz, C., Hester, D., Pickett, N., Vervaert, C., Barber, J. R., et al. (1997) A Phase I clinical trial of immunotherapy with interferon-gamma gene-modified autologous melanoma cells: monitoring the humoral immune response. *Cancer* **80**:401–412.

148. DeBruyne, L. (1996) Treatment of malignancy by direct gene transfer of a foreign MCH class I molecule. *Cancer Immunol. Immunother.* **43**:189–189.

149. Nabel, G. J., Gordon, D., Bishop, D. K., Nickoloff, B. J., Yang, Z. Y., Aruga, A., et al. (1996) Immune response in human melanoma after transfer of an allogeneic class I major histocompatibility complex gene with DNA-liposome complexes. *Proc. Natl. Acad. Sci. USA* **93**:15,388–15,393.

150. Stopeck, A. T., Hersh, E. M., Akporiaye, E. T., Harris, D. T., Grogan, T., Unger, E., et al. (1997) Phase I study of direct gene transfer of an allogeneic histocompatibility antigen, HLA-B7, in patients with metastatic melanoma. *J. Clin. Oncol.* **15**:341–349.

151. Sartor, W. M., Kyprianou, N., Fabian, D. F., and Lefor, A. T. (1995) Enhanced expression of ICAM-1 in a murine fibrosarcoma reduces tumor growth rate. *J. Surg. Res.* **59**:66–74.

152. Wei, K., Wilson, J. G., Jurgensen, C. H., Iannone, M. A., Wolberg, G., and Huber, B. E. (1996) Xenogeneic ICAM-1 gene transfer suppresses tumorigenicity and generates protective antitumor immunity. *Gene Ther.* **3**:531–541.

153. Wang, R. F. (1997) Tumor antigens discovery: perspectives for cancer therapy. *Mol. Med.* **3**:716–731.

154. Taupier, M. A., Kearney, J. F., Leibson, P. J., Loken, M. R., and Schreiber, H. (1983) Nonrandom escape of tumor cells from immune lysis due to intraclonal fluctuations in antigen expression *Cancer Res.* **43**:4050–4056.

155. Welch, W. R., Niloff, J. M., Anderson, D., Battaile, A., Emery, S., Knapp, R. C., et al. (1990) Antigenic heterogeneity in human ovarian cancer. *Gynecol. Oncol.* **38**:12–16.

156. Fenton, R. G. and Longo, D. L. (1997) Danger versus tolerance: paradigms for future studies of tumor-specific cytotoxic T lymphocytes. *J. Natl. Cancer Inst.* **89**:272–275.

157. Staveley-O'Carroll, K., Sotomayor, E., Montgomery, J., Borrello, I., Hwang, L., Fein, S., et al. (1998) Induction of antigen-specific T cell anergy: An early event in the course of tumor progression. *Proc. Natl. Acad. Sci. USA* **95**:1178–1183.

158. Morel, A., de La Coste, A., Fernandez, N., Berson, A., Kaybanda, M., Molina, T., et al. (1998) Does preventive vaccination with engineered tumor cells work in cancer-prone transgenic mice? *Cancer Gene Ther.* **5**:92–100.

159. Miller, R. and Curiel, D. T. (1996) Towards the use of replicative adenoviral vectors for cancer gene therapy. *Gene Ther.* **3**:557–559.

160. Bilbao, G., Feng, M., Rancourt, C., Jackson, W. H. J., and Curiel, D. T. (1997) Adenoviral/retroviral vector chimeras: a novel strategy to achieve high- efficiency stable transduction in vivo. *FASEB J.* **11**:624–634.

161. Kirn, D. H. and McCormick, F. (1996) Replicating viruses as selective cancer therapeutics. *Mol. Med. Today* **2**:519–527.

162. Rodriguez, R., Schuur, E. R., Lim, H. Y., Henderson, G. A., Simons, J. W., and Henderson, D. R. (1997) Prostate attenuated replication competent adenovirus (ARCA) CN706: a selective cytotoxic for

prostate-specific antigen-positive prostate cancer cells. *Cancer Res.* **57**:2559–2563.

163. Bischoff, J. R., Kirn, D. H., Williams, A., Heise, C., Horn, S., Muna, M., et al. (1996) An adenovirus mutant that replicates selectively in p53-deficient human tumor cells. *Science* **274**:373–376.

164. Dion, L. D., Goldsmith, K. T., and Garver, R. I., Jr. (1996) Quantitative and in vivo activity of adenoviral-producing cells made by cotransduction of a replication-defective adenovirus and a replication- enabling plasmid. *Cancer Gene Ther.* **3**:230–237.

165. Gomez-Navarro, J., Rancourt, C., Wang, M. H., Siegal, G. P., Alvarez, R. D., Garver, R. I., Jr., et al. (1998) Transcomplementation of a replication-incompetent adenovirus expressing herpes simplex virus thymidine kinase in ovarian carcinoma cells produces progeny virus capable of killing after treatment with ganciclovir. *Tumor Targeting* **3**:169–177.

166. Kramm, C. M., Chase, M., Herrlinger, U., Jacobs, A., Pechan, P. A., Rainov, N. G., et al. (1997) Therapeutic efficiency and safety of a second-generation replication-conditional HSV1 vector for brain tumor gene therapy. *Human Gene Ther.* **8**:2057–2068.

167. Vile, R. G. (1997) A marriage of viral vectors. *Nature Biotechnol.* **15**:840–841.

168. Zufferey, R., Nagy, D., Mandel, R .J., Naldini, L., and Trono, D. (1997) Multiply attenuated lentiviral vector achieves efficient gene delivery in vivo. *Nature Biotechnol.* **15**:871–875.

169. Gahery-Segard, H., Farace, F., Godfrin, D., Gaston, J., Lengagne, R., Tursz, T., et al. (1998) Immune response to recombinant capsid proteins of adenovirus in humans: antifiber and anti-penton base antibodies have a synergistic effect on neutralizing activity. *J. Virol.* **72**:2388–2397.

170. Zinkernagel, R. M. and Hengartner, H. (1997) Antiviral immunity. *Immunol. Today* **18**:258–260.

171. Worgall, S., Wolff, G., Falck-Pedersen, E., and Crystal, R. G. (1997) Innate immune mechanisms dominate elimination of adenoviral vectors following in vivo administration. *Human Gene Ther.* **8**:37–44.

172. Bilbao, G., Gomez-Navarro, J., Contreras, J. L., and Curiel, D. T. (1998) Improving adenoviral vectors for cancer gene therapy. *Tumor Targeting* **3**:59–79.

173. Michael, S. I., Hong, J. S., Curiel, D. T., and Engler, J. A. (1995) Addition of a short peptide ligand to the adenovirus fiber protein. *Gene Ther.* **2**:660–668.

174. Douglas, J. T., Rogers, B. E., Rosenfeld, M. E., Michael, S. I., Feng, M. Z., and Curiel, D. T. (1996) Targeted gene delivery by tropism-modified adenoviral vector. *Nature Biotechnol.* **14**:1574–1578

175. Wickham, T. J., Segal, D. M., Roelvink, P. W., Carrion, M. E., Lizonova, A., Lee, G. M., et al. (1996) Targeted adenovirus gene transfer to endothelial and smooth muscle cells by using bispecific antibodies. *J. Virol.* **70**:6831–6838.

176. Krasnykh, V. N., Mikheeva, G. V., Douglas, J. T., and Curiel, D. T. (1996) Generation of recombinant adenovirus vectors with modified fibers for altering viral tropism. *J. Virol.* **70**:6839–6846.

177. Rogers, B. E., Douglas, J. T., Sosnowski, B. A., Ying, W., Pierce, G., Buchsbaum, D. J., et al. (1998) Enhanced in vivo gene delivery to human ovarian cancer xenografts utilizing a tropsim-modified adenovirus vector. *Tumor Targeting* **3**:25–31

178. Wickham, T. J., Tzeng, E., Shears, L. L., Roelvink, P. W., Li, Y., Lee, G. M., et al. (1997) Increased in vitro and in vivo gene transfer by adenovirus vectors containing chimeric fiber proteins. *J. Virol.* **71**:8221–8229.

179. Stevenson, S. C., Rollence, M., Marshall-Neff, J., and McClelland, A. (1997) Selective targeting of human cells by a chimeric adenovirus vector containing a modified fiber protein. *J. Virol.* **71**:4782–4790.

180. Krasnykh, V., Dmitriev, I., Mikheeva, G., Miller, C. R., Belousova, N., and Curiel, D. T. (1998) Characterization of an adenovirus vector containing a heterologous peptide epitope in the HI loop of the fiber knob. *J. Virol.* **72**:1844–1852.

181. Scott, J. K. and Smith, G. P. (1990) Searching for peptide ligands with an epitope library. *Science* **249**:386–390.

182. Pasqualini, R., Koivunen, E., and Ruoslahti, E. (1997) Alpha v integrins as receptors for tumor targeting by circulating ligands. *Nature Biotechnol.* **15**:542–546.

183. Conry, R. M., LoBuglio, A. F., and Curiel, D. T. (1996) Polynucleotide-mediated immunization therapy of cancer. *Semin. Oncol.* **23**:135–147.

184. Banchereau, J. and Steinman, R. M. (1998) Dendritic cells and the control of immunity. *Nature* **392**:245–252.

185. Schuler, G. and Steinman, R. M. (1997) Dendritic cells as adjuvants for immune-mediated resistance to tumors. *J. Exp. Med.* **186**:1183–1187.

186. Nestle, F. O., Alijagic, S., Gilliet, M., Sun, Y., Grabbe, S., Dummer, R., et al. (1998) Vaccination of melanoma patients with peptide- or tumor lysate-pulsed dendritic cells. *Nat. Med.* **4**:328–332.

187. Gilboa, E., Nair, S. K., and Lyerly, H. K. (1998) Immunotherapy of cancer with dendritic-cell-based vaccines. *Cancer Immunol. Immunother.* **46**:82–87.

188. Gong, J., Chen, D., Kashiwaba, M., Li, Y., Chen, L., Takeuchi, H., et al. (1998) Reversal of tolerance to human MUC1 antigen in MUC1 transgenic mice immunized with fusions of dendritic and carcinoma cells. *Proc. Natl. Acad. Sci. USA* **95**:6279–6283.

189. Danks, M. K., Morton, C. L., Pawlik, C. A., and Potter, P. M. (1998) Overexpression of a rabbit liver carboxylesterase sensitizes human tumor cells to CPT-11. *Cancer Res.* **58**:20–22.

190. Kojima, A., Hackett, N. R., Ohwada, A., and Crystal, R. G. (1998) In vivo human carboxylesterase cDNA gene transfer to activate the prodrug CPT-11 for local treatment of solid tumors. *J. Clin. Invest.* **101**:1789–1796.

191. Marais, R., Spooner, R. A., Light, Y., Martin, J., and Springer, C. J. (1996) Gene-directed enzyme prodrug therapy with a mustard prodrug/carboxypeptidase G2 combination. *Cancer Res.* **56**:4735–4742.

192. Chen, L., Yu, L. J., and Waxman, D. J. (1997) Potentiation of cytochrome P450/cyclophosphamide-based cancer gene therapy by coexpression of the P450 reductase gene. *Cancer Res.* **57**:4830–4837.

193. Huber, B. E., Richards, C. A., and Austin, E. A. (1993) Gene therapy for primary and metastatic tumors in the liver (meeting abstract). Gene Therapy for Neoplastic Diseases. June 26–29, 1993, Washington, DC, A10.

194. Consalvo, M., Mullen, C. A., Modesti, A., Musiani, P., Allione, A., Cavallo, F., et al. (1995) 5-fluorocytosine-induced eradication of murine adenocarcinomas engineered to express the cytosine deaminase suicide gene requires host immune competence and leaves an efficient memory. *J. Immunol.* **154**:5302–5312.

195. Manome, Y., Wen, P. Y., Dong, Y., Tanaka, T., Mitchell, B. S., Kufe, D. W., et al. (1996) Viral vector transduction of the human deoxycytidine kinase cDNA sensitizes glioma cells to the cytotoxic effects of cytosine arabinoside in vitro and in vivo. *Nature Med.* **2**:567–573.

196. Hapke, D. M., Stegmann, A. P., and Mitchell, B. S. (1996) Retroviral transfer of deoxycytidine kinase into tumor cell lines enhances nucleoside toxicity. *Cancer Res.* **56**:2343–2347.

197. Green, N. K., Youngs, D. J., Neoptolemos, J. P., Friedlos, F., Knox, R. J., Springer, C. J., et al. (1997) Sensitization of colorectal and pancreatic cancer cell lines to the prodrug 5-(aziridin-1-yl)-2,4-dinitrobenzamide (CB1954) by retroviral transduction and expression of the E. coli nitroreductase gene. *Cancer Gene Ther.* **4**:229–238.

198. Bridgewater, J. A., Knox, R. J., Pitts, J. D., Collins, M. K., and Springer, C. J. (1997) The bystander effect of the nitroreductase/CB1954 enzyme/prodrug system is due to a cell-permeable metabolite. *Human Gene Ther.* **8**:709–717.

199. Bailey, S. M. and Hart, I. R. (1997) Nitroreductase activation of CB1954: an alternative "suicide" gene system. *Gene Ther.* **4**:80–81.

200. Friedlos, F., Court, S., Ford, M., Denny, W. A., and Springer, C. (1998) Gene-directed enzyme prodrug therapy: quantitative bystander cytotoxicity and DNA damage induced by CB1954 in cells expressing bacterial nitroreductase. *Gene Ther.* **5**:105–112.

201. Parker, W. B., King, S. A., Allan, P. W., Bennett, L. L. J., Secrist, J. A., Montgomery, J. A., et al. (1997) In vivo gene therapy of cancer with E. coli purine nucleoside phosphorylase. *Human Gene Ther.* **8**:1637–1644.

202. Mroz, P. J. and Moolten, F. L. (1993) Retrovirally transduced Escherichia coli gpt genes combine selectability with chemosensitivity capable of mediating tumor eradication. *Human Gene Ther.* **4**:589–595.

203. Tamiya, T., Ono, Y., Wei, M. X., Mroz, P. J., Moolten, F. L., and Chiocca, E. A. (1996) Escherichia coli gpt gene sensitizes rat glioma cells to killing by 6- thioxanthine or 6-thioguanine. *Cancer Gene Ther.* **3**:155–162.

204. Ono, Y., Ikeda, K., Wei, M. X., Harsh, G. R., Tamiya, T., and Chiocca, E. A. (1997) Regression of experimental brain tumors with 6-thioxanthine and Escherichia coli gpt gene therapy. *Human Gene Ther.* **8**:2043–2055.

205. Nabel, E. G. and Nabel, G. J. (1993) Direct gene transfer: basic studies and human therapies. *Thrombosis Haemostasis* **70**:202–203.

206. Isner, J. M., Pieczek, A., Schainfeld, R., Blair, R., Haley, L., Asahara, T., et al. (1996) Clinical evidence of angiogenesis after arterial gene transfer of phVEGF165 in patient with ischaemic limb. *Lancet* **348**:370–374.

207. Rosenfeld, M. E., Wang, M., Siegal, G. P., Alvarez, R. D., Mikheeva, G., Krasnykh, V., et al. (1996) Adenoviral-mediated delivery of herpes simplex virus thymidine kinase results in tumor reduction and prolonged survival in a SCID mouse model of human ovarian carcinoma. *J. Mol. Med.* **74**:455–462.

208. Culver, K. W., Ram, Z., Wallbridge, S., Ishii, H., Oldfield, E. H., and Blaese, R. M. (1992) In vivo gene transfer with retroviral vector-producer cells for treatment of experimental brain tumors. *Science* **256**:1550–1552

209. Carroll, N. M., Chiocca, E. A., Takahashi, K., and Tanabe, K. K. (1996) Enhancement of gene therapy specificity for diffuse colon carcinoma liver metastases with recombinant herpes simplex virus. *Ann. Surg.* **224**:323–329

210. Boviatsis, E. J., Park, J. S., Sena-Esteves, M., Kramm, C. M., Chase, M., Efird, J. T., et al. (1994) Long-term survival of rats harboring brain neoplasms treated with ganciclovir and a herpes simplex virus vector that retains an intact thymidine kinase gene. *Cancer Res.* **54**:5745–5751.

211. Burns, J. C., Friedmann, T., Driever, W., Burrascano, M., and Yee, J. K. (1993) Vesicular stomatitis virus G glycoprotein pseudotyped retroviral vectors: concentration to very high titer and efficient gene transfer into mammalian and nonmammalian cells. *Proc. Natl. Acad. Sci. USA* **90**:8033–8037.

212. Kasahara, N., Dozy, A. M., and Kan, Y. W. (1994) Tissue-specific targeting of retroviral vectors through ligand- receptor interactions. *Science* **266**:1373–1376.

213. Marin, M., Noel, D., Valsesia-Wittman, S., Brockly, F., Etienne-Julan, M., Russell, S., et al. (1996) Targeted infection of human cells via major histocompatibility complex class I molecules by Moloney murine leukemia virus-derived viruses displaying single-chain antibody fragment-envelope fusion proteins. *J. Virol.* **70**:2957–2962.

214. Konishi, H., Ochiya, T., Chester, K. A., Begent, R. H., Muto, T., Sugimura, T., et al. (1998) Targeting strategy for gene delivery to carcinoembryonic antigen- producing cancer cells by retrovirus displaying a single-chain variable fragment antibody. *Human Gene Ther.* **9**:235–248.

215. Wu, G. Y., Wilson, J. M., Shalaby, F., Grossman, M., Shafritz, D. A., and Wu, C. H. (1991) Receptor-mediated gene delivery in vivo. partial correction of genetic analbuminemia in nagase rats. *J Biol. Chem.* **266**:14,338–14,342.

216. Curiel, D. T., Wagner, E., Cotten, M., Birnstiel, M. L., Agarwal, S., Li, C. M., et al. (1992) High-efficiency gene transfer mediated by adenovirus coupled to DNA-polylysine complexes. *Human Gene Ther.* **3**:147–154.

217. Citro, G., Perrotti, D., Cucco, C., D'Agnano, I., Sacchi, A., Zupi, G., et al. (1992) Inhibition of leukemia cell proliferation by receptor-mediated uptake of c-myb antisense oligodeoxynucleotides. *Proc. Natl. Acad. Sci. USA* **89**:7031–7035.

218. Mizuno, M., Yoshida, J., Sugita, K., Inoue, I., Seo, H., Hayashi, Y., et al. (1990) Growth inhibition of glioma cells transfected with the human beta- interferon gene by liposomes coupled with a monoclonal antibody. *Cancer Res.* **50**:7826–7829.

219. Kaneko, S., Hallenbeck, P., Kotani, T., Nakabayashi, H., McGarrity, G., Tamaoki, T., et al. (1995) Adenovirus-mediated gene therapy of hepatocellular carcinoma using cancer-specific gene expression. *Cancer Res.* **55**:5283–5287.

220. Chen, L., Chen, D., Manome, Y., Dong, Y., Fine, H. A., and Kufe, D. W. (1995) Breast cancer selective gene expression and therapy mediated by recombinant adenoviruses containing the DF3/MUC1 promoter. *J. Clin. Invest.* **96**:2775–2782.

221. Richards, C. A., Austin, E. A., and Huber, B. E. (1995) Transcriptional regulatory sequences of carcinoembryonic antigen: identification and use with cytosine deaminase for tumor-specific gene therapy. *Human Gene Ther.* **6**:881–893.

222. Garver, R. I., Jr., Goldsmith, K. T., Rodu, B., Hu, P. C., Sorscher, E. J., and Curiel, D. T. (1994) Strategy for achieving selective killing of carcinomas. *Gene Ther.* **1**:46–50.

223. Harris, J. D., Gutierrez, A. A., Hurst, H. C., Sikora, K., and Lemoine, N. R. (1994) Gene therapy for cancer using tumor-specific prodrug activation. *Gene Ther.* **1**:170–175.

224. Vile, R. G. and Hart, I. R. (1993) Use of tissue-specific expression of the herpes simplex virus thymidine kinase gene to inhibit growth of established murine melanomas following direct intratumoral injection of DNA. *Cancer Res.* **53**:3860–3864.

Index

RIT - WALLACE LIBRARY
CIRCULATING LIBRARY BOOKS

OVERDUE FINES AND FEES FOR <u>ALL</u> BORROWERS

*Recalled = $1/ day overdue (no grace period)
*Billed = $10.00/ item when returned 4 or more weeks overdue
*Lost Items = replacement cost+$10 fee
*All materials must be returned or renewed by the duedate.